STEM CELLS – LABORATORY AND CLINICAL RESEARCH

ENCYCLOPEDIA OF STEM CELL RESEARCH (2 VOLUME SET)

VOLUME 1

STEM CELLS – LABORATORY AND CLINICAL RESEARCH

Additional books in this series can be found on Nova's website under the Series tab.

Additional E-books in this series can be found on Nova's website under the E-books tab.

STEM CELLS AND REGENERATIVE MEDICINE

Additional books in this series can be found on Nova's website under the Series tab.

Additional E-books in this series can be found on Nova's website under the E-books tab.

STEM CELLS – LABORATORY AND CLINICAL RESEARCH

ENCYCLOPEDIA OF STEM CELL RESEARCH (2 VOLUME SET)

VOLUME 1

ALEXANDER L. GREENE
EDITOR

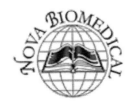

Nova Science Publishers, Inc.
New York

Copyright ©2012 by Nova Science Publishers, Inc.

All rights reserved. No part of this book may be reproduced, stored in a retrieval system or transmitted in any form or by any means: electronic, electrostatic, magnetic, tape, mechanical photocopying, recording or otherwise without the written permission of the Publisher.

For permission to use material from this book please contact us:
Telephone 631-231-7269; Fax 631-231-8175
Web Site: http://www.novapublishers.com

NOTICE TO THE READER

The Publisher has taken reasonable care in the preparation of this book, but makes no expressed or implied warranty of any kind and assumes no responsibility for any errors or omissions. No liability is assumed for incidental or consequential damages in connection with or arising out of information contained in this book. The Publisher shall not be liable for any special, consequential, or exemplary damages resulting, in whole or in part, from the readers' use of, or reliance upon, this material.

Independent verification should be sought for any data, advice or recommendations contained in this book. In addition, no responsibility is assumed by the publisher for any injury and/or damage to persons or property arising from any methods, products, instructions, ideas or otherwise contained in this publication.

This publication is designed to provide accurate and authoritative information with regard to the subject matter covered herein. It is sold with the clear understanding that the Publisher is not engaged in rendering legal or any other professional services. If legal or any other expert assistance is required, the services of a competent person should be sought. FROM A DECLARATION OF PARTICIPANTS JOINTLY ADOPTED BY A COMMITTEE OF THE AMERICAN BAR ASSOCIATION AND A COMMITTEE OF PUBLISHERS.

Additional color graphics may be available in the e-book version of this book.

LIBRARY OF CONGRESS CATALOGING-IN-PUBLICATION DATA

Encyclopedia of stem cell research / editor, Alexander L. Greene.
    p. ; cm.
  Includes bibliographical references and index.
  ISBN 978-1-61761-835-2 (hardcover)
  1. Stem cells--Encyclopedias. I. Greene, Alexander L.
  [DNLM: 1. Stem Cells. 2. Stem Cell Transplantation. QU 325]
  QH588.S83E532 2010
  616'.02774--dc22
                        2010034298

Published by Nova Science Publishers, Inc. † New York

CONTENTS

Volume 1

Preface xiii

Expert Comm A Stem Cell Therapy for Alzheimer's Disease   1
Philippe Taupin

Expert Comm B Adult Neurogenesis and Depression:
A Novel Theory for Depression?   7
Philippe Taupin

Expert Comm C Mannan-Binding Lectin and Stem Cell Transplantation   11
David C. Kilpatrick

Expert Comm D Sexuality of Men Treated by Means of Haematopoietic
Stem Cell Transplantation   17
Ladislav Slovacek and Birgita Slovackova

Short Comm A Therapeutic Potential of the Newly Characterized Human
Blood-Derived Stem Cell in Type 1 Diabetes   25
Yong Zhao and Lijun Yang

Short Comm B Recent Progress of Radiation Research: Cancer Stem Cells
and ncRNAs   37
Hideshi Ishii and Toshiyuki Saito

Short Comm C Recruitment of Transplanted Dermal Multipotent Cells
to the Injured Sites of Rats with Combined Radiation
and Wound Injury by SDF-1/CXCR4 Interaction   49
Zong Zhaowen, Ran Xinze, Cheng Tianmin and Su Yongping

Short Comm D Neural Cell Differentiation from Embryonic Stem Cell
by the Neural Stem Sphere Method   59
Takashi Nakayama, Masahiro Otsu and Nobuo Inoue

Chapter I	Stem Cell Applications in Disease Research: Recent Advances in Stem Cell and Cancer Stem Cell Biology and Their Therapeutic Implications *Murielle Mimeault and Surinder K. Batra*	67
Chapter II	Stem Cell Applications in Diabetes *Hirofumi Noguchi*	109
Chapter III	Stem Cells in Kidney Diseases *María José Soler and José Tomas Ortiz-Pérez*	131
Chapter IV	Role of Survivin in Adult Stem Cells and Cancer *Seiji Fukuda and Louis M. Pelus*	153
Chapter V	Cancer Stem Cells *Saranya Chumsri and Angelika M. Burger*	167
Chapter VI	Mesenchymal Stem Cells in Bone Diseases: State of the Art and Future Prospects *Gael Y. Rochefort and C. L. Benhamou*	181
Chapter VII	Radial Glia in the Repair of Central Nervous System Injury *I. Kulbatski and C.H. Tator*	211
Chapter VIII	A Review of Corneal Epithelial Stem Cell Therapy *David Hui-Kang Ma, Arvin Chi-Chin Sun, Jui-Yang Lai and Jan-Kan Chen*	239
Chapter IX	Towards Image-Guided Stem Cell Therapy *Kimberly J. Blackwood, Eric Sabondjian, Donna E. Goldhawk, Michael S. Kovacs, Gerald Wisenberg, Peter Merrifield, Frank S. Prato, Janice M. DeMoor and Robert Z. Stodilka*	281
Chapter X	Human Post-Natal Stem Cells in Organs Produced by Tissue Engineering for Clinical Applications *Lucie Germain, Danielle Larouche, François A. Auger and Julie Fradette*	309
Chapter XI	Cell Differentiation: Therapeutical Challenges in Diabetes *Enrique Roche, Nestor Vicente-Salar, Maribel Arribas and Beatriz Paredes*	337
Chapter XII	Mesenchymal Stem Cell Based Therapy in Liver Disease *I. Aurich, M. Sgodda and H. Aurich*	363
Chapter XIII	Recent Advancements towards the Derivation of Immune-Compatible Patient-Specific Human Pluripotent Stem Cell Lines *Micha Drukker*	393

Chapter XIV	Oxidative Damage in Age-Related Neurodegenerative Diseases and Interventions *H. Fai Poon and Sara C. Doore*	405
Chapter XV	The Activation of Adult Endogenous Neural Stem Cells by Neurodegenerative Process within the Striatum in an Animal Model of Huntington's Disease *Yvona Mazurová, Emil Rudolf, Ivana Gunčová and Ivan Látr*	417
Chapter XVI	Corneal Epithelial Stem Cells: A Biological and Clinical Approach *Maria Notara and Julie T. Daniels*	445
Chapter XVII	Immunological Responses of CD34+ Stem Cells to Bacterial Products *Jung Mogg Kim*	463
Chapter XVIII	Endothelial Progenitor Cells: From Bench to Bedside *Jeremy Ben-Shoshan and Jacob George*	489
Chapter XIX	Mesenchymal Stem Cells in Vascular Therapy *Gael Y. Rochefort*	509
Chapter XX	Human Embryonic Stem Cells: Key Characteristics and Main Applications in Disease Research *Kathryn Cherise Davidson, Mirella Dottori and Alice Pébay*	593
Chapter XXI	Establishment of Individual-Specific ES Cells from Adult Somatic Cells by Nuclear Transfer *Sayaka Wakayama and Teruhiko Wakayama*	625
Chapter XXII	Ocular Limbal Stem Cell Biology and Transplantation *Ali R. Djalilian, Nariman Nassiri and Chi-Chao Chan*	651
Chapter XXIII	Paracrine, Autocrine and Intracrine Patterning for Cardiovascular Repair with Human Mesenchymal Stem Cells: Role of New Chemistry for Regenerative Medicine *Carlo Ventura, Silvia Cantoni, Francesca Bianchi and Claudia Cavallini*	665
Chapter XXIV	Yin and Yang of Adult Stem Cells: Cure-All for Therapy or Roots for Cancer? *Christian Dani, Cédric Darini and Annie Ladoux*	687

Volume 2

Chapter XXV	Stem Cell Transplantation in Leukemia The Kidney *Terje Forslund*	705

Chapter XXVI	New Insights in the Development of Biological Chimeras: Genomic Instability and Epithelial Chimerism after Hematopoietic Stem Cell Transplantation *Alexandros Spyridonidis, Yannis Metaxas, Maria Themeli, Hartmut Bertz, Nicholas Zoumbos and Juergen Finke*	761
Chapter XXVII	The Evolving Role of Hematopoietic Stem Cell Transplantation in Non-Hodgkin Lymphoma *Koji Kato, Smitha Mellacheruvu and Shin Mineishi*	785
Chapter XXVIII	Efficient in vivo Gene Transfer into Rat Bone Marrow Progenitor Cells Using SV40-Derived Viral Vectors: Migration and Differentiation of Transduced Bone Marrow-Resident Cells to Other Organs *Jean-Pierre Louboutin, Alena A. Chekmasova, Bianling Liu and David S. Strayer*	823
Chapter XXIX	Stem Cells and Their Use in Regenerative Therapy of the Retina *Abed Namavari*	851
Chapter XXX	Vascular Tissue Engineering: Current Approaches and Strategies *Shannon L. M. Dahl*	873
Chapter XXXI	Skeletal Muscle Tissue Engineering Using Adipose Tissue Derived Stem Cells *MiJung Kim and Yu Suk Choi*	899
Chapter XXXII	Olfactory Neuroblastoma *Zhichun Lu and Honggang Liu*	915
Chapter XXXIII	Does Neural Phenotypic Plasticity from Non-Neural Cells Really Exist? *S. Wislet-Gendebien, F. Wautier, E. Laudet and B. Rogister*	937
Chapter XXXIV	Central Nervous System Lymphoma *Andrew Lister, Lauren E. Abrey and John T. Sandlund*	965
Chapter XXXV	Background and Legal Issues Related to Stem Cell Research *Jon O. Shimabukuro*	991
Chapter XXXVI	Bone Marrow-Derived Stem Cells: Homing and Rescue of Injury in the Lung *Donatella Piro, Silvia Lepore, Angela Bruna Maffione and Massimo Conese*	997
Chapter XXXVII	Role of Platelet Derived Factors for the Protection Against Graft-Versus-Host Disease *Tsuyoshi Iwasaki*	1025
Chapter XXXVIII	Stem Cell Plasticity *Suraksha Agrawal, Piyush Tripathi and Sita Naik*	1051

Chapter XXXIX	Dental Management before Hematopoietic Stem Cell Transplantation for Adult and Pediatric Patients with Hematological Disease *Kenji Yamagata, Kojiro Onizawa and Hiroshi Yoshida*	1095
Chapter XL	Haematopoietic Stem Cell Transplantation and Quality of Life *Ladislav Slovacek and Birgita Slovackova*	1115
Chapter XLI	Risk Factors for Survival in Pediatric Patients Undergoing Allogeneic Cord Blood Transplantation *Marta Gonzalez-Vicent, Julian Sevilla, Alvaro Lassaletta, Manuel Ramírez, Luis Madero, and Miguel A. Diaz*	1139
Chapter XLII	Multipoptent Mesenchymal Stromal Cells for Skin Wound Healing and Skeletal Muscle Repair *Ying Zhu, Chunmeng Shi, Xinze Ran, Yongping Su, Chengji Luo and Tianmin Cheng*	1155
Chapter XLIII	Normal and Pathological Development of Pluripotent Stem Cells *Olga F. Gordeeva*	1167
Chapter XLIV	Molecular Mechanism Involved in the Maintenance of Pluripotent Stem Cells *Raymond Ching-Bong Wong, Peter J Donovan and Alice Pébay*	1201
Chapter XLV	Generation of Clinically Relevant "Induced Pluripotent Stem" (iPS) Cells *Corey Heffernan, Huseyin Sumer and Paul J. Verma*	1227
Chapter XLVI	Amniotic Fluid and Placental Stem Cells *Emily C. Moorefield, Dawn M. Delo, Paolo De Coppi and Anthony Atala*	1253
Chapter XLVII	Exploring a Stem Cell Basis to Identify Novel Treatment for Human Malignancies *Shyam A. Patel and Pranela Rameshwar*	1271
Chapter XLVIII	Outstanding Questions Regarding Induced Pluripotent Stem (iPS) Cell Research *Miguel A. Esteban, Jiekai Chen, Jiayin Yang, Feng Li, Wen Li, and Duanqing Pei*	1285
Chapter XLIX	Lepidopteran Midgut Stem Cells in Culture: A New Tool for Cell Biology and Physiological Studies *Gianluca Tettamanti and Morena Casartelli*	1299
Chapter L	Are Embryonic Stem Cells Really Needed for Regenerative Medicine? *David T. Harris*	1309

Chapter LI	Genetic Stability of Murine Pluripotent and Somatic Hybrid Cells may be Affected by Conditions of Their Cultivation *Shramova Elena Ivanovna, Larionov Oleg Alekseevich, Khodarovich Yurii Mikhailovich and Zatsepina Olga Vladimirovna*	1315
Chapter LII	Recent Advancements towards the Derivation of Immune-Compatible Patient-Specific Human Pluripotent Stem Cell Lines *Micha Drukker*	1333
Chapter LIII	Pluripotent Cells in Embryogenesis and in Teratoma Formation *O. F. Gordeeva*	1345
Chapter LIV	Legal Issues Related to Human Embryonic Stem Cell Research *Edward C. Liu*	1361
Chapter LV	Stem Cell Research: Ethical Issues *Erin D. Williams and Judith A. Johnson*	1369
Chapter LVI	Stem Cell Research: Federal Research Funding and Oversight *Judith A. Johnson and Erin D. Williams*	1387
Chapter LVII	Testimony to be Presented to the House Committee on Energy and Commerce's Subcommittee on Health *Joseph R. Bertino*	1411
Chapter LVIII	Testimony to House Committee on Energy and Commerce, Subcommittee on Health "Stem Cell Science: The Foundation for Future Cures" *George Q. Daley*	1415
Chapter LIX	Testimony of John K. Fraser	1419
Chapter LX	Testimony on Stem Cell Science: The Foundation for Future Cures before the U.S. House of Representatives Subcommittee on Health of the Committee on Energy and Commerce *John Gearhart and C. Michael Armstron*	1425
Chapter LXI	Written Testimony of Weyman Johnson, Individual Living with Multiple Sclerosis, Chairman of the Board, National Multiple Sclerosis Society, Energy and Commerce Committee Subcommittee on Health U.S. House of Representatives	1431
Chapter LXII	Testimony for "Stem Cell Science: The Foundation for Future Cures" before the Subcommittee on Health of the Committee on Energy and Commerce *Amit N Patel*	1435
Chapter LXIII	Adult Stem Cell Recipient for the Heart *Douglas T. Rice*	1439

Chapter LXIV	Testimony Before the Subcommittee on Health Committee on Energy and Commerce United States House of Representatives Stem Cell Science: The Foundation of Future Cures. Statement of Elais A. Zerhouni *Elias A. Zerhouni*	**1443**
Chapter Sources		**1449**
Index		**1451**

PREFACE

This book presents important research advances in the study of stem cell research, as well as stem cell applications in diseases; stem cell transplantation; and pluripotent stem cells. Topics discussed herein include stem cell therapy for alzheimer's disease; cancer stem cells and ncRNAs; stem cell applications in diabetes; image-guided stem cell therapy; cancer stem cells; stem cell transplantation; vascular tissue engineering; bone marrow-derived stem cells; and stem cell plasticity.

Expert Commentary A - Alzheimer's disease (AD) is a neurodegenerative disease. It is the most common form of dementia among older people for which there is at present no cure. Current treatments for AD consist mainly in drug therapy. The recent confirmation that neurogenesis occurs in the adult brain and neural stem cells (NSCs) reside in the adult central nervous system (CNS) provide new opportunities for cellular therapy in the CNS, particularly for AD. Besides its therapeutic potential, neurogenesis is increased in the hippocampus of patients with AD and animal models of AD. The effect of drugs used to treat AD on neurogenesis is currently being investigated, to identify whether neurogenesis contributes to their therapeutic activities. In all, adult NSCs not only provide a promising model to treat AD, but also provide the opportunity to better understand the pathogenesis of AD and its pharmacology.

Expert Commentary B - The recent confirmation that neurogenesis occurs throughout adulthood in mammals raises the question of the function of newly generated neuronal cells in the adult brain.

The hippocampus is an important memory center of the brain. It is also involved in pathological processes, like Alzheimer's disease and epilepsy. Several lines of evidence further suggest that the hippocampus is involved in the etiology of major depressive disorders, like chronic stress and depression.

Short Communication A - Stem cell-derived insulin-producing cells may provide a rational tool for treatment of both type 1 (T1D) and type 2 (T2D) diabetes. Previous studies suggest that either embryonic or adult stem cells can serve as potential sources of β cell surrogates for therapeutic applications. However, the immune system will recognize and attack any foreign cells utilized for the restoration of euglycemia due to the immune surveillance, even the application of allogeneic embryonic stem (ES) cells. To circumvent these barriers, many novel approaches are being investigated, including those directed at manipulating the host immune responses, altered nuclear transfer, and other aspects directed at modulating disease pathogenesis. However, despite these efforts, no suitable solution has been achieved. Therefore, application of autologous stem cells-derived insulin-producing cells is a potentially attractive strategy and may serve as a means to overcome many of the major issues that can complicate cell-based therapies.

Recently, the authors have identified a unique stem cell population from adult human blood, designated peripheral blood-derived stem cells (PB-SC). PB-SC were expandable and displayed embryonic stem (ES) cell characteristics, along with hematopoietic markers; but lacked expression of hematopoietic stem cell marker CD34 as well as lymphocyte and monocyte/macrophage markers. Notably, PB-SC showed the high potential to give rise to functional insulin-producing cells, as demonstrated the authentic insulin production at different levels by *in vitro* and *in vivo* characterizations. Using the same technology, the authors have found a similar type of stem cells from human umbilical cord blood. Their current studies have revealed that these newly characterized human blood-derived stem cells not only act as stem cells giving rise to insulin-producing cells, but also as immune modulator cells. In conclusion, application of PB-SC is easy to access, culture, expand, differentiate, and is safe, without any ethical issues or immune rejection. These findings may lead to developing new approaches for autologous transplantation of these blood insulin-producing cells to treat diabetes.

Short Communication B - For over three decades, stem cells have been used in the replenishment of hematological and immune systems damaged by genotoxins or during treatment of malignant cells by chemotherapy or radiotherapy. The cancer stem cell hypothesis suggests that a tumor can be viewed as an aberrant organ that is sustained, in a way similar to normal tissues, by a stem cell that drives tumorigenesis, as well as giving rise to a large population of differentiated progeny. The cancer stem cells, controlled by the micro-environmental conditions in the cancer tissue structures, may be involved in the process of relapse, metastasis and resistance to therapy. The strategy of targeting a small fraction of cancer stem cells would be efficient and would minimize the side-effects of the total kill strategy. The aim of this mini-review is to focus on recent developments in radiation research on cancer stem cells and transcriptome of noncoding (nc) RNA molecules, as well as their role in carcinogenesis and their implications in the development of new cancer treatments in the future.

Short Communication C - Systemic transplantation of dermal multipotent cells (dMSCs) has been shown to accelerate both hematopoietic recovery and wound healing in rats with combined radiation and wound injury. In the present study, the authors explored the the mechanisms governing the recruitment of dMSCs to the injured sites of combine-injured rats. Male dMSCs were transplanted into female rats, and by employing quantitative real-time PCR for the sex-determining region of Y chromosome, it was found that the amount of dMSCs in bone marrow and wounded skin of rats with combined injury were about 2 times more than those of normal rats ($P<0.01$). Incubation dMSCs with AMD3100 before transplantation, which specifically blocks binding of stromal cell-derived factor-1 (SDF-1) to its receptor CXCR4, diminished dMSCs recruitment to the injured sites by $57.5\pm4.2\%$ and $59.5\pm3.8\%$ respectively ($P<0.05$). In addition, it was confirmed that the expression of SDF-1 in injured bone marrow and wound was up-regulated when compared with normal rats, and *in vitro* analysis revealed that bone marrow extracts and wound fluid obtained from combine-injured rats had strong chemotactic effect on dMSCs, but decreased significantly when dMSCs was pre-incubated by AMD3100 ($P<0.05$). These data suggest that transplanted dMSCs were recruited more frequently to bone marrow and wounded skin in combine-injured rats than normal rats and the interactions of SDF-1/CXCR4 played an important role in this process.

Short Communication D - The authors have established a novel method to efficiently produce a large number of neural stem cells from mouse, monkey, and human embryonic stem (ES) cells. The procedure requires only free-floating culture of ES colonies in astrocyte-conditioned medium (ACM) for differentiation into neural stem cells. These ES cell-derived neural stem cells can proliferate easily on an adhesive substrate in the presence of fibroblast growth factor-2 (FGF-2). They can be preserved by freezing, and can proliferate again after thawing. Furthermore, the authors have succeeded in unidirectional differentiation of ES cell-derived neural stem cells into neurons or astrocytes by choosing culture conditions. Neurogenesis of ES cell-derived neural stem cells can be induced by changing the medium from FGF-2-containing proliferation medium to ACM containing inductive factors. In contrast, withdrawing FGF-2 from the medium can induce differentiation of these cells into astrocytes, indicating that astrocytogenesis does not require any additional signals, such as humoral factors. Here, they describe the characteristics of their method applicable to cell transplantation therapy.

Chapter I - Recent advances in embryonic, fetal, umbilical cord, placental, amniotic and tissue-resident adult stem/progenitor cell research is of great clinical interest due to their potential therapeutic applications in regenerative medicine and gene therapies. The tissue-resident adult stem/progenitor cells, which possess several characteristics common with embryonic stem cells (ESCs) but generally display more limited self-renewal ability and restricted differentiating potential, are emerging as promising sources of immature cells. The presence of a rare population of adult stem/progenitor cells in most tissues and organs offers the possibility to stimulate their *in vivo* differentiation or to use their *ex vivo* expanded progenies for cell replacement-based therapies with multiple applications in humans. Among the human diseases that could be treated by the stem cell-based therapies, the hematopoietic and immune disorders, cardiovascular disorders, multiple degenerative disorders such as Parkinson's and Alzeimeher's diseases, type 1 or 2 diabetes mellitus as well as eye, liver, lung, gastrointestinal and skin disorders and aggressive and metastatic cancers deserve immediate attention. In addition, the genetically-modified adult stem/progenitor cells could also be used as a delivery system for expressing the therapeutic molecules in specific damaged areas of different tissues in humans. Recent progress in cancer stem/progenitor cell research also offers the possibility to target these undifferentiated and malignant cells that provide critical functions in cancer initiation and progression and disease relapse for treating patients diagnosed with advanced and metastatic cancers which remain incurable in clinics with the current therapies.

Chapter II - Diabetes mellitus is a devastating disease and the World Health Organization (WHO) expects that the number of diabetic patients will increase to 300 million by the year 2025. Patients with diabetes experience decreased insulin secretion that is linked to a significant reduction in the number of islet cells. Type 1 diabetes is characterized by the selective destruction of pancreatic β cells caused by an autoimmune attack. Type 2 diabetes is a more complex pathology that, in addition to β cell loss caused by apoptotic programs, includes β cell de-differentiation and peripheric insulin resistance. The success achieved over the last few years with islet transplantation suggests that diabetes can be cured by the replenishment of deficient β cells. These observations are proof of the concept and have intensified interest in treating diabetes or other diseases not only by cell transplantation but also by stem cells. An increasing body of evidence indicates that, in addition to embryonic stem cells, several potential adult stem/progenitor cells derived from the pancreas, liver, spleen, and bone marrow could differentiate into insulin-producing cells *in vitro* or *in vivo*. However, significant controversy currently exists in this field. Pharmacological approaches aimed at stimulating the *in vivo/ex vivo* regeneration of β cells have been proposed as a way of augmenting islet cell mass. Overexpression of embryonic transcription factors in stem cells could efficiently induce their differentiation into insulin-expressing cells. A new technology, known as protein transduction, facilitates the differentiation of stem cells into insulin-producing cells. Recent progress in the search for new sources of β cells has opened up several possibilities for the development of new treatments for diabetes.

Chapter III - Circulating bone marrow-derived endothelial progenitor cells (EPCs) seem to play a crucial role in both vasculogenesis and vascular homeostasis. Chronic kidney disease is a state of endothelial dysfunction, accelerated progression of atherosclerosis and high cardiovascular risk. As a consequence, cardiovascular disorders are the main cause of death in end-stage renal disease (ESRD). It has been shown that patients with advanced renal failure have decreased number of bone marrow-derived endothelial progenitor cells and impaired EPCs function. Moreover, in kidney transplant patients, renal graft function significantly correlated with EPC number. The reduced number of EPCs in patients with ESRD has been ascribed to the uremia. Therefore, therapies that improve the uremic status in dialysis patients such as nocturnal hemodialysis are associated with restoration of impaired EPCs number and migratory function. In fact, some of the common treatments for patients with chronic kidney disease such as erythropoietin, statins and angiotensin II receptor antagonist increase the number of EPCs. Nowadays, there is growing evidence indicating that, under pathophysiological conditions, stem cells (SCs) derived from bone marrow are able to migrate in the injured kidney, and they seem to play a role in glomerular and tubular regeneration. After acute tubular renal injury, surviving tubular epithelial cells and putative renal stem cells proliferate and differentiate into tubular epithelial cells to promote structural and functional repair. Moreover, bone marrow stem cells, including hematopoietic stem cells and mesenchymal stem cells can also participate in the repair process by proliferation and differentiation into renal lineages. For instance, mesenchymal SCs have been shown to decrease inflammation and enhance renal regeneration. The administration of *ex vivo* expanded bone marrow-derived mesenchymal SCs have been proved to be beneficial in various experimental models of acute renal failure. The mechanisms underlining this beneficial effect are still a matter of debate. Thus, therapeutic strategies aimed at correcting the regenerative potential of stem cells based on the administration of *ex vivo* expanded SCs or stimulating expansion and differentiation of local progenitor/SC populations are another exciting area of future research.

Chapter IV - The inhibitor of apoptosis protein (IAP), Survivin regulates apoptosis, cell cycle and cell division. Its expression in normal tissue is developmentally regulated and becomes barely detectable in most terminally differentiated adult tissues. Survivin has been proposed as a potential cancer target because the vast majority of the human tumors express high levels of Survivin in contrast to limited expression in most normal adult tissues. However, recent studies have demonstrated that Survivin regulates adult stem cell physiology, such as hematopoietic stem cells, neuronal precursor cells, keratinocyte stem cells and intestinal crypt stem cells. Furthermore, mouse embryonic stem cells express Survivin and homozygous gene deletion in mice leads to embryonic death at E4.5, indicating that Survivin is required for totipotent stem cell function. It is believed that cancer stem cells are primarily responsible for the development and dissemination of cancer. The authors' recent data suggests that Survivin regulates not just normal hematopoietic stem and progenitor cell (HSPC) proliferation but transformed HSPC with self-renewal capability. Since cancer stem cells share biological phenotypes with normal adult stem cells and almost all cancer cells over-express Survivin, it is likely that Survivin regulates leukemia and/or cancer stem cell fate. Although targeting Survivin in leukemia/cancer stem cells may be an effective treatment modality, ablation of Survivin may have adverse consequences *in vivo*, as a result of toxicity to normal stem cells. In this review, the authors will summarize and compare the roles of Survivin in normal adult stem cells and leukemia/cancer cells. Investigating mechanisms responsible for differentially regulating Survivin expression and function in cancer and normal adult stem cells will help to identify critical differences in Survivin behavior between neoplastic and normal tissues that can be utilized to develop innovative strategies for selectively antagonizing Survivin. In addition, manipulating pathways associated with Survivin may identify novel stem cell therapies with application for regenerative medicine.

Chapter V - Emerging evidence suggests that cancers contain a rare and biologically distinct subpopulation of cells with the ability to self-renew and to sustain tumor growth, termed "cancer stem cells". Cancer stem cells share many characteristics with normal stem cells including self-renewal, asymmetric division, indefinite proliferative capacity, and self-protection mechanisms. The cancer stem cell concept is best understood in hematologic malignancies. In solid tumors, breast cancer stem cells have been the most explored. Several techniques have been described, allowing the identification or isolation of cancer stem cells by either expression of specific cell surface markers, their differential ability to efflux dyes, or by a distinct enzymatic activity. More recent studies also established the crucial role of cancer stem cells in multistage cancer progression and metastasis which has important implications for the design of novel targeted therapies. Since most of the conventional chemotherapies only affect differentiated cancer cells, initial reduction in tumor mass is often followed by a rapid relapse. In order to achieve durable remissions, it will be imperative to eradicate cancer stem cells.

Chapter VI - Bone remodeling is a physiological process determined by the sequential and coordinated interaction of osteoclasts, osteoblasts and angiogenesis. During bone repair, osteoblastic cells, originated from mesenchymal stem cells (MSCs), are highly regulated to proliferate and to produce an osteogenic matrix, thus forming a new bone. MSCs are multipotential and undifferentiated cells that are present in the adult bone marrow. They serve *in vitro* and *in vivo* as precursors for bone marrow stroma, bone, fat, cartilage, muscle (smooth, cardiac and skeletal) and neural cells. MSCs are usually isolated from adult bone marrow but can also be isolated from several other tissues, such as fetal liver, adult circulating blood, umbilical cord blood, placenta or adipose tissue. In the bone marrow, MSCs give rise to mesenchymal cells residing in the bone (osteogenic, chondrogenic and adipogenic cells) and also support hematopoiesis. Therefore, MSCs regulate both osteogenesis and hematopoiesis, and they are responsible in part for the regenerative capacity of bone tissue. Osteoporosis, resulting of an imbalance between resorption and formation of endosteal and trabecular bone surfaces, is a systemic disorder characterized by a low bone mass and an altered bone quality with a consistent increase in bone fragility and susceptibility to fracture correlated to functional aberrations in MSCs. This chapter highlights current status and progresses in the use of MSCs to treat or attenuate bone diseases, including osteoporosis.

Chapter VII - During central nervous system (CNS) development, radial glia function as specialized scaffold cells that guide migrating neurons. Radial glia also proliferate during neurogenesis, give rise to oligodendrocytes and astrocytes, and guide migrating glial precursors. In most cases, radial glia are only present for as long as they function during CNS development; however, some radial glia remain into adulthood. In lower vertebrates such as birds and amphibians in which there is continual neurogenesis into adulthood, radial glia are always present, and may play a role in regeneration. In the adult rat, radial glia emerge following spinal cord injury and likely play a role in neural regeneration. It was recently shown that embryonic rat radial glia transplanted into the injured rat spinal cord formed bridges and promoted functional recovery.

Radial glia comprise the majority of precursors in the ventricular zones in most areas of the CNS, especially in the brain. Radial glia in neonates and radial glia-derived cells in the adult lateral ventricle exhibit neural stem/precursor cell (NSPC) properties, since they generate self-renewing multipotent neurospheres in vitro. The authors recently showed that NSPCs isolated from the adult rat spinal cord and propagated in vitro differentiate into large numbers of radial glia, and appear to function as guidance scaffolds. This suggests a recapitulation of their developmental role *in vitro*. This role may extend to reflect their capacity to act as NSPCs within the adult CNS, and highlights their potential for transplantation therapies.

This chapter focuses on the function of radial glia in the CNS, with particular emphasis on their role as NSPCs, their endogenous response following CNS injury, and the potential of therapies that enhance the endogenous radial glial response or supply an exogenously expanded source of radial glia in the form of a cellular transplant strategy for CNS regeneration.

Chapter VIII - Owing to the rapid progress in biomedical science and the highly anticipated therapeutic potentials, stem cell-related research has boomed since the beginning of the new millennium. However, in contrast to enormous basic research papers that have been published, clinical applications of stem cells, except hematopoietic stem cell transplantation, are still in infancy. Nevertheless, during the last decade we have witnessed a remarkable success in corneal epithelial stem cell therapy, which merits special attention to what has been found regarding corneal epithelial biology, and what has been reported regarding the therapeutic modalities.

The corneal epithelial stem cells are located in the basal layer of limbus (therefore are called limbal stem cells – LSCs), and are pivotal for the maintenance of corneal transparency and avascularity. In event of LSC deficiency that is caused by burns or autoimmune diseases, conjunctival epithelial cell invasion is accompanied by pannas ingrowth and persistent inflammation. Transplantation of autologous or allogeneic healthy limbal tissue restores corneal epithelium and therefore improves vision.

In recent years, LSC transplantation has evolved to become a successful example of tissue engineering. Corneal, conjunctival, and oral mucosal epithelial cells (as an alternative source of corneal epithelium) can be harvested in small size, cultured and expanded in vitro. Preserved human amniotic membrane (AM) is the natural biomaterial that most widely used as the carrier for cultivated epithelium. It has been well documented that AM preserves epithelial progenitor cells during cultivation, and inhibits corneal inflammation and angiogenesis after transplantation. Fibrin has also been used to transport the cultivated epithelium, but was less reported.

However, either with AM or fibrin, the graft transparency may be affected, and in order to further improve vision, penetrating or lamellar keratoplasty is sometimes needed after epithelial transplantation.

Thermo-responsive culture surface (TRCS) is a newly developed intelligent interface that enables complete detachment of the epithelial sheet upon lowering of temperature without the use of proteolytic enzymes. Because the integrity of basement membrane was maintained, the epithelial sheet graft can attach to the recipient bed readily without the need for laborious suturing procedure, while the graft transparency is optimal. TRCS has been used for cultivated oral mucosal and corneal epithelial cell transplantation, and in the near future, it may even facilitate cultivated corneal endothelial cell transplantation, which may eventually solve the problem of global shortage of donor corneas.

Chapter IX - Cellular imaging is the non-invasive and repetitive imaging of targeted cells and cellular processes in living organisms. Previously, lack of technology prevented *in vivo* study of cell populations; studies of cellular dynamics relied on "snapshot" images from *ex vivo* histology. With the emergence of cell tracking technologies, it may become possible to study *in vivo* cell distribution, migration, gene expression, differentiation, proliferation, engraftment, and death. Cellular imaging has been used to monitor migration of transplanted cells in therapies for neurodegenerative, cerebral ischemic, cardiac, and oncologic disorders, and to characterize cell migration during the developmental stages of an organism. Many imaging modalities are being evaluated for application to cell tracking and monitoring of regenerative therapy - with no clear leading contender. This article discusses the advantages and disadvantages among leading modalities, including MRI, SPECT, PET, optical, as well as "hybrid" modalities such as SPECT/CT and PET/MRI. The authors also describe cell labeling strategies such as *ex vivo* labeling with radioactivity (for SPECT), superparamagnetic iron oxide nanoparticles (for MRI), reporter gene expression, and their associated challenges such as toxicity, contrast dilution, and non-specific uptake. From a clinical perspective, the authors focus on cardiology applications due to the importance of myocardial regeneration, and finally feature two in-depth examples of cell tracking using imaging: SPECT imaging of radiolabeled cells for monitoring myocardial stem cell therapy, and a magnetosome gene-based contrast agent for cell tracking and molecular imaging with MRI.

Chapter X - This chapter will focus on the clinical applications of post-natal stem cells. Massive tissue loss frequently requires grafting for proper healing. Considering that there is a shortage of organ donors, the expansion of cells *in vitro* and the reconstruction of tissues or organs constitute a very valuable alternative solution. The first clinical application of such tissues has been the autologous culture of epidermal cells for the treatment of burn patients, and will be presented herein. Since the cutaneous epithelium forms squames that are lost, it is continuously renewed every 28 days and its long-term regeneration depends on stem cells. The importance of preserving stem cells during *in vitro* expansion and after grafting will thus be discussed. Clinical applications of cultured cells from other tissues, such as limbal stem cells for corneal epithelium (surface of the eye) replacement, will also be reviewed. Finally, the development of new promising technologies and methods taking advantage of other sources of stem cells that could be isolated after birth from tissues such as adipose depots will also be presented.

Chapter XI - Stem cells, derived from either embryonic or adult tissues, are considered to be potential sources of insulin-secreting cells to be transplanted into type 1 and advanced stages of type 2 diabetic patients. Many laboratories have considered this possibility, resulting in a large amount of published protocols, with a wide degree of complexity among them. The authors' group was the first to report that it was possible to obtain insulin-secreting cells from mouse embryonic stem cells, proving the feasibility of this new challenge. The same observation was immediately reported using human embryonic stem cells. However, the resulting cell product was not properly characterised, affecting the reproducibility of the protocol by other groups. A more elaborated protocol was developed by Lumelsky and co-workers, demonstrating that neuroectodermal cells could be an alternative source for insulin-producing cells. However, the resulting cells of this protocol produced low amounts of the hormone. This directed other groups to perform key changes in order to improve the insulin content of the resulting cells. Recently, Baetge's group has published a new protocol based on the knowledge accumulated in pancreatic development. In this protocol, human embryonic stem cells were differentiated into islet-like structures through a five step protocol, emulating the key steps during embryonic development of the endocrine pancreas. The final cell product, however, seemed to be in an immature state, thus further improvement is required. Despite this drawback, the protocol represents the culmination of work performed by different groups and offers new research challenges for the investigators in this exciting field. Concerning adult stem cells, the possibility of identifying pancreatic precursors or of reprogramming extrapancreatic derived cells are key possibilities that may circumvent the problems that appear when using embryonic stem cells, such as immune rejection and tumour formation.

Chapter XII - The use of primary human hepatocytes for cell therapy of liver diseases is limited because of the restricted availability of marginal donor organs. Hence, novel cell sources are required to gain hepatocytes of adequate quality and quantity for clinical use. Due to the plasticity and potential to proliferate, stem cells isolated from various origins may be an alternative source to generate functional hepatocytes suitable for clinical use. Within the last decade, different protocols have been published to investigate the potential of adult stem cells to differentiate into hepatocyte-like cells. In contrast, protocols using embryonic stem cells (ESC) still struggle with the problem of tumorigenicity, and major ethical concerns restrict the applicability of human embryonic stem cells. Hence, research focused on adult hematopoietic (HSC) and mesenchymal stem cells (MSC). Regarding availability, in vitro proliferation, cultivation and differentiation, MSC are usually prefered over HSC. The specific surface expression pattern (CD34, CD45, CD105) is clearly different in the two types of stem cells. After expansion of MSC in vitro, the differentiation into hepatocyte-like cells proceeds with treatment applying specific growth factors and supplements. The level of hepatogenic differentiation is indicated by the loss of progenitor cell markers (CX43, CK7, CK19, alpha fetoprotein) and the increase in expression of hepatogenic markers (CK18, CX32, HepPar I, CD26, CYP) as well as hepatocyte-specific functions (urea synthesis, detoxification, albumin expression, storage of polyhydrocarbons). Different animal models have been used to investigate the integration and repopulation of transplanted MSC into injured livers. The hepatogenic differentiated MSC results in an improved integration into the liver parenchyma. After transplantation into regenerating mouse livers, MSC continue to express hepatocyte-specific functions. Besides others, the detection of human serum albumin in the mouse serum and the activation of liver specific promoters indicate a functionality of transplanted human stem cell-derived hepatocytes in the host mouse liver. Thus it is expected that MSC may become a useful source for hepatocyte regeneration in liver-cell therapy.

Chapter XIII - The derivation of human embryonic stem cell lines from blastocyst stage embryos, first achieved almost a decade ago, demonstrated the potential to prepare virtually unlimited numbers of therapeutically beneficial cells *in vitro*. Assuming that large-scale production of differentiated cells is attainable, it is imperative to develop strategies to prevent immune responses towards the grafted cells following transplantation. This paper presents recent advances in the production of pluripotent cell lines using three emerging techniques: somatic cell nuclear transfer into enucleated oocytes and zygotes, parthenogenetic activation of unfertilized oocytes and induction of pluripotency in somatic cells. These techniques have a remarkable potential for generation of patient-specific pluripotent cells that would be tolerated by the immune system.

Chapter XIV - Aging, a universal process of all organisms, is defined as a functional decline of systems, to which the dysregulation of the redox signaling pathway contributes. The brain is not excluded from the aging process, and the aged brain is more susceptible to neurodegenerative diseases than the young one. Much research is being conducted to examine the variables involved in age-related neurodegeneration, as well as its interventions. One potential method of treatment may incorporate stem cells, which could provide a renewed resource for aged neurons or aberrant genes and/or proteins in the degenerated brain. Here, the authors will examine the biological processes that are affected by the dysregualtion of the redox signaling pathway in age-related degenerative central nervous systems. Furthermore, the authors will discuss how stem cell research and other treatments could provide potential intervention for these biological processes.

Chapter XV - Studies, carried out in the last decade, have demonstrated a continuous postnatal neurogenesis in the subependymal zone (SEZ) of lateral brain ventricles in the normal adult brain. However, some morphological and functional relationships, especially under pathological conditions, remain unclear. Crucial for endogenous neural stem cells (NSCs) is believed to be a specialized microenvironment – neurogenic niche. The glial nature of adult NSCs is already well documented, indicating that SEZ stem/niche cells are GFAP-positive astrocytes. But some other properties and relationships remain to be investigated.

The neurodegenerative process within the striatum, a hallmark of Huntington's disease (HD), represents severe damage of the brain parenchyma. In an animal model of HD, induced by intrastriatal injection of quolinic acid (QA), neurodegenerative process initiates immediate intensive cell proliferation, resulting in characteristic enlargement of the SEZ. For that reason, the authors were interested in a reaction of the neurogenic niche in the SEZ at 7 days after the QA lesion. The reaction of the SEZ changed over time. Therefore, a protracted reaction of the SEZ in the ongoing neurodegenerative process within the striatum was observed after 6 months.

The authors have described the compartmentalization of the SEZ: (1) In the R-SEZ, i.e., in a rostral part of anterior horn of lateral brain ventricles (AP 1.4-1.5 from bregma), related to the rostral migratory stream and olfactory bulb, the generation of new neuronal cell typically prevails, whereas (2) in the more posterior region (AP 1.1-1.2 from bregma), the lateral part of the SEZ (L-SEZ) opposite the degenerated striatum was characteristic by proliferation of both types of cells, with neuronal and mainly with astrocytic properties. Accompanied angiogenesis was also obvious as an integral morphological and functional component of activated SEZ.

The authors' results show some new morphological features, particularly a wide plasticity of endogenous astrocyte-like stem/niche cells in immediate response to an extensive pathological process in the adult brain but also their inability to become mature neurons in the region of L-SEZ. Their further findings document that astrocyte-like cells in the adult SEZ, during their extensive proliferation, retain some features of embryonic stem cells, including the reexpression of vimentin intermediate filaments which contributes to the suggestion that these astrocyte-like cells are derivatives of radial glia. On the other hand, their following differentiation is limited by the microenvironment of the adult neurogenic niche.

Chapter XVI - The clinical use of stem cells is a promising alternative treatment of life threatening and dehabilitating conditions such as leukaemia, diabetes, heart disease and spinal cord injury. The ethical and scientific debates regarding the appropriate stem cell source e.g. embryonic versus adult, autologous versus allogeneic etc are ongoing. In this review, the authors will describe limbal epithelial stem cells (LESC), a population of cells believed to be residing in the vascularised corneoscleral junction (i.e. the limbus) which are responsible for the maintenance and repair of the corneal epithelium. Partial or total depletion of the LESC population can have devastating effects including vision impairment, pain and ultimately blindness. LESCs are already successfully used clinically to treat blinding conditions of the cornea such as chemical burns, Stevens Johnson syndrome or aniridia. The function, properties and cytokine signalling of the LESC-corneal stroma as well as the potentials in exploiting their therapeutic uses will be discussed.

Chapter XVII - Since umbilical cord blood contains a significantly higher number of $CD34^+$ stem cells than adult peripheral blood, umbilical cord blood is proposed as an ideal alternative to bone marrow and peripheral blood for the hematopoietic stem cell transplantation. However, the sepsis induced by bacterial infection has known to be one of the complications after cord blood transplantation. Therefore, it is important to evaluate immunological responses of $CD34^+$ stem cells to bacterial infection. The authors found that

CD34$^+$ cells and their cultured cells infected with *Escherichia coli* induced expression of proinflammatory cytokines, such as IL-1α, IL-6, IL-8, and TNF-α, via NF-κB pathway. Expression of the proinflammatory cytokines was mainly generated from granulocytes-macrophage lineages. CD34$^+$ cells may recognize the molecular patterns associated with pathogens and subsequently initiate the transcription of inflammatory genes. These molecular patterns may be specifically conserved components of microbes such as CpG DNA. Exposure of the cells to synthetic oligodeoxynucleotides containing unmethylated CpG motifs (CpG ODN) resulted in a time- and dose-dependent increase of IL-8 expression and activation of phosphorylated mitogen-activated protein kinase (MAPK) such as ERK1/2 and p38. In addition, CpG ODN stimulated AP-1, but not NF-κB signals. Moreover, inhibition of MAPK reduced the IL-8 production, while inhibition of NF-κB did not affect the IL-8 expression increased by CpG ODN. Blocking Toll-like receptor 9 (TLR9) in CD34$^+$ cells decreased CpG ODN-induced up-regulation of IL-8, indicating that CpG DNA, acting on TLR9, activates CD34$^+$ cells to express IL-8 through MAPK-dependent and NF-κB-independent pathways, although whole Gram-negative *E. coli* can activate NF-κB and up-regulate IL-8 in CD34+ cells. Moreover, co-stimulation with lipopolysaccharide and CpG synergistically up-regulates IL-8 in CD34$^+$ cells. Results obtained from the authors' studies may have important implications in host defense and gene therapy strategies. In particular, a new role of CpG DNA and CD34$^+$ cells in systemic bacterial infection is possible. Furthermore, attention should be paid to distinguish the therapeutic gene-mediated biological effect from the CpG-mediated nonspecific effect.

Chapter XVIII - Cell-based restoration of tissue blood supply for the treatment of ischemic cardiovascular diseases has been profoundly examined during the last decade. The recent discovery of a bone marrow-derived scarce population of endothelial progenitor cells (EPCs), capable of participating in postnatal formation of new blood vessels, has thus gained considerable attention. Substantial efforts are still being made in order to identify the phenotype of these putative cells. Meanwhile, growing evidence obtained from both animal and primary human studies point to the tremendous potential of bone marrow-derived progenitor cells as diagnostic and therapeutic tools. Nevertheless, the long term clinical benefits of progenitor cell mobilization or delivery still remain to be further elucidated. In the present chapter, the authors describe the phenotypical and functional characterization of EPCs known so far, as well as their value as diagnostic markers of vascular dysfunction. Additionally, they review the data accumulated from animal studies and pilot clinical trials regarding cell-based angiogenic therapy. Eventually, they discuss the potential hurdles to be taken into account as well as potential strategies for the amelioration of the angiogenic properties of EPCs.

Chapter IXX - Mesenchymal stem cells (MSCs) constitute a heterogeneous population of undifferentiated and committed multipotential cells. They serve *in vitro* and *in vivo* as precursors for bone marrow stroma, bone, fat, cartilage, muscle (smooth, cardiac and skeletal) and neural cells. They are able to home upon engraftment to a number of microenvironments, capable of extensive proliferation and of producing large number of differentiated progenitors to repair functionally tissue after injury. MSCs are usually isolated from adult bone marrow but can also be isolated from several other tissues, such as fetal liver, adult circulating blood, umbilical cord blood, placenta or adipose tissue. Furthermore, MSCs present several immuno-regulatory characteristics with immuno-suppressive effects that induce a tolerance and could be therapeutic for reduction of graft-versus-host disease, rejection and modulation of inflammation. Since MSCs follow a vascular smooth muscle differentiation pathway, their therapeutic potential has been widely investigated in the treatment of vascular diseases. Indeed, MSCs can participate in the development of new vessels from pre-existing vascular walls (angiogenesis), in the induction of new vascular networks (vasculogenesis), in the collateral artery growth (arteriogenesis) or in plastic and reconstructive surgery applications. These cells can promote vascular growth by incorporating into vessels' wall, but they also may function as supporting factors by producing paracrine vascular promoting factors. In this chapter, the mesenchymal stem cells isolation, culture and characterization, but also their potential use in vascular therapy, in both human and animal models, are reported and discussed, whereas perspectives in angiogenesis, vasculogenesis, arteriogenesis or vascular engineering are explored.

Chapter XX - Embryonic stem cells (ESC), derived from the inner cell mass of pre-implantation mammalian embryos, are primordial, pluripotent cells capable of both self-renewal and further differentiation into the three primary germ lineages, ectoderm, endoderm, and mesoderm, which give rise to all cells types found within an adult organism. Once established in culture, ESC lines can be propagated indefinitely without undergoing a restriction in developmental potential and thereby can provide an unlimited source of cells for exploitation. Since ESC were first isolated from mouse blastocysts in 1981, they have become a vital tool for the study of development and diseases. The derivation of human ESC (hESC) nearly twenty years later generated considerable interest and excitement as researchers predicted their broad utility for human studies and cellular therapies. Understanding the mechanisms that govern stem cell self-renewal and differentiation is of fundamental significance to cellular and developmental biology. The knowledge gained from such research is anticipated to lead to major biomedical outcomes. This review aims to summarize the current knowledge on hESC characterization, and will discuss the potential applications of hESC in disease research.

Chapter XXI - Cloning methods are now well described and becoming routine. Yet the frequency at which cloned offspring are produced still remains below 10%, irrespective of the nucleus donor species or cell type. Especially in the mouse, only a few laboratories have obtained clones from adult somatic cells, and most mouse strains never succeed in producing cloned mice. On the other hand, nuclear transfer can be used to generate embryonic stem (ntES) cell lines from a subject's own somatic cells. The authors have shown that ntES cells can be generated relatively easily from a variety of mouse genotypes and cell types of both sexes, even though it may be more difficult to generate clones directly. Several reports have already demonstrated that ntES cells can be used in regenerative medicine in order to rescue immunodeficient or infertile phenotypes. This technique can also be applied for preservation of genetic resource of mouse strains instead of embryos, oocytes or spermatozoa. However, if ntES cells have abnormalities, such as those associated with the offspring produced by reproductive cloning, then their scientific and medical utilities could prove to be limited. Fortunately, turned out to be a groundless fear, for these ntES cells were able to differentiate into all functional embryonic tissues *in vivo*. Moreover, they were identical to fertilized - derived ES cells in terms of their expression of pluripotency markers, pattern of tissue-dependent differentially DNA methylated regions and global gene expression. These similarities of ntES cells and ES cells indicate that murine therapeutic cloning by somatic cell nuclear transfer can provide a reliable model for preclinical stem cell research. Nuclear transfer requires a large number of fresh oocytes, which gives rise to fundamental ethical concerns surrounding its potential applications in human cells, as fresh oocytes must be obtained from a healthy female donor. This review seeks to describe the phenotype, application, possible abnormalities and resolution of ethical problem of cloned mice and ntES cell lines.

Chapter XXII - The cornea is covered by a continuous renewing stratified squamous epithelium. Like stem cells of other epithelial surfaces that reside in a special region (niche) throughout adulthood, the corneal epithelial stem cells are localized in the basal layer of the corneoscleral junction, known as the limbus. These stem cells are important prerequisite for corneal epithelial homeostasis. Meanwhile, the ocular surface is an ideal site to conduct epithelial stem cell research due to the unique compartmentalization of the corneal stem cells in the limbus allowing the study of the proliferative and nonproliferative population of cells, regulatory factors (growth or inhibitor), and mechanism of the differentiation and migration of epithelial cells. Elucidation of the biology of stem cells of corneal epithelia has led to better therapeutic strategies in treatment of patients with a group of ocular surface diseases caused by limbal stem cell deficiency, manifesting with abnormal conjunctival epithelial ingrowths (conjunctivalization) over the cornea, vascularization, and ultimately visual loss. The objective of this chapter is to review the basic biology of corneal epithelial stem cells and their clinical application in limbal stem cell transplantation.

Chapter XXIII - Acute myocardial infarction and extensive loss of cardiomyocytes may progress toward heart failure despite revascularization procedures and pharmacological treatments. Initial studies supported the concept that bone marrow cells may hold the promise of rebuilding the injured heart from its component elements, offering a valid alternative to the ultimate resort of heart transplantation. However, stem cell biology turned out to be considerably more complex that initially expected. Different stem cell populations, including mesenchymal stem cells, adipose- and amniotic fluid-derived stem cells, and cardiac-resident stem cells have been progressively characterized. It is increasingly becoming evident that secretion of specific growth factors from transplanted stem cells may activate angiogenic, antiapoptotic and antifibrotic paracrine patterning, playing a major role in cardiac repair. Released growth factors may also act in an autocrine fashion on cell surface receptors to prime differentiating decisions and orchestrate a complex interplay with the recipient tissue. The stem cell nucleus itself harbors the potential for intrinsic signal transduction pathways. The term "intracrine" has been proposed for growth regulatory peptides acting within their cell of synthesis on the nuclear envelope, or subnuclear components to drive targeted lineage commitment.

Multiple randomized clinical trials of autologous bone marrow cells are on the way in acute myocardial infarction. However, based on the complexity of stem cell biology, it is not surprising that the results of these trials showed modest, transient, or no improvement in cardiac performance. These hurdles raise the larger question as to whether their efforts to provide mechanistic basis for cardiovascular cell therapy should be more closely related to the biology of wound healing than regenerative medicine. Cardiovascular commitment and secretion of trophic mediators are extremely low-yield processes in both adult and embryonic stem cells. Cell-based phenotypic- and pathway-specific screens of natural and synthetic compounds will provide a number of molecules achieving selective control of stem cell growth and differentiation. Novel hyaluronan mixed esters of butyric and retinoic acids have been recently synthesized, emerging as new tools for manipulation of cardio/vasculogenic gene expression through the modulation of targeted signaling pathways and chromatin-remodeling enzymes. These molecules have coaxed both murine embryonic and human mesenchymal stem cells towards cardiovascular decision and paracrine secretion of bioactive factors, remarkably enhancing the rescuing potential of human stem cells in in vivo animal models of myocardial infarction. This new chemistry may ultimately pave the way to promising approaches in tissue engineering and cardiovascular repair.

Chapter XXIV - Stem cells have raised hope for patients and doctors to cure diseases devoid of any appropriate treatment. Adult stem cells have been identified in several organs including bone marrow, brain, skin, muscle, intestine, liver and adipose tissue where they interact with their micro environment to maintain specific properties such as the capacity to seemingly indefinitely self-renew, i.e., divide and create additional stem cells. They also retain the ability to differentiate along, at least, one or multiple lineages to generate and to properly control the turnover of cells bearing an assigned function.

Thus, they play a critical role to maintain and repair organ systems, but when their ability to divide and/or differentiate is disrupted, certain diseases such as cancers may result.

Considerable efforts have been put in the identification of markers that specifically define stem cells within an organ and cancer stem cells within a population of tumor cells, allowing prospective isolation and evaluation of their potential either to regenerate a functional organ or to drive a terrible disease.

This review will focus on the characterization and the isolation of mesenchymal stem cells. They represent invaluable tools to regenerate an accurate biological function within an organ and thus display a great therapeutic potential if carefully monitored.

The authors will then consider the concept of cancer stem cells, evaluate their implication in the progression of solid tumors and will propose tools designed specifically to target and kill this population.

Chapter XXV - Haematopoietic stem cell transplantation (HSCT) and bone marrow transplantation (BMT) is often used to treat different types of leukaemia (L) like acute myelogenous (AML), chronic myelogenous (CML), acute lymphoblastic (ALL), chronic lymphocytic leukaemia (CLL), and juvenile myelomonocytic leukaemia (JML). In 2002 approximately 17.700 such stem cell transplantations (SCT) were performed in the USA. The total number of HSCTs carried out in Europe in 2004 was 22 216 of which 33 % were allogenic and 67 % autologous. Major differences in transplant rates between the European countries have been reported, however. CLL represents 22-30% of all leukaemia cases worldwide, and the incidence was assumed to be between <1 to 5.5 cases per 100.000 habitants with the highest rates in USA, Ireland and Italy. Further, CML was reported to occur at an incidence of 1-2 cases per 100.000 habitants per year.

During the years 1997 to 2002 Yamamoto and Goodman identified a total of 144,559 leukaemia patients, including 66,067 (46%) acute and 71,860 (50%) chronic leukaemia cases. While the highest rates of AML were observed in Asian-Pacific Islanders (API) the incidence of ALL and promyelocytic leukaemia occurred more often in Hispanics than non-Hispanics, and African-Americans had the highest rates of HTLV-1 positive adult T-cell leukaemia/lymphoma. A sharp increase in the incidence of CML was observed in subjects over 85 years-of-age. Known risk factors could not explain the observed disparities in leukaemia incidence. Lately HSCT treatment has also become available for subjects with advanced age and for patients with co-morbidities.

A new concept for the treatment of CML has emerged with the development of the specific tyrosine kinase inhibitor imatinib mesylate (Gleevec®, USA; Glivec®, Europe), which blocks the BCR/ ABL expression. As a result of these new treatment modalities the number of HSCT performed for CML has declined somewhat during the last years. Still, HSCT remains an important treatment option for patients with CML and long-term results with imatinib mesylate are still lacking.

Kidney complications associated to conventional treatment of leukaemia may occur in different ways and was recognized as early as 1943. Later, after the introduction of BMT treatment, acute renal failure (ARF) and chronic renal failure (CRF), among many other complications, was acknowledged as one of the most frequent and a potentially life-threatening complication. Following BMT, renal failure developed in approximately 40 % of cases, of which 50% required dialysis. With this in mind, pre-existent kidney diseases, previously known or undiscovered, could be present and should be searched for prior to HSCT. Leukaemia may also contribute by producing infiltrations or induce immunological responses within the kidney causing renal failure. In some of these cases the leukemic infiltrates may give the impression of or mimic other diseases including Wegener's granulomatosis or sarcoidosis as demonstrated in the kidney biopsy material. Intrarenal granulomas might be found, and together with leukaemia renal failure may develop. Moreover, renal disease may be a direct complication associated to the conditional treatment of leukaemia (see later), occurring shortly after or later in the course after HSCT treatment.

Chapter XXVI - Allogeneic hematopoietic stem cell transplantation (allo-HSCT) in humans results in true biological chimeras. While circulating hematopoietic and immune cells and their tissue derivatives (e.g., Kupffer cells, Langerhans cells) become donor genotype after transplantation, other cells remain recipient in origin. This unphysiological formation of biological chimeras is not free of consequences. The first sequel which has been recognized in the development of chimerical organisms after allo-HSCT is the graft versus host reaction, in which the new developed immune cells from the graft recognize the host's epithelial cells as foreign and kill them. There is now accumulating evidence that there are also other consequences in the co-existence of two genetically distinct populations in the transplant recipient. First, epithelial cells with donor-derived genotype emerge. Second, epithelial tissues of the host acquire genomic alterations. The current chapter discusses existing data on these recently discovered phenomena and focuses on their pathogenesis, clinical significance and therapeutic implications.

Chapter XXVII - Autologous hematopoietic stem cell transplantation (auto-HSCT) is widely accepted as an effective therapy for patients with relapsed diffuse large B-cell lymphoma (DLBL). Although some of these patients can expect to be cured, many patients will relapse. In addition, follicular lymphoma (FL) and mantle cell lymphoma (MCL) are rarely cured with auto-HSCT. To reduce the incidence of relapse after auto-HSCT, more and more attempts have been made to combine the transplantation with so-called "targeted therapy" such as rituximab before, during, and after HSCT. The other approach to reduce relapse is allogeneic HSCT (allo-HSCT) through graft-versus-lymphoma (GVL) effect. The GVL effect may be prominent in FL and MCL, while it is much less in DLBL. Allo-HSCT has been increasingly used in patients with non-Hodgkin lymphoma (NHL), although it is associated with high non-relapse mortality (NRM). Recently, reduced-intensity stem cell transplantation (RIST) has opened a new era for allo-HSCT. It was developed based on the knowledge that GVL effect is the main anti-tumor effect in allo-HSCT. Because RIST is associated with less morbidity and mortality, it can be applied to many patients with NHL who could not undergo myeloablative allogeneic stem cell transplantation (MAST).

Although HSCT has been developing in NHL with the introduction of new treatment and improvements of supportive care, there are still many unsolved questions, especially regarding optimal timing and optimal types for each disease categories in NHL. In this review, the authors would like to attempt to evaluate the efficacy of HSCT for NHL and also to provide future perspectives.

Chapter XXVIII - Gene transfer to hematopoietic stem cells (HSCs) has been mainly attempted *ex vivo* and has been limited by transplantation-related problems in homing and engraftment, as well as by cytokine-induced loss of self-renewal capacity. The goal is usually to provide long-term gene expression in the differentiated progeny of HSCs. We attempted to circumvent such limitations by transducing HSCs directly in their native environment, the bone marrow (BM). To do this, an efficient method of gene transfer to resting HSCs is needed. Tag-deleted SV40-derived vectors (rSV40s) fit this description. Rats received direct injection of SV(Nef-FLAG) into the femoral BM cavities. The vector is a rSV40 carrying a marker gene (FLAG epitope). Control rats received an unrelated rSV40 or saline. Peripheral blood cells (5%) and femoral marrow cells (25%) expressed FLAG for the entire study (16 months). Flow cytometry analysis demonstrated transgene expression in multiple hematopoietic cell lineages, including granulocytes, CD3+ T lymphocytes and CD45R+ B lymphocytes, indicating successful gene transfer to long-lived progenitor cells with multilineage capacity. FLAG expression was also assessed in different organs at 1, 4 and 16 months. FLAG+ macrophages were detected throughout the body, and were very prominent in the spleen. FLAG+ cells were also common in pulmonary alveoli. The latter included immunologically identifiable alveolar macrophages and type II pneumocytes. FLAG+ pneumocytes were not detected at 1 month, infrequent at 4 months and common at 16 months after intramarrow injection. Rare liver cells were positive for both FLAG and ferritin, indicating that some hepatocytes also expressed this BM-delivered transgene. In the CNS, FLAG-expressing cells were mainly detected in the dentate gyrus (DG) of the hippocampus and in the periventricular subependymal zone (PSZ). These areas are involved in spontaneous adult neurogenesis. DG and PSZ FLAG+ cells were virtually nonexistant before 1 month and were rare at 4 months, but they were abundant 16 months after BM injection. Approximately 5% of DG cells were FLAG+. Of these, 48.6% were neurons, 49.7% were microglial cells and 1.6% were astrocytes, as determined by double immunostaining for FLAG and CNS lineage markers. DG and PSZ studies of control animals were negative. Thus: (a) direct intramarrow administration of rSV40 vectors provides efficient gene transfer to rat BM progenitor cells; (b) fixed tissue phagocytes may be accessible to gene delivery by intramarrow transduction of their progenitors; (c) transduced BM-resident cells or their derivatives may migrate to other organs (lungs, brain) and may differentiate into cells specific of these organs and (d) intramarrow injection of rSV40s does not detectably transduce parenchymal cells of other organs.

Chapter XXIX - Sight is one of the most crucial senses for patient quality of life. Indeed, many patients consider their quality of vision to be more important than many other essential physical functions. As such, the role of ophthalmic pathology in a growing geriatric population and the limitations of current vision therapies have gained profound significance. In particular, diseases of the retina have a notable impact on elderly patients and progress in therapies for retinal impairments have become increasingly important over the past decade.

In this context, it is understandable why the novel possibility of stem cell tissue engineering for retinal repair has garnered much excitement in the scientific community. Tissue engineered therapies and stem cell technologies are rapidly becoming more clinically applicable, and accordingly, the use of such treatments for the retina has gained prominence.

In this chapter, the authors discuss the current state of progress in the retinal application of stem cell therapies and tissue engineering technologies. The authors begin with a brief review of clinical pathologies that are applicable for regeneration therapies, discuss the regeneration of the various cell types that compose the retina, delineate the issues affecting current transplantation modalities, and conclude with a brief discussion of necessary future progress.

Chapter XXX - A myriad of approaches have been used to create tissue engineered blood vessels over the past 20 years. In this chapter, current approaches and strategies for culturing blood vessels are reviewed. First, scaffold choices are discussed with respect to their impact on vessel strength; persistence or degradation; and ability to facilitate cellular attachment, growth, and extracellular matrix production. Cell sourcing strategies are reviewed with respect to their impact on vessel strength, ability to adhere to scaffolds, and feasibility for translation to clinical use. Culture strategies also are discussed, and where possible, compositional characteristics of tissue engineered blood vessels cultured are highlighted. Implantation of tissue engineered blood vessels into large animal models is reviewed with an emphasis on graft functionality, cellular retention or infiltration, remodeling of extracellular matrix, and remaining challenges. Two human clinical trials focused on tissue engineered blood vessels are described. Future directions are proposed based on the advantages and roadblocks of different strategies. The topics reviewed within this chapter are applicable not only to the development of tissue engineered blood vessels, but also to other engineered tissues.

Chapter XXXI - The use of adult stem cells for cell-based tissue engineering and regeneration represents a promising approach for repairing damaged tissue. This emerging field of regenerative medicine will require a reliable source of stem cells in addition to biomaterial scaffolds and growth factors. Recent studies have shown that stem cells can be isolated from a wide variety of tissues including bone marrow, muscle, and adipose tissue. The cellular component of this regenerative approach will play a key role in bringing tissue-engineered constructs from the laboratory bench to the clinical bedside. An ideal source of stem cells still remains undefined, however, and may differ depending upon the required application.

Muscle tissue engineering approaches could revolutionize current therapies for irreversible skeletal muscle damage and muscular dystrophies, and may significantly improve the quality of life of millions of patients. Skeletal muscle tissue engineering approaches rely mainly on myoblasts and biomaterials; however, myoblasts lack expansion capability. Cells from other sources, including adult stem cells, are being investigated to overcome this problem. Several cell sources have been proposed for creation of engineered skeletal tissue, but the literature to date unfortunately does not assist in the identification of an ideal cell source. We describe here the advantages and limitations of candidate cell sources for skeletal muscle tissue engineering.

As with bone marrow, adipose tissue is a mesoderm-derived organ that contains a stromal population including microvascular endothelial cells, smooth muscle cells, and stem cells. This population shares many characteristics with its bone marrow counterpart including extensive proliferative potential and an ability to undergo multilinear differentiation. Adipose tissue also has the ability to dynamically expand and shrink throughout the life of an adult. This capacity is mediated by the presence of vascular and non-vascular cells that provide a pool of stem and progenitor cells with unique regenerative capacities. Human adipose tissue-derived adult stem cells (ASCs) therefore meet many of the requirements of "ideal" cells for stem cell therapy and tissue engineering. ASCs have been used in cell-based tissue engineering of hard tissues such as bone and cartilage, but their capacity to assist in regeneration of damaged muscle has not yet been investigated in detail.

Here the authors review recent progress in the muscle tissue engineering field and describe one of our experiments as an example of successful skeletal muscle tissue engineering. The aothors engineered skeletal muscle tissue using a combination of ASCs and injectable PLGA spheres. These findings suggest that mixtures of ASCs and injectable scaffolds may provide excellent tools for muscle tissue engineering and that such combinations may find applications in clinical settings requiring muscle tissue regeneration therapy.

Chapter XXXII - Olfactory neuroblastoma (ONB), also known as esthesioneuroblastoma, is a rare malignant neoplasm arising from the olfactory neuroepithelium in the upper nasal cavity. It accounts for 3% of all intranasal tumors. The ONB incidence is reported at 4 cases per ten million inhabitants. There are more than 1000 cases being reported in the literature since it was first described in 1924.

This chapter provides an overview of the disease and highlights the updates in physiology, anatomy, histopathology, molecular biology, clinical feature, treatment, prognosis and predictive factors based on the literature reviews.

Chapter XXXIII - Cellular therapies are promising approaches in the treatment of several neurological diseases such as Parkinson's disease or Huntington's disease, but also for spinal cord injury. One main problem concerns the origin and nature of the cells to be used for such procedures. In this context, recent studies suggest that somatic stem cells (stem cells from foetal or adult tissues) might be able to exhibit more plasticity than previously thought as they seem able to differentiate into many cell types, including cell types which are not encountered in their tissue origin. This last property, named phenotypic plasticity of somatic stem cells, is thus the capacity for a stem cell to develop in several phenotypes depending on their environment. Several recent reports suggest that bone marrow mesenchymal stem cells

(MSC) could be a source of somatic stem cells suitable for cell replacement strategies in the treatment of central nervous system (CNS) disorders. MSC can differentiate into many types of mesenchymal cells, i.e. osteocytes, chondrocytes and adipocytes, but can also differentiate into non-mesenchymal cell, i.e. neural cells in appropriate *in vivo* and *in vitro* experimental conditions. Some works have attributed the neural phenotypic plasticity to "transdifferentiation", while some other works suggested that this neural plasticity could be explained by cell fusion. These observations could suggest that mesenchymal cells are heterogeneous and there are two cell populations able to adopt a neural phenotype: one which is able to fuse with already-present neurons and a second one which is really able to differentiate in neurons. In the first part of this chapter, we will review the studies realized on the potential neural phenotypic plasticity of the mesenchymal stem cells. The second part of this chapter will focus on recent studies demonstrating that stem cells isolated from adipose, skin and umbilical cord cells have the ability to differentiate into neural. This ability could be attributed to the presence of neural crest stem cells in those tissue. Consequently, we will address the question of the potential presence of neural crest stem cells in bone marrow.

Chapter XXXIV - Central nervous system involvement with malignant lymphoma whether primary or secondary is an uncommon but not rare complication observed in the management. Importance lies in the considerable morbidity and mortality with which it is associated and the inadequacy of therapy.

In Section I, Dr. Lauren Abrey addresses the totality of the problem of primary central nervous system lymphoma, with emphasis on strategies increasingly dependent on systemic chemotherapy.

In Section II, Dr. John Sandlund reviews the success of sequential clinical trials of overall therapy for acute lymphoblastic leukemia in child-hood, identifying those patients at high risk of central nervous system leukemia and the development of a rational therapeutic strategy for prevention.

In Section III, Dr. Andrew Lister discusses the issue of secondary central nervous system involvement with lymphoma and the indications for prophylaxis.

Chapter XXXV - In August 2001, President Bush announced that federal funds, with certain restrictions, may be used to conduct research on human embryonic stem cells. Federal research is limited to "the more than 60" existing stem cell lines that were derived (1) with the informed consent of the donors; (2) from excess embryos created solely for reproductive purposes; and (3) without any financial inducements to the donors. No federal funds may be used for the derivation or use of stem cell lines derived from newly destroyed embryos; the creation of any human embryos for research purposes; or cloning of human embryos for any purposes. Legislation that responds to the limitations imposed by the President's 2001 announcement has been introduced in the last two Congresses. During the 110th Congress, at least 10 bills, including the Stem Cell Research Enhancement Act of 2007 (H.R. 3/S. 5/S. 997), have been introduced.

Chapter XXXVI - Bone marrow contains hematopoietic stem cells (HSCs), which differentiate into every type of mature blood cells, endothelial cell progenitors (EPCs), and marrow stromal cells, also called mesenchymal stem cells (MSCs), which can differentiate into mature cells of multiple mesenchymal tissues including fat, bone and cartilage. Moreover, a bone marrow-borne circulating cell with fibroblast-like features, termed fibrocyte, has been described. Numerous studies have demonstrated the ability of HSCs, MSCs, EPCs and fibrocytes to home to the lung and differentiate into a variety of cells types, including epithelial, endothelial, fibroblasts and myofibroblast cells. Injury is an essential catalyst that enables the production of lung cells from bone marrow; however, the degree of organ injury, the mode of injury used, and characteristics of the donor marrow cells may be among the multitude of factors that influence the extent of tissue replacement and the phenotype of newly produced cells. Moreover, engraftment of bone marrow-derived stem cells into the airways is a very inefficient process. Studies on the molecular network (i.e., chemokine/chemokine receptor axis) governing the homing of circulating stem cells to the airways will reveal the mechanism(s) by which stem cells home to the airways. Better knowledge of the local stem cells in the respiratory tract will aid to understand the 'plasticity' of bone marrow-derived stem cells. Some lung disease treatable by stem cell transplantation, like for example cystic fibrosis, will need gene transfer into stem cells, with possible immunological reactions to gene products inserted to replace a deficiency or to down-regulate a hyper-expressed protein. An intensive research effort is therefore necessary before acute and chronic lung diseases can benefit from this stem cell approach.

Chapter XXXVII - Platelets exhibit the ability to release considerable quantities of secretory products such as proinflammatory mediators and growth factors and to express immune receptors on their membrane. These secretory products and immune receptors play significant roles in inflammation, immune reactions, and tissue regeneration. This review summarizes the secretory products and immune receptors of platelets and their roles for the pathogenesis of graft-versus-host disease (GVHD), focusing on mechanisms responsible for protection against GVHD by platelet derived factors such as hepatocyte growth factor and sphingosine 1-phosphate.

Chapter XXXVIII - Although hematopoetic stem cell (HSC) transplantation has been in practice for almost half a century, the improved understanding of stem cells over past two decades has revolutionized this field making it as most promising aspect of translational medicine. HSC are found in small numbers in peripheral blood as compared to bone marrow. However, use of growth factors has opened new avenues to successfully use peripheral blood as source of CD 34+ HSC. These are pluripotent cells that are competent for self renewal and differentiation to a variety of specialized cells and are replenished with fresh cells every day. Recent understanding about their mobilization, homing and plasticity suggest that they can be useful for the maintenance and regeneration of various specialized tissues. This provides an opportunity to explore the specific niche responsible for stem cell plasticity, their trans-differentiation into specific cellular lineages as well the kinetics of their recovery whenever required. The normal physiological microenvironment may be unable to provide a suitable environment for the rapid regeneration of HSC required for coping with tissue damage and may need some external interventions. The autologous stem –cell transplantation (SCT), has decreased risk of graft –versus –host disease, and provides opportunities of external interventions in terms of ex vivo manipulation. In the diseases of hematopoietic and immune system allogeneic transplant remains a better modality but is associated with grave risk of graft –versus –host disease (GVHD). However, in these cases it is needed to engineer the hematopoietic stem cell (HSC) graft to remove the cells which cause GVHD or relapse to improve graft functions. Hematopoetic stem cell transplantations have been successful in a variety of diseases including leukemia and other hematopoetic disorders. Though results of HSCT are promising, developing a more mechanistic approach to plasticity and improving the external interventions and ex vivo manipulations may lead to improving the efficiency and speed of regeneration of transplanted cells. This could result in better use and wider application of stem cell based therapies.

Chapter XXXIX - Hematopoietic stem cell transplantation (HSCT) has become an essential treatment for many patients with hematological diseases. Their immunosuppressed status during HSCT makes the patients more susceptible to infection and leads to an increased risk of infectious complications, including the development of severe septicemia that may be life-threatening. The oral cavity is a potential source for such complications in patients receiving HSCT therapy, because it is an important port of entry for agents that can cause systemic infections. To prevent these oral complications, pre-transplant comprehensive oral care has been incorporated into the preparatory steps for patients scheduled to receive HSCT therapy. Pre-HSCT dental treatments are expected to decrease the risk of local and systemic odontogenic infections during immunosuppression. This approach is supported by the National Institutes of Health consensus statement on oral complications of cancer therapy. Although in the best-case scenario all sources of potential infection would be identified upon pre-HSCT dental screening and treated appropriately, the period available for pre-HSCT dental treatment is limited, sometimes precluding complete treatment. Therefore, the authors constructed protocols that define the appropriate minimal treatment modality for dental disorders in adults and children scheduled for HSCT to treat hematological malignancies. The protocols were constructed with the intent of preserving the patients' teeth whenever possible, and taking into account the severity of the disorder and the treatment time available.

In this chapter the authors describe these protocols, their application, and the patient outcomes. They also discuss the treatment modalities chosen for the protocols in the context of findings in the published literature and their own studies.

For their studies, patients scheduled for HSCT were given a pre-treatment clinical and radiological oral examination. Treatment modalities for potentially complicating or conditions were chosen according to the protocols. In adults, these oral conditions were dental caries, pulpitis, periapical and marginal periodontitis, and partially erupted third molars. In pediatric patients, they were dental caries, pulpitis, periapical periodontitis, simple gingivitis, loose primary teeth, and gingivitis associated with tooth eruption. In their studies, following their dental treatment, all the patients received their scheduled HSCT therapy without alteration, interruption, or delay, and none of the patients showed any signs or symptoms of odontogenic infection while they were immunosuppressed. These protocols, therefore, appear to be appropriate for the pre-HSCT dental treatment of adult and pediatric patients with hematological diseases.

Chapter XL - Haematopoietic stem cell transplantation (HSCT) is a modern therapeutic method used for biomodulation antitumour therapy of haematological malignancies (acute and chronic leukemia, malignant Hodgkin's and non-Hodgkin's lymphoma, multiple myeloma, aplastic anaemia, etc.) and of the selected solid tumours (Grawitz's tumour of the kidney, breast carcinoma, testicular tumours, neuroblastoma, small-cellular lung carcinoma). It is also used for the therapy of non-tumour and hereditary diseases (demyelinization disease – sclerosis multiplex, systemic disease - systemic lupus erythematodes, systemic sclerodermia and hereditary disease – Fanconi's anaemia). It is divided into the bone marrow transplantation (BMT), the transplantation of stem (progenitor) cells (PSCT) and the umbilical cord blood transplantation (UCBT). From a donor's point of view there are three kinds of transplantations: syngenic transplantation (the donor is a monozygotic twin), allogeneic transplantation (HLA from a compatible sibling or parent or HLA from a compatible donor) and autologous transplantation (patient is the donor). The aim of the HSCT is to replace a patient's pathological bone marrow which contains tumorous cells with haematopoietic cells from a healthy donor and to restore haematopoiesis which is damaged by an intensive antitumour therapy.

Chapter XLI - The presence of primitive and committed hematopoietic progenitor cells (HPC) in the cord blood was initially described in the early seventies. Broxmeyer et al, later in experimental studies showed the potential application of umbilical cord blood (UCB) stem cells for clinical transplantation. However it was in the late eighties when for the first time was reported the success of a cord blood transplant (CBT). It was performed in a child with Fanconi anemia, and it provided both hematological and immunological reconstitution after myeloablative therapy. Since then, umbilical cord blood (UCB) is being increasingly used as an alternative source for hematopoietic stem cell transplantation. To further analyze the clinical outcome and survival, the authors report results of CB transplants performed in their center for both malignant and nonmalignant diseases in 34 pediatric patients. The median follow-up for survivors was 36 months (range:2-96).

Median age was 6 years (range: 1-18). There were nineteen male. Four cases were HLA-identical sibling CB donors and the others were unrelated CB donors. The diagnosis was malignancy in 27 patients and non malignancy in 7 patients. Disease status was early in 5 patients, intermediate in 2 patients and advanced disease in 27 patients. For 13 patients, it was the second stem cell transplant.

The conditioning regimen was chemotherapy based in all cases. Tymoglobulin was added in 28 patients. Graft versus-host disease (GVHD) prophylaxis consisted on cyclosporine A (CsA) and steroids in unrelated and CsA alone in related CB transplants.

The median number of total nucleated cells (TNC) and CD34+ cells infused was 4.64×10^7 /Kg (range:1.4-44) and 1.4×10^5 /Kg (range:0.1-7.5), respectively.

HLA match was as follows: 6/6 in eight patients, 5/6 in eight, 4/6 in fifteen and 3/3 in three.

The cumulative incidence for neutrophil and platelet engraftment at day +60 was 81% and 51% respectively. The probability of develop acute GVHD grade $\geq$ II was 31±11% and chronic GVHD 19±10%.

The 3-year event-free survival (EFS) for whole group was 34±8%. The variables associated with improved survival by multivariate analysis were early disease status at transplant and a higher number of CD34+ cells infused ($>1.5 \times 10^5$/Kg). If we analyze separately these results, the EFS in children transplanted in early phase of disease and with higher number of CD34+ cells was 100% whereas for patients transplanted in advanced phase of disease and with a lower number of CD34+ cells was of 7±6%. The patients with only one of these favorable factors had an EFS of 46±13%.

These results strongly suggest that the main factor to select the CB unit for stem cell transplant should be the $CD34^+$ cell dose.

Available data show that umbilical cord blood offer at least comparable results to other sources of progenitor cells for hematopoietic transplantation. In the author's experience, the CD34+ cell dose is the main factor related to overall results in this clinical setting.

Chapter XLII - Skin and skeletal muscle are frequently damaged tissues after trauma due to their localization and constant turn-over. Large skin or skeletal muscle defects are also sometimes life threatening. Bone marrow-derived multipotent mesenchymal stromal cells have the potential to differentiate into various cell lineages that participating in wound healing and skeletal muscle repair. One of the present goals in the author's lab is to promote the skin wound healing and skeletal muscle repair after traumatic events, particular for the impaired-healing wounds after radiation. Mesenchymal stromal cells can effectively accelerate the speed and improve the quality of skin wound healing and skeletal muscle repair after topical implantation. Pathological studies confirm that mesenchymal stem cells differentiate into fibroblasts, vascular endothelial cells, epidermal cells and skeletal muscle cells in regenerated tissues. Transplantation of mesenchymal stromal cells over-expressing healing-promoting factors such as vascular endothelial growth factor (VEGF), platelet derived growth factor (PDGF) for skin wound healing and muscle differentiation-initiating gene MyoD for skeletal further improves the therapeutic effects. Taken together, bone marrow multipotent mesenchymal stromal cells appear to provide a very promising tool for cell-based therapeutic strategies in skin and skeletal muscle regeneration.

Chapter XLIII - Pluripotent cells of the early embryo originate all types of somatic cells and germ cells of adult organism. Pluripotent stem cell lines were derived from mammalian embryos and adult tissues using different techniques and from different sources—inner cell mass of the blastocyst, primordial germ cells, parthenogenetic oocytes, and mature spermatogonia — as well as by transgenic modification of various adult somatic cells. Despite different origin, all pluripotent stem cell lines demonstrate considerable similarity of the major biological properties: unlimited self-renewal and differentiation into various somatic and germ cells in vitro and in vivo, similar gene expression profiles, and similar cell cycle structure. Their malignant counterpart embryonal teratocarcinoma stem cell lines have restricted developmental potentials caused by genetic disturbances that result in deregulation of proliferation and differentiation balance. Numerous studies on the stability of different pluripotent stem cell lines demonstrated that, irrespective of their origin, long-term in vitro cultivation leads to the accumulation of chromosomal and gene mutations as well as epigenetic changes that can cause oncogenic transformation of cells. Our research of signaling pathways and pattern of specific gene expression in pluripotent stem cells and teratocarcinoma cells is focused on discovery of fundamental mechanisms that regulate normal development of pluripotent cells into different lineages and are disrupted in cancer initiating cells. Analysis gene expression profiles, differentiation potentials and cell cycle of normal and mutant pluripotent stem cells provide new data to search molecular targets to eliminate malignant cells in tumors.

Chapter XLIV - The idea of growing human cells *in vitro* to yield a renewable source of cells for transplantation has captured the imagination of scientists for many years. The derivation of human embryonic stem cells (hESC) represented a major milestone in achieving this goal. hESC are pluripotent and can proliferate *in vitro* indefinitely, rendering them an ideal source for cell replacement therapy. Moreover, recent advances in reprogramming somatic cells into induced pluripotent stem cells (iPS cells) have enabled us to unravel some of the key master regulators of stem cell pluripotency. By integrating recent findings of molecular mechanism involved in maintenance of these different pluripotent stem cell types, we aim to present a global picture of how extracellular signals, intracellular signal transduction pathways and transcriptional networks cooperate together to determine the cell fate of pluripotent stem cells. Unraveling the signaling networks that control stem cell pluripotency will be helpful in deriving novel methods to maintain these pluripotent stem cells *in vitro*.

Chapter XLV - Proviral expression of early development genes Oct4 and Sox2, in concert with cMyc and Klf4 or Nanog and Lin28, can induce differentiated cells to adopt morphological and functional characteristics of pluripotency indistinguishable from embryonic stem cells. Termed induced pluripotent stem (iPS) cells, in mice the pluripotency of these cells was confirmed by altered gene/surface antigen expression, remodeling of the epigenome, ability to contribute to embryonic lineages following blastocyst injection and commitment to all three germ layers in teratomas and liveborn chimeras. Importantly, *in vitro* directed differentiation of iPS cells yield cells capable of treating mouse models of humanized disease. Despite these impressive results, iPS cell conversion is frustratingly inefficient. Also, the unpredictable and random mutagenesis imposed on the host cell genome, inherent with integrative viral methodologies, continues to hamper use of these cells in a therapeutic setting. This has initiated exploration of non-integrating strategies for generating iPS cells. Here, we review mechanisms that drive conversion of somatic cells to iPS cells and the strategies adopted to circumvent integrative viral strategies. Finally, we discuss practical, ethical and legal considerations that require addressing before iPS cells can realize their potential as patient-specific cells for treatment of degenerative disease.

Chapter XLVI - Human amniotic fluid has been used in prenatal diagnosis for more than 70 years. It has proven to be a safe, reliable, and simple screening tool for a wide variety of developmental and genetic diseases. However, there is now evidence that amniotic fluid may be used as more than simply a diagnostic tool. It may be the source of a powerful therapy for a multitude of congenital and adult disorders. A subset of cells found in amniotic fluid and placenta has been isolated and found to be capable of maintaining prolonged undifferentiated proliferation as well as able to differentiate into multiple tissue types encompassing the three germ layers. It is possible that in the near future, we will see the development of therapies using progenitor cells isolated from amniotic fland and placenta for the treatment of newborns with congenital malformations, as well as adults with various disorders, using cryopreserved amniotic fluid and placental stem cells. In this chapter, we describe a number of experiments that have isolated and characterized pluripotent progenitor cells from amniotic fland and placenta. We also discuss various cell lines derived from amniotic fluid and placenta and future directions for this area of research.

Chapter XLVII - Research investigations on various sources of stem cells have been conducted for potential to exert tissue regeneration, reverse immune-enhancement, and protect against tissue insult. At a more distant goal, it is likely that stem cells could be applied to medicine via organogenesis. However, the field of stem cells is not new since immune replacement via bone marrow transplantation is considered a successful form of cell therapy. There is evidence that stem cell therapies are close for several disorders such as neurodegeneration, immune hyperactivity, and functional insufficiencies such as Type I diabetes mellitus. The field of stem cell biology is gaining a strong foothold in science and medicine as the molecular mechanisms underlying stem cell behavior are gradually being unraveled. Although stem cells have tremendous therapeutic applicability in the aforementioned conditions, their uniqueness may also confer adverse properties, rendering them a double-edged sword. The discovery that stem cells have immortal and resilient characteristics has shed insight into the link between stem cells and tumorigenesis. Specifically, recent advancements in cancer research have implicated that a stem cell may be responsible for the refractoriness of cancers to conventional treatment such as chemotherapy and radiation. Here, we summarize the recent advancements in the cancer stem cell hypothesis and present the challenges associated with targeting resistant cancers in the context of stem cell microenvironments.

Chapter - XLVIII - Terminal somatic cell differentiation is not irreversible. The same route that transforms embryonic stem cells (ESCs) into specific lineages can be walked backwards, e.g. by means of the "induced pluripotent stem (iPS) cell" technology discovered by Shinya Yamanaka in 2006. The implications of iPS are out of proportion and its ease and reproducibility has made it a favorite option compared to other existing approaches including cell fusion or somatic cell nuclear transfer (SCNT). iPS allows the generation of patient specific embryonic-like stem cells that are devoid of ethical concerns and may be used for transplantation. iPS has also proven useful to create *in vitro* models that mimic human diseases and this could be used for high throughput drug screening. Besides, thanks to iPS we are now compelled to think of differentiation processes in a bidirectional way, which may be as well cell type and transcription factor specific. Therefore, knowledge is flourishing that will benefit Stem Cell Biology as much as unrelated disciplines. But the pace of discovery has been so quick that every technical advance has raised new issues, creating confusion. Here we will briefly define and try to answer some key questions that in our opinion will shape iPS research and application in following years.

Chapter XLIX - Holometabolous insects recruit a wide array of stem cell types to fulfil the growth of larval organs at moulting and their remodelling at metamorphosis, thus achieving the final body organization of the adult.

Over the years a large number of different stem cells, with specific roles in growth and renewal of insect tissues, have been identified in Lepidoptera and Diptera. A particular interest for the stem cells residing within the insect gut is now emerging and the early morphological studies that analyzed the behaviour of these cells are progressively supported by new cellular and molecular data.

After a brief summary of the current knowledge on insect intestinal stem cells, here we will focus on some characteristics of the stem cells in culture of the larval midgut of *Bombyx mori*. These cells can be released from the midgut just before the fourth moult and, once placed in an appropriate medium, they multiply and differentiate in mature cells that are able to perform normal absorptive and digestive functions *in vitro*.

Thereafter we will discuss the use of this reliable *in vitro* system as a tool to study intestinal morphogenesis and differentiation, to investigate the specific roles and reciprocal relationships of autophagy and apoptosis during midgut remodelling, and to analyze physiological functions of midgut cells, such as their ability to internalize different substrates and the mechanisms involved. Studies on midgut stem cells appear of key importance in consideration of the extensive similarities evidenced among mammalian and insect intestinal epithelia in their development, organization and molecular regulatory mechanisms.

Chapter L - It is estimated that as many as 1 in 3 individuals in the United States might benefit from regenerative medicine therapy. Most regenerative medicine therapies have been postulated to require the use of embryonic stem (ES) cells for optimal effect. Unfortunately, ES cell therapies are currently limited by ethical, political, regulatory, and most importantly biological hurdles. These limitations include the inherent allogenicity of this stem cell source and the accompanying threat of immune rejection. Even with use of the rapidly developing iPS technology, the issues of low efficiency of ES/iPS derivation and the threat of teratoma formation limit ES applications directly in patients. The time and cost of deriving and validating mature, differentiated tissues for clinical use further restricts its use to a small number of well-to-do patients with a limited number of afflictions. Thus, for the foreseeable future, the march of regenerative medicine to the clinic for widespread use will depend upon the development of non-ES cell therapies. Current sources of non-ES cells easily available in large numbers can be found in the bone marrow, adipose tissue and umbilical cord blood. Each of these types of stem cells has already begun to be utilized to treat a variety of diseases.

Chapter LI – It is estimated that as many as 1 in 3 individuals in the United States might benefit from regenerative medicine therapy. Most regenerative medicine therapies have been postulated to require the use of embryonic stem (ES) cells for optimal effect. Unfortunately, ES cell therapies are currently limited by ethical, political, regulatory, and most importantly biological hurdles. These limitations include the inherent allogenicity of this stem cell source and the accompanying threat of immune rejection. Even with use of the rapidly developing iPS technology, the issues of low efficiency of ES/iPS derivation and the threat of teratoma formation limit ES applications directly in patients. The time and cost of deriving and validating mature, differentiated tissues for clinical use further restricts its use to a small number of well-to-do patients with a limited number of afflictions. Thus, for the foreseeable future, the march of regenerative medicine to the clinic for widespread use will depend upon the development of non-ES cell therapies. Current sources of non-ES cells easily available in large numbers can be found in the bone marrow, adipose tissue and umbilical cord blood. Each of these types of stem cells has already begun to be utilized to treat a variety of diseases.

Chapter LII - The derivation of human embryonic stem cell lines from blastocyst stage embryos, first achieved almost a decade ago, demonstrated the potential to prepare virtually unlimited numbers of therapeutically beneficial cells *in vitro*. Assuming that large-scale production of differentiated cells is attainable, it is imperative to develop strategies to prevent immune responses towards the grafted cells following transplantation. This paper presents recent advances in the production of pluripotent cell lines using three emerging techniques: somatic cell nuclear transfer into enucleated oocytes and zygotes, parthenogenetic activation of unfertilized oocytes and induction of pluripotency in somatic cells. These techniques have a remarkable potential for generation of patient-specific pluripotent cells that would be tolerated by the immune system.

Chapter LIII - Pluripotent cells of the early preimplantation embryo originate all types of somatic cell and germ cells of the adult organism. Permanent pluripotent cell lines (ES and EG cells) that were derived from an inner cell mass of blastocysts and primordial germ cells have a high proliferative potential and ability to differentiate in vitro into a wide variety of somatic and extraembryonic tissues as well as germ cells and to contribute to different organs of chimeric animals. In some cases pluripotent cells and primordial germ cells can generate teratomas, teratocarsinomas and some kinds of seminomas as the results of damages of differentiation programme of these cells. Experimental teratomas which formed after transplantation of undifferentiated ES and EG cells into immunocompromiced mice may provide a unique opportunity to study pluripotent cell specification and to develop novel approaches in carcinogenesis investigations. Research of signaling and metabolic pathways regulating the pluripotent cell maintenance and their multilineage differentiation are essential to search molecular targets to eliminate undifferentiated cells in tumors. Analysis of interactions between pluripotent cells and differentiated cells of the recipient animals, identification of the factors that may drive differentiation ES and EG cells in vivo contribute in understanding the mechanisms involved in the determination of cell fate during normal development and tumorigenesis. These data are important for development of effective and safe stem cell based technologies for prospective clinical treatment.

Chapter LIV - Human embryonic stem cells are often described as "master cells," able to develop into any other type of cell in the human body. Research on embryonic stem cells has given rise to ethical debates, as the removal of an embryonic stem cell from an embryo typically involves the destruction of that embryo. In 2007, researchers in Japan and the United States published reports that they had successfully induced adult human somatic cells to exhibit characteristics similar to embryonic stem cells. Some have argued that these new induced pluripotent stem cells render embryonic stem cell research unnecessary, while others contend that continued embryonic stem cell research is still important.

Restrictions on the federal funding of research using stem cell lines were recently lifted by an executive order issued by President Obama. Pursuant to that order, the National Institutes of Health is directed to issue guidance on human stem cell research within 120 days. This change reversed an existing executive branch policy that limited federal funds to stem cell lines that were already in existence on August 9, 2001, and were derived with the informed consent of the donors; from excess embryos created solely for reproductive purposes; and without any financial inducements to the donors.

In contrast, the federal funding of most methods of human embryonic stem cell procurement is still prohibited by federal legislation. No federal funds may be used for the derivation of stem cell lines from newly destroyed embryos; the creation of any human embryos for research purposes; or cloning of human embryos for any purposes. Recipients of federal funds may also be prohibited from discriminating against individuals who are opposed to stem cell research.

Several bills have been introduced in the 111th Congress that would direct the Secretary of Health and Human Services to conduct and support stem cell research. Some of these bills would appear to sanction continued federal funding of human embryonic stem cell research, while others would not.

Chapter LV - The central question before Congress in the debate over human stem cell research is how to treat human embryonic stem cell research (ESR), which may lead to lifesaving treatments, but which requires the destruction of embryos. Current federal law and policy address this question primarily through restrictions on federal funding for ESR. The

Dickey amendment prohibits the use of Department of Health Human Services (HHS) funds for the creation of human embryos for research purposes or research in which a human embryo or embryos are destroyed, discarded, or knowingly subjected to certain risks of injury or death. The Dickey amendment thus prohibits the use of HHS funds to establish ES lines (line establishment involves embryo destruction), but not to conduct research using established lines. President Obama established current federal ESR policy with a March 9, 2009, executive order: *Removing Barriers to Responsible Scientific Research Involving Human Stem Cells* (Obama policy). The Obama policy authorizes HHS's National Institutes of Health (NIH) to support and conduct responsible, scientifically worthy human stem cell research, including ESR, to the extent permitted by law. It also requires NIH to issue a guidance consistent with the order. The Obama policy reversed one established by President George W. Bush, which had been the first to allow federal ESR funding, but only for a limited number of ES lines.

Congress has several sets of policy options, each one prompting a set of ethical dilemmas. The first set of options involves permitting or expanding federal ESR funding, as proposed in H.R. 872, H.R. 873, and S. 487. One such option is to take no action, allowing the Obama policy to persist. This option would permit federal funding for ESR with a range of lines, and would allow the executive branch to change the ESR policy in the future. Another such option is to enact a law permitting ESR. Even if consistent with the Obama policy, this course would limit the opportunity for the executive branch to change the policy in the future. A final such option involves expanding ESR by eliminating the Dickey amendment, thus allowing the use of federal funds for the establishment of ES lines, and/or for the creation of embryos for ESR. Some supporters this set of options assert that unused frozen embryos that are created for in vitro fertilization (IVF) could be used for federally regulated research instead of being destroyed. Other supporters seek federally regulated and funded research on embryos created specifically for research purposes, which might help to facilitate more targeted research. Critics seek to protect embryos and/or egg donors, and assert that federal funds should not be used for such purposes.

Congress's second set of options involves funding additional research that may eventually generate embryonic stem cells without destroying embryos, as proposed in H.R. 877. Supporters assert that this facilitates research without ethical dilemmas. Critics characterize it as unnecessary, costly, and a diversion from developing treatments. Congress's third set of options involves discouraging ESR via tax measures, or limiting or eliminating it by restricting research funding, banning certain cloning techniques, or giving embryos the Constitutional right to life. Examples include H.R. 110, H.R. 227, H.R. 881, H.R. 1050, H.R. 1654, S. 99, and S. 346. Supporters claim their approaches respect human dignity; critics claim they harm people already living.

Chapter LVI - Embryonic stem cells have the ability to develop into virtually any cell in the body, and may have the potential to treat injuries as well as illnesses, such as diabetes and Parkinson's disease. In January 2009, the Food and Drug Administration approved a request from Geron, a California biotechnology company, to begin a clinical trial involving safety tests of embryonic stem cells in patients with recent spinal cord injuries.

Currently, most human embryonic stem cell lines used in research are derived from embryos produced via in vitro fertilization (IVF). Because the process of removing these cells destroys the embryo, some individuals believe the derivation of stem cells from human embryos is ethically unacceptable. In November 2007, research groups in Japan and the United States announced the development of embryonic stem cell-like cells, called induced pluripotent stem (iPS) cells, via the introduction of four genes into human skin cells. Those concerned about the ethical implications of deriving stem cells from human embryos argue that researchers should use iPS cells or adult stem cells (from bone marrow or umbilical cord blood). However, many scientists believe research should focus on all types of stem cells.

On March 9, 2009, President Barack Obama signed an executive order that reversed the nearly eight-year old Bush Administration restriction on federal funding for human embryonic stem cell research. In August 2001, President George W. Bush had announced that for the first time, federal funds would be used to support research on human embryonic stem cells, but funding would be limited to "existing stem cell lines." NIH established a registry of 78 human embryonic stem cell lines eligible for use in federally funded research, but only 21 cell lines were available due to technical reasons and other limitations. Over time scientists became increasingly concerned about the quality and longevity of these 21 stem cell lines. These scientists believe that research advancement requires access to new human embryonic stem cell lines.

H.R. 873 (DeGette), the Stem Cell Research Enhancement Act of 2009, was introduced on February 4, 2009. The text of H.R. 873 is identical to legislation introduced in the 110th Congress, H.R. 3 (DeGette), and the 109th Congress, H.R. 810 (Castle). The bill would allow federal support of research that utilizes human embryonic stem cells regardless of the date on which the stem cells were derived from a human embryo. Stem cell lines must meet ethical guidelines established by the NIH, which would be issued within 60 days of enactment. H.R. 872 (DeGette), the Stem Cell Research Improvement Act of 2009, was also introduced on February 4, 2009. It is similar to H.R. 873 in that it adds the same Section 498D, "Human Embryonic Stem Cell Research," to the PHS Act, but it also adds another Section 498E, "Guidelines on Research Involving Human Stem Cells," which would require the Director of NIH to issue guidelines on research involving human embryonic stem cell within 90 days of enactment; updates of the guidelines would be required every three years. S. 487 (Harkin), introduced on February 26, 2009, is the same as H.R. 873, except it has an additional section supporting research on alternative human pluripotent stem cells. It is identical to a bill introduced in the 110th Congress, S. 5 (Reid).

During the 110th Congress, the Senate passed legislation (S. 5) in April 2007 that would have allowed federal support of research that utilizes human embryonic stem cells regardless of the date on which the stem cells were derived from a human embryo. The bill would have also provided support for research on alternatives, such as iPS cells. The House passed the bill in June 2007, and President Bush vetoed it on June 20, 2007. (The 109th Congress passed a similar bill, which also was vetoed by President Bush, the first veto of his presidency; an attempt to override the veto in the House failed.) On the related issue of human cloning, in June 2007 the House failed to pass a bill (H.R. 2560) that would have imposed penalties on anyone who cloned a human embryo and implanted it in a uterus.

Chapter LVII – This is a testimony of Joseph R. Bertino, presented to the House Committee on Energy and Commerce's Subcommittee on Health.

Chapter LVIII – This is a testimony of George Q. Daley, presented to House Committee on Energy and Commerce, Subcommittee on Health "Stem cell science: the foundation for future cures."

Chapter LIX – This is a testimony of John K. Fraser, Principal Scientist, Cytori Therapeutics Inc.

Chapter LX – This is a testimony of John Gearhart, Institute for Cell Engineering, Johns Hopkins Medicine, given before the United States House of Representatives Subcommittee on Health of the Committee on Energy and Commerce.

Chapter LXI – This is a written testimony of Weyman Johnson, Individual living with Multiple Sclerosis, Chairman of the Board, National Multiple Sclerosis Society to Energy and Commerce Committee Subcommittee on Health, United States House of Representatives.

Chapter LXII – This is a testimony of Amit N Patel, Director of Cardiovascular Cell Therapies, before the Subcommittee on Health of the Committee on Energy and Commerce.

Chapter LXIII – This is a statement of Douglas T. Rice, Adult Stem Cell Recipient for the heart.

Chapter LXIV – This is a testimony of Elias A. Zerhouni, Director, National Institutes of Health, before the Subcommittee on Health Committee on Energy and Commerce, United States House of Representatives.

In: Encyclopedia of Stem Cell Research (2 Volume Set) ISBN: 978-1-61761-835-2
Editor: Alexander L. Greene © 2012 Nova Science Publishers, Inc.

Expert Commentary A

STEM CELL THERAPY FOR ALZHEIMER'S DISEASE

*Philippe Taupin**
National Neuroscience Institute, Singapore
National University of Singapore
Nanyang Technological University, Singapore

ABSTRACT

Alzheimer's disease (AD) is a neurodegenerative disease. It is the most common form of dementia among older people for which there is at present no cure. Current treatments for AD consist mainly in drug therapy. The recent confirmation that neurogenesis occurs in the adult brain and neural stem cells (NSCs) reside in the adult central nervous system (CNS) provide new opportunities for cellular therapy in the CNS, particularly for AD. Besides its therapeutic potential, neurogenesis is increased in the hippocampus of patients with AD and animal models of AD. The effect of drugs used to treat AD on neurogenesis is currently being investigated, to identify whether neurogenesis contributes to their therapeutic activities. In all, adult NSCs not only provide a promising model to treat AD, but also provide the opportunity to better understand the pathogenesis of AD and its pharmacology.

INTRODUCTION

AD is a progressive neurodegenerative disease characterized in the brain by amyloid plaque deposits and neurofibrillary tangles [1]. It is associated with the loss of nerve cells in areas of the brain that are vital to memory and other mental abilities, like the hippocampus.

---

* Correspondence: 11 Jalan Tan Tock Seng, Singapore 308433. Tel. (65) 6357 - 7533. Fax (65) 6256 - 9178. Email obgpjt@nus.edu.sg

AD is a slow disease, starting with mild memory problems and ending with severe brain damage. The early-onset form of the disease is primarily genetic in origin and inherited. It is a very rare form of the disease, referred to as a familial form of AD [2]. The late-onset, over age 65, is not inherited and is the most common type of dementia among older people. It is also referred to as a sporadic form of AD. Mutations in the β-amyloid precursor protein (APP) and presenilin 1 (PSEN1) underlie the pathogenesis of most cases of early-onset AD [3]. AD is the fourth highest cause of death in the developed world.

There is currently no cure for AD. Current treatments for AD consist mainly in drug therapy. Two classes of drugs are currently used to treat patients with AD: acetylcholinesterase inhibitors, like tacrine, donepezil, galantamine and rivastigmine, and N-methyl-D-aspartate-glutamate receptor antagonist, like memantine. These drugs produce improvements in cognitive and behavioral symptoms [4].

Contrary to a long-held dogma, neurogenesis, the generation of new nerve cells, occurs throughout adulthood in the mammalian brain [5, 6]. Neurogenesis occurs primarily in two regions of the adult brain, the subventricular zone (SVZ), along the ventricles, and the dentate gyrus (DG) of the hippocampus [7], in various species including human [8, 9]. In the DG, newly generated neuronal cells in the subgranular zone (SGZ) migrate to the granular layer, extend axonal projection to the CA3 region of hippocampal Ammon's horn and establish functional connections with neighboring cells [10-12]. The SGZ is a layer beneath the granular layer. The confirmation that neurogenesis occurs in the adult brain and neural stem cells (NSCs) reside in the adult brain in mammals, has tremendous implications, not only for cellular therapy, but also for our understanding of the development and physiopathology of the CNS [13]. New opportunities for cellular therapy involve the stimulation of endogenous neural progenitor or stem cells and the grafting of isolated and characterized neural progenitor and stem cells in vitro, to restore the damaged neuronal network [14].

Because neurodegenerative diseases are associated with the loss of nerve cells in areas of the brain, cellular therapy offers a promising strategy for restoring a damaged network, particularly in AD.

ADULT NSC THERAPY FOR ALZHEIMER'S DISEASE

Experimental studies reveal that adult derived-neural progenitor and stem cells, isolated and cultured in vitro, engraft the host tissues and express mature neuronal and glial phenotypes, when administered by intracerebral injection [15-17]. When administered intravenously, neural progenitor and stem cells migrate to diseased and injured sites of the brain [18, 19]. Intravenous administration of adult-derived neural progenitor and stem cells promote functional recovery in animal models of neurodegenerative diseases, like multiple sclerosis [20]. Systemic injection provides a non-invasive strategy for delivering neural progenitor and stem cells in the adult CNS. In all, systemic injection provides a model of choice for delivering adult derived-neural progenitor and stem cells for the treatment of neurological diseases and injuries, like neurodegenerative diseases, cerebral strokes, traumatic and spinal cord injuries.

Particularly, in AD, like multiple sclerosis, the degeneration is widespread, therefore direct transplantation of neural progenitor and stem cells in the brain may not offer an optimum strategy for treating these diseases. Systemic administration of adult derived-neural progenitor and stem cells may represent a promising strategy for the treatment of AD. The stimulation and recruitment of endogenous neural progenitor and stem cells at the sites of degeneration provides an alternative strategy for the treatment of AD, but proof-of-principle and data supporting the feasibility of such strategy remain to be demonstrated and validated.

ADULT NEUROGENESIS AND ALZHEIMER'S DISEASE

Neurogenesis is increased in the hippocampus of brains of patients with AD, as revealed by an increase in the expression of markers for immature neuronal cells, like doublecortin and polysialylated nerve cell adhesion molecule, in the SGZ and granular layer of the DG, as well as the CA1 region of hippocampal Ammon's horn [21]. In animal models of AD, neurogenesis is increased in the DG of transgenic mice that express the Swedish and Indiana APP mutations, a mutant form of human APP [22], and decreased in the DG and SVZ of knock-out mice for PSEN1 and APP [23, 24].

The discrepancies between the studies could be explained by the limitation of the transgenic animal models as representative of complex diseases and to study adult phenotypes, like adult neurogenesis [25]. Particularly, mutant or deficient mice for single genes, like PSEN1 and APP, may not fully reproduce the features of AD, associated with loss of multiple cell types. Furthermore, these animal studies were performed using bromodeoxyurine (BrdU) labeling. BrdU is a thymidine analog that incorporates into the DNA of dividing cells during the S-phase of the cell cycle and is used for birthdating cells and monitoring cell proliferation [26]. Four to 10% of nerve cells in regions in which degeneration occurs in AD, like the hippocampus, are tetraploids [27]. Nerve cells may have entered the cell cycle and undergone DNA replication, but did not complete the cell cycle. It is proposed that cell cycle re-entry and DNA duplication precedes neuronal death in degenerating regions of the CNS [28]. As BrdU incorporates DNA of dividing cells during the S-phase of the cell cycle, BrdU labeling will not allow discriminate cell proliferation versus cell cycle re-entry and DNA duplication without cell division [29, 30]. The existence of aneuploid cells may account for some of the newly generated neuronal cells observed using BrdU-labeling in experimental models of AD.

In all, though reports suggest that neurogenesis is enhanced in AD. This remains to be further confirmed. Particularly, in light of recent data showing the existence of tetraploid cells in regions in which degeneration occurs in AD and taking into account the limitation of animal models to study complex diseases and adult neurogenesis, as well as limitation of BrdU to study adult neurogenesis [29, 30].

Interestingly, drugs used to treat AD, like galantamine and memantine, increase adult neurogenesis in the DG and SVZ of rodents, by 26-45%, as revealed by BrdU labeling [31]. The significance of an increase of neurogenesis in AD and of neurogenesis mediated by drugs used to treat AD remains to be understood. On the one hand, it may represent a regenerative attempt by the CNS, to compensate for the loss of nerve cells [13]. On the other hand, it may represent a compensatory process to increase CNS plasticity in the diseased brain [13, 32]. The increase of neurogenesis mediated by drugs used to treat AD may contribute to their therapeutic effects.

CONCLUSION

The confirmation that neurogenesis occurs in the adult brain and NSCs reside in the adult CNS suggests that the brain has the potential to self-repair, and that adult-derived neural progenitor and stem cells may be isolated and cultured in vitro, providing a source of material for the treatment of neurological diseases and injuries. The property of adult-derived neural progenitor and stem cells to migrate to diseased and injured sites of the brain, when administered intravenously, provide an opportunity to treat neurodegenerative diseases, like AD, with non-invasive surgical procedures. Future studies will aim at devising strategies for the transplantation of neural progenitor and stem cells and identifying factors that promote neurogenesis in animal models of AD, as candidates for cellular therapy.

Beside its therapeutic potential, adult neurogenesis has also tremendous implications for our understanding of the development and physiopathology of the CNS. Neurogenesis is increased in AD, and drugs used to treat AD increase adult neurogenesis. However, the increase of neurogenesis in AD is a source of controversy and remains to be confirmed. Further studies will aim at evaluating neurogenesis in AD and its significance and role in the pathogenesis of the disease. The observation that drugs used to treat AD increase adult neurogenesis may prove to be keys for the understanding of their activities and lead to new drug design and strategies to treat AD. The mechanism underlying the involvement of adult neurogenesis in the pathogenesis of AD and the activity of drugs used to treat AD remain to be fully understood.

REFERENCES

[1] Caselli RJ, Beach TG, Yaari R, Reiman EM. (2006) Alzheimer's disease a century later. *J. Clin. Psychiatry.* 67, 1784-800.
[2] St George-Hyslop PH, Petit A. (2005) Molecular biology and genetics of Alzheimer's disease. *C. R. Biol.* 328, 119-30.
[3] Hardy J, Selkoe DJ. (2002) The amyloid hypothesis of Alzheimer's disease: progress and problems on the road to therapeutics. *Science.* 297, 353-6. Erratum in: (2002) Science. 297, 2209.
[4] Scarpini E, Scheltens P, Feldman H. (2003) Treatment of Alzheimer's disease: current status and new perspectives. *Lancet Neurol.* 2, 539-47.
[5] Gage FH. (2000) Mammalian neural stem cells. *Science.* 287, 1433-8.
[6] Gross CG. (2000) Neurogenesis in the adult brain: death of a dogma. *Nat. Rev. Neurosci.* 1, 67-73.
[7] Taupin P, Gage FH. (2002) Adult neurogenesis and neural stem cells of the central nervous system in mammals. *J. Neurosci. Res.* 69, 745-9.

[8] Eriksson PS, Perfilieva E, Bjork-Eriksson T, Alborn AM, Nordborg C, Peterson DA, Gage FH. (1998) Neurogenesis in the adult human hippocampus. *Nat. Med.* 4, 1313-7.

[9] Curtis MA, Kam M, Nannmark U, Anderson MF, Axell MZ, Wikkelso C, Holtas S, van Roon-Mom WM, Bjork-Eriksson T, Nordborg C, Frisen J, Dragunow M, Faull RL, Eriksson PS. (2007) Human neuroblasts migrate to the olfactory bulb via a lateral ventricular extension. *Science.* 315, 1243-9.

[10] Cameron HA, Wolley CS, McEwen BS, Gould E. (1993) Differentiation of newly born neurons and glia in the dentate gyrus of the adult rat. *Neurosci.* 56, 337-44.

[11] Markakis EA, Gage FH. (1999) Adult-generated neurons in the dentate gyrus send axonal projections to field CA3 and are surrounded by synaptic vesicles. *J. Comp. Neurol.* 406, 449-60.

[12] Van Praag H, Schinder AF, Christie BR, Toni N, Palmer TD, Gage FH. (2002) Functional neurogenesis in the adult hippocampus. *Nature.* 415, 1030-4.

[13] Taupin P. *Adult neurogenesis and neural stem cells in mammals.* Nova Science Publishers; 1 edition (January 2007).

[14] Taupin P. (2006) The therapeutic potential of adult neural stem cells. *Curr. Opin. Mol. Ther.* 8, 225-31.

[15] Gage FH, Coates PW, Palmer TD, Kuhn HG, Fisher LJ, Suhonen JO, Peterson DA, Suhr ST, Ray J. (1995) Survival and differentiation of adult neuronal progenitor cells transplanted to the adult brain. *Proc. Natl. Acad. Sci. USA.* 92, 11879-83.

[16] Suhonen JO, Peterson DA, Ray J, Gage FH. (1996) Differentiation of adult hippocampus-derived progenitors into olfactory neurons in vivo. *Nature.* 383, 624-27.

[17] Shihabuddin LS, Horner PJ, Ray J, Gage FH. (2000) Adult spinal cord stem cells generate neurons after transplantation in the adult dentate gyrus. *J. Neurosci.* 20, 8727-35.

[18] Macklis JD. (1993) Transplanted neocortical neurons migrate selectively into regions of neuronal degeneration produced by chromophore-targeted laser photolysis. *J. Neurosci.* 13, 3848-63.

[19] Fujiwara Y, Tanaka N, Ishida O, Fujimoto Y, Murakami T, Kajihara H, Yasunaga Y, Ochi M. (2004) Intravenously injected neural progenitor cells of transgenic rats can migrate to the injured spinal cord and differentiate into neurons, astrocytes and oligodendrocytes. *Neurosci. Lett.* 366, 287-91.

[20] Pluchino S, Quattrini A, Brambilla E, Gritti A, Salani G, Dina G, Galli R, Del Carro U, Amadio S, Bergami A, Furlan R, Comi G, Vescovi AL, Martino G. (2003) Injection of adult neurospheres induces recovery in a chronic model of multiple sclerosis. *Nature.* 422, 688-94.

[21] Jin K, Peel AL, Mao XO, Xie L, Cottrell BA, Henshall DC, Greenberg DA. (2004) Increased hippocampal neurogenesis in Alzheimer's disease. *Proc. Natl. Acad. Sci. USA.* 101, 343-7.

[22] Jin K, Galvan V, Xie L, Mao XO, Gorostiza OF, Bredesen DE, Greenberg DA. (2004) Enhanced neurogenesis in Alzheimer's disease transgenic (PDGF-APPSw,Ind) mice. *Proc. Natl. Acad. Sci. USA.* 101, 13363-7.

[23] Feng R, Rampon C, Tang YP, Shrom D, Jin J, Kyin M, Sopher B, Miller MW, Ware CB, Martin GM, Kim SH, Langdon RB, Sisodia SS, Tsien JZ. (2001) Deficient

neurogenesis in forebrain-specific presenilin-1 knockout mice is associated with reduced clearance of hippocampal memory traces. *Neuron.* 32, 911-26. Erratum in: (2002) Neuron. 33, 313.

[24] Wen PH, Shao X, Shao Z, Hof PR, Wisniewski T, Kelley K, Friedrich VL, Ho L, Pasinetti GM, Shioi J, Robakis NK, Elder GA. (2002) Overexpression of wild type but not an FAD mutant presenilin-1 promotes neurogenesis in the hippocampus of adult mice. *Neurobiol. Dis.* 10, 8-19.

[25] Dodart JC, Mathis C, Bales KR, Paul SM. (2002) Does my mouse have Alzheimer's disease? *Genes Brain Behav.* 1, 142-55.

[26] Miller MW, Nowakowski RS. (1988) Use of bromodeoxyuridine-immunohistochemistry to examine the proliferation, migration and time of origin of cells in the central nervous system. *Brain Res.* 457, 44-52.

[27] Yang Y, Geldmacher DS, Herrup K. (2001) DNA replication precedes neuronal cell death in Alzheimer's disease. *J. Neurosci.* 21, 2661-8.

[28] Herrup K, Neve R, Ackerman SL, Copani A. (2004) Divide and die: cell cycle events as triggers of nerve cell death. *J. Neurosci.* 24, 9232-9.

[29] Taupin P. (2007) BrdU Immunohistochemistry for Studying Adult Neurogenesis: paradigms, pitfalls, limitations, and validation. *Brain Research Reviews.* 53, 198-214.

[30] Taupin P. (2007) Protocols for Studying Adult Neurogenesis: Insights and Recent Developments. *Regenerative Medicine.* 2, 51-62.

[31] Jin K, Xie L, Mao XO, Greenberg DA. (2006) Alzheimer's disease drugs promote neurogenesis. *Brain Res.* 1085, 183-8.

[32] Taupin P. (2006) Adult neurogenesis and neuroplasticity. *Restor. Neurol. Neurosci.* 24, 9-15.

In: Encyclopedia of Stem Cell Research (2 Volume Set) ISBN: 978-1-61761-835-2
Editor: Alexander L. Greene © 2012 Nova Science Publishers, Inc.

Expert Commentary B

ADULT NEUROGENESIS AND DEPRESSION: A NOVEL THEORY FOR DEPRESSION?

Philippe Taupin[*]
National Neuroscience Institute, Singapore
National University of Singapore
Nanyang Technological University, Singapore

The recent confirmation that neurogenesis occurs throughout adulthood in mammals raises the question of the function of newly generated neuronal cells in the adult brain [1-2].

The hippocampus is an important memory center of the brain [3]. It is also involved in pathological processes, like Alzheimer's disease and epilepsy [4, 5]. Several lines of evidence further suggest that the hippocampus is involved in the etiology of major depressive disorders, like chronic stress and depression [6].

In the adult brain, neurogenesis occurs primarily in two regions, the subventricular zone (SVZ) and the dentate gurus (DG) hippocampus, in various species including human [7-9]. The hippocampus of patients with depression show signs of atrophy and neuronal loss [11-13]. This suggests that adult hippocampal neurogenesis may contribute to the etiology of depression.

Various classes of drugs are currently prescribed for the treatment of depression, like the selective serotonin reuptake inhibitors fluoxetine, the monoamine oxidase inhibitors tranylcypromine, the specific norepinephrine reuptake inhibitors reboxetine and the phosphodiesterase-IV inhibitors rolipram [14]. Chronic administration of these antidepressants increases neurogenesis in the DG, but not the SVZ in adult rats [15, 16]. This suggests that hippocampal neurogenesis contributes to the therapeutic effects of antidepressants. X-irradiation of the hippocampal region, but not other brain regions, like the SVZ or the cerebellar region, prevents the behavioral effect of the antidepressants, like

---

[*] Correspondence: 11 Jalan Tan Tock Seng, Singapore 308433. Tel. (65) 6357 - 7533. Fax (65) 6256 - 9178. Email obgpjt@nus.edu.sg

fluoxetine, in adult mice [17]. As X-irradiation of the hippocampal area in adult rats causes long-term reductions in cell proliferation in the DG [18]. These data show that adult hippocampal neurogenesis mediates the activity of antidepressants, like fluoxetine, in adult mice.

Stress is an important causal factor in precipitating episodes of depression, and decreases hippocampal neurogenesis in adult monkeys [19]. It is proposed that the waning and waxing of hippocampal neurogenesis are important causal factors in the precipitation and recovery from episodes of clinical depression [20]. In all, neurogenesis plays an important role in the etiology of depression and the activity of antidepressants [17, 21].

There are however controversies and debates over the involvement of the hippocampus and adult neurogenesis in the etiology of depression. Among them, 1) a link between neurogenesis, loss of nerve cells, atrophy and decrease of hippocampal volume in patients with depression or animal models remains to be demonstrated, 2) some studies show that hippocampal volume remains unchanged in depressive patients [22], 3) the hippocampal formation may not be the brain region primarily involved in depressive episodes, as other areas may play a critical role in depression [23], 4) there are questions over the validity of animal models of depression as representative of the human disorder, and 5) neurogenesis may be more a contributing factor of plasticity of the central nervous system, rather than of specific physiological or pathological processes [24]. The involvement of adult neurogenesis in depression remains therefore speculative [25, 26].

In all these data involved with the hippocampus, a structure classically involved in learning and memory, and adult neurogenesis in depression, anxiety disorders and the activity of antidepressants. However, the neurogenic theory of depression remains the source of controversies and debates, and must be further confirmed. More data and evidence are needed to confirm the involvement of adult neurogenesis in depression. Nonetheless, the evidence that increased neurogenesis contributes to the effects of antidepressants may hold the key for the understanding of the long-term consequences of the effects of antidepressants of the physiopathology of the central nervous system. It may lead to new drug design and new strategies to treat depressive disorders. To this aim, the mechanism underlying the involvement of adult neurogenesis in the etiology of depression and the activity of antidepressants remain to be fully understood [27].

REFERENCES

[1] Gage FH. (2000) Mammalian neural stem cells. *Science.* 287, 1433-8.
[2] Kaplan MS. (2001) Environment complexity stimulates visual cortex neurogenesis: death of a dogma and a research career. *Trends Neurosci.* 24, 617-20.
[3] Sweatt JD. (2004) Hippocampal function in cognition. *Psychopharmacology* (Berl). 174, 99-110.
[4] Panegyres PK. (2004) The contribution of the study of neurodegenerative disorders to the understanding of human memory. *QJM.* 97, 555-67.
[5] Sloviter RS. (2005) The neurobiology of temporal lobe epilepsy: too much information, not enough knowledge. *C. R .Biol.* 328, 143-53.

[6]   Campbell S, Macqueen G. (2004) The role of the hippocampus in the pathophysiology of major depression. *J. Psychiatry Neurosci.* 29, 417-26.
[7]   Taupin P, Gage FH. (2002) Adult neurogenesis and neural stem cells of the central nervous system in mammals. *J. Neurosci Res.* 69, 745-9.
[8]   Eriksson PS, Perfilieva E, Bjork-Eriksson T, Alborn AM, Nordborg C, Peterson DA, Gage FH. (1998) Neurogenesis in the adult human hippocampus. *Nat. Med.* 4, 1313-7.
[9]   Curtis MA, Kam M, Nannmark U, Anderson MF, Axell MZ, Wikkelso C, Holtas S, van Roon-Mom WM, Bjork-Eriksson T, Nordborg C, Frisen J, Dragunow M, Faull RL, Eriksson PS. (2007) Human neuroblasts migrate to the olfactory bulb via a lateral ventricular extension. *Science.* 315, 1243-9.
[10] Sheline YI, Wang PW, Gado MH, Csernansky JG, Vannier MW. (1996) Hippocampal atrophy in recurrent major depression. *Proc. Natl. Acad. Sci. USA.* 93, 3908-13.
[11] Campbell S, Marriott M, Nahmias C, MacQueen GM. (2004) Lower hippocampal volume in patients suffering from depression: a meta-analysis. *Am. J. Psychiatry.* 161, 598-607.
[12] Colla M, Kronenberg G, Deuschle M, Meichel K, Hagen T, Bohrer M, Heuser I. (2007) Hippocampal volume reduction and HPA-system activity in major depression. *J. Psychiatr. Res.* 41, 553-60.
[13] Brunello N, Mendlewicz J, Kasper S, Leonard B, Montgomery S, Nelson J, Paykel E, Versiani M, Racagni G. (2002) The role of noradrenaline and selective noradrenaline reuptake inhibition in depression. *Eur. Neuropsychopharmacol.* 12, 461-75.
[14] Malberg JE, Eisch AJ, Nestler EJ, Duman RS. (2000) Chronic antidepressant treatment increases neurogenesis in adult rat hippocampus. *J. Neurosci.* 20, 9104-10.
[15] Malberg JE, Duman RS. (2003) Cell proliferation in adult hippocampus is decreased by inescapable stress: reversal by fluoxetine treatment. *Neuropsychopharmacology.* 28, 1562-71.
[16] Santarelli L, Saxe M, Gross C, Surget A, Battaglia F, Dulawa S, Weisstaub N, Lee J, Duman R, Arancio O, Belzung C, Hen R. (2003) Requirement of hippocampal neurogenesis for the behavioral effects of antidepressants. *Science.* 301, 805-9.
[17] Tada E, Parent JM, Lowenstein DH, Fike JR. (2000) X-irradiation causes a prolonged reduction in cell proliferation in the dentate gyrus of adult rats. *Neurosci.* 99, 33-41.
[18] Gould E, Tanapat P, McEwen BS, Flugge G, Fuchs E. (1998) Proliferation of granule cell precursors in the dentate gyrus of adult monkeys is diminished by stress. *Proc. Natl. Acad. Sci. USA.* 95, 3168-71.
[19] Jacobs BL, Praag H, Gage FH. (2000) Adult brain neurogenesis and psychiatry: a novel theory of depression. *Mol. Psychiatry.* 5, 262-9.
[20] Malberg JE. (2004) Implications of adult hippocampal neurogenesis in antidepressant action. *J. Psychiatry Neurosci.* 29, 196-205.
[21] Campbell S, MacQueen G. (2006) An update on regional brain volume differences associated with mood disorders. *Curr. Opin. Psychiatry.* 19, 25-33.
[22] Ebmeier KP, Donaghey C, Steele JD. (2006) Recent developments and current controversies in depression. *Lancet.* 367, 153-67.
[23] Taupin P. (2006) Adult neurogenesis and neuroplasticity. *Restor. Neurol. Neurosci.* 24, 9-15.

[24] Taupin P. (2006) Neurogenesis and the Effects of Antidepressants. *Drug Target Insights*. 1, 13-17.

[25] Feldmann RE Jr, Sawa A, Seidler GH. (2007) Causality of stem cell based neurogenesis and depression - To be or not to be, is that the question? *J. Psychiatr. Res.* 41, 713-23.

[26] Djavadian RL. (2004) Serotonin and neurogenesis in the hippocampal dentate gyrus of adult mammals. *Acta Neurobiol. Exp.* (Wars). 64, 189-200.

In: Encyclopedia of Stem Cell Research (2 Volume Set) ISBN: 978-1-61761-835-2
Editor: Alexander L. Greene © 2012 Nova Science Publishers, Inc.

Expert Commentary C

MANNAN-BINDING LECTIN AND STEM CELL TRANSPLANTATION

David C. Kilpatrick
Scottish National Blood Transfusion Service, Edinburgh, Scotland, UK

Mannan-binding (or mannose-binding) lectin (MBL) belongs to the small collectin subfamily of C-type animal lectins [1]. In humans, it is synthesised by the liver and secreted into the bloodstream. The plasma/serum concentration is largely determined by genetic polymorphisms although it is known that other factors can influence its level in the circulation [2]. Mutations at any of three sites (named B, C and D at codons 54, 57 and 52, respectively, and collectively designated "O") in the structural gene influence the level of functional MBL by hindering the oligomerization of the basic tripeptide subunit. Another point mutation in the promoter region (-221; Y to X) has a similar, if less pronounced effect on concentration. It is now apparent that what is usually measured as serum MBL is in fact functional or oligomeric MBL. Oligomeric MBL differs from other collectins in being able to activate complement, a quality it shares with the structurally-distinct family of ficolins. Most of the typical properties of MBL (complement activation etc) are those possessed by oligomeric MBL: there is some evidence, however, that monomeric MBL (the basic triplet subunit) has some biological activity [3,4].

In 2001, two independent research reports appeared in the same issue of Lancet [5,6], suggesting that low concentrations of MBL conferred an additional risk of infection in patients experiencing iatrogenic neutropenia. This appeared to confirm the widely held belief that MBL insufficiency is only of real significance in association with another immune system defect, and carried the important promise that MBL replacement therapy could have a major influence on oncology patients being treated with chemotherapy.

Two subsequent studies failed to confirm these initial findings and seemed to refute the possibility that MBL had a universally protective influence in patients rendered susceptible to infections through neutropenia. Bergmann et al [7] studied acute myeloid leukaemia (AML) patients. There were only a few with very low MBL levels, but no influence whatsoever of

MBL concentration on infection incidence could be discerned. Kilpatrick et al [8] did obtain positive results to some extent, but any influence of MBL was much weaker than expected and only at much lower concentrations.

At this point it could be concluded that MBL was not always strongly influential in neutropenic patients and that the role of MBL, if any, must vary markedly in different clinical contexts [9]. In the last few years several other studies on this topic have been published with widely varying results and conclusions [10-17]. The challenge is now to try to explain how, if at all, these disparate investigations can be reconciled.

Before returning to the later studies it is worth critically comparing the two seminal papers that initiated this debate. They seemed to point to the same conclusion and are often cited together, but in fact they are very different in almost every respect. Peterslund et al [6] described a small number (n=54) of adults with various haematological malignancies receiving chemotherapy who were followed up for only 3 weeks. Neth et al [5] studied 100 children (mean age 5 years) receiving chemotherapy, but not stem cell transplants, for "cancer" (including 4 with aplastic anaemia!), most of whom had acute lymphoblastic leukaemia (ALL) and who were followed up for six months. The results of Peterlund and coworkers were very straightforward: there was a very strong and statistically significant association between serum MBL <500 ng/ml and serious infections defined by bacteraemia and/or pneumonia. This was true if the data from the entire heterogeneous cohort were analysed or simply those of a subgroup of just 18 myeloma patients. In contrast, Neth et al reported an increased duration of febrile neutropenia (a rather indirect indicator of morbidity) in patients with serum MBL < 1000 ng/ml, but more importantly, no relationship between frequency of bacterial or fungal infections and MBL genotype. No allowance was made for the proportion of neutropenic time spent with fever. It is possible that if the quotient, duration of fever/ duration of neutropenia, had been calculated, entirely negative results might have been obtained.

Why the differences in those and subsequent reports in the literature? Is it because of differences in the patient populations studied? If so, is the important consideration the specific disease involved, age (children v adults), treatment (chemotherapy alone v stem cell transplantation), or what?

Series with a high proportion of acute myeloid leukaemia patients have yielded broadly negative results [7, 8], but MBL may have a greater influence in patients with non-Hodgkin's lymphoma [12, 13]. Exclusively childhood ALL patients were not influenced by *MBL-2* genotype, at least during a rather short 2-month follow-up period [14]. Two studies on the same group of myeloma patients [16, 17] concluded that while *MBL-2* genotype had no appreciable influence on serious infections generally, the wild-type (A/A) genotype conferred some protection against septicaemia. This modest influence contrasts starkly with the strong protection MBL afforded against pneumonia in the report of Peterslund et al [6]. Unfortunately, Molle and coworkers [16, 17] had no serum MBL data so a direct comparison was not possible. In conclusion, therefore, MBL seems unlikely to confer protection in the context of AML, but some beneficial influence in the context of myeloma and NHL is possible if unproven.

MBL is popularly thought to be more clinically relevant in children compared to adults, but for chemotherapy patients that does not seem to be true. Two of the largest series, a mixed oncology group (about half with solid tumours) of 110 children followed up for 2 to 46 (median 13) months [15], and the homogeneous group of 137 patients with childhood ALL referred to above [14] provided entirely negative results. To those studies could be added the results of Neth et al already discussed. Where a clear positive role for MBL has been found, however, the patients concerned have been adults [6, 12, 13].

Some of those studies were of patients given chemotherapy as conditioning followed by some form of stem cell transplantation. The first two reports in that category were typically contradictory [10, 11]. Rocha et al [11] investigated 107 HLA-identical allogeneic bone marrow transplants in unspecified "leukaemia" patients (both chronic and acute leukaemias); Mullighan et al [10] studied 97 patients mainly (~70%) with leukaemias treated with either bone marrow or peripheral blood allogeneic stem cell preparations. Both studies analysed *MBL-2* haplotypes, not serum MBL; there was only one recipient (and 4 donors) homozygous for variant alleles in the former series.

Rocha found no relationship beween variant alleles and infections over a six month follow-up period; Mullighan et al found variant alleles in both recipients and donors to be associated with increased risk of major infection over a longer (median >1 year) follow-up. Arguably, the most obvious factor that could be responsible for the conflicting results was the length of follow-up, but the lack of serum MBL data makes a full comparison very difficult.

Kilpatrick et al [8] obtained modestly positive results with a serum MBL cut-off level of 100 ng/ml with a series in which a substantial proportion of the patients received either allogeneic or autologous stem cell transplants. A very much stronger relationship was apparent in a series of exclusively autologous stem cell transplants for haematological malignancies, mostly non-Hodgkin's lymphoma but also some acute leukaemias [12]. Both studies used similar follow-up periods of 3-4 months. The previously-mentioned myeloma study [17] also exclusively involved autologous stem cell transplantation and perhaps indicated that MBL confers some protection from serious infections in those patients, some of whom were followed up for 6 months.

Perhaps the most intriguing aspect of the studies involving stem cell transplantation was the observation that a stronger and more significant association with infections was obtained with the *MBL-2* genotype of the donor compared to that of the recipient [10]. Relative strength apart, the observation that the MBL status of a donor had any prognostic value for his recipient was remarkable and opened up the possibility that MBL replacement therapy could be achieved by stem cell therapy, a permanent cure in contrast to infusions of MBL formulations that have biological half-lives of only 2 [18] or 3 [19] days. Certainly, the most obvious explanation for donor variant alleles (circulating MBL protein was not measured) having an independent association with infection in multivariant analysis would be that some leukocytes could synthesize and secrete MBL. Some direct evidence was indeed found that monocytes and monocyte-derived dendritic cells express MBL on their cell surfaces [20], suggesting that stem cells and monocytes might differentiate into MBL-secreting tissue macrophages post-transplant. This exciting possibility was examined by identifying two MBL deficient patients treated with marrow transplants from donors with high MBL concentrations [21]. Although both patients engrafted successfully, neither seroconverted to the MBL sufficient status of his donor over the following two years or more during which period both recipients remained in complete remission. Subsequently, a study on liver transplantation clearly demonstrated that the liver is the only significant source of circulating MBL [22]. Seyfarth et al [23] found traces of *MBL-2* transcription (specific mRNA) in human small intestine and testis tissue as well as in cord blood mononuclear cells and a differentiated cultured monocytic cell line. No evidence for translation into protein was offered, nor is it clear how closely their observations reflect relative transcription patterns in vivo. Those findings provided no evidence for an appreciable contribution of extra-hepatic synthesis towards circulating MBL, but raised the possibility of local MBL synthesis and secretion in extra-hepatic tissues. If the *MBL-2* status of a stem cell donor really affects the susceptibility to infection of his recipient, we have to consider whether this is due to an unknown gene in linkage disequilibrium with *MBL-2* or whether MBL affects cells in some unknown manner that those cells retain when transferred to another person.

The direct evidence concerning MBL after stem cell transplantation is inconclusive but some indirect evidence may be considered helpful. In the context of human renal transplantation, Manuel et al [24] found that a MBL level below 500ng/ml was a significant risk factor for cytomegalovirus (CMV) infection after discontinuation of valganciclovir prophylaxis. Since CMV infection is obviously a potential problem after stem cell transplantation, this observation has important implications for MBL replacement therapy.

Animal experimentation has also provided indirect evidence of interest. Shi et al [25] studied MBL null (A^-/C^-) mice infected with *Staphylococcus aureas*. These mice were susceptible to *S. aureas* administered intravenously but not if administered intra-peritoneally. However, the mice were rendered susceptible to intraperitonal *S.aureas* infection with cyclophosphamide-induced neutropenia. This susceptibility could be reversed by recombinant human MBL prophylaxis. In a separate series of investigations with those MBL null mice, it was found the mice succumbed to *Pseudomonas aeruginosa* septicaemia only if the bacteria were inoculated at a burn site [26]. Collectively, these studies not only support the concept that MBL is more influencial in immunocompromised hosts, but indicate that the site of infection may be important.

On balance, the rather inconclusive data we have at present supports the view that MBL insufficiency may have some influence in some patients following stem cell transplantation. The magnitude of the influence is likely to vary greatly with different clinical contexts. Large, prospective studies of well-defined and homogeneous sets of patients followed up for a substantial period are now needed.

REFERENCES

[1] Kilpatrick, DC. (2000) Handbook of Animal Lectins: properties and biomedical applications. Chichester, England: John Wiley and Sons.

[2] Kilpatrick, DC. (2002) Mannan-binding lectin and its role in innate immunity. *Transfusion Medicine*. 12, 335-351

[3] Kase T, Suzuki Y, Kawai T et al (1999). Human mannan-binding lectin inhibits the infection of influenza A virus without complement. *Immunology*. 97, 385-392

[4] Takahashi K, Shi L, Gowda LD, Ezekowitz RAB (2005). Relative roles of complement factor 3 and mannose-binding lectin in host defense against infection. *Infection and Immunity.* 73, 8188- 8193

[5] Neth O, Hann I, Turner MW, Klein NJ. (2001) Deficiency of mannose-binding lectin and burden of infection in children with malignancy: a prospective study. *Lancet.* 358, 614-618

[6] Peterlund N, Koch C, Jensenius JC, Thiel S. (2001) Association between deficiency of mannose-binding lectin and severe infections after chemotherapy. *Lancet.* 358, 637-638

[7] Bergmann OJ, Christiansen M, Laursen I et al (2003). Low levels of mannose-binding lectin do not affect occurrence of severe infections or duration of fever in acute myeloid leukaemia during remission induction therapy. *European Journal of Haematology.* 70, 91-97

[8] Kilpatrick DC, Mclintock LA, Allan EK et al (2003). No strong relationship between mannan binding lectin or plasma ficolins and chemotherapy-related infections. *Clinical and Experimental Immunology.* 134, 279-284

[9] Klein NJ, Kilpatrick DC (2004). Is there a role for mannan/mannose-binding lectin in defence against infection following chemotherapy for cancer? *Clinical and Experimental Immunology.* 138, 202-204

[10] Mullighan CG, Heatley S, Doherty K et al (2002). Mannose-binding lectin gene polymorphisms are associated with major infection following allogeneic hemopoietic stem cell transplantation. *Blood.* 99, 3524-3529

[11] Rocha V, Franco RF, Porcher R et al (2002). Host defense and inflammatory gene polymorphisms are associated with outcomes after HLA-identical sibling bone marrow transplantation. *Blood.* 100, 3908-3918

[12] Horiuchi T, Gondo H, Miyagawa H et al (2005). Association of MBL gene polymorphisms with major bacterial infection in patients treated with high-dose chemotherapy and autologous PBSCT. *Genes and Immunity.* 6, 162-166

[13] Vekemans M, Georgala A, Heymans C et al (2005) Influence of mannan binding lectin serum levels on the risk of infection during chemotherapy-induced neutropenia in adult haematological cancer patients. *Clinical Microbiology and Infection.* 11, Supplement 2, 20

[14] Lausen B, Schmiegelow K, Andreassen, B, Madsen HO, Garred, P (2006) infections during induction therapy of childhood acute lymphoblastic leukaemia - no association to mannose-binding lectin deficiency. *European Journal of Haematology.* 76, 481-487

[15] Frakking FNJ, van de Wetering, Brouwer N et al (2006). The role of mannose-binding lectin (MBL) in paediatric oncology patients with febrile neutropenia. *European Journal of Cancer.* 42, 909-916

[16] Molle I, Steffensen R, Thiel S, Peterslund NA (2006). Chemotherapy-related infections in patients with multiple myeloma: associations with mannan-binding lectin genotypes (2006). *European Journal of Haematology.* 77, 19-26

[17] Molle I, Peterslund NA, Thiel S, Steffensen R (2006). MBL2 polymorphism and risk of severe infections in multiple myeloma patients receiving high-dose melphalan and autologous stem cell transplantation. *Bone Marrow Transplantation.* 38, 555-560

[18] Petersen KA, Matthiesen F, Agger T et al (2006). Phase I safety, tolerability, and pharmacokinetic study of recombinant human mannan-binding lectin. *Journal of Clinical Immunology.* 26, 465-475

[19] Valdimarsson H, Vikingsdottir T, Bang P et al (2004). Human plasma-derived mannose-binding lectin: a phase I safety and pharmacokinetic study. *Scandinavian Journal of Immunology.* 59, 97-102

[20] Downing I, Koch C, Kilpatrick DC (2003). Immature dendritic cells possess a sugar-sensitive receptor for human mannan-binding lectin. *Immunology.* 109, 360-364

[21] Kilpatrick DC, Stewart K, Allan EK, McLintock LA, Holyoake TL, Turner ML (2005). Successful haemopoietic stem cell transplantation does not correct mannan-binding lectin deficiency. *Bone Marrow Transplantation.* 35, 179-181

[22] Bouwman LH, Roos A, Terpstra OT et al (2005) Mannose binding lectin gene polymorphisms confer a major risk for severe infections after liver transplantation. *Gastroenterology.* 129, 408-414

[23] Seyfarth J, Garred P, Madsen HO (2006). Extra-hepatic transcription of the human mannose-binding gene (mbl2) and the MBL-associated serine protease 1-3 genes. *Molecular Immunology.* 43, 962-971

[24] Manuel O, Pascual M, Trendelenburg M, Meylan PR (2007). Association between mannose-binding lectin deficiency and cytomegalovirus infection after kidney transplantation. *Transplantation.* 83, 359-362

[25] Shi L, Takahashi K, Dundee et al (2004). Mannose-binding lectin-deficient mice are susceptible to infection with Staphylococcus aureus. *Journal of Experimental Medicine.* 199, 1379-1390

[26] Moller-Kristensen M, Ip WKI, Shi L et al (2006). Deficiency of mannose-binding lectin greatly increases susceptibility to postburn infection with Pseudomonas aeruginosa. *Journal of Immunology.* 176, 1769-1775

Expert Commentary D

SEXUALITY OF MEN TREATED BY MEANS OF HAEMATOPOIETIC STEM CELL TRANSPLANTATION

Ladislav Slovacek[1,2,3] *and Birgita Slovackova*[4]

[1]Department of Field Internal Medicine, Faculty of Military Health Sciences, University of Defence, Hradec Kralove, Czech Republic
[2]Department of Clinical Haematology, Department of Medicine, Charles University Hospital and Faculty of Medicine, Hradec Kralove, Czech Republic
[3]Department of Clinical Oncology and Radiotherapy, Charles University Hospital and Faculty of Medicine, Hradec Kralove, Czech Republic
[4]Department of Psychiatry, Charles University Hospital and Faculty of Medicine, Hradec Kralove, Czech Republic

INTRODUCTION

Haematopoietic stem cell transplantation (HSCT) is a therapeutic modality used in antitumorous treatment of haematological malignancies as well as solid tumors. Apart from that it is also used in therapy of non-malignant and hereditary diseases [1]. Own process of SCT is for quite challenging patients, and that's for several reasons. First of all there are unwanted effects of systematic chemotherapy, repetitive invasive performances - central and peripheral vein catheterization, diagnostic aspiration of bone marrow and so on. In men it is also sperm taking followed by cryoconservation of seminal fluid because of the possibility of reproductive organs dysfunction caused by intensive antitumorous therapy (permanent or temporary infertility). Hormonal substitutional therapy is indicated in young females, because of the possibility of damaging the reproductive organs. Also we have to consider several weeks of isolation in a sterile box. There is increased sensibility to opportunistic infections (bacterial, viral, fungal, mycoplasmatic etc.) as an affect of bone marrow toxicity caused by high-dose chemotherapy. Besides those symptoms, the patient is loaded with results of toxicity caused by high dose chemotherapy (mucositis, gastroenteritis, dermatitis, alveolitis, signs of cardiotoxicity and neurotoxicity). Serious complication is acute or chronic Graft-Versus-Host Disease (GVHD), which is the result of allogeneic transplantation (from relative or non-relative donor). Acute GVHD affects especially the liver, mucosa of intestinal tract and skin. Serious forms can cause death. Chronic GVHD damage particularly intestinal tract and skin and can handicap the patient. By listing all possible risks and complications it is necessary to mention, that high-dose chemotherapy followed by SCT cannot insure by 100% that all malignant cells will be eliminated. There is a possibility of relapse and as an optional treatment, we can again choose high dose chemotherapy followed by HSCT [1].

As well as all the other treatments SCT also affects the disease process and with that also the quality of a patient's life. In the last decade of the 20th century several studies about quality of life (QoL) in patients after HSCT were undertaken and there was influence at particular dimensions of QoL observed. One of the closely watched aspects was sexuality in the patient after HSCT.

SEXUALITY, SEXUAL MOTIVATION AND SEXUAL DYSFUNCTION

Sexual health is defined by the *World Health Organization* as "a state of physical, emotional, mental and social well-being related to sexuality; not merely the absence of disease, dysfunction or infirmity." All those aspects enrich and advance personality, communication and love of humans [2].

Human sexual behavior is a result of a long evolution process. Therefore, behavior that *human* beings use when seeking sexual or relational partners, gaining approval of possible partners, forming *relationships*, showing affection and *mating*. It could be quite imperative, to some level not depending on rational control mechanisms [3]. Because of didactic reason we suggest to see 4 components in human sexuality, which are [4]: (1). sexual identity (sexual role), (2). sexual orientation (erotic preference), (3). sexual emotion (sexual excitement, orgasm, love), (4). sexual behavior. Sexual identity based on sexual orientation is the headstone for sexual motivation. A sign of sexual identity is the ability of an individual to take a correspondent social role. The basic dimorphism in sexual orientation results from the principle of bisexual differentiation. Normal sexual orientation means that is related to a sexually mature person with the opposite sex. To sexual emotions belong: sexuality, sensational top (orgasm) and emotion of love (erotic fascination). Sexual behavior has a pair character. Determined sexual pair has a certain stickiness and shows restriction in sexual behavior to other members of the unit. In a well-functioning pair sexuality is lived more naturally and more intensively [4].

Sexual dysfunctions are known as quantitative disorders of sexual performance [3]. Behaviorist conception of sexual dysfunctions result from the conception of four basal components of human sexual behavior [3, 4]: (1). sexual appetence, (2). sexuality, (3). orgasm, (4). sexual satisfaction. Etiology of sexual dysfunctions is multiplex, it's composed of constitutional, biological, psychological and social factors [3, 4].

CHANGES IN SEXUALITY OF MEN TREATED BY MEANS OF HSCT AND INFLUENCE OF HSCT ON QoL

Diagnosis of malignancy, subsequent treatment with high dose chemotherapy followed by HSCT and its complications and their treatment, all according to Ferrell [7], can lead to changes in a patient's sexual life, particularly in accordance with sexual dysfunctions and sexual frustration. Sexual dysfunctions and sexual frustration are often mentioned as the factors, which negatively influence QoL in patients after HSCT [9, 10]. According to Marks [11], Molassiotis [12, 13] and Schubert [14] loss of desire for sex, ejaculation disorders, erectile dysfunction and infertility are the most common sexual problems in men after HSCT. Incidence of sexual dysfunctions or dissatisfaction in men after HSCT is high, as evidenced by results of Andersen's study [15]. The study observed sexual dysfunctions in more than 90% of patients with neoplasia. Wigard's [16] and Chiodi's [17] study shows a range of 22-70% patients after HSCT with sexual dysfunctions. Watson [18] noticed deterioration in sexual life in 55% patients after allogenic HSCT and in 42% patients after autologous HSCT.

Physical and Psychological Aspects Affecting the Male Sexual Condition after HSCT

Physical and biological changes in the male after HSCT treatment are determined by gonadal function and hypothalamo-pituitary-gonadal axis [19]. Physiological changes include at most neurovascular disorders, erectile dysfunction, ejaculation praecox and infertility [19, 20]. Those changes could affect negatively one or more phases of sexual motivation and at the same time could affect adversely sexual behavior and satisfaction. In the period of preparation before transplantation (often high dose chemotherapy with/without whole-body radiation) is deletion or reduction of male sexual hormone production, and that's because of negative feedback absence [20]. Gonadal dysfunction and changes of endocrinal functions (defect at hypothalamo-pituitary-gonadal axis level) in men after HSCT can lead to their infertility and potential changes in their sexual functioning [19]. Reduced reply to gonadoliberines (GnRH) can in some men show the potential dysfunction at hypothalamo-pituitary level [21]. Elevated serum levels of prolactin can in some men after HSCT point out the defect on hypothalamic level. Hyperprolactinemia is one of the reasons for infertility, erectile dysfunction and loss of sexual desire in men after HSCT [21]. Grade of gonadal and endocrinal dysfunction is determined by age, intercurrent diseases, total dose of radiation, type of cytostatic schedule used in preparation before transplantation and it is also determined by the type of HSCT (autologous, allogeneic) [20, 22]. Alkylating agents are often used in HSCT, their side effect is infertility [23]. External radiotherapy and chemotherapy damage germinal sexual cells and seminiferous tubules. The result of that is azoosperm, testicular atrophy and infertility. Kaupilla's [21] study from 1998 was concerned with longterm influence of allogeneic transplantation of steam cells on hypophysal, gonadal, thyroidal and epinephral function. One of the main results of this study is depletion of germinal sexual cells by men after HSCT, which is explained by small size of testes and reduction of testicular volume [21]. Kaupilla [21] tried to quantify those discrepancies, so he shows that the average size of testicles in healthy men is 5x3cm comparing to average size 3.7x2.3 in men after HSCT. He also makes a point about average testicular volume, which is 16-30cm3 in healthy men and 8-15cm3 in men after HSCT. The other outcome from this study are the changes of endocrinal production in men after HSCT, the serum values are (in parentheses are listed physiological values): FSH (follicle-stimulating hormone) 25-90mIU/ml (4-25 mIU/ml), LH (luteinizing hormone) 8-25 mIU/ml (4-20 mIU/ml), testosterone 200-700 mg/100ml (250-1200 mg/100ml), daily production of testosterone 3.5 mg/per day (7.5 mg per day), free testosterone 8.6 ng/100ml (15.3 ng/100ml) [21].

One of the negative effects on sexuality in men after HSCT is chronic GVHD according to Fiedner [24] and Muir [25]. Authors like Barton-Burke [26], Inder [27] and Toy [28] sympathize with this statement.

Psychological Aspects Affecting the Sexual Condition of a Male Treated by Means of HSCT

Sexual motivation in patients after HSCT is negatively affected by: changes in physical condition, changes of self-perception, depression, anxiety, weak self-confidence, somatisation, fear of relapse, anger, desperation and infertility [18, 29]. Playing an essential role in all psychological aspects is infertility, because it could be the reason for relationship disturbances, not only in family, but also among friends and at work [18, 30]. Psychological aspects like depression and anxiety could significantly influence more than one phase of human sexual motivation. Higher incidence of sexual disorders was described in men with a rigid perspective on sexuality, with restricted range of sexual behavior and also in men with a pessimistic future outlook [15, 16].

Social Aspects Affecting the Sexual Condition of a Male Treated by Means of HCT

The most important role from all social aspects is having a faithful partner [9]. The negative affects at the social dimension of QoL could be caused by partner's insecurity, lability, anxiety, faithlessness and communication difficulties during the treatment. Social encouragement is important to the patient during and after HSCT. It also affects psychosocial adaptation of the patient after HSCT [9, 10, 31].

CONCLUSION

The dimensional module of QoL represents a multiple approach to a number of life aspects [1]. The effect of several aspects could vary, because they depend on the phase of the disease and treatment. These findings bring our knowledge about the patients needs into a different perspective and so they could significantly contribute to improvement of health care. They also can discover mechanisms, which modify the disease origin and process [1].

Sexuality is one of the closely watched aspects of QoL in patients after HSCT. Sexuality and its expression belong to a very important aspect of human behavior. It is also very sensitive and a sensible aspect, so with no doubt it is affected by a diagnosis of neoplasm and cancer treatment [7]. Physical and psychosocial factors of HSCT do affect a patient's sexuality and sexual functioning, with that also the QoL. They remain in focus because of the complex care of a patient after HSCT [32].

REFERENCES

[1] Slovacek, L., Slovackova, B., Jebavy, L. Global Quality of Life in Patients Who Have Undergone the Hematopoietic Stem Cell Transplantation: Finding from Transversal and Retrospective Study. *Exp. Oncol.* 2005, 27 (3): 238-242.

[2] World Health Organization. Education and Treatment in Human Sexuality. Technical Report. Geneva World Health Organization, 1975.

[3] Zverina, J. Medical Sexuology. 1st edc. Prague HaH, 1991.

[4] Zbytovsky, J., Balon, R., Prasko, J., Seifertova, D. Sexual dysfunction. 1st edc. Prague Academia Medica Pragensis, 2004.

[5] Ferrell, B. R., Grant, M. M. Quality of Life Scale: Bone Marrow Transplant. In.: Quality of Life from Nursing and Patient Perspectives: Theory, Research, Practice. Jones and Bartlett Publishers, 2nd Edition, 2003.

[6] Grant, M. M., Ferrell, B. R, Schmidt, G. M., Fonbuena, P., Niland, J. C. Measurement of quality of life in bone marrow transplantat survivors. *Qual. Life Res.* 1992, 1: 375-384.

[7] Ferrell, B. R. et al. Quality of life among long-term cancer survivors. *Oncology* 1997, 11: 565-576.

[8] Haas, B. K. Clarification and integration of similar quality of life concepts. *J. Nursing. Scholarship* 1999, 31: 215-220.

[9] Baker, F. et al. Quality of life of bone marrow transplant long-term survivors. *Bone Marrow Transplant.* 1994, 13: 589-596.

[10] Bush, N. E. et al. Quality of life of 125 adults surviving 6-18 years after bone marrow transplantation. *Soc. Sci. Med.* 1995, 40: 479-490.

[11] Marks, D. et al. A prospective study of the effects of hig-dose chemotherapy and bone marrow transplantation on sexual function in the first year after transplant. *Bone Marrow Transplant.* 1997, 19: 819-822.

[12] Molassiotis, A. et al. Comparison of the overall quality of life in 50 long-term survivors of autologous and allogeneic bone marrow transplantation. *J. Adv. Nurs.* 1995, 22: 509-516.

[13] Molassiotis, A. et al. Quality of life in long-term survivors of marrow transplantation: comparison with a matched group receiving maintenance chemotherapy. *Bone Marrow Transplant.* 1996, 17: 249-258.

[14] Schubert, M. A. et al. Gynecological abnormalities following allogeneic bone marrow transplantation. *Bone Marrow Transplant.* 1990, 5: 425-430.
[15] Andersen, B. L. Sexual functioning morbidity among cancer survivors. Current status and future research directions. *Cancer* 1985, 55: 425-430.
[16] Wingard, J. R. et al. Sexual satisfaction in survivors of bone marrow transplantation. *Bone Marrow Transplant.* 1992, 9: 185-190.
[17] Chiodi, S. et al. Cyclic sex hormone replacement therapy in women undergoing allogeneic bone marrow transplantation: aims and results. *Bone Marrow Transplant.* 1991, 8 (Suppl. 1): 47-49.
[18] Watson, M. et al. Severe adverse impact on sexual functioning and fertility of bone marrow transplantation, either allogeneic or autologous, compared with consolidation cheotherapy alone: analysis of the MRC AML 10 trial. *Cancer* 1999, 86: 1231-1236.
[19] Brook, C. G. D., Marshall, N. J. (eds). Essential Endocrinology. London Blackwell Science, 2001.
[20] Klein, C. E. et al. Gonadal complications. In: Armitage JO, Antman KH, eds. High-Dose Cancer Therapy. Pharmacology, Hematopoientins, Stem Cells. Williams and Wilkins, 1992.
[21] Kauppila, M. et al. Long-term effects of allogeneic bone marrow transplantation (BMT) on pituitary, gonad, thyreoid and adrenal function in adults. *Bone Marrow Transplant.* 1998, 22: 331-337.
[22] Sherins, R. J. Gonadal dysfunction. In: Devita VT, Hellman S, Rosenberg SA, eds. Cancer, Principles and Practice of Oncology, 4th edc. Philadelphia: Lippincott, 1993.
[23] Averette, H. E. et al. Effects of cancer chemotherapy on gonadal function and reproductive capacity. *CA Cancer J. Clin.* 1990, 40: 199-209.
[24] Fliedner, M. C. A European Perspective on Quality of Life of Stem Cell Transplantation Patients. In.: Quality of Life from Nursing and Patient Perspectives: Theory, Research, Practice. Jones and Bartlett Publishers, 2nd Edition, 2003.
[25] Muir, A. Sexuality and Bone Marrow Transplantation (BMT) – Considerations for Nursing Care. *EBMT Nurses Group Journal* 2000, 1: 7-11.
[26] Barton-Burke, M. Fatigue and Quality of Life – A Question of Balance. In. King, C. R., Hinds, P. S.: Quality of Life from Nursing nad Pateint Perspectives – Theory – Research – Practice, Jones and Bartlett Publishers, 2nd Edition, 2003.
[27] Inder, A. Long-term effects of bone marrow transplantation at Christchuch Hospital. Proceedings of the 6th Meeting of the EBMT Nurses Group 1990, Hague, Netherlands: 81-86.
[28] Toy, A. Out pateint care following bone marrow transplantation. Proceedings of the 5th Meeting of the EBMT Nurses Group 1989, Badgastein, Austria, 143-148.
[29] Mumma, G. H. et al. Long-term psychosexual adjustment of acute leukemia survivors: impact of marrow transplantation versus conventional chemotherapy. *General Hosp. Psychiatry* 1992, 14: 43-55.
[30] Sutherland, H. J. et al. Quality of life following bone marrow transplantation: a comparison of patient reports with population norms. *Bone Marrow Transplant.* 1997, 19: 1129-1136.

[31] Dobkin, P. L. et al. Assessement of sexual dysfunction in oncology patients: review, critique, and suggestions. *J. Psychosocial Oncol.* 1991, 9: 43-74.

[32] Prieto, J. M. et al. Physical and psychosocial functioning of 117 survivors of bone marrow transplantation. *Bone Marrow Transplant.* 1996, 17: 1133-1142.

Short Communication A

THERAPEUTIC POTENTIAL OF THE NEWLY CHARACTERIZED HUMAN BLOOD-DERIVED STEM CELL IN TYPE 1 DIABETES

Yong Zhao[1] and Lijun Yang[2]

[1]Section of Endocrinology, Diabetes and Metabolism,
Department of Medicine, University of Illinois at Chicago, IL, US
[2]Department of Pathology, Immunology, and Laboratory Medicine,
University of Florida College of Medicine, FL, US

ABSTRACT

Stem cell-derived insulin-producing cells may provide a rational tool for treatment of both type 1 (T1D) and type 2 (T2D) diabetes. Previous studies suggest that either embryonic or adult stem cells can serve as potential sources of β cell surrogates for therapeutic applications. However, the immune system will recognize and attack any foreign cells utilized for the restoration of euglycemia due to the immune surveillance, even the application of allogeneic embryonic stem (ES) cells. To circumvent these barriers, many novel approaches are being investigated, including those directed at manipulating the host immune responses, altered nuclear transfer, and other aspects directed at modulating disease pathogenesis. However, despite these efforts, no suitable solution has been achieved. Therefore, application of autologous stem cells-derived insulin-producing cells is a potentially attractive strategy and may serve as a means to overcome many of the major issues that can complicate cell-based therapies.

Recently, we have identified a unique stem cell population from adult human blood, designated peripheral blood-derived stem cells (PB-SC). PB-SC were expandable and displayed embryonic stem (ES) cell characteristics, along with hematopoietic markers; but lacked expression of hematopoietic stem cell marker CD34 as well as lymphocyte and monocyte/macrophage markers. Notably, PB-SC showed the high potential to give rise to functional insulin-producing cells, as demonstrated the authentic insulin production at different levels by *in vitro* and *in vivo* characterizations. Using the same technology, we have found a similar type of stem cells from human umbilical cord blood. Our current studies have revealed that these newly characterized human blood-derived stem cells not only act as stem cells giving rise to insulin-producing cells, but also as immune modulator cells. In conclusion, application of PB-SC is easy to access, culture, expand, differentiate, and safe, without any ethical issues and immune rejection. These findings may lead to develop new approaches for autologous transplantation of these blood insulin-producing cells to treat diabetes.

INTRODUCTION

Diabetes and its complications are posing one of the major public health problems worldwide. Recently, significant progresses have been made in the prevention and treatment of diabetes. To overcome the shortage of insulin-producing cells in both type 1 (T1D) and overt type 2 (T2D) diabetes patients, pancreas and islet transplantations have offered the potential treatments that obliterate the dependence on insulin injections [1-3]. However, the scarcity of donor islets and pancreas severely hinders their wide-spread applications. Stem cell-derived insulin-producing cells hold a promise to provide the beta cell surrogates. To date, insulin-producing cells have been generated from embryonic stem (ES) cells, umbilical cord blood stem cells, liver and pancreatic progenitor cells, and other tissues [1-3]. Recent reseach findings in stem cell biology have indicated that ES cells and ES cell-derived cells can be rejected post transplantation due to the immune surveillance of the human body, in addition to the ethical and safety issues [4]. Thus, application of autologous stem cells is a potentially attractive strategy for clinical therapeutics and may serve as a means to overcome many of the major issues that complicate cell-based therapies such as immune rejection and shortage of suitable donors [5, 6].

Currently, autologous adult stem cells are usually taken from bone marrow or blood for clinical applications. Although stem cells derived from bone marrow normally possess higher potential of proliferation than those obtained from peripheral blood, it remains problematic to obtain bone marrow cells in comparison to that of peripheral blood, for example painful operations and potential infections. To this end, peripheral blood is easy to access and represents a valuable source for provision of autologous stem cells [5]. Here, we focus on adult blood stem cell-derived insulin-producing cells. Immune regulation of stem cells is also discussed in relevance to their potential of treating type 1 diabetes.

1. BLOOD STEM CELLS PB-SC DISPLAY EMBRYONIC STEM (ES) CELL-RELATED MARKERS

Our previous works have characterized a novel type of stem cells from human umbilical cord blood [7, 8], displaying embryonic stem (ES) cell markers [7, 9]. Based on these studies, we hypothesized that adult human peripheral blood may contain similar cells. To test this hypothesis, we cultured peripheral blood mononuclear cells (PBMC) from healthy donors by adhering PBMC to the plastic Petri dishes (not vacuum gas-treated tissue culture dishes) as previously reported [7]; consequently, we examined the expression of embryonic stem (ES) cell-related transcription factors Oct-4, Nanog, and Sox-2 (associated with the self renewal of embryonic stem cells [10]), in comparison with human embryonic stem cells. Notably, Western blot showed the strong expression of Oct-4, Nanog and Sox-2 in PB-SC (figure 1A).

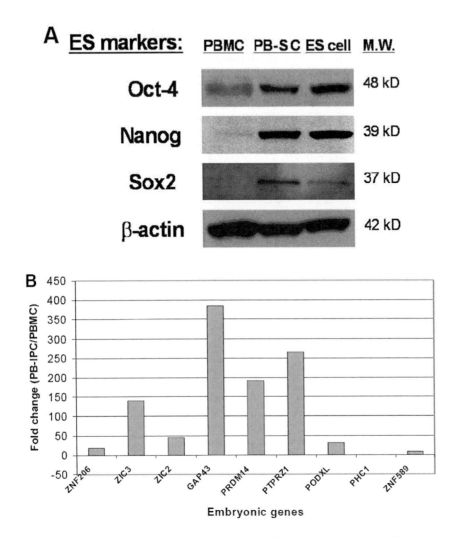

Figure 1. Characterization of PB-SC with embryonic stem cell-related markers. (A) Western blot shows the three ES cell-specific transcription factors. Human ES cell lysate served as positive controls. Freshly isolated PBMC served as negative controls. (B) Real time PCR analysis for other ES cell-related genes. Data represent their expression levels of three experiments after amplification for 40 cycles.

Additionally, we examined other embryonic stem (ES) cell-related markers by real time quantitative PCR (figure 1B), including zinc finger and SCAN domain containing 10 (ZNF206, also named ZSCAN10), Zic family member 3 heterotaxy 1 (ZIC3), Zic family member 2 (ZIC2), Growth associated protein 43 (GAP43), PR domain containing 14 (PRDM14), Protein tyrosine phosphatase, receptor-type, Z polypeptide 1 (PTPRZ1), Podocalyxin-like (PODXL), Polyhomeotic homolog 1 (PHC1), and Zinc finger protein 589 (ZNF589). Collectively, these data demonstrated that PB-SC displayed embryonic stem cell characteristics. Application of autologous PB-SC may provide the best solution overcoming the ethical issues by using human embryonic stem cells.

2. BLOOD STEM CELLS PB-SC DISPLAY UNIQUE PHENOTYPE AND DISCRIMINATE FROM REGULAR BLOOD CELL LINEAGES

Phenotypic analysis showed that PB-SC highly expressed leukocyte common antigen CD45, along with hematopoietic cell antigens including tetraspanin CD9 and stem cell factor receptor CD117 (figure 2); around 60% of cells was positive for endothelial progenitor marker CD31; but PB-SC were negative for hematopoietic stem cell marker CD34, lymphocyte markers CD3, CD20, and CD90, monocyte/macrophage antigens CD11b/Mac-1 and CD14, dendritic cell marker CD11c (figure 2). Especially, high expression of CD45 indicates that PB-SC are hematopoietic ($CD45^+$) origin, not mesenchymal ($CD45^-$) cells circulating in peripheral blood [11].

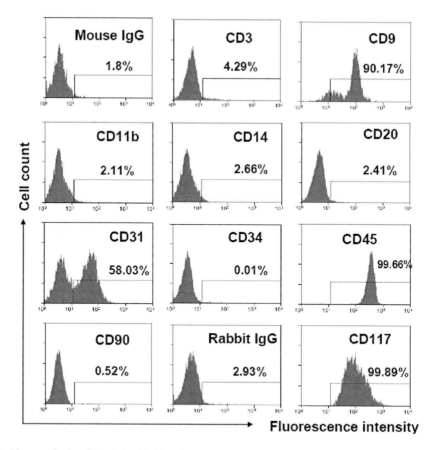

Figure 2. Flow analysis of PB-SC with blood cell lineage markers. Isotype-matched IgG served as controls. Data represent from one of four experiments with similar results.

Attached cells in blood are usually regarded as "macrophages". However, PB-SC failed to express human monocyte/macrophage specific antigens [6] CD14 and CD11b/Mac-1 (figure 2). To further distinguish PB-SC from monocytes/macrophages, we examined PB-SC for monocyte/macrophage-related phenotypes [6] such as human leukocyte antigens (HLA): HLA-DR, HLA-DQ, and HLA-ABC, along with costimulating molecules: CD40, CD80, and CD86. Compared with monocytes, PB-SC were negative for HLA-DR, CD40, and CD80 [5]; Less than 10% of cells were positive for CD86 and HLA-DQ; but strongly expressed HLA-ABC (usually expressed on all nucleated adult cells) [5].

To further substantiate that PB-SC were different from monocytes/macrophages, we performed cell sorting. After removal of monocyte ($CD14^+$), PB-SC could still be generated from $CD14^-$ cell population of peripheral blood mononuclear cells. Immunostaining showed that they were double positive for PB-SC markers: CD45 and transcription factors Oct-4 or Nanog (figure 3). Thus, these results indicate generation of PB-SC is independent of monocytes.

To further evaluate their percentage in peripheral blood, we performed flow analysis using CD45 and transcription factors Oct-4 or Nanog as indicators. Results showed that $0.1 \pm 0.01‰$ of mononuclear cells were positive for $CD45^+Oct-4^+$, $1.9 \pm 0.02‰$ of mononuclear cells were for $CD45^+Nanog^+$. Taken together, these results suggest that PB-SC may represent a unique cell population.

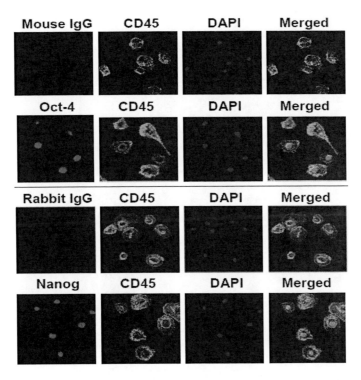

Figure 3. Double immunostaining of cultured $CD14^-$ cell population after cell sorting. The sorted $CD14^-$ cell population was planted in the 8-well Lab-Tek chamber slides in 7% FBS-RPMI1640 culture medium. After culture for 10-14 days, cells stained with antibodies to embryonic stem (ES) cell markers Oct-4 (red), Nanog (red), and leukocyte common antigen CD45 (green), along with DAPI nuclear staining (blue). Cells were photographed using Zeiss LSM 510 META confocal microscope.

3. PB-SC ACTS AS ISLET BETA CELL PROGENITORS

Insulin-producing cells are the highly specialized cell populations and are usually located in pancreatic islets after differentiation and maturation during the embryonic development. Notably, we demonstrated that a very small number of insulin-producing cells are present in healthy human circulating blood [5]. By virtue of their capability to attach to plastic surface, PB-SC could be isolated and their potential for insulin production could be preserved, as proved by their expression of the β cell-specific transcription factors (figure 4A), insulin synthesis-related converting enzymes (figure 4A), insulin production at protein and mRNA levels (figure 4B), C-peptide production (a by-product of insulin, figure 4C) and formation of insulin granules [5]. Our findings provide a novel approach for the generation of the autologous insulin-producing cells from patients themselves to treat diabetes. In comparison with the generation of insulin-producing cells from embryonic stem (ES) cells [12], this technology can efficiently make insulin-producing cells from their own blood stem cells, without any ethical issues and the hazards of immune rejection [5].

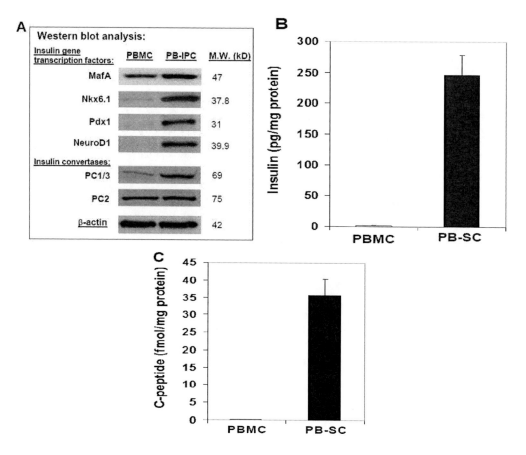

Figure 4. Characterization of PB-SC for insulin production. *A:* Western blot for transcription factors including PDX-1, NeuroD, and NKX6.1, along with prohormone convertases PC-1 and PC-2. Freshly isolated peripheral blood mononuclear cells (PBMC) served as controls. *B:* Quantification of insulin and *C:* C-peptide levels per total cell protein by ELISA. Zhao Y, et al. 2007.BBRC.360:205-211.

Insulin-producing cells that exist in circulating blood may naturally function as a bank and contribute to insulin production under the diabetic situations. It is important to note that extrapancreatic insulin-producing cells have been found in multiple organs of the diabetic rodent animal models (e.g., liver, adipose tissues, spleen, bone marrow, and thymus) [13]. The potential mechanism for this compensatory phenomenon may be associated with the replication and expansion of PB-SC in blood which are then distributed via blood circulation into different organs in order to produce more insulin and meet the body's insulin need. Recently, Voltarelli and colleagues performed small clinical trials in newly diagnosed type 1 diabetes by autologous nonmyeloablative hematopoietic stem cell transplantation (AHST) and achieved the prolonged insulin independence in the majority of the trial participants [14].

4. PB-SC Reduces Hyperglycemia and Migrates into Pancreatic Islets in the Chemical STZ-Induced Type 1 Diabetes Model

Deficit of insulin-producing cells is the crucial issue for type 1 and overt type 2 diabetes. Increasing lines of evidence demonstrate that insulin-producing beta cells can physiologically compensate for the beta cells lost by reproducing themselves and/or differentiation from the pancreatic duct progenitors or pancreatic acinar cells [3, 15]. Due to the limited compensatory effects and continuous reduction of beta cell numbers, pancreatic islet can not produce enough insulin to meet the body' daily needs and the development of diabetes ensues. How to provide the beta cell surrogates and restore the functions of islet beta cells?

In vitro experiments have demonstrated that PB-SC displayed high potential producing insulin [5]. Next, we want to evaluate whether PB-SC can give rise to functional insulin-producing cells; we therefore transplanted PB-SC into the chemical streptozotocin (STZ)-induced diabetic NOD-scid mice. Results demonstrated that PB-SC transplantation could reduce about 20-30% of severe hyperglycemia in comparison with the untransplanted diabetic mice. Importantly, we utilized an assay that is specific for human C-peptide (does not recognize mouse C-peptide) to evaluate human insulin secretion [7, 16-18]. Data showed that human C-peptide level was significantly increased after transplantation ($p<0.01$). However, human C-peptide was undetectable in mouse sera of PB-SC-untransplanted diabetic mice and normal mice [5].

Stem cell homing to diabetic islets is the critical step and may provide new seeds for regeneration of beta cells. Notably, PB-SC possessed the ability to migrate into pancreatic islets after transplantation into the diabetic mice, as proved by the identification of human C-peptide-positive cells in pancreatic islets were also positive for human chromosome karyotyping [5]. Interestingly, we found that homing of PB-SC to diabetic pancreatic islets was not a random process [5]. Accumulated evidence has defined that chemokines and their receptors can control trafficking of blood stem cells into bone marrow post transplantation. This is an emerging field for investigation of the stem cells homing to pancreatic islets. Our mechanistic studies revealed that a chemokine stromal cell-derived factor-1 (SDF-1) and its receptor CXCR-4 may contribute to the homing of PB-SC into the diabetic islets [5]. Further understanding of the mechanisms involved in stem cell homing to islets should facilitate stem cell mobilization and improve their therapeutic potential for diabetes.

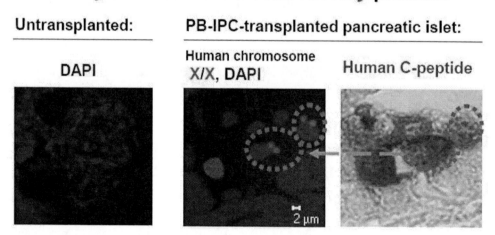

Figure 5. Homing of PB-SC into diabetic pancreatic islets following transplantation into the streptozotocin (STZ)-induced diabetic NOD-scid mice. Fluorescence in situ hybridization (FISH) for human chromosome X/Y after immunostaining for human C-peptide. A human C-peptide-positive cell (brown, in green circle) is also positive for human chromosome x/x (red, pointed by green dashed arrow, female karyotype). *Zhao Y, et al. 2007.BBRC.360:205-211.*

5. IMMUNE REGULATION OF BLOOD STEM CELLS

Clinical transplantation of tissues and organs between two unrelated individuals results almost invariably in graft rejection, unless immunosuppressive therapy is given to control the immune response. Similarly, immune rejection is also challenging stem cell-based therapy [4, 19]. How to develop strategies to overcome the inevitable immunological barriers of host that will achieve long-term therapeutics post transplantation of stem cells and/or stem cell-derived cells? This is an emerging area for stem cell-based therapy and must be addressed before clinical application can realize its full potential. To circumvent these barriers, several approaches [20-23] are being investigated including immunosuppressive drugs, encapsulation, manipulation of host immune responses, constitution of immune chimerism, in *vitro* fertilization (IVF) and altered nuclear transfer (ANT). Currently no final solution has achieved. The use of human embryonic stem (ES) cells as an attractive mean to deal with immune rejection issues has been limited by ethical and safety issues (for example, formation of teratoma) [24]. Therefore, new strategies are needed. Recently, we have characterized a similar type of stem cell from human umbilical cord blood, designated cord blood-stem cells (CB-SC) [25]. CB-SC displayed immune regulations on lymphocyte proliferation and T cell subsets (figure 6) [25]. Thus, blood stem cells CB-SC may provide an ideal stem cell model for therapeutics.

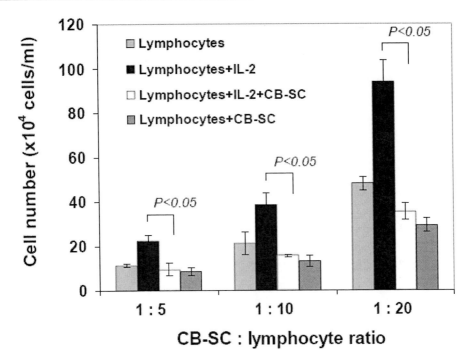

Figure 6. Inhibitory effects of CB-SC on the lymphocyte proliferation. CB-SC inhibited the proliferation of IL-2-stimulated lymphocytes. Allogeneic lymphocytes were quantified after coculture with CB-SC for 4-5 days at ratios 1:5, 1:10, and 1:20 of CB-SC: lymphocytes, in the presence or absence of 500U/ml IL-2. Data represent mean (± SD) of three experiments. *Zhao Y, et al. 2007.Immunology Letters.108:78-87.*

Application of autologous blood stem cells PB-SC may provide a potential approach for beta cell-replacement therapy without immune rejection. However, for treatment of human autoimmune disease like type 1 diabetes, it is important to control the autoimmune cells in addition to providing beta cell surrogates. Type 1 diabetes is a disease in which the pancreatic islet beta-cells are selectively destroyed by auto-reactive T lymphocytes. These T cells may also attack the stem cell-derived insulin-producing cells. Therefore, to radically cure type 1 diabetes, it is very important to manage autoimmune responses and protect the stem cells and/or stem cell-derived cells from immune attack post transplantation, without the need for long-term immunosuppressive drug therapies. Based on our previous studies in human umbilical cord blood-derived stem cells [25], our ongoing studies have demonstrated that PB-SC may function not only as stem cells giving rise to insulin-producing cells, but also as immunomodulatory cells to control the autoimmune cells.

Additionally, mesenchymal stem cells (MSC) are a rare population residing in postnatal tissues and organs, such as bone marrow, adipose tissue, fetal liver, or spleen, and passing through the blood. They are negative for leukocyte common antigen CD45 and therefore are different from blood stem cells [5, 7]. Recently, MSC have shown unique immunological properties, including failure to stimulate alloreactivity and suppress activation of T cells both in *vitro* and in *vivo*. Results from animal studies demonstrate that the mesenchymal stem cells can contribute to initiating the regeneration of islet β cells, albeit with a very low frequency to transdifferentiate into insulin-producing cells by themselves [26].

In conclusion, identification of insulin-producing cells from adult blood brings a new hope for treatment of diabetes patients by using their own blood stem cells, without immune rejection and ethical issues. Further characterization and optimization with inducers that can differentiate these brand-new stem cells into the beta cell-like insulin-producing cells holds great promise for diabetes cure.

REFERENCES

[1] Bonner-Weir S, Weir GC. 2005. New sources of pancreatic beta-cells. *Nat. Biotechnol.* 23:857-861.
[2] Nanji SA, Shapiro AM. 2006. Advances in pancreatic islet transplantation in humans. *Diabetes Obes Metab.* 8:15-25.
[3] Trucco M. 2005. Regeneration of the pancreatic beta cell. *J. Clin. Invest.* 115:5-12.
[4] Bradley JA, Bolton EM, Pedersen RA. 2002. Stem cell medicine encounters the immune system. *Nat. Rev. Immunol.* 2: 859-871.
[5] Zhao Y, Huang Z, Lazzarini P, Wang Y, Di A, Chen M. 2007. A unique human blood-derived cell population displays high potential for producing insulin. *Biochem. Biophys. Res. Commun.* 360: 205-211.
[6] Zhao Y, Glesne D, Huberman E. 2003. A human peripheral blood monocyte-derived subset acts as pluripotent stem cells. *Proc. Natl. Acad. Sci. U. S. A.* 100: 2426-2431.
[7] Zhao Y, H. Wang, T. Mazzone. 2006. Identification of stem cells from human umbilical cord blood with embryonic and hematopoietic characteristics. *Exp. Cell Res.* 312: 2454-2464.
[8] Zhao Y, Huang Z, Qi M, Lazzarini P, Mazzone T. 2007. Immune regulation of T lymphocyte by a newly characterized human umbilical cord blood stem cell. *Immunology Letters.* 108:78-87.
[9] Ian Rogers, Nobuko Yamanaka, Ryszard Bielecki, Christine J. Wong, Shawn Chua, Shelia Yuen and Robert F. Casper. 2007. Identification and analysis of in vitro cultured CD45-positive cells capable of multi-lineage differentiation. *Experimental Cell Research*, 313: 1839-1852.
[10] Takahashi K, Yamanaka S. 2006. Induction of pluripotent stem cells from mouse embryonic and adult fibroblast cultures by defined factors. *Cell.* 126:663-676.
[11] da Silva Meirelles L, Chagastelles PC, Nardi NB. 2006. Mesenchymal stem cells reside in virtually all post-natal organs and tissues. *J. Cell Sci.* 119: 2204-2213.
[12] D'Amour KA, Bang AG, Eliazer S, Kelly OG, Agulnick AD, Smart NG, Moorman MA, Kroon E, Carpenter MK, Baetge EE. 2006. Production of pancreatic hormone-expressing endocrine cells from human embryonic stem cells. *Nat. Biotechnol.* 24: 1392-1401.
[13] Kojima H, Fujimiya M, Matsumura K, Nakahara T, Hara M, Chan L. 2004. Extrapancreatic insulin-producing cells in multiple organs in diabetes. *Proc. Natl. Acad. Sci. U. S. A.* 101: 2458-2463.
[14] Voltarelli JC, Couri CE, Stracieri AB, Oliveira MC, Moraes DA, Pieroni F, Coutinho M, Malmegrim KC, Foss-Freitas MC, Simoes BP, Foss MC, Squiers E, Burt RK. 2007.

Autologous nonmyeloablative hematopoietic stem cell transplantation in newly diagnosed type 1 diabetes mellitus. *JAMA.* 297: 1568-1576.

[15] Dor Y, Brown J, Martinez OI, Melton DA. 2004. Adult pancreatic beta-cells are formed by self-duplication rather than stem-cell differentiation. *Nature.* 429: 41-46.

[16] Hori Y, Gu X, Xie X, Kim SK. 2005. Differentiation of insulin-producing cells from human neural progenitor cells. *PLoS Med.* 2: 347-356.

[17] Hayek A, Beattie GM. 1997Experimental transplantation of human fetal and adult pancreatic islets. *J. Clin. Endocrinol. Metab.* 82: 2471-2475.

[18] Zalzman M, Gupta S, Giri RK, Berkovich I, Sappal BS, Karnieli O, Zern MA, Fleischer N, Efrat S. 2003. Reversal of hyperglycemia in mice by using human expandable insulin-producing cells differentiated from fetal liver progenitor cells. *Proc. Natl. Acad. Sci. U. S. A.* 100: 7253-7258.

[19] Drukker M. 2002. Characterisation of MHC protein expression in human embryonic stem cells. *Proc. Natl. Acad. Sci.* 99: 9864–9869.

[20] Bonde J, Hess DA, Nolta JA. 2004. Recent advances in hematopoietic stem cell biology, *Curr. Opin. Hematol.* 11: 392-398.

[21] Melton DA, Daley GQ, Jennings CG. 2004. Altered nuclear transfer in stem-cell research - a flawed proposal, *N. Engl. J. Med.* 351: 2791-2792.

[22] Draper J S Pigott C, Thomson JA, Andrews PW. 2002. Surface antigens of human embryonic stem cells: changes upon differentiation in culture. *J. Anat.* 200: 249–258.

[23] Roche E, Reig JA, Campos A, Paredes B, Isaac JR, Lim S. 2005. Insulin-secreting cells derived from stem cells: clinical perspectives, hypes and hopes. *Transpl. Immunol.* 15:113-129.

[24] Evans M. 2005. Ethical sourcing of human embryonic stem cells--rational solutions? *Nat. Rev. Mol. Cell Biol.* 6: 663-667.

[25] Zhao Y, Mazzone T. 2005. Human umbilical cord blood-derived f-macrophages retain pluripotentiality after thrombopoietin expansion. *Exp. Cell Res.* 310: 311-318.

[26] Chong AS, Shen J, Tao J, Yin D, Kuznetsov A, Hara M, Philipson LH. 2006. Reversal of diabetes in non-obese diabetic mice without spleen cell-derived beta cell regeneration. *Science.* 311:1774-1775.

In: Encyclopedia of Stem Cell Research (2 Volume Set)   ISBN: 978-1-61761-835-2
Editor: Alexander L. Greene   © 2012 Nova Science Publishers, Inc.

Short Communication B

RECENT PROGRESS OF RADIATION RESEARCH: CANCER STEM CELLS AND NCRNAS

Hideshi Ishii[1,2] *and Toshiyuki Saito*[*,2]
[1]Center for Molecular Medicine,
Jichi Medical School, Tochigi, Japan
[2]Research Center for Charged Particle Therapy,
National Institute for Radiological Science,
Chiba, Japan

ABSTRACT

For over three decades, stem cells have been used in the replenishment of hematological and immune systems damaged by genotoxins or during treatment of malignant cells by chemotherapy or radiotherapy. The cancer stem cell hypothesis suggests that a tumor can be viewed as an aberrant organ that is sustained, in a way similar to normal tissues, by a stem cell that drives tumorigenesis, as well as giving rise to a large population of differentiated progeny. The cancer stem cells, controlled by the micro-environmental conditions in the cancer tissue structures, may be involved in the process of relapse, metastasis and resistance to therapy. The strategy of targeting a small fraction of cancer stem cells would be efficient and would minimize the side-effects of the total kill strategy. The aim of this mini-review is to focus on recent developments in radiation research on cancer stem cells and transcriptome of noncoding (nc) RNA molecules, as well as their role in carcinogenesis and their implications in the development of new cancer treatments in the future.

---

[*] Correspondence should be addressed to H.I. (e-mail: hishii@ms.jichi.ac.jp) or T.S. (e-mail: t_saito@nirs.go.jp)

1. INTRODUCTION

Epithelial tumors, including environmental carcinogen-induced cancers, such as those of the esophagus, stomach, colon, bladder and lung, contain cellular heterogeneity, which is accounted for by ongoing mutations with accumulating genomic instability. The complex structures can reflect multiple factors, including DNA damage checkpoints, repairs and apoptosis of epithelial cancerous cells, as well as microenvironmental factors such as epithelial-mesenchymal interactions, angiogenesis and infiltrations of lymphocytes, which surround cancer cells. The cancer stem cell hypothesis suggests that a tumor can be viewed as an aberrant organ that is sustained by a stem cell that drives tumorigenesis and accumulates genomic instability, as well as giving rise to a large population of differentiated progeny that make up the bulk of a tumor but that lack tumorigenic potential [1]. The strategy of targeting a small fraction of cancer stem cells would be efficient. We note the recent progress in radiation research mainly on cancer stem cells, which are supposed to be involved in the process of relapse, metastasis and resistance to therapy, and note their implications in the future development of new cancer treatments.

2. NORMAL STEM CELLS

Normal stem cells can be divided into three main categories: embryonic, germinal, and somatic [2]. The classification depends mainly on the origin of the cells.

Embryonic stem (ES) cells originate from the inner cell mass of the blastocyst. ES cells were first derived from mice and are now derived from various mammalian cells [3, 4]. ES cells are characterized by indefinite self-renewal in an undifferentiated, pluri-potential state [5]. Because of their ability to differentiate into various somatic cell types, ES cells have the potential for clinical and biotechnological applications [5]. Several molecules are known to participate in the regulation of self-renewal and pluri-potency of mouse ES cells, including POU family transcription factor Oct4 [6], leukemia inhibitory factor (LIF), Stat3 [7], Sox2 [8], FoxD3 [9], and Nanog [10, 11]. Germinal stem cells are derived from primary germinal layers of the embryo. They differentiate into progenitor cells to produce specific organ cells [2].

In contrast, somatic or adult stem cells are progenitor cells that are less totipotent than ES cells [2]. Somatic or adult stem cells are found in mature tissues such as hematopoietic, neural, gastrointestinal and mesenchymal tissues. These cells are commonly used in clinical applications, including bone marrow transplantation with hemopoietic stem cells and other primitive progenitor cells including mesenchymal stem cells [12]. Certain micro(mi)RNAs, subgroups of ncRNAs, must be expressed in order to bypass checkpoints for the self-renewal of stem cells [13].

3. NONCODING TRANSCRIPTOME

Although ncRNA molecules have been known for quite a while, their importance was not fully appreciated until recent genome-wide searches discovered thousands of these molecules and their genes in a variety of model organisms [14].

3.1. ncRNAs (Including miRNAs)

Cellular RNAs that do not function as messenger RNAs (mRNAs), transfer RNAs (tRNAs) or ribosomal RNAs (rRNAs) comprise a diverse class of molecules that are commonly referred to as ncRNAs. Over the last few years, the importance of this surprisingly diverse class of molecules has been widely recognized [15]. ncRNAs have been identified in unexpectedly large numbers using bioinformatical approaches [16]. Previous research has shown that ncRNAs are involved in many biological functions: chromosome maintenance, regulation of stability and translocation of proteins, DNA replication, regulation of transcription and translation, and RNA processing, including RNA cleavage, religation, modification editing and stability, directly hampering the function of targets by binding to their surfaces [15, 16]. Another class of small ncRNA, aptamers, act as high-affinity ligands and potential antagonists of disease-associated proteins [17, 18].

Among these ncRNAs, it is well known that small RNA molecules play multiple roles in regulating gene expression, including transcriptional gene silencing [19, 20], targeted degradation of mRNA by small interfering RNAs (siRNAs) (posttranscriptional gene silencing) [21], and developmentally regulated, sequence-specific translational repression of mRNA [22].

The miRNAs, which are an abundant class of ncRNAs of about 21-25 nucleotides in length, are part of a phylogenetically extensive family of small RNAs with potential roles in gene regulation [23]. The first identified miRNA, *lin-4*, is required for the appropriate timing of post-embryonic development in *Caenorhabditis elegans* [24, 25]. Since this discovery, miRNAs have been identified in diverse animals and plants and it now seems likely that all multicellular eukaryotes, and perhaps some unicellular eukaryotes, use these small RNAs to regulate gene expression [26, 27]. Gene expression can be regulated at the posttranscriptional or translational level [28, 29]. Recent work has identified over 450 human miRNA genes, but more recent research has predicted that the number is closer to 1000 [30-32] and that miRNAs repress more than one-third of human genes [33]. 474 miRNAs in humans, 373 miRNAs in mice, and 234 miRNAs in rats are listed in the NCBI data-base (January, 2007). It has been suggested that miRNA genes are one of the most abundant classes of regulatory genes in mammals [31, 33]. Currently, about 2% of the known human genes encode miRNAs, which are essential for development [26].

3.2. miRNAs and Cancer

The most compelling evidence for a gene's involvement in human cancer is the observation of acquired genetic mutations in patient tumors. Such alterations can occur through point mutations or through larger chromosomal changes, including amplifications or deletions. Calin GA *et al* reported that miRNAs frequently reside in hot spots for chromosomal abnormalities in human cancer [34]. They initiated the study of bioinformatics by cloning 'in silico' and generated several databases containing the exact genomic positions of markers used for cloning cancer-associated genomic regions, including 157 minimal regions of loss-of-heterozygosity (LOH), suggestive of the presence of tumor suppressor genes, 37 minimal regions of amplification, suggestive of the presence of oncogenes, and 29 fragile sites [34]. The study indicated that more than half of miRNA genes were located in cancer-associated genomic regions, including 65 miRNAs located exactly in minimal regions of LOH and 15 miRNAs in minimal regions of amplification, in a variety of tumors, and that 61 miRNAs are located in the same cytogenetic positions as fragile sites [35].

Fragile sites are chromosome regions that exhibit gaps or breaks, visible in metaphase chromosomes, when cells are exposed to replicative stress conditions [36-39]. A substantial body of evidence supports the proposal that at least some common chromosomal fragile sites are predisposed to DNA instability in cancer cells [40, 41]. Fragile sites are preferential sites of sister chromatid exchange, translocation, deletion, amplification or integration of plasmid DNA and tumor-associated viruses such as human papilloma virus. Thus the studies of Calin GA *et al* strongly suggest a larger involvement of miRNAs in cancer than previously thought [35].

3.3. Radiation and ncRNAs

Radiation induces various types of DNA damage, including double stranded breaks, but also replication folk stalling, single stranded breaks, and oxidative stress. Reactive oxygen species are a major source of DNA damage, suggesting that stress defense in stem cells is superior to that of various differentiated cells [42]. It has been shown that the activity of ataxia-telangiectasia mutated- and Rad3-related kinase, Atr, is essential for normal cell cycle progression of exponentially proliferating stem cells even in the absence of exogenously-introduced DNA damage, and Atr deregulation triggers p38alpha-dependent cell-cycle checkpoint and apoptotic responses, supporting the DNA damage-induced response [43].

Radiation can induce genomic alterations, leading to deregulation of ncRNAs and resultant carcinogenesis. For example, recent reports indicate that mouse tumors with a provirus at the Kis2 common retrovirus integration site, located on mouse chromosome X, in radiation leukemia virus induced T cell leukemia, overexpress a novel ncRNA with a complex splicing pattern and no polyA tail [44, 45]. It has been shown that Kis2 ncRNAs are the pri-miRNA of miR-106-363, and that Kis2 ncRNA overexpression in mouse tumors results in miR-106a, miR-19b-2, miR-92-2, and miR-20b accumulation, showing the oncogenic potential of those miRNAs, and furthermore that pri-miR-106-363 overexpresses in 46% of human T-cell leukemias, which establishes a link with alterations of miRNAs and T-cell leukemias [45].

Another study using *A thaliana* reported that, in response to UV-B radiation, an important adverse abiotic stress, 21 microRNA genes in 11 microRNA families are upregulated under UV-B stress conditions, suggesting putative transcriptional downregulation pathways triggered by the induction of these miRNA genes [46].

A study of human lymphoblastoid cells grown under various conditions or treatments indicated that folate deficiency induced a pronounced global increase in miRNA expression, such as miR-222, whereas no significant alteration was found in miRNA expression in cells treated with irradiation [47]. A study of murine stem cells detected alterations of miRNA expression in response to radiation exposure [48], suggesting that miRNA expression plays a role in the regulation of undifferentiated stem cells and it responds to conditions of growth and differentiation. The exact mechanism and function of the miRNA response remains to be understood.

4. CANCER STEM CELLS

Normal stem cells are characterized as having: 1) capability of self-renewal; 2) potential to divide and differentiate to generate all functional elements of a particular tissue; and 3) strict control over stem cell numbers [2, 49]. Since cancer stem cells can be defined as cells in the tumor growth with tumor initiating potential [1, 2], the cancer stem cells are believed to have no control over cell numbers [2]. Cancer stem cells are present in very small numbers in whole tumors and are responsible for the growth of the tumor cells [2]. According to a recent theory of cancer stem cells, the involvement of a small fraction of cancer stem cells in tumor tissues is an attractive explanation for the observation that higher numbers of cancer cells from tissues are needed to maximize the probability of injecting cancer stem cells into an animal model, and that the tumor often shrinks in size in response to treatment only to recur again [2]. It is suggested that treatments targeting cancer cells may not be able to target the cancer stem cells [2].

The implication of cancer stem cells is shown first in a non-epithelial tumor, leukemia [2]. Heterogeneity was observed in leukemia [50-52], but also in cancers of the head and neck [53], gastro-intestinal system [54], colon [55, 56], breast [57] and brain [58, 59]. Cancer stem cells may play a role in the resistance to chemotherapy or radiation therapy and seem be responsible for recurrence after cancer treatment, even when most of the cancer cells appear to be killed and few cancer stem cells remain [60].

Epithelial cancer stem cells and their daughter cells of epithelial tumors, including environmental carcinogen-induced cancers, provide a complex structure composed of epithelial and mesenchymal cells. Epithelial stem cells are specified during development and are controlled by epithelial-mesenchymal interactions [61]. Epithelial tumors contain cellular heterogeneity, which is accounted for by ongoing mutations with accumulating genomic instability. The complex mechanism can reflect multiple factors, including DNA damage checkpoints, repairs and apoptosis of epithelial cancerous cells, but also microenvironmental factors such as epithelial-mesenchymal interactions, angiogenesis and infiltrations of lymphocytes, which surround cancer cells. The strategy of targeting the small fraction of cancer stem cells would be useful for efficient treatment and for minimization of any side-effects in therapy.

4.1. Breast Cancer

Breast cancer is the most common type of carcinoma in women. Recent studies indicate that breast cancer tissues are composed of heterogeneous cells with distinct phenotypes, some with stem-cell-like properties, *i.e.* self-renewing cells with potent tumorigenicity [62, 63]. Recent studies show that CD44+/CD24(-/low) breast cancer cells exhibit enhanced invasive properties [57, 64]. Our knockdown study of Notch3, rather than Notch1, resulted in the sensitization of CD44+ cells to deionizing radiation, which was more apparent in CD44+ cells than in CD44- cells (data not shown).

Notch proteins are members of the conserved transmembrane receptor family and play a role in cell fate decisions such as stem cell proliferation, differentiation and cell death [65]. There are four receptors, Notch 1 to 4, and five ligands, Jagged1 and 2 and Delta-like 1, 3 and 4. Notch signaling is activated by ligand-receptor interaction and triggers proteolytic cleavages by the gamma-secretase complex, which releases the Notch intracellular domain into the nucleus. The Notch intracellular domain binds to the CBF1 DNA binding protein of the transcriptional activator complex, the activation of which can lead to the expression of target genes such as Hes family genes involved in cell growth and differentiation. We thus propose a preferential role for the Notch family in the protection of breast cancer-initiating cells from radiation-dependent tumor regression, which may lead to promising candidates for therapeutic targets to induce radiation sensitivity.

4.2. Brain Cancer

A subset of cells called neurospheres in paediatric brain tumors such as medulloblastomas and gliomas has been shown to have self-renewal capability [2]. In differentiation promoting conditions, the neuospheres gave rise to neurones and glia in proportions that reflect the amount in the tumor [66].

A recent study demonstrated that cancer stem cells contribute to glioma radio-resistance through preferential activation of the DNA damage checkpoint response and an increase in DNA repair capacity in the fraction of tumor cells expressing CD133, a marker for both neural stem cells and brain cancer stem cells [59]. The radio-resistance of CD133-positive glioma stem cells can be reversed with a specific inhibitor of the Chk1 and Chk2 checkpoint kinases [59]. The study indicates that CD133-positive tumor cells represent the cellular population that confers glioma radio-resistance and could be the source of tumor recurrence after radiation [59]. Considering that ionizing radiation represents the most effective therapy for glioblastoma, one of the most lethal human malignancies, it is important to know if we can target the DNA damage checkpoint response in cancer stem cells in order to overcome the radio-resistance of malignant brain cancers [59, 67].

4.3. Perspective

All life on earth must cope with constant exposure to environmental or endogenous genotoxic insults such as the sun's radiation, ionizing or ultraviolet radiation, various chemicals and drugs, and reactive cellular metabolites [68, 69]. In the case of radiation, both protection and use are important. Here we noted our use of radiation as cancer therapy, especially focusing on cancer stem cells. Radiation research on cancer stem cells raises many questions about the details of the radiobiology of cancer cells with stem-ness in their native environment within tumors *in vivo*, and the answers to those questions may lead to better optimization of radiation treatments and schedules for patients.

REFERENCES

[1] Reya, T., Morrison, S.J., Clarke, M.F., and Weissman, I.L. (2001). Stem cells, cancer, and cancer stem cells. *Nature, 414*, 105-111.

[2] Sagar, J., Chaib, B., Sales, K., Winslet, M., and Seifalian, A. (2007). Role of stem cells in cancer therapy and cancer stem cells: a review. *Cancer Cell Intern., 7*, 9.

[3] Evans, M.J., and Kaufman, M.H. (1981). Establishment in culture of pluripotential cells from mouse embryos. *Nature, 292*, 154-156.

[4] Martin, G.R. (1981). Isolation of a pluripotent cell line from early mouse embryos cultured in medium conditioned by teratocarcinoma stem cells. *Proc. Natl. Acad. Sci. U S A., 78*, 7634-7638.

[5] Smith, A. Embryonic stem cells. New York: Cold Spring Harbor Laboratory Press; 2001.

[6] Palmieri, S.L., Peter, W., Hess, H., and Scholer, H.R. (1994). Oct-4 transcription factor is differentially expressed in the mouse embryo during establishment of the first two extraembryonic cell lineages involved in implantation. *Dev. Biol., 166*, 259-267.

[7] Matsuda, T., Nakamura, T., Nakao, K., Arai, T., Katsuki, M., Heike, T., and Yokota, T. (1999). STAT3 activation is sufficient to maintain an undifferentiated state of mouse embryonic stem cells. *EMBO J., 18*, 4261-4269.

[8] Avilion, A.A., Nicolis, S.K., Pevny, L.H., Perez, L., Vivian, N., and Lovell-Badge, R. (2003). Multipotent cell lineages in early mouse development depend on SOX2 function. *Gene. Dev., 17*, 126-140.

[9] Hanna, L.A., Foreman, R.K., Tarasenko, I.A., Kessler, D.S., and Labosky, P.A. (2002). Requirement for Foxd3 in maintaining pluripotent cells of the early mouse embryo. *Gene. Dev., 16*, 2650-2661.

[10] Chambers, I., Colby, D., Robertson, M., Nichols, J., Lee, S., Tweedie, S., and Smith, A. (2003). Functional expression cloning of Nanog, a pluripotency sustaining factor in embryonic stem cells. *Cell, 113*, 643-655.

[11] Mitsui, K., Tokuzawa, Y., Itoh, H., Segawa, K., Murakami, M., Takahashi, K., Maruyama, M., Maeda, M., and Yamanaka, S. (2003). The homeoprotein Nanog is required for maintenance of pluripotency in mouse epiblast and ES cells. *Cell, 113*, 631-642.

[12] Jiang, Y., Jahagirdar, B.N., Reinhardt, R.L., Schwartz, R.E., Keene, C.D., Ortiz-Gonzalez, X.R., Reyes, M., Lenvik, T., Lund, T., Blackstad, M., Du, J., Aldrich, S., Lisberg, A., Low, W.C., Largaespada, D.A., and Verfaillie, C.M. (2002). Pluripotency of mesenchymal stem cells derived from adult marrow. *Nature, 418*, 41-49.

[13] Hatfield, S.D., Shcherbata, H.R., Fischer, K.A., Nakahara, K., Carthew, R.W., and Ruohola-Baker, H. (2005). Stem cell division is regulated by the microRNA pathway. *Nature, 435,* 974-978.

[14] Huttenhofer, A., and Vogel, J. (2006). Experimental approaches to identify non-coding RNAs. *Nucl. Acid. Res., 34*, 635–646.

[15] Storz, G. (2002). An expanding universe of noncoding RNAs. *Science, 296*, 1260–1263.

[16] Washietl, S., Hofacker, I.L., Lukasser, M., Huttenhofer, A., and Stadler, P.F. (2005). Mapping of conserved RNA secondary structures predicts thousands of functional noncoding RNAs in the human genome. *Nat. Biotechnol., 23*, 1383–1390.

[17] Ellington, A.D., and Szostak JW. (1990). In vitro selection of RNA molecules that bind specific ligands. *Nature, 346*, 818–822.

[18] Tuerk, C., and Gold, L. (1990). Systemic evolution of ligands by exponential enrichment: RNA ligands to bacteriophage T4 DNA polymerase. *Science, 249*, 505–510.

[19] Pal-Bhadra, M., Bhadra, U., and Birchler, J.A. (2002). RNAi related mechanisms affect both transcriptional and posttranscriptional transgene silencing in Drosophila. *Mol. Cell, 9*, 315-327.

[20] Birchler, J.A., Pal-Bhadra, M., and Bhadra, U. RNAi, *A Guide to Gene Silencing.* In: E. G. J. Hannon, editor. New York: Cold Spring Harbor Laboratory Press; 2003.

[21] Hammond, S.M., Caudy, A.A., and Hannon, G.J. (2001). Post-transcriptional gene silencing by double-stranded RNA. *Nat. Rev. Genet., 2,* 110-119.

[22] Carrington, J.C., and Ambros, V. (2003). Role of MicroRNAs in Plant and Animal Development. *Science, 301*, 336-338.

[23] Lim, L.P., Glasner, M.E., Yekta, S., Burge, C.B., and Bartel, D.P. (2003). Vertebrate microRNA genes. *Science, 299*, 1540.

[24] Lee, R.C., Feinbaum, R.L., and Ambros, V. (1993). The C. elegans heterochronic gene lin-4 encodes small RNAs with antisense complementarity to lin-14. *Cell, 75*, 843-54.

[25] Wightman, B., Ha, I., and Ruvkun, G. (1993). Posttranscriptional regulation of the heterochronic gene lin-14 by lin-4 mediates temporal pattern formation in C. elegans. *Cell, 75*, 855–862.

[26] Alvarez-Garcia, I., and Miska, E.A. (2005). MicroRNA functions in animal development and human disease. *Development, 132*, 4653-62.

[27] Kent, O.A., and Mendell, J.T. (2006). A small piece in the cancer puzzle: microRNAs as tumor suppressors and oncogenes. *Oncogene,* 25, 6188–6196.

[28] Bartel, D.P. (2004). MicroRNAs: genomics, biogenesis, mechanism, and function. *Cell, 116*, 281-97.

[29] Ambros, V. (2004). The functions of animal microRNAs. *Nature, 431*, 350-355.

[30] Bentwich, I., Avniel, A., Karov, Y., Aharonov, R., Gilad, S., Barad, O., Barzilai, A., Einat, P., Einav, U., Meiri, E., Sharon, E., Spector, Y., and Bentwich, Z. (2005).

Identification of hundreds of conserved and nonconserved human microRNAs. *Nat. Genet., 37,* 766–770.

[31] Berezikov, E., Guryev, V., van de Belt, J., Wienholds, E., Plasterk, R.H., and Cuppen, E. (2005). Phylogenetic shadowing and computational identification of human microRNA genes. *Cell, 120,* 21-4.

[32] Griffiths-Jones, S., Grocock, R.J., van Dongen, S., Bateman, A., and Enright, A.J. (2006). miRBase: microRNA sequences, targets and gene nomenclature. *Nucl. Acid. Res., 34,* D140–D144.

[33] Lewis, B.P., Burge, C.B., and Bartel, D.P. (2005). Conserved seed pairing, often flanked by adenosines, indicates that thousands of human genes are microRNA targets. *Cell, 120,* 15-20.

[34] Calin, G.A., Sevignani, C., Dumitru, C.D., Hyslop, T., Noch, E., Yendamuri, S., Shimizu, M., Rattan, S., Bullrich, F., Negrini, M., and Croce, C.M. (2004). Human microRNA genes are frequently located at fragile sites and genomic regions involved in cancers. *Proc. Natl. Acad. Sci. U S A., 101,* 2999-3004.

[35] Calin, G.A., and Croce, C.M. (2006). MicroRNAs and chromosomal abnormalities in cancer cells. *Oncogene, 25,* 6202-6210.

[36] Glover, T.W., Berger, C., Coyle, J., and Echo, B. (1984). DNA polymerase alpha inhibition by aphidicolin induces gaps and breaks at common fragile sites in human chromosomes. *Hum. Genet., 67,* 136-142.

[37] Glover, T.W., and Stein, C.K. (1988). Chromosome breakage and recombination at fragile sites. *Am. J. Hum. Genet., 43,* 265-273.

[38] Huebner, K., and Croce, C.M. (2001). FRA3B and other common fragile sites: the weakest link. *Nat. Rev. Cancer, 1,* 214-221.

[39] Zlotorynski, E., Rahat, A., Skaug, J., Ben-Porat, N., Ozeri, E., Hershberg, R., Levi, A., Scherer, S.W., Margalit, H., and Kerem, B. (2003). Molecular basis for expression of common and rare fragile sites. *Mol. Cell. Biol., 23,* 7143-7151.

[40] Richards, R.I. (2001). Fragile and unstable chromosomes in cancer: causes and consequences. *Trend. Genet., 17,* 339-345.

[41] Arlt, M.F., Casper, A.M., and Glover, T.W. (2003). Common fragile sites. *Cytogenet. Genome. Res., 100,* 92-100.

[42] Saretzki, G., Armstrong, L., Leake, A., Lako, M., and von Zglinicki, T. (2004). Stress defense in murine embryonic stem cells is superior to that of various differentiated murine cells. *Stem. Cell., 22,* 962-971.

[43] Jirmanova, L., Bulavin, D.V., and Fornace, A.J. Jr. (2005). Inhibition of the ATR/Chk1 Pathway Induces a p38-Dependent S-phase Delay in Mouse Embryonic Stem Cells. *Cell Cycle, 4,* 1428-1434.

[44] Landais, S., Quantin, R., and Rassart, E. (2005). Radiation leukemia virus common integration at the Kis2 locus: simultaneous overexpression of a novel non-coding RNA and of the proximal Phf6 gene. *J. Virol., 79,* 11443–11456.

[45] Landais, S., Landry, S., Legault, P., and Rassart, E. (2007). Oncogenic Potential of the miR-106-363 Cluster and Its Implication in Human T-Cell Leukemia. *Cancer Res., 67,* 5699-5707.

[46] Zhou, X., Wang, G., and Zhang, W. (2007). UV-B responsive microRNA genes in Arabidopsis thaliana. *Mol. Syst. Biol., 3,* 103.

[47] Marsit, C.J., Eddy, K., and Kelsey, K.T. (2006). MicroRNA responses to cellular stress. *Cancer Res., 66,* 10843-10848.

[48] Ishii, H., and Saito, T. (2006). Radiation-induced response of micro RNA expression in murine embryonic stem cells. *Med. Chem., 2,* 555-563.

[49] Bixby, S., Kruger, G.M., Mosher, J.T., Joseph, N.M., and Morrison, S.J. (2002). Cell-intrinsic differences between stem cells from different regions of the peripheral nervous system regulate the generation of neural diversity. *Neuron, 35,* 643-656.

[50] Wulf, G.G., Wang, R.Y., Kuehnle, I., Weidner, D., Marini, F., Brenner, M.K., Andreeff, M., and Goodell, M.A. (2001). A leukemic stem cell with intrinsic drug efflux capacity in acute myeloid leukemia. *Blood, 98,* 1166–1173.

[51] Lapidot, T., Sirard, C., Vormoor, J., Murdoch, B., Hoang, T., Caceres-Cortes, J., Minden, M., Paterson, B., Caligiuri, M.A., and Dick, J.E. (1994). A cell initiating human acute myeloid leukemia after transplantation into SCID mice. *Nature, 367,* 645–648.

[52] Bonnet, D., and Dick, J.E. (1997). Human acute leukemia is organized as a hierarchy that originates from a primitive hematopoietic cell. *Nat. Med., 3,* 730–737.

[53] Prince, M.E., Sivanandan, R., Kaczorowski, A., Wolf, G.T., Kaplan, M.J., Dalerba, P., Weissman, I.L., Clarke, M.F., and Ailles, L.E. (2007). Identification of a subpopulation of cells with cancer stem cell properties in head and neck squamous cell carcinoma. *Proc. Natl. Acad. Sci. U S A. 104,* 973-978.

[54] Haraguchi, N., Utsunomiya, T., Inoue, H., Tanaka, F., Mimori, K., Barnard, G.F., and Mori, M. (2006). Characterization of a side population of cancer cells from human gastrointestinal system. *Stem Cell., 24,* 506-513.

[55] .Ricci-Vitiani, L., Lombardi, D.G., Pilozzi, E., Biffoni, M., Todaro, M., Peschle, C., and De Maria, R. (2007). Identification and expansion of human colon-cancer-initiating cells. *Nature, 445,* 111-5.

[56] O'Brien, C.A., Pollett, A., Gallinger, S., and Dick, J.E. (2007). A human colon cancer cell capable of initiating tumour growth in immunodeficient mice. *Nature., 445,* 106-110.

[57] Al-Hajj, M., Wicha, M.S., Benito-Hernandez, A., Morrison, S.J., and Clarke, M.F. (2003). Prospective identification of tumorigenic breast cancer cells. *Proc. Natl. Acad. Sci. U S A, 100,* 3983–3988.

[58] Piccirillo, S.G., Reynolds, B.A., Zanetti, N., Lamorte, G., Binda, E., Broggi, G., Brem, H., Olivi, A., Dimeco, F., and Vescovi, A.L. (2006). Bone morphogenetic proteins inhibit the tumorigenic potential of human brain tumour-initiating cells. *Nature, 444,* 761-765.

[59] Bao, S., Wu, Q., McLendon, R.E., Hao, Y., Shi, Q., Hjelmeland, A.B,, Dewhirst. M,W., Bigner, D.D., and Rich, J.N. (2006). Glioma stem cells promote radioresistance by preferential activation of the DNA damage response. *Nature, 444,* 756-760.

[60] Tan, B.T., Park, C.Y., Ailles, L.E., and Weissman, I.L. (2006). The cancer stem cell hypothesis: a work in progress. *Lab. Invest., 86,* 1203-1207.

[61] Blanpain, C., Horsley, V., and Fuchs, E. (2007). Epithelial stem cells: turning over new leaves. *Cell, 128,* 445-458.

[62] Dontu, G., Liu, S., and Wicha, M.S. (2005). Stem cells in mammary development and carcinogenesis: implications for prevention and treatment. *Stem Cell Rev., 1,* 207-213.

[63] Ponti, D., Zaffaroni, N., Capelli, C., and Daidone, M.G. (2006). Breast cancer stem cells: an overview. *Eur. J. Cancer, 42,* 1219-1224.

[64] Sheridan, C., Kishimoto, H., Fuchs, R.K., Mehrotra, S., Bhat-Nakshatri, P., Turner, C.H., Goulet, R. Jr., Badve, S., and Nakshatri, H. (2006). CD44+/CD24- breast cancer cells exhibit enhanced invasive properties: an early step necessary for metastasis. *Breast Cancer Res., 8,* R59.

[65] Bray, S. (2006). Notch signalling: a simple pathway becomes complex. *Nat. Rev. Mol. Cell Biol., 7,* 678-689.

[66] Hemmati, H.D., Nakano, I., Lazareff, J.A., Masterman-Smith, M., Geschwind, D.H., Bronner-Fraser, M., and Kornblum, H.I. (2003). Cancerous stem cells can arise from pediatric brain tumors. *Proc. Natl. Acad. Sci. USA*, 100, 15178-15183.

[67] Hambardzumyan, D., Squatrito, M., and Holland, E.C. (2006). Radiation resistance and stem-like cells in brain tumors. *Cancer Cell, 10,* 454-456.

[68] Kastan, M.B., and Bartek, J. (2004)., Cell-cycle checkpoints and cancer. *Nature, 432*, 316-323.

[69] Sancar, A., Lindsey-Boltz, L.A., Unsal-Kacmaz, K., and Linn, S. (2004). Molecular mechanisms of mammalian DNA repair and the DNA damage checkpoints. *Annu. Rev. Biochem., 73,* 39-85.

Short Communication C

Recruitment of Transplanted Dermal Multipotent Cells to the Injured Sites of Rats with Combined Radiation and Wound Injury by SDF-1/CXCR4 Interaction

Zong Zhaowen[*], Ran Xinze, Cheng Tianmi and Su Yongping

Institute of combined injury, State Key Laboratory of Trauma,
Burns and combined injury, School of Military Preventive Medicine,
Third Military Medical University, ChongQing, China

Abstract

Systemic transplantation of dermal multipotent cells (dMSCs) has been shown to accelerate both hematopoietic recovery and wound healing in rats with combined radiation and wound injury. In the present study, we explored the the mechanisms governing the recruitment of dMSCs to the injured sites of combine-injured rats. Male dMSCs were transplanted into female rats, and by employing quantitative real-time PCR for the sex-determining region of Y chromosome, it was found that the amount of dMSCs in bone marrow and wounded skin of rats with combined injury were about 2 times more than those of normal rats ($P<0.01$). Incubation dMSCs with AMD3100 before transplantation, which specifically blocks binding of stromal cell-derived factor-1 (SDF-1) to its receptor CXCR4, diminished dMSCs recruitment to the injured sites by 57.5±4.2% and 59.5±3.8% respectively ($P<0.05$). In addition, it was confirmed that the expression of SDF-1 in injured bone marrow and wound was up-regulated when

---

[*] Address: Institute of combined injury, State Key Laboratory of Trauma, Burns and combined injury, School of Military Preventive Medicine, Third Military Medical University, 30 GaoTan Yan Street, Shapingba District, Chongqing, 400038, china. Pnone: +86-2368752278; Fax: +86-2368752009; E-mail: zongzhaowen2004@sina.com

compared with normal rats, and *in vitro* analysis revealed that bone marrow extracts and wound fluid obtained from combine-injured rats had strong chemotactic effect on dMSCs, but decreased significantly when dMSCs was pre-incubated by AMD3100 ($P<0.05$). These data suggest that transplanted dMSCs were recruited more frequently to bone marrow and wounded skin in combine-injured rats than normal rats and the interactions of SDF-1/CXCR4 played an important role in this process.

INTRODUCTION

Combined injury of radiation and wound injury often occurs after severe nuclear accidents that accompany explosions in peacetime and nuclear attacks in war [1, 2]. High doses of ionizing radiation can cause bone marrow aplasia and delay wound healing [3]. Disorder of hematopoietic function could affect the wound healing process and open wound influence overall recovery. All these make combined radiation and wound injury is difficult to manage. In our previous study, dermal multipotent cells (dMSCs) were isolated from the enzymatically dissociated dermal cells of newborn rats by their adherence to culture dish plastic and the isolated dMSCs demonstrated multipotent differentiation capacity. After systemic transplantation, dMSCs could accelerate both hematopoietic recovery and wound healing in rats with combined radiation and wound injury, and promote the survival of rats. Also, fluorescence in situ hybridization (FISH) analysis, using Y-chromosome specific probe, showed that dMSCs could engraft into bone marrow and wound of injured rats [4]. In the present study, great interests being given to the mechanisms governing the recruitment of dMSCs to the injured sites (irradiation-injured bone marrow and wounded skin) in combine-injured rats since it is the first step when transplanted dMSCs exert its repair effect. Also, exploration of the mechanism may help us find new measures to enhance the recruitment of transplanted cells to the injured sites and thus improve the repair effect of grafted stem cells.

Stromal cell-derived factor-1 (SDF-1), also termed as CXCL12, the powerful chemoattractant of hematopoietic stem cells of both human and murine origin, is widely expressed in many tissues during development and adulthood, such as bone marrow, liver, central nervous system, and skin, et al. Its interaction with CXCR4, the only known receptor of SDF-1, is essential during the BM-dereived stem cells homing to BM [5]. SDF-1/CXCR4 interaction is also reported to involving in recruiting transplanted stem cells to injured sites and participate repair of the injured tissue [6-10]. So in the present study, we tested the role of SDF-1/CXCR4 interaction in recruiting transplanted dMSCs to the injured sites in combined radiation and wound injury. Using the chemokine receptor CXCR4 antagonist AMD3100, we firstly assessed the effect of blocking the SDF-1/CXCR4 interaction on the recruitment of delivered dMSCs. Then we compared the expression level of SDF-1 in injured bone marrow and skin with their normal counterparts by RT-PCR and Western Blot. In addition, *in vitro* chemotactic analysis was used to observe the chemotactic effect of bone marrow and skin extracts on dMSCs, with or without AMD 3100 pre-incubation.

MATERIALS AND METHODS

Experimental Animals

Wistar rats were purchased from the Center of Laboratory Animals of the Third Military Medical University (Qualified certification number: SCXKYU2002002). The experimental protocol was reviewed and approved by the Animal Ethical Committee of the Third Military Medical University, P. R. China and were carried out in compliance with the "Guide for the Care and Use of Laboratory Animals" published by the National Institute of Health.

Isolation and Culture of Male dMSCs

Isolation and culture of dMSCs were carried out as described previously [4], and the expression of CXCR4 in dMSCs was examined by RT-PCR and fluorescent immunocytochemistry. For RT-PCR, total RNA was isolated form cultured dMSCs using TripureTM (Promega Corp., Wisconsin, USA) according to the manufacture's instructions and was spectrophotometrically quantified. The cDNA was prepared from 1.0 μg RNA in the presence of 2.5 μM oligo (dT) primer and 200 U moloney murine leukemia virus reverse transcriptase (TaKaRa BIO INC., Kyoto, Japan) in a total volume of 10 μl. The reaction mixture was incubated for 1 hour at 42°C and stopped by heating for 5 minutes at 99°C. Aliquots (1 μl) of cDNA were subsequently amplified using specific primers for CXCR4 (forward primer was 5'-AGT GGG CAA TGG GTT GGT AAT-3' and reverse primer was 5'-TCA GGG ATA GTC AGG AGG AGG G-3'). The PCR cycles consist of denaturation at 94°C fro 45 s, annealing at 56°C for 45 s, and extension at 72°C for 45 s. The PCR product was 354 bp. A 10 μl aliquot of each PCR product was size-separated by electrophoresis on a 2% ethidium-bromide-containing agarose gel and photographed. Sterile water and 293 cells served as control.

For fluorescent immunocytochemistry, dMSCs were plated and cultured on ploylysine-coated coverslips and then the coverslips were blocked with normal serum for 30 minutes, followed by incubation with anti-CXCR4 rabbit polyclonal antibody (Santa Cruz Biotech, California, USA) at 4°C overnight. Subsequently, coverslips were incubated wtih phycoerythrin-conjugated anti-rabbit secondary antibody (Sigma-Aldrich, Missouri, USA) for 1 hour, and the reaction products were visualized under fluorescent reverse microscope. Control coverslips were incubated as above but without the primary antibody.

Sex-genotype of dMSCs was determined by PCR for SRY. Oligonucleotide primers used to detect the rat SRY were 5'-ATA CTG GCT CTG CTC CTA CCT-3' (forward) and 5'-GCT GTT TGC TGC CTT TGA-3' (reverse). The PCR was run for 35 cycles under cycling condition of 94 °C for 30 s, 52 °C for 30 s and 72 °C for 45 s. The product was 328 bp. Sterile water and DNA isolated from female rats' liver served as control.

Animal Group and Transplantation Procedure

Sixty female Wistar rats, six-week-old and weighing about 150 g, were divided randomly into three groups: group N (normal rats accepted dMSCs transplantation, n=20), group CI (combine-injured rats accepted dMSCs transplantation, n=20) and group AMD3100 (combine-injured rats accepted transplantation of dMSCs incubated by AMD3100, n=20).

Injury model was carried out as as described previously [4]. Briefly, rats in group CI and group AMD3100 were irradiated over the whole body with a sublethal dose of 5 Gy of gamma rays from a ^{60}Co source, and the absorption rate was 31.02-31.98 cGy/min. Thirty minutes after irradiation, rats were anaesthetized and a circular wound with full-thickness skin tissue was made surgically on the back. The area of the wound corresponded 2.5% of the rats' surface area. Then rats of group N and group CI received 5×10^6 dMSCs in 1 ml saline. For group AMD3100, the same dose of dMdCs were incubated for 30 minutes at 37°C with 5 µg/mL AMD3100 (Sigma-Aldrich, Missouri, USA), then were washed in phosphate buffered saline and transplanted. All animals were fed with commercial laboratory food and purified tap water and housed under standard conditions. Three days after transplantation, rats were sacrificed and four rats from each group were used in one of the following experiments.

Quantitative Real-Time TaqMan PCR

The amount of transplanted male dMSCs in bone marrow and skin of female recipient was determined by quantitative real-time TaqMan PCR for rat SRY. DNA of dMSCs or tissues (100 mg) was prepared and dissolved in water. DNA concentration was determined by spectrophotometry, and the total amount of recovered DNA was calculated as [concentration]×[resuspension volume].

Real-time PCR was carried out on DNA Engine Opticon (MJ Research, Inc) by using the above-mentioned PCR primers to SRY and the TaqMan probe 5'-FAM- TGC CAA CAC TCC CCT TGC TGC TGT AAT T- TAMRA-3'. The thermal cycle was configured as follows: incubation at 95°C for 5 min, 40 cycles of de-naturation at 95°C for 30 s, and annealing and extension at 60°C for 60 s. In the procedure of real-time TaqMan PCR, amplification resulted in a fluorescent signal proportional to the amount of PCR product. The template quantity was inversely proportional to the cycle number at which the fluorescent signal crossed a threshold in the exponential phase of the reaction. In present study, standard curves was generated by serially diluting male dMSCs DNA into female rat genomic DNA as follows: DNA prepared from 0, 5, 50, 100, 500, 1000, 5000, 50 000 or 100 000 dMSCs were diluted into DNA prepared from 100 mg femaleliver. The amount of dMSCs in bone marrow and skin were determined by cycle number in the standard curve.

Examination of the Expression of SDF-1 in Bone Marrow and Skin

The expression of SDF-1 in bone marrow and skin were determined by RT-PCR and Western Blot.

RT-PCR. One-hundred microgram normal skin and wounded skin, along with bone marrow obtained by flushing the BM cavity of the femurs and tibiae with a 21-gauge syringe filled with PBS was used to isolate total RNA by using Tripure reagent. RT-PCR was performed as above-mentioned method, except the primers used for SDF-1 were 5'-CCA ATC AGA AAT GGG AAC AAG A-3' (forward) and 5'-GAG GCT TAC AGC ACG AAA CAG-3' (reverse), with the product of which was 377 bp. Also, primers (forward primer was 5'-TCA TCA GCG AAA GTG GAA A-3' and reverse primer was 5'-TGT CTG TCT CAC AAG GGA AGT-3') to detect hypoxanthine guanine phosphoribosyl transferase (HPRT) were added to each reaction tube as internal control. The RT-PCR product of HPRT was 270 bp.

Western Blot. Samples were obtained as the above-mentioned method in the procedure of RT-PCR, and 1 ml T-PER™ reagent (Pierce, Illinois, USA) was added. After homogenization, the sample was centrifuged 10,000 rpm for 5 minutes. The supernatant was collected and were run on 15% SDS-PAGE gels. Proteins were then transferred onto PVDF membrane using the Trans-Blot Semi-Dry Transfer Cell (Bio-Rad Laboratories Inc., California, USA), blocked in 5% skim milk, and probed with anti-SDF-1 rabbit polyclonal antibody (diluted 1:500 in blocking buffer) followed by biotinylated goat anti-rabbit IgG (Boster, Wuhan, China). Then the PVDF membrane were developed with avidin:biotinylated enzyme complex and were visualized by diaminobenzidine.

In Vitro Chemotaxis Assay

Preparation of bone marrow and skin extracts. One-hundred microgram normal skin, wounded skin, normal bone marrow and injured bone marrow were obtained as above-mentioned method and was then homogenized by adding IMDM (150 mg tissue/ml IMDM) and was incubated on ice for 10 minutes. The homogenate was centrifuged at 10,000 g for 20 minutes at 4°C and the supernant was extracted.

Chemotaxis assay. Chemotactic activity of bone marrow and skin extracts and recombinant human SDF-1 (rhSDF-1) toward dMSCs was evaluated using 12-well microchemotaxis Transwell chamber (Costar, Miami, USA) according to the manufacture's instructions. To observe the chemotactic effect of recombinant human SDF-1 (rhSDF-1, PEPROTECH, London, UK) toward dMSCs, twenty-five microlitres rhSDF-1 at various concentrations (50,100,150 ng/ml) was placed in the lower wells, and 50 µl re-suspended normal dMSCs or AMD3100 pre-incubated dMSCs (containing 1×10^4 cells) were placed in the upper wells. To observe the chemotactic effect of bone marrow and skin extracts, twenty-five microlitres bone marrow and skin extracts from each group was placed in the lower wells, and cells the same as above-mentioned were placed in the upper wells. The contents of the upper and lower well were separated by a polycarbonate filter (8-µm pore size). After 6 hours incubation at 37°C in 5% CO2, the upper surface of the membrane was scraped free of cells and debris. The membrane was then fixed and stained using hematoxylin staining. Cells that had migrated though pores and adhered to the lower surface of the membrane were analyzed under high-power (×400) light microscopy and counted in five random high-power fields (HPF). Experiments were performed in triplicate, and data were expressed as means of the numbers of cells per high-power field (cells/HPF) ±standard error (SE).

Statistical Analysis

All data were expressed as means ±standard error. Statistical significance was evaluated with an unpaired Student's t test for comparison between 2 groups or by ANOVA for multiple comparisons. A value of $P<0.05$ was considered significant.

RESULTS

Biological Characterization of Cultured dMSCs

Dermal multipotent stem cells were obtained by the methods as described previously [4]. Then the sex-genotype of dMSCs was determined by PCR for SRY. As shown in Figure 1A, DNA from female rats' liver and sterile water produced no detectable PCR products, while DNA from isolated male dMSCs produced specific PCR products. We also examined the expression of CXCR4, the only known receptor of SDF-1, in isolated dMSCs by using RT-PCR and fluorescent immunocytochemistry. Most of the cultured dMSCs reacted positively to CXCR4 antibody (Figure 1B), and expression of CXCR4 at mRNA level also could be detected by RT-PCR (Figure 1C). These data indicated that the isolated dMSCs were male-derived and expressed CXCR4.

Recruitment of Transplanted dMSCs to Bone Marrow and Skin

The amount of transplanted dMSCs in bone marrow and skin was obtained by real-time TaqMan PCR for rat SRY.

Three days after transplantation, the amount of dMSCs in bone marrow and wounded skin of group CI rats was $(1.67±0.20) ×10^4$ and $(1.53±0.15) ×10^4$ respectively, about 2 times greater than that of group N rats $((0.52±0.09) × 10^4$ and $(0.49±0.12) × 10^4)$ $(P<0.01)$. For group AMD3100, the number is $(0.71±0.52) × 10^4$ and $(0.62±0.07) ×10^4$ respectively. That is to say, incubation dMSCs with AMD3100 before transplantation reduced the recruitment of dMSCs to irradiation injured BM and wounded skin by 57.5±4.2% and 59.5±3.8% respectively ($P<0.05$), suggesting that SDF-1/CXCR4 interaction played a crucial role in dMSCs recruitment to injured BM. Of note, although the amount of dMSCs in injured bone marrow and skin was greater than that of normal bone marrow and skin, the absolute amount of dMSCs in every 100 mg injured bone marrow and wounded skin account only about 0.33% and 0.31% of the total transplanted dMSCs tissues respectively.

The Expression of SDF-1 in Irradiation Injured Bone Marrow and Wounded Skin Were Up-Regulated

By employing RT-PCR and Western Blot, we investigated the expression of SDF-1 in bone marrow and skin in each group (Figure 2). The signals of RT-PCR products on agarose gel in group CI and group AMD3100 were stronger than those in Group N (Figure 2A). The results of Western Blot also demonstrated that the signals on PVDF membrane in group CI and group AMD3100 were stronger than those in Group N (Figure 2B). These data indicated that the expression of SDF-1 in irradiation-injured bone marrow and wounded skin were up-regulated than that in normal bone marrow and normal skin.

In Vitro Chemotaxis Assay

The structure of SDF-1 is very conservative and the similarity between rat's and human SDF-1 is above 99%, so rhSDF-1 can be used to observe the chemotactic effect on rat-derived dMSCs. The results showed that the chemotactic effect of rhSDF-1 toward dMSCs was does-dependent. The optimal effect was observed at 150 ng/ml, but when dMSCs were pre-incubated by AMD3100, the chemotactic effect of rhSDF-1 was almost abolished ($P<0.01$) (Figure 3A).

When bone marrow extracts from group CI and group AMD3100 were placed in the lower chamber, the number of dMSCs migrate to the lower surface of the filter were 119.8±4.8 and 124.6±6.8 cells/HPF respectively, significantly greater than that of group N rats (25.2±2.4, $P<0.01$). However, when dMSCs were pre-incubated by AMD3100, the chemotactic effect of bone marrow extracts of group CI and group AMD3100 decreased significantly ($P<0.05$), but didn't abolish (Figure 3B). Similar chemotactic effect was observed when normal skin and wounded skin extracts were tested (Figure 3C).

DISCUSSION

Adult stem cells have been isolated in various tissues and showed promising prospects in regenerative medicine. Among various kinds of adult stem cells, bone marrow mesenchymal stem cells or hematopoietic stem cells transplantation have been shown excellent repair effect on central nervous system disorders [10], osteogenesis imperfecta [11] and osteochondral defect [12]. In the case of irradiation-induced BM injury, however, auto-transplantation of bone marrow stem cells is limited since BM is injured itself. Under such conditions, stem cells of alternative sources are needed. In our previous study [4], we reported that dMSCs could be isolated from newborn rats demonstrated multipotent differentiation capacity, and after systemic transplantation into rats with combined radiation and wound injury, it could accelerate both hematopoietic recovery and wound healing. But the mechanisms governing the transplanted dMSCs recruiting to the injured sites, which is the crucial first step of the repair process by transplanted dMSCs, are poorly understood.

SDF-1, which is widely expressed in many tissues during development and adulthood, have been found to increase its expression after tissue injuries in bone marrow, central nervous system, blood vessel and heart, and its interaction with CXCR4 was found to involve in recruiting transplanted bone marrow-derived mesenchymal stem cells [6], CD34+ hematopoietic progenitors [7], neural stem cells [8] and endothelial progenitor cells [9] to the above-mentioned injured sites and participate repair process. In the present study, we tested the role of SDF-1/CXCR4 interaction in recruiting transplanted dMSCs to irradiation-injured BM. We firstly found increased SDF-1 expression in wounded skin and irradiation-injured bone marrow of rats with combined injury by employing RT-PCR and Western Blot, and then by sex-mismatched transplantation and quantitative Real-Time PCR, we found that the amount of dMSCs in wounded skin and irradiation-injured bone marrow were 2 times more than those of normal rats ($P < 0.01$), but the recruitment were reduced by almost 60% ($P<0.05$) when dMSCs were incubated with AMD3100 before transplantation, suggesting that SDF-1/CXCR4 interaction play a crucial role in recruiting transplanted dMSCs to wounded skin and irradiation-injured bone marrow. This is further supported by in vitro chemotactic analysis. Bone marrow and wounded skin extracts from combine-injured rats had strong chemotactic effect on normal dMSCs, but decreased significantly when dMSCs was pre-incubated with AMD3100 ($P<0.05$).

Of note, stem cells recruitment to the injured sites is a 2-step process that begins with binding of circulating stem cells to adhesive complexes in the vasculature around an injury zone, followed by local chemotaxis to the site of engraftment. Increased expression of intercellular adhesion molecule-1, and vascular cell adhesion molecule-1, matrix metalloproteinase-9, vascular endothelial growth factor, monocyte chemoattractant protein-1 and stem cell factor in the injured sites might in concert with SDF-1 to recruit transplanted stem cells to the injured sites [6, 13, 14]. That is why when the interaction of SDF-1/CXCR4 was blocked by AMD3100 incubation, there were still dMSCs recruited to irradiation-injured BM although the number was significantly reduced (Figure 3B).

In summary, the present study showed that transplanted dMSCs were recruited more frequently to irradiation-injured bone marrow and wounded skin than normal bone marrow and normal skin, and the interactions of SDF-1/CXCR4 played an important role in this process. However, there are many other issues needed to be further studied, such as the fate of dMSCs recruited to the injured sites, and measures to increase dMSCs recruit to injured sites should also be investigated to enhance the repair effect of transplanted dMSCs, which is the main purpose of the present study, that is to find meaningful measures to enhance dMSCs recruit to injured sites through the mechanisms governing recruitment. In our unpublished data, dMSCs overexpressed CXCR4 by transfected with CXCR4 adenovirus expression vector was found to be recruited 3.1 times more than the normal dMSCs to the irradiation injured BM.

ACKNOWLEDGMENTS

This study was supported by Special Fund for National Key Project "973" for Development of Basic Research (2005CB522605), and National Science Foundation of China (30500141).

REFERENCES

[1] V. Vegesna, H.R. Withers, F.E. Holly and W.H. McBride, The effect of local and systemic irradiation on impairment of wound healing in mice. *Radiat. Res. 135*, 431-433 (1993).

[2] T. Ishii, S. Futami, M. Nishida, T. Suzuki, T. Sakamoto, N. Suzuki and K. Maekawa, Brief note and evaluation of acute-radiation syndrome and treatment of a Tokai-mura criticality accident patient. *J. Radiat. Res. 42* (Suppl.), S167-S182 (2001).

[3] M. Schaffer, W. Weimer, S. Wider, C. Stulten, M. Bongartz, W. Budach and H.D. Becker, Differential expression of inflammatory mediators in radiation-impaired wound healing. *J. Surg. Res. 107*, 93-100 (2002).

[4] CM. Shi, T.M. Cheng, Y.P. Su, Y. Mai, J.F. Qu, S.F. Lou, X.Z. Ran, H. Xu, and C.J. Luo, Transplantation of dermal multipotent cells promotes survival and wound healing in rats with combined radiation and wound injury. *Radiat. Res. 162*, 56-63 (2004).

[5] Peled, I. Petit, O. Kollet, M. Magid, T. Ponomaryov, T. Byk, A. Nagler, H. Ben-Hur, A. Many, L. Shultz, O. Lider, R. Alon, D. Zipori, and T. Lapidot, Dependence of human stem cell engraftment and repopulation of NOD/SCID mice on CXCR4, *Science 283*, 845–848. (1999).

[6] J.D. Abbott, Y. Huang, D. Liu, R. Hickey, D.S. Krause, F.J. Giordano, Stromal cell-derived factor-1alpha plays a critical role in stem cell recruitment to the heart after myocardial infarction but is not sufficient to induce homing in the absence of injury. *Circulation 110*, 3300-3305 (2004).

[7] Kollet, S. Shivtiel, Y.Q. Chen, J. Suriawinata, S.N. Thung, M.D. Dabeva, J. Kahn, A. Spiegel, A. Dar, S. Samira, P. Goichberg, A. Kalinkovich, F. Arenzana-Seisdedos, A. Nagler, I. Hardan, M. Revel, D.A. Shafritz, and T, Lapidot. HGF, SDF-1, and MMP-9 are involved in stress-induced human CD34+ stem cell recruitment to the liver. *J Clin Invest 112*, 160–169 (2003)

[8] J. Imitola, K. Raddassi, K.I. Park, F.J. Mueller, M. Nieto, Y.D. Teng, D.Frenkel, J.X. Li, R.L. Sidman, C.A. Walsh, E.Y. Snyder and S.J.Khoury, Directed migration of neural stem cells to sites of CNS injury by the stromal cell-derived factor 1alpha/CXC chemokine receptor 4 pathway. *Proc Natl Acad Sci U S A 101*, 18117-18122 (2004).

[9] J. Yamaguchi, K.F.Kusano, O.Masuo, A. Kawamoto, M. Silver, S. Murasawa, M. Bosch-Marce, H. Masuda, D.W. Losordo, JM. Isner, T. and Asahara, Stromal cell-derived factor-1 effects on ex vivo expanded endothelial progenitor cell recruitment for ischemic neovascularization. *Circulation 107*, 1322-1328 (2003).

[10] J.S. Bae, S. Furuya, Y. Shinoda, S. Endo, E.H. Schuchman, Y. Hirabayashi, and H.K. Jin, Neurodegeneration augments the ability of bone marrow-derived mesenchymal

stem cells to fuse with Purkinje neurons in Niemann-Pick type C mice. *Hum Gene Ther.16*: 1006-1011 (2005).

[11] C. Lange, F. Togel, H. Ittrich, F. Clayton, C. Nolte-Ernsting, A.R. Zander, and C. Westenfelder, Administered mesenchymal stem cells enhance recovery from ischemia/reperfusion-induced acute renal failure in rats. *Kidney Int. 68*:1613-1617 (2005).

[12] M. Tatebe, R. Nakamura, H. Kagami, K. Okada, and M. Ueda, Differentiation of transplanted mesenchymal stem cells in a large osteochondral defect in rabbit. *Cytotherapy. 7*:520-30 (2005).

[13] J.F. Ji, B.P. He, S.T. Dheen, and S.S. Tay, Interactions of chemokines and chemokine receptors mediate the migration of mesenchymal stem cells to the impaired site in the brain after hypoglossal nerve injury. *Stem cells 22*, 415-427 (2004).

[14] L. Wang, Y. Li, X. Chen, S.C. Gautam, Z.G. Zhang, M. Lu and M. Chopp, Ischemic cerebral tissue and MCP-1 enhance rat bone marrow stromal cell migration in interface culture. *Hematology 30*, 831-836 (2002).

In: Encyclopedia of Stem Cell Research (2 Volume Set) ISBN: 978-1-61761-835-2
Editor: Alexander L. Greene © 2012 Nova Science Publishers, Inc.

Short Communication D

NEURAL CELL DIFFERENTIATION FROM EMBRYONIC STEM CELL BY THE NEURAL STEM SPHERE METHOD

Takashi Nakayama[*1], *Masahiro Otsu*[2] *and Nobuo Inoue*[2]

[1]Department of Biochemistry,
Yokohama City University School of Medicine, Yokohama, Japan
[2]Laboratory of Regenerative Neurosciences,
Graduate School of Human Health Sciences,
Tokyo Metropolitan University, Tokyo, Japan

ABSTRACT

We have established a novel method to efficiently produce a large number of neural stem cells from mouse, monkey, and human embryonic stem (ES) cells. The procedure requires only free-floating culture of ES colonies in astrocyte-conditioned medium (ACM) for differentiation into neural stem cells. These ES cell-derived neural stem cells can proliferate easily on an adhesive substrate in the presence of fibroblast growth factor-2 (FGF-2). They can be preserved by freezing, and can proliferate again after thawing. Furthermore, we have succeeded in unidirectional differentiation of ES cell-derived neural stem cells into neurons or astrocytes by choosing culture conditions. Neurogenesis of ES cell-derived neural stem cells can be induced by changing the medium from FGF-2-containing proliferation medium to ACM containing inductive factors. In contrast, withdrawing FGF-2 from the medium can induce differentiation of these cells into astrocytes, indicating that astrocytogenesis does not require any additional signals, such as humoral factors. Here, we describe the characteristics of our method applicable to cell transplantation therapy.

---

[*] Correspondence to Takashi Nakayama, Department of Biochemistry, Yokohama City University School of Medicine, Fukuura 3-9, Kanazawa-ku Yokohama 236-0004, Japan

INTRODUCTION

In neurodegenerative disorders, such as Parkinson's disease, Huntington's disease, amyotrophic lateral sclerosis, *etc.*, serious dysfunction of the central nervous system results from the death of specific neuronal cell types. Regenerative therapy by cell transplantation is considered an effective therapeutic strategy to ameliorate these dysfunctions. In this case, neural stem cells suitable for cell transplantation are required for establishment of replacement therapy. Unfortunately, somatic neural stem cells present in both the embryonic and adult brain are inadequate for this purpose, because they only show limited proliferation and differentiation capabilities. Embryonic stem (ES) cells derived from the inner cell mass in the blast stage embryo are pluripotent and thus able to differentiate into any cell type, including neural stem cells and neural cells. ES cells can also proliferate easily and differentiate directly into neural stem cells. Therefore, neural stem cells developed from ES cells can be supplied sufficiently in cell transplantation therapy, and so are highly suitable as donor cells compared with brain-derived neural stem cells. ES cell-derived neural stem cells can be prepared from monkey and human ES cells as well as mouse ES cells. Thus, ES cell-derived neural stem cells are useful in screening and toxicity testing for the developing central nervous system in humans where species specificity is crucial.

COMMENTARY

1. Conventional Method of Differentiation From ES Cells into Neural Cells (Embryoid Body Method)

The embryoid body method has generally been used for differentiation of neural cells from ES cells. One to several ES cells, cultured in serum-containing medium, form floating aggregates called embryoid bodies (EB). The EB mimics an implantation germ and differentiates into endoderm, ectoderm, and mesoderm within an aggregate [1]. However, this differentiation is not organized in a spatiotemporal manner, and therefore neural differentiation is rare. To overcome this problem, retinoic acid, a teratogenic agent, is added to the culture medium at a low concentration to improve neuronal differentiation [2]. It was found, however, that retinoic acid induces limited caudalization of neural progenitor cells in EB [3]. Alternatively, fibroblast growth factor (FGF)-2 is added to culture medium to promote the proliferation of neural stem cells selectively from EB, which caused an increase of neural stem cell number, but non-neural cells remain within the culture [4]. In addition, differentiation from aggregates of ES cells, not identical to EB, into neuronal cells was also attempted without using serum, retinoic acid, or FGF-2 [5]. This method, serum-free floating culture of embryoid body-like aggregates, generated telencephalic precursor neurons straightway.

2. DIRECT DIFFERENTIATION FROM ES CELLS INTO NEURAL CELLS BY THE NEURAL STEM SPHERE METHOD

2.1. Free-Floating Culture in Astrocyte-Conditioned Medium

In EB methods, one to several ES cells are cultured to form aggregates in culture medium with or without serum. In our method, however, colonies of undifferentiated ES cells grown on a mouse fibroblast feeder layer are picked up whole and transferred into non-adhesive bacteriological dishes. In addition, direct differentiation from ES cells into neural stem cells is induced by astrocyte-conditioned medium (ACM) in free-floating culture [6]. Astrocytes secrete humoral factors into the culture medium, which can provoke ES cell differentiation into neuronal stem cells. After cultivation under free-floating conditions in ACM for 3 to 4 days, colonies of undifferentiated ES cells formed floating spheres with a cored structure, which we named the Neural Stem Sphere (NSS). The NSS exhibits a concentric stratiform structure composed of a periphery of nestin-positive neural stem cells, a core of proliferating BrdU-positive ES cells, and an intermediate layer (Figure 1, A).

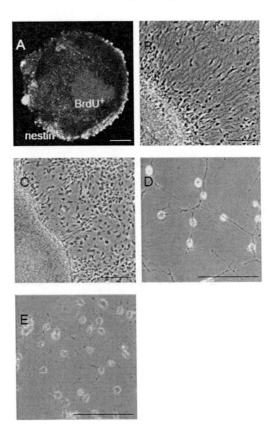

Figure 1. Morphological changes with differentiation. (A) Immunofluorescence analysis of Neural Stem Spheres (NSS). Nestin$^+$ neural stem cells were seen at the periphery, while BrdU$^+$ ES cells were present at the core. (B) Neurites extended from the NSS. (C) Neural stem cells migrated from NSS. (D) Neurons differentiated from ES cell-derived neural stem cells. (E) Astrocytes differentiated from ES cell-derived neural stem cells. Bars represent 100 μm.

This structure resembles the configuration of the earth in which the neural stem cells, ES cells, and intermediate layer cells correspond to the earth's crust, the centrosphere, and the mantle, respectively. Furthermore, ES cells enzymatically dispersed from ES colonies did not differentiate into neural stem cells even when cultured in ACM. These observations indicate that cell-to-cell interactions within the ES colony are required for the formation of NSS. When NSS culture was continued in ACM, neural stem cells differentiated further into neurons and extended their neurites within the sphere. Changes in gene expression during differentiation evoked by the NSS method were analyzed quantitatively for each mRNA by real-time reverse transcription-polymerase chain reaction (RT-PCR) (Figure 2, A).

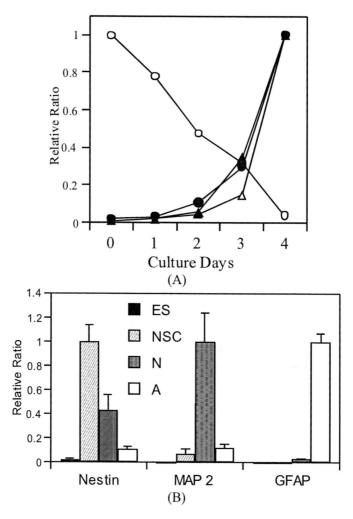

Figure 2. Changes in gene expression with differentiation. (A) Time course of changes in gene expression during floating culture in astrocyte-conditioned medium. Results of real-time RT-PCR analysis are shown as normalized values relative to the maximum. Oct4 (open circles) decreased. Pax6 (closed circles), nestin (open triangles), and NF-M (closed triangles) increased. (B) Expression of nestin, microtubule-associated protein 2 (MAP2), and glial fibrillary acidic protein (GFAP) mRNA normalized to expression of GAPDH mRNA. ES, ES cells; NSC, neural stem cells; N, neurons; A, astrocytes.

Expression of Oct4, a transcription factor involved in maintenance of totipotency of ES cells, decreased and disappeared almost completely by day 4. These observations clearly indicate that the properties of ES cells were altered during culture in ACM. Pax6, a transcription factor in neuroprogenitor cells, and nestin, intermediate filament protein expressed in neural stem cells, showed the same gene expression pattern; both increased gradually at 2 days and then increased rapidly at 4 days in floating culture. Gene expression of NF-M, a neuronal marker, was also up-regulated at 3 days, which indicated that differentiation of neural stem cells into neurons occurred in NSS during culture.

2.2. Expansion of Neural Stem Cells in Adhesion Culture and Cryopreservation

After floating for 4 days, the NSS was transferred to an adhesive dish and cultured continuously in ACM. Neural stem cells within the NSS differentiated into neurons and extended their neurites the following day (Figure 1, B). Further cultivation in ACM resulted in complete progression of neurogenesis of neural stem cells. To suppress neurogenesis and promote the proliferation of neural stem cells, culture medium was changed from ACM to Neurobasal B-27 supplemented with FGF-2 after attachment of the NSS to the adhesive substrate [7]. Following the switch in culture medium, many of the neural stem cells migrated from the attached NSS to the surrounding area forming a circular monolayer (Figure 1, C). After one week, the circular area of monolayer culture had spread 300–500 μm in diameter and included more than 100,000 neural stem cells. Thus, neural stem cells differentiated from one ES colony can be expanded by about 1,000-fold after only 11 days. After removing the attached NSS cluster that may have included undifferentiated cells, only the migrated neural stem cells were harvested from the dishes by trypsinization and cryopreserved in liquid nitrogen [8]. The purity of neural stem cells was confirmed by gene expression analysis (Figure 2, B). Furthermore, these cells differentiated easily into dopaminergic neurons.

3. DIFFERENTIATION OF ES CELL-DERIVED NEURAL STEM CELLS INTO NEURONS

The cryopreserved neural stem cells were thawed and expanded again in Neurobasal B-27 medium supplemented with FGF-2. These cells could be induced to differentiate into neurons by changing the medium to ACM for several days (Figure 1, D). Characterization of neurons differentiated from ES cell-derived neural stem cells was confirmed by immunohistochemistry and electrophysiology. These cells expressed neurofilament protein, a neuronal cell marker, and also acquired electrical excitability [7]. In addition, they specifically expressed MAP2, a neuronal marker gene (Figure 2, B). Differentiation evoked by ACM is unidirectional, so almost all ES cell-derived neural stem cells gave rise to neurons. Neural stem cells prepared by the NSS method can be stored by cryopreservation, which is an essential requirement for cell transplantation therapy. Cryopreserved neural stem cells can be shipped in dry ice as donor cells for cell transplantation. In addition, cryopreservation was also successful with monkey- and human-derived ES cells.

4. Differentiation of ES Cell-Derived Neural Stem Cells into Astrocytes

How do astrocytes, another neural cell type, develop from neural stem cells? Somatic neural stem cells present in the adult subventricular zone and hippocampus appear to differentiate mainly into neurons. In fact, cultured somatic neural stem cells taken from hippocampus differentiated into neurons when used in orthotopic transplantation, whereas they differentiated into astrocytes when they transplanted into ectopic sites [9]. Furthermore, neurospheres, cultured as aggregates of neural stem cells, exhibit wide differentiation capability, and can develop into neurons, astrocytes, and oligodendrocytes [10]. From these observations, it was suggested that adult neural stem cells are affected by humoral factors in neuron-producing loci, and then differentiate into neurons. In contrast, neural stem cells may be able to differentiate into astrocytes in ectopic transplantation sites and in culture, where they escape from the influence of neurogenesis factors. An equivalent phenomenon was observed in our system. ES cell-derived neural stem cells proliferating in medium containing FGF-2 differentiated unidirectionally into astrocytes only with the withdrawal of FGF-2 (Figure 1, E) [11]. Glial fibrillary acidic protein (GFAP) gene expression, an astrocytic marker, was markedly up-regulated (Figure 2, B). This astrocytogenesis did not require any humoral factors. These observations indicated that differentiation along the astrocyte lineage is the default fate of ES cell-derived neural stem cells. Recently, Radial glial cells have been shown to give rise to neurons in the neuroepithelial layer. Furthermore, differentiated astrocytes expressing GFAP have been identified as neural stem cells in the adult subventricular zone [12]. In the conventional theory of neural development, neural stem cells differentiate into neurons at first along the temporal axis, and then into astrocytes and oligodendrocytes. However, there is another possible explanation based on our results indicating that differentiation of ES cell-derived neural stem cells into astrocytes is the default fate of these cells, taken together with the observation that Radial glia and astrocytes act as neural stem cells. The roles of neural stem cells present in the neuroepithelium during early development are inherited by the astrocytic lineage. Neurons differentiate along this cell lineage due to the effects of some neurogenesis factors [13]. Therefore, astrocytes play an important role in neural development.

5. Differentiation of Primate ES Cells

Unlike mouse ES cells, those of monkeys do not pile up but rather form planar colonies during proliferation. However, human ES cells form colonies more like mouse ES cells. The culture conditions used for primate ES cells are different from these used for mouse ES cells. The major difference is that primate ES cells do not require leukemia inhibitory factor, which is essential for mouse ES cells to maintain their totipotency. In addition, primate ES cells require 2 to 3 times longer in floating culture in ACM to differentiate into neural stem cells as compared with mouse ES cells. The gene expression pattern of primate ES cells during floating culture is also slightly different from that of mouse ES cells (manuscript in preparation). Although some differences were observed, primate ES cells could be induced to differentiate into neural stem cells by the NSS method. These primate ES cell-derived neural stem cells could be cryopreserved and again could be induced to differentiate into neurons after thawing. Next, we attempted to transplant monkey ES cell-derived neural stem cells as donor cells. We generated a monkey model of Parkinson's disease with selective and irreversible loss of dopaminergic neurons in the substantia nigra by administration of 1-methyl-4-phenyl-1,2,3,6-tetrahydropyridine. In this Parkinson's disease model, congeneric ES cell-derived neural stem cells were transplanted in the corpus striatum on one side, and the therapeutic effects were investigated. The incorporation of isotope-labeled L-3,4-dihydroxyphenylalanine (L-dopa) was examined with positron emission tomography, and a significant difference was found in the graft side as compared to the control side one month after transplantation [14]. Furthermore, neurons that were immunoreactive for tyrosine hydroxylase, a marker of dopaminergic neurons, were observed in the graft side three months after transplantation. These results confirmed that ES cell-derived neural stem cells produced by the NSS method were effective in cell transplantation therapy. In future, this may become a true alternative form of therapy if a projection circuit is seen to be formed to the corpus striatum as well as lost dopaminergic neurons when ES cell-derived neural stem cells are actually transplanted into the substantia nigra.

CONCLUSION

In this report, we described the NSS method using ACM to differentiate ES cells into neural stem cells directly. It is likely that this method succeeded by preserving cell-to-cell interactions in the NSS during floating culture with the aid of humoral factors. We are currently attempting to develop specialized neurons with specific phenotypes, including dopaminergic neurons, by addition of various factors into the culture medium. In the near future, these approaches will be applied to human ES cell-derived neural stem cells that may show ameliorating effects in various neurodegenerative diseases.

REFERENCES

[1] O'Shea KS. (1999): Embryonic stem cell models of development. *Anat. Rec.,* 257:32–41.

[2] Bain G, Kitchens D, Yao M, Huettner JE, Gottlieb DI. (1995): Embryonic stem cells express neuronal properties *in vitro*. *Dev. Biol.,* 168:342–57.

[3] Wichterle H, Lieberam I, Porter JA, Jessell TM. (2002): Directed differentiation of embryonic stem cells into motor neurons. *Cell,* 110:385–97.

[4] Okabe S, Forsberg-Nilsson K, Spiro AC, Segal M, McKay RD. (1996): Development of neuronal precursor cells and functional postmitotic neurons from embryonic stem cells in vitro. *Mech. Dev.*, 59:89–102.

[5] Watanabe K, Kamiya D, Nishiyama A, Katayama T, Nozaki S, Kawasaki H, Watanabe Y, Mizuseki K, Sasai Y. (2005): Directed differentiation of telencephalic precursors from embryonic stem cells. *Nat. Neurosci,* 8288–96.

[6] Nakayama T, Momoki-Soga T, Inoue N. (2003): Astrocyte-derived factors instruct differentiation of embryonic stem cells into neurons. *Neurosci. Res.*, 46:241–9.

[7] Nakayama T, Momoki-Soga T, Yamaguchi K, Inoue N. (2004): Efficient production of neural stem cells and neurons from embryonic stem cells. *Neuroreport*, 15:487–91.

[8] Nakayama T, Inoue N. (2006): Neural stem sphere method: induction of neural stem cells and neurons by astrocyte-derived factors in embryonic stem cells in vitro. *Methods Mol. Biol.*, 330:1–13.

[9] Gage FH, Coates PW, Palmer TD, Kuhn HG, Fisher LJ, Suhonen JO, Peterson DA, Suhr ST, Ray J. (1995): Survival and differentiation of adult neuronal progenitor cells transplanted to the adult brain. *Proc. Natl. Acad. Sci. USA*, 92:11879–83.

[10] Nait-Oumesmar B, Decker L, Lachapelle F, Avellana-Adalid V, Bachelin C, Van Evercooren AB. (1999): Progenitor cells of the adult mouse subventricular zone proliferate, migrate and differentiate into oligodendrocytes after demyelination. *Eur. J. Neurosci.*, 11:4357–66.

[11] Nakayama T, Sai T, Otsu M, Momoki-Soga T, Inoue N. (2006): Astrocytogenesis of embryonic stem-cell-derived neural stem cells: Default differentiation. *Neuroreport*, 17:1519–23.

[12] Doetsch F. (2003): The glial identity of neural stem cells. *Nat. Neurosci.*, 6:1127–1134.

[13] Alvarez-Buylla A, Garcia-Verdugo JM, Tramontin AD. (2001): A unified hypothesis on the lineage of neural stem cells. *Nat. Rev. Neurosci.*, 2:287–93.

[14] Muramatsu S, Nakayama T, Nara Y, Suzuki Y, Nagata M, Ono F, Kondo Y, Terao K, Tsukada H, Inoue N, Nakano I. (2004): Restoration of dopamine function in a primate model of Parkinson's disease after transplantation of primate ES cell-derived neuronal stem cell. *Keystone Symposium on Stem Cells*: 110.

In: Encyclopedia of Stem Cell Research (2 Volume Set)
Editor: Alexander L. Greene

ISBN: 978-1-61761-835-2
© 2012 Nova Science Publishers, Inc.

Chapter I

STEM CELL APPLICATIONS IN DISEASE RESEARCH: RECENT ADVANCES IN STEM CELL AND CANCER STEM CELL BIOLOGY AND THEIR THERAPEUTIC IMPLICATIONS

Murielle Mimeault and Surinder K. Batra

Department of Biochemistry and Molecular Biology, Eppley Institute of Cancer and Allied Diseases, University of Nebraska Medical Center, Omaha, NE, US

ABSTRACT

Recent advances in embryonic, fetal, umbilical cord, placental, amniotic and tissue-resident adult stem/progenitor cell research is of great clinical interest due to their potential therapeutic applications in regenerative medicine and gene therapies. The tissue-resident adult stem/progenitor cells, which possess several characteristics common with embryonic stem cells (ESCs) but generally display more limited self-renewal ability and restricted differentiating potential, are emerging as promising sources of immature cells. The presence of a rare population of adult stem/progenitor cells in most tissues and organs offers the possibility to stimulate their *in vivo* differentiation or to use their *ex vivo* expanded progenies for cell replacement-based therapies with multiple applications in humans. Among the human diseases that could be treated by the stem cell-based therapies, the hematopoietic and immune disorders, cardiovascular disorders, multiple degenerative disorders such as Parkinson's and Alzeimeher's diseases, type 1 or 2 diabetes mellitus as well as eye, liver, lung, gastrointestinal and skin disorders and aggressive and metastatic cancers are of immediate attention. In addition, the genetically-modified adult stem/progenitor cells could also be used as a delivery system for expressing the therapeutic molecules in specific damaged areas of different tissues in humans. Recent progress in cancer stem/progenitor cell research also offers the possibility to target these undifferentiated and malignant cells that provide critical functions in cancer initiation and progression and disease relapse for treating patients diagnosed with advanced and metastatic cancers which remain incurable in the clinics with the current therapies.

ABBREVIATIONS

ABC	ATP-binding cassette;
ADSCs	adipose tissue-derived stem cells;
ATP	adenosine triphosphate;
BM,	bone marrow;
BMP	bone morphogenic protein;
bESCs	bulge epithelial stem cells;
CESCs	corneal epithelial stem cells;
CNS	central nervous system;
EGF	epidermal growth factor;
eNCSCs	epidermal neural crest stem cells,
EPCs	endothelial progenitor cells;
ESCs	embryonic stem cells;
hAECs	human amniotic epithelial cells;
hESCs	human embryonic stem cells;
HGF	hepatocyte growth factor;
HSCs	hematopoietic stem cells;
IGF-I	insulin-like growth factor-I;
KSCs	keratinocyte stem cells;
MDSCs	muscle-derived stem cells;
MSCs	mesenchymal stem cells;
NCSCs	neural crest stem cells;
NSCs	neural stem cells;
Oct-3/4	octamer-binding protein;
SDF-1	stromal cell-derived factor-1;
TA	transit-amplifying; umbilical cord;
SHH	sonic hedgehog ligand,
UCB	umbilical cord blood;
PSCs	pancreatic stem cells;
PDMSCs	placenta-derived multipotent stem/progenitor cells;
RSCs	retinal stem cells;
VEGF	vascular endothelial growth factor;
Wnt	Wingless ligand.

INTRODUCTION

Stem cell field is a rapidly advancing area of biomedical research. Recent advances in stem cell biology, especially on the embryonic, fetal, umbilical cord (UC), placenta, amniotic and adult stem cell-based therapies have suspired great interest and given new hopes. The possibility to use the undifferentiated stem cells or their further differentiated progenies for cell replacement in regenerative medicine and cancer therapy is immense importance [1-14]. The multipotent adult stem/progenitor cell populations, which have been identified in the most tissues and organs in human, notably represent the attractive sources of immature cells with important implications for cell replacement-based therapies [5,6,8,9,14-26]. Normal tissue-resident adult stem/progenitor cells are able to give rise to further differentiated cell lineages in tissues from which they originate, and regenerate the tissues and organs throughout the lifespan of an individual. Several efforts have permitted to identify the unique features of each tissue-resident adult stem/progenitor cells and their specialized local microenvironment designated as niche as well as their critical functions in homeostasis state maintenance and tissue regeneration [6-9,14,20,22,26-28]. The activation of aberrant molecular signaling pathways in adult stem/progenitor cells and their deregulated interactions with the niche components resulting to their acquisition of a dysfunctional behavior have also been associated with the occurrence of particular human degenerative disorders and diseases [6-8,14,15,18,20,22,27-30]. Importantly, certain adult stem cells including bone marrow (BM)-derived stem cells may also be attracted at distant extramedullary peripheral sites after intense injuries and participate to the tissue repair through remodeling and regeneration process of damaged areas [8,12,14,15,21,31-36]. Hence, the adult stem cells offer great therapeutic potentials for regenerating damaged tissues and serving as gene delivery vehicle for treating and even curing diverse degenerative diseases and aggressive cancers. Among the human diseases that could be treated by stem cell-based therapies, there are hematopoietic and immune disorders, type 1 or 2 diabetes mellitus, cardiovascular and neurodegenerative diseases, lung, skin, liver, gastrointestinal and eye disorders and aggressive and recurrent cancers [8,12,14,21,22,24,26,33-67].

Numerous recent investigations revealed that the accumulation of genetic and/or epigenic alterations occurring in stem/progenitor cells during aging and severe injuries including chronic inflammatory atrophy could trigger their malignant transformation into cancer stem/progenitor cells [8,14,18,29,37,68-79]. Thus, the targeting of the deregulated signaling pathways in the cancer stem/progenitor cells, which may contribute to their sustained growth, survival, invasion, metastasis and/or treatment resistance during cancer progression, is also of particular therapeutic interest for eradicating these cancer-initiating cells [8,14,37,75,77-80]. The elimination of cancer stem/progenitor cells should permit to counteract the cancer progression and disease recurrence. Thereby, the targeting of cancer stem/progenitor cells and their local microenvironment should lead to a complete remission of patients diagnosed with advanced and metastatic cancers which remain lethal in the clinics with the current surgical, hormonal, radiation and/or chemotherapeutic treatments. We describe here the available sources and types of human stem/progenitor cells with a description of their known specific biomarkers, functional characteristics and therapeutic potentials to give rise to particular cell lineages in the well-defined culture conditions *in vitro* and *ex vivo* as well as in animal models *in vivo* and clinical settings. The emphasis is on the recent research on adult stem/progenitor cells and their niches in term of their functions in the tissue regeneration in physiological and pathophysiological conditions. We also summarize and discuss the major advances in the field of the research on the diseases that may be associated with a dysfunctional behavior of adult stem/progenitor cells including the implication of cancer stem/progenitor cells in cancer progression. The provided information should help to develop novel therapeutic strategies that could be translated into clinical applications for treating and curing the patients with diverse degenerative disorders and lethal diseases including the metastatic and recurrent cancers.

STEM CELL SOURCES AND TYPES

All of the stem cells have the unique capacity to self-renew and to give rise in a specific microenvironment to more committed cell lineages [1-3,5,7,8,12,14,16,19,22-26,33,36,38,40,48,50,56,61,75,81-89]. The supply of the specific growth factors and cytokines and maintenance or restoring a local microenvironment resembling to the specialized niche of stem cells is also essential for their successful *ex vivo* and *in vivo* expansion and/or differentiation into a specific cell lineage with the normal functional properties. Several feeder layer types have been developed and used as vital support systems of stem cells for these purposes. There are the serum- containing and serum-free feeders, consisting of stromal cells, such as mouse NIH 3T3 fibroblasts or human mesenchymal cells, human amniotic epithelial cells (hAECs), amniotic membranes, cell-free feeders and diverse culture mediums containing of extracellular matrix components such as the collagen, gelatin, fibrinogen and laminin [8,81,90-93]. Among the most studied stem cells, there are the embryonic, fetal, umbilical, placental, amniotic and tissue-resident adult stem cells which may constitute the potential sources of functional cells for regenerative medicine and cancer therapy.

Embryonic Stem Cells

Pluripotent embryonic stem cells (ESCs) are derived from inner cell mass of the blastocyst in embryos and may differentiate into all cell types of three germ layers including endoderm, mesoderm and ectoderm *in vitro* and *in vivo* in appropriate conditions (figure 1) [8,12,14,81,94]. Human ESCs (hESCs) express telomerase activity and many specific biomarkers such as CD9, CD24, octamer-binding protein (Oct-3/4), Nanog, alkaline phosphatase, LIN28, Rex-1, Cripto/TDGF1, DNA methyltransferase 3B (DNMT3B), SRY-box containing gene 2 (SOX2), endometrial bleeding associated factor (EBAF) and Thy-1 as well as the stage-specific embryonic antigen-3 and -4 (SSEA-3 and -4) and tumor-rejection antigen-1-60 and -1-81 (TRA-1-60 and -1-81) [81,94,95]. The pluripotency of mammalian ESCs, including hESCs, is associated with a complex network of developmental intracellular signaling cascades initiated by diverse growth factors, cytokines and chemokines including EGFR, hedgehog, Wnt/β-catenin and Notch systems, RNA-binding proteins, musashi-1 and -2 (Msi-1 and Msi-2) and transcription factors such as Nanog, Oct-3/4 and Pou homeodomain that control their self-renewal ability and/or promote their differentiation into any cell types of the body [8,14,81]. Numerous recent works revealed that the loss of pluripotency and differentiation of ESCs into functional differentiated cells as well as the engineering tissues may be accomplished using specific culture medium and composite support, which may provide the differentiative factors necessary for their commitment into the particular cell lineages. Among the cell types that can be derived from ESCs, there are the hematopoietic cell lineages, dendritic cells, mesenchymal cells, neural and glial cells including motor neurons and dopaminergic neurons, cardiomyocytes, muscular and adipose cells, hepatocytes, pancreatic islet-like cells, lung, skin and retinal cell-like cells (figure 1) [1,5,8,12,14,21, 22,40,48,81,82,90,91,96-98]. In addition, cranial neural crest-derived ectomesenchymal cells, which represent the multipotent progenitors that contribute to various tissue types during embryogenesis also may be isolated from first branchial arch in embryos, expanded in culture as a monolayer and further differentiated into different cell lineages including adipogenic, osteogenic, chondrogenic myogenic, odontogenic, neurogenic and endothelial cells in appropriate media *in vitro* and *in vivo* [99,100]. It is noteworthy that several congenital diseases including certain innate cancers have been proposed to derive from an aberrant developmental process that affects the pluripotent neural crest stem cells (NCSCs) [77,101]. Interestingly, it has been reported that the gut NCSCs from the enteric nervous system can represent a potential source of stem cells for treating the Hirschsprung disease which is a rare congenital abnormality that leads in an absence of ganglion cells in the intestine after the birth [101]. Although these advances, the ethic associated with the necessity to use the embryos as well as the possibility of graft rejection due to their immunogenecity and potential tumorigenic properties of ESC-derived cell progenitors yet represent a major obstacle that limits their clinical therapeutic applications [1,8,14,81,98,102-105]. Particularly, the persistence of undifferentiated hESCs in transplant may result in the formation of teratocarcinomas *in vivo*.

Investigations of functional properties of hESCs and their progenies appear to be necessary before their eventual use for treating the patients in the clinical practice in safe conditions. These studies can be performed using both different derivation and differentiation strategies *in vitro* culture systems and *in vivo* pre-clinical animal models. These additional studies should also help to shed the light on the early and late molecular events associated with the proliferation and cell lineage specification of hESCs during the embryonic development. Another alternative approach may also consist to use the stem cells and their progenies established from human fetal tissues, term placenta and umbilical cord tissues which are less immunogenic that the hESCs and non-tumorigenic *in vivo* [3,4,8,14,47, 48,83,84,106-112].

Fetal, Placental and Amniotic Stem/Progenitor Cells

The stem cells and their progenies derived from fetal tissues obtained up until week 12 have considerable applications in numerous clinics in regenerative medicine. For instance, the fetal stem/progenitor cells may constitute a source to obtain the functional cells including the hematopoietic cells, cardiomyocytes, hepatocytes, insulin-secreting β cells, lung progenitor cells, muscles and neural cells including dopaminergic neurons that may be used for the cell replacement and tissue engineering-based therapies in regenerative medicine [8,14,47,83,84,106,110-112]. More recently, the use of the human placenta-derived multipotent stem/progenitor cells (PDMSCs), such as amniotic and chorionic mesenchymal stem cells (MSCs), and MSCs from villous stroma, hematopoietic, trophoblastic and pluripotent AECs derived from amniotic membrane have suspired great interest [3,4,8,14,47,48,83,84,106-114]. In fact, the natural biologic properties of these cells that are present *in utero* and their ability to differentiate into different mature cell lineages *in vitro* made them the promising sources for cell replacement therapies (table 1) [3,14,115]. For instance, it has been reported that MSCs from chorion, amnion, and villous stroma expressing CD166, CD105, CD90, CD73, CD49e, CD44, CD29, CD13, MHC I phenotype, which present unique features as compared to BM-derived stem cells, can be differentiated into neurogenic, chondrogenic, osteogenic, adipogenic, and myogenic lineages [113,114]. Moreover, the use of amniotic membrane, which is the innermost lining of the placenta that serves as a natural barrier to protect the fetus from potential bacterial and viral infections, also presents several therapeutic advantages. Among them, there are the release of growth factors and cytokines by amniotic membrane that may reduce inflammation, prevent the formation of blood vessels, and promote wound repair and healing process [116-119]. All of these above functional properties associated with amniotic membrane make it an ideal composite for its therapeutic use in surgical transplantation procedures in the clinics, and more particularly in the eye surgery [117-119]. Furthermore, pluripotent hAECs derived from amniotic membrane, which did not form the teratomas or teratocarcinomas in human, may generate diverse functional progenies including neuronal and glial cells, keratinocytes, pancreatic and hepatic cells, cardiomyocytes, myocytes, osteocytes and adipocytes in culture *in vitro* that could be used in cell replacement therapies for treating diverse human diseases (table 1) [3,4,8,14,47,48,83,84,106-109,111,112,120].

Umbilical Cord-Derived Stem Cells

The establishment of umbilical cord (UC) and umbilical cord blood (UCB) banks offers the possibility to rapidly obtain them for their use in the stem cell-based therapies in the clinics [2,8,14,121,122]. Several works have revealed the possibility of differentiating the UC-derived stem cells into diverse functional progenitors, including hematopoietic cell lineages, dendritic cells, cardiomyocytes, MSC progenitors, neural stem cell (NSC) progenitors, keratinocytes, hepatocytes, pancreatic β cells and endothelial cells in specific culture conditions *in vitro* and *in vivo* [2,8,14,41,85-87,122-126]. Hence, these stem/progenitor cells or their differentiated progenies may be used in autograft or allograft transplantations without or with a low rate of graft-rejection for treating the patients with neuronal degenerative diseases, heart failure, hepatic disorders or type 1 or 2 diabetes (table 1) [2,8,14,121,122].

Adult Stem/Progenitor Cells

Diverse poorly-differentiated adult stem/progenitor cell types, which have generally small size relative to the terminally differentiated cells, have recently been identified and

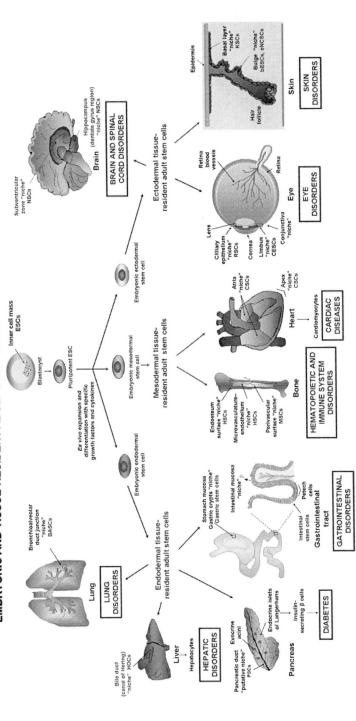

Figure 1. Schematic diagram showing the possible differentiation pathways of ESCs and tissue-resident adult stem cells into mature cell lineages and the disorders that could be treated by stem cell-based therapies. The ESCs can give rise to three germ layers, endoderm, mesoderm, and ectoderm during embryonic development. Similarly, ESC progenitors derived through the formation of EBs might also give rise to all the adult stem cells and mature cell types constituting the tissues/organs of endodermal, mesodermal, or ectodermal origin after their *ex vivo* expansion and differentiation in the presence of the specific growth factors and cytokines in culture medium. Abbreviations: BASCs, bronchioalveolar stem cells; bESCs, bulge epithelial stem cells; CESCs, corneal epithelial stem cells; CSCs, cardiac stem cells; EB, embryoid body; EPCs, endothelial progenitor cells; eNCSCs, epidermal neural crest stem cells; ESCs, human embryonic stem cells; HOCs, hepatic oval cells; HSCs, hematopoietic stem cells; KSCs, keratinocyte stem cells; MDSCs, muscle-derived stem cells; MSCs, mesenchymal stem cells; NSCs, neural stem cells; PSCs, pancreatic stem cells; RSCs, retinal stem cells.

isolated by fluorescence-activated cell sorting (FACS) with the specific antibodies directed against specific stem cell markers as well as by side population (SP) technique based on their ability to efflux Hoechst 33342 dye due to their high expression of ATP-binding cassette (ABC) transporters such as ABCG2 in the most mammalian tissues/organs [8,14,37,127].

Table 1. Tissue-Resident Adult Stem/Progenitor Cells and Their Therapeutic Applications in Disease Treatment

Adult stem cell/progenitor cell source and type	Differentiated cells	Treated degenerative disorders and diseases
BM and vascular walls		
HSCs	Myeloid and lymphoid cells, Platelets	Autoimmune diseases, anemias, thrombocytopenia, Leukemias, aggressive solide tumors
MSCs	Osteoblasts	Osteoporosis, Osteogenesis imperfecta
	Chondrocytes	Cartilage disorders, osteoarthritis
	Muscular cells	Muscular disorders
HSCs, MSCs	Neural cells	Nervous system disorders
	Cardiomyocytes	Heart disorders
	Insulin-producing β cells	Type 1 or 2 diabetes mellitus
	Hepatocytes	Liver disorders
EPCs	Endothelial cells	Vascular disorders
Adipose tissue/Skeletal muscle		
ADSCs and MDSCs	Muscle cells	Muscular disorders (muscular Duchenne and Becker dystrophies, neuromuscular disorders)
	Osteoblasts	Osteoporosis, Osteogenesis imperfecta
	Chondrocytes	Cartilage disorders, osteoarthritis
	Endothelial cells	Vascular disorders
	Cardiomyocytes	Heart disorders
	Neural cells	Nervous system disorders
ADSCs	Insulin-producing β cells	Type 1 or 2 diabetes mellitus
	Hepatocytes	Liver disorders
Heart		
CSCs	Cardiomyocytes	Heart disorders
Brain		
NSCs	Neurons, Astrocytes	Nervous system disorders
	Oligodendrocytes	Myelin disorders
	Insulin-producing β cells	Type 1 or 2 diabetes mellitus
Eye		
CESCs	Corneal epithelial cells	Corneal disorders
Conjunctival SCs	Conjunctival epithelial cells	Cunjunctival epithelial injury
CE-RSCs	Retinal progenitor cells	Retinal disorders
Skin		
KSCs, bESCs and eNCSCs	Skin cells	Skin and hair disorders
Gastrointestinal tract		
ISCs and GSCs	Intestinal and stomach cells	Chronic inflammatory bowel diseases, ulcers
Pancreas		
PSCs	Insulin-producing β cells	Type 1 or 2 diabetes mellitus
	Hepatocytes	Liver disorders
Liver		
HOCs,	Hepatocytes, cholangiocytes	Hepatitis, acute liver failure, cirrhosis
	Cardiomyocytes	Heart failures
Lung		
BASCs	Lung cells (Bronchiolar Clara Cells and alveolar cells)	Interstitial lung diseases, cystic fibrosis, asthma, chronic bronchitis, emphysema

BASCs, bronchioalveolar stem cells; bESCs, bulge epithelial stem cells; CE-RSCs, ciliary epithelium-retinal stem cells; CESCs, corneal epithelial stem cells; CSCs, cardiac stem cells; EPCs, endothelial progenitor cells; eNCSCs, epidermal neural crest stem cells; GSCs, gastric stem cells; HOCs, hepatic oval cells; HSCs, hematopoietic stem cells; ISCs, intestinal stem cells; KSCs, keratinocyte stem cells; MDSCs, muscle-derived stem cells; MSCs, mesenchymal stem cells; NSCs, neural stem cells; PSCs, pancreatic stem cells; SCs, stem cells.

Among the tissues and organs harboring a very small number of specific multipotent and undifferentiated adult stem/progenitor cells, there are BM, vascular walls, heart, skeletal muscles, adipose tissues, brain as well as epithelium of lung, liver, pancreas, digestive tract, skin, limbus, retina, breast, ovaries, prostate and testis (figure 1) [6,8,14-17,19-25,38,56,75,77,78,88,128-130]. In general, the adult stem/progenitor cells are localized within a specialized microenvironment designated as niche consisting of the nearboring cells such as fibroblasts, endothelial cells and/or stromal components that tightly regulate their functions through the direct interactions and release of specific soluble factors [6-9,14,20,26-28,30,77,78]. All of the multipotent or bi-potent adult stem/progenitor cell types display a long-term self-renewing capacity and can give rise in appropriate conditions including after intense injury to all of mature and specialized cell types of distinct lineages in the tissue/organ from which they originate or in certain cases to cell lineages at distant sites (figure 2) [6,8,9,14,15,17-26,29,68,71,73,75,77,78]. Despite certain adult stem/progenitor cells found in BM, skin and gastrointestinal tract usually show a rapid turnover to replenish the cell loss along lifespan, other adult stem/progenitor cell types remain under a quiescent state and rarely divide in normal conditions, and undergo only a sustained proliferation after intense tissue injuries [8,14-16,27]. The expansion of adult stem/progenitor cell pool within niche is accomplished though a symmetric cell division that gives rise to two identical stem cell daughters (figure 2). The generation of differentiated cell lineages rather generally implicates an asymmetric division of a stem cell that gives rise to one stem cell daughter and one cell termed early transit-amplifying (TA)/intermediate cell (figure 2) [7,8,14,15,27,77,78,88]. The early TA/intermediate cells, which possess a high proliferative potential and migratory ability, may exit the stem cell niche and give rise to late TA cells. The changes in the local environmental of early and late TA/intermediate cells during amplification process and their migration at distant sites from niche may also influence the phenotype of their further and terminally differentiated progenies, and thereby contribute to the populational asymmetry and cellular diversity characterizing each tissue and organ (figure 2) [8,14,131].

The tissue regeneration mediated *via* adult stem/progenitor cells is usually accompanied by environmental changes in the niche and orchestrated by several growth factors and cytokines such as epidermal growth factor (EGF), sonic hedgehog ligand (SHH), Wnt/β-catenin, Notch, bone morphogenic protein (BMP), stromal cell-derived factor-1 (SDF-1) [8,14,78]. These soluble factors may be released by tissue-resident activated stem/progenitor cells and stromal cells including the myofibroblasts, endothelial cells and immune cells such as macrophages attracted at the injured areas (figure 2). In certain pathological conditions including intense wound and chronic inflammatory atrophies, certain adult stem/progenitor cells, and more particularly, BM derived-stem/progenitor cells, may also be attracted to distant injured tissues [8,12,14,21,31-36,77,78]. BM-derived cells may thereby contribute to the tissue repair by the release of diverse factors and/or to transdifferentiate into specific cell types within the host tissue. Hence, the tissue-resident adult stem/progenitor cells are unique as compared with other embryonic, UC, fetal and placenta-derived stem cell sources, in being enriched in an anatomic location that may be easy to access. Thus, in that way the adult stem cells may be stimulated *in vivo* in their respective environment by the exogenous application of specific growth factors and cytokines in the damaged areas that restores the endogenous tissue regeneration program. We describe here in more detailed manner, the specific biomarkers and functional properties of tissue-resident adult stem cells and their niches, with a particular emphasis on the adult stem/progenitor cells localized in BM, adipose tissues, muscles, heart, brain and pancreas as well as their potential therapeutic applications in cell replacement-based therapies for treating diverse degenerative disorders and diseases in human.

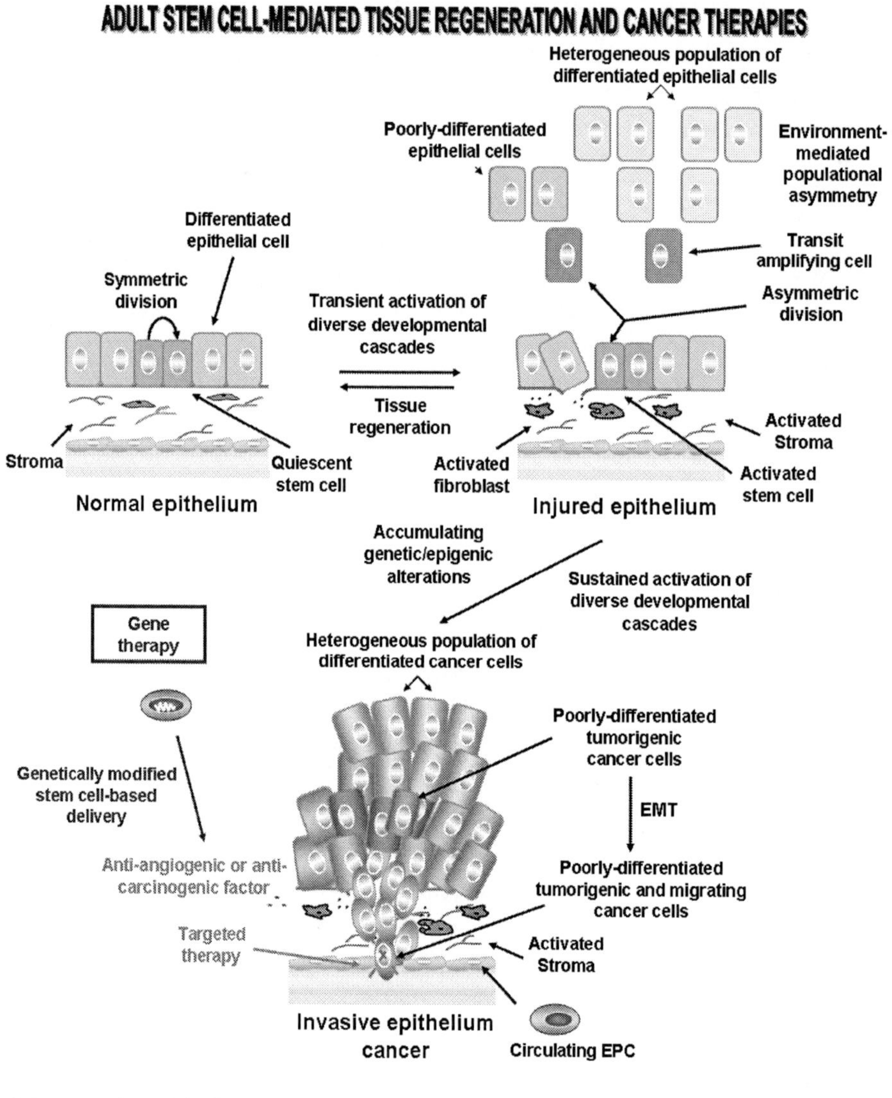

Figure 2. Proposed model of the molecular events associated with the epithelium regeneration *via* adult stem/progenitor cells after tissue injury and cancer initiation and progression through their malignant transformation. This scheme shows the asymmetric division of adult stem cells into transit-amplifying/intermediate cells that in turn may regenerate the bulk mass of further differentiated epithelial cells during the repair of injured tissue. The malignant transformation of adult stem/progenitor cells into tumorigenic and migrating cancer stem/progenitor cells, which may be induced through the genetic and/or epigenetic alterations leading to the sustained activation of distinct tumorigenic cascades and triggering epithelial-mesenchymal transition program during cancer progression to the invasive and metastatic disease stages is also illustrated.

TISSUE-RESIDENT ADULT STEM/PROGENITOR CELLS AND THEIR THERAPEUTIC APPLICATIONS

BM-Derived Stem/Progenitor Cells and Their Therapeutic Applications

Hematopoietic Stem Cells and Their Therapeutic Applications

The BM-derived hematopoietic stem cells (HSCs) provide a critical role by generating all of the new mature and differentiated white and red blood cell lineages along lifespan of an individual [7,8,12,14,132]. The most immature and quiescent multipotent HSCs, which are characterized by the expression of specific biomarkers including $CD34^-$ or $CD34^+/CD38^{-/low}$/*Thy1$^+$/CD90$^+$/C-kit*$^{/lo}$/Lin$^-$/CD133$^+$/vascular endothelial growth factor receptor 2 (VEGFR2$^+$) are co-localized with the osteoblasts in a specialized niche within a BM region designated as endosteum (figure 1) [7,8,14,27,133]. Moreover, another subpopulation of HSCs, which is found in a BM microvasculature-sinusoidal endothelium niche, appears to represent the stem cells that may rapidly supply new mature blood cell lineages cells which have a short live into peripheral circulation (figure 1) [7,14,30,133].

HSCs may be used in autologous or allogenic transplantations for the treatment of patients with inherited immunodeficient and autoimmune diseases and diverse hematopoietic disorders to reconstitute the hematopoietic cell lineages and immune system defense [8-10,14,134]. Among them, HSC aging related-intrinsic functional defects, autoimmune diseases, refractory and severe aplastic anemias, congenital thrombocytopenia, osteoporosis, cardiovascular disorders, chronic inflammatory Bowel disorders (IBD) including Crohn's disease and ulcerative colitis, diabetes, leukemias, multiple myelanomas and Hodgkin's and non-Hodgkin's lymphomas and aggressive tumors may be treated by HSC transplants, alone or in combination therapies [8,14,15,62-67,134,135].

Mesenchymal Stem Cells and Endothelial Progenitor Cells and Their Therapeutic Applications

The BM stroma as well as the walls of large and small blood vessels in most tissues/organs including brain, spleen, liver, kidney, lung, muscle, thymus and pancreas also contain the multipotent MSCs and endothelial progenitor cells (EPCs) [8,12,14,35,36,136-140]. Much of the work conducted on adult stem/progenitor cells has focused on MSCs found within the BM stroma. More particularly, the MSCs expressing CD49a and CD133 markers are localized in a perivascular niche in BM, and may give rise to the osteoblasts that are co-localized with HSCs, and which may support the hematopoieises by producing the growth factors and cytokines that promote the expansion and/or differentiation of HSCs (figure 1) [8,12,14,83,141]. The BM-derived or tissue-resident MSCs can generate diverse mesodermal cell lineages involved in osteogenesis, adipogenesis, cartilage and muscle formation including the osteoblasts, osteocytes, adipocytes, chondrocytes, myoblasts and myocytes under appropriate culturing conditions *ex vivo* and *in vivo*. Moreover, MSCs may also be induced to differentiate into fibroblasts, neuronal cells, pulmonary cells, pancreatic islet β cells, corneal epithelial cells and cardiomyocytes *ex vivo* and/or *in vivo* using specific growth factors and cytokines [8,14,83,84,87,88,108,109,140,142-148]. In the case of EPCs, which are derived like HSCs from the embryonic hemangioblasts, they may be distinguished by the expression of different biomarkers, including CD34$^+$ or CD34$^-$, CD133, vascular endothelial growth factor receptor-2 (VEGFR-2), also designated as Flk-1 (fetal liver kinase-1), SCF receptor (KIT) and CXC chemokine receptor-4 (CXCR4) [77]. EPCs may contribute in a significant manner to give rise to mature endothelial cells that form new vascular walls of vessels after intense injury and vascular diseases as well as the new vessel formation in tumors as described in a more detailed manner in below section (figures 2 and 3) [8,12,14,35,36,137,139,149-155]. The critical role of circulating EPCs in endothelial cell maintenance after tissue injury is notably supporting by the observation that their number and function is inversely associated with the progression of atherosclerosis and an enhanced risk of cardiovascular diseases.

All of the above functional properties of MSCs and EPCs made them the promising sources of immature cells for treating numerous degenerative and vascular disorders in human. The autologous or allogeneic transplantation of BM or peripheral blood (PB) can lead to the homing and engraftment of functional HSCs, MSCs and EPCs and/or their differentiated progenies at BM and distant damaged tissues. Thus, this support the feasibility of this strategy for improving the tissue remodeling and healing processes after severe injury as well as in the treatment of diverse human disorders including osteogenesis imperfecta, atherosclerotic lesions, ischemic cardiovascular and muscular diseases (figure 3) [8,14,137,139,143,144,147]. It has been reported that MSCs, EPCs and their progenies can contribute to the regenerative process of several tissues including bone, cartilage, tendon, muscle, adipose, brain, lung, heart, pancreas, kidney and eye [156,157]. Importantly, adult BM-derived and tissue-resident MSCs are little immunogenic and display immunomodulatory and anti-inflammatory effects in host *in vivo* [134,157-159]. Therefore, these therapeutic properties of MSCs also support their possible clinical applications to prevent the tissue/organ allograft rejection and severe acute graft-versus-host diseases as well as to treat the autoimmune disorders such as inflammatory bowel disease and inflammation of the heart muscle walls associated with autoimmune myocarditis in which immunomodulation and tissue repair are required [134,157,158,160]. Indeed, MSCs can prolong skin allograft survival and reverse severe acute graft-versus-host disease *in vivo* supporting their use in treating skin diseases as well as in the maxillofacial surgery [157,161].

In counterpart, the migration and proliferation of vascular smooth-muscle cells (SMCs) derived BM cells including HSCs and MSCs in vascular injured area leading an excessive cell accumulation may however contribute to the development of vascular pathologies such as intimal hyperplasia and atherosclerotic lesions (figure 3) [162,163]. The recruited SMCs may mediated their detrimental effects through the synthesis of the extracellular matrix components such as collagen and fibronectin that accumulate on the luminal side of the damaged vessel walls and thereby induce an occlusive vascular remodeling that may result in an ischemic heart attack or restenosis (figure 3) [162]. Therefore, future studies to optimize the BM-derived cell transplantation strategies and establish the specific mechanism(s) of action and physiological effects of HSCs, MSCs and EPCs at long term is essential in order to improve their therapeutic and curative benefits and prevent their detrimental clinical effects in treated patients.

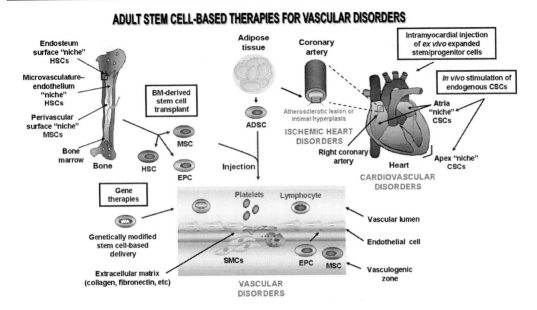

Figure 3. Scheme showing the possible molecular events and cellular changes associated with the development of vascular disorders and the potent cellular and gene therapies for restoring the damaged walls of blood vessels. The recruitment of smooth muscle cells (SMCs) which may participate to the vascular disorder formation by the release of extracellular matrix components such as collagen and fibronectin and immune cells including macrophage in injury area is shown. The stem cell-based therapy using genetically- modified stem/progenitor cells or BM-derived stem/progenitor cell transplant is also illustrated. Abbreviations: ADSCs, adipose tissue-derived stem cells; CSCs, cardiac stem cells; EPCs, endothelial progenitor cells; HSCs, hematopoietic stem cells; MSCs, mesenchymal stem cells.

Adipose Tissue-Derived Stem Cells and their Therapeutic Applications

Adipose tissue is a highly specialized, complex and active metabolic and endocrine structure that contributes to the energy storage under form of fat. In mammals, the adipose-tissues are found in diverse anatomic compartments and designed as subcutaneous adipose tissue, internal organ-surrounding adipose tissue and interstitial adipose tissue [164]. Adipose tissue, like BM, is derived from the embryonic mesenchyme and contains a stroma-vascular fraction. More specifically, adipose tissue is mainly constituted of mature adipocytes, loose connective tissue matrix, nerve tissue and stromal host cells including immature MSC-like cells, fibroblasts, vascular smooth muscle cells, endothelial cells, and immune cells such as the resident hematopoietic progenitor cells and macrophages [165]. Recent studies have permitted to identify a putative adult stem/progenitor cell population termed as processed lipoaspirate (PLA) cells or adipose tissue-derived stem cells (ADSC), within the human adipose compartment [24,165-172]. The stromal immature cell population, termed processed lipoaspirate (PLA) cells can be easily isolated from human lipoaspirates and, like BM-derived hMSCs express the CD29, CD44, CD71, CD90, CD105/SH2 and SH3 [166]. Importantly, it has also been noticed that the PLA cells could be distinguished from BM-derived stromal hMSCs by its unique expression of antigen CD49d (α4-integrin) and CD106 (VCAM) while they did not express hMSC marker, CD106[166]. Moreover, it has been shown that the

ADSCs may be differentiated into functional cells expressing the specific markers of mesodermal (adipocytes, chondrocytes, osteocytes, myocytes, cardiomyocytes and endothelial/vascular cells, endodermal (hepatocytes and endocrine pancreatic cells) or ectodermal (neurons) tissue origin *in vitro* and/or *in vivo* under well definite culture containing specific differentiation factors [24,57-59,165-172]. Since human adipose tissues containing ADSCs can be easily obtained by surgical resection, tumescent lipoaspiration, or ultrasound-assisted lipoaspiration, it constitutes another promising source enriched in immature cells for cellular therapy for diverse human diseases. Among them, there are the clinical management of diverse bone, cartilage and musculoskeletal disorders, cardiovascular and liver disorders, neuronal diseases and diabetes as well as the bioengineering of fat and musculoskeletal tissue reconstitution (table 1) [24,57-59,167,168,173].

Muscle-Derived Stem Cells and their Therapeutic Applications

Adult skeletal muscles contain two distinct stem/progenitor cells, the muscle-derived stem cells (MDSCs) and satellite cell population that may actively participate to myofiber regenerative process and repair of injured or diseased musculoskeletal tissues [56,174]. Muscle-committed satellite cells expressing the markers such as M-cadherin, Pax7, transcription factors, Myf5, and neural cell adhesion molecule-1, are quiescent progenitor cells located at the periphery of skeletal myofibers under homeostatic conditions [56,175]. The satellite cells endowed with self-renewal ability may be activated and to trigger a migration and differentiation into myogenic cells *in vitro* and after muscle injury *in vivo* [56,175]. In addition, the multipotent MDSCs, which may correspond to the more immature progenitor cells relative to satellite cells, can give rise to satellite cells and more committed progenies such as musculoskeletal, osteogenic, chondrogenic, vascular, cardiac and peripheral nerve (Schwann cells and perineurium) cell lineages *in vitro* under specific conditions and induce new myofiber formation in animal models *in vivo* [55,56,129,174,176-179]. Muscle stem/progenitor cells-based regenerative therapy and orthopaedic tissue engineering using *ex vivo* gene therapy, are promising approaches for the treatment of muscle atrophy with aging, muscle wasting (cachexia) and various musculoskeletal and neuromuscular degenerative disorders such as muscular Duchenne and Becker dystrophies and amyotrophic lateral sclerosis as well as the urological degenerative disorders and cardiovascular disorders (table 1) [13,56,174,180,181]. More specifically, Duchenne muscular dystrophy (DMS) is a severe X-linked recessive muscle disease occurring majoritly in boys, which is associated with a defect on the gene encoding protein dystrophin on the sarcolemma of muscle fiber, and that results in a rapidly progressive weakness of the body's muscles [182,183]. At present time, no curative treatment for DMS exists and the current therapies principally consist to delay its progression and provide palliative cares that will result to the death of young patients. Importantly, the results from a phase I trial have revealed that the autologous transplantation of $CD133^+$ MDSCs was safe, without systemic secondary effects and improved the symptoms of DMS in treated patients[182]. Recently, MDSC or ADSC injection based-therapies have also emerging as a potent alternative therapeutic option for the remedial treatment of deficient urethral functions such as the repair of the damaged urethral sphincter associated with the stress urinary incontinence [180].

The genetic and/or epigenetic alterations and changes in the microenvironment "niche" of adult MDSCs and/or satellite cells or the embryonic muscle precursors may however lead to defective skeletal muscle differentiation and rhabdomyosarcoma development [184-187]. The metastatic forms of embryonal, alveolar and pleomorphic rhabdomyosarcomas have a poor clinical management and prognosis. Thus, among the possible therapeutic approaches to treat the rhabdomyosarcomas, the targeted therapies consisting to the toxic gene product delivery in satellite tumor cells by the carriers such as MSCs may represent a promising strategy (figure 2) [184-187]. In addition, it has also been observed that the injection of MDSCs or MDSC engineered to overexpress VEGF into an animal model of acute myocardial infraction induced angiogenesis and improved cardiac function suggesting that the MDSCs could constitute an adjuvant therapy for treating the cardiovascular disorders (figure 3) [188].

Cardiac Stem Cells and their Therapeutic Applications

The heart is a vital muscular organ that by its repeated and rhythmic contractions is responsible for pumping the blood through the circulatory system and delivering the oxygenated blood *via* the systemic circulation to all parts of the body. The heart muscle is constituted by the cardiac involuntary striated muscle cells also called cardiomyocytes or cardiac myocytes. Importantly, the cell renewal in the adult myocardium may be accomplished along lifespan *via* the activation of cardiac stem/progenitor cells (CSCs) found within the specialized niches localized at the apex and atria of the heart (figure 1) [8,14,22,38,128,189,190]. CSCs are able to give rise to three major cell types constituting the myocardium including cardiomyocytes, smooth muscles and vascular endothelial cells in physiological and pathological conditions. With this regard, in infracted myocardium of patients with heart failure or animal models, the regenerative process appears notably to occur through the differentiation of resident small interstitial cells expressing nestin, c-kit, Sca-1, Mdr-1 and ABCG2 into cardiomyocytes, endothelial cells, smooth muscle cells, neuronal cells and fibroblasts [191]. Therefore, the *in vivo* stimulation of these endogenous CSCs or the intravascular, intramyocardial or catheter-based delivery of *ex vivo* expanded CSCs or their further differentiated progenies may constitute the therapeutic strategies for the cardiac cell replacement-based therapies (figure 3; table 1) [8,14,22,38,128,192-195]. Particularly, the CSC-based therapies could be used to replace the aged, dysfunctional or loosed CSCs by new functional cardiomyocytes and regenerate coronary vessels after cardiac injury [196]. The transplantation of genetically modified cells also offer great promise by permitting to delivery a specific therapeutic gene product such as angiogenic factors or survival agents of endogenous cardiomyocytes in the ischemic or non-ischemic heart disease areas (figure 3) [196]. For instance, it has been observed that the transplantation of tumor necrosis factor receptor (TNFR) gene-modified MSCs induced an anti-inflammatory effect and inhibited the apoptotic death of resident cardiomyocytes, and thereby improved the left ventricular function in rat with acute myocardial infraction [197]. Similarly, the transplantation of adenovirus carrying human vascular endothelial growth factor 165 (Ad-hVEGF) (165) gene-transfected

MSCs into rats with ischemic heart disease significantly promoted the host-derived angiogenesis and produced effective myogenesis as compared to MSCs transplant[198]. The transplantation of angiogenin-overexpressing human MSCs obtained after infection adenovirus containing angiogenin gene (AdAng) also improved the heart perfusion and function in a porcine model of chronic ischemia as compared to hMSC (AdNull) [199]. These treatment types, alone or in conjunction with the conventional medical therapies by using pharmaceutical agents such as angiotensin-converting enzyme (ACE) inhibitors, β-adrenergic blockers, and nitroglycerin, should permit to improving the myocardiac regeneration and long-term outcome of patients diagnosed with heart failures resulting from ischemic heart disease, hypertension and myocardial infarction [8,14,22,38,39,128,192-196].

In addition, several lines of evidence have also revealed that the functional and contractile cardiomyocytes and/or vascular endothelial cells could be derived from other stem/progenitor cell sources including ESCs, UCB-derived stem cells ($CD133^+$ cells, HSCs or MSCs), AECs, BMSCs ($CD133^+$ cells, HSCs, MSCs or EPCs), ADSCs, MDSCs, PSCs and adult testicular stem cells or their progenies *in vitro* and/or *in vivo* under specific differentiation conditions [3,8,14,22,24,38-40,85-87,105,126,143,144,169,189,194,200-204]. Interestingly, it has been observed that the co-culture of adult rat liver stem cells or hPSCs in a cardiomyocyte microenvironment consisting to the rat neonatal cardiac cells or human myocardial biopsies, respectively promoted their differentiation into autonomously contracting cardiomyocyte-like cells *in vitro* [202]. Hence, these stem/progenitor cell types or their further differentiated progenies could be used for improving the myocardial and vascular regeneration and cardiac function. In support with this, the results from several experiments carried out on animal injury models *in vivo* have revealed the potential benefit to use these stem cell types or their further differentiated progenies with the cardiomyogenic properties to repair the damaged myocardium [14,24,39,40,85-87,105,128,143,144,169,192-194,201,205]. For instance, it has been observed that the transplantation of *ex vivo* differentiated cardiomyocytes derived from hESCs resulted in a stable cardiomyocyte engraftment and improvement of myocardial performance in rat with extensive myocardial infraction [98]. The data from small clinical trials consisting to the transplantation of human BMSC, mobilized PB cells or purified $CD133^+$ BMSCs into patients with advanced ischemic heart diseases have also indicated that this treatment generally improves the vascularization process and/or myocardial function [39,195,200,203,206]. More specifically, the BM-derived cells, ADSCs and MDSCs may contribute to the repair of the injured cardiovascular system *via* multiple molecular mechanisms. Among them, there are the transdifferentiation of these adult stem cells into new cardiomyocytes, smooth muscle cells and/or endothelial cells as well as their release of diverse paracrine factors such as hepatocyte growth factor (HGF), insulin-like growth factor (IGF-I) and vascular endothelial growth factor (VEGF) that may in turn stimulates the angiogenesis and endogenous CSCs and inhibit their apoptotic/necrotic cell death (figure 3) [105,149,188,207-209]. More specifically, BM-derived MSCs recruited to the infracted heart in animal model *in vivo* seem principally to mediate their therapeutic cardioprotective effects through the releasing of paracrine growth factors and cytokines including HGF that promotes the repair of cardiac lesion by inducing re-vascularization of diseased vessels and stimulating resident CSCs that contribute to repair of damaged cardiac lesion [105,160,207,210,211].

Unfortunatley, in certain cases, MSCs may also differentiate into aortic smooth muscle cells and contribute to intimal hyperplasia development after coronary vascular injury whose pathological effect may be attenuated by co-culture with late-outgrowth endothelial cells (figure 3) [163]. Moreover, it has also been observed that MSCs may display cytogenic instability and may differentiate toward progenies endowed with unwanted phenotype *in vivo* such as osteocytes and adipocytes that are not undesirable for their therapeutic application in the cardiac repair [210]. All of these above detrimental effects of MSCs must be considered before their use to treat cardiovascular diseases in clinical setting.

There are great therapeutic potential and clinical interests of using these diverse stem/progenitor cell types for curing cardiovascular diseases in humans, and more particularly for treating late-stage heart failure patients that have little hope of survival without an opportunity of heart transplantation due to a massive loss of functional cardiomyocyte mass. In counterbalance, additional work appears however necessary for establish more precisely the specific biomarkers and anatomic localization, niche of endogeneous CSCs within heart and the intrinsic and extrinsic factors that regulate their self-renewal and differentiation ability. Moreover, the functional properties of transplanted stem/progenitor cells and the progenies, their cytogenetic stability at long-term, and the molecular mechanisms at the basis of observed effects in the animal models *in vivo* and clinical setting also require additional studies. Particularly, it will be important to ascertain the therapeutic effects on cardiac function associated with each stem/progenitor cell type found in BM-derived transplants. An optimization of cell delivery methods and number of cell injected as well as the establishment of possible interactions between the cardiac cell-replacement therapies and conventional pharmacotherapies currently used to treat the ischemic and non-ischemic heart diseases in the clinics and their specific therapeutic potential after long-term treatment also merit further investigations. These future works are necessary for minimizing the potential clinical risks associated with cell replacement therapy before their possible applications as effective cellular or gene therapies of cardiovascular diseases in the safe conditions in humans.

Neuronal Stem Cells and their Therapeutic Applications

Although the mammalian adult central and peripheral nervous systems have been considered during long time as non-renewal tissues, accumulating body of evidence over the past few years to reverse this dogma by showing that the neurogenesis may occur in adult life through self-renewal and multipotent adult neural stem/progenitor cells present in central and peripheral nervous tissues. More specifically, NSCs found in the adult human brain are localized within two specific neurogenic regions designated as the lateral subventricular zone of lateral ventricle in the forebrain and dentate gyrus in hippocampus (figure 1) [6,8,14,26,96]. Multipotent $CD133^+$/nestin NSCs with an astroglia-like cell phenotype are endowed with a self-renewal potential and capable to give rise to the progenitors that can proliferate and migrate at distant damaged areas of brain where they can generate further differentiated and functional progenies [6,8,14,26,96,212]. More particularly, NSCs found in the subraventricular zone, can give rise to three principal neural cell lineages, including mature neurons and glial cells, astrocytes and oligodentrocytes while them localized in the subgranular cell layer of hippocampus may generate the granule cell projection neurons [6,8,14,26,96]. Hence, NSCs and their progenitors can participate to regenerate and repair the injuried tissues after neurological damages and trauma in human. NSCs may notably give rise to diverse neural and glial cell lineages in appropriate conditions *ex vivo* and *in vivo* [8,14,41,81,92,96,112,212-214]. Numerous developmental signaling cascades [EGF-EGFR, sonic hedgehog (SHH)-patched receptor (PTCH)-GLI, Wnt/β-catenin, Notch, basic fibroblast growth factor (bFGF), nerve growth factor (NGF), neureguins, BMPs, platelet-derived growth factors (PDGFs), ciliary neutrophic factor, vascular endothelial growth factor (VEGF), thyroid hormone T3, dopamine, TGF-β, integrins, Ephrins/Ephs, leukemia inhibitory factor (LIF) and/or RNA-binding proteins, Musashi (Msi-1 and Msi-2)] may contribute to the stringent regulation of the proliferation and cell fate decision of NSCs and astroglial progenitor cells in developing and adult CNS [6,14]. In regard with this, the sustained activation of these mitotic cascades including EGF-EGFR and SHH-patched receptor (PTCH) pathways in NSCs may also result in their malignant transformation and brain tumor formation [14,29,37,73,77-79]. The local microenvironment of NSCs also may influence their behavior. The changes in the niche components including nearboring endothelial cells co-localized with NSCs in the subraventricular zone may assume a critical function during regeneration process as well as during the progression of several neuropathologic diseases including the brain cancers which may arise from the alterations occurring in NSCs and their microenvironments [6,8,14,26,96]. More recently, the adult stem/progenitor cells derived from neural crest-derived stem cells have also been identified in peripheral nervous system within a germinal center designated carotid body (CB) [215]. Multipotent CB-resident adult stem cells, which represent the glia-like sustentacular cells expressing the glial markers can give rise to the dopaminergic glomus cells that produce the glial cell line-derived neurotrophic factor [215].

The identification of NSCs has important therapeutic repercussions by offering the possibilities to stimulate them *in vivo* or replace these immature cells by new one for treating diverse CNS degenerative disorders including Parkinson's, Alzheiher's, Lou Gehrig's and Huntington's diseases, temporal lobe epilepsy, stroke, multiple sclerosis and amyotrophic lateral sclerosis (table 1) [8,14,26,41-44,96,216-222]. Several lines of evidence revealed that the *ex vivo* expanded NSCs or their progenies may be transplanted in damaged areas of brain where they can proliferate, survive, migrate, and differentiate into functional neural and glial cell *in vivo* [8,14,219-223]. For instance, it has been reported that the transplantation of adult neural precursor cells (aNPCs) from the brain of adult transgenic mice into the spinal cords of adult Shiverer (shi/shi) mice with congenitally dysmyelinated adult CNS axons, give rise to the cells expressing the oligodendrocyte markers and resulted in formation of nodes of Ranvier and improved axonal conduction[219]. Importantly, it has also been reported that the transplanted dopaminergic neurons derived from mouse ES cells survived for more than 32 weeks and displayed the functional properties into an animal model of Parkinson's disease [222]. In regard with this, the intrastriatal transplantation of CB-stem/progenitor cells or their progenies also offers great promising as antiparkinsonian therapy [215]. Additionally, ESCs, fetal stem/progenitor cells, UC-derived stem cells, AECs, BMSCs including MSCs, ADSCs, and pluripotent epidermal neural crest stem cells (eNCSCs) found in bulge areas within the hair follicle of the skin may also be induced to differentiate or trans-differentiate into functional neurons (tubulin-β and Tuj1), astrocytes (glial fibrillary acidic protein, GFAP) or oligodendrocytes (O4) *in vitro* and/or *in vivo* [8,14,24,41,112,120,125,224,225]. These observatiosn support the feasibility to use these immature cells or their further differentiated progenies for treating diverse incurable neurodegenerative diseases. Nevertheless, before the clinical applications of NSCs, CB-resident stem/progenitor cells and other stem/progenitor cell sources for neurorestoration therapies, future investigations are required in order to more precisely establish the extrinsic and intrinsic factors that control their behavior within the niche *in vivo* as well as their therapeutic advantages at long term after treatment initiation.

Pancreatic Stem/Progenitor Cells and their Therapeutic Applications

The pancreas is a glandular organ constituted of three tissue types including the ductal tree, the exocrine acinar cells that produce digestive enzymes, and the endocrine islets of Langerhans containing four different types of cells: insulin-producing β cells, glucagon-releasing α cells, somatostatin-producing δ cells and pancreatic polypeptide-containing cells (figure 1) [8,14,226]. The pancreatic β cells, which represent the major type of endocrine cells, are co-localized near at a vascular basement membrane and produce the insulin that is released into bloodstream, and which in turn controls the level of blood glucose in the peripheral circulation [227]. Recent lines of evidences have revealed that the human and rodent mature insulin-producing islet β cells could arise from adult pancreatic stem/progenitor cells (PSCs) expressing ductal epithelial cell markers, cytokeratin 19 ($CK19^{high}$), neural (nestin) and endocrine nuclear pancreatic and duodenal homeobox factor-1 (PDX-1) markers and/or more committed $nestin^+/PDX-1^+/CD19^{low}$ islet precursors localized in the ductal regions and/or within islet compartment (figure 1) [5,8,14,23,226,228-233]. Therefore, these poorly differentiated adult PSCs or their early progenies within the adult pancreas could represent a potential source of β cells for cell replacement or gene therapy for treating the type 1 or 2 diabetes mellitus [234,235]. More particularly, the stimulation of PSCs *in vivo* or transplantation of *ex vivo* expanded pancreatic β cells in the host diseased recipient may constitute a therapeutic strategy for restoring the β cell mass and treating the type 1 or 2 diabetes mellitus [5,8,14,23,24,51-54,110,236-238]. For instance, it has also been reported that the transplantation of purified pancreatic duct cells from islet-depleted human pancreatic tissue plus stromal cell preparation generated the insulin-producing cells in normoglycemic NOD/SCID mice [1].

In addition, the differentiation of embryonic, fetal and UCB stem/progenitor cells, hAECs, PDMSCs, and adult stem cells including HSCs, MSCs, HOCs, NSCs, hAECs, ADSCs into pancreatic insulin-producing β cell-like progenitors has been performed *in vitro* by using specific growth factors such as basic FGF, SCF, nicotinamide, betacellulin, glucagon-like peptide, or activin A (table 1) [3,5,8,14,24,53,54,81,82,92,115,122, 140,148,239-241]. Moreover, the results from numerous *in vitro* pre-clinical investigations and β cell-based transplantation studies in diabetic animal models *in vivo* have also revealed the potential to use these stem /progenitor cells for generating insulin-producing β cells for the treatment of type 1 or 2 diabetes mellitus[1,8,14,81,82,115,238,241]. For instance, it has also been observed that the activation of the hepatic oval cells by treatment of C57BL/6 mice with a diet containing 0.1% 3,5-diethoxycarbonyl-1,4-dihydrocollidine (DDC) for 4 weeks following by inducing hyperglycemia with streptozotocin (STZ) leaded to a reversal of hyperglycemia in this *in vivo* animal model [242]. It has been proposed that the reverasal of hyperglycemia may be due in part to a hepatic transdifferentiation followed by endogenous β-cell regeneration in the pancreas [242]. Furthermore, the transplantation of BM-derived cells plus syngenic or allogenic MSCs has also been observed to promote the pancreatic tissue regeneration and restore the blood glucose and insulin at normal levels in irradiated diabetic mice models *in vivo* while the single injection was ineffective [243]. On the basis of these observation, it has been proposed that the therapeutic effects associated with this treatment type could be mediated *via* a stimulation of the regeneration of endogenous insulin-secreting β cells in recipient combined with an inhibition of T-cell-mediated immune response against the newly formed β cells [243]. In spite of these significance advancements, additional *in vivo* studies appear to be necessary for establishing the beneficial effects to use these stem cell types and their further differentiated progenies for treating patients suffering from type 1 or 2 diabetes mellitus or other human pancreatic diseases in the clinics. Particularly, it will be essential to establish the effects of insulin-producing progenitors on the restoration and normalization of blood sugar levels after long-term treatment.

Other Adult Stem/Progenitor Cells and their Therapeutic Applications

Among the other tissues/organs harboring an adult stem/progenitor cell population, there are lung (bronchioalveolar stem cells "BASCs") [19,88,130], liver (hepatic oval cells "HOCs") [21,25,48,244-248], intestinal crypts and gastic glands [15,16,18,50,248-251], eye (corneal epithelial stem cells "CESCs', retinal stem cells "RSCs" and conjunctival stem cells) [17,61,252-258] and skin (keratinocyte stem cells "KSCs", bulge epithelial stem cells "bESCs" and epithelial neural crest stem cells "eNCSCs") [89,259,260]. Hence, the *in vivo* stimulation of these adult stem/progenitor cells and/or the replacement of their dysfunctional counterparts and/or their further differentiated progenies, also constitute potential stem cell-based strategies and gene therapy for the treatment of numerous pathological disorders in human (figure 1; table 1)[8,11,12,20,261]. This could result in the restoration of the regeneration program, and thereby prevent the progressive loss of functions of these adult stem cells with aging and lead to treatment of diverse human disorders. Amongst them, there are lung disorders (interstitial lung diseases, cystic fibrosis, asthma, chronic bronchitis and emphysema) [31,45-47,88,130], chronic liver injuries (hepatitis and liver cirrhosis) [21,25,32,34,48,49,246,247], gastrointestinal disorders (chronic inflammatory bowel diseases and ulcers) [15,16,50,135,262], eye diseases (partial or total limbal and/or conjunctival stem cell deficiency, bullous keratopathy, glaucoma and retinal damages) [17,60,61,93, 111,117,119,254,263] and skin and hair disorders [147,259,264]. Moreover, the targeting of their malignant counterparts, cancer stem/progenitor cells and their local microenviroment involved in cancer development also offers great promises for the development of new therapeutic approaches for treating the aggressive and metastatic cancer derived from these tissue-resident adult stem cells.

NEW CONCEPTS ON CANCER STEM/PROGENITOR CELLS AND THEIR THERAPEUTIC IMPLICATIONS FOR CANCER TREATMENT

The cancer stem/progenitor cell concepts are based on the accumulating lines of evidence that the most of cancers including leukemias, lymphomas, multiple myeloma, melanoma, head and neck, eye, brain, breast, ovary, prostate, liver, pancreas and gastrointestinal cancers may arise from the malignant transformation of embryonic or adult stem cells into cancer stem/progenitor cells also designated cancer-initiating cells (figure 2) [8,14,18,29,37,68-79,265]. Cancer stem/progenitor cells, which are endowed with self-renewal potential and multilineage differentiating ability can generate the total bulk mass of further differentiated cancer cells *in vitro* and *in vivo*, and thereby drive tumorigenesis and metastases at distant tissues/organs [8,14,37,68-72,74,77-79]. Moreover, the modest efficacy of current clinical therapies against aggressive and metastaic cancers, which often result to disease relapse and mortality of patients, also suggest that the highly tumorigenic and migrating cancer stem/progenitor cells may to be more resistance or insensitive to convential treatments [8,14,18,28,37,77-80]. Thereby, they could persist at the primary and secondary neoplasms and be responsible for the metastases and disease recurrence. In support with these new concepts on the leukemic and tumorigenic and migrating cancer stem/progenitor cells, numerous data have revealed their critical implications in the initiation and progression of the most the aggressive and recurrent cancers and treatment resistance [8,14,37,68-72,74,77-79,266]. Furthermore, further differentiated tumor cells and activated stromal cells including myofibroblasts as well as BM-derived cells including immune cells, macrophages, HSCs and EPCs attracted at the tumoral sites, also may actively collaborate during each step of the tumor formation at primary and secondary sites (figure 2) [14,37,77-79,150-155,267,268]. Therefore, the targeting of the cancer stem/progenitor cells and their local microenviroment involved in the cancer development offers great promises for the development of new therapeutic approaches for treating the aggressive, metastatic and recurrent cancers in the clinics [14,37,74,77-79]. More specifically, the molecular targeting of the tumorigenic cascades such as EGFR, hedgehog and/or Wnt/β-catenin, oncogenic signaling elements (telomerase, Scr, Bcl-2, NF-kB, PI$_3$K/AKT, COX-2) and ABC multidrug efflux pumps that assume a critical function in regulating the stem cell self-renewal, differentiation, survival and/or drug resistance of cancer stem/progenitor cells, in certain leukemia subtypes, multiple myeloma and numerous solid cancers is of particular therapeutic interest for eradicating the cancer-initiating cells (figure 2) [8,14,18,29,37,77-80,269,270]. The targeting of the microenvironment of cancer stem/progenitor cells including the host cells such as myofibroblasts that support their malignant transformation as well as the use of anti-angionegic agents also may constitute an adjuvant treatment for counteracting the cancer progression to metastatic and lethal disease states [14,37,77-79].

In addition, the recent development of diverse enhanced delivery techniques for administration of anti-carcinogenic drugs may constitute promising approaches for targeting cancer stem/progenitor cells, which express specific biomarkers, and thereby reverse their multi-drug resistance phenotype *in vivo*. Among the available strategies, there are the targeted delivered of therapeutic agents into tumors by using the conjugation/fusion of drugs to tumor-specific antibodies, encapsulation of chemotherapeutic drugs in liposomes, or other carriers such as nanoparticles as well as use of genetically-engineered stem/progenitor cells as vehicles [271-274]. More specifically, the gene therapies by using genetically-modified stem cells as carriers for the delivery of anti-angiogenic or cytotoxic agents at specific tumoral sites represent promising strategies for treating numerous aggressive and metastatic cancers (figure 2) [8,275-278]. For instance, it has been observed that genetically-modified migrating NSCs, which are able to migrate through the CNS and reach the extracranial neoplastic sites, may be transplanted in the animal models *in vivo* and specifically attracted to tumoral sites due to the release of chemotactic signals such as VEGF and SDF-1 [275,278,279]. Importantly, the combined treatment with 5-fluorocytosine plus engineered NSCs expressing cytosine deaminase, which acts as a pro-drug activating enzyme, resulted in significant cytotoxic effects on melanoma cells as well as a reduction in tumor border in animal models with established melanoma brain metastasis *in vivo* [279]. Additionally, the combined used of HSC transplant, alone or in combination therapies with high-dose chemotherapy or ionizing radiation, also constitute a major advance by offering an alternative therapeutic strategy to treat and cure several high-risk patients with advanced, metastatic and/or relapsed/refractory leukemias, multiple myelanomas and Hodgkin's and non-Hodgkin's lymphomas and aggressive non-hematological cancers such as melanoma, retinoblastoma, kidney, lung, brain, pancreatic, breast and ovarian and prostatic cancers [8,14,62,65-67,134,280-282]. The data of a recent study have also indicated that BM-resident MSCs isolated from patients with acute myeloid leukemia (AML) may exhibit abnormal biological properties including a limited proliferation capacity and impaired differentiation ability [283]. These observations underline the importance to also provide new functional MSCs endowed with the immunomodulatory properties in BM-derived cell-based transplantation therapies for restoring the normal hematopoiesis in patients with AML [134].

CONCLUSION

Taken together, these advancements in the research on embryonic, fetal, placental, amniotic, umbilical and diverse tissue-resident adult stem cells/progenitors have provided experimental evidence supporting their therapeutic potential for the cell replacement therapies in regenerative medicine and gene therapies for treating numerous human disorders. More specifically, the recent progress in the field of tissue-resident adult stem/progenitor cell research suggests their major implications in tissue homeostatic state maintenance under physiologic conditions as well as their malignant counterparts including the cancer stem/progenitor cells in the development of numerous human disorders and aggressive and recurrent cancers. Thus, these results support the feasibility to replace or target the malignant adult stem/progenitor cells endowed with a self-renewal potential for treating diverse incurable human disorders. Further research is however necessary to more precisely establish the gene expression patterns of normal and malignant embryonic, fetal and adult stem/progenitor cell *versus* their differentiated progenies in order to identify the specific biomarkers as well as the molecular mechanisms that may regulate their biological behavior *in vivo* and after their *ex vivo* expansion. The identification of the specific intrinsic factors that govern the decision between the self-renewal *versus* differentiation of tissue-resident adult stem cells as well as the influence of the extracelllular signals from their local microenvironment "niche" on their behavior is notably of immense interest for the design of new therapeutic strategies. These future studies should lead to the identification of the specific growth factors, cytokines and/or chemokines and host cells that control the expansion and commitment of these immature cells into the specific differentiated cell lineages. Hence, these studies should aid to optimize the methods for the *ex vitro* and *in vivo* expansion of pluripotent and multipotent stem cells and differentiation into wanted cell lineages as well as the most appropriate administration mode for their delivery in the specific damaged tissue areas *in vivo*. These additional investigations on the establishment of specific properties of embryonic, fetal and diverse tissue-resident adult stem cells/progenitors is essential for the successful formulation of therapeutic stem cell-based approaches that could be translated for treating and even curing diverse human inherited diseases, degenerative disorders and agressive and recurrent cancers which remain incurable in the clinics with the current conventional therapies.

ACKNOWLEDGMENTS

This work was supported by the grants from the U.S. Department of Defense (PC04502, OC04110) and the National Institutes of Health (CA78590, CA111294). We thank Ms. Kristi L. Berger for editing the manuscript.

REFERENCES

[1] Aboody,K.S., Bush,R.A., Garcia,E., Metz,M.Z., Najbauer,J., Justus,K.A., Phelps,D.A., Remack,J.S., Yoon,K.J., Gillespie,S., Kim,S.U., Glackin,C.A., Potter,P.M., and Danks,M.K. (2006) Development of a tumor-selective approach to treat metastatic cancer. *PLoS.ONE.*, 1, e23.

[2] Ahmad,I., Das,A.V., James,J., Bhattacharya,S., and Zhao,X. (2004) Neural stem cells in the mammalian eye: types and regulation. *Semin.Cell Dev.Biol.*, 15, 53-62.

[3] Ahmadi,H., Baharvand,H., Ashtiani,S.K., Soleimani,M., Sadeghian,H., Ardekani,J.M., Mehrjerdi,N.Z., Kouhkan,A., Namiri,M., Madani-Civi,M., Fattahi,F., Shahverdi,A., and Dizaji,A.V. (2007) Safety analysis and improved cardiac function following local autologous transplantation of CD133(+) enriched bone marrow cells after myocardial infarction. *Curr.Neurovasc.Res.*, 4, 153-160.

[4] Al-Hajj,M. and Clarke,M.F. (2004) Self-renewal and solid tumor stem cells. *Oncogene*, 23, 7274-7282.

[5] Alison,M.R., Brittan,M., Lovell,M.J., and Wright,N.A. (2006) Markers of adult tissue-based stem cells. *Handb.Exp.Pharmacol.*, 185-227.

[6] Alison,M.R., Vig,P., Russo,F., Bigger,B.W., Amofah,E., Themis,M., and Forbes,S. (2004) Hepatic stem cells: from inside and outside the liver? *Cell Prolif.*, 37, 1-21.

[7] Alviano,F., Fossati,V., Marchionni,C., Arpinati,M., Bonsi,L., Franchina,M., Lanzoni,G., Cantoni,S., Cavallini,C., Bianchi,F., Tazzari,P.L., Pasquinelli,G., Foroni,L., Ventura,C., Grossi,A., and Bagnara,G.P. (2007) Term amniotic membrane is a high throughput source for multipotent mesenchymal stem cells with the ability to differentiate into endothelial cells *in vitro*. *BMC.Dev.Biol.*, 7, 11.

[8] Andrade,C.F., Wong,A.P., Waddell,T.K., Keshavjee,S., and Liu,M. (2007) Cell-based tissue engineering for lung regeneration. *Am.J.Physiol.Lung Cell Mol.Physiol.*, 292, L510-L518.

[9] Andrews,P.W., Matin,M.M., Bahrami,A.R., Damjanov,I., Gokhale,P., and Draper,J.S. (2005) Embryonic stem (ES) cells and embryonal carcinoma (EC) cells: opposite sides of the same coin. *Biochem.Soc.Trans.*, 33, 1526-1530.

[10] Anton,R., Kuhl,M., and Pandur,P. (2007) A molecular signature for the "master" heart cell. *Bioessays*, 29, 422-426.

[11] Arai,F. and Suda,T. (2007) Maintenance of quiescent hematopoietic stem cells in the osteoblastic niche. *Ann.N.Y.Acad.Sci.*.

[12] Asahara,T. and Kawamoto,A. (2004) Endothelial progenitor cells for postnatal vasculogenesis. *Am.J.Physiol.Cell.Physiol.*, 287, C572-C579.

[13] Atsma,D.E., Fibbe,W.E., and Rabelink,T.J. (2007) Opportunities and challenges for mesenchymal stem cell-mediated heart repair. *Curr.Opin.Lipidol.*, 18, 645-649.

[14] Avramova,B., Jordanova,M., Michailov,G., Konstantinov,D., Christosova,I., and Bobev,D. (2006) Myeloablative chemotherapy with autologous peripheral blood stem cell transplantation in patients with poor-prognosis solid tumors - Bulgarian experience. *J.BUON.*, 11, 433-438.

[15] Balbarini,A., Barsotti,M.C., Di,S.R., Leone,A., and Santoni,T. (2007) Circulating endothelial progenitor cells characterization, function and relationship with cardiovascular risk factors. *Curr.Pharm.Des.*, 13, 1699-1713.

[16] Banas,A., Teratani,T., Yamamoto,Y., Tokuhara,M., Takeshita,F., Quinn,G., Okochi,H., and Ochiya,T. (2007) Adipose tissue-derived mesenchymal stem cells as a source of human hepatocytes. *Hepatology*, 46, 219-228.

[17] Banerjee,M., Kanitkar,M., and Bhonde,R.R. (2005) Approaches towards endogenous pancreatic regeneration. *Rev.Diabet.Stud.*, 2, 165-176.

[18] Banin,E., Obolensky,A., Idelson,M., Hemo,I., Reinhardtz,E., Pikarsky,E., Ben-Hur,T., and Reubinoff,B. (2006) Retinal incorporation and differentiation of neural precursors derived from human embryonic stem cells. *Stem Cells*, 24, 246-257.

[19] Bao,C., Guo,J., Lin,G., Hu,M., and Hu,Z. (2007) TNFR gene-modified mesenchymal stem cells attenuate inflammation and cardiac dysfunction following MI. *Scand.Cardiovasc.J.*, 1-7.

[20] Bapat,S.A., Mali,A.M., Koppikar,C.B., and Kurrey,N.K. (2005) Stem and progenitor-like cells contribute to the aggressive behavior of human epithelial ovarian cancer. *Cancer Res.*, 65, 3025-3029.

[21] Barfield,R.C., Hale,G.A., Burnette,K., Behm,F.G., Knapp,K., Eldridge,P., and Handgretinger,R. (2007) Autologous transplantation of CD133 selected hematopoietic progenitor cells for treatment of relapsed acute lymphoblastic leukemia. *Pediatr.Blood Cancer*, 48, 349-353.

[22] Barker,N., van Es,J.H., Kuipers,J., Kujala,P., van den,B.M., Cozijnsen,M., Haegebarth,A., Korving,J., Begthel,H., Peters,P.J., and Clevers,H. (2007) Identification of stem cells in small intestine and colon by marker gene Lgr5. *Nature*, 449, 1003-1007.

[23] Barrilleaux,B., Phinney,D.G., Prockop,D.J., and O'Connor,K.C. (2006) Review: *ex vivo* engineering of living tissues with adult stem cells. *Tissue Eng.*, 12, 3007-3019.
[24] Bartunek,J., Vanderheyden,M., Vandekerckhove,B., Mansour,S., De,B.B., De,B.P., Van,H., I, Lootens,N., Heyndrickx,G., and Wijns,W. (2005) Intracoronary injection of CD133-positive enriched bone marrow progenitor cells promotes cardiac recovery after recent myocardial infarction: feasibility and safety. *Circulation*, 112, I178-I183.
[25] Beachy,P.A., Karhadkar,S.S., and Berman,D.M. (2004) Tissue repair and stem cell renewal in carcinogenesis. *Nature*, 432, 324-331.
[26] Bearzi,C., Rota,M., Hosoda,T., Tillmanns,J., Nascimbene,A., De,A.A., Yasuzawa-Amano,S., Trofimova,I., Siggins,R.W., Lecapitaine,N., Cascapera,S., Beltrami,A.P., D'Alessandro,D.A., Zias,E., Quaini,F., Urbanek,K., Michler,R.E., Bolli,R., Kajstura,J., Leri,A., and Anversa,P. (2007) Human cardiac stem cells. *Proc.Natl.Acad.Sci.U.S.A.*, 104, 14068-14073.
[27] Behfar,A., Perez-Terzic,C., Faustino,R.S., Arrell,D.K., Hodgson,D.M., Yamada,S., Puceat,M., Niederlander,N., Alekseev,A.E., Zingman,L.V., and Terzic,A. (2007) Cardiopoietic programming of embryonic stem cells for tumor-free heart repair. *J.Exp.Med.*, 204, 405-420.
[28] Beltrami,A.P., Barlucchi,L., Torella,D., Baker,M., Limana,F., Chimenti,S., Kasahara,H., Rota,M., Musso,E., Urbanek,K., Leri,A., Kajstura,J., Nadal-Ginard,B., and Anversa,P. (2003) Adult cardiac stem cells are multipotent and support myocardial regeneration. *Cell*, 114, 763-776.
[29] Bernardo,M.E., Emons,J.A., Karperien,M., Nauta,A.J., Willemze,R., Roelofs,H., Romeo,S., Marchini,A., Rappold,G.A., Vukicevic,S., Locatelli,F., and Fibbe,W.E. (2007) Human mesenchymal stem cells derived from bone marrow display a better chondrogenic differentiation compared with other sources. *Connect.Tissue Res.*, 48, 132-140.
[30] Bobis,S., Jarocha,D., and Majka,M. (2006) Mesenchymal stem cells: characteristics and clinical applications. *Folia Histochem.Cytobiol.*, 44, 215-230.
[31] Bonanno,G., Mariotti,A., Procoli,A., Corallo,M., Rutella,S., Pessina,G., Scambia,G., Mancuso,S., and Pierelli,L. (2007) Human cord blood CD133+ cells immunoselected by a clinical-grade apparatus differentiate *in vitro* into endothelial- and cardiomyocyte-like cells. *Transfusion*, 47, 280-289.
[32] Bonner-Weir,S. and Weir,G.C. (2005) New sources of pancreatic beta-cells. *Nat.Biotechnol.*, 23, 857-861.
[33] Bouwens,L. and Rooman,I. (2005) Regulation of pancreatic beta-cell mass. *Physiol.Rev.*, 85, 1255-1270.
[34] Bregni,M., Bernardi,M., Ciceri,F., and Peccatori,J. (2004) Allogeneic stem cell transplantation for the treatment of advanced solid tumors. *Springer Semin.Immunopathol.*, 26, 95-108.
[35] Brittan,M. and Wright,N.A. (2002) Gastrointestinal stem cells. *J.Pathol.*, 197, 492-509.
[36] Brunstein,C.G., Setubal,D.C., and Wagner,J.E. (2007) Expanding the role of umbilical cord blood transplantation. *Br.J.Haematol.*, 137, 20-35.
[37] Bryder,D., Rossi,D.J., and Weissman,I.L. (2006) Hematopoietic stem cells: the paradigmatic tissue-specific stem cell. *Am.J.Pathol.*, 169, 338-346.
[38] Burke,Z.D., Thowfeequ,S., Peran,M., and Tosh,D. (2007) Stem cells in the adult pancreas and liver. *Biochem.J.*, 404, 169-178.
[39] Cantz,T., Manns,M.P., and Ott,M. (2007) Stem cells in liver regeneration and therapy. *Cell Tissue Res.*.

[40] Caspi,O., Huber,I., Kehat,I., Habib,M., Arbel,G., Gepstein,A., Yankelson,L., Aronson,D., Beyar,R., and Gepstein,L. (2007) Transplantation of human embryonic stem cell-derived cardiomyocytes improves myocardial performance in infarcted rat hearts. *J.Am.Coll.Cardiol.*, 50, 1884-1893.

[41] Ceschel,S., Casotto,V., Valsecchi,M.G., Tamaro,P., Jankovic,M., Hanau,G., Fossati,F., Pillon,M., Rondelli,R., Sandri,A., Silvestri,D., Haupt,R., and Cuttini,M. (2006) Survival after relapse in children with solid tumors: a follow-up study from the Italian off-therapy registry. *Pediatr.Blood Cancer*, 47, 560-566.

[42] Chan,J., Waddington,S.N., O'Donoghue,K., Kurata,H., Guillot,P.V., Gotherstrom,C., Themis,M., Morgan,J.E., and Fisk,N.M. (2007) Widespread distribution and muscle differentiation of human fetal mesenchymal stem cells after intrauterine transplantation in dystrophic mdx mouse. *Stem Cells*, 25, 875-884.

[43] Chang,C.M., Kao,C.L., Chang,Y.L., Yang,M.J., Chen,Y.C., Sung,B.L., Tsai,T.H., Chao,K.C., Chiou,S.H., and Ku,H.H. (2007a) Placenta-derived multipotent stem cells induced to differentiate into insulin-positive cells. *Biochem.Biophys.Res.Commun.*, 357, 414-420.

[44] Chang,Y.C., Shyu,W.C., Lin,S.Z., and Li,H. (2007b) Regenerative therapy for stroke. *Cell Transplant.*, 16, 171-181.

[45] Chang,Y.J., Shih,D.T., Tseng,C.P., Hsieh,T.B., Lee,D.C., and Hwang,S.M. (2006) Disparate mesenchyme-lineage tendencies in mesenchymal stem cells from human bone marrow and umbilical cord blood. *Stem Cells*, 24, 679-685.

[46] Chen,Y.T., Li,W., Hayashida,Y., He,H., Chen,S.Y., Tseng,D.Y., Kheirkhah,A., and Tseng,S.C. (2007) Human amniotic epithelial cells as novel feeder layers for promoting *ex vivo* expansion of limbal epithelial progenitor cells. *Stem Cells*, 25, 1995-2005.

[47] Chen,Z., de Paiva,C.S., Luo,L., Kretzer,F.L., Pflugfelder,S.C., and Li,D.Q. (2004) Characterization of putative stem cell phenotype in human limbal epithelia. *Stem Cells*, 22, 355-366.

[48] Christoforou,N. and Gearhart,J.D. (2007) Stem cells and their potential in cell-based cardiac therapies. *Prog.Cardiovasc.Dis.*, 49, 396-413.

[49] Corsi,K.A., Schwarz,E.M., Mooney,D.J., and Huard,J. (2007) Regenerative medicine in orthopaedic surgery. *J.Orthop.Res.*, 25, 1261-1268.

[50] D'Alessandro,J.S., Lu,K., Fung,B.P., Colman,A., and Clarke,D.L. (2007) Rapid and efficient *in vitro* generation of pancreatic islet progenitor cells from nonendocrine epithelial cells in the adult human pancreas. *Stem Cells Dev.*, 16, 75-89.

[51] D'Amour,K.A., Agulnick,A.D., Eliazer,S., Kelly,O.G., Kroon,E., and Baetge,E.E. (2005) Efficient differentiation of human embryonic stem cells to definitive endoderm. *Nat.Biotechnol.*, 23, 1534-1541.

[52] da Silva,M.L., Chagastelles,P.C., and Nardi,N.B. (2006) Mesenchymal stem cells reside in virtually all post-natal organs and tissues. *J.Cell Sci.*, 119, 2204-2213.

[53] Das,A.V., James,J., Rahnenfuhrer,J., Thoreson,W.B., Bhattacharya,S., Zhao,X., and Ahmad,I. (2005) Retinal properties and potential of the adult mammalian ciliary epithelium stem cells. *Vision Res.*, 45, 1653-1666.

[54] Davidoff,A.M., Ng,C.Y., Brown,P., Leary,M.A., Spurbeck,W.W., Zhou,J., Horwitz,E., Vanin,E.F., and Nienhuis,A.W. (2001) Bone marrow-derived cells contribute to tumor neovasculature and, when modified to express an angiogenesis inhibitor, can restrict tumor growth in mice. *Clin. Cancer Res.*, 7, 2870-2879.

[55] Dawn,B., Stein,A.B., Urbanek,K., Rota,M., Whang,B., Rastaldo,R., Torella,D., Tang,X.L., Rezazadeh,A., Kajstura,J., Leri,A., Hunt,G., Varma,J., Prabhu,S.D.,

Anversa,P., and Bolli,R. (2005) Cardiac stem cells delivered intravascularly traverse the vessel barrier, regenerate infarcted myocardium, and improve cardiac function. *Proc.Natl.Acad.Sci.U.S.A.*, 102, 3766-3771.

[56] de Macedo Braga,L.M., Rosa,K., Rodrigues,B., Malfitano,C., Camassola,M., Chagastelles,P., Lacchini,S., Fiorino,P., De,A.K., D'Agord,S.B., Irigoyen,M.C., and Beyer,N.N. (2007) Systemic delivery of adult stem cells improves cardiac function in spontaneously hypertensive rats. *Clin. Exp.Pharmacol.Physiol.*

[57] de Paiva,C.S., Pflugfelder,S.C., and Li,D.Q. (2006) Cell size correlates with phenotype and proliferative capacity in human corneal epithelial cells. *Stem Cells*, 24, 368-375.

[58] Dean,M., Fojo,T., and Bates,S. (2005) Tumour stem cells and drug resistance. *Nat.Rev.Cancer*, 5, 275-284.

[59] Delorme,B., Chateauvieux,S., and Charbord,P. (2006) The concept of mesenchymal stem cells. *Regen.Med.*, 1, 497-509.

[60] Dhar,S., Yoon,E.S., Kachgal,S., and Evans,G.R. (2007) Long-term maintenance of neuronally differentiated human adipose tissue-derived stem cells. *Tissue Eng.*, 13, 2625-2632.

[61] Dhawan,J. and Rando,T.A. (2005) Stem cells in postnatal myogenesis: molecular mechanisms of satellite cell quiescence, activation and replenishment. *Trends Cell Biol.*, 15, 666-673.

[62] Domanska-Janik,K., Habich,A., Sarnowska,A., and Janowski,M. (2006) Neural commitment of cord blood stem cells (HUCB-NSC/NP): therapeutic perspectives. *Acta Neurobiol.Exp.(Wars.)*, 66, 279-291.

[63] Dragoo,J.L., Carlson,G., McCormick,F., Khan-Farooqi,H., Zhu,M., Zuk,P.A., and Benhaim,P. (2007) Healing full-thickness cartilage defects using adipose-derived stem cells. *Tissue Eng.*, 13, 1615-1621.

[64] Dua,H.S., Shanmuganathan,V.A., Powell-Richards,A.O., Tighe,P.J., and Joseph,A. (2005) Limbal epithelial crypts: a novel anatomical structure and a putative limbal stem cell niche. *Br.J.Ophthalmol.*, 89, 529-532.

[65] Eftekharpour,E., Karimi-Abdolrezaee,S., Wang,J., El,B.H., Morshead,C., and Fehlings,M.G. (2007) Myelination of congenitally dysmyelinated spinal cord axons by adult neural precursor cells results in formation of nodes of Ranvier and improved axonal conduction. *J.Neurosci.*, 27, 3416-3428.

[66] Elabd,C., Chiellini,C., Massoudi,A., Cochet,O., Zaragosi,L.E., Trojani,C., Michiels,J.F., Weiss,P., Carle,G., Rochet,N., Dechesne,C.A., Ailhaud,G., Dani,C., and Amri,E.Z. (2007) Human adipose tissue-derived multipotent stem cells differentiate *in vitro* and *in vivo* into osteocyte-like cells. *Biochem.Biophys.Res.Commun.*, 361, 342-348.

[67] Fang,D., Nguyen,T.K., Leishear,K., Finko,R., Kulp,A.N., Hotz,S., Van Belle,P.A., Xu,X., Elder,D.E., and Herlyn,M. (2005) A tumorigenic subpopulation with stem cell properties in melanomas. *Cancer Res.*, 65, 9328-9337.

[68] Fausto,N., Campbell,J.S., and Riehle,K.J. (2006) Liver regeneration. *Hepatology*, 43, S45-S53.

[69] Feldmann,G., Dhara,S., Fendrich,V., Bedja,D., Beaty,R., Mullendore,M., Karikari,C., Alvarez,H., Iacobuzio-Donahue,C., Jimeno,A., Gabrielson,K.L., Matsui,W., and Maitra,A. (2007) Blockade of hedgehog signaling inhibits pancreatic cancer invasion and metastases: a new paradigm for combination therapy in solid cancers. *Cancer Res.*, 67, 2187-2196.

[70] Fellous,T.G., Guppy,N.J., Brittan,M., and Alison,M.R. (2007) Cellular pathways to beta-cell replacement. *Diabetes Metab.Res.Rev.*, 23, 87-99.

[71] Fiegel,H.C., Lange,C., Kneser,U., Lambrecht,W., Zander,A.R., Rogiers,X., and Kluth,D. (2006) Fetal and adult liver stem cells for liver regeneration and tissue engineering. *J.Cell.Mol.Med.*, 10, 577-587.

[72] Fox,J.G. and Wang,T.C. (2007) Inflammation, atrophy, and gastric cancer. *J.Clin.Invest.*, 117, 60-69.

[73] Friedrich,E.B., Walenta,K., Scharlau,J., Nickenig,G., and Werner,N. (2006) CD34-/CD133+/VEGFR-2+ endothelial progenitor cell subpopulation with potent vasoregenerative capacities. *Circ.Res.*, 98, E20-E25.

[74] Fujikawa,T., Oh,S.H., Pi,L., Hatch,H.M., Shupe,T., and Petersen,B.E. (2005) Teratoma formation leads to failure of treatment for type I diabetes using embryonic stem cell-derived insulin-producing cells. *Am.J.Pathol.*, 166, 1781-1791.

[75] Furst,G., Schulte am,E.J., Poll,L.W., Hosch,S.B., Fritz,L.B., Klein,M., Godehardt,E., Krieg,A., Wecker,B., Stoldt,V., Stockschlader,M., Eisenberger,C.F., Modder,U., and Knoefel,W.T. (2007) Portal vein embolization and autologous $CD133^{+}$ bone marrow stem cells for liver regeneration: initial experience. *Radiology*, 243, 171-179.

[76] Furuta,A., Jankowski,R.J., Pruchnic,R., Yoshimura,N., and Chancellor,M.B. (2007) The potential of muscle-derived stem cells for stress urinary incontinence. *Expert.Opin.Biol.Ther.*, 7, 1483-1486.

[77] Galderisi,U., Cipollaro,M., and Giordano,A. (2006) Stem cells and brain cancer. *Cell Death.Differ.*, 13, 5-11.

[78] Gangaram-Panday,S.T., Faas,M.M., and de Vos P. (2007) Towards stem-cell therapy in the endocrine pancreas. *Trends Mol.Med.*, 13, 164-173.

[79] Ganss,R. (2006) Tumor stroma fosters neovascularization by recruitment of progenitor cells into the tumor bed. *J.Cell.Mol.Med.*, 10, 857-865.

[80] Gao,F., He,T., Wang,H., Yu,S., Yi,D., Liu,W., and Cai,Z. (2007) A promising strategy for the treatment of ischemic heart disease: Mesenchymal stem cell-mediated vascular endothelial growth factor gene transfer in rats. *Can.J.Cardiol.*, 23, 891-898.

[81] Gao,J., Prough,D.S., McAdoo,D.J., Grady,J.J., Parsley,M.O., Ma,L., Tarensenko,Y.I., and Wu,P. (2006) Transplantation of primed human fetal neural stem cells improves cognitive function in rats after traumatic brain injury. *Exp.Neurol.*, 201, 281-292.

[82] Garbuzova-Davis,S., Willing,A.E., Saporta,S., Bickford,P.C., Gemma,C., Chen,N., Sanberg,C.D., Klasko,S.K., Borlongan,C.V., and Sanberg,P.R. (2006) Novel cell therapy approaches for brain repair. *Prog.Brain Res.*, 157, 207-222.

[83] Geraerts,M., Krylyshkina,O., Debyser,Z., and Baekelandt,V. (2007) Concise review: therapeutic strategies for Parkinson disease based on the modulation of adult neurogenesis. *Stem Cells*, 25, 263-270.

[84] Gharaee-Kermani,M., Gyetko,M.R., Hu,B., and Phan,S.H. (2007) New insights into the pathogenesis and treatment of idiopathic pulmonary fibrosis: a potential role for stem cells in the lung parenchyma and implications for therapy. *Pharm.Res.*, 24, 819-841.

[85] Ghods,A.J., Irvin,D., Liu,G., Yuan,X., Abdulkadir,I.R., Tunici,P., Konda,B., Wachsmann-Hogiu,S., Black,K.L., and Yu,J.S. (2007) Spheres isolated from 9L gliosarcoma rat cell line possess chemoresistant and aggressive cancer stem-like cells. *Stem Cells*, 25, 1645-1653.

[86] Gimble,J.M., Katz,A.J., and Bunnell,B.A. (2007) Adipose-derived stem cells for regenerative medicine. *Circ.Res.*, 100, 1249-1260.

[87] Gindraux,F., Selmani,Z., Obert,L., Davani,S., Tiberghien,P., Herve,P., and Deschaseaux,F. (2007) Human and rodent bone marrow mesenchymal stem cells that express primitive stem cell markers can be directly enriched by using the CD49a molecule. *Cell Tissue Res.*, 327, 471-483.

[88] Goessler,U.R., Riedel,K., Hormann,K., and Riedel,F. (2006) Perspectives of gene therapy in stem cell tissue engineering. *Cells Tissues.Organs*, 183, 169-179.

[89] Griffiths,M.J., Bonnet,D., and Janes,S.M. (2005) Stem cells of the alveolar epithelium. *Lancet*, 366, 249-260.

[90] Guettier,C. (2005) Which stem cells for adult liver? *Ann.Pathol.*, 25, 33-44.

[91] Guldner,N.W., Kajahn,J., Klinger,M., Sievers,H.H., and Kruse,C. (2006) Autonomously contracting human cardiomyocytes generated from adult pancreatic stem cells and enhanced in co-cultures with myocardial biopsies. *Int.J.Artif.Organs*, 29, 1158-1166.

[92] Haider,H.K., Elmadbouh,I., Jean-Baptiste,M., and Ashraf,M. (2007) Non-viral vector gene modification of stem cells for myocardial repair. *Mol.Med.*.

[93] Halban,P.A. (2004) Cellular sources of new pancreatic beta cells and therapeutic implications for regenerative medicine. *Nat.Cell Biol.*, 6, 1021-1025.

[94] Hale,G.A. (2005) Autologous hematopoietic stem cell transplantation for pediatric solid tumors. *Expert Rev.Anticancer Ther.*, 5, 835-846.

[95] Hattan,N., Kawaguchi,H., Ando,K., Kuwabara,E., Fujita,J., Murata,M., Suematsu,M., Mori,H., and Fukuda,K. (2005) Purified cardiomyocytes from bone marrow mesenchymal stem cells produce stable intracardiac grafts in mice. *Cardiovasc.Res.*, 65, 334-344.

[96] Helder,M.N., Knippenberg,M., Klein-Nulend,J., and Wuisman,P.I. (2007) Stem cells from adipose tissue allow challenging new concepts for regenerative medicine. *Tissue Eng.*, 13, 1799-1808.

[97] Hemmoranta,H., Hautaniemi,S., Niemi,J., Nicorici,D., Laine,J., Yli-Harja,O., Partanen,J., and Jaatinen,T. (2006) Transcriptional profiling reflects shared and unique characters for $CD34^+$ and $CD133^+$ cells. *Stem Cells Dev.*, 15, 839-851.

[98] Herrera,M.B., Bruno,S., Buttiglieri,S., Tetta,C., Gatti,S., Deregibus,M.C., Bussolati,B., and Camussi,G. (2006) Isolation and characterization of a stem cell population from adult human liver. *Stem Cells*, 24, 2840-2850.

[99] Herzog,E.L. and Krause,D.S. (2006) Engraftment of marrow-derived epithelial cells: the role of fusion. *Proc.Am.Thorac.Soc.*, 3, 691-695.

[100] Hoogduijn,M.J., Crop,M.J., Peeters,A.M., Van Osch,G.J., Balk,A.H., Ijzermans,J.N., Weimar,W., and Baan,C.C. (2007) Human heart, spleen, and perirenal fat-derived mesenchymal stem cells have immunomodulatory capacities. *Stem Cells Dev.*, 16, 597-604.

[101] Hope,K.J., Jin,L., and Dick,J.E. (2004) Acute myeloid leukemia originates from a hierarchy of leukemic stem cell classes that differ in self-renewal capacity. *Nat.Immunol.*, 5, 738-743.

[102] Huang,S.D., Lu,F.L., Xu,X.Y., Liu,X.H., Zhao,X.X., Zhao,B.Z., Wang,L., Gong,D.J., Yuan,Y., and Xu,Z.Y. (2006) Transplantation of angiogenin-overexpressing mesenchymal stem cells synergistically augments cardiac function in a porcine model of chronic ischemia. *J.Thorac.Cardiovasc.Surg.*, 132, 1329-1338.

[103] Ilancheran,S., Michalska,A., Peh,G., Wallace,E.M., Pera,M., and Manuelpillai,U. (2007) Stem cells derived from human fetal membranes display multi-lineage differentiation potential. *Biol.Reprod.*, 77, 577-588.

[104] Iwaguro,H. and Asahara,T. (2005) Endothelial progenitor cell culture and gene transfer. *Methods Mol.Med.*, 112, 239-247.
[105] Janssens,S., Dubois,C., Bogaert,J., Theunissen,K., Deroose,C., Desmet,W., Kalantzi,M., Herbots,L., Sinnaeve,P., Dens,J., Maertens,J., Rademakers,F., Dymarkowski,S., Gheysens,O., Van,C.J., Bormans,G., Nuyts,J., Belmans,A., Mortelmans,L., Boogaerts,M., and Van de,W.F. (2006) Autologous bone marrow-derived stem-cell transfer in patients with ST-segment elevation myocardial infarction: double-blind, randomised controlled trial. *Lancet*, 367, 113-121.
[106] Jiang,J., Au,M., Lu,K., Eshpeter,A., Korbutt,G., Fisk,G., and Majumdar,A.S. (2007) Generation of insulin-producing islet-like clusters from human embryonic stem cells. *Stem Cells*, 25, 1940-1953.
[107] Jin,C.Z., Park,S.R., Choi,B.H., Lee,K.Y., Kang,C.K., and Min,B.H. (2007) Human amniotic membrane as a delivery matrix for articular cartilage repair. *Tissue Eng.*, 13, 693-702.
[108] Jo,J., Nagaya,N., Miyahara,Y., Kataoka,M., Harada-Shiba,M., Kangawa,K., and Tabata,Y. (2007) Transplantation of genetically engineered mesenchymal stem cells improves cardiac function in rats with myocardial infarction: benefit of a novel nonviral vector, cationized dextran. *Tissue Eng.*, 13, 313-322.
[109] Ju,Z., Jiang,H., Jaworski,M., Rathinam,C., Gompf,A., Klein,C., Trumpp,A., and Rudolph,K.L. (2007) Telomere dysfunction induces environmental alterations limiting hematopoietic stem cell function and engraftment. *Nat.Med.*, 13, 742-747.
[110] Kajstura,J., Rota,M., Whang,B., Cascapera,S., Hosoda,T., Bearzi,C., Nurzynska,D., Kasahara,H., Zias,E., Bonafe,M., Nadal-Ginard,B., Torella,D., Nascimbene,A., Quaini,F., Urbanek,K., Leri,A., and Anversa,P. (2005) Bone marrow cells differentiate in cardiac cell lineages after infarction independently of cell fusion. *Circ.Res.*, 96, 127-137.
[111] Kalluri,R. and Zeisberg,M. (2006) Fibroblasts in cancer. *Nat.Rev.Cancer*, 6, 392-401.
[112] Kaplan,R.N., Riba,R.D., Zacharoulis,S., Bramley,A.H., Vincent,L., Costa,C., MacDonald,D.D., Jin,D.K., Shido,K., Kerns,S.A., Zhu,Z., Hicklin,D., Wu,Y., Port,J.L., Altorki,N., Port,E.R., Ruggero,D., Shmelkov,S.V., Jensen,K.K., Rafii,S., and Lyden,D. (2005) VEGFR1-positive haematopoietic bone marrow progenitors initiate the pre-metastatic niche. *Nature*, 438, 820-827.
[113] Kawamoto,A., Murayama,T., Kusano,K., Ii,M., Tkebuchava,T., Shintani,S., Iwakura,A., Johnson,I., von,S.P., Hanley,A., Gavin,M., Curry,C., Silver,M., Ma,H., Kearney,M., and Losordo,D.W. (2004) Synergistic effect of bone marrow mobilization and vascular endothelial growth factor-2 gene therapy in myocardial ischemia. *Circulation*, 110, 1398-1405.
[114] Khalil,P.N., Weiler,V., Nelson,P.J., Khalil,M.N., Moosmann,S., Mutschler,W.E., Siebeck,M., and Huss,R. (2007) Nonmyeloablative stem cell therapy enhances microcirculation and tissue regeneration in murine inflammatory bowel disease. *Gastroenterology*, 132, 944-954.
[115] Kiel,M.J., Yilmaz,O.H., Iwashita,T., Yilmaz,O.H., Terhorst,C., and Morrison,S.J. (2005) SLAM family receptors distinguish hematopoietic stem and progenitor cells and reveal endothelial niches for stem cells. *Cell*, 121, 1109-1121.
[116] Kim,C.F., Jackson,E.L., Woolfenden,A.E., Lawrence,S., Babar,I., Vogel,S., Crowley,D., Bronson,R.T., and Jacks,T. (2005) Identification of bronchioalveolar stem cells in normal lung and lung cancer. *Cell*, 121, 823-835.

[117] Kim,S., Shin,J.S., Kim,H.J., Fisher,R.C., Lee,M.J., and Kim,C.W. (2007a) Streptozotocin-induced diabetes can be reversed by hepatic oval cell activation through hepatic transdifferentiation and pancreatic islet regeneration. *Lab. Invest.*, 87, 702-712.

[118] Kim,S.E., Kim,B.K., Gil,J.E., Kim,S.K., and Kim,J.H. (2007b) Comparative analysis of the developmental competence of three human embryonic stem cell lines *in vitro*. *Mol.Cells*, 23, 49-56.

[119] Koblas,T., Harman,S.M., and Saudek,F. (2005) The application of umbilical cord blood cells in the treatment of diabetes mellitus. *Rev. Diabet.Stud.*, 2, 228-234.

[120] Koblas,T., Zacharovova,K., Berkova,Z., Mindlova,M., Girman,P., Dovolilova,E., Karasova,L., and Saudek,F. (2007) Isolation and characterization of human CXCR4-positive pancreatic cells. *Folia Biol.(Praha)*, 53, 13-22.

[121] Kondo,T., Case,J., Srour,E.F., and Hashino,E. (2006) Skeletal muscle-derived progenitor cells exhibit neural competence. *Neuroreport*, 17, 1-4.

[122] Kornblum,H.I. (2007) Introduction to neural stem cells. *Stroke*, 38, 810-816.

[123] Kuroda,R., Usas,A., Kubo,S., Corsi,K., Peng,H., Rose,T., Cummins,J., Fu,F.H., and Huard,J. (2006) Cartilage repair using bone morphogenetic protein 4 and muscle-derived stem cells. *Arthritis Rheum.*, 54, 433-442.

[124] Kuznetsov,S.L., Nikolaeva,L.R., Spivak,I.A., Chentsova,E.V., Poltavtseva,R.A., Marei,M.V., and Sukhikh,G.T. (2006) Effect of transplantation of cultured human neural stem and progenitor cells on regeneration of the cornea after chemical burn. *Bull.Exp.Biol.Med.*, 141, 129-132.

[125] Langenau,D.M., Keefe,M.D., Storer,N.Y., Guyon,J.R., Kutok,J.L., Le,X., Goessling,W., Neuberg,D.S., Kunkel,L.M., and Zon,L.I. (2007) Effects of RAS on the genesis of embryonal rhabdomyosarcoma. *Genes Dev.*, 21, 1382-1395.

[126] Latella,G., Fiocchi,C., and Caprilli,R. (2007) Late-breaking news from the "4th International Meeting on Inflammatory Bowel Diseases" Capri, 2006. *Inflamm.Bowel.Dis.*, 13, 1031-1050.

[127] Lavker,R.M., Tseng,S.C., and Sun,T.T. (2004) Corneal epithelial stem cells at the limbus: looking at some old problems from a new angle. *Exp.Eye Res.*, 78, 433-446.

[128] Le Blanc K. and Ringden,O. (2006) Mesenchymal stem cells: properties and role in clinical bone marrow transplantation. *Curr.Opin.Immunol.*, 18, 586-591.

[129] Le Blanc K. and Ringden,O. (2007) Immunomodulation by mesenchymal stem cells and clinical experience. *J.Intern.Med.*, 262, 509-525.

[130] Lee,M.W., Moon,Y.J., Yang,M.S., Kim,S.K., Jang,I.K., Eom,Y.W., Park,J.S., Kim,H.C., Song,K.Y., Park,S.C., Lim,H.S., and Kim,Y.J. (2007) Neural differentiation of novel multipotent progenitor cells from cryopreserved human umbilical cord blood. *Biochem.Biophys.Res.Commun.*, 358, 637-643.

[131] Lees,J.G. and Tuch,B.E. (2006) Conversion of embryonic stem cells into pancreatic beta-cell surrogates guided by ontogeny. *Regen.Med.*, 1, 327-336.

[132] Leri,A., Kajstura,J., and Anversa,P. (2005) Cardiac stem cells and mechanisms of myocardial regeneration. *Physiol.Rev.*, 85, 1373-1416.

[133] Levy,V., Lindon,C., Zheng,Y., Harfe,B.D., and Morgan,B.A. (2007) Epidermal stem cells arise from the hair follicle after wounding. *FASEB J.*, 21, 1358-1366.

[134] Li,C., Heidt,D.G., Dalerba,P., Burant,C.F., Zhang,L., Adsay,V., Wicha,M., Clarke,M.F., and Simeone,D.M. (2007a) Identification of pancreatic cancer stem cells. *Cancer Res.*, 67, 1030-1037.

[135] Li,L. and Xie,T. (2005) Stem cell niche: Structure and function. *Annu.Rev.Cell Dev.Biol.*, 21, 605-631.

[136] Li,W., Hayashida,Y., He,H., Kuo,C.L., and Tseng,S.C. (2007b) The fate of limbal epithelial progenitor cells during explant culture on intact amniotic membrane. *Invest. Ophthalmol.Vis.Sci.*, 48, 605-613.

[137] Li,Y., Zhang,R., Qiao,H., Zhang,H., Wang,Y., Yuan,H., Liu,Q., Liu,D., Chen,L., and Pei,X. (2007c) Generation of insulin-producing cells from PDX-1 gene-modified human mesenchymal stem cells. *J.Cell.Physiol.*, 211, 36-44.

[138] Lim,D.A., Huang,Y.C., and Alvarez-Buylla,A. (2007) The adult neural stem cell niche: lessons for future neural cell replacement strategies. *Neurosurg.Clin.N.Am.*, 18, 81-92.

[139] Limb,G.A., Daniels,J.T., Cambrey,A.D., Secker,G.A., Shortt,A.J., Lawrence,J.M., and Khaw,P.T. (2006) Current prospects for adult stem cell-based therapies in ocular repair and regeneration. *Curr.Eye Res.*, 31, 381-390.

[140] Lin,H.T., Chiou,S.H., Kao,C.L., Shyr,Y.M., Hsu,C.J., Tarng,Y.W., Ho,L.L., Kwok,C.F., and Ku,H.H. (2006a) Characterization of pancreatic stem cells derived from adult human pancreas ducts by fluorescence activated cell sorting. *World J.Gastroenterol.*, 12, 4529-4535.

[141] Lin,Y., Chen,X., Yan,Z., Liu,L., Tang,W., Zheng,X., Li,Z., Qiao,J., Li,S., and Tian,W. (2006b) Multilineage differentiation of adipose-derived stromal cells from GFP transgenic mice. *Mol.Cell. Biochem.*, 285, 69-78.

[142] Lin,Y., Liu,L., Li,Z., Qiao,J., Wu,L., Tang,W., Zheng,X., Chen,X., Yan,Z., and Tian,W. (2006c) Pluripotency potential of human adipose-derived stem cells marked with exogenous green fluorescent protein. *Mol.Cell. Biochem.*, 291, 1-10.

[143] Lin,Y., Yan,Z., Liu,L., Qiao,J., Jing,W., Wu,L., Chen,X., Li,Z., Tang,W., Zheng,X., and Tian,W. (2006d) Proliferation and pluripotency potential of ectomesenchymal cells derived from first branchial arch. *Cell Prolif.*, 39, 79-92.

[144] Lindvall,O., Kokaia,Z., and Martinez-Serrano,A. (2004) Stem cell therapy for human neurodegenerative disorders-how to make it work. *Nat.Med.*, 10, S42-S50.

[145] Liu,F., Pan,X., Chen,G., Jiang,D., Cong,X., Fei,R., and Wei,L. (2006) Hematopoietic stem cells mobilized by granulocyte colony-stimulating factor partly contribute to liver graft regeneration after partial orthotopic liver transplantation. *Liver Transpl.*, 12, 1129-1137.

[146] Liu,X., Driskell,R.R., and Engelhardt,J.F. (2004) Airway glandular development and stem cells. *Curr.Top.Dev.Biol.*, 64, 33-56.

[147] Liu,Y., Yan,X., Sun,Z., Chen,B., Han,Q., Li,J., and Zhao,R.C. (2007) Flk-1(+) Adipose-derived mesenchymal stem cells differentiate into skeletal muscle satellite cells and ameliorate muscular dystrophy in MDX mice. *Stem Cells Dev.*, 16, 695-706.

[148] Lock,L.T. and Tzanakakis,E.S. (2007) Stem/Progenitor cell sources of insulin-producing cells for the treatment of diabetes. *Tissue Eng.*, 13, 1399-1412.

[149] Lovell,M.A., Geiger,H., Van Zant,G.E., Lynn,B.C., and Markesbery,W.R. (2006) Isolation of neural precursor cells from Alzheimer's disease and aged control postmortem brain. *Neurobiol.Aging*, 27, 909-917.

[150] Lu,P., Liu,F., Yan,L., Peng,T., Liu,T., Yao,Z., and Wang,C.Y. (2007) Stem cells therapy for type 1 diabetes. *Diabetes Res.Clin.Pract.*, 78, 1-7.

[151] Ma,Y., Xu,Y., Xiao,Z., Yang,W., Zhang,C., Song,E., Du,Y., and Li,L. (2006) Reconstruction of chemically burned rat corneal surface by bone marrow-derived human mesenchymal stem cells. *Stem Cells*, 24, 315-321.

[152] MacLaren,R.E., Pearson,R.A., MacNeil,A., Douglas,R.H., Salt,T.E., Akimoto,M., Swaroop,A., Sowden,J.C., and Ali,R.R. (2006) Retinal repair by transplantation of photoreceptor precursors. *Nature*, 444, 203-207.

[153] Maharajan,V.S., Shanmuganathan,V., Currie,A., Hopkinson,A., Powell-Richards,A., and Dua,H.S. (2007) Amniotic membrane transplantation for ocular surface reconstruction: indications and outcomes. *Clin. Experiment.Ophthalmol.*, 35, 140-147.

[154] Mapara,K.Y., Stevenson,C.B., Thompson,R.C., and Ehtesham,M. (2007) Stem cells as vehicles for the treatment of brain cancer. *Neurosurg.Clin. N.Am.*, 18, 71-80.

[155] McMullen,N.M. and Pasumarthi,K.B. (2007) Donor cell transplantation for myocardial disease: does it complement current pharmacological therapies? *Can.J.Physiol. Pharmacol.*, 85, 1-15.

[156] Mercer,S.E., Ewton,D.Z., Shah,S., Naqvi,A., and Friedman,E. (2006) Mirk/Dyrk1b mediates cell survival in rhabdomyosarcomas. *Cancer Res.*, 66, 5143-5150.

[157] Metcalfe,A.D. and Ferguson,M.W. (2006) Tissue engineering of replacement skin: the crossroads of biomaterials, wound healing, embryonic development, stem cells and regeneration. *J.R.Soc.Interface.*

[158] Miki,T., Lehmann,T., Cai,H., Stolz,D.B., and Strom,S.C. (2005) Stem cell characteristics of amniotic epithelial cells. *Stem Cells*, 23, 1549-1559.

[159] Miki,T., Mitamura,K., Ross,M.A., Stolz,D.B., and Strom,S.C. (2007) Identification of stem cell marker-positive cells by immunofluorescence in term human amnion. *J.Reprod.Immunol.*, 75, 91-96.

[160] Millar,S.E. (2005) An ideal society? Neighbors of diverse origins interact to create and maintain complex mini-organs in the skin. *PLoS.Biol.*, 3, 1873-1877.

[161] Mimeault,M., Hauke,R., and Batra,S.K. (2007b) Stem cells -- A revolution in therapeutics--Recent advances on the stem cell biology and their therapeutic applications in regenerative medicine and cancer therapies. *Clin.Pharmacol.Ther.*, 82, 252-264.

[162] Mimeault,M., Hauke,R., and Batra,S.K. (2007a) Recent advances on the molecular mechanisms involved in drug-resistance of cancer cells and novel targeting therapies. *Clin.Pharmacol.Ther..*

[163] Mimeault,M., Hauke,R., Mehta,P.P., and Batra,S.K. (2007c) Recent advances on cancer stem/progenitor cell research: therapeutic implications for overcoming resistance to the most aggressive cancers. *J.Mol.Cell.Med.*, 11, 981-1011.

[164] Mimeault,M. and Batra,S.K. (2006b) Recent advances on the significance of stem cells in tissue regeneration and cancer therapies. *Stem Cells*, 24, 2319-2345.

[165] Mimeault,M. and Batra,S.K. (2006a) Recent advances on multiple tumorigenic cascades involved in prostatic cancer progression and targeting therapies. *Carcinogenesis*, 27, 1-22.

[166] Mimeault,M. and Batra,S.K. (2007d) Functions of tumorigenic and migrating cancer progenitor cells in cancer progression and metastasis and their therapeutic implications. *Cancer Metastasis Rev.*, 26, 203-214.

[167] Mimeault,M. and Batra,S.K. (2007e) Interplay of distinct growth factors during epithelial-mesenchymal transition of cancer progenitor cells and molecular targeting as novel cancer therapies. *Ann.Oncol.*, 18, 1605-1619.

[168] Modlin,I.M., Kidd,M., Lye,K.D., and Wright,N.A. (2003) Gastric stem cells: an update. *Keio J.Med.*, 52, 134-137.

[169] Moore,K.A. and Lemischka,I.R. (2006) Stem cells and their niches. *Science*, 311, 1880-1885.

[170] Morris,R.J., Liu,Y., Marles,L., Yang,Z., Trempus,C., Li,S., Lin,J.S., Sawicki,J.A., and Cotsarelis,G. (2004) Capturing and profiling adult hair follicle stem cells. *Nat.Biotechnol.*, 22, 411-417.

[171] Mosher,J.T., Yeager,K.J., Kruger,G.M., Joseph,N.M., Hutchin,M.E., Dlugosz,A.A., and Morrison,S.J. (2007) Intrinsic differences among spatially distinct neural crest stem cells in terms of migratory properties, fate determination, and ability to colonize the enteric nervous system. *Dev.Biol.*, 303, 1-15.

[172] Moshiri,A., Close,J., and Reh,T.A. (2004) Retinal stem cells and regeneration. *Int.J.Dev.Biol.*, 48, 1003-1014.

[173] Muller,F.J., Snyder,E.Y., and Loring,J.F. (2006) Gene therapy: can neural stem cells deliver? *Nat. Rev. Neurosci.*, 7, 75-84.

[174] Muller,P., Beltrami,A.P., Cesselli,D., Pfeiffer,P., Kazakov,A., and Bohm,M. (2005) Myocardial regeneration by endogenous adult progenitor cells. *J.Mol.Cell Cardiol.*, 39, 377-387.

[175] Napoli,C., Maione,C., Schiano,C., Fiorito,C., and Ignarro,L.J. (2007) Bone marrow cell-mediated cardiovascular repair: potential of combined therapies. *Trends Mol.Med.*, 13, 278-286.

[176] Neiva,K., Sun,Y.X., and Taichman,R.S. (2005) The role of osteoblasts in regulating hematopoietic stem cell activity and tumor metastasis. *Braz.J.Med.Biol.Res.*, 38, 1449-1454.

[177] Niemela,S.M., Miettinen,S., Konttinen,Y., Waris,T., Kellomaki,M., Ashammakhi,N.A., and Ylikomi,T. (2007) Fat tissue: views on reconstruction and exploitation. *J.Craniofac.Surg.*, 18, 325-335.

[178] Nikolova,G., Jabs,N., Konstantinova,I., Domogatskaya,A., Tryggvason,K., Sorokin,L., Fassler,R., Gu,G., Gerber,H.P., Ferrara,N., Melton,D.A., and Lammert,E. (2006) The vascular basement membrane: a niche for insulin gene expression and Beta cell proliferation. *Dev.Cell*, 10, 397-405.

[179] Ning,H., Lin,G., Lue,T.F., and Lin,C.S. (2006) Neuron-like differentiation of adipose tissue-derived stromal cells and vascular smooth muscle cells. *Differentiation*, 74, 510-518.

[180] Nobili,S., Landini,I., Giglioni,B., and Mini,E. (2006) Pharmacological strategies for overcoming multidrug resistance. *Curr.Drug Targets.*, 7, 861-879.

[181] Oh,S.H., Witek,R.P., Bae,S.H., Zheng,D., Jung,Y., Piscaglia,A.C., and Petersen,B.E. (2007) Bone marrow-derived hepatic oval cells differentiate into hepatocytes in 2-acetylaminofluorene/partial hepatectomy-induced liver regeneration. *Gastroenterology*, 132, 1077-1087.

[182] Ohnishi,S., Ohgushi,H., Kitamura,S., and Nagaya,N. (2007) Mesenchymal stem cells for the treatment of heart failure. *Int.J.Hematol.*, 86, 17-21.

[183] Okada,H., Suzuki,J., Futamatsu,H., Maejima,Y., Hirao,K., and Isobe,M. (2007) Attenuation of autoimmune myocarditis in rats by mesenchymal stem cell transplantation through enhanced expression of hepatocyte growth factor. *Int.Heart J.*, 48, 649-661.

[184] Okada,T. and Ozawa,K. (2008) Vector-producing tumor-tracking multipotent mesenchymal stromal cells for suicide cancer gene therapy. *Front. Biosci.*, 13, 1887-1891.

[185] Ookura,N., Fujimori,Y., Nishioka,K., Kai,S., Hara,H., and Ogawa,H. (2007) Adipocyte differentiation of human marrow mesenchymal stem cells reduces the supporting capacity for hematopoietic progenitors but not for severe combined immunodeficiency repopulating cells. *Int.J.Mol. Med.*, 19, 387-392.

[186] Orimo,A. and Weinberg,R.A. (2006) Stromal fibroblasts in cancer: A novel tumor-promoting cell type. *Cell Cycle*, 5, 1597-1601.

[187] Ourednik,J., Ourednik,V., Lynch,W.P., Schachner,M., and Snyder,E.Y. (2002) Neural stem cells display an inherent mechanism for rescuing dysfunctional neurons. *Nat. Biotechnol.*, 20, 1103-1110.

[188] Pardal,R., Ortega-Saenz,P., Duran,R., and Lopez-Barneo,J. (2007) Glia-like stem cells sustain physiologic neurogenesis in the adult mammalian carotid body. *Cell*, 131, 364-377.

[189] Pasquinelli,G., Tazzari,P., Ricci,F., Vaselli,C., Buzzi,M., Conte,R., Orrico,C., Foroni,L., Stella,A., Alviano,F., Bagnara,G.P., and Lucarelli,E. (2007) Ultrastructural characteristics of human mesenchymal stromal (stem) cells derived from bone marrow and term placenta. *Ultrastruct.Pathol.*, 31, 23-31.

[190] Payne,T.R., Oshima,H., Okada,M., Momoi,N., Tobita,K., Keller,B.B., Peng,H., and Huard,J. (2007) A relationship between vascular endothelial growth factor, angiogenesis, and cardiac repair after muscle stem cell transplantation into ischemic hearts. *J.Am.Coll.Cardiol.*, 50, 1677-1684.

[191] Peault,B., Rudnicki,M., Torrente,Y., Cossu,G., Tremblay,J.P., Partridge,T., Gussoni,E., Kunkel,L.M., and Huard,J. (2007) Stem and progenitor cells in skeletal muscle development, maintenance, and therapy. *Mol.Ther.*, 15, 867-877.

[192] Pessina,A. and Gribaldo,L. (2006) The key role of adult stem cells: therapeutic perspectives. *Curr.Med.Res.Opin.*, 22, 2287-2300.

[193] Peters,B.A., Diaz,L.A., Polyak,K., Meszler,L., Romans,K., Guinan,E.C., Antin,J.H., Myerson,D., Hamilton,S.R., Vogelstein,B., Kinzler,K.W., and Lengauer,C. (2005) Contribution of bone marrow-derived endothelial cells to human tumor vasculature. *Nat. Med.*, 11, 261-262.

[194] Pollett,J.B., Corsi,K.A., Weiss,K.R., Cooper,G.M., Barry,D.A., Gharaibeh,B., and Huard,J. (2007) Malignant transformation of multipotent muscle-derived cells by concurrent differentiation signals. *Stem Cells*, 25, 2302-2311.

[195] Portmann-Lanz,C.B., Schoeberlein,A., Huber,A., Sager,R., Malek,A., Holzgreve,W., and Surbek,D.V. (2006) Placental mesenchymal stem cells as potential autologous graft for pre- and perinatal neuroregeneration. *Am.J.Obstet.Gynecol.*, 194, 664-673.

[196] Potten,C.S. and Ellis,J.R. (2006) Adult small intestinal stem cells: identification, location, characteristics, and clinical applications. *Ernst.Schering.Res.Found.Workshop*, 60, 81-98.

[197] Prunet-Marcassus,B., Cousin,B., Caton,D., Andre,M., Penicaud,L., and Casteilla,L. (2006) From heterogeneity to plasticity in adipose tissues: site-specific differences. *Exp.Cell Res.*, 312, 727-736.

[198] Qiao,H., Zhao,T., Wang,Y., Yang,C.R., Xiao,M., and Dou,Z.Y. (2007) Isolation, purification and identification of epithelial cells derived from fetal islet-like cell clusters. *Sheng Wu Gong.Cheng Xue.Bao.*, 23, 246-251.

[199] Rafii, S and Lyden, D. Contribution of hematopoietic and vascular progenitor cells to the neoangiogenic niche. 181-185. 2006.

[200] Rafii,S., Lyden,D., Benezra,R., Hattori,K., and Heissig,B. (2002) Vascular and haematopoietic stem cells: novel targets for anti-angiogenesis therapy? *Nat.Rev.Cancer*, 2, 826-835.

[201] Ramaswamy,S., Shannon,K.M., and Kordower,J.H. (2007) Huntington's disease: pathological mechanisms and therapeutic strategies. *Cell Transplant.*, 16, 301-312.

[202] Reya,T. and Clevers,H. (2005) Wnt signalling in stem cells and cancer. *Nature*, 434, 843-850.

[203] Richards,M., Tan,S.P., Tan,J.H., Chan,W.K., and Bongso,A. (2004) The transcriptome profile of human embryonic stem cells as defined by SAGE. *Stem Cells*, 22, 51-64.
[204] Ringden,O. (2007) Immunotherapy by allogeneic stem cell transplantation. *Adv.Cancer Res.*, 97C, 25-60.
[205] Rizo,A., Vellenga,E., de Haan G., and Schuringa,J.J. (2006) Signaling pathways in self-renewing hematopoietic and leukemic stem cells: do all stem cells need a niche? *Hum.Mol.Genet.*, 15, R210-R219.
[206] Rodriguez-Gomez,J.A., Lu,J.Q., Velasco,I., Rivera,S., Zoghbi,S.S., Liow,J.S., Musachio,J.L., Chin,F.T., Toyama,H., Seidel,J., Green,M.V., Thanos,P.K., Ichise,M., Pike,V.W., Innis,R.B., and McKay,R.D. (2007) Persistent dopamine functions of neurons derived from embryonic stem cells in a rodent model of Parkinson disease. *Stem Cells*, 25, 918-928.
[207] Rollini,P., Kaiser,S., Faes-van't,H.E., Kapp,U., and Leyvraz,S. (2004) Long-term expansion of transplantable human fetal liver hematopoietic stem cells. *Blood*, 103, 1166-1170.
[208] Roskams,T. (2006) Liver stem cells and their implication in hepatocellular and cholangiocarcinoma. *Oncogene*, 25, 3818-3822.
[209] Rossi,D.J., Bryder,D., and Weissman,I.L. (2007) Hematopoietic stem cell aging: Mechanism and consequence. *Exp.Gerontol.*, 42, 385-390.
[210] Rouger,K., Fornasari,B., Armengol,V., Jouvion,G., Leroux,I., Dubreil,L., Feron,M., Guevel,L., and Cherel,Y. (2007) Progenitor cell isolation from muscle-derived cells based on adhesion properties. *J.Histochem.Cytochem.*, 55, 607-618.
[211] Roy,N.S., Cleren,C., Singh,S.K., Yang,L., Beal,M.F., and Goldman,S.A. (2006) Functional engraftment of human ES cell-derived dopaminergic neurons enriched by coculture with telomerase-immortalized midbrain astrocytes. *Nat.Med.*, 12, 1259-1268.
[212] Sadat,S., Gehmert,S., Song,Y.H., Yen,Y., Bai,X., Gaiser,S., Klein,H., and Alt,E. (2007) The cardioprotective effect of mesenchymal stem cells is mediated by IGF-I and VEGF. *Biochem.Biophys.Res.Commun.*, 363, 674-679.
[213] Santana,A., Ensenat-Waser,R., Arribas,M.I., Reig,J.A., and Roche,E. (2006) Insulin-producing cells derived from stem cells: recent progress and future directions. *J.Cell.Mol.Med.*, 10, 866-883.
[214] Sata,M., Saiura,A., Kunisato,A., Tojo,A., Okada,S., Tokuhisa,T., Hirai,H., Makuuchi,M., Hirata,Y., and Nagai,R. (2002) Hematopoietic stem cells differentiate into vascular cells that participate in the pathogenesis of atherosclerosis. *Nat.Med.*, 8, 403-409.
[215] Schaffler,A. and Buchler,C. (2007) Concise review: adipose tissue-derived stromal cells--basic and clinical implications for novel cell-based therapies. *Stem Cells*, 25, 818-827.
[216] Schatteman,G.C., Dunnwald,M., and Jiao,C. (2007) Biology of bone marrow-derived endothelial cell precursors. *Am.J.Physiol.Heart Circ.Physiol.*, 292, H1-18.
[217] Schatzlein,A.G. (2006) Delivering cancer stem cell therapies - a role for nanomedicines? *Eur.J.Cancer*, 42, 1309-1315.
[218] Schrama,D., Reisfeld,R.A., and Becker,J.C. (2006) Antibody targeted drugs as cancer therapeutics. *Nat.Rev.Drug Discov.*, 5, 147-159.
[219] Schuldiner,M., Yanuka,O., Itskovitz-Eldor,J., Melton,D.A., and Benvenisty,N. (2000) Effects of eight growth factors on the differentiation of cells derived from human embryonic stem cells. *Proc.Natl.Acad.Sci.U.S.A.*, 97, 11307-11312.

[220] Schwarzkopf,M., Coletti,D., Sassoon,D., and Marazzi,G. (2006) Muscle cachexia is regulated by a p53-PW1/Peg3-dependent pathway. *Genes Dev.*, 20, 3440-3452.

[221] Scobioala,S., Klocke,R., Kuhlmann,M., Tian,W., Hasib,L., Milting,H., Koenig,S., Stelljes,M., El-Banayosy,A., Tenderich,G., Michel,G., Breithardt,G., and Nikol,S. (2007) Up-regulation of nestin in the infarcted myocardium potentially indicates differentiation of resident cardiac stem cells into various lineages including cardiomyocytes. *FASEB J.*.

[222] Seaberg,R.M., Smukler,S.R., Kieffer,T.J., Enikolopov,G., Asghar,Z., Wheeler,M.B., Korbutt,G., and van der,K.D. (2004) Clonal identification of multipotent precursors from adult mouse pancreas that generate neural and pancreatic lineages. *Nat.Biotechnol.*, 22, 1115-1124.

[223] Seeberger,K.L., Dufour,J.M., Shapiro,A.M., Lakey,J.R., Rajotte,R.V., and Korbutt,G.S. (2006) Expansion of mesenchymal stem cells from human pancreatic ductal epithelium. *Lab. Invest.*, 86, 141-153.

[224] Sell,S. (2004) Stem cell origin of cancer and differentiation therapy. *Crit.Rev.Oncol.Hematol.*, 51, 1-28.

[225] Shanti,R.M., Li,W.J., Nesti,L.J., Wang,X., and Tuan,R.S. (2007) Adult mesenchymal stem cells: biological properties, characteristics, and applications in maxillofacial surgery. *J.Oral Maxillofac.Surg.*, 65, 1640-1647.

[226] Sharma,A.D., Cantz,T., Manns,M.P., and Ott,M. (2006) The role of stem cells in physiology, pathophysiology, and therapy of the liver. *Stem Cell Rev.*, 2, 51-58.

[227] Shen,W., Wang,Z., Punyanita,M., Lei,J., Sinav,A., Kral,J.G., Imielinska,C., Ross,R., and Heymsfield,S.B. (2003) Adipose tissue quantification by imaging methods: a proposed classification. *Obes.Res.*, 11, 5-16.

[228] Shetty,A.K. and Hattiangady,B. (2007) Concise review: prospects of stem cell therapy for temporal lobe epilepsy. *Stem Cells*, 25, 2396-2407.

[229] Shih,C.C., Forman,S.J., Chu,P., and Slovak,M. (2007) Human embryonic stem cells are prone to generate primitive, undifferentiated tumors in engrafted human fetal tissues in severe combined immunodeficient mice. *Stem Cells Dev.*.

[230] Shim,J.H., Kim,S.E., Woo,D.H., Kim,S.K., Oh,C.H., McKay,R., and Kim,J.H. (2007) Directed differentiation of human embryonic stem cells towards a pancreatic cell fate. *Diabetologia*, 50, 1228-1238.

[231] Shinin,V., Gayraud-Morel,B., Gomes,D., and Tajbakhsh,S. (2006) Asymmetric division and cosegregation of template DNA strands in adult muscle satellite cells. *Nat. Cell Biol.*, 8, 677-687.

[232] Singh,S.K., Hawkins,C., Clarke,I.D., Squire,J.A., Bayani,J., Hide,T., Henkelman,R.M., Cusimano,M.D., and Dirks,P.B. (2004) Identification of human brain tumour initiating cells. *Nature*, 432, 396-401.

[233] Siu,C.W., Moore,J.C., and Li,R.A. (2007) Human embryonic stem cell-derived cardiomyocytes for heart therapies. *Cardiovasc.Hematol.Disord.Drug Targets.*, 7, 145-152.

[234] Small,T.N., Young,J.W., Castro-Malaspina,H., Prockop,S., Wilton,A., Heller,G., Boulad,F., Chiu,M., Hsu,K., Jakubowski,A., Kernan,N.A., Perales,M.A., O'Reilly,R.J., and Papadopoulos,E.B. (2007) Intravenous busulfan and melphalan, tacrolimus, and short-course methotrexate followed by unmodified HLA-matched related or unrelated hematopoietic stem cell transplantation for the treatment of advanced hematologic malignancies. *Biol.Blood Marrow Transplant.*, 13, 235-244.

[235] Smidt,M.P. and Burbach,J.P. (2007) How to make a mesodiencephalic dopaminergic neuron. *Nat.Rev. Neurosci.*, 8, 21-32.

[236] Sohn,R.L., Jain,M., and Liao,R. (2007) Adult stem cells and heart regeneration. *Expert.Rev. Cardiovasc.Ther.*, 5, 507-517.

[237] Sora,F., Piccirillo,N., Chiusolo,P., Laurenti,L., Marra,R., Bartolozzi,F., Leone,G., and Sica,S. (2006) Mitoxantrone, carboplatin, cytosine arabinoside, and methylprednisolone followed by autologous peripheral blood stem cell transplantation: a salvage regimen for patients with refractory or recurrent non-Hodgkin lymphoma. *Cancer*, 106, 859-866.

[238] Sueblinvong,V., Suratt,B.T., and Weiss,D.J. (2007) Novel therapies for the treatment of cystic fibrosis: new developments in gene and stem cell therapy. *Clin.Chest Med.*, 28, 361-379.

[239] Suen,P.M. and Leung,P.S. (2005) Pancreatic stem cells: a glimmer of hope for diabetes? *J.O.P.*, 6, 422-424.

[240] Sun,Y., Chen,L., Hou,X.G., Hou,W.K., Dong,J.J., Sun,L., Tang,K.X., Wang,B., Song,J., Li,H., and Wang,K.X. (2007) Differentiation of bone marrow-derived mesenchymal stem cells from diabetic patients into insulin-producing cells *in vitro*. *Chin. Med.J.(Engl.)*, 120, 771-776.

[241] Taguchi,M. and Otsuki,M. (2004) Co-localization of nestin and PDX-1 in small evaginations of the main pancreatic duct in adult rats. *J.Mol. Histol.*, 35, 785-789.

[242] Tamaki,T., Okada,Y., Uchiyama,Y., Tono,K., Masuda,M., Wada,M., Hoshi,A., and Akatsuka,A. (2007) Synchronized reconstitution of muscle fibers, peripheral nerves and blood vessels by murine skeletal muscle-derived CD34(-)/45 (-) cells. *Histochem.Cell Biol.*, 128, 349-360.

[243] Tejwani,S., Kolari,R.S., Sangwan,V.S., and Rao,G.N. (2007) Role of amniotic membrane graft for ocular chemical and thermal injuries. *Cornea*, 26, 21-26.

[244] Thorne,S.H. (2007) Strategies to achieve systemic delivery of therapeutic cells and microbes to tumors. *Expert.Opin.Biol.Ther.*, 7, 41-51.

[245] Torrente,Y., Belicchi,M., Marchesi,C., Dantona,G., Cogiamanian,F., Pisati,F., Gavina,M., Giordano,R., Tonlorenzi,R., Fagiolari,G., Lamperti,C., Porretti,L., Lopa,R., Sampaolesi,M., Vicentini,L., Grimoldi,N., Tiberio,F., Songa,V., Baratta,P., Prelle,A., Forzenigo,L., Guglieri,M., Pansarasa,O., Rinaldi,C., Mouly,V., Butler-Browne,G.S., Comi,G.P., Biondetti,P., Moggio,M., Gaini,S.M., Stocchetti,N., Priori,A., D'Angelo,M.G., Turconi,A., Bottinelli,R., Cossu,G., Rebulla,P., and Bresolin,N. (2007) Autologous transplantation of muscle-derived CD133^{+} stem cells in Duchenne muscle patients. *Cell Transplant.*, 16, 563-577.

[246] Tropepe,V., Coles,B.L., Chiasson,B.J., Horsford,D.J., Elia,A.J., McInnes,R.R., and van der,K.D. (2000) Retinal stem cells in the adult mammalian eye. *Science*, 287, 2032-2036.

[247] Trounson,A. (2006) The production and directed differentiation of human embryonic stem cells. *Endocr.Rev.*, 27, 208-219.

[248] Trzaska,K.A. and Rameshwar,P. (2007) Current advances in the treatment of Parkinson's disease with stem cells. *Curr.Neurovasc.Res.*, 4, 99-109.

[249] Urban,V.S., Kiss,J., Kovacs,J., Gocza,E., Vas,V., Monostori,E., and Uher,F. (2007) Mesenchymal stem cells cooperate with bone marrow cells in therapy of diabetes. *Stem Cells*.

[250] Urbanek,K., Cesselli,D., Rota,M., Nascimbene,A., De,A.A., Hosoda,T., Bearzi,C., Boni,A., Bolli,R., Kajstura,J., Anversa,P., and Leri,A. (2006) Stem cell niches in the adult mouse heart. *Proc.Natl.Acad.Sci.U.S.A.*, 103, 9226-9231.

[251] Urbanek,K., Rota,M., Cascapera,S., Bearzi,C., Nascimbene,A., De,A.A., Hosoda,T., Chimenti,S., Baker,M., Limana,F., Nurzynska,D., Torella,D., Rotatori,F., Rastaldo,R., Musso,E., Quaini,F., Leri,A., Kajstura,J., and Anversa,P. (2005) Cardiac stem cells possess growth factor-receptor systems that after activation regenerate the infarcted myocardium, improving ventricular function and long-term survival. *Circ.Res.*, 97, 663-673.

[252] Usas,A. and Huard,J. (2007) Muscle-derived stem cells for tissue engineering and regenerative therapy. *Biomaterials*, 28, 5401-5406.

[253] Valina,C., Pinkernell,K., Song,Y.H., Bai,X., Sadat,S., Campeau,R.J., Le Jemtel,T.H., and Alt,E. (2007) Intracoronary administration of autologous adipose tissue-derived stem cells improves left ventricular function, perfusion, and remodelling after acute myocardial infarction. *Eur.Heart J.*, 28, 2667-2677.

[254] van de Ven,C., Collins,D., Bradley,M.B., Morris,E., and Cairo,M.S. (2007) The potential of umbilical cord blood multipotent stem cells for nonhematopoietic tissue and cell regeneration. *Exp.Hematol..*

[255] van Vliet P., Sluijter,J.P., Doevendans,P.A., and Goumans,M.J. (2007) Isolation and expansion of resident cardiac progenitor cells. *Expert.Rev.Cardiovasc.Ther.*, 5, 33-43.

[256] Vendrame,M., Cassady,J., Newcomb,J., Butler,T., Pennypacker,K.R., Zigova,T., Sanberg,C.D., Sanberg,P.R., and Willing,A.E. (2004) Infusion of human umbilical cord blood cells in a rat model of stroke dose-dependently rescues behavioral deficits and reduces infarct volume. *Stroke*, 35, 2390-2395.

[257] Vescovi,A.L., Galli,R., and Reynolds,B.A. (2006) Brain tumour stem cells. *Nat.Rev.Cancer*, 6, 425-436.

[258] Wagner,W., Wein,F., Seckinger,A., Frankhauser,M., Wirkner,U., Krause,U., Blake,J., Schwager,C., Eckstein,V., Ansorge,W., and Ho,A.D. (2005) Comparative characteristics of mesenchymal stem cells from human bone marrow, adipose tissue, and umbilical cord blood. *Exp.Hematol.*, 33, 1402-1416.

[259] Walton,N.M., Sutter,B.M., Chen,H.X., Chang,L.J., Roper,S.N., Scheffler,B., and Steindler,D.A. (2006) Derivation and large-scale expansion of multipotent astroglial neural progenitors from adult human brain. *Development*, 133, 3671-3681.

[260] Wang,C.H., Cherng,W.J., Yang,N.I., Kuo,L.T., Hsu,C.M., Yeh,H.I., Lan,Y.J., Yeh,C.H., and Stanford,W.L. (2007) Late-outgrowth endothelial cells attenuate ntimal hyperplasia contributed by mesenchymal stem cells after vascular injury. *Arterioscler.Thromb.Vasc.Biol..*

[261] Wang,G.S., Rosenberg,L., and Scott,F.W. (2005) Tubular complexes as a source for islet neogenesis in the pancreas of diabetes-prone BB rats. *Lab.Invest*, 85, 675-688.

[262] Watts,C., McConkey,H., Anderson,L., and Caldwell,M. (2005) Anatomical perspectives on adult neural stem cells. *J.Anat.*, 207, 197-208.

[263] Weiss,M.L. and Troyer,D.L. (2006) Stem cells in the umbilical cord. *Stem Cell Rev.*, 2, 155-162.

[264] Wilshaw,S.P., Kearney,J.N., Fisher,J., and Ingham,E. (2006) Production of an acellular amniotic membrane matrix for use in tissue engineering. *Tissue Eng.*, 12, 2117-2129.

[265] Wilson,A. and Trumpp,A. (2006) Bone-marrow haematopoietic-stem-cell niches. *Nat.Rev.Immunol.*, 6, 93-106.

[266] Wolbank,S., Peterbauer,A., Fahrner,M., Hennerbichler,S., van,G.M., Stadler,G., Redl,H., and Gabriel,C. (2007) Dose-dependent immunomodulatory effect of human stem cells from amniotic membrane: A comparison with human mesenchymal stem cells from adipose tissue. *Tissue Eng.*, 13, 1173-1183.

[267] Woodward,W.A., Chen,M.S., Behbod,F., and Rosen,J.M. (2005) On mammary stem cells. *J.Cell Sci.*, 118, 3585-3594.

[268] Wu,D.C., Byod,A.S., and Wood,K.J. (2007a) Embryonic stem cell transplantation: potential applicability in cell replacement therapy and regenerative medicine. *Front. Biosci.*, 12, 4525-4535.

[269] Wu,K.H., Zhou,B., Yu,C.T., Cui,B., Lu,S.H., Han,Z.C., and Liu,Y.L. (2007b) Therapeutic potential of human umbilical cord derived stem cells in a rat myocardial infarction model. *Ann.Thorac.Surg.*, 83, 1491-1498.

[270] Wu,Z.Y., Hui,G.Z., Lu,Y., Wu,X., and Guo,L.H. (2006) Transplantation of human amniotic epithelial cells improves hindlimb function in rats with spinal cord injury. *Chin. Med.J.(Engl.)*, 119, 2101-2107.

[271] Xu,H., Sta Iglesia,D.D., Kielczewski,J.L., Valenta,D.F., Pease,M.E., Zack,D.J., and Quigley,H.A. (2007) Characteristics of progenitor cells derived from adult ciliary body in mouse, rat, and human eyes. *Invest. Ophthalmol.Vis.Sci.*, 48, 1674-1682.

[272] Yamada,Y., Yokoyama,S., Wang,X.D., Fukuda,N., and Takakura,N. (2007) Cardiac stem cells in brown adipose tissue express CD133 and induce bone marrow nonhematopoietic cells to differentiate into cardiomyocytes. *Stem Cells*, 25, 1326-1333.

[273] Yan,Z., Lin,Y., Jiao,X., Li,Z., Wu,L., Jing,W., Qiao,J., Liu,L., Tang,W., Zheng,X., and Tian,W. (2006) Characterization of ectomesenchymal cells isolated from the first branchial arch during multilineage differentiation. *Cells Tissues.Organs*, 183, 123-132.

[274] Yao,S., Chen,S., Clark,J., Hao,E., Beattie,G.M., Hayek,A., and Ding,S. (2006) Long-term self-renewal and directed differentiation of human embryonic stem cells in chemically defined conditions. *Proc.Natl.Acad.Sci.U.S.A.*, 6907-6912.

[275] Yen,T.H. and Wright,N.A. (2006) The gastrointestinal tract stem cell niche. *Stem Cell Rev.*, 2, 203-212.

[276] Yoon,Y.S., Wecker,A., Heyd,L., Park,J.S., Tkebuchava,T., Kusano,K., Hanley,A., Scadova,H., Qin,G., Cha,D.H., Johnson,K.L., Aikawa,R., Asahara,T., and Losordo,D.W. (2005) Clonally expanded novel multipotent stem cells from human bone marrow regenerate myocardium after myocardial infarction. *J.Clin.Invest.*, 115, 326-338.

[277] Yu,J.J., Sun,X., Yuan,X., Lee,J.W., Snyder,E.Y., and Yu,J.S. (2006) Immuno-modulatory neural stem cells for brain tumour therapy. *Expert.Opin.Biol.Ther.*, 6, 1255-1262.

[278] Zengin,E., Chalajour,F., Gehling,U.M., Ito,W.D., Treede,H., Lauke,H., Weil,J., Reichenspurner,H., Kilic,N., and Ergun,S. (2006) Vascular wall resident progenitor cells: a source for postnatal vasculogenesis. *Development*, 133, 1543-1551.

[279] Zhang,L., Hong,T.P., Hu,J., Liu,Y.N., Wu,Y.H., and Li,L.S. (2005) Nestin-positive progenitor cells isolated from human fetal pancreas have phenotypic markers identical to mesenchymal stem cells. *World J.Gastroenterol.*, 11, 2906-2911.

[280] Zhao,Z.G., Liang,Y., Li,K., Li,W.M., Li,Q.B., Chen,Z.C., and Zou,P. (2007) Phenotypic and functional comparison of mesenchymal stem cells derived from the bone marrow of normal adults and patients with hematologic malignant diseases. *Stem Cells Dev.*, 16, 637-648.

[281] Zuba-Surma,E.K., bdel-Latif,A., Case,J., Tiwari,S., Hunt,G., Kucia,M., Vincent,R.J., Ranjan,S., Ratajczak,M.Z., Srour,E.F., Bolli,R., and Dawn,B. (2006) Sca-1 expression is associated with decreased cardiomyogenic differentiation potential of skeletal muscle-derived adult primitive cells. *J.Mol.Cell. Cardiol.*, 41, 650-660.

[282] Zuk,P.A., Zhu,M., Ashjian,P., De Ugarte,D.A., Huang,J.I., Mizuno,H., Alfonso,Z.C., Fraser,J.K., Benhaim,P., and Hedrick,M.H. (2002) Human adipose tissue is a source of multipotent stem cells. *Mol. Biol.Cell*, 13, 4279-4295.

[283] Zulewski,H., Abraham,E.J., Gerlach,M.J., Daniel,P.B., Moritz,W., Muller,B., Vallejo,M., Thomas,M.K., and Habener,J.F. (2001) Multipotential nestin-positive stem cells isolated from adult pancreatic islets differentiate *ex vitro* into pancreatic endocrine, exocrine, and hepatic phenotypes. *Diabetes*, 50, 521-533.

Chapter II

STEM CELL APPLICATIONS IN DIABETES

Hirofumi Noguchi[*1, 2]
[1] Baylor Institute for Immunology Research, Baylor Research Institute,
Dallas, Texas, US
[2] Institute of Biomedical Studies, Baylor University,
Waco, TX, US

ABSTRACT

Diabetes mellitus is a devastating disease and the World Health Organization (WHO) expects that the number of diabetic patients will increase to 300 million by the year 2025. Patients with diabetes experience decreased insulin secretion that is linked to a significant reduction in the number of islet cells. Type 1 diabetes is characterized by the selective destruction of pancreatic β cells caused by an autoimmune attack. Type 2 diabetes is a more complex pathology that, in addition to β cell loss caused by apoptotic programs, includes β cell de-differentiation and peripheral insulin resistance. The success achieved over the last few years with islet transplantation suggests that diabetes can be cured by the replenishment of deficient β cells. These observations are proof of the concept and have intensified interest in treating diabetes or other diseases not only by cell transplantation but also by stem cells. An increasing body of evidence indicates that, in addition to embryonic stem cells, several potential adult stem/progenitor cells derived from the pancreas, liver, spleen, and bone marrow could differentiate into insulin-producing cells *in vitro* or *in vivo*. However, significant controversy currently exists in this field. Pharmacological approaches aimed at stimulating the *in vivo/ex vivo* regeneration of β cells have been proposed as a way of augmenting islet cell mass. Overexpression of embryonic transcription factors in stem cells could efficiently induce their differentiation into insulin-expressing cells. A new technology, known as protein transduction, facilitates the differentiation of stem cells into insulin-producing cells. Recent progress in the search

---

[*] Address correspondence to: Hirofumi Noguchi MD, PhD; Baylor Institute for Immunology Research, Baylor Research Institute; 3434 Live Oak St., Dallas, Texas 75204, USA; Tel.: 214-820-8794; Fax: 214-820-4952; E-mail: hirofumn@baylorhealth.edu

for new sources of β cells has opened up several possibilities for the development of new treatments for diabetes.

Keywords: diabetes, stem cell, pancreatic β cells, islet regeneration, protein transduction

INTRODUCTION

Diabetes mellitus and its devastating effects, such as retinopathy, neuropathy, and nephropathy, afflict more than 194 million people worldwide. Type 1 diabetic patients are insulin dependent as a result of autoimmune-mediated destruction of insulin-secreting β cells in the islets of Langerhans of the pancreas. In contrast, type 2 diabetes is mainly caused by a combination of systemic insulin resistance and inadequate insulin secretion by pancreatic β cells. In later stages of type 2 diabetes, β cell mass is reduced by about 50%, and oral hypoglycemic agents fail in 20-30% of these patients, requiring exogenous insulin to control hyperglycemia. Surgical resection of the pancreas may also cause insulin-dependent diabetes depending on the size of the remaining pancreas. It is now well established that the risk of diabetic complications is dependent on the degree of glycemic control in diabetic patients. Clinical trials such as the Diabetes Control and Complications Trial (DCCT) [1, 2, 3], the UK Prospective Diabetes Study (UKPDS) [4], and Kumamoto study [5] have demonstrated that tight glycemic control achieved with intensive insulin regimens can reduce the risk of developing or progressing retinopathy, nephropathy or neuropathy in patients with all types of diabetes. However, the Third National Health and Nutrition Examination Survey (NHANES III) showed that only 50% of diabetics have been able to achieve a HbA_{1C} level of less than 7%; therefore, the only way to ensure the long-term health of diabetic patients is to maintain constant normoglycemia.

Although the most advanced insulin preparations and intensified insulin regimens can improve blood glucose levels, exogenous insulin administration cannot ensure continuous blood glucose control and satisfactory prevention of diabetes complications. Moreover, intensive glycemic control with insulin therapy is associated with an increased incidence of hypoglycemia, which is the major barrier to the implementation of intensive treatment from the perspective of both physicians and patients. In fact, investigators are exploring alternative treatments to substitute exogenous insulin therapy. The successes achieved over the last few decades by the transplantation of whole pancreas and isolated islets suggest that diabetes can be cured by the replenishment of deficient β cells. It seems logical that replacement of the islet tissue itself offers a better approach than simply replacing insulin that has been lost. Islet allotransplantation can achieve insulin independence in patients with type 1 diabetes [6-20]. Since the Edmonton protocol was announced, more than 600 type 1 diabetics in more than fifty institutions have undergone islet transplantation to cure their disease; however, the clinical benefit of this protocol can be provided only to a small minority of patients and is not lasting [21]. Nonetheless, the promising results afforded by transplantation of whole pancreata and isolated islets, coupled with the shortage of cadaver pancreata relative to the potential demand, have lent strong impetus to the search for new sources of insulin-producing cells [22].

Here we review the most relevant work currently conducted in this exciting area.

ISLET TRANSPLANTATION

The DCCT showed that intensive insulin therapy improved HbA_{1C} and protected against diabetic triopathy [2], but the penalty was a three-fold-increased risk of serous hypoglycemic events including recurrent seizures and coma [3]. Islet transplantation is one feasible approach to reverse type 1 diabetes mellitus [6-20]. Islet transplantation can avoid major surgery, general anesthesia and complications related to exocrine enzymes. Although the first human islet allograft transplant was performed in 1974 [23], the clinical success rates were not outstanding until 2000 [24]. At this time, dramatic improvement was achieved with the Edmonton Protocol [6]. Since the Edmonton protocol was announced, islet transplantation technology has advanced considerably, including improvements in islet after kidney transplantation, utilization of non-heart-beating donors [8, 15, 16], single-donor islet transplantation [11], and living-donor islet transplantation [7, 17, 18]. These advances were based on revised immunosuppression protocols [25, 26], improved pancreas procurement strategies [27, 28], improved islet isolation methods [8, 9, 15], and enhanced islet engraftment [29-31]. However, islet transplantation efforts have limitations including the short supply of donor pancreata, the paucity of experienced islet isolation teams, side effects of immunosuppressants and poor long-term results [32-34]. Further improvements are necessary to make islet transplantation a routine and effective clinical treatment. The results obtained through human pancreatic islet transplantation were an encouraging advancement in the efforts to generate new sources of insulin producing cells.

EMBRYONIC STEM CELLS

Embryonic stem cells (ES cells) are pluripotent diploid cells, derived from the inner mass of the mammalian blastocyst. ES cells indefinitely proliferate in an undifferentiated state and can be induced to differentiate into cells of all three germ layers both *in vivo* and *in vitro* [35, 36]. It has been reported that ES cells from mouse [37-44], monkey [45], and human [38, 46] were able to differentiate into insulin-positive cells, a potential source of new β cells. However, this has proven more difficult than expected. Beginning in 2000, it was reported by many groups that ES cells can differentiate into insulin-producing cells *in vitro* [37-39]. Several approaches have been used to obtain enriched populations: selection by manipulating culture conditions [39, 40, 46, 47]; overexpression of key transcription factors such as paired box gene 4 (Pax4) and the pancreatic and duodenal homeobox factor-1 (PDX-1) [41, 42, 48]; and cell trapping with antibiotic resistance driven by the Nkx6.1 or insulin promoter to select cells [37, 43]. In particular, the selection of ES cells expressing nestin, an intermediate filament protein thought to be a marker of neural stem cells, has been used to obtain insulin-producing cells efficiently in several articles [39-42].

However, recent reports demonstrated that ES cells give rise to a population of cells that contain insulin, not as a result of biosynthesis but from the uptake of exogenous insulin by cell apoptosis [49-51]. Melton's group took five ES cell lines (both murine and human) and differentiated them into insulin-producing cells. Their results agreed with the previous findings that 10 to 30% of the cells stain with antibodies to insulin and that fifty-micrometer clusters of insulin-staining cells were produced as described [39]. However, they did not detect insulin 1 mRNA by reverse transcription-polymerase chain reaction (RT-PCR) and insulin 2 mRNA detection was weak. Only about 1/100,000 cells had insulin gene expression despite insulin antibody staining in 10 to 30% of cells. Moreover, they showed that the insulin-positive cells did not stain with an antibody for C-peptide, a byproduct of de novo insulin synthesis. They ultimately concluded that most of the insulin-staining cells were apoptotic cells and insulin in the culture medium affected staining [49]. Therefore, the measurement of not only insulin but also C-peptide is needed to prove that insulin has been synthesized. Also, considering that several articles have shown the selection of nestin and that human neural stem cells are capable of producing small amounts of insulin [52], it is possible that the insulin found in ES cell-derived cells arises from aberrant neuronal differentiation. However, these cells have no more than a tiny fraction of the insulin content of normal β cells and exhibit incomplete expression of β cell markers.

The lack of success of these early attempts at differentiating ES cells has focused attention on the fundamentals of normal embryonic development to better understand the early stages of endoderm formation. D'Amour *et al.* recently developed a differentiation process that converts human ES cells to endocrine cells capable of synthesizing the pancreatic hormones insulin, glucagon, somatostatin, pancreatic polypeptide and ghrelin. Using a five-step protocol cleverly designed to mimic pancreatic development, they succeeded in differentiating a substantial fraction of an initial population of human ES cells into pancreatic islet-like cells, including cells that produce high levels of insulin [53]. The protocol's success depends entirely on efficient initial production of definitive endoderm. As the authors showed, mesoderm or neuroectoderm induced in the first step does not form insulin-producing cells when subjected to the same subsequent differentiation steps. The high efficiency of definitive-endoderm production may be due to complete block of human ES cell self-renewal (by low serum) combined with activin A/Wnt treatment. Although the differentiated cells do not reliably release insulin in response to glucose, with further optimization this approach may yield fully mature β-cells that are suitable for transplantation. In addition, this study demonstrates how a detailed understanding of developmental biology can be applied to achieve efficient differentiation of human ES cells to a desired cell type.

A significant number of problems remain unsolved in terms of their clinical application, such as the risk of tumorigenicity. The ethical issue is another major obstacle to the clinical use of ES cells.

PANCREATIC STEM/PROGENITOR CELLS

Since damaged tissues are repaired even in elderly people, adult stem/progenitor cells seem to be present and active within our body throughout life. Adult stem/progenitor cells play central roles in maintenance, repair, and reconstitution of tissues, regulated by homeostatic and regenerative signals [54]. Adult stem cells have initially been identified in tissues with high turnover, namely skin and gut [55]. More recently, adult stem cells were also identified in tissues with low regeneration potential, such as brain [56], kidney [57], and pancreas [58-60].

Islet neogenesis, the budding of new islets from pancreatic stem/progenitor cells located in or near ducts, has long been assumed to be an active process in the postnatal pancreas. Several *in vitro* studies have shown that insulin-producing cells can be generated from adult pancreatic ductal tissues [61-68]. Bonner-Weir *et al*. cultured human adult ductal tissues with Matrigel and observed the formation of islet-like buds consisting of cytokeratin 19 (CK19)-positive duct cells and insulin-positive cells [64]. Gao *et al*. used the same protocol as Bonner-Weir *et al*. and showed that some CK19-positive duct epithelial cells differentiated into endocrine cells. A serum-free, nicotinamide, Matrigel culture was an absolute requirement for differentiation [65]. Bonner-Weir's group recently showed differentiation of affinity-purified human pancreatic duct cells to insulin producing cells [69]. Pancreatic duct cells were purified from dispersed islet-depleted human pancreatic tissue using CA19-9 antibody. The purified fraction was almost entirely CK19 positive cells. Some of these cells transplanted into normoglycemic NOD/SCID mice differentiated into insulin producing cells. The addition of 0.1% cultured stromal cells improved percentage of insulin positive cells. Some insulin-positive cells coexpressed duct markers (CK19 and CA19-9) and heat shock protein (HSP)27, a marker of non-islet cells, suggesting the transition from ductal cells. Such interesting results suggest the possibility of multipotent progenitors in adult pancreatic ducts.

Some studies have investigated the clonal source of pancreatic stem/progenitor cells. Using a serum-free, colony-forming assay, Seaberg *et al*. reported the clonal identification of multipotent precursor cells from the adult mouse pancreas [70]. These cells proliferate *in vitro* to form clonal colonies that coexpress neural and pancreatic precursor markers. These pancreas-derived cells appear to have limited capacity for self-renewal, lack the stem cell markers Oct4 and Nanog, and are of neither mesodermal nor neural crest origin. Upon differentiation, individual clonal colonies produce distinct populations of neurons and glial cells; pancreatic endocrine β, α, and δ cells; and pancreatic exocrine and stellate cells. Pancreas-related proteins were expressed in 4−6% of these cells. Taniguchi's group showed the isolation of multipotent pancreatic progenitors from both neonatal and adult pancreata using flow-cytometric cell sorting [67, 68]. By combining flow cytometry and clonal analysis, they showed that a possible pancreatic stem/progenitor cell candidate that resides in the developing and adult mouse pancreata expresses the receptor for the hepatocyte growth factor (HGF) c-Met, but does not express hematopoietic and vascular endothelial antigens such as CD45, TER119, c-Kit, and Flk-1. Moreover, they identified a newly specific marker for ductal cells, CD133 [68]. The cells purified with CD133 (+), CD34(-), CD45(-), Ter199(-) could not only differentiate into pancreatic endocrine and acinar cells but also expressed multiple markers of nonpancreatic organs including the liver, stomach, and intestine. The expanded colonies also expressed the duct marker, CK-19, and nestin. As the duct cells replicated, they transiently expressed the protein PDX-1, a transcription factor expressed widely in embryonic pancreatic progenitors but by birth restricted to β and δ cells [71]. Yamamoto *et al*. showed a method for isolating pancreatic ductal epithelial cells from adult mice by stimulation of cAMP signaling [58]. Pancreatic ductal cells were grown in medium containing cholera toxin or 8-bromo-cyclic adenosine monophosphate, which is known to be an intracellular cAMP generator and then cloned by limiting dilution. The isolated clonal cells were maintained for more than a year under the medium condition. The cells expressed high levels of CK and PDX-1 and were differentiated into insulin- and somatostatin-producing cells by adenovirus-mediated expression of ngn3. Furthermore, albumin production was induced by dexamethasone or by long-term culture in serum-containing medium. These cells are able to partially differentiate into pancreatic endocrine cells and hepatocyte-like cells and are therefore considered to have the characteristics of endodermal progenitor cells. Our group also has succeeded isolation of pancreatic stem/progenitor cells which are similar morphology to these cells [unpublished data].

A recent study showed that pre-existing β cells, rather than pancreatic stem cells, are the major source of new β cells in mice after birth or following 70% pancreatectomy [72]. Genetic marking for lineage tracing with the insulin promoter showed that adult pancreatic β cells are formed by self-duplication rather than stem-cell differentiation. Although this study supports the concept that β cell replication is the dominant mechanism for β cell expansion in adult mice, it remains controversial because it does not convincingly prove that new islets are not formed during neonatal life or after regeneration-inducing maneuvers, such as duct ligation or a 90% partial pancreatectomy. This is a well-established model in which regeneration occurs by two pathways: replication of pre-existing endocrine or exocrine cells, and proliferation of ductules and their subsequent differentiation into whole new lobes of pancreas that become indistinguishable from pre-existing ones.

The transdifferentiation of acinar cells to islets has also been championed [73-75]. Minami *et al.* showed that pancreatic acinar cells could trans-differentiate into insulin-secreting cells with secretory properties similar to those of native pancreatic β cells [75]. The frequency of insulin-positive cells was only 0.01% in the initial preparation and increased to approximately 5% under culture conditions. Analysis by the Cre/loxP-based direct cell lineage tracing system indicates that these newly made cells originate from amylase/elastase-expressing pancreatic acinar cells. Bouwens' group found evidence for acinar-to-islet conversion under the form of transitional cells co-expressing amylase and insulin, suggesting that fully differentiated exocrine pancreatic cells retain the capacity to undergo important phenotypic switches [73]. However, using alloxan diabetic mice treated *in vivo* with epidermal growth factor (EGF) and gastrin, the same group concluded that the observed normalization of blood glucose and increased islet mass resulted from increased neogenesis from ducts [76]. This conclusion was based on the findings of transitional cells expressing both CK and insulin and increased ductal proliferation without increased β cell proliferation.

The Edmonton group followed eighty-three human islet grafts transplanted using the Edmonton Protocol since 1999 [77]. They attempted to define a correlation between graft cellular composition and long-term transplant success. A significant positive correlation was observed between the number of ductal-epithelial cells transplanted and long-term metabolic success as assessed by an intravenous glucose tolerance test at approximately two years post-transplantation, while no significant correlation was observed between the total islet equivalents and long-term metabolic success. The data showed that the presence of ductal cells in clinical islet transplantation may improve the long-term metabolic outcome (table 1).

Table 1. Clinical Application of Stem Cell Therapy in Diabetes

Authors		Reference
Street CN *et al.*	A significant positive correlation between the number of ductal cells transplanted and long-term metabolic success	[77]
Voltarelli JC *et al.*	High-dose immunosuppression and AHST* induced prolonged insulin independence in newly diagnosed type 1 diabetes.	[87]
DeFronzo RA *et al.* Kendall DM *et al.*	Exendin-4 treatment in type 2 diabetes significantly improved glycemic control and reduced HbA1$_c$	[119] [120]
Ghofaili KA *et al.*	Exendin-4 treatment improved glycemic control of type 1 diabetes patients after islet transplantation.	[121]

HEMATOPOIETIC STEM CELLS/BONE MARROW CELLS

Bone marrow-derived stem cells can reconstitute the hematopoietic system and a significant number of bone marrow transplantations have been performed over many years. Recent studies suggest that transplanted bone marrow-derived stem cells can generate into multiple lineage cells, including liver, brain, lung, gastrointestinal tract, and skin [78-80]. If bone marrow cells are multipotent stem cells, there is no ethical issue in their clinical use. An appealing report suggested that cells derived from bone marrow have the capacity to differentiate into functionally competent pancreatic endocrine β cells *in vivo* without evidence of cell fusion [81]. Moreover, clonal cell lines from murine bone marrow cultured in high glucose for four months *in vitro* were reported to contain cells expressing a number of β cell genes, although their insulin content was less than 1% that of a normal β cells [82]. However, several other laboratories showed no evidence in this model that bone marrow-derived cells differentiated into insulin-expressing cells [83-85].

On the other hand, some recent studies showed that bone marrow-derived stem cells could initiate pancreatic regeneration. Although adult bone marrow-derived cells reduce hyperglycemia in mice with streptozotocin (STZ)-induced pancreatic damage, many of these bone marrow-derived cells were found to have an endothelial phenotype, but there was little evidence of them becoming β cells [83, 84]. Hess *et al.* showed that transplantation of adult bone marrow-derived cells expressing c-kit reduces hyperglycemia in mice with STZ-induced pancreatic damage, although quantitative analysis of the pancreas revealed an extremely low frequency of insulin-producing cells derived from donor bone marrow [83]. The majority of transplanted bone marrow cells were localized to ductal and islet structures, and their presence was accompanied by a proliferation of recipient pancreatic cells that resulted in insulin production. Hasegawa *et al.* showed that lethal irradiation and subsequent bone marrow cell infusion improved STZ-induced hyperglycemia, nearly normalizing glucose levels and partially restoring pancreatic islet number and size [86]. Donor bone marrow cells were detected around islets and were CD45 positive but not insulin positive. Homing of donor cells in bone marrow and subsequent mobilization into the injured periphery were required for recipient β cell regeneration after bone marrow transplantation.

Voltarelli *et al.* showed that the safety and metabolic effects of high-dose immunosuppression followed by autologous nonmyeloablative hematopoietic stem cell transplantation (AHST) in newly diagnosed type 1 diabetes [87]. They performed a prospective study of fifteen patients with type 1 diabetes (aged 14-31 years) diagnosed within the previous six weeks by clinical findings and hyperglycemia and confirmed with positive antibodies against glutamic acid decarboxylase. Hematopoietic stem cells were mobilized with cyclophosphamide (2.0 g/m^2) and granulocyte colony-stimulating factor (10 μg/kg per day) and then collected from peripheral blood by leukapheresis and cryopreserved. The cells were injected intravenously after conditioning with cyclophosphamide (200 mg/kg) and rabbit antithymocyte globulin (4.5 mg/kg). During a seven to thirty-six month follow-up (mean 18.8 months), fourteen patients became insulin free (one for thirty-five months, four for at least twenty-one months, seven for at least six months, and two with late response were insulin-free for one and five months). Among those, one patient resumed insulin use one year after AHST. At six months after AHST, the mean total area under the C-peptide response curve was significantly greater than the pretreatment values and at twelve and twenty-four months it did not change. Anti-glutamic acid decarboxylase antibody levels decreased after six months and stabilized between twelve and twenty-four months. Serum levels of HbA1$_C$ were maintained at less than 7% in thirteen of fourteen patients. Although the mechanism of these effects is unknown, high-dose immunosuppression and AHST certainly improved β cell function in all but one patient and induced prolonged insulin independence in the majority of the patients (table 1).

In summary, the infusion of bone marrow cells facilitates islet regeneration and/or replication, although the mechanism is unknown. β cell neogenesis from only bone marrow-derived cells might be rare, but the existence of multipotent adult stem cells that can differentiate into β cells has not been disproved.

OTHER STEM/PROGENITOR CELLS

Another approach to the generation of β cells is the differentiation of stem/progenitor cells in other organs derived from endoderm. The pancreas, liver, and gastrointestinal tract are all derived from the anterior endoderm and some articles show that their stem/ progenitor cells can differentiate into insulin-producing cells [88-93]. *In vivo* transduction of mice with an adenovirus expressing PDX-1 [88, 89], or both betacellulin and BETA2/NeuroD [91], or a modified form of PDX-1 carrying the VP16 transcriptional activation domain [93] markedly increases insulin biosynthesis and induces various pancreas-related factors in the liver. The question of which liver cell adopts the insulin-producing phenotype remains unanswered. Highly purified adult rat hepatic oval cells, which are capable of differentiation to hepatocytes and bile duct epithelium, can trans-differentiate into pancreatic endocrine hormone-producing cells when cultured in a high glucose environment [94]. In a follow-up study using a stably transfected rat hepatic cell line (WB-1) that expresses an active form of PDX-1 along with a reporter gene, RIP-eGFP, many endocrine pancreatic development genes were induced. An even more mature islet expression profile was obtained after exposure to high glucose levels

[95]. However, even after 4 weeks of *ex vivo* culture with high glucose, the insulin content was less than 1% that of normal β cells.

PDX-1 and/or Isl-1 induction of immature rat intestinal stem cells (IEC-6) into insulin-producing cells has been reported [96, 97]. It was also shown that GLP-1-(1-37) induces insulin production in developing and, to a lesser extent, adult intestinal epithelial cells *in vitro* and *in vivo*. This process is mediated by the up-regulation of the Notch-related gene, *ngn3*, and its downstream targets, which are involved in pancreatic endocrine differentiation [98]. These adult intestinal stem cells are also probable candidates for a new therapeutic approach to diabetes mellitus.

Recent reports suggested the existence of mesenchymal stem/progenitor cells in not only bone marrow [99, 100] but also human umbilical cord blood [101, 102], pancreatic tissue [103-105] and adipose tissue [106]. Mononucleated adherent cells displayed a similar immunophenotype and, under appropriate conditions, these cells differentiated into the same variety of mesenchymal lineages such as osteoblasts, chondrocytes, adipocytes and skeletal myoblasts. It has been also reported that some of these mesenchymal stem/progenitor cells have the potential to differentiate into insulin-producing cells.

A 2003 study reported the achievement of both advances in the NOD mouse model by coupling the injection of Freund's complete adjuvant with the infusion of allogeneic spleen cells [107]. It was concluded that the adjuvant eliminated anti-islet autoimmunity and the donor splenocytes differentiated into insulin-producing (presumably β) cells, culminating in islet regeneration. However, three separate groups recently reported that, although this treatment indeed allowed for the survival of transplanted islets and recovery of endogenous β cell function in a proportion of mice, there was no evidence of allogeneic splenocyte-derived differentiation of new islet β cells [108-110].

Other stem cells such as salivary gland progenitor cells [111, 112], amnion cells [113], brain [52], and dermis [114] were reported for differentiation into insulin-producing cells. However, multiple studies have been claiming differentiation capacity of adult extra-pancreatic stem populations into insulin-producing cells from not only these tissues but also liver, intestine, and adipose tissue [115]. Interpretation of data proposing such plasticity of adult stem cells remains controversial and mechanisms underlying stem cell plasticity must be clarified. Recent work suggests that most of these "transdifferentiations" may correspond to cell-fusion events, such as in epithelium repair [116] and hepatocyte experiments [117], or initiation of pancreatic stem cell differentiation.

INDUCTION OF INSULIN-PRODUCING CELLS FROM STEM CELLS

Some agents are shown to stimulate islet neogenesis. GLP-1/exendin-4 has incretin effects, enhancing insulin secretion; they also stimulate β cell replication and neogenesis and have anti-apoptotic effects [118]. Exendin-4 has recently received FDA approval for clinical use since successful trials of exendin-4 treatment in type 2 diabetes have been reported [119, 120], and patients had a significant improvement in glycemic control associated with weight loss [119] (table 1). DeFronzo *et al.* showed that a triple-blind, placebo-controlled, thirty-week study at eighty-two U.S. sites was performed with 336 randomized patients. After four weeks of placebo, subjects self-administered 5 μg exendin-4 or placebo subcutaneously twice daily for four weeks followed by 5 μg or 10 μg exendin-4, or placebo subcutaneously twice daily for twenty-six weeks. At week thirty, $HbA1_C$ changes from baseline ± SE for each group were -0.78 ± 0.10% (10 μg), -0.40 ± 0.11% (5 μg), and +0.08 ± 0.10% (placebo). Of evaluable subjects, 46% (10 μg), 32% (5 μg), and 13% (placebo) achieved $HbA1_C \leq 7\%$. There are significant differences between 5 μg or 10 μg exendin-4 group and placebo group [119]. Kendall *et al.* showed that a thirty-week, double-blind, placebo-controlled study was performed in 733 patients with type 2 diabetes unable to achieve adequate glycemic control with maximally effective doses of combined metformin-sulfonylurea therapy and that exendin-4 significantly reduced $HbA1_C$ [120]. Ghofaili *et al.* evaluated the effect of exendin-4 on insulin secretion after islet transplantation [121]. Eleven C-peptide positive islet cell recipients with elevated glucose levels were treated with exendin-4 for three months and ten patients responded to exendin-4. Two patients who had not restarted insulin achieved good glycemic control and one patient who had received 5,500 IE/kg in a first islet infusion was able to stop insulin. Seven other patients decreased their insulin dose by 39% on exendin-4. These data suggest that exendin-4 also improves glycemic control of type 1 diabetes patients after islet transplantation (table 1).

In addition to exendin-4, inhibitory compounds of dipeptidyl peptidase IV, which inhibits GLP-1 breakdown in blood, have been examined by multiple companies. The compounds can be taken orally. Plans are underway to examine the effects of enhanced GLP-1 action on β cell regeneration at various stages of type 1 diabetes, including the prediabetic phase before clinical onset, just after diagnosis, after a long duration of diabetes and with islet transplantation. Trials are also being initiated with various combinations of gastrin, EGF and GLP-1 agonists. No doubt other approaches to increasing β cell mass will soon be developed.

Some other agents, such as INGAP [122], the combination of betacellulin and activin A [123], conophylline [124], and the combination of EGF and gastrin [76] are shown to stimulate islet neogenesis. INGAP, a peptide fragment of pancreatic REG protein, has been associated with regeneration in rodents [122]. Betacellulin is a member of the EGF family that stimulates β cell proliferation [123]. Conophylline is useful in inducing the differentiation of pancreatic β cells both *in vivo* and *in vitro* [124]. Both activin A, a member of the TGFβ family [123], and gastrin [76] are thought to promote β cell differentiation.

It has also been shown that overexpression of embryonic transcription factors, such as PDX-1, Ngn3, BETA2/NeuroD and Pax4, in stem cells could efficiently induce their differentiation into insulin-expressing cells. Overexpression of PDX-1 induced insulin expression in pancreatic ductal cells [61, 125] or the liver [88, 93], and improved the glucose tolerance of STZ-induced diabetic mice [88, 93]. The ability of PDX-1 protein to both regulate its own gene expression through an A-box element in its promoter [126] and to induce the expression of other β cell genes is thought to be the basis of this induced insulin expression. When the expression of the class B basic helix-loop-helix (bHLH) transcription factor Ngn3 is directed ectopically into the embryonic epithelium, pancreas precursor cells develop prematurely and exclusively into glucagon-producing cells [127, 128]. Overexpression of Ngn3 in ductal progenitor cells induced differentiation into insulin-producing cells [61, 66]. BETA2/NeuroD protein, one of the class B bHLH factors, was cloned both as a transcriptional activator of the insulin gene [129] and as a neurogenic factor in *Xenopus* embryos [130]. Adenoviral-mediated introduction of BETA2/NeuroD induced β cell neogenesis in the liver and reversed diabetes in mice with betacellulin gene therapy [91] or PDX-1/VP16 gene therapy [93]. The constitutive expression of Pax4 in combination with histotypic lineage leads to the formation of islet-like spheroid structures that produce increased levels of insulin [48]. We examined which embryonic transcription factors in adult mouse and human duct cells could efficiently induce their differentiation into insulin-expressing cells [61]. Infection with the adenovirus expressing PDX-1, Ngn3, NeuroD, or Pax4 induced the insulin gene expression and NeuroD was the most effective inducer of insulin expression in primary duct cells. These data suggest that the overexpression of transcription factors, especially NeuroD, facilitates pancreatic stem/progenitor cell differentiation into insulin-producing cells.

We and other groups recently showed that a novel protein delivery system into cells, known as protein transduction technology, is an effective method for the induction of insulin-producing cells from stem cells. Although proteins and peptides are primary targets in drug development, the hydrophobic nature of these lipids makes it impossible for the vast majority to cross the membrane. Major advances have recently been made through protein and peptide delivery into cells using protein transduction technology. Proteins and peptides can be directly internalized into cells when covalently linked to protein transduction domains (PTDs), also known as cell-penetrating peptides (CPPs) [60-63, 131-140]. PTDs attach to cell membrane heparan sulfate proteoglycans and penetrate cells by macropinocytosis, a form of endocytosis. They are released from the endosome homogeneously into the cytoplasm and carried to the nucleus by retrograde transport [62, 63, 141-143]. We reported that PDX-1 protein has an Antennapedia-like PTD sequence in its structure and can permeate cells without extra PTD addition. Moreover, PDX-1 protein transduced into cultures of pancreatic ducts, thought to be islet progenitor cells, induces insulin gene expression [61]. We also reported that BETA2/NeuroD protein could be transduced into several cells, including pancreatic islets, due to an arginine- and lysine-rich PTD sequence in its structure. Furthermore, BETA2/NeuroD protein transduced into cultures of pancreatic progenitor cells induces insulin gene expression [141]. *In vivo*-transduced NeuroD in the small intestine remained functionally active and could ameliorate the non-fasting glucose levels of STZ-induced, diabetic mice by inducing enteric insulin expression [144]. Internalization of BETA2/NeuroD and PDX-1 proteins is extremely interesting because the *pdx-1* gene has A-boxes and PDX-1 protein positively autoregulates its expression [126]. Furthermore, the *BETA2/NeuroD* gene has E-boxes and BETA2/NeuroD protein stimulates its own transcription [145]. Once BETA2/NeuroD and PDX-1 proteins are transduced into stem/progenitor cells, endogenous *BETA2/NeuroD* and *pdx-1* gene transcription is amplified by these proteins, insulin transcription is stimulated and differentiation to insulin-producing cells may be facilitated. These data suggest that PDX-1 and BETA2/NeuroD protein transduction could be a safe and valuable strategy for enhancing insulin gene transcription and for facilitating the differentiation of stem/progenitor cells into insulin-producing cells without requiring gene transfer technology.

Edlund's group reported that the administration of Ngn3 fused TAT-PTD to cultured pancreatic explants, resulted in efficient uptake, nuclear translocation, and stimulation of the downstream reporter and endogenous genes. Consistent with the predicted activity of the protein, e9.5 and e13.5 mouse pancreatic explants cultured in the presence of TAT-Ngn3 showed an increased level of endocrine differentiation compared with control samples [146]. These results also raised the possibility of differentiating stem/progenitor cells into insulin-producing cells by using the appropriate sequence and combination of TAT-fused transcription factors.

Graslund's group reported that the third helix of the homeodomain of transcription factor Isletl-1 (Isl-1) internalized into cells [147]. Prochiantz's group reported in their review article that transcription factor Pax6 internalized into cells [148]. Isl-1 and Pax6 are also key regulators of pancreatic development and evidence of their transduction suggests the differentiation of stem cells into insulin-producing or other endocrine cells may be obtained by using Isl-1 and/or Pax6 protein as has been shown with PDX-1 and BETA2/NeuroD protein.

Conclusion

Although stem cell research is one of the most promising fields for therapeutic potential in biomedical research, we need to know the molecular mechanisms and signaling pathways that control the expansion and differentiation of stem cells. The most difficult and yet unsolved issue is how to differentiate stem/progenitor cells and acquire fully functional islets. The possibility that pharmacological agents might increase β cell mass is tantalizing because a decrease in β cell mass is the root cause of both types of diabetes. Because of the intensity with which new agents are being tested in clinical trials, answers should emerge in the very near future. Protein transduction technology could also offer a novel therapeutic approach for diabetes. Further investigations to understand the regenerative process of the adult pancreas and the appropriate induction of stem/progenitor cell differentiation will help to establish cell-based therapies in diabetes.

Acknowledgments

The author wishes to thank Dr. Shinichi Matsumoto for his valuable suggestions and Dr. Carson Harrod for editing the manuscript.

References

[1] DCCT Research Group (1993) The effect of intensive treatment of diabetes on the development and progression of long-term complications in insulin-dependent diabetes mellitus. *N. Engl. J. Med.* 329, 977-986.
[2] DCCT Research Group (1990) Diabetes control and complications trial (DCCT). Update. *Diabetes Care.* 13, 427-433.

[3] DCCT Research Group (1995) Adverse events and their association with treatment regimens in the diabetes control and complications trial. *Diabetes Care.* 18, 1415-1427.

[4] UK Prospective Diabetes Study (UKPDS) Group (1998) Intensive blood-glucose control with sulphonylureas or insulin compared with conventional treatment and risk of complications in patients with type 2 diabetes (UKPDS 33). *Lancet.* 352, 837-853.

[5] Ohkubo Y, Kishikawa H, Araki E, Miyata T, Isami S, Motoyoshi S, Kojima Y, Furuyoshi N, Shichiri M (1995) Intensive insulin therapy prevents the progression of diabetic microvascular complications in Japanese patients with non-insulin-dependent diabetes mellitus: a randomized prospective 6-year study. *Diabetes Res. Clin. Pract.* 28, 103-117.

[6] Shapiro AM, Lakey JR, Ryan EA, Korbutt GS, Toth E, Warnock GL, Kneteman NM, Rajotte RV (2000) Islet transplantation in seven patients with type 1 diabetes mellitus using a glucocorticoid-free immunosuppressive regimen. *N. Engl. J. Med.* 343, 230-238.

[7] Matsumoto S, Okitsu T, Iwanaga Y, Noguchi H, Nagata H, Yonekawa Y, Yamada Y, Fukuda K, Tsukiyama K, Suzuki H, Kawasaki Y, Shimodaira M, Matsuoka K, Shibata T, Kasai Y, Maekawa T, Shapiro J, Tanaka K (2005) Insulin independence after living-donor distal pancreatectomy and islet allotransplantation. *Lancet.* 365, 1642-1644.

[8] Matsumoto S, Okitsu T, Iwanaga Y, Noguchi H, Nagata H, Yonekawa Y, Yamada Y, Fukuda K, Shibata T, Kasai Y, Maekawa T, Wada H, Nakamura T, Tanaka K (2006) Successful Islet Transplantation from Nonheartbeating Donor Pancreata Using Modified Ricordi Islet Isolation Method. *Transplantation.* 82, 460-465.

[9] Noguchi H, Ueda M, Nakai Y, Iwanaga Y, Okitsu T, Nagata H, Yonekawa Y, Kobayashi N, Nakamura T, Wada H, Matsumoto S (2006) Modified two-layer preservation method (M-Kyoto/PFC) improves islet yields in islet isolation. *Am. J. Transplant.* 6, 496-504.

[10] Froud T, Ricordi C, Baidal DA, Hafiz MM, Ponte G, Cure P, Pileggi A, Poggioli R, Ichii H, Khan A, Ferreira JV, Pugliese A, Esquenazi VV, Kenyon NS, Alejandro R (2005) Islet transplantation in type 1 diabetes mellitus using cultured islets and steroid-free immunosuppression: Miami experience. *Am. J. Transplant.* 5, 2037-2046.

[11] Hering BJ, Kandaswamy R, Ansite JD, Eckman PM, Nakano M, Sawada T, Matsumoto I, Ihm SH, Zhang HJ, Parkey J, Hunter DW, Sutherland DE (2005) Single-donor, marginal-dose islet transplantation in patients with type 1 diabetes. *JAMA.* 293, 830-835.

[12] Hering BJ, Matsumoto I, Sawada T, Nakano M, Sakai T, Kandaswamy R, Sutherland DE (2002) Impact of two-layer pancreas preservation on islet isolation and transplantation. *Transplantation.* 74, 1813-1816.

[13] Onaca N, Naziruddin B, Matsumoto S, Noguchi H, Klintmalm GB, Levy MF (2007) Pancreatic islet cell transplantation: update and new developments. *Nutr. Clin. Pract.* 22, 485-493.

[14] Ryan EA, Lakey JR, Rajotte RV, Korbutt GS, Kin T, Imes S, Rabinovitch A, Elliott JF, Bigam D, Kneteman NM, Warnock GL, Larsen I, Shapiro AM (2001) Clinical outcomes and insulin secretion after islet transplantation with the Edmonton protocol. *Diabetes.* 50, 710-719.

[15] Noguchi H, Iwanaga Y, Okitsu T, Nagata H, Yonekawa Y, Matsumoto S (2006) Evaluation of islet transplantation from non-heart beating donors. *Am. J. Transplant.* 6, 2476-2482.

[16] Matsumoto S, Tanaka K (2005) Pancreatic islet cell transplantation using non-heart-beating donors (NHBDs). *J. Hepatobiliary Pancreat. Surg.* 12: 227-230.
[17] Matsumoto S, Okitsu T, Iwanaga Y, Noguchi H, Nagata H, Yonekawa Y, Liu X, Kamiya H, Ueda M, Hatanaka N, Kobayashi N, Yamada Y, Miyakawa S, Seino Y, Shapiro AM, Tanaka K (2006) Follow-up Study of the First Successful Living Donor Islet Transplantation. *Transplantation.* 82, 1629-1633.
[18] Iwanaga Y, Matsumoto S, Okitsu T, Noguchi H, Nagata H, Yonekawa Y, Yamada Y, Fukuda K, Tsukiyama K, Tanaka K (2006) Living donor islet transplantation, the alternative approach to overcome the obstacles limiting transplant. *Ann. N. Y. Acad. Sci.* 1079, 335-339.
[19] Sassa M, Fukuda K, Fujimoto S, Toyoda K, Fujita Y, Matsumoto S, Okitsu T, Iwanaga Y, Noguchi H, Nagata H, Yonekawa Y, Ohara T, Okamoto M, Tanaka K, Seino Y, Inagaki N, Yamada Y (2006) A single transplantation of the islets can produce glycemic stability and reduction of basal insulin requirement. *Diabetes Res. Clin. Pract.* 73, 235-240.
[20] Matsumoto S, Noguchi H, Yonekawa Y, Okitsu T, Iwanaga Y, Liu X, Nagata H, Kobayashi N, Ricordi C (2006) Pancreatic islet transplantation for treating diabetes. *Expert Opin. Biol. Ther.* 6, 23-37.
[21] Robertson RP (2004) Islet transplantation as a treatment for diabetes - a work in progress. *N. Engl. J. Med.* 350, 694-705.
[22] Bonner-Weir S, Weir GC (2005) New sources of pancreatic beta-cells. *Nat. Biotechnol.* 23, 857-861.
[23] Najarian JS, Sutherland DE, Matas AJ, Steffes MW, Simmons RL, Goetz FC (1977) Human islet transplantation: a preliminary report. *Transplant. Proc.* 9, 233-236.
[24] Ricordi C, Strom TB (2004) Clinical islet transplantation: Advances and immunological challenges. *Nat. Rev. Immuunol.* 4: 259-268.
[25] Noguchi H, Matsumoto S, Matsushita M, Kobayashi N, Tanaka K, Matsui H, Tanaka N (2006) Immunosuppression for islet transplantation. *Acta Med. Okayama.* 60, 71-76.
[26] Sato E, Shimomura M, Masuda S, Yano I, Katsura T, Matsumoto S, Okitsu T, Iwanaga Y, Noguchi H, Nagata H, Yonekawa Y, Inui K (2006) Temporal decline in sirolimus elimination immediately after pancreatic islet transplantation. *Drug Metab. Pharmacokinet.* 21, 492-500.
[27] Noguchi H, Ueda M, Hayashi S, Kobayashi N, Nagata H, Iwanaga Y, Okitsu T, Matsumoto S (2007) Comparison of M-Kyoto Solution and Histidine-Tryptophan-Ketoglutarate Solution With a Trypsin Inhibitor for Pancreas Preservation in Islet Transplantation. *Transplantation.* 84, 655-658.
[28] Nagata H, Matsumoto S, Okitsu T, Iwanaga Y, Noguchi H, Yonekawa Y, Kinukawa T, Shimizu T, Miyakawa S, Shiraki R, Hoshinaga K, Tanaka K (2006) Procurement of the Human Pancreas for Pancreatic Islet Transplantation from Marginal Cadaver Donors. *Transplantation.* 82, 327-331.
[29] Noguchi H (2007) Activation of c-Jun NH2-terminal Kinase during Islet Isolation. *Endocr. J.* 54, 169-176.
[30] Noguchi H, Nakai Y, Ueda M, Masui Y, Futaki S, Kobayashi N, Hayashi S, Matsumoto S (2007) Activation of c-Jun NH(2)-terminal kinase (JNK) pathway during islet transplantation and prevention of islet graft loss by intraportal injection of JNK inhibitor. *Diabetologia.* 50, 612-619.
[31] Rivas-Carrillo JD, Soto-Gutierrez A, Navarro-Alvarez N, Noguchi H, Okitsu T, Chen Y, Yuasa T, Haruo M, Tabata Y, Jun HS, Matsumoto S, Fox IJ, Tanaka N, Kobayashi

N (2007) Cell-permeable Pentapeptide V5 Inhibits Apoptosis and Enhances Insulin Secretion, Allowing Experimental Single-donor Islet Transplantation In Mice. *Diabetes.* 56, 1259-1267.

[32] Rother KI, Harlan DM (2004) Challenges facing islet transplantation for the treatment of type 1 diabetes mellitus. *J. Clin. Invest.* 114, 877-83.

[33] Rivas-Carrillo JD, Navarro-Alvarez N, Soto-Gutierrez A, Okitsu T, Chen Y, Tabata Y, Misawa H, Noguchi H, Matsumoto S, Tanaka N, Kobayashi N (2006) Amelioration of diabetes in mice after single-donor islet transplantation using the controlled release of gelatinized FGF-2. *Cell Transplant.* 15, 939-944.

[34] Narushima M, Kobayashi N, Okitsu T, Tanaka Y, Li SA, Chen Y, Miki A, Tanaka K, Nakaji S, Takei K, Gutierrez AS, Rivas-Carrillo JD, Navarro-Alvarez N, Jun HS, Westerman KA, Noguchi H, Lakey JR, Leboulch P, Tanaka N, Yoon JW (2005) A human beta-cell line for transplantation therapy to control type 1 diabetes. *Nat. Biotechnol.* 23, 1274-1282.

[35] Hoffman LM, Carpenter MK (2005) Characterization and culture of human embryonic stem cells. *Nat. Biotechnol.* 23, 699-708.

[36] Soto-Gutierrez A, Kobayashi N, Rivas-Carrillo JD, Navarro-Alvarez N, Zhao D, Okitsu T, Noguchi H, Basma H, Tabata Y, Chen Y, Tanaka K, Narushima M, Miki A, Ueda T, Jun HS, Yoon JW, Lebkowski J, Tanaka N, Fox IJ (2006) Reversal of mouse hepatic failure using an implanted liver-assist device containing ES cell-derived hepatocytes. *Nat. Biotechnol.* 24, 1412-1419.

[37] Soria B, Roche E, Berna G, Leon-Quinto T, Reig JA, Martin F (2000) Insulin-secreting cells derived from embryonic stem cells normalize glycemia in streptozotocin-induced diabetic mice. *Diabetes.* 49, 157-162.

[38] Assady S, Maor G, Amit M, Itskovitz-Eldor J, Skorecki KL, Tzukerman M (2001) Insulin production by human embryonic stem cells. *Diabetes.* 50, 1691-1697.

[39] Lumelsky N, Blondel O, Laeng P, Velasco I, Ravin R, McKay R (2001) Differentiation of embryonic stem cells to insulin-secreting structures similar to pancreatic islets. *Science.* 292, 1389-1394.

[40] Hori Y, Rulifson IC, Tsai BC, Heit JJ, Cahoy JD, Kim SK (2002) Growth inhibitors promote differentiation of insulin-producing tissue from embryonic stem cells. *Proc. Natl. Acad. Sci. U. S. A.* 99, 16105-16110.

[41] Blyszczuk P, Asbrand C, Rozzo A, Kania G, St-Onge L, Rupnik M, Wobus AM (2004) Embryonic stem cells differentiate into insulin-producing cells without selection of nestin-expressing cells. *Int. J. Dev. Biol.* 48, 1095-1104.

[42] Miyazaki S, Yamato E, Miyazaki J (2004) Regulated expression of pdx-1 promotes in vitro differentiation of insulin-producing cells from embryonic stem cells. *Diabetes.* 53, 1030-1037.

[43] Leon-Quinto T, Jones J, Skoudy A, Burcin M, Soria B (2004) In vitro directed differentiation of mouse embryonic stem cells into insulin-producing cells. *Diabetologia.* 47, 1442-1451.

[44] Moritoh Y, Yamato E, Yasui Y, Miyazaki S, Miyazaki J (2003) Analysis of insulin-producing cells during in vitro differentiation from feeder-free embryonic stem cells. *Diabetes.* 52, 1163-1168.

[45] Lester LB, Kuo HC, Andrews L, Nauert B, Wolf DP (2004) Directed differentiation of rhesus monkey ES cells into pancreatic cell phenotypes. *Reprod. Biol. Endocrinol.* 2, 42.

[46] Segev H, Fishman B, Ziskind A, Shulman M, Itskovitz-Eldor J (2004) Differentiation of human embryonic stem cells into insulin-producing clusters. *Stem Cells.* 22, 265-274.
[47] Kahan BW, Jacobson LM, Hullett DA, Ochoada JM, Oberley TD, Lang KM, Odorico JS (2003) Pancreatic precursors and differentiated islet cell types from murine embryonic stem cells: an in vitro model to study islet differentiation. *Diabetes.* 52, 2016-2024.
[48] Blyszczuk P, Czyz J, Kania G, Wagner M, Roll U, St-Onge L, Wobus AM (2003) Expression of Pax4 in embryonic stem cells promotes differentiation of nestin-positive progenitor and insulin-producing cells. *Proc. Natl. Acad. Sci. U. S. A.* 100, 998-1003.
[49] Rajagopal J, Anderson WJ, Kume S, Martinez OI, Melton DA (2003) Insulin staining of ES cell progeny from insulin uptake. *Science.* 299, 363.
[50] Hansson M, Tonning A, Frandsen U, Petri A, Rajagopal J, Englund MC, Heller RS, Hakansson J, Fleckner J, Skold HN, Melton D, Semb H, Serup P (2004) Artifactual insulin release from differentiated embryonic stem cells. *Diabetes.* 53, 2603-2609.
[51] Sipione S, Eshpeter A, Lyon JG, Korbutt GS, Bleackley RC (2004) Insulin expressing cells from differentiated embryonic stem cells are not beta cells. *Diabetologia.* 47, 499-508.
[52] Hori Y, Gu X, Xie X, Kim SK (2005) Differentiation of insulin-producing cells from human neural progenitor cells. *PLoS Med.* 2, e103.
[53] D'Amour KA, Bang AG, Eliazer S, Kelly OG, Agulnick AD, Smart NG, Moorman MA, Kroon E, Carpenter MK, Baetge EE (2006) Production of pancreatic hormone-expressing endocrine cells from human embryonic stem cells. *Nat. Biotechnol.* 24, 1392-401.
[54] Weissman IL (2000) Translating stem and progenitor cell biology to the clinic: barriers and opportunities. *Science.* 287, 1442-1446.
[55] Potten CS, Grant HK (1998) The relationship between ionizing radiation-induced apoptosis and stem cells in the small and large intestine. *Br. J. Cancer.* 78, 993-1003.
[56] Galli R, Gritti A, Bonfanti L, Vescovi AL (2003) Neural stem cells: an overview. *Circ. Res.* 92, 598-608.
[57] Oliver JA (2004) Adult renal stem cells and renal repair. *Curr. Opin. Nephrol. Hypertens.* 13, 17-22.
[58] Yamamoto T, Yamato E, Taniguchi H, Shimoda M, Tashiro F, Hosoi M, Sato T, Fujii S, Miyazaki JI (2006) Stimulation of cAMP signalling allows isolation of clonal pancreatic precursor cells from adult mouse pancreas. *Diabetologia.* 49, 2359-2367.
[59] Noguchi H, Xu G, Matsumoto S, Kaneto H, Kobayashi N, Bonner-Weir S, Hayashi S (2006) Induction of pancreatic stem/progenitor cells into insulin-producing cells by adenoviral-mediated gene transfer technology. *Cell Transplant.* 15, 929-938.
[60] Noguchi H (2007) Stem cells for the treatment of diabetes. *Endocr. J.* 54, 7-16.
[61] Noguchi H, Kaneto H, Weir GC, Bonner-Weir S (2003) PDX-1 protein containing its own antennapedia-like protein transduction domain can transduce pancreatic duct and islet cells. *Diabetes.* 52, 1732-1737.
[62] Noguchi H, Matsushita M, Matsumoto S, Lu YF, Matsui H, Bonner-Weir S (2005) Mechanism of PDX-1 protein transduction. *Biochem. Biophys. Res. Commun.* 332, 68-74.
[63] Noguchi H, Matsumoto S, Okitsu T, Iwanaga Y, Yonekawa Y, Nagata H, Matsushita M, Wei FY, Matsui H, Minami K, Seino S, Masui Y, Futaki S, Tanaka K (2005) PDX-

1 protein is internalized by lipid raft-dependent macropinocytosis. *Cell Transplant.* 14, 637-645.

[64] Bonner-Weir S, Taneja M, Weir GC, Tatarkiewicz K, Song KH, Sharma A, O'Neil JJ (2000) In vitro cultivation of human islets from expanded ductal tissue. *Proc. Natl. Acad. Sci. U. S. A.* 97, 7999-8004.

[65] Gao R, Ustinov J, Pulkkinen MA, Lundin K, Korsgren O, Otonkoski T (2003) Characterization of endocrine progenitor cells and critical factors for their differentiation in human adult pancreatic cell culture. *Diabetes.* 52, 2007-2015.

[66] Heremans Y, Van De Casteele M, in't Veld P, Gradwohl G, Serup P, Madsen O, Pipeleers D, Heimberg H (2002) Recapitulation of embryonic neuroendocrine differentiation in adult human pancreatic duct cells expressing neurogenin 3. *J. Cell Biol.* 159, 303-312.

[67] Suzuki A, Nakauchi H, Taniguchi H (2004) Prospective isolation of multipotent pancreatic progenitors using flow-cytometric cell sorting. *Diabetes.* 53, 2143-2152.

[68] Oshima Y, Suzuki A, Kawashimo K, Ishikawa M, Ohkohchi N, Taniguchi H (2007) Isolation of mouse pancreatic ductal progenitor cells expressing CD133 and c-Met by flow cytometric cell sorting. *Gastroenterology.* 132, 720-732.

[69] Yatoh S, Dodge R, Akashi T, Omer A, Sharma A, Weir GC, Bonner-Weir S (2007) Differentiation of affinity-purified human pancreatic duct cells to beta-cells. *Diabetes.* 56, 1802-1809.

[70] Seaberg RM, Smukler SR, Kieffer TJ, Enikolopov G, Asghar Z, Wheeler MB, Korbutt G, van der Kooy D (2004) Clonal identification of multipotent precursors from adult mouse pancreas that generate neural and pancreatic lineages. *Nat. Biotechnol.* 22, 1115-1124.

[71] Bonner-Weir S, Toschi E, Inada A, Reitz P, Fonseca SY, Aye T, Sharma A (2004) The pancreatic ductal epithelium serves as a potential pool of progenitor cells. *Pediatr. Diabetes.* 5 Suppl. 2, 16-22.

[72] Dor Y, Brown J, Martinez OI, Melton DA (2004) Adult pancreatic beta-cells are formed by self-duplication rather than stem-cell differentiation. *Nature.* 429, 41-46.

[73] Lardon J, Huyens N, Rooman I, Bouwens L (2004) Exocrine cell transdifferentiation in dexamethasone-treated rat pancreas. *Virchows Arch.* 444, 61-65.

[74] Baeyens L, De Breuck S, Lardon J, Mfopou JK, Rooman I, Bouwens L (2005) In vitro generation of insulin-producing beta cells from adult exocrine pancreatic cells. *Diabetologia.* 48, 49-57.

[75] Minami K, Okuno M, Miyawaki K, Okumachi A, Ishizaki K, Oyama K, Kawaguchi M, Ishizuka N, Iwanaga T, Seino S (2005) Lineage tracing and characterization of insulin-secreting cells generated from adult pancreatic acinar cells. *Proc. Natl. Acad. Sci. U. S. A.* 102, 15116-15121.

[76] Rooman I, Bouwens L (2004) Combined gastrin and epidermal growth factor treatment induces islet regeneration and restores normoglycaemia in C57Bl6/J mice treated with alloxan. *Diabetologia.* 47, 259-265.

[77] Street CN, Lakey JR, Shapiro AM, Imes S, Rajotte RV, Ryan EA, Lyon JG, Kin T, Avila J, Tsujimura T, Korbutt GS (2004) Islet graft assessment in the Edmonton Protocol: implications for predicting long-term clinical outcome. *Diabetes* 53, 3107-3114.

[78] Krause DS, Theise ND, Collector MI, Henegariu O, Hwang S, Gardner R, Neutzel S, Sharkis SJ (2001) Multi-organ, multi-lineage engraftment by a single bone marrow-derived stem cell. *Cell.* 105, 369-377.

[79] Brazelton TR, Rossi FM, Keshet GI, Blau HM (2000) From marrow to brain: expression of neuronal phenotypes in adult mice. *Science.* 290, 1775-1779.

[80] Jiang Y, Jahagirdar BN, Reinhardt RL, Schwartz RE, Keene CD, Ortiz-Gonzalez XR, Reyes M, Lenvik T, Lund T, Blackstad M, Du J, Aldrich S, Lisberg A, Low WC, Largaespada DA, Verfaillie CM (2002) Pluripotency of mesenchymal stem cells derived from adult marrow. *Nature.* 418, 41-49.

[81] Ianus A, Holz GG, Theise ND, Hussain MA (2003) In vivo derivation of glucose-competent pancreatic endocrine cells from bone marrow without evidence of cell fusion. *J. Clin. Invest.* 111, 843-850.

[82] Tang DQ, Cao LZ, Burkhardt BR, Xia CQ, Litherland SA, Atkinson MA, Yang LJ (2004) In vivo and in vitro characterization of insulin-producing cells obtained from murine bone marrow. *Diabetes.* 53, 1721-1732.

[83] Hess D, Li L, Martin M, Sakano S, Hill D, Strutt B, Thyssen S, Gray DA, Bhatia M (2003) Bone marrow-derived stem cells initiate pancreatic regeneration. *Nat. Biotechnol.* 21, 763-770.

[84] Mathews V, Hanson PT, Ford E, Fujita J, Polonsky KS, Graubert TA (2004) Recruitment of bone marrow-derived endothelial cells to sites of pancreatic beta-cell injury. *Diabetes.* 53, 91-98.

[85] Choi JB, Uchino H, Azuma K, Iwashita N, Tanaka Y, Mochizuki H, Migita M, Shimada T, Kawamori R, Watada H (2003) Little evidence of transdifferentiation of bone marrow-derived cells into pancreatic beta cells. *Diabetologia.* 46, 1366-1374.

[86] Hasegawa Y, Ogihara T, Yamada T, Ishigaki Y, Imai J, Uno K, Gao J, Kaneko K, Ishihara H, Sasano H, Nakauchi H, Oka Y, Katagiri H (2007) Bone marrow (BM) transplantation promotes beta-cell regeneration after acute injury through BM cell mobilization. *Endocrinology.* 148, 2006-2015.

[87] Voltarelli JC, Couri CE, Stracieri AB, Oliveira MC, Moraes DA, Pieroni F, Coutinho M, Malmegrim KC, Foss-Freitas MC, Simoes BP, Foss MC, Squiers E, Burt RK (2007) Autologous nonmyeloablative hematopoietic stem cell transplantation in newly diagnosed type 1 diabetes mellitus. *JAMA.* 297, 1568-1576.

[88] Ferber S, Halkin A, Cohen H, Ber I, Einav Y, Goldberg I, Barshack I, Seijffers R, Kopolovic J, Kaiser N, Karasik A (2000) Pancreatic and duodenal homeobox gene 1 induces expression of insulin genes in liver and ameliorates streptozotocin-induced hyperglycemia. *Nat. Med.* 6, 568-572.

[89] Ber I, Shternhall K, Perl S, Ohanuna Z, Goldberg I, Barshack I, Benvenisti-Zarum L, Meivar-Levy I, Ferber S (2003) Functional, persistent, and extended liver to pancreas transdifferentiation. *J. Biol. Chem.* 278, 31950-31957.

[90] Kaneto H, Matsuoka TA, Nakatani Y, Miyatsuka T, Matsuhisa M, Hori M, Yamasaki Y (2005) A crucial role of MafA as a novel therapeutic target for diabetes. *J. Biol. Chem.* 280, 15047-15052.

[91] Kojima H, Fujimiya M, Matsumura K, Younan P, Imaeda H, Maeda M, Chan L (2003) NeuroD-betacellulin gene therapy induces islet neogenesis in the liver and reverses diabetes in mice. *Nat. Med.* 9, 596-603.

[92] Zalzman M, Gupta S, Giri RK, Berkovich I, Sappal BS, Karnieli O, Zern MA, Fleischer N, Efrat S (2003) Reversal of hyperglycemia in mice by using human expandable insulin-producing cells differentiated from fetal liver progenitor cells. *Proc. Natl. Acad. Sci. U. S. A.* 100, 7253-7258.

[93] Kaneto H, Nakatani Y, Miyatsuka T, Matsuoka TA, Matsuhisa M, Hori M, Yamasaki Y (2005) PDX-1/VP16 fusion protein, together with NeuroD or Ngn3, markedly

induces insulin gene transcription and ameliorates glucose tolerance. *Diabetes.* 54, 1009-1022.

[94] Yang L, Li S, Hatch H, Ahrens K, Cornelius JG, Petersen BE, Peck AB (2002) In vitro trans-differentiation of adult hepatic stem cells into pancreatic endocrine hormone-producing cells. *Proc. Natl. Acad. Sci. U. S. A.* 99, 8078-8083.

[95] Cao LZ, Tang DQ, Horb ME, Li SW, Yang LJ (2004) High glucose is necessary for complete maturation of Pdx1-VP16-expressing hepatic cells into functional insulin-producing cells. *Diabetes.* 53, 3168-3178.

[96] Kojima H, Nakamura T, Fujita Y, Kishi A, Fujimiya M, Yamada S, Kudo M, Nishio Y, Maegawa H, Haneda M, Yasuda H, Kojima I, Seno M, Wong NC, Kikkawa R, Kashiwagi A (2002) Combined expression of pancreatic duodenal homeobox 1 and islet factor 1 induces immature enterocytes to produce insulin. *Diabetes.* 51, 1398-1408.

[97] Yoshida S, Kajimoto Y, Yasuda T, Watada H, Fujitani Y, Kosaka H, Gotow T, Miyatsuka T, Umayahara Y, Yamasaki Y, Hori M (2002) PDX-1 induces differentiation of intestinal epithelioid IEC-6 into insulin-producing cells. *Diabetes.* 51, 2505-2513.

[98] Suzuki A, Nakauchi H, Taniguchi H (2003) Glucagon-like peptide 1 (1-37) converts intestinal epithelial cells into insulin-producing cells. *Proc. Natl. Acad. Sci. U. S. A.* 100, 5034-5039.

[99] Pittenger MF, Mackay AM, Beck SC, Jaiswal RK, Douglas R, Mosca JD, Moorman MA, Simonetti DW, Craig S, Marshak DR (1999) Multilineage potential of adult human mesenchymal stem cells. *Science.* 284, 143-147.

[100] Eckfeldt CE, Mendenhall EM, Verfaillie CM (2005) The molecular repertoire of the 'almighty' stem cell. *Nat. Rev. Mol. Cell Biol.* 6, 726-737.

[101] Erices A, Conget P, Minguell JJ (2000) Mesenchymal progenitor cells in human umbilical cord blood. *Br. J. Haematol.* 109, 235-242.

[102] Pessina A, Eletti B, Croera C, Savalli N, Diodovich C, Gribaldo L (2004) Pancreas developing markers expressed on human mononucleated umbilical cord blood cells. *Biochem. Biophys. Res. Commun.* 323, 315-322.

[103] Eberhardt M, Salmon P, von Mach MA, Hengstler JG, Brulport M, Linscheid P, Seboek D, Oberholzer J, Barbero A, Martin I, Muller B, Trono D, Zulewski H (2006) Multipotential nestin and Isl-1 positive mesenchymal stem cells isolated from human pancreatic islets. *Biochem. Biophys. Res. Commun.* 345, 1167-1176.

[104] Seeberger KL, Dufour JM, Shapiro AM, Lakey JR, Rajotte RV, Korbutt GS (2006) Expansion of mesenchymal stem cells from human pancreatic ductal epithelium. *Lab. Invest.* 86, 141-153.

[105] Choi KS, Shin JS, Lee JJ, Kim YS, Kim SB, Kim CW (2005) In vitro trans-differentiation of rat mesenchymal cells into insulin-producing cells by rat pancreatic extract. *Biochem. Biophys. Res. Commun.* 330, 1299-1305.

[106] Timper K, Seboek D, Eberhardt M, Linscheid P, Christ-Crain M, Keller U, Muller B, Zulewski H (2006) Human adipose tissue-derived mesenchymal stem cells differentiate into insulin, somatostatin, and glucagon expressing cells. *Biochem. Biophys. Res. Commun.* 341, 1135-1140.

[107] Kodama S, Kuhtreiber W, Fujimura S, Dale EA, Faustman DL (2003) Islet regeneration during the reversal of autoimmune diabetes in NOD mice. *Science.* 302: 1223-1227.

[108] Suri A, Calderon B, Esparza TJ, Frederick K, Bittner P, Unanue ER (2006) Immunological reversal of autoimmune diabetes without hematopoietic replacement of beta cells. *Science.* 311, 1778-1780.

[109] Nishio J, Gaglia JL, Turvey SE, Campbell C, Benoist C, Mathis D (2006) Islet recovery and reversal of murine type 1 diabetes in the absence of any infused spleen cell contribution. *Science.* 311, 1775-1778.

[110] Chong AS, Shen J, Tao J, Yin D, Kuznetsov A, Hara M, Philipson LH (2006) Reversal of diabetes in non-obese diabetic mice without spleen cell-derived beta cell regeneration. *Science.* 311, 1774-1775.

[111] Okumura K, Nakamura K, Hisatomi Y, Nagano K, Tanaka Y, Terada K, Sugiyama T, Umeyama K, Matsumoto K, Yamamoto T, Endo F (2003) Salivary gland progenitor cells induced by duct ligation differentiate into hepatic and pancreatic lineages. *Hepatology.* 38, 104-113.

[112] Hisatomi Y, Okumura K, Nakamura K, Matsumoto S, Satoh A, Nagano K, Yamamoto T, Endo F (2004) Flow cytometric isolation of endodermal progenitors from mouse salivary gland differentiate into hepatic and pancreatic lineages. *Hepatology.* 39, 667-675.

[113] Wei JP, Zhang TS, Kawa S, Aizawa T, Ota M, Akaike T, Kato K, Konishi I, Nikaido T (2003) Human amnion-isolated cells normalize blood glucose in streptozotocin-induced diabetic mice. *Cell Transplant.* 12, 545-552.

[114] Shi CM, Cheng TM (2004) Differentiation of dermis-derived multipotent cells into insulin-producing pancreatic cells in vitro. *World J. Gastroenterol.* 10, 2550-2552.

[115] Limbert C, Path G, Jakob F, Seufert J (2008) Beta-cell replacement and regeneration: Strategies of cell-based therapy for type 1 diabetes mellitus. *Diabetes Res. Clin. Pract.* 79, 389-399

[116] Spees JL, Olson SD, Ylostalo J, Lynch PJ, Smith J, Perry A, Peister A, Wang MY, Prockop DJ (2003) Differentiation, cell fusion, and nuclear fusion during ex vivo repair of epithelium by human adult stem cells from bone marrow stroma. *Proc. Natl. Acad. Sci. U. S. A.* 100, 2397-2402.

[117] Wang X, Willenbring H, Akkari Y, Torimaru Y, Foster M, Al-Dhalimy M, Lagasse E, Finegold M, Olson S, Grompe M (2003) Cell fusion is the principal source of bone-marrow-derived hepatocytes. *Nature.* 422, 897-901.

[118] Brubaker PL, Drucker DJ (2004) Minireview: Glucagon-like peptides regulate cell proliferation and apoptosis in the pancreas, gut, and central nervous system. *Endocrinology.* 145, 2653-2659.

[119] DeFronzo RA, Ratner RE, Han J, Kim DD, Fineman MS, Baron AD (2005) Effects of exenatide (exendin-4) on glycemic control and weight over 30 weeks in metformin-treated patients with type 2 diabetes. *Diabetes Care.* 28, 1092-1100.

[120] Kendall DM, Riddle MC, Rosenstock J, Zhuang D, Kim DD, Fineman MS, Baron AD (2005) Effects of exenatide (exendin-4) on glycemic control over 30 weeks in patients with type 2 diabetes treated with metformin and a sulfonylurea. *Diabetes Care.* 28, 1083-1091.

[121] Ghofaili KA, Fung M, Ao Z, Meloche M, Shapiro RJ, Warnock GL, Elahi D, Meneilly GS, Thompson DM (2007) Effect of exenatide on beta cell function after islet transplantation in type 1 diabetes. *Transplantation.* 83, 24-28.

[122] Rosenberg L, Lipsett M, Yoon JW, Prentki M, Wang R, Jun HS, Pittenger GL, Taylor-Fishwick D, Vinik AI (2004) A pentadecapeptide fragment of islet neogenesis-associated protein increases beta-cell mass and reverses diabetes in C57BL/6J mice. *Ann. Surg.* 240, 875-884.

[123] Li L, Yi Z, Seno M, Kojima I (2004) Activin A and betacellulin: effect on regeneration of pancreatic beta-cells in neonatal streptozotocin-treated rats. *Diabetes.* 53, 608-615.

[124] Kojima I, Umezawa K (2006) Conophylline: a novel differentiation inducer for pancreatic beta cells. *Int. J. Biochem. Cell Biol.* 38, 923-930.
[125] Taniguchi H, Yamato E, Tashiro F, Ikegami H, Ogihara T, Miyazaki J (2003) beta-cell neogenesis induced by adenovirus-mediated gene delivery of transcription factor pdx-1 into mouse pancreas. *Gene Ther.* 10, 15-23.
[126] Marshak S, Benshushan E, Shoshkes M, Havin L, Cerasi E, Melloul D (2000) Functional conservation of regulatory elements in the pdx-1 gene: PDX-1 and hepatocyte nuclear factor 3beta transcription factors mediate beta-cell-specific expression. *Mol. Cell Biol.* 20, 7583-7590.
[127] Apelqvist A, Li H, Sommer L, Beatus P, Anderson DJ, Honjo T, Hrabe de Angelis M, Lendahl U, Edlund H (1999) Notch signalling controls pancreatic cell differentiation. *Nature.* 400, 877-881.
[128] Schwitzgebel VM, Scheel DW, Conners JR, Kalamaras J, Lee JE, Anderson DJ, Sussel L, Johnson JD, German MS (2000) Expression of neurogenin3 reveals an islet cell precursor population in the pancreas. *Development.* 127, 3533-3542.
[129] Naya FJ, Stellrecht CM, Tsai MJ (1995) Tissue-specific regulation of the insulin gene by a novel basic helix-loop-helix transcription factor. *Genes Dev.* 9, 1009-1019.
[130] Lee JE, Hollenberg SM, Snider L, Turner DL, Lipnick N, Weintraub H (1995) Conversion of Xenopus ectoderm into neurons by NeuroD, a basic helix-loop-helix protein. *Science.* 268, 836-844.
[131] Noguchi H, Matsumoto S (2006) Protein transduction technology: a novel therapeutic perspective. *Acta. Med. Okayama.* 60, 1-11.
[132] Noguchi H, Matsumoto S (2006) Protein transduction technology offers a novel therapeutic approach for diabetes. *J. Hepatobiliary Pancreat. Surg.* 13, 306-313.
[133] Joliot A, Prochiantz A (2004) Transduction peptides: from technology to physiology. *Nat. Cell Biol.* 6, 189-196.
[134] Matsushita M, Noguchi H, Lu YF, Tomizawa K, Michiue H, Li ST, Hirose K, Bonner-Weir S, Matsui H (2004) Photo-acceleration of protein release from endosome in the protein transduction system. *FEBS Lett.* 572, 221-226.
[135] Elliott G, O'Hare P (1997) Intercellular trafficking and protein delivery by a herpesvirus structural protein. *Cell.* 88, 223-233.
[136] Schwarze SR, Ho A, Vocero-Akbani A, Dowdy SF (1999) In vivo protein transduction: delivery of a biologically active protein into the mouse. *Science.* 285, 1569-1572.
[137] Noguchi H, Matsushita M, Okitsu T, Moriwaki A, Tomizawa K, Kang S, Li ST, Kobayashi N, Matsumoto S, Tanaka K, Tanaka N, Matsui H (2004) A new cell-permeable peptide allows successful allogeneic islet transplantation in mice. *Nat. Med.* 10, 305-309.
[138] Noguchi H, Nakai Y, Matsumoto S, Kawaguchi M, Ueda M, Okitsu T, Iwanaga Y, Yonekawa Y, Nagata H, Minami K, Masui Y, Futaki S, Tanaka K (2005) Cell permeable peptide of JNK inhibitor prevents islet apoptosis immediately after isolation and improves islet graft function. *Am. J. Transplant.* 5, 1848-1855.
[139] Matsushita M, Tomizawa K, Moriwaki A, Li ST, Terada H, Matsui H (2001) A high-efficiency protein transduction system demonstrating the role of PKA in long-lasting long-term potentiation. *J. Neurosci.* 21, 6000-6007.
[140] Futaki S, Suzuki T, Ohashi W, Yagami T, Tanaka S, Ueda K, Sugiura Y (2001) Arginine-rich peptides. An abundant source of membrane-permeable peptides having potential as carriers for intracellular protein delivery. *J. Biol. Chem.* 276, 5836-5840.

[141] Noguchi H, Bonner-Weir S, Wei FY, Matsushita M, Matsumoto S (2005) BETA2/NeuroD protein can be transduced into cells due to an arginine- and lysine-rich sequence. *Diabetes.* 54, 2859-2866.

[142] Wadia JS, Stan RV, Dowdy SF (2004) Transducible TAT-HA fusogenic peptide enhances escape of TAT-fusion proteins after lipid raft macropinocytosis. *Nat. Med.* 10, 310-315.

[143] Noguchi H, Ueda M, Matsumoto S, Kobayashi N, Hayashi S (2007) BETA2/NeuroD protein transduction requires cell surface heparan sulfate proteoglycans. *Hum. Gene Ther.* 18, 10-17.

[144] Huang Y, Chen J, Li G, Cheng TY, Jiang MH, Zhang SY, Lu J, Yan S, Fan WW, Lu DR (2007) Reversal of hyperglycemia by protein transduction of NeuroD in vivo. *Acta Pharmacol. Sin.* 28, 1181-1188.

[145] Miyachi T, Maruyama H, Kitamura T, Nakamura S, Kawakami H (1999) Structure and regulation of the human NeuroD (BETA2/BHF1) gene. *Brain Res. Mol. Brain Res.* 69, 223-231.

[146] Dominguez-Bendala J, Klein D, Ribeiro M, Ricordi C, Inverardi L, Pastori R, Edlund H (2005) TAT-mediated neurogenin 3 protein transduction stimulates pancreatic endocrine differentiation in vitro. *Diabetes.* 54, 720-726.

[147] Kilk K, Magzoub M, Pooga M, Eriksson LE, Langel U, Graslund A (2001) Cellular internalization of a cargo complex with a novel peptide derived from the third helix of the islet-1 homeodomain. Comparison with the penetratin peptide. *Bioconjug. Chem.* 12, 911-916.

[148] Prochiantz A, Joliot A (2003) Can transcription factors function as cell-cell signalling molecules? *Nat. Rev. Mol. Cell Biol.* 4, 814-819.

Chapter III

STEM CELLS IN KIDNEY DISEASES

María José Soler[*1] *and José Tomas Ortiz-Pérez*[2],
[1]Nephrology Department, Hospital del Mar,
Universitat Autònoma de Barcelona, Barcelona, Spain
[2]Cardiology Department, Hospital Clínic i Provincial,
Universitat de Barcelona, Barcelona, Spain

ABSTRACT

Circulating bone marrow-derived endothelial progenitor cells (EPCs) seem to play a crucial role in both vasculogenesis and vascular homeostasis. Chronic kidney disease is a state of endothelial dysfunction, accelerated progression of atherosclerosis and high cardiovascular risk. As a consequence, cardiovascular disorders are the main cause of death in end-stage renal disease (ESRD). It has been shown that patients with advanced renal failure have decreased number of bone marrow-derived endothelial progenitor cells and impaired EPCs function. Moreover, in kidney transplant patients, renal graft function significantly correlated with EPC number. The reduced number of EPCs in patients with ESRD has been ascribed to the uremia. Therefore, therapies that improve the uremic status in dialysis patients such as nocturnal hemodialysis are associated with restoration of impaired EPCs number and migratory function. In fact, some of the common treatments for patients with chronic kidney disease such as erythropoietin, statins and angiotensin II receptor antagonist increase the number of EPCs. Nowadays, there is growing evidence indicating that, under pathophysiological conditions, stem cells (SCs) derived from bone marrow are able to migrate in the injured kidney, and they seem to play a role in glomerular and tubular regeneration. After acute tubular renal injury, surviving tubular epithelial cells and putative renal stem cells proliferate and differentiate into tubular epithelial cells to promote structural and functional repair. Moreover, bone marrow stem cells, including hematopoietic stem cells and mesenchymal stem cells can also participate in the repair process by proliferation and differentiation into renal lineages. For instance,

---

[*] CORRESPONDENCE: María José Soler Romeo; Nephrology department. Hospital del Mar. Universitat Autònoma de Barcelona. Passeig Marítim 25-29; 08003 Barcelona- Spain; e-mail address: MSoler@imas.imim.es

mesenchymal SCs have been shown to decrease inflammation and enhance renal regeneration. The administration of ex vivo expanded bone marrow-derived mesenchymal SCs have been proved to be beneficial in various experimental models of acute renal failure. The mechanisms underlining this beneficial effect are still a matter of debate. Thus, therapeutic strategies aimed at correcting the regenerative potential of stem cells based on the administration of *ex vivo* expanded SCs or stimulating expansion and differentiation of local progenitor/SC populations are another exciting area of future research.

1. INTRODUCTION

Stem or progenitor cells have been found in various tissues, including bone marrow (BM), peripheral blood (BC), brain, and reproductive organs, in adult animals as well as in humans[1-4]. These stem cells are retained locally or released to the systemic circulation and activated by environmental stimuli for physiological and pathological tissue regeneration[5]. Bone marrow-derived circulating endothelial progenitor cells (EPCs) have been isolated from the mononuclear cell fraction of the adult peripheral blood by magnetic beams or Ficoll density-gradient[6, 7]. Flk-1, CD34 or AC133 antigens were used to detect putative EPCs from the mononuclear cell fraction of peripheral blood[8]. Available evidence suggests that hematopoietic stem cells (HSCs) and EPCs are derived from a common precursor (hemangioblast) (figure 1)[9, 10]. This was supported by former findings that embryonic HSCs and EPCs share certain antigenic determinants, including Flk-1, Tie-2, c-Kit, Sca-1, CD133, and CD34[9, 10].

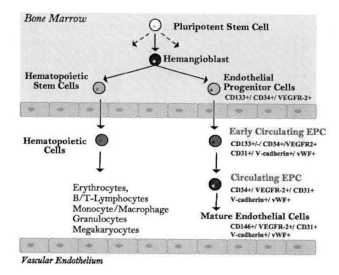

Figure 1. Cascade and expressional profiles of human bone marrow-derived endothelial progenitor cell differentiation. Hematopoietic stem cells and endothelial progenitor cells (EPCs) are derived from a common precursor (hemangioblast). EPCs in the bone marrow are positive for CD133/CD34/VEGFR-2. Circulating EPCs lose CD133 and are positive for CD34/VEGFR-2/CD31/VE-cadherin/von Willebrand factor (vWF).

It has been demonstrated that circulating endothelial progenitor cells (EPCs) promote vascular repair and maintain integrity of the endothelial monolayer[11]. Several groups have studied the relationship between EPCs and the cumulative cardiovascular risk[12, 13]. Hill et al. found a strong inverse correlation between the number of EPC and the overall cumulative cardiovascular risk assessed by the Framinghan risk score in healthy men, being EPCs counts a better predictor of flow-mediated brachial reactivity than other traditional risk factors for coronary disease[12]. In addition, patients with coronary artery disease (CAD) have both reduced levels of EPCs which suffer from functional impairment[13]. A reduction in both the levels and migratory capacity of EPCs were inversely correlated with the number of risk factors[13]. Moreover, in the same study, smoking and hypertension were found to be independent predictors of EPCs levels and migration, respectively[13]. In agreement with these findings, the number of circulating EPCs was significantly lower in patients with cerebrovascular disease than in control subjects[14, 15]. Smoking, aging and diabetes, which are well-known risk factors for coronary artery disease, lead to reduced number and EPCs dysfunction[16-22]. In two previous studies, patients with type 1 or type 2 diabetes revealed lower numbers of EPCs as assessed by outgrowth assays. Both studies have shown that the number of EPCs inversely correlated with hemoglobin A1c in type 1 and type 2 diabetes[16, 19]. Moreover, among patients with type 2 diabetes, EPCs show impaired adhesion to the endothelium, proliferation and tubulization capabilities. Taking together, EPC dysfunction resulting in incompetent vascular repair is thought to contribute to the increased risk of atherosclerosis and the prolonged and often complicated recovery from ischemic events. It has been demonstrated that the number of circulating EPCs predicts the occurrence of cardiovascular events and death from cardiovascular causes in patients with coronary artery disease and may help identify patients at increased cardiovascular risk[23, 24]. On the other hand, it should be noted that spontaneous mobilization of EPCs occurs in response to tissue ischemia and seems to be a repairing process mechanism[25-27]. However, further studies are needed to elucidate the exact role of EPCs in acute coronary syndromes, including myocardial infarction.

Broadly, this chapter discusses and reviews the mobilization, differentiation and homing processes in which stem/ progenitor cells are involved in patients with kidney disease. We also expound on the effect of the classical risk factors on EPCs in those patients. Lastly, we explore the regenerative potential of stem cells for therapeutic strategies in the setting of renal insufficiency.

2. EPCs and Kidney Disease

Patients with chronic kidney disease (CKD) have increased risk of cardiovascular disease, and consequently increased morbidity and mortality as a result of cardiovascular events[28, 29]. Go et al. showed in a large-scale study an independent progressive inverse correlation between the levels of the estimated glomerular filtration rate (GFR) and the risks of death, cardiovascular events and hospitalization. These risks were evident at an estimated GFR of less than 60 ml per minute per 1.73 m^2 and substantially increased with an estimated GFR of less than 45 ml per minute per 1.73 m^2 [30]. Moreover, renal subclinical dysfunction is highly prevalent and is independently associated with classical cardiovascular risk factors and metabolic syndrome[31]. CKD promotes hypertension and dyslipidemia, which in turn can contribute to the progression of renal failure. In addition, diabetic nephropathy is the leading cause of renal failure in developing countries. As a whole, hypertension, dyslipidemia, and diabetes are major risk factors for the development of endothelial dysfunction and progression of atherosclerosis[32, 33]. The impairment of endothelial function is well-recognized as one of the initial key mechanisms leading to atherosclerosis. Endothelial dysfunction, which occurs in both large and small arteries, is present at early stages in renal disease[34]. The pathophysiology of endothelial dysfunction includes abnormal vasomotor function, proinflammatory and prothrombotic states. A variety of invasive and non-invasive techniques are available for the assessment and quantification of endothelial dysfunction. Initially, these techniques focused on the study of: 1) the release of molecules into the plasma (i.e., nitric oxide and prostacyclin), 2) the vasodilator responses to an specific stimulus, and 3) the number of circulating endothelial cells present in the plasma[35]. Currently, new evolving and fascinating concepts about endothelial function are emerging from ongoing research on endothelial progenitor cells. As a result, studying the number and functional properties of EPCs in renal patients may help to detect the mechanisms involved in the endothelial dysfunction in the next future.

2.1. Endothelial Progenitor Cells and End-Stage Renal Disease

As well as with other clinical diseases, the number and functional properties of EPCs in patients with end-stage renal disease (ESRD) have been studied in hemodialysis and peritoneal dialysis patients [36-42]. Table 1 shows the clinical studies estimating circulating, clonogenic growth and function of EPCs in patients with ESRD. In patients with ESRD undergoing hemodialysis, the number of circulating EPCs is significantly decreased as compared to control subjects[36, 38, 41]. The number of circulating EPCs inversely correlates with predialysis urea concentration, left ventricular hypertrophy (LVH) and systolic blood pressure (SBP) in hemodialysis patients[36]. Cardiovascular diseases account for more than 50% mortality in uremic patients undergoing dialysis and the incidence of cardiac death is 10 to 20-fold greater in hemodialysis patients than in the age-matched general population[43]. As previously mentioned, the number of circulating EPCs inversely correlates with the number of cardiovascular risk factors in healthy subjects and in patients with CAD[12, 13]. In contrast to these findings, in hemodialysis patients there is no association between the numbers of circulating ECPs and the presence of concomitant risk factors for cardiovascular disease such as diabetes, hypertension, hypercholesterolemia or smoking[38, 41], and there is no association with gender and age either[38, 41]. Interestingly, the dose of recombinant erythropoietin in hemodialysis patients correlated positively with the number of circulating EPCs[41].

Table 1. Circulating EPC number, clonogenic growth and function in patients with ESRD

ESRD Treatment	Study	Sample size	Circulating precursor populations	Cultured EPCs (Lectin Dil-LDL)	EPCs functional capacity	Blood levels of VEGF	Other findings
HEMODIALYSIS	Eizawa et al.	50	CD45+CD34+↓ CD45+AC133+↓	↓	ND	NS	No relation between atherosclerosis risk factors and circulating EPCs.
	Choi et al.	44	ND	↓	MC↓ TF↓	ND	Correlation between Framingham's risk factor score and cultured EPCs. Correlation between dialysis dose and EPCs incorporation into HUVEC.
	Westerweel et al.	30	CD45+CD34+KDR+↓	↓	TF↓	NS	The hemodialysis procedure itself induces acute depletion of circulating EPCs.
	Chan et al.	12 CHD	CD34+VE-cadherin+↓	ND	MC↓	ND	EPC number and function inversely correlated with predialysis urea, LVMI and systolic BP.
		10 NHD	CD34+VE-cadherin+↑[a]		MC↑[a]		
PERITONEAL DIALYSIS	Steiner et al.	38	CD34+KDR+CD133+(NS)	NS	ND	ND	Association between history of familiar disease and cultured EPC.

ND: Not done, MC: Migratory capacity, TF: Tube formation, CHD: conventional hemodialysis, NHD: Nocturnal hemodialysis, LVMI: left ventricular mass index, BP: blood pressure, NS: no significant differences. [a] Nocturnal hemodialysis vs. conventional hemodialysis.

In one report, the direct effect of a dialysis session on the number of circulating EPCs was investigated. They found that the levels of these cells were reduced once the dialysis session was completed as compared with the levels before the start of dialysis. This observation may be attributed to different mechanisms including circulating EPCs sequestration, increased apoptosis or the unexpected impairment of endothelial function occurring during hemodialysis[44].

The levels of EPCs *in vitro* culture assays are also decreased in ESRD patients ongoing conventional hemodialysis (table 1) [37, 38, 41]. The reduction of cultured EPCs inversely correlates with Framingham's risk factor score in hemodialysis patients as well as in control subjects[37]. In contrast, the cultured vascular smooth muscle/myofibroblast progenitor cells (SPC) are not affected in hemodialysis patients[41]. This EPC-SPC imbalance may contribute to the acceleration of cardiovascular diseases in ESRD patients and could offer novel therapeutic targets.

The EPCs migration in response to vascular endothelial growth factor (VEGF), which is essential for angiogenesis, was examined using a modified Boyden chamber technique and a Transwell chamber[36, 37]. Patients treated with conventional hemodialysis have impaired EPCs migratory function as compared with healthy subjects[36, 37]. In consonance with the above mentioned findings in the EPCs pool, the EPCs function inversely correlates with predialysis urea concentration, left ventricular hypertrophy (LVH) and systolic blood pressure (SBP) in hemodialysis patients[36].

The ability of EPCs to incorporate into vascular structures which is believed to be important in new vessel formation was studied using a Matrigel tube formation assay[45]. The EPCs from ESRD patients are significantly less effective in stimulating human umbilical vein endothelial cells (HUVEC) angiogenesis as compared with the EPCs from normal controls (table 1)[37, 41]. Interestingly, when the impact of dialysis dose on EPC incorporation into HUVEC was studied, patients receiving lower doses of dialysis (Kt/V<1.3) showed a significantly impaired incorporation into endothelial cells as compared to that of patients receiving higher doses of dialysis (Kt/V≥1.3)[37]. This interesting finding suggests that higher doses of dialysis may be related to improved angiogenic function of EPCs. Further studies carried out by Chan et al. showed that restoration of impaired endothelial progenitor cell biology in ESRD can be achieved by increasing the dose and frequency of dialysis with nocturnal home hemodialysis (NHD), [36]. NHD, which provides 8-10 h of renal replacement therapy during sleep, five to six nights per week, increases the dialysis time per week. NHD permits a dialysis time about 30 hours per week, whereas in conventional hemodialysis the dialysis time is about 12 hours for a usual three 4 hours-dialysis sessions per week. This results in an augmented uremia clearance using NHD, which in turn is associated with restoration of EPC number and migratory function in ESRD patients[36]. In agreement with these findings, it is not surprising that uremic serum from ESRD patients impairs EPCs culture *in vitro* as compared with serum from healthy controls[41]. However, the aberrant outgrowth of EPCs is not accompanied by changes in SPC outgrowth[41], suggesting that the regenerative capacity of progenitor cells may be impaired in ESRD, while the capacity of smooth muscle progenitor cells to contribute to fibrosis and adverse remodeling of vascular lesions is unaffected.

VEGF contributes to postnatal neovascularization by mobilizing bone marrow-derived EPCs and it is present in the circulation[46]. VEGF plasma levels measured in hemodialysis patients were not different than those in controls[37, 38, 41]. This finding suggests that the reduced EPC levels present in hemodialysis patients are not related to the lack of VEGF.

In patients with ESRD treated with peritoneal dialysis, the number of cultured EPCs are similar than in healthy controls[42]. Interestingly, there is an inverse association between the presence of vascular disease with the number of cultured EPC in erythropoietin-treated peritoneal patients, whereas this was not the case for other conventional cardiovascular disease risk factors such as smoking, serum cholesterol level, diabetes and blood pressure[42]. Moreover, there is no association of endothelial-independent forearm blood flow reactivity with either circulating or cultured EPCs in peritoneal dialysis patients[42].

2.2. Endothelial Progenitor Cells and Chronic Kidney Disease

As previously mentioned, the number of circulating and *in vitro* cultured EPCs is significantly decreased in patients with CKD, as compared with control subjects[40,47-49]. There is a positive correlation between the absolute number of circulating CD34+ hematopoietic progenitor cells and EPCs both in healthy subjects as well as in renal patients[49]. It has been shown that uremic solutes, such as P-cresol and indoxyl sulfate, decrease endothelial proliferation and wound repair *in vitro*[50, 51]. These substances at concentrations commonly found in uremia, induce an inhibition of endothelial proliferation[50]. The inhibition of endothelial proliferation induced by p-cresol is dose-dependent[50]. On the contrary, the inhibition of endothelial proliferation induced by indoxyl sulfate is not dose-dependent[50]. To study the adverse effect of uremia on EPCs, these cells were cultured with uremic serum from patients with CKD and control serum from healthy subjects. Uremic serum inhibited EPCs differentiation and functional activity *in vitro* as compared with control serum[49]. This suggests that uremia may impair cardiovascular repair mechanisms by decreasing EPCs in patients with renal failure. Moreover, the amelioration of uremia after instauration of renal replacement therapy in patients with end-stage renal failure increases the number of EPCs[49]. Taken these results together, it seems that uremia milieu worsens EPCs differentiation and activity, and the therapies aimed at decreasing the uremic status will help to improve the endothelial dysfunction.

2.3. Endothelial Progenitor Cells after Kidney Transplantation

In the setting of kidney transplantation, many contradictory results have been reported on the levels of EPCs number and *in vitro* culture assays[52-55]. Steiner et al.[55] and de Groot et al.[52] reported no changes or increased number of circulating precursors of EPCs, respectively. These two studies reported no differences in cultured EPCs among kidney transplant patients as well. These findings are in contrast with those from Soler et al.[54] who found a significant reduction in both circulating and cultured EPCS in this population (figure 2). The last was also reproduced by Herbrig et al.[53]. There are several explanations for this discrepancy. First, Herbrig et al. [53] studied patients immediately after kidney transplantation who discontinued the therapy with erythropoietin. In this context, the absence of erythropoietin treatment and the high doses of immunosuppressive therapy might have played a role in the decreased number of cultured EPCs. Soler et al. [54] studied long-term renal transplant recipients with worse graft function than the other groups (see table 2). Hence, in this study with renal transplant patients with advanced chronic kidney disease the uremia might have played a significant impact on EPCs concentration and proliferation.

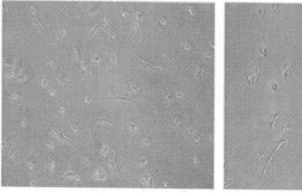
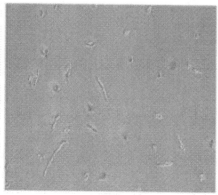

Figure 2. Endothelial progenitor cells after 7 days in culture from control subjects (left panel) and kidney transplant patients (right panel). The *in vitro* proliferation of endothelial progenitor cells in kidney transplant patients is reduced as compared with healthy controls (X200).

The potential impact of graft function on EPCs concentration and proliferation after *in vitro* culture have been assessed in diverse cross-sectional studies[52, 54]. GFR has been found to be an independent predictor of ciculating EPCs in kidney transplanted patients[54]. Those patients with reduced graft function (GFR < 30 mL/min) have lower EPCs concentration than those with GFR above 30 mL/min[54]. Interestingly, serum obtained from renal transplant recipients with poor graft function (GFR < 30 mL/min) inhibits EPC differentiation *in vitro* as compared with serum from patients with GFR above 50 mL/min[52] supporting the hypothesis that EPC differentiation is affected by the uremic environment. The effect of kidney transplant (KTx) on EPCs dysfunction in patients with ESRD has been further investigated. Herbrig et al. demonstrated that KTx ameliorates EPCs function, namely migratory and adhesion capabilities, as compared to patients with ESRD[53] despite the fact that in this study the number of circulating and cultured EPCs did not increased after KTx.

In KTx patients with stable graft function, there is no association between several recognized cardiovascular risk factors (hyperlipidemia, hyperglycemia, smoking and inflammation) and EPCs concentration or *in vitro* cultured counts[54, 55]. However, there are independent inverse associations between the number of cultured EPCs and the body mass index, the mean arterial pressure, and a positive history of cardiovascular disease[55]. In concordance with these results, another study found HDL, LDL and body weight to be independent predictors of EPCs concentration in KTx[52].

Table 2. Circulating EPC number, clonogenic growth and function in patients with renal transplantation

Study	Sample size	Age (Mean ± SD)	GFR (Mean ± SD) (mL/min/1.73m^2)	Circulating precursor populations	Cultured EPCs (Lectin DiI-LDL)	EPCs functional capacity
de Groot et al.	74	51.6 ± 11.5	55 ± 21	CD45+CD34+↑	NS	ND
Soler et al.	94	53.7 ± 12.5	36.0 ± 15.4	CD45+CD34+CD133+↓	↓	ND
Steiner et al.	105	45.4 ± 6.0	45.2 ± 21.4	CD34+ (NS) CD34+CD133+ (NS)	NS	ND
Herbrig et al.	20	45.5 ± 2.9	UK	CD34+ (NS) CD34+CD133+ (NS)	↓	MC↑* AD↑*

ND: Not done, MC: Migratory capacity, AD: Adhesion capacity, UK: Unknown, NS: no significant differences.
*after-kidney transplantation as compared to pre-kidney transplantation (dialysis patients).

Finally, it should be noted that KTx recipients should be considered patients with CKD at different degrees of kidney function, treated with a wide variety of drugs and with an overall increased CV risk as compared with healthy individuals. Thus, in these patients there are multiple mechanisms involved in the maintenance of the integrity of the endothelium.

3. THE EFFECT OF DRUG THERAPIES ON EPCs

The traditional risk factors for the progression of CVD in CKD include diabetes, proteinuria/albuminuria, hypertension, and hyperlipidemia[56]. A non-traditional factor that increases CV risk in CKD patients, perhaps by enhancing some of the traditional risk factors, is anemia. For this reason, appropriate management strategies of traditional, non-traditional risk factors and comorbidities can result in increased quality of life and a decreased rate of progression to ESRD.

Several sources of evidence have shown that antihypertensive drugs targeted to the renin-angiotensin system (RAS) can reduce proteinuria, preserve GFR and kidney function, and consequently reduce CV morbidity and mortality as well[57, 58]. In patients with CAD, ramipril therapy is associated with an increase in the number of cultured EPCs, which is obvious as early as 1 week after the initiation of ramipril treatment[59]. The increased number of cultured EPCs is paralleled by an enhancement of the migratory, proliferative, adhesive and *in vitro* vasculogenesis capabilities of isolated EPCs[59].

In response to ischemic stress (severe unilateral hind limb ischemia), enalapril specifically activates CD26/dipeptidylpeptidase IV (DPP IV) within the bone marrow microenvironment, but downregulates CD26/DPP IV activity in the peripheral blood primarily through an anti-inflammatory effect by reducing the number of CD26+ cells in peripheral blood[60]. The increased stroma-derived factor-1α (SDF-1α) concentration gradient between the bone marrow and the peripheral blood significantly mobilizes EPCs from the bone marrow into the circulation. Thus, the CD26/DPP IV system provides a possible target for enhancing EPC mobilization for use in therapeutic applications[60]. On the other hand, in patients with type 2 diabetes, angiotensin II subtype 1-receptor blockade increases the number of cultured EPCs[61]. The effect seems to be a class effect of angiotensin II receptor antagonists, because this effect has been demonstrated with standard daily doses of 2 long-acting substances, namely olmesartan and irbesartan[61]. Therefore, it seems reasonable that the increased number and mobilization of circulating EPCs with enhanced functional activity may contribute to the well-established beneficial effects of ACEI and ARB in patients with CAD.

Among the traditional risk factors, a high level of cholesterol has long been identified as especially deleterious regarding cardiovascular morbidity and mortality in non-renal patients[62]. Lipid-lowering therapy with statins not only has the potential to lower cardiovascular morbidity and mortality in patients with CKD through an improvement in lipids profile but also to slow the progression of renal disease[63, 64]. In the other hand, statins induce the differentiation of endothelial progenitor cells and upregulate EPC numbers *in vitro* and *in vivo*[65]. In this regard, the PI3K/Akt pathway appears to play a major role for statin-induced increases in EPC proliferation, migration and differentiation[65, 66]. In addition, in a murine model of acute myocardial infarction, atorvastatin markedly improved myocardial neovascularization at the infarct border zone and substantially enhanced mobilization of EPCs in wild-type but not in endothelial nitric oxide synthase knockout mice, suggesting a critical role for restored endothelial nitric oxide production in statin-induced myocardial neovascularization and EPC mobilization[67]. In the clinical scenario, it should be noted that in patients with chronic heart failure, treatment with simvastatin for four weeks improves endothelial function independently of LDL cholesterol levels, suggesting that simvastatin may exert important pleiotropic effects in humans[68].

Anemia is common in CKD due to a state of erythropoietin deficiency. It worsens as renal function declines and is an important CVD risk factor in those patients with CKD[69-72]. Indeed, anemia has been recognized as the "fifth CV risk factor," along with smoking, hypercholesterolemia, diabetes and hypertension in those with CKD[73]. Currently anemia is a modifiable risk factor, and correction of anemia with recombinant human erythropoietin (EPO) or analogues is the treatment of choice for patients with anemia and chronic renal failure due to EPO deficiency[28]. In the pre-dialysis population, the treatment with recombinant human EPO may decrease the progression of CKD, delay subsequent renal failure, improve quality of life, and improve overall cardiac function [74, 75]. EPO or analogues also appears to have direct biologic effects on endothelial cells. For instance, in healthy subjects and in renal patients, erythropoietin analogue darbepoetin alpha stimulates EPCs *in vitro* and *in vivo* via the Akt tyrosine kinase signaling pathway[76]. Furthermore, the EPO analogue darbepoetin stimulates endothelial progenitor cell proliferation and differentiation in renal patients. Importantly, this effect of darbapoetin on EPCs was achieved with a standard therapeutic dose[76]. Since EPO stimulates EPCs, treatment with rhEPO or analogues may open new therapeutic strategies in patients with cardiovascular disease.

Finally, kidney transplanted patients are under immunosuppression therapy to avoid the rejection of the graft. Immunosuppressive therapy has been shown to have an inhibitory effect on EPCs proliferation[77]. Buztal et al. studied the anti-angiogenic effect of rapamycin. These authors showed that rapamycin inhibited the proliferation and differentiation of human EPCs *in vitro*. They also observed that rapamycin induced apoptosis of EPCs[77]. The anti-proliferative effect of mycophenolate on vascular smooth muscle cells in experimental models, in rat and human mesangial cells *in vitro* has also been documented[78, 79].

4. BONE-MARROW-DERIVED CELLS AND ACUTE KIDNEY DISEASE

It has been shown that the induction of an experimental model of glomerulonephritis by a single injection of anti-Thy-1, caused a significant, more than 4-fold increase in the number of Bone-Marrow (BM) derived glomerular endothelial cells as compared to chimeric rats without glomerular injury. This finding suggests that BM derived cells have the capacity to participate in glomerular endothelial and mesangial repair[80]. Moreover, it seems that the chemokine RANTES (regulated upon activation normal T-cell expressed and secreted; CCL5) stimulates the homing and participation of EPC in renal vascular regeneration and glomerular repair in experimental glomerulonephritis[81].

In another model of experimental acute ischemic renal failure following unilateral renal artery ligation, Patschan et al. described EPCs mobilization which transiently reside in the splenic niche and later accumulate in the kidney. Ischemic preconditioning facilitated the traffic of EPCs from the splenic niche to the kidney, and subsequent accumulation of EPCs in the late phase was at least partly responsible for the beneficial effects of ischemic preconditioning[82]. In addition, it has been shown that acute elevation of uric acid acts as "physiologic" fast-acting endogenous mediator of EPC mobilization and renoprotection in response to tissue ischemia (bilateral renal artery clamping in FVB/NJ mice), consistent with its novel function in pharmacologic preconditioning[83]. The stimulatory effects of uric acid, reflected by splenic accumulation of EPCs, are detectable as early as 3 h after a single injection of uric acid as well as 3 h after indirect elevation of uric acid by treatment with oxonic acid, an uricase inhibitor[83]. However, both of these actions do not occur in mice with chronic hyperuricemia[83]. Thus, a transient surge in uric acid concentration may serve as an effective universal herald of tissue injury to accelerate the recruitment of EPCs[83]. In addition, Togel and colleagues demonstrated that another stem cell-mobilizing factor, stromal cell-derived factor-1 (SDF-1), is upregulated in the kidney after ischemic injury and decreases in the bone marrow, thereby reversing the normal gradient between bone marrow and the peripheral circulation[84]. This causes stem cell (CD34-positive cell) mobilization and homing via activation of its receptor CXCR4[84].

During active Wegener's granulomatosis, the amount of inflammatory endothelial cells (IEC) is significantly increased, whereas vasculitis treatment results in a significant reduction of IEC[85]. These observations suggest that circulating IEC may be cells detached from sites of injury, a reflection of the functional capacity of the cells at these sites. IEC are defined as endothelial cells that express the two inflammatory-associated markers, namely vascular-adhesion protein-1 and MHC class I-related chain A (MICA)[85]. These cells express high levels of inducible nitric oxide synthase and produce chemokines that are known to recruit and activate neutrophils[85]. Moreover, patients with active Wegener's disease have decreased numbers of EPC colony-forming units and a high expression of vascular-adhesion protein-1 and MICA in kidney endothelium as compared with those who were in remission[85]. In addition, IEC produce soluble factors, which have a significant negative effect on the proliferation, migration, and endothelial-nitric oxide synthase expression of EPCs[85]. On the basis of these results, circulating IEC may contribute to the pathogenesis/progression of Wegener's granulomatosis by preventing from vascular wall repair induced by endothelial progenitor cells.

5. ADULT STEM CELLS AND RENAL REPAIR

5.1. Kidney Adult Stem Cells

The presence of stem cells in the kidney and their potential benefits in renal repair have been widely studied. In normal conditions, tubule cell turnover in the kidney is exceedingly low, and the turnover that can be detected appears to occur by division of terminally differentiated tubular epithelial cells[86]. By contrast, after kidney injury, there is diffuse tubular proliferation[86]. This may reflect the intrinsic ability of surviving epithelial cells to adapt to the loss of neighboring cells by differentiation and proliferation, and ultimately replace those cells that have died as a result of the insult[86]. Based on the high proliferative capacity of injured kidney, one longstanding model holds that tubular cells themselves are the source of nephron repair[87]. In 2003, Maeshima et al. demonstrated the presence of renal progenitor tubular cells (label-retaining cells [LRC]) in normal rat kidneys by *in vivo* bromodeoxyuridine (BrdU)[88]. During tubular regeneration, LRC act as a source of regenerating cells that have an immature phenotype, actively proliferate, and consequently differentiate into epithelial tubular cells[88]. From the scope of regenerative medicine, identification of the factors regulating cell growth and differentiation of LRC is likely to be a very important issue, and such factors may become effective therapeutic agents that accelerate tubular regeneration[88].

The renal adult papilla contains large numbers of slowly cycling cells (i.e., BrdU-retaining cells) that persist throughout the life of Sprague-Dawley rats, but quickly enter the cell cycle and disappear from the papilla during recovery from a transient episode of ischemia, suggesting that these cells participate in renal repair[89]. The disappearance of these cells from the papilla could not be explained by their death in response to ischemia; apoptosis was absent from the papilla but was abundant in other renal regions after ischemia. This suggests that, as in other organs[90], proliferating cells may migrate toward the site of maximal injury (i.e., the medulla). In addition, renal papillary cells grown *in vitro* were capable of incorporating into other parts of the renal parenchyma, including renal tubules[89]. Isolation and *in vitro* culture of papillary cells allowed derivation of clones capable of generating more than one cell type, which, like metanephric mesenchymal stem cells[91], showed remarkable plasticity and co-expressed epithelial and mesenchymal markers. Furthermore, these cells were capable of forming spheres, a characteristic of many organ-specific adult stem cells *in vitro*[92, 93]. As an aggregate, these data indicate that adult kidney stem cells reside in the papilla[89].

Other studies were able to detect small numbers of CD133+ cells in the interstitium of adult human kidneys—approximately 1% of the total cell population—and isolate these cells in culture[94]. *In vitro* studies showed that CD133+ cells isolated from the kidney interstitium, might be pluripotent, having the capacity to differentiate into either tubular cells or vascular cells if presented with the appropriate cues[94]. In an experimental model of rhabdomyolysis and subsequent myoglobin-mediated acute renal failure, the injection of CD133+ labeled cells into mice, revealed that these transplanted cells proliferated and were incorporated into cortical proximal and distal tubules[94].

5.2. Stem Cell Transplantation and Renal Repair

There is evidence indicating that, under pathophysiological conditions, SCs derived from bone marrow are able to migrate to the injured kidney[94], including the vascular and interstitial compartments of renal allografts suffering chronic rejection[94, 95]. It should be noted that the administration of ex vivo expanded bone marrow-derived mesenchymal stem cells (MSCs) have been proven to be beneficial in various experimental models of acute renal failure[96-98]. Intravenous injection of the lineage-negative BM fraction prior to injury, part of which contains MSCs, attenuates the initial rise in BUN after ischemia reperfusion injury (IRI)[99], whereas whole BM injection has no protective effect[100]. Injection of purified MSCs almost completely protects against the cisplatin-induced rise in BUN, whereas injection of purified HSCs has virtually no protective effect[97]. In this study, MSCs markedly accelerated tubular proliferation in response to cisplatin-induced damage, as revealed by higher numbers of Ki-67–positive cells within the tubuli with respect to cisplatin-treated mice that were given saline[97]. Similar protection from injected MSCs was found in a glycerol pigment-induced nephropathy model [96]. Green fluorescent protein (GFP)-positive MSCs injected intravenously homed to the kidney of mice with glycerol-induced acute renal failure but not to the kidney of normal mice[96]. MSC GFP-positive cells localized in the tubular epithelial lining and expressed cytokeratin, indicating that MSCs engrafted in the damaged kidney, differentiated into tubular epithelial cells and promoted the recovery of morphological and functional alterations[96]. Moreover, MSCs enhanced tubular proliferation as detected by the increased number of proliferating nuclear antigen (PCNA) positive cells[96]. Importanlty, infused MSCs have been shown to enhance recovery of rodents subjected to IRI even if administered 24 h after the injury, suggesting active participation of these cells in the repair process[98, 101, 102]. In summary, there is strong evidence that MSCs protect against acute kidney injury and accelerate the recovery process in toxic and ischemic rodent models. The mechanisms responsible for their protective and regenerative effects remain incompletely understood.

Morigi et al.[97] and Herrera et al.[96] reported that exogenous MSCs can engraft into injured tubules and proposed that the ability to transdifferentiate explained their protective effect. Yokoo et al. injected exogenous MSCs directly into developing kidney, and after subsequent embryonic and organ culture observed MSC incorporation into glomerulus, tubules, and interstitium, which support the possibility of direct engraftment[103]. This is highly controversial, however, and even those who argue there is engraftment acknowledge that the primary means of repair by these cells most likely involves paracrine and endocrine effects, including mitogenic, antiapoptotic, anti-inflammatory, and angiogenic influences[104]. Whether the higher local concentrations of paracrine factors released from intrarenal MSCs *vs.* lower systemic concentrations relased from extrarenal MSCs are critical factors in their therapeutic effect requires careful follow-up studies.

In conclusion, stem cells transplantation seems to play a key role in kidney regeneration following acute renal injury. Therapeutic strategies to explore the regenerative potential of stem cells based on the administration of *ex vivo* expanded SCs or stimulating expansion and differentiation of local progenitor/SC populations will become an additional exciting area of future research.

REFERENCES

[1] Bartlett PF: Pluripotential hemopoietic stem cells in adult mouse brain. *Proc. Natl. Acad. Sci. U. S. A.* 1982;79:2722-2725.

[2] Clermont Y, Hermo L: Spermatogonial stem cells in the albino rat. *Am. J. Anat.* 1975;142:159-175.

[3] Erslev AJ: Erythropoietin in Vitro. Ii. Effect on "Stem Cells". *Blood.* 1964;24:331-342.

[4] Reyners H, Gianfelici de Reyners E, Regniers L, Maisin JR: A glial progenitor cell in the cerebral cortex of the adult rat. *J. Neurocytol.* 1986;15:53-61.

[5] Isner JM, Asahara T: Angiogenesis and vasculogenesis as therapeutic strategies for postnatal neovascularization. *J. Clin. Invest.* 1999;103:1231-1236.

[6] Asahara T, Murohara T, Sullivan A, Silver M, van der Zee R, Li T, Witzenbichler B, Schatteman G, Isner JM: Isolation of putative progenitor endothelial cells for angiogenesis. *Science.* 1997;275:964-967.

[7] Rehman J, Li J, Orschell CM, March KL: Peripheral blood "endothelial progenitor cells" are derived from monocyte/macrophages and secrete angiogenic growth factors. *Circulation.* 2003;107:1164-1169.

[8] Asahara T, Masuda H, Takahashi T, Kalka C, Pastore C, Silver M, Kearne M, Magner M, Isner JM: Bone marrow origin of endothelial progenitor cells responsible for postnatal vasculogenesis in physiological and pathological neovascularization. *Circ. Res.* 1999;85:221-228.

[9] Flamme I, Risau W: Induction of vasculogenesis and hematopoiesis in vitro. *Development.* 1992;116:435-439.

[10] Weiss MJ, Orkin SH: In vitro differentiation of murine embryonic stem cells. New approaches to old problems. *J. Clin. Invest.* 1996;97:591-595.

[11] Hristov M, Erl W, Weber PC: Endothelial progenitor cells: mobilization, differentiation, and homing. *Arterioscler. Thromb. Vasc. Biol.* 2003;23:1185-1189.

[12] Hill JM, Zalos G, Halcox JP, Schenke WH, Waclawiw MA, Quyyumi AA, Finkel T: Circulating endothelial progenitor cells, vascular function, and cardiovascular risk. *N. Engl. J. Med.* 2003;348:593-600.

[13] Vasa M, Fichtlscherer S, Aicher A, Adler K, Urbich C, Martin H, Zeiher AM, Dimmeler S: Number and migratory activity of circulating endothelial progenitor cells inversely correlate with risk factors for coronary artery disease. *Circ. Res.* 2001;89:E1-7.

[14] Ghani U, Shuaib A, Salam A, Nasir A, Shuaib U, Jeerakathil T, Sher F, O'Rourke F, Nasser AM, Schwindt B, Todd K: Endothelial progenitor cells during cerebrovascular disease. *Stroke.* 2005;36:151-153.

[15] Lau KK, Chan YH, Yiu KH, Li SW, Tam S, Lau CP, Kwong YL, Tse HF: Burden of carotid atherosclerosis in patients with stroke: relationships with circulating endothelial progenitor cells and hypertension. *J. Hum. Hypertens.* 2007;21:445-451.

[16] Loomans CJ, de Koning EJ, Staal FJ, Rookmaaker MB, Verseyden C, de Boer HC, Verhaar MC, Braam B, Rabelink TJ, van Zonneveld AJ: Endothelial progenitor cell dysfunction: a novel concept in the pathogenesis of vascular complications of type 1 diabetes. *Diabetes.* 2004;53:195-199.

[17] Michaud SE, Dussault S, Haddad P, Groleau J, Rivard A: Circulating endothelial progenitor cells from healthy smokers exhibit impaired functional activities. *Atherosclerosis.* 2006;187:423-432.

[18] Schatteman GC, Hanlon HD, Jiao C, Dodds SG, Christy BA: Blood-derived angioblasts accelerate blood-flow restoration in diabetic mice. *J. Clin. Invest.* 2000;106:571-578.

[19] Tepper OM, Galiano RD, Capla JM, Kalka C, Gagne PJ, Jacobowitz GR, Levine JP, Gurtner GC: Human endothelial progenitor cells from type II diabetics exhibit impaired proliferation, adhesion, and incorporation into vascular structures. *Circulation.* 2002;106:2781-2786.

[20] Hoetzer GL, Van Guilder GP, Irmiger HM, Keith RS, Stauffer BL, DeSouza CA: Aging, exercise, and endothelial progenitor cell clonogenic and migratory capacity in men. *J. Appl. Physiol.* 2007;102:847-852.

[21] Tao J, Wang Y, Yang Z, Tu C, Xu MG, Wang JM: Circulating endothelial progenitor cell deficiency contributes to impaired arterial elasticity in persons of advancing age. *J. Hum. Hypertens.* 2006;20:490-495.

[22] Heiss C, Keymel S, Niesler U, Ziemann J, Kelm M, Kalka C: Impaired progenitor cell activity in age-related endothelial dysfunction. *J. Am. Coll Cardiol.* 2005;45:1441-1448.

[23] Werner N, Kosiol S, Schiegl T, Ahlers P, Walenta K, Link A, Bohm M, Nickenig G: Circulating endothelial progenitor cells and cardiovascular outcomes. *N. Engl. J. Med.* 2005;353:999-1007.

[24] Schmidt-Lucke C, Rossig L, Fichtlscherer S, Vasa M, Britten M, Kamper U, Dimmeler S, Zeiher AM: Reduced number of circulating endothelial progenitor cells predicts future cardiovascular events: proof of concept for the clinical importance of endogenous vascular repair. *Circulation.* 2005;111:2981-2987.

[25] Gill M, Dias S, Hattori K, Rivera ML, Hicklin D, Witte L, Girardi L, Yurt R, Himel H, Rafii S: Vascular trauma induces rapid but transient mobilization of VEGFR2(+)AC133(+) endothelial precursor cells. *Circ. Res.* 2001;88:167-174.

[26] Massa M, Rosti V, Ferrario M, Campanelli R, Ramajoli I, Rosso R, De Ferrari GM, Ferlini M, Goffredo L, Bertoletti A, Klersy C, Pecci A, Moratti R, Tavazzi L: Increased circulating hematopoietic and endothelial progenitor cells in the early phase of acute myocardial infarction. *Blood.* 2005;105:199-206.

[27] Shintani S, Murohara T, Ikeda H, Ueno T, Honma T, Katoh A, Sasaki K, Shimada T, Oike Y, Imaizumi T: Mobilization of endothelial progenitor cells in patients with acute myocardial infarction. *Circulation.* 2001;103:2776-2779.

[28] K/DOQI clinical practice guidelines for chronic kidney disease: evaluation, classification, and stratification. *Am. J. Kidney Dis.* 2002;39:S1-266.

[29] Schiffrin EL, Lipman ML, Mann JF: Chronic kidney disease: effects on the cardiovascular system. *Circulation.* 2007;116:85-97.

[30] Go AS, Chertow GM, Fan D, McCulloch CE, Hsu CY: Chronic kidney disease and the risks of death, cardiovascular events, and hospitalization. *N. Engl. J. Med.* 2004;351:1296-1305.

[31] Cordero A, Laclaustra M, Leon M, Casasnovas JA, Grima A, Najar M, Luengo E, del Rio A, Ferreira I, Alegria E: [Cardiovascular risk factors and metabolic syndrome associated with subclinical renal failure]. *Med. Clin.* (Barc) 2005;125:653-658.

[32] Tobe SW, Burgess E, Lebel M: Atherosclerotic renovascular disease. *Can. J. Cardiol.* 2006;22:623-628.

[33] Morris ST, Jardine AG: The vascular endothelium in chronic renal failure. *J. Nephrol.* 2000;13:96-105.

[34] Endemann DH, Schiffrin EL: Endothelial dysfunction. *J. Am. Soc. Nephrol.* 2004;15:1983-1992.
[35] Blann AD: Assessment of endothelial dysfunction: focus on atherothrombotic disease. *Pathophysiol. Haemost. Thromb.* 2003;33:256-261.
[36] Chan CT, Li SH, Verma S: Nocturnal hemodialysis is associated with restoration of impaired endothelial progenitor cell biology in end-stage renal disease. *Am. J. Physiol. Renal. Physiol.* 2005;289:F679-684.
[37] Choi JH, Kim KL, Huh W, Kim B, Byun J, Suh W, Sung J, Jeon ES, Oh HY, Kim DK: Decreased number and impaired angiogenic function of endothelial progenitor cells in patients with chronic renal failure. *Arterioscler. Thromb. Vasc. Biol.* 2004;24:1246-1252.
[38] Eizawa T, Murakami Y, Matsui K, Takahashi M, Muroi K, Amemiya M, Takano R, Kusano E, Shimada K, Ikeda U: Circulating endothelial progenitor cells are reduced in hemodialysis patients. *Curr. Med. Res. Opin.* 2003;19:627-633.
[39] Herbrig K, Pistrosch F, Oelschlaegel U, Wichmann G, Wagner A, Foerster S, Richter S, Gross P, Passauer J: Increased total number but impaired migratory activity and adhesion of endothelial progenitor cells in patients on long-term hemodialysis. *Am. J. Kidney Dis.* 2004;44:840-849.
[40] Rodriguez-Ayala E, Yao Q, Holmen C, Lindholm B, Sumitran-Holgersson S, Stenvinkel P: Imbalance between detached circulating endothelial cells and endothelial progenitor cells in chronic kidney disease. *Blood Purif.* 2006;24:196-202.
[41] Westerweel PE, Hoefer IE, Blankestijn PJ, de Bree P, Groeneveld D, van Oostrom O, Braam B, Koomans HA, Verhaar MC: End-stage renal disease causes an imbalance between endothelial and smooth muscle progenitor cells. *Am. J. Physiol. Renal. Physiol.* 2007;292:F1132-1140.
[42] Steiner S, Schaller G, Puttinger H, Fodinger M, Kopp CW, Seidinger D, Grisar J, Horl WH, Minar E, Vychytil A, Wolzt M, Sunder-Plassmann G: History of cardiovascular disease is associated with endothelial progenitor cells in peritoneal dialysis patients. *Am. J. Kidney Dis.* 2005;46:520-528.
[43] Raine AE, Margreiter R, Brunner FP, Ehrich JH, Geerlings W, Landais P, Loirat C, Mallick NP, Selwood NH, Tufveson G, et al.: Report on management of renal failure in Europe, XXII, 1991. *Nephrol. Dial. Transplant.* 1992;7 Suppl 2:7-35.
[44] Miyazaki H, Matsuoka H, Itabe H, Usui M, Ueda S, Okuda S, Imaizumi T: Hemodialysis impairs endothelial function via oxidative stress: effects of vitamin E-coated dialyzer. *Circulation.* 2000;101:1002-1006.
[45] Rafii S, Lyden D: Therapeutic stem and progenitor cell transplantation for organ vascularization and regeneration. *Nat. Med.* 2003;9:702-712.
[46] Asahara T, Takahashi T, Masuda H, Kalka C, Chen D, Iwaguro H, Inai Y, Silver M, Isner JM: VEGF contributes to postnatal neovascularization by mobilizing bone marrow-derived endothelial progenitor cells. *Embo J.* 1999;18:3964-3972.
[47] Bahlmann FH, De Groot K, Spandau JM, Landry AL, Hertel B, Duckert T, Boehm SM, Menne J, Haller H, Fliser D: Erythropoietin regulates endothelial progenitor cells. *Blood.* 2004;103:921-926.
[48] Bahlmann FH, DeGroot K, Duckert T, Niemczyk E, Bahlmann E, Boehm SM, Haller H, Fliser D: Endothelial progenitor cell proliferation and differentiation is regulated by erythropoietin. *Kidney Int.* 2003;64:1648-1652.
[49] de Groot K, Bahlmann FH, Sowa J, Koenig J, Menne J, Haller H, Fliser D: Uremia causes endothelial progenitor cell deficiency. *Kidney Int.* 2004;66:641-646.

[50] Dou L, Bertrand E, Cerini C, Faure V, Sampol J, Vanholder R, Berland Y, Brunet P: The uremic solutes p-cresol and indoxyl sulfate inhibit endothelial proliferation and wound repair. *Kidney Int.* 2004;65:442-451.

[51] Cerini C, Dou L, Anfosso F, Sabatier F, Moal V, Glorieux G, De Smet R, Vanholder R, Dignat-George F, Sampol J, Berland Y, Brunet P: P-cresol, a uremic retention solute, alters the endothelial barrier function in vitro. *Thromb. Haemost.* 2004;92:140-150.

[52] de Groot K, Bahlmann FH, Bahlmann E, Menne J, Haller H, Fliser D: Kidney graft function determines endothelial progenitor cell number in renal transplant recipients. *Transplantation.* 2005;79:941-945.

[53] Herbrig K, Gebler K, Oelschlaegel U, Pistrosch F, Foerster S, Wagner A, Gross P, Passauer J: Kidney transplantation substantially improves endothelial progenitor cell dysfunction in patients with end-stage renal disease. *Am. J. Transplant.* 2006;6:2922-2928.

[54] Soler MJ, Martinez-Estrada OM, Puig-Mari JM, Marco-Feliu D, Oliveras A, Vila J, Mir M, Orfila A, Vilaro S, Lloveras J: Circulating endothelial progenitor cells after kidney transplantation. *Am. J. Transplant.* 2005;5:2154-2159.

[55] Steiner S, Winkelmayer WC, Kleinert J, Grisar J, Seidinger D, Kopp CW, Watschinger B, Minar E, Horl WH, Fodinger M, Sunder-Plassmann G: Endothelial progenitor cells in kidney transplant recipients. *Transplantation.* 2006;81:599-606.

[56] Basile JN: Recognizing the link between CKD and CVD in the primary care setting: accurate and early diagnosis for timely and appropriate intervention. *South. Med. J.* 2007;100:499-505.

[57] Parving HH, Andersen AR, Smidt UM, Hommel E, Mathiesen ER, Svendsen PA: Effect of antihypertensive treatment on kidney function in diabetic nephropathy. *Br. Med. J.* (Clin Res Ed) 1987;294:1443-1447.

[58] Parving HH, Andersen S, Jacobsen P, Christensen PK, Rossing K, Hovind P, Rossing P, Tarnow L: Angiotensin receptor blockers in diabetic nephropathy: renal and cardiovascular end points. *Semin. Nephrol.* 2004;24:147-157.

[59] Min TQ, Zhu CJ, Xiang WX, Hui ZJ, Peng SY: Improvement in endothelial progenitor cells from peripheral blood by ramipril therapy in patients with stable coronary artery disease. *Cardiovasc. Drugs Ther.* 2004;18:203-209.

[60] Wang CH, Verma S, Hsieh IC, Chen YJ, Kuo LT, Yang NI, Wang SY, Wu MY, Hsu CM, Cheng CW, Cherng WJ: Enalapril increases ischemia-induced endothelial progenitor cell mobilization through manipulation of the CD26 system. *J. Mol. Cell. Cardiol.* 2006;41:34-43.

[61] Bahlmann FH, de Groot K, Mueller O, Hertel B, Haller H, Fliser D: Stimulation of endothelial progenitor cells: a new putative therapeutic effect of angiotensin II receptor antagonists. *Hypertension.* 2005;45:526-529.

[62] Levine GN, Keaney JF, Jr., Vita JA: Cholesterol reduction in cardiovascular disease. Clinical benefits and possible mechanisms. *N. Engl. J. Med.* 1995;332:512-521.

[63] Diamond JR, Karnovsky MJ: Focal and segmental glomerulosclerosis: analogies to atherosclerosis. *Kidney Int.* 1988;33:917-924.

[64] Heusinger-Ribeiro J, Fischer B, Goppelt-Struebe M: Differential effects of simvastatin on mesangial cells. *Kidney Int.* 2004;66:187-195.

[65] Dimmeler S, Aicher A, Vasa M, Mildner-Rihm C, Adler K, Tiemann M, Rutten H, Fichtlscherer S, Martin H, Zeiher AM: HMG-CoA reductase inhibitors (statins) increase endothelial progenitor cells via the PI 3-kinase/Akt pathway. *J. Clin. Invest.* 2001;108:391-397.

[66] Llevadot J, Murasawa S, Kureishi Y, Uchida S, Masuda H, Kawamoto A, Walsh K, Isner JM, Asahara T: HMG-CoA reductase inhibitor mobilizes bone marrow--derived endothelial progenitor cells. *J. Clin. Invest.* 2001;108:399-405.

[67] Landmesser U, Engberding N, Bahlmann FH, Schaefer A, Wiencke A, Heineke A, Spiekermann S, Hilfiker-Kleiner D, Templin C, Kotlarz D, Mueller M, Fuchs M, Hornig B, Haller H, Drexler H: Statin-induced improvement of endothelial progenitor cell mobilization, myocardial neovascularization, left ventricular function, and survival after experimental myocardial infarction requires endothelial nitric oxide synthase. *Circulation.* 2004;110:1933-1939.

[68] Landmesser U, Bahlmann F, Mueller M, Spiekermann S, Kirchhoff N, Schulz S, Manes C, Fischer D, de Groot K, Fliser D, Fauler G, Marz W, Drexler H: Simvastatin versus ezetimibe: pleiotropic and lipid-lowering effects on endothelial function in humans. *Circulation.* 2005;111:2356-2363.

[69] Levin A: How should anaemia be managed in pre-dialysis patients? *Nephrol. Dial. Transplant.* 1999;14 Suppl 2:66-74.

[70] Levin A: Anaemia in the patient with renal insufficiency: documenting the impact and reviewing treatment strategies. *Nephrol. Dial. Transplant.* 1999;14:292-295.

[71] Levin A, Singer J, Thompson CR, Ross H, Lewis M: Prevalent left ventricular hypertrophy in the predialysis population: identifying opportunities for intervention. *Am. J. Kidney Dis.* 1996;27:347-354.

[72] Levin A, Thompson CR, Ethier J, Carlisle EJ, Tobe S, Mendelssohn D, Burgess E, Jindal K, Barrett B, Singer J, Djurdjev O: Left ventricular mass index increase in early renal disease: impact of decline in hemoglobin. *Am. J. Kidney Dis.* 1999;34:125-134.

[73] Silverberg D, Wexler D: Anemia, the Fifth Major Cardiovascular Risk Factor. *Transfus. Med. Hemother.* 2004;31:175-179.

[74] McCullough PA, Lepor NE: Piecing together the evidence on anemia: the link between chronic kidney disease and cardiovascular disease. *Rev. Cardiovasc. Med.* 2005;6 Suppl 3:S4-12.

[75] Serrano A, Huang J, Ghossein C, Nishi L, Gangavathi A, Madhan V, Ramadugu P, Ahya SN, Paparello J, Khosla N, Schlueter W, Batlle D: Stabilization of glomerular filtration rate in advanced chronic kidney disease: a two-year follow-up of a cohort of chronic kidney disease patients stages 4 and 5. *Adv. Chronic. Kidney Dis.* 2007;14:105-112.

[76] Bahlmann FH, Song R, Boehm SM, Mengel M, von Wasielewski R, Lindschau C, Kirsch T, de Groot K, Laudeley R, Niemczyk E, Guler F, Menne J, Haller H, Fliser D: Low-dose therapy with the long-acting erythropoietin analogue darbepoetin alpha persistently activates endothelial Akt and attenuates progressive organ failure. *Circulation.* 2004;110:1006-1012.

[77] Butzal M, Loges S, Schweizer M, Fischer U, Gehling UM, Hossfeld DK, Fiedler W: Rapamycin inhibits proliferation and differentiation of human endothelial progenitor cells in vitro. *Exp. Cell Res.* 2004;300:65-71.

[78] Gregory CR, Pratt RE, Huie P, Shorthouse R, Dzau VJ, Billingham ME, Morris RE: Effects of treatment with cyclosporine, FK 506, rapamycin, mycophenolic acid, or deoxyspergualin on vascular muscle proliferation in vitro and in vivo. *Transplant. Proc.* 1993;25:770-771.

[79] Hauser IA, Renders L, Radeke HH, Sterzel RB, Goppelt-Struebe M: Mycophenolate mofetil inhibits rat and human mesangial cell proliferation by guanosine depletion. *Nephrol. Dial. Transplant.* 1999;14:58-63.

[80] Rookmaaker MB, Smits AM, Tolboom H, Van 't Wout K, Martens AC, Goldschmeding R, Joles JA, Van Zonneveld AJ, Grone HJ, Rabelink TJ, Verhaar MC: Bone-marrow-derived cells contribute to glomerular endothelial repair in experimental glomerulonephritis. *Am. J. Pathol.* 2003;163:553-562.

[81] Rookmaaker MB, Verhaar MC, de Boer HC, Goldschmeding R, Joles JA, Koomans HA, Grone HJ, Rabelink TJ: Met-RANTES reduces endothelial progenitor cell homing to activated (glomerular) endothelium in vitro and in vivo. *Am. J. Physiol. Renal. Physiol.* 2007;293:F624-630.

[82] Patschan D, Krupincza K, Patschan S, Zhang Z, Hamby C, Goligorsky MS: Dynamics of mobilization and homing of endothelial progenitor cells after acute renal ischemia: modulation by ischemic preconditioning. *Am. J. Physiol. Renal. Physiol.* 2006;291:F176-185.

[83] Patschan D, Patschan S, Gobe GG, Chintala S, Goligorsky MS: Uric acid heralds ischemic tissue injury to mobilize endothelial progenitor cells. *J. Am. Soc. Nephrol.* 2007;18:1516-1524.

[84] Togel F, Isaac J, Hu Z, Weiss K, Westenfelder C: Renal SDF-1 signals mobilization and homing of CXCR4-positive cells to the kidney after ischemic injury. *Kidney Int.* 2005;67:1772-1784.

[85] Holmen C, Elsheikh E, Stenvinkel P, Qureshi AR, Pettersson E, Jalkanen S, Sumitran-Holgersson S: Circulating inflammatory endothelial cells contribute to endothelial progenitor cell dysfunction in patients with vasculitis and kidney involvement. *J. Am. Soc. Nephrol.* 2005;16:3110-3120.

[86] Humphreys BD, Bonventre JV: The contribution of adult stem cells to renal repair. *Nephrol. Ther.* 2007;3:3-10.

[87] Bonventre JV: Dedifferentiation and proliferation of surviving epithelial cells in acute renal failure. *J. Am. Soc. Nephrol.* 2003;14 Suppl 1:S55-61.

[88] Maeshima A, Yamashita S, Nojima Y: Identification of renal progenitor-like tubular cells that participate in the regeneration processes of the kidney. *J. Am. Soc. Nephrol.* 2003;14:3138-3146.

[89] Oliver JA, Maarouf O, Cheema FH, Martens TP, Al-Awqati Q: The renal papilla is a niche for adult kidney stem cells. *J. Clin. Invest.* 2004;114:795-804.

[90] Lavker RM, Sun TT: Epidermal stem cells: properties, markers, and location. *Proc. Natl. Acad. Sci. U. S. A.* 2000;97:13473-13475.

[91] Oliver JA, Barasch J, Yang J, Herzlinger D, Al-Awqati Q: Metanephric mesenchyme contains embryonic renal stem cells. *Am. J. Physiol. Renal. Physiol.* 2002;283:F799-809.

[92] Bodine DM, Crosier PS, Clark SC: Effects of hematopoietic growth factors on the survival of primitive stem cells in liquid suspension culture. *Blood.* 1991;78:914-920.

[93] Reynolds BA, Weiss S: Clonal and population analyses demonstrate that an EGF-responsive mammalian embryonic CNS precursor is a stem cell. *Dev. Biol.* 1996;175:1-13.

[94] Bussolati B, Bruno S, Grange C, Buttiglieri S, Deregibus MC, Cantino D, Camussi G: Isolation of renal progenitor cells from adult human kidney. *Am. J. Pathol.* 2005;166:545-555.

[95] Grimm PC, Nickerson P, Jeffery J, Savani RC, Gough J, McKenna RM, Stern E, Rush DN: Neointimal and tubulointerstitial infiltration by recipient mesenchymal cells in chronic renal-allograft rejection. *N. Engl. J. Med.* 2001;345:93-97.

[96] Herrera MB, Bussolati B, Bruno S, Fonsato V, Romanazzi GM, Camussi G: Mesenchymal stem cells contribute to the renal repair of acute tubular epithelial injury. *Int. J. Mol. Med.* 2004;14:1035-1041.

[97] Morigi M, Imberti B, Zoja C, Corna D, Tomasoni S, Abbate M, Rottoli D, Angioletti S, Benigni A, Perico N, Alison M, Remuzzi G: Mesenchymal stem cells are renotropic, helping to repair the kidney and improve function in acute renal failure. *J. Am. Soc. Nephrol.* 2004;15:1794-1804.

[98] Togel F, Hu Z, Weiss K, Isaac J, Lange C, Westenfelder C: Administered mesenchymal stem cells protect against ischemic acute renal failure through differentiation-independent mechanisms. *Am. J. Physiol. Renal Physiol.* 2005;289:F31-42.

[99] Kale S, Karihaloo A, Clark PR, Kashgarian M, Krause DS, Cantley LG: Bone marrow stem cells contribute to repair of the ischemically injured renal tubule. *J. Clin. Invest.* 2003;112:42-49.

[100] Lin F, Moran A, Igarashi P: Intrarenal cells, not bone marrow-derived cells, are the major source for regeneration in postischemic kidney. *J. Clin. Invest.* 2005;115:1756-1764.

[101] Bi B, Schmitt R, Israilova M, Nishio H, Cantley LG: Stromal Cells Protect against Acute Tubular Injury via an Endocrine Effect. *J. Am. Soc. Nephrol.* 2007;18:2486-2496.

[102] Lange C, Togel F, Ittrich H, Clayton F, Nolte-Ernsting C, Zander AR, Westenfelder C: Administered mesenchymal stem cells enhance recovery from ischemia/reperfusion-induced acute renal failure in rats. *Kidney Int.* 2005;68:1613-1617.

[103] Yokoo T, Ohashi T, Shen JS, Sakurai K, Miyazaki Y, Utsunomiya Y, Takahashi M, Terada Y, Eto Y, Kawamura T, Osumi N, Hosoya T: Human mesenchymal stem cells in rodent whole-embryo culture are reprogrammed to contribute to kidney tissues. *Proc. Natl. Acad. Sci. U. S. A.* 2005;102:3296-3300.

[104] Togel F, Weiss K, Yang Y, Hu Z, Zhang P, Westenfelder C: Vasculotropic, paracrine actions of infused mesenchymal stem cells are important to the recovery from acute kidney injury. *Am. J. Physiol. Renal. Physiol.* 2007;292:F1626-1635.

In: Encyclopedia of Stem Cell Research (2 Volume Set) ISBN: 978-1-61761-835-2
Editor: Alexander L. Greene © 2012 Nova Science Publishers, Inc.

Chapter IV

ROLE OF SURVIVIN IN ADULT STEM CELLS AND CANCER

Seiji Fukuda[*,1,2] and Louis M. Pelus[2]

[1]Department of Pediatrics, Shimane University Faculty of Medicine,
Enya-cho, Izumo, Shimane, Japan
[2]Department of Microbiology and Immunology, Walther Oncology Center,
Indiana University School of Medicine, Indianapolis, IN, US

ABSTRACT

The inhibitor of apoptosis protein (IAP) Survivin regulates apoptosis, cell cycle and cell division. Its expression in normal tissue is developmentally regulated and becomes barely detectable in most terminally differentiated adult tissues. Survivin has been proposed as a potential cancer target because the vast majority of the human tumors express high levels of Survivin in contrast to limited expression in most normal adult tissues. However, recent studies have demonstrated that Survivin regulates adult stem cell physiology, such as hematopoietic stem cells, neuronal precursor cells, keratinocyte stem cells and intestinal crypt stem cells. Furthermore, mouse embryonic stem cells express Survivin and homozygous gene deletion in mice leads to embryonic death at E4.5, indicating that Survivin is required for totipotent stem cell function. It is believed that cancer stem cells are primarily responsible for the development and dissemination of cancer. Our recent data suggests that Survivin regulates not just normal hematopoietic stem and progenitor cell (HSPC) proliferation but transformed HSPC with self-renewal capability. Since cancer stem cells share biological phenotypes with normal adult stem cells and almost all cancer cells over-express Survivin, it is likely that Survivin regulates leukemia and/or cancer stem cell fate. Although targeting Survivin in leukemia/cancer stem cells may be an effective treatment modality, ablation of Survivin may have adverse consequences in vivo, as a result of toxicity to normal stem cells. In this review, we will

---

[*] Corresponding author: Seiji Fukuda, M.D., Ph.D.; Department of Pediatrics, Shimane University Faculty of Medicine, 89-1 Enya-cho, Izumo, Shimane 693-8501, Japan; sfukuda@med.shimane-u.ac.jp; Tel: 81-853-20-2219; Fax: 81-853-20-2215

summarize and compare the roles of Survivin in normal adult stem cells and leukemia/cancer cells. Investigating mechanisms responsible for differentially regulating Survivin expression and function in cancer and normal adult stem cells will help to identify critical differences in Survivin behavior between neoplastic and normal tissues that can be utilized to develop innovative strategies for selectively antagonizing Survivin. In addition, manipulating pathways associated with Survivin may identify novel stem cell therapies with application for regenerative medicine.

INTRODUCTION

Stem cells are unspecialized cells able to generate themselves through self-renewal and also give rise to mature cells of a particular tissue through differentiation. The most important clinical application of human stem cells is the generation of cells and tissues that can be used for cell based therapies. The most striking example of the utility and curative potential of adult stem cells is hematopoietic stem cell transplantation. Recently, embryonic stem cells have been recognized as source of pluripotent stem cells with unlimited curative potential. The specific factors and conditions that allow stem cells to remain unspecialized and to direct their lineage differentiation are the primary focus of stem cell research and are required to realize their true potential for regenerative medicine. Recent studies indicate that tumors often originate through the transformation of normal stem cells [1]. Since striking parallels can be found between stem cells and cancer cells and similar signaling pathways may regulate self-renewal in stem cells and cancer cells that include 'cancer stem cells' — rare cells with indefinite potential for self-renewal that drive tumorigenesis. A number of studies show that many pathways that are associated with cancer also regulate normal stem cell development. In this regard, understanding mechanisms responsible for self-renewal versus differentiation in stem cells will provide profound insight into cancer stem cell renewal and proliferation. For instance, Wnt [1], Shh[2-4] and Notch pathways [5-7] have all been shown to contribute to the stem cell self-renewal of stem cells and/or progenitors in a variety of organs, and that these pathways can contribute to oncogenesis when deregulated.

One of the genes that is strongly associated with aberrant cancer cell proliferation and poor overall prognosis is Survivin. This inhibitor of apoptosis protein (IAP) family member blocks apoptosis through inhibiting caspases and/or by interacting with Stat3 [8-10], $p21^{WAF1/Cip1}$[11; 12], CDK4 [12], Cdc2(CDK1) [13], Smac/Diablo [14], XIAP [14], NFkB [15], Rb/E2F[16], HSP90 [17], or p53 [18-20]. All IAPs share a common domain of ~75 amino acids termed the Baculoviral IAP Repeat (BIR) domain, characterized by a $CX_2CX_{16}HX_{6-8}C$ motif with one invariant histidine and three cysteines. Survivin contains just a single BIR domain [13; 20]. Phosphorylation of Survivin on Threonine 34 by CDK1 is crucial for stability and activity of Survivin, which in turn contributes to proliferation and cell division in the majority of cancer cells [13; 21; 22]. Survivin is highly over-expressed primarily during G_2/M phase of the cell cycle in most transformed cells, solid tumors and leukemias and lymphomas [23-25]. Survivin was originally shown to be developmentally regulated [26]; expressed in fetal tissues with no detectable expression in adult differentiated tissues except thymus and placenta [25]. Limited cancer specific expression and function in loss of apoptosis and cell cycle regulation has made Survivin an attractive candidate for cancer therapy [27]. More recently, studies have clearly shown that Survivin is expressed in vascular endothelial cells [28; 29], keratinocyte stem cells [30], neural precursor cells [31], mature blood cells such as the megakaryocytes [32], neutrophils [33] and T-lymphocytes [34; 35], hematopoietic stem and progenitor cells [36; 37] and ES cells [38], where it most likely plays a physiologic role in development. Identification of specific differences in Survivin regulation and function between normal stem cells and cancer cells will be critical for the development of novel strategies for selectively targeting Survivin, while minimizing toxicity to normal stem cells. This review will focus on comparative expression and function of Survivin between normal stem cells and cancer cells.

EXPRESSION AND POTENTIAL ROLE OF SURVIVIN IN ADULT STEM CELLS

Mouse embryonic stem cells express Survivin [38] and homozygous gene deletion in mice leads to embryonic death at E4.5 [39], indicating that Survivin expression/function is required in totipotent stem cells. While expression of Survivin and its function in malignant cells has been extensively studied; its emerging role in normal adult cells, in particular in adult stem cells, has only recently been appreciated. The first observation that implicated Survivin in normal adult stem cells was the finding that it is expressed and growth factor regulated in normal human $CD34^+$ cells, the immunophenotypically-defined cell population that contains hematopoietic stem cells (HSC)[36; 37] capable of long-term hematopoietic reconstitution.

Survivin is expressed in freshly isolated normal human $CD34^+$ cells [36; 37] and hematopoietic growth factors, such as Thrombopoietin, Stem Cell Factor and Flt3 ligand, which stimulate proliferation, cell cycle progression and survival of $CD34^+$ cells, up-regulate Survivin mRNA and protein expression in these cells [36; 37], as well as mRNA for the Survivin splice variants $\Delta Ex3$ and 2B (S Fukuda and LM Pelus, unpublished). Among the 7 known IAPs, Survivin is the only IAP up-regulated by cytokines in $CD34^+$ cells and therefore is the only likely IAP mediating suppression of apoptosis by hematopoietic cytokines. In contrast, growth factor deprivation down-regulates Survivin expression that correlates with elevated active caspase-3 and $CD34^+$ cell apoptosis [36]. Although Survivin expression is associated with cell cycle progression, Survivin was up-regulated in all phases of the cell cycle in $CD34^+$ cells after cytokine stimulation [36], suggesting both cell cycle dependent and independent regulation, which is in contrast to cell cycle dependent and selective expression of Survivin during G_2/M in the majority of cancer cells. Using freshly isolated fluorescently labeled G_0 $CD34^+$ cells, Survivin was shown to be up-regulated during G_0, before cells enter G_1 and that Survivin expression was a function of growth factor stimulation not cytokine driven cell cycle progression [37]. Expression and regulation of Survivin in G_0 cells, the quiescent stage in which most HSC normally reside, suggests that Survivin is required for HSC function.

Over-expression of wild-type Survivin induces hyper-proliferation of hematopoietic progenitor cells and reduces apoptosis induced upon growth factor withdrawal. However, neither of these effects is observed when the cyclin dependent kinase inhibitor $p21^{WAF/Cip1}$

gene is deleted [40]. Apoptosis measured by active caspase-3 and hypodiploid DNA content are reduced by ectopic Survivin in p21$^{+/+}$ but not in p21$^{-/-}$ cells. In contrast, elevated S-phase induced by ectopic Survivin is unaffected by p21 status, indicating that Survivin blocks apoptosis of hematopoietic progenitor cells via a p21-dependent mechanism but promotes S-phase progression in a p21-independent manner. Furthermore, aberrant Survivin expression induces polyploidy in progenitor cells, which is enhanced in the absence of p21, suggesting a functional link between Survivin and p21 in regulating hematopoietic cell division. [40]. Consistent with findings in human CD34$^+$ cells, Survivin mRNA is expressed in freshly isolated normal mouse marrow c-kit$^+$, Sca-1$^+$, lin^{neg} (KSL) cells and more primitive CD34^{neg}KSL cells, cell populations that identify long-term repopulating hematopoietic stem cells in mice. In vitro, conditional Survivin gene deletion significantly reduces the number of myeloid hematopoietic progenitor cells concomitant with increased apoptosis [41] and impairs production of marrow erythroid (BFU-E) or megakaryocytic (CFU-Mk) colonies *in vitro* [32]. These findings suggest that Survivin regulates hematopoietic progenitor cell proliferation, at least in vitro.

In adult Survivin$^{flox/flox}$ mice expressing a Tamoxifen-inducible Cre transgene, conditional Survivin gene deletion significantly decreased lin^{neg} cells, c-kit$^+$, lin^{neg} cells, CFU-GM, common myeloid progenitor cells, KSL cells and CD34^{neg}KSL cells in bone marrow and CFU-GM in spleen compared to control mice. In transplantation studies, marrow stem cells derived from Mx1-Cre Survivin$^{flox/flox}$ mice showed significant reduced contribution to hematopoietic chimerism [42]. In chimeric mice in which only the hematopoietic system contained the Mx1-Cre inducible Survivin$^{flox/flox}$ gene, transplantation of Survivin gene deleted HSC showed significant reduction in stem cell function upon competitive transplant into primary recipients (Fukuda S and Pelus LM, unpublished observation). In addition, haploinsufficiency of Survivin in mice leads to defects in erythropoiesis, suggesting that Survivin deletion alters hematopoietic cell commitment [42]. This finding is supported by the fact that Survivin expression is down-regulated in patients with Aplastic Anemia where the absolute numbers of HSC are significantly reduced [43; 44]. Overall, these data strongly suggest that Survivin plays a physiological role in maintaining normal adult hematopoiesis through regulation of the self-renewal and proliferation of primitive hematopoietic stem cells.

Expression of Survivin in normal murine CD34^{neg}KSL cells is consistent with Survivin expression in G_0 CD34$^+$ cells that contain human HSC [37] and conditional Survivin deletion in vivo with the sequela of reduction in the number of HSPC is consistent with inhibition of hematopoietic cell proliferation by anti-sense or dominant-negative strategies in vitro [37; 40]. However, while these studies suggest that Survivin is indispensable for HSC maintenance; it does not necessarily imply that ectopic Survivin over-expression leads to HSC expansion. Survivin expression is cell cycle regulated and its expression is low during G_0/G_1 phase but up-regulated during S-G_2/M phase in CD34$^+$ cells [36; 37]. While our previous data indicates that forced expression of Survivin can increase the proliferation of HPC and their entry into S-phase [37], it is unlikely that ectopic Survivin results in HSC expansion/self-renewal since HSC would likely exit quiescence and commit to differentiation as a result of S-phase enhancement. In this regard, cell cycle dependent regulation of Survivin, i.e. reduction of its expression and increase at appropriate stages of cell cycle, is likely critical for HSC maintenance.

SURVIVIN IN OTHER ADULT STEM AND PROGENITOR CELLS

Recent studies indicate that Survivin is expressed and plays a regulatory role in adult stem and progenitor cells in various tissues. Full-length Survivin is highly expressed in keratinocyte stem cells (KSCs), whereas its transcript decreases in transit amplifying (TA) cells and disappears in postmitotic cells [30]. Blocking β1 integrin signal down regulates full-length Survivin mRNA and protein expression and induces apoptosis in KSCs, while up-regulating Survivin-2α mRNA. These results suggest that expression of Survivin may be an identifying feature of human KSCs. Moreover, nuclear Survivin dominates in KSC, while cytosolic Survivin predominates in TA cells, suggesting a correlation between Survivin localization and proliferative capacity [30].

Survivin is up-regulated by WNT/β-catenin in intestinal progenitor cells upon UV-B irradiation [45]. β-Catenin is an essential component of both intercellular junctions and the canonical Wnt signaling pathway that has been implicated in stem cell survival [46]. Survivin mRNA expression was selectively enhanced in stem cell antigen 1-positive (Sca-1$^+$) mammary epithelial cells in response to radiation. Furthermore, irradiated Sca-1$^+$ cells showed selective increases in active β-catenin and Survivin expression compared with Sca-1neg cells [47]. A functional association between Survivin and WNT/β-catenin signaling in mammary stem cells is consistent with the important role of WNT signaling in stem cells and substantiates the physiological role of Survivin in stem cell function.

Survivin is expressed in gastrointestinal tract mucosa in humans, which like the hematopoietic system, undergoes continuous cell renewal [48]. This suggests that Survivin may be important in regulating self-renewal and differentiation of crypt stem cells. Survivin is expressed in neurons, astrocytes, oligodendrocytes, ependymal cells and choroid plexus in the human brain [49]. In a mouse model, neuronal Survivin expression was significantly up-regulated by hypoxia [50] and conditional Survivin deletion in neuronal precursor cells resulted in significant apoptosis in cerebrum, cerebellum, brain stem, spinal cord and retina, indicating that Survivin functions as an anti-apoptotic protein in neuronal development in vivo [51]. Lack of endothelial cell Survivin causes embryonic defects in angiogenesis, cardiogenesis, and neural tube closure, suggesting that regulation of endothelial cell survival, and maintenance of vascular integrity by Survivin are crucial for normal embryonic angiogenesis, cardiogenesis, and neurogenesis [52].

In addition to adult progenitor/precursor or stem cells, Survivin expression has also been reported in melanocytes [53], testes [54] and ovary [55] in humans. Stem Cell Factor and human chorionic gonadotropin also induce Survivin expression in testes [54] and in ovarian granulosa cells [55], suggesting that Survivin may have a role in the regulation of spermatogenesis and oogenesis. Survivin expression is detected in adult liver and is down regulated by ischemia [56] but up-regulated by hepatectomy [57]. Furthermore, the Fas agonistic antibody Jo2 induces Survivin expression in liver, while Survivin haploinsufficiency sensitizes hepatocytes to Jo2 antibody-mediated apoptosis via the mitochondrial pathway [58], indicating that hepatocyte proliferation and apoptosis are regulated by Survivin.

SURVIVIN AND MALIGNANT HSPC WITH SELF-RENEWAL CAPABILITY

When leukemic cells are transplanted *in vivo*, only 1–4% of cells are able to form spleen colonies [59] [60]. In general, most leukemia cells are unable to proliferate extensively and only a small subset of cells is clonogenic. In patients with acute myeloid leukemia (AML), leukemic stem cells can be identified prospectively and purified as $CD34^+CD38^-$ cells [61]. These results indicate that leukemia stem cells are responsible for disease and that identification of mechanisms responsible for leukemia stem cells proliferation will be necessary to eradicate cells that are refractory to conventional therapies.

Recent reports by us [62] and others demonstrate that Survivin expression provides resistance of chronic myeloid leukemia (CML) cells to Imatinib and that activation of β-catenin in CML granulocyte–macrophage progenitor cells enhances their self-renewal activity and leukemic potential [63]. As described earlier, Survivin has been shown to be up-regulated by WNT/β-catenin in intestinal progenitor cells upon UV-B irradiation [47]. These findings suggest that WNT/β-catenin-Survivin signaling may regulate CML stem cells.

Recently, we have also found that Survivin is associated with deregulated proliferation of HSPC, with self-renewal capability, induced by Internal Tandem Duplication mutations of the fetal liver tyrosine kinase receptor (Flt3) gene (ITD-Flt3) frequently found in patients with AML and associated with extremely poor prognosis [64]. Over expression of ITD-Flt3 results in a significant increase in the number of $Sca-1^+$, $c-kit^+$, lin^{neg} cells able to proliferate in the absence of hematopoietic growth factors, while conditional Survivin deletion significantly reduces the effects, which could be further attenuated by a Flt3 kinase inhibitor. The effect of Survivin deletion is associated with increased apoptosis measured by Annexin V, sub-G1 content and G_0/G_1 arrest. Over expressing ITD-Flt3 also reduced the proportion of lin^+ cells derived from lin^{neg} marrow cells cultured with GM-CSF plus Stem Cell Factor compared to wild-type Flt3, while Survivin deletion in ITD-Flt3 expressing cells partially abrogated the effect. Survivin deletion dramatically diminishes secondary CFU formation induced by ITD-Flt3 in the absence of hematopoietic growth factors, a measure of self-renewal. In addition, progression of acute leukemia induced by transplantation of hematopoietic cell lines expressing ITD-Flt3 was significantly delayed by co-expression of a dominant-negative Survivin construct that inhibits endogenous Survivin function. These results suggest that Survivin regulates the expansion of HSPC with self-renewal capability transformed by ITD-Flt3 and the development of ITD-Flt3 positive acute leukemia.

DIFFERENCES OF SURVIVIN EXPRESSION AND FUNCTION BETWEEN CANCER AND STEM CELLS

Survivin is expressed in many cancer cells, adult stem cells and ES cells and regulates proliferation and resistance to apoptosis of these cells. It seems reasonable therefore that cancer cells utilize the same machinery for self-renewal as normal stem cells. In quiescent $CD34^+$ cells that contain HSC, as well as in AML cells, Survivin expression is regulated by hematopoietic cytokines, although its expression is significantly higher in AML cells than normal $CD34^+$ cells [65]. This may be due to autocrine or paracrine mechanisms resulting from co-expression of cytokines and their receptors that stimulate leukemic cell proliferation and/or to the fact that normal stem cells are primarily quiescent, i.e. in G_0, where Survivin expression normally remains low [36; 37]. Although one may conclude that Survivin expression may be higher in cancer cells, simply because they proliferate faster, a growing of body of evidence suggest that the intracellular pathways that activate Survivin transcription or block Survivin sequestration may be more active in malignant cells than in normal tissues. Oncogenes such as Bcr-abl [62] and activated H-Ras [66] significantly increase Survivin expression. Survivin expression is also associated with Stat3 [8-10], NFkB[15] and association with HSP90 [17]. Furthermore, Rb/E2F and p53 pathways may contribute to aberrant Survivin expression [16] since wild-type p53 [18; 19] and RB [16] can transcriptionally repress Survivin, but are mutated and inactivated in variety of cancer cells.

Forced Survivin over expression increases the number of hematopoietic progenitor cells in S-phase [37; 40], while Survivin disruption reduces the number of cells in S-phase [35; 37; 67], suggesting that Survivin regulates their G_1/S transition. Similarly, Survivin expression in Ki-67^{neg} breast cancer cells [13], Survivin-mediated enhancement of Rb phosphorylation resulting from its interaction with CDK4/p16^{INK4a} and activation of CDK2/CyclinE complex in hepatoma cells [12] and resistance to Vitamin-D mediated G_1 arrest associated with increased $S+G_2/M$ phase observed upon ectopic Survivin over expression in MCF7 breast cancer cells [68], suggest that Survivin may also regulate G_1/S transition in some cancer cells. However, disrupting Survivin in HeLa cells failed to initiate G_1/S arrest [17], although this may be due to inactivation of Rb or p53 in HeLa cells [17].

Survivin can regulate apoptosis, cell cycle and cytokinesis through functional or physical interactions with HSP90 [17], Smac/Diablo [14], XIAP [14], p21$^{WAF1/Cip1}$[11; 12], CDK4 [12], Cdc2(CDK1) [13], Rb/E2F[16], NFkB [15], Stat3 [8-10] or p53 [18-20; 69]. Although crucial differences in the mechanisms of action of Survivin between cancer cells and normal stem cells is poorly understood, cancer cells and normal somatic cells share some of the same signaling pathways associated with Survivin. Survivin regulates proliferation of normal hematopoietic progenitor cells through p21-dependent pathways [40], which is consistent with the requirement of p21 for HSC maintenance and suppression of apoptosis in hepatoma cells resulting from the interaction of Survivin with the pro-caspase-3/p21 complex [12]. Induction of apoptosis in hematopoietic progenitor cells [40], HUVEC [28] and several cancers cells [13] by the phosphorylation dead T34A-Survivin mutant suggests that phosphorylation of Survivin on Threonine-34 by Cdc2 is required for survival in both normal and cancer cells. In contrast to the common pathways through which Survivin regulates normal somatic cells and cancer cells, mitochondrial Survivin is exclusively expressed in cancer cells, and may be associated with transformation [70].

Our recent findings demonstrate that disrupting Survivin in mouse HSC populations leads to alteration of several genes associated with apoptosis, cytokine signaling and stem cell function. Of particular interest, GATA2 mRNA, which is known to regulate HSC proliferation/self-renewal [71; 72], was coincidently down regulated upon Survivin deletion (S Fukuda and LM Pelus, unpublished). Significant reduction in HOXA5 an important regulator of hematopoietic lineage commitment [73] and a 2-fold increase in HIF1α, a transcription factor that regulates oxidative responses [74; 75] were also observed. Egr1, also known as a tumor suppressor and promoter [76; 77], and which also controls hematopoietic cell differentiation [78; 79], was also differentially regulated. These findings suggest that Survivin may regulate HSC proliferation through these signaling pathways and manipulation of these pathways may increase the number of somatic stem cells that may be used for regenerative medicine. It remains to be determined if these same signaling pathways are down-stream targets of Survivin in cancer cells. Identifying pathways down-stream of Survivin selectively utilized in cancer versus stem cells will likely prove importance for the development of selective and minimally toxic anti-Survivin therapies.

POTENTIAL ADVERSE EFFECTS OF ANTI-SURVIVIN THERAPY

The observations described above clearly indicate that Survivin should not be considered a cancer specific protein but rather a regulatory protein deregulated in cancer but which plays significant roles in normal adult stem cell function. Although studies using in vivo anti-Survivin therapy clearly indicate that disrupting Survivin in cancers may be clinically beneficial without obvious toxicity, no studies have specifically examined toxicity to adult stem cells, particularly HSC, since most models did not utilize systemic administration. Studies using Survivin peptide-activated cytotoxic T-cells showed little effect on normal CFU [80], but likewise have shown little effect on cancer cells. Shepherdin, a small peptide that blocks the interaction of Survivin with HSP90 shows significant reduction of human breast and prostate cancer cell growth without apparent toxicity in a mouse xenograft model [81]. However, treatment of $CD34^+$ cells in vitro, dose dependently inhibited CFU-GM and CFU-GEMM at concentrations only moderately higher than required for inhibition of cancer cell growth [81]. The concern over potential hematotoxicity of anti-Survivin therapies is supported by the findings that ablation of Survivin reduces the number of CFU-GM, BFU-E and CFU-Mk [37] [40] [32] as well as $c\text{-}kit^+$ $Sca1^+$ lin^{neg} (KSL) cells and $CD34^{neg}$ KSL cells and impairs hematopoietic reconstitution in mouse transplantation models [42] [41]. In light of recent new information that several normal adult stem and precursor cell populations, major organ systems will have to be carefully monitored for toxicity, particularly under conditions of dose escalation/multiple round therapy or combination therapy with traditional chemotherapeutic compounds. An intriguing potential utilization brought out by these studies however, is the concept of manipulating Survivin in normal stem cell populations as a means to increase their number for use in stem cell transplantation and regenerative medicine. It is clear that Survivin over-expression alone is not sufficient to cause transformation; however, since normal stem cells and cancer cells share Survivin-mediated pathways, Survivin overexpression may be associated with an increased risk of transformation. Manipulating pathways involving Survivin that are specific to normal stem cells but not malignant cells may provide selective stem cell expansion strategies without risk of cancer.

CONCLUSION

Molecular dissection of genes associated with aberrant proliferation of cancer cells has identified Survivin as a candidate gene responsible for cancer progression and an attractive molecular target for cancer therapy. However, Survivin is not a cancer specific molecule; rather it is involved in regulating normal stem cell function necessary for long-term tissue maintenance and regeneration and Survivin disruption can have toxicity to these normal tissue stem cells. These findings also suggest that selective/differential manipulation of Survivin signaling pathways may help to develop novel strategies to expand somatic stem cells that can be used for tissue regeneration. While expression of Survivin in cancer cells is significantly enhanced compared to normal cells, including HSC, suggesting the presence of crucial differences in mechanisms, studies have not yet identified down-stream targets or molecular mechanisms differentially regulating Survivin expression and function in normal versus transformed cells. Studies that pinpoint the crucial difference of Survivin behavior in cancers versus normal stem cells will be required to develop innovative anti-Survivin cancer strategies with limited normal stem cell toxicities and Survivin over expression strategies in normal stem cells without increasing the risk of cancer.

ACKNOWLEDGMENTS

Supported by US Public Health Service grants HL69669 and HL079654 from the National Institutes of Health (to LMP), Biomedical Research Grant from Indiana University School of Medicine, Research Support Funds Grant from Indiana University, Purdue University, Indianapolis, the Mochida Memorial Foundation for Medical and Pharmaceutical Research, Japan Leukemia Research Foundation, Sankyo Biomedical Research Foundation and Mitsubishi Pharma Research Foundation (to SF)

REFERENCES

[1] Reya T, Morrison SJ, Clarke MF, Weissman IL. Stem cells, cancer, and cancer stem cells. *Nature.* 2001;414:105-111.
[2] Bhardwaj G, Murdoch B, Wu D et al. Sonic hedgehog induces the proliferation of primitive human hematopoietic cells via BMP regulation. *Nature Immunol.* 2001;2:172-180.
[3] Wechsler-Reya RJ, and Scott MP. Control of neuronal precursor proliferation in the cerebellum by Sonic Hedgehog. *Neuron.* 1999;22:103-114.

[4] Zhang Y, Kalderon D. Hedgehog acts as a somatic stem cell factor in the *Drosophila* ovary. *Nature.* 2001;410:599-604.
[5] Varnum-Finney B, Xu L, Brashem-Stein C et al. Pluripotent, cytokine-dependent, hematopoietic stem cells are immortalized by constitutive Notch1 signaling. *Nature Med.* 2000;6:1278-1281.
[6] Henrique D, Hirsinger E, Adam J et al. Maintenance of neuroepithelial progenitor cells by Delta-Notch signalling in the embryonic chick retina. *Curr. Biol.* 1997;7:661-670.
[7] Austin J, Kimble J. glp-1 is required in the germ line for regulation of the decision between mitosis and meiosis in *C. elegans*. *Cell.* 1987;51:589-599.
[8] Abu-El-Asrar AM, Dralands L, Missotten L, Al-Jadaan IA, Geboes K. Expression of apoptosis markers in the retinas of human subjects with diabetes. *Invest. Ophthalmol. Vis. Sci.* 2004;45:2760-2766.
[9] Fulda S, Debatin KM. Sensitization for anticancer drug-induced apoptosis by the chemopreventive agent resveratrol. *Oncogene.* 2004;23:6702-6711.
[10] Aoki Y, Feldman GM, Tosato G. Inhibition of STAT3 signaling induces apoptosis and decreases survivin expression in primary effusion lymphoma. *Blood.* 2003;101:1535-1542.
[11] Li F, Ackermann EJ, Bennett CF et al. Pleiotropic cell-division defects and apoptosis induced by interference with survivin function. *Nat. Cell Biol.* 1999;1:461-466.
[12] Suzuki A, Shiraki K. Tumor cell "dead or alive": caspase and survivin regulate cell death, cell cycle and cell survival. *Histol. Histopathol.* 2001;16:583-593.
[13] Altieri DC. Validating survivin as a cancer therapeutic target. *Nat. Rev. Cancer.* 2003;3:46-54.
[14] Song Z, Yao X, Wu M. Direct interaction between survivin and Smac/DIABLO is essential for the anti-apoptotic activity of survivin during taxol-induced apoptosis. *J. Biol. Chem.* 2003;278:23130-23140.
[15] Tracey L, Perez-Rosado A, Artiga MJ et al. Expression of the NF-kappaB targets BCL2 and BIRC5/Survivin characterizes small B-cell and aggressive B-cell lymphomas, respectively. J. Pathol. 2005;206:123-134.
[16] Jiang Y, Saavedra HI, Holloway MP, Leone G, Altura RA. Aberrant regulation of survivin by the RB/E2F family of proteins. *J. Biol. Chem.* 2004;279:40511-40520.
[17] Fortugno P, Beltrami E, Plescia J et al. Regulation of survivin function by Hsp90. *Proc. Natl. Acad. Sci. U. S. A.* 2003;100:13791-13796.
[18] Hoffman WH, Biade S, Zilfou JT, Chen J, Murphy M. Transcriptional repression of the anti-apoptotic survivin gene by wild type p53. *J. Biol. Chem.* 2002;277:3247-3257.
[19] Mirza A, McGuirk M, Hockenberry TN et al. Human survivin is negatively regulated by wild-type p53 and participates in p53-dependent apoptotic pathway. *Oncogene.* 2002;21:2613-2622.
[20] Altieri DC. Survivin, versatile modulation of cell division and apoptosis in cancer. *Oncogene.* 2003;22:8581-8589.
[21] O'Connor DS, Grossman D, Plescia J et al. Regulation of apoptosis at cell division by p34cdc2 phosphorylation of survivin. *Proc. Natl. Acad. Sci. U. S. A.* 2000;97:13103-13107.
[22] O'Connor DS, Wall NR, Porter AC, Altieri DC. A p34(cdc2) survival checkpoint in cancer. *Cancer Cell.* 2002;2:43-54.
[23] Adida C, Recher C, Raffoux E et al. Expression and prognostic significance of survivin in de novo acute myeloid leukaemia. *Br. J. Haematol.* 2000;111:196-203.

[24] Adida C, Haioun C, Gaulard P et al. Prognostic significance of survivin expression in diffuse large B-cell lymphomas. *Blood.* 2000;96:1921-1925.

[25] Ambrosini G, Adida C, Altieri DC. A novel anti-apoptosis gene, survivin, expressed in cancer and lymphoma. *Nat. Med.* 1997;3:917-921.

[26] Adida C, Crotty PL, McGrath J et al. Developmentally regulated expression of the novel cancer anti-apoptosis gene survivin in human and mouse differentiation. *Am. J. Pathol.* 1998;152:43-49.

[27] Fukuda S, Pelus LM. Survivin, a cancer target with an emerging role in normal adult tissues. *Mol. Cancer Ther.* 2006;5:1087-1098.

[28] Blanc-Brude OP, Mesri M, Wall NR et al. Therapeutic targeting of the survivin pathway in cancer: initiation of mitochondrial apoptosis and suppression of tumor-associated angiogenesis. *Clin. Cancer Res.* 2003;9:2683-2692.

[29] Mesri M, Morales-Ruiz M, Ackermann EJ et al. Suppression of vascular endothelial growth factor-mediated endothelial cell protection by survivin targeting. *Am. J. Pathol.* 2001;158:1757-1765.

[30] Marconi A, Dallaglio K, Lotti R et al. Survivin identifies keratinocyte stem cells and is downregulated by anti-beta1 integrin during anoikis. *Stem Cells.* 2007;25:149-155.

[31] Pennartz S, Belvindrah R, Tomiuk S et al. Purification of neuronal precursors from the adult mouse brain: comprehensive gene expression analysis provides new insights into the control of cell migration, differentiation, and homeostasis. *Mol. Cell Neurosci.* 2004;25:692-706.

[32] Gurbuxani S, Xu Y, Keerthivasan G, Wickrema A, Crispino JD. Differential requirements for survivin in hematopoietic cell development. *Proc. Natl. Acad. Sci. U. S. A.* 2005;102:11480-11485.

[33] Altznauer F, Martinelli S, Yousefi S et al. Inflammation-associated cell cycle-independent block of apoptosis by survivin in terminally differentiated neutrophils. *J. Exp. Med.* 2004;199:1343-1354.

[34] Xing Z, Conway EM, Kang C, Winoto A. Essential role of survivin, an inhibitor of apoptosis protein, in T cell development, maturation, and homeostasis. *J. Exp. Med.* 2004;199:69-80.

[35] Okada H, Bakal C, Shahinian A et al. Survivin loss in thymocytes triggers p53-mediated growth arrest and p53-independent cell death. *J. Exp. Med.* 2004;199:399-410.

[36] Fukuda S, Pelus LM. Regulation of the inhibitor-of-apoptosis family member survivin in normal cord blood and bone marrow CD34(+) cells by hematopoietic growth factors: implication of survivin expression in normal hematopoiesis. *Blood.* 2001;98:2091-2100.

[37] Fukuda S, Foster RG, Porter SB, Pelus LM. The antiapoptosis protein survivin is associated with cell cycle entry of normal cord blood CD34(+) cells and modulates cell cycle and proliferation of mouse hematopoietic progenitor cells. *Blood.* 2002;100:2463-2471.

[38] Coumoul X, Li W, Wang RH, Deng C. Inducible suppression of Fgfr2 and Survivin in ES cells using a combination of the RNA interference (RNAi) and the Cre-LoxP system. *Nucleic Acids Res.* 2004;32:e85.

[39] Uren AG, Wong L, Pakusch M et al. Survivin and the inner centromere protein INCENP show similar cell-cycle localization and gene knockout phenotype. *Curr. Biol.* 2000;10:1319-1328.

[40] Fukuda S, Mantel CR, Pelus LM. Survivin regulates hematopoietic progenitor cell proliferation through p21$^{WAF1/Cip1}$-dependent and -independent pathways. *Blood.* 2004;103:120-127.

[41] Fukuda S, Conway EM, Pelus LM. Survivin regulates proliferation of normal hematopoietic stem and progenitor cells in vivo. *Blood.* 2006;108:859.

[42] Leung CG, Xu Y, Mularski B et al. Requirements for survivin in terminal differentiation of erythroid cells and maintenance of hematopoietic stem and progenitor cells. *J. Exp. Med.* 2007;204:1603-11.

[43] Zeng W, Chen G, Kajigaya S et al. Gene expression profiling in CD34 cells to identify differences between aplastic anemia patients and healthy volunteers. *Blood.* 2004;103:325-32.

[44] Badran A, Yoshida A, Wano Y et al. Expression of the anti-apoptotic gene survivin in myelodysplastic syndrome. *Int. J. Oncol.* 2003;22:59-64.

[45] Kim PJ., Plescia J, Clevers H, Fearon ER, Altieri DC. Survivin and molecular pathogenesis of colorectal cancer. *Lancet.* 2003;362:205-209.

[46] Polakis P. Wnt signaling and cancer. *Genes Dev.* 2000;14:1837-1851.

[47] Woodward WA, Chen MS, Behbod F et al. WNT/-catenin mediates radiation resistance of mouse mammary progenitor cells. *Proc. Natl. Acad. Sci. U. S. A.* 2007;104:618-623.

[48] Chiou SK, Moon WS, Jones MK, Tarnawski AS. Survivin expression in the stomach: implications for mucosal integrity and protection. *Biochem. Biophys. Res. Commun.* 2003;305:374-379.

[49] Sasaki T, Lopes MB, Hankins GR, Helm GA. Expression of survivin, an inhibitor of apoptosis protein, in tumors of the nervous system. *Acta Neuropathol.* 2002;104:105-109.

[50] Conway EM, Zwerts F, Van E, V et al. Survivin-dependent angiogenesis in ischemic brain: molecular mechanisms of hypoxia-induced up-regulation. *Am. J. Pathol.* 2003;163:935-946.

[51] Jiang Y, de Bruin A, Caldas H et al. Essential role for survivin in early brain development. *J. Neurosci.* 2005;25:6962-6970.

[52] Zwerts F, Lupu F, De Vriese A et al. Lack of endothelial cell survivin causes embryonic defects in angiogenesis, cardiogenesis, and neural tube closure. *Blood.* 2007;109:4742-4752.

[53] Vetter CS, Muller-Blech K, Schrama D, Brocker EB, Becker JC. Cytoplasmic and nuclear expression of survivin in melanocytic skin lesions. *Arch. Dermatol. Res.* 2005;297:26-30.

[54] Wang Y, Suominen JS, Hakovirta H et al. Survivin expression in rat testis is upregulated by stem-cell factor. *Mol. Cell Endocrinol.* 2004;218:165-174.

[55] Kumazawa Y, Kawamura K, Sato T et al. HCG up-regulates survivin mRNA in human granulosa cells. *Mol. Hum. Reprod.* 2005;11:161-166.

[56] Lu QP, Cao TJ, Zhang ZY, Liu W. Multiple gene differential expression patterns in human ischemic liver: safe limit of warm ischemic time. *World J. Gastroenterol.* 2004;10:2130-2133.

[57] Deguchi M, Shiraki K, Inoue H et al. Expression of survivin during liver regeneration. *Biochem. Biophys. Res. Commun.* 2002;297:59-64.

[58] Conway EM, Pollefeyt S, Steiner-Mosonyi M et al. Deficiency of survivin in transgenic mice exacerbates Fas-induced apoptosis via mitochondrial pathways. *Gastroenterology.* 2002;123:619-631.

[59] Bruce WR, Van Der Gaag H. A quantitative assay for the number of murine lymphoma cells capable of proliferation in vivo. *Nature.* 1963;199:79-80.

[60] Wodinsky I, Swiniarski J, Kensler CJ. Spleen colony studies of leukemia L1210. I. Growth kinetics of lymphocytic L1210 cells in vivo as determined by spleen colony assay. *Cancer Chemother. Rep.* 1967;51:415-421.

[61] Bonnet D, Dick JE. Human acute myeloid leukemia is organized as a hierarchy that originates from a primitive hematopoietic cell. *Nature Med.* 1997;3:730-737.

[62] Wang Z, Sampath J, Fukuda S, Pelus LM. Disruption of the inhibitor of apoptosis protein survivin sensitizes Bcr-abl-positive cells to STI571-induced apoptosis. *Cancer Res.* 2005;65:8224-8232.

[63] Jamieson CH, Ailles LE, Dylla SJ et al. Granulocyte macrophage progenitors as candidate leukemic stem cells in blast-crisis CML. *N. Engl. J. Med.* 2004;351:657-667.

[64] Fukuda S, Singh P, Conway EM, Yamaguchi S, Pelus LM. Survivin regulates aberrant proliferation of hematopoietic progenitor cells with self renewal capability and development of acute leukemia induced by Internal Tandem Duplication of Flt3. *Blood.* 2007;110: 599

[65] Carter BZ, Milella M, Altieri DC, Andreeff M. Cytokine-regulated expression of survivin in myeloid leukemia. *Blood.* 2001;97:2784-2790.

[66] Sommer KW, Schamberger CJ, Schmidt GE, Sasgary S, Cerni C. Inhibitor of apoptosis protein (IAP) survivin is upregulated by oncogenic c-H-Ras. *Oncogene.* 2003;22:4266-4280.

[67] Song J, So T, Cheng M, Tang X, Croft M. Sustained survivin expression from OX40 costimulatory signals drives T cell clonal expansion. *Immunity.* 2005;22:621-631.

[68] Li F, Ling X, Huang H et al. Differential regulation of survivin expression and apoptosis by vitamin D3 compounds in two isogenic MCF-7 breast cancer cell sublines. *Oncogene.* 2005;24:1385-1395.

[69] Wang Z, Fukuda S, Pelus LM. Survivin regulates the p53 tumor suppressor gene family. *Oncogene.* 2004;23:8146-8153.

[70] Dohi T, Beltrami E, Wall NR, Plescia J, Altieri DC. Mitochondrial survivin inhibits apoptosis and promotes tumorigenesis. *J. Clin. Invest.* 2004;114:1117-1127.

[71] Tsai FY, Keller G, Kuo FC et al. An early haematopoietic defect in mice lacking the transcription factor GATA-2. *Nature.* 1994;371:221-226.

[72] Rodrigues NP, Janzen V, Forkert R et al. Haploinsufficiency of GATA-2 perturbs adult hematopoietic stem-cell homeostasis. *Blood.* 2005;106:477-484.

[73] Crooks GM, Fuller J, Petersen D et al. Constitutive HOXA5 expression inhibits erythropoiesis and increases myelopoiesis from human hematopoietic progenitors. *Blood.* 1990;94:519-28.

[74] Semenza GL. Regulation of mammalian O2 homeostasis by hypoxia-inducible factor 1. *Annu. Rev. Cell Dev. Biol.* 1999;15:551-578.

[75] Kirito K, Fox N, Komatsu N, Kaushansky K. Thrombopoietin enhances expression of vascular endothelial growth factor (VEGF) in primitive hematopoietic cells through induction of HIF-1alpha. *Blood.* 2005;105:4258-4263.

[76] Krones-Herzig A, Mittal S, Yule K et al. Early growth response 1 acts as a tumor suppressor in vivo and in vitro via regulation of p53. *Cancer Res.* 2005;65:5133-5143.

[77] Joslin JM, Fernald AA, Tennant TR et al. Haploinsufficiency of EGR1, a candidate gene in the del(5q), leads to the development of myeloid disorders. *Blood.* 2007;110:719-726.

[78] Dinkel A, Warnatz K, Ledermann B et al. The transcription factor early growth response 1 (Egr-1) advances differentiation of pre-B and immature B cells. *J. Exp. Med.* 1998;188:2215-2224.
[79] Krishnaraju K, Hoffman B, Liebermann DA. The zinc finger transcription factor Egr-1 activates macrophage differentiation in M1 myeloblastic leukemia cells. *Blood.* 1998;92:1957-1966.
[80] Pisarev V, Yu B, Salup R et al. Full-length dominant-negative survivin for cancer immunotherapy. *Clin. Cancer Res.* 2003;9:6523-6533.
[81] Plescia J, Salz W, Xia F et al. Rational design of shepherdin, a novel anticancer agent. *Cancer Cell.* 2005;7:457-468.

Chapter V

CANCER STEM CELLS

Saranya Chumsri[1] and Angelika M. Burger[1,2]
[1]Marlene and Stewart Greenebaum Cancer Center, Maryland, US
[2]Department of Pharmacology and Experimental Therapeutics,
University of Maryland, School of Medicine, Baltimore, Maryland, US

ABSTRACT

Emerging evidence suggests that cancers contain a rare and biologically distinct subpopulation of cells with the ability to self-renew and to sustain tumor growth, termed "cancer stem cells". Cancer stem cells share many characteristics with normal stem cells including self-renewal, asymmetric division, indefinite proliferative capacity, and self-protection mechanisms. The cancer stem cell concept is best understood in hematologic malignancies. In solid tumors, breast cancer stem cells have been the most explored. Several techniques have been described, allowing the identification or isolation of cancer stem cells by either expression of specific cell surface markers, their differential ability to efflux dyes, or by a distinct enzymatic activity. More recent studies also established the crucial role of cancer stem cells in multistage cancer progression and metastasis which has important implications for the design of novel targeted therapies. Since most of the conventional chemotherapies only affect differentiated cancer cells, initial reduction in tumor mass is often followed by a rapid relapse. In order to achieve durable remissions, it will be imperative to eradicate cancer stem cells.

INTRODUCTION

Cancer is the third leading cause of death worldwide and only preceded by cardiovascular disease and infection [1]. Despite improvements of existing and the development of novel treatment modalities, the majority of cancer patients still have a poor prognosis. Although chemotherapy and/or radiation can induce initial tumor shrinkage, a high proportion of cancer patients will inevitably relapse and ultimately die of their disease. It was not until recently that advances in molecular biology and embryonic stem cell research have shed more light on the biology of cancer recurrence. There is emerging evidence that a rare and biologically distinct population of cancer cells exists that has exclusive self-renewal ability and limitless proliferative capacity. These characteristics are analogous to those of normal stem cells and hence this population was termed "cancer stem cells". Most conventional chemotherapies affect differentiated cancer cells that make up the bulk of a tumor, but are often ineffective against cancer stem cells [2,3]. Thus, a critical challenge in anti-cancer drug development is to target and eradicate cancer stem cells together with the bulk tumor mass. In this chapter, we will review the discovery of cancer stem cells, the available evidence of their origin, and novel strategies to target cancer stem cells [4].

STEM CELLS

While the concept of a stem cell has been proposed since the early 1900s, stem cells were actually identified in the early 1960's by two Canadian scientists, Ernest A. McCulloch and James E. Till. They pioneered the field by injecting bone marrow cells into sub-lethally irradiated mice and noticed that visible nodules formed in the spleens. These nodules were described as "spleen colonies". Initially, they postulated that each nodule arose from a single marrow cell and perhaps a stem cell. Subsequently, they were able to demonstrate that each nodule did indeed arise from a single cell [5,6]. This work illustrated the fundamental characteristics of stem cells, namely their ability to self-renew and to differentiate into multiple lineages [7]. Self-renewal is a unique characteristic of stem cells and is distinct from proliferation (figure 1). Unlike progenitor cells which have extensive proliferative capacity, stem cells are mostly quiescent (long term stem cells). Owing to their self-renewal gene signature, stem cells can produce the identical daughter cells that preserve stem cell properties [8]. Moreover, stem cells are capable of dividing asymmetrically and possess an axis of polarity. Polarity is the unequal spatial distribution of cellular constituents. For example, there are two types of polarity in simple epithelia: planar cell polarity and apicobasal polarity. After asymmetric division, one daughter cell will retain stem cell characteristics and the other daughter cell will become a committed progenitor which will give rise to differentiated cells. There is evidence that disruption of the process of asymmetric cell division and loss of polarity induces a cancer-like state in neuronal stem cells [9,10].

CANCER STEM CELLS

The stochastic model of cell division assumes that cancer cells are homogenous and that each cancer cell can give rise to the entire tumor [7]. However, recent studies have provided strong evidence that cancer cells are in fact heterogeneous and exhibit a hierarchical arrangement similar to their normal counterparts, and that only a rare and biologically distinct subset of cancer cells is capable of recapitulation of the entire tumor [2]. Prior to the molecular definition of cancer stem cells, experiments in the 1960s [11] have shown that only a small fraction (0.77%) of murine lymphoma cells was able to form colonies in the spleens of mice and that 1 in 10,000 mouse myeloma cells was capable of forming colonies in clonal *in vitro* colony-forming assays [10,12]. It was further proposed that for successful control of tumor growth, these tumor stem cells must be eradicated. In absence of means to isolate and classify cancer stem cells, it still remained possible that all cells have clonogenic capacity, but that they were unable to proliferate under the assay conditions used. In order to demonstrate that cancer cells are in fact heterogeneous and that only a distinct subset of cells has clonogenic capacity, it was essential to separate the different populations and define one subset of cancer cells that has extensive proliferating capacity. This was accomplished in 1997, when it was demonstrated that only cells with a $CD34^+/CD38^-$ phenotype were able to initiate human acute myelogenous leukemia in non-obese diabetic/severe combined immunodeficient (NOD/SCID) mice [13]. These cells were capable of self-renewal and recapitulation of the leukemia, similar to the parental tumor phenotype *in vivo*. It was further demonstrated that leukemic stem cells are not functionally homogeneous but consist of a distinct hierarchically arranged class similar to normal hematopoietic stem cells [14].

Likewise, solid tumors have been demonstrated to possess a phenotypically distinct and rare population of cancer cells with self-renewal capacity [15]. Al-Hajj and colleagues[16] were the first to isolate and describe a distinct cell population in solid cancers and demonstrated self-renewal properties, namely for $CD44^+/CD24^{-/low}$/lineage$^-$ cells in breast cancer. As few as 100 cells of this particular phenotype were capable of generating a phenotypically diverse breast tumor similar to the original patient tumor in NOD/SCID mice, whereas as many as 20,000 cells with the $CD44^+/CD24^+$ phenotype were unable to generate a tumor [16,17]. NOD/SCID mouse repopulation capabilities were also demonstrated for $CD133^+$/Nestin$^+$/Lineage$^-$ cells from human brain tumors [18,19], a $CD138^-$ population in multiple myeloma [20], and cells with a $CD44^+/\alpha_2\beta_1^{hi}/CD133^+$ phenotype in prostate cancers [21]. Most recently, cancer stem cells exhibiting a $CD44^+/CD24^+/ESA^+$ phenotype were also described in pancreatic cancer.

Since the discovery of cancer stem cells some decades ago, their existence and significance have been continously debated. Work that has been accepted as proof of cancer stem cell properties was based on the ability of a distinct subpopulation of cancer cells that can form a tumor in sublethally irradiated NOD/SCID mice. The latter is complicated however by the interactions between cancer cells and their microenvironment. It is possible that only a rare subpopulation of cancer cells can acclimatize and grow in a foreign or mouse microenvironment. Kelly *et al [22]* have recently demonstrated that as few as 10 of primary pre-B/B lymphoma cells from Eμ-*myc* transgenic mice of every phenotype can form a tumor in non-irradiated congenic mice. This observation challenges the concept that only a rare cancer stem cell subpopulation can sustain the tumor growth. Moreover, Kern and Shibata suggested that the mathematical model for the concept of cancer stem cells in solid tumor is weak and even may be invalid [23].

In February 2006, the American Association for Cancer Research (AACR) had a workshop on cancer stem cells to discuss the definition, importance, and implications of this rapid emerging field. Currently, cancer stem cells have been defined as "a small subset of cancer cells within a cancer that constitute a reservoir of self-sustaining cells with the exclusive ability to self-renew and to cause the heterogeneous lineages of cancer cells that comprise the tumor" [24,25]. While a normal stem cell is considered to be multipotent or capable of differentiating into different cell phenotypes across all lineages, the current definition of a cancer stem cell does not include multipotency. In fact, the extent to which cancer stem cells share the characteristics of normal stem cells, including self-renewal properties, remains unclear. Therefore, although the term "cancer stem cell" may be attractive, it may be illusory and suitable only in a limited sense. Some groups have proposed that it may be more appropriate to use a functional definition such as "tumor-initiating cell" or "cancer-initiating cell" [26-28].

ORIGIN OF CANCER STEM CELLS

Cancer stem cells and "normal" (embryonic and adult) stem cells share several common features. At the molecular level, distinct sets of genes have emerged that can be associated with "stemness". In particular the Wnt- (Wnt-3, β-catenin), Notch- (Notch-1) and Hedgehog- (Gli1 and 2, PTCH1, SMO) signaling pathways, the polycomb family transcriptional repressor Bmi1, octamer-binding transcription factor Oct-4, the drug efflux pump breast cancer resistance protein (BCRP), and human telomerase reverse transcriptase (hTERT) have been associated with stem cells [17,29-32]. Biological similarities that are governed by these genes include the ability to self-renew, the ability to differentiate, limitless proliferative capacity, the ability to activate anti-apoptotic pathways, resistance to cytotoxic agents, and the ability to migrate [33]. This has led to the thought that cancer stem cells may derive from mutated and/or dysregulated stem cells.

Most of the published data regarding the origin of cancer stem cells has been described in leukemia. Leukemic stem cells (LSCs) express CD34 and lack markers of lineage commitment such as CD38. In addition, LSCs can develop at each step in the hierarchy of the hematopoietic stem cell system; it has therefore been hypothesized that most human leukemias arise from transformation of HSCs [13,34]. For example it has been demonstrated that transduction of the MLL-ENL or MOZ-TIF2 fusion genes into HSCs, common myeloid progenitors (CMPs), and granulocyte-macrophage progenitors (GMPs) resulted in identical leukemia [35]. These results indicate that committed progenitors with little long-term replicative potential may acquire self-renewal capability and transform into LSCs. Nevertheless, it is currently uncertain what proportion of human myeloid leukemia arise from committed progenitors or a single oncogenic event such as MLL-ENL and MOZ-TIF2 tanslocations.

Further support of the hypothesis that tumors may derive from the transformation of a progenitor and/or stem cell are studies which showed that soft-tissue sarcoma cells and bone marrow derived mesenchymal progenitor cells share a common phenotype [36,37]. By transfecting the oncogenic fusion protein ETS–FLI-1, mesenchymal progenitor cells could be converted into Ewing's sarcoma [38]. There is also evidence suggesting an epithelial tumor type, namely gastric cancer, may arise from progenitor cells of non-epithelial origin [39]. Together, these results raise the possibility that a small subset of cancer stem cells may originate from normal stem cells, progenitor cells, or even different cell lineages as illustrated in figure 1.

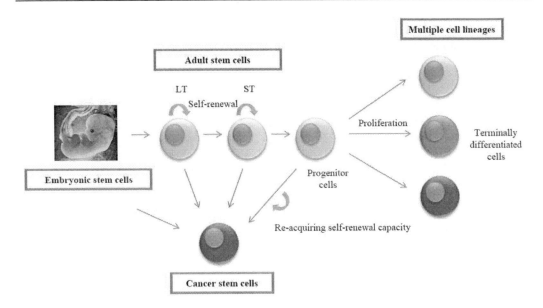

Figure 1. The origin of cancer stem cells. Embryonic stem cells (ES) are pluripotent and capable of recapitulating multiple lineages of adult stem cells. Long-term repopulating stem cells (LT) are slowly cycling and long-lasting through the life span. Short-term repopulating stem cells (ST) mobilize out of the niches and become more rapidly cycling. ST can give rise to progenitor cells which are actively proliferating. Unlike LT and ST, progenitor cells lost self-renewal capacity and are only able to produce terminally differentiated cells. Recent evidence suggests that cancer stem cells may derive from either ES, LT, ST or progenitor cells that re-acquire self-renewal capacity.

IDENTIFICATION AND ISOLATION OF CANCER STEM CELLS

Self-renewal and lineage capacity are the hallmarks of any stem cell, including cancer stem cells. Assays for identifying cancer stem cells are thus based on both self-renewal capability and tumor recapitulation. The current assay that is considered as the "gold standard", and that tests these cancer stem cell criteria best, is serial transplantation in animal models, most commonly NOD/SCID mice. Limiting dilutions of selected cancer cells are injected into sublethally irradiated immunodeficient mice to evaluate which phenotype of cancer cells can best recapitulate the tumor *in vivo*.

Cell Surface Markers

The majority of the described methods for the identification and isolation of viable cancer stem cells are based on the ability in the cell surface markers between stem and bulk cancer cells. The basis for detecting the different subtype of cancer cells by cell surface markers was pioneered by John E. Dick and colleagues in leukemia [13]. As described earlier, only the $CD34^+/CD38^-$ phenotype was able to initiate human AML in NOD/SCID mice. Subsequently, several other groups also used differences in cell surface markers between stem and differentiated cells to identify cancer stem cells in solid tumor types. These markers include CD44, $α_6$ integrin, $β_6$ integrin, and CD133.

Side Population

The side population (SP) is a particular cell population enriched in primitive stem/progenitor cells and undifferentiated cells [40-42]. The work was originally pioneered by Goodell *et al.* in 1996 [40]. The assay is based on the capability of stem cells to efflux the vital dye, Hoechst 33342. This particular dye simultaneously emits at two wavelengths (red 675 nm and blue 450 nm). A distinct, small, non-stained cell population, which comprises approximately 0.1% of all cells in bone marrow from mice, and which resides in the left lower quadrant of a Flow Activated Cell Sorter (FACS) profile, was first described as the side population. This population expressed bone marrow stem cells markers ($Sca1^+lin^{neg/low}$) and was enriched at least 1,000-fold for *in vivo* reconstitution activity. The differential ability of stem cells to efflux the vital dye H33342 is based on the high expression level of several members of the ABC transporter family, such as MDR1 (multidrug resistance 1, or P-glycoprotein) and BCRP (breast cancer resistance protein), which are also responsible for drug resistance. Although the SP is not "pure", but only enriched for putative stem cells, it is considered as an alternative assay, particularly in situations where stem cells molecular markers are unknown [43]. However, some authors remain skeptical about the existence of stem cells in the SP. Triel et al. [44] demonstrated that the SP of dermal epithelial cells did not express stem cells markers and identified high expression of BCRP in the secretory duct epithelium of the sweat glands instead of the basal layer of the epidermis.

Aldehyde Dehydrogenase (ALDH)

Aldehyde dehydrogenases (ALDH) are a family of enzymes involved in the oxidization of intracellular aldehydes. ALDH are thought to have an important role in oxidation of alcohol and vitamin A as well as in resistance to cyclophosphamide [45,46]. Cytosolic ALDH1 is highly expressed in human and murine hematopoietic stem and progenitor cells [47,48]. More recently, a technique has been developed for the assessment of ALDH activity in viable cells by flow cytometric analysis and has been made commercially available as ALDEFLUOR® kit (StemCell Technologies). This non cytotoxic method uses a cell-permeable fluorescent substrate to identify cells with high ALDH activity [49]. The substrate converted by ALDH is a charged molecule and is unable to leave the cell as freely as the parent substrate. Therefore, the cells with high ALDH activity will accumulate fluorescent ALDH substrate which can be quantified by FACS and used for FACS sorting of viable cells for functional studies. This method has been used mainly to study hematopoietic and leukemic stem cells. $CD34^+ALDH^{bright}$ ($ALDH^{br}$) cells from human umbilical cord blood (UCB) have been shown to contain all the NOD/SCID engrafting cells in the $CD34^+$ fraction [49]. In leukemia, the $ALDH^{br}$ cell population was found to coexpress $CD34^+$ and engraft significantly better in NOD/SCID mice [50].

Tumor Spheres

In 1996, Reynolds and Weiss described a method to culture undifferentiated multipotent neural cells in suspension or on non-adherent surfaces with growth factors, termed the "neurosphere assay".[51] Neurospheres were shown to consist of 4%–20% stem cells, the rest of the population representing progenitor cells in various stages of differentiation. A similar concept was also applied to normal human mammary epithelial cells and is known as the mammosphere assay. Mammospheres have been shown to be enriched in early progenitor/stem cells and are able to differentiate along all three mammary epithelial lineages and to clonally generate complex functional structures in reconstituted 3D culture systems. Furthermore, gene expression analysis of cells isolated from these mammospheres seems to be similar to genetic programs in other stem and progenitor cells.[17] This technique is frequently used as a model to enrich a cancer stem cell population *in vitro* for functional and molecular studies.

Although there are several described methods to identify and isolate cancer stem cells, most of the current methods are flow cytometry-based assays that often require fresh and substantial amounts of tumor tissue, which clearly limits their clinical application for example as a diagnostic tool. Hence, novel methods to identify cancer stem cells by other techniques such as blood based stem cell markers and ultra-sensitive assays that can measure low-abundance proteins are urgently needed. The identification of circulating cancer stem cell markers would allow the monitoring of the efficacy of therapy and disease relapse.

More recently, a gene expression analysis by Clarke and colleagues [52] identified a 186-gene signature differentially expressed in $CD44^+CD24^{-/low}$ breast cancer cells that can serve as a better prognostic marker for both overall survival and metastasis-free survival in patients with breast cancer independent of conventional clinical and pathological factors. Furthermore, several groups demonstrated that self-renewal pathways as well as multiple "stemness" genes are highly expressed in $CD44^+CD24^{-/low}$ breast cancer cells. These include hedgehog signaling components such as *PTCH1*, *Gli1*, *Gli2*, the polycomb gene *Bmi1*, Notch homolog3, Msh homeobox homolog 1, cyclin-dependent kinase inhibitor 1A, Chordin, H19, and Insulin-like growth factor binding protein 7 (IGFBP-7/IGFBP-rP1) [29,53].

CANCER STEM CELL-TARGETED THERAPIES

The vast majority of the over 100 registered and clinically utilized anticancer drugs are "classical" cytotoxic agents. Their common mechanism of action is the preferential killing of rapid dividing bulk tumor cells by either interruption of their cytoskeletal integrity or targeting of DNA-synthesis. To date, only about 4% of advanced cancers that require systemic treatment are curable [33]. The failure of cytotoxic chemotherapy could best be explained by the inability to eradicate cancer stem cells. Similar to their normal counterparts, cancer stem cells are quiescent and primarily persist in the G_0 phase; therefore, cancer stem cells are resistant to cell cycle specific drugs such as those targeting DNA-synthesis [54]. In addition, the over expression of drug efflux pumps in cancer stem cells limits a drug's ability to achieve cell kill.

In an approach similar to the culture and sensitivity assays used in infectious disease, Salmon and Hamburger pioneered the concept of targeting cancer stem cells and concomitantly individualizing cancer therapy in the late 1970s [55]. Single cell suspensions from patients' tumor tissues or malignant effusions were cultured in multilayered soft agar and treated with anticancer drugs. This technique was termed "clonogenic assay" or "human tumor stem cell assay" (HTCA) and was based on the observation that only 0.001-0.1% of tumor cells grow in soft agar comparable to the extent of colony formation by pluripotent cells in bone marrow. Additionally, the homogenous appearance of tumor colonies as well as the staining of these colonies with cell type specific dyes was consistent with a hypothesis that they were stem cells [55,56]. The HTCA was used in a first approach to personalize cancer medicine by assessing a patient's prognosis and response to chemotherapy. However, in prospective clinical studies and a meta analysis of all available data, the HTCA was found to be a better predictor for clinical resistance than sensitivity [55,57]. This outcome could perhaps be explained by the fact that the HTCA was largely used to test drugs (standard chemotherapy) that are substrates of drug efflux pumps expressed on the cell surface by cancer stem cells.

Owing to the limitations of standard chemotherapy, pathways that regulate the self-renewal of normal stem cells [17,58], including Wnt, Notch, and Hedgehog, and that have also been found to play an important role in human carcinogenesis offer interesting new targets for anticancer therapies [17]. Deregulation of developmental pathways has been reported in colon, pancreatic, gastric, prostate [59], cervical, leukemia, skin [60] and breast [61] cancers [17,62]. Several groups are now focusing their efforts on targeting these self-renewal pathways in cancer stem cells. Whilst these essential pathways are shared by normal stem cells and cancer stem cells alike, multiple studies in animal models have shown that interdicting a particular self-renewal pathways may selectively target cancer stem cells [17]. Inhibitors of the Hedgehog pathway, such as cyclopamine, were identified and have a therapeutic window with remarkable activity against a wide range of human cancer cell lines and tumor xenografts including ovarian cancer [45], medulloblastoma [63], gastrointestinal neuroendocrine carcinomas [64], and prostate cancer [59]. Similarly, gamma secretase inhibitors such as LY-411,575, which block Notch activation, were found to have activity in Kaposi's sarcoma [65], breast cancers [66], and melanoma [67].

Another possibility to target the self-renewal capacity of cancer stem cells is to force them to differentiate [68]. Retinoic acid can induce differentiation in embryonic stem cells [69]. All-trans retinoic acid (ATRA) has been used with great success in combination chemotherapy in acute promyelocytic leukemia (APL), a disease with a cure rate of more than 70 %. This suggests that cancer stem cells are being successfully eliminated in this particular disease [70-72]. Arsenic trioxide, an agent that may function through telomere targeting, has recently been demonstrated to further improve the rate of cure in patients with APL. Histone deacetylases (HDACs) regulate transcriptional gene activity. HDAC inhibitors can be used for epigenetic reprogramming of silenced genes and thus, induce cell differentiation. The HDAC inhibitor, vorinostat (SAHA), has been found to have activity in multiple malignancies including leukemia [24], lymphoma [73], thyroid cancer [74], myeloma [75], and hepatocellular carcinoma [76].

Vascular endothelial growth factor (VEGF) has been validated as a target for anti-cancer therapeutics and demonstrated clinical efficacy in colon, lung and breast cancers when the monoclonal anti-VEGF antibody bevacizumab was combined with cytotoxic chemotherapy [77-79]. Initially, the driving hypothesis for this approach was that tumors could not grow beyond a certain size without generating a new blood supply and therefore inhibition of the blood supply would destroy the malignancy. Another hypothesis is that anti-VEGF therapy results in "normalization " of blood supply to the tumor by decreasing interstitial pressures and ultimately by increasing the flow of chemotherapy to the tumor [80]. More recently, a third, stem cell-related hypothesis has emerged. It has become apparent that cancer stem cells live in vascularized lacunae and that anti-VEGF therapy may destroy these sites and consequently improve outcome [81].

Finally, cancer stem cells within a tumor may change their phenotype as the tumor progresses, and also may exhibit a hierarchy, in which different populations of stem cells have a different response to treatment. Treatments targeted against a certain phenotype of cancer stem cells may not be effective against another type of cancer stem cell in a tumor. Thus, multifaceted approaches may be required similar to polychemotherapy of bulk tumor masses in order to eradicate "all" cancer stem cells [25].

CONCLUSION

Recent evidence strengthens the hypothesis that cancer stem cells exist. Further investigations into the origin and characteristics of cancer stem cells will increase our understanding of tumor initiation and progression and provide selective drug targets. Future development of new drugs that target cancer stem cells will require the implementation of new paradigms in investigating these agents in a clinical setting since we may not be able to determine their effectiveness by using currently employed tumor regression endpoints. Because chronic treatment of cancer patients is likely to be necessary for the eradication of cancer stem cells, long-term toxicity studies will also be necessary that determine whether side effects are associated with the depletion of a particular stem cell pool in normal tissues.

REFERENCES

[1] Mathers CD, Shibuya K, Boschi-Pinto C, et al: Global and regional estimates of cancer mortality and incidence by site: I. Application of regional cancer survival model to estimate cancer mortality distribution by site. *BMC Cancer.* 2:36, 2002

[2] Al-Hajj M, Becker MW, Wicha M, et al: Therapeutic implications of cancer stem cells. *Curr. Opin. Genet. Dev.* 14:43-7, 2004

[3] Jordan CT: Targeting the most critical cells: approaching leukemia therapy as a problem in stem cell biology. *Nat. Clin. Pract. Oncol.* 2:224-5, 2005

[4] Abbott A: Cancer: the root of the problem. *Nature.* 442:742-3, 2006

[5] Wikipedia tfe: Ernest McCulloch, 2006

[6] Becker AJ, Mc CE, Till JE: Cytological demonstration of the clonal nature of spleen colonies derived from transplanted mouse marrow cells. *Nature.* 197:452-4, 1963

[7] Reya T, Morrison SJ, Clarke MF, et al: Stem cells, cancer, and cancer stem cells. *Nature.* 414:105-11, 2001
[8] Ramalho-Santos M, Yoon S, Matsuzaki Y, et al: "Stemness": transcriptional profiling of embryonic and adult stem cells. *Science.* 298:597-600, 2002
[9] Clevers H: Stem cells, asymmetric division and cancer. *Nat. Genet.* 37:1027-8, 2005
[10] Caussinus E, Gonzalez C: Induction of tumor growth by altered stem-cell asymmetric division in Drosophila melanogaster. *Nat. Genet.* 37:1125-9, 2005
[11] Bruce WR, Van Der Gaag H: A Quantitative Assay for the Number of Murine Lymphoma Cells Capable of Proliferation in Vivo. *Nature.* 199:79-80, 1963
[12] Park CH, Bergsagel DE, McCulloch EA: Mouse myeloma tumor stem cells: a primary cell culture assay. *J. Natl. Cancer Inst.* 46:411-22, 1971
[13] Bonnet D, Dick JE: Human acute myeloid leukemia is organized as a hierarchy that originates from a primitive hematopoietic cell. *Nat. Med.* 3:730-7, 1997
[14] Hope KJ, Jin L, Dick JE: Acute myeloid leukemia originates from a hierarchy of leukemic stem cell classes that differ in self-renewal capacity. *Nat. Immunol.* 5:738-43, 2004
[15] Fidler IJ, Hart IR: Biological diversity in metastatic neoplasms: origins and implications. *Science.* 217:998-1003, 1982
[16] Al-Hajj M, Wicha MS, Benito-Hernandez A, et al: Prospective identification of tumorigenic breast cancer cells. *Proc. Natl. Acad. Sci. U. S. A.* 100:3983-8, 2003
[17] Dontu G, Abdallah WM, Foley JM, et al: In vitro propagation and transcriptional profiling of human mammary stem/progenitor cells. *Genes Dev.* 17:1253-70, 2003
[18] Singh SK, Hawkins C, Clarke ID, et al: Identification of human brain tumour initiating cells. *Nature.* 432:396-401, 2004
[19] Singh SK, Clarke ID, Hide T, et al: Cancer stem cells in nervous system tumors. *Oncogene.* 23:7267-73, 2004
[20] Matsui W, Huff CA, Wang Q, et al: Characterization of clonogenic multiple myeloma cells. *Blood.* 103:2332-6, 2004
[21] Collins AT, Berry PA, Hyde C, et al: Prospective identification of tumorigenic prostate cancer stem cells. *Cancer Res.* 65:10946-51, 2005
[22] Kelly PN, Dakic A, Adams JM, et al: Tumor growth need not be driven by rare cancer stem cells. *Science.* 317:337, 2007
[23] Kern SE, Shibata D: The fuzzy math of solid tumor stem cells: a perspective. *Cancer Res.* 67:8985-8, 2007
[24] Clarke MF, Dick JE, Dirks PB, et al: Cancer Stem Cells--Perspectives on Current Status and Future Directions: AACR Workshop on Cancer Stem Cells. *Cancer Res.* 66:9339-44, 2006
[25] Hill RP, Perris R: "Destemming" cancer stem cells. *J. Natl. Cancer Inst.* 99:1435-40, 2007
[26] Neuzil J, Stantic M, Zobalova R, et al: Tumour-initiating cells vs. cancer 'stem' cells and CD133: what's in the name? *Biochem. Biophys. Res. Commun.* 355:855-9, 2007
[27] Phillips TM, McBride WH, Pajonk F: The response of CD24(-/low)/CD44+ breast cancer-initiating cells to radiation. *J. Natl. Cancer Inst.* 98:1777-85, 2006
[28] Ricci-Vitiani L, Lombardi DG, Pilozzi E, et al: Identification and expansion of human colon-cancer-initiating cells. *Nature.* 445:111-5, 2007
[29] Liu S, Dontu G, Mantle ID, et al: Hedgehog signaling and Bmi-1 regulate self-renewal of normal and malignant human mammary stem cells. *Cancer Res.* 66:6063-71, 2006

[30] Doyle LA, Yang W, Abruzzo LV, et al: A multidrug resistance transporter from human MCF-7 breast cancer cells. *Proc. Natl. Acad. Sci. U. S. A.* 95:15665-70, 1998
[31] Patrawala L, Calhoun T, Schneider-Broussard R, et al: Highly purified CD44+ prostate cancer cells from xenograft human tumors are enriched in tumorigenic and metastatic progenitor cells. *Oncogene.* 25:1696-708, 2006
[32] Ponti D, Costa A, Zaffaroni N, et al: Isolation and in vitro propagation of tumorigenic breast cancer cells with stem/progenitor cell properties. *Cancer Res.* 65:5506-11, 2005
[33] Chumsri S, Phatak P, Edelman MJ, et al: Cancer stem cells and individualized therapy. *Cancer Genomics Proteomics.* 4:165-74, 2007
[34] Ravandi F, Estrov Z: Eradication of leukemia stem cells as a new goal of therapy in leukemia. *Clin. Cancer Res.* 12:340-4, 2006
[35] Cozzio A, Passegue E, Ayton PM, et al: Similar MLL-associated leukemias arising from self-renewing stem cells and short-lived myeloid progenitors. *Genes Dev.* 17:3029-35, 2003
[36] Gazziola C, Cordani N, Wasserman B, et al: Malignant fibrous histiocytoma: a proposed cellular origin and identification of its characterizing gene transcripts. *Int. J. Oncol.* 23:343-51, 2003
[37] Tirode F, Laud-Duval K, Prieur A, et al: Mesenchymal stem cell features of Ewing tumors. *Cancer Cell.* 11:421-9, 2007
[38] Riggi N, Cironi L, Provero P, et al: Development of Ewing's sarcoma from primary bone marrow-derived mesenchymal progenitor cells. *Cancer Res.* 65:11459-68, 2005
[39] Houghton J, Stoicov C, Nomura S, et al: Gastric cancer originating from bone marrow-derived cells. *Science.* 306:1568-71, 2004
[40] Goodell MA, Brose K, Paradis G, et al: Isolation and functional properties of murine hematopoietic stem cells that are replicating in vivo. *J. Exp. Med.* 183:1797-806, 1996
[41] Hadnagy A, Gaboury L, Beaulieu R, et al: SP analysis may be used to identify cancer stem cell populations. *Exp. Cell Res.* 312:3701-10, 2006
[42] Camargo FD, Chambers SM, Drew E, et al: Hematopoietic stem cells do not engraft with absolute efficiencies. *Blood.* 107:501-7, 2006
[43] Challen GA, Little MH: A side order of stem cells: the SP phenotype. *Stem Cells.* 24:3-12, 2006
[44] Triel C, Vestergaard ME, Bolund L, et al: Side population cells in human and mouse epidermis lack stem cell characteristics. *Exp. Cell Res.* 295:79-90, 2004
[45] Wang JS, Fang Q, Sun DJ, et al: Genetic modification of hematopoietic progenitor cells for combined resistance to 4-hydroperoxycyclophosphamide, vincristine, and daunorubicin. *Acta Pharmacol. Sin.* 22:949-55, 2001
[46] Duester G: Families of retinoid dehydrogenases regulating vitamin A function: production of visual pigment and retinoic acid. *Eur. J. Biochem.* 267:4315-24, 2000
[47] Kastan MB, Schlaffer E, Russo JE, et al: Direct demonstration of elevated aldehyde dehydrogenase in human hematopoietic progenitor cells. *Blood.* 75:1947-50, 1990
[48] Storms RW, Trujillo AP, Springer JB, et al: Isolation of primitive human hematopoietic progenitors on the basis of aldehyde dehydrogenase activity. *Proc. Natl. Acad. Sci. U. S. A.* 96:9118-23, 1999
[49] Storms RW, Green PD, Safford KM, et al: Distinct hematopoietic progenitor compartments are delineated by the expression of aldehyde dehydrogenase and CD34. *Blood.* 106:95-102, 2005

[50] Cheung AM, Wan TS, Leung JC, et al: Aldehyde dehydrogenase activity in leukemic blasts defines a subgroup of acute myeloid leukemia with adverse prognosis and superior NOD/SCID engrafting potential. *Leukemia.* 21:1423-30, 2007
[51] Weiss S, Reynolds BA, Vescovi AL, et al: Is there a neural stem cell in the mammalian forebrain? *Trends Neurosci.* 19:387-93, 1996
[52] Liu R, Wang X, Chen GY, et al: The prognostic role of a gene signature from tumorigenic breast-cancer cells. *N. Engl. J. Med.* 356:217-26, 2007
[53] Shipitsin M, Campbell LL, Argani P, et al: Molecular definition of breast tumor heterogeneity. *Cancer Cell.* 11:259-73, 2007
[54] Venezia TA, Merchant AA, Ramos CA, et al: Molecular signatures of proliferation and quiescence in hematopoietic stem cells. *PLoS Biol.* 2:e301, 2004
[55] Salmon SE, Hamburger AW, Soehnlen B, et al: Quantitation of differential sensitivity of human-tumor stem cells to anticancer drugs. *N. Engl. J. Med.* 298:1321-7, 1978
[56] Schrag D, Garewal HS, Burstein HJ, et al: American Society of Clinical Oncology Technology Assessment: chemotherapy sensitivity and resistance assays. *J. Clin. Oncol.* 22:3631-8, 2004
[57] Fiebig HH, Maier A, Burger AM: Clonogenic assay with established human tumour xenografts: correlation of in vitro to in vivo activity as a basis for anticancer drug discovery. *Eur. J. Cancer.* 40:802-20, 2004
[58] Liu S, Dontu G, Wicha MS: Mammary stem cells, self-renewal pathways, and carcinogenesis. *Breast Cancer Res.* 7:86-95, 2005
[59] Karhadkar SS, Bova GS, Abdallah N, et al: Hedgehog signalling in prostate regeneration, neoplasia and metastasis. *Nature.* 431:707-12, 2004
[60] Gailani MR, Stahle-Backdahl M, Leffell DJ, et al: The role of the human homologue of Drosophila patched in sporadic basal cell carcinomas. *Nat. Genet.* 14:78-81, 1996
[61] Dievart A, Beaulieu N, Jolicoeur P: Involvement of Notch1 in the development of mouse mammary tumors. *Oncogene.* 18:5973-81, 1999
[62] Olsen CL, Hsu PP, Glienke J, et al: Hedgehog-interacting protein is highly expressed in endothelial cells but down-regulated during angiogenesis and in several human tumors. *BMC Cancer.* 4:43, 2004
[63] Romer JT, Kimura H, Magdaleno S, et al: Suppression of the Shh pathway using a small molecule inhibitor eliminates medulloblastoma in Ptc1(+/-)p53(-/-) mice. *Cancer Cell.* 6:229-40, 2004
[64] Shida T, Furuya M, Nikaido T, et al: Sonic Hedgehog-Gli1 Signaling Pathway Might Become an Effective Therapeutic Target in Gastrointestinal Neuroendocrine Carcinomas. *Cancer Biol. Ther.* 5, 2006
[65] Lan K, Choudhuri T, Murakami M, et al: Intracellular activated Notch1 is critical for proliferation of Kaposi's sarcoma-associated herpesvirus-associated B-lymphoma cell lines in vitro. *J. Virol.* 80:6411-9, 2006
[66] Pece S, Serresi M, Santolini E, et al: Loss of negative regulation by Numb over Notch is relevant to human breast carcinogenesis. *J. Cell Biol.* 167:215-21, 2004
[67] Nickoloff BJ, Hendrix MJ, Pollock PM, et al: Notch and NOXA-related pathways in melanoma cells. *J. Investig. Dermatol. Symp. Proc.* 10:95-104, 2005
[68] Massard C, Deutsch E, Soria JC: Tumour stem cell-targeted treatment: elimination or differentiation. *Ann. Oncol.* 17:1620-4, 2006
[69] Motohashi T, Aoki H, Chiba K, et al: Multipotent cell fate of neural crest-like cells derived from embryonic stem cells. *Stem Cells.* 2006

[70] Sanz MA, Lo Coco F, Martin G, et al: Definition of relapse risk and role of nonanthracycline drugs for consolidation in patients with acute promyelocytic leukemia: a joint study of the PETHEMA and GIMEMA cooperative groups. *Blood.* 96:1247-53, 2000

[71] Sanz MA, Martin G, Gonzalez M, et al: Risk-adapted treatment of acute promyelocytic leukemia with all-trans-retinoic acid and anthracycline monochemotherapy: a multicenter study by the PETHEMA group. *Blood.* 103:1237-43, 2004

[72] Sanz MA, Martin G, Rayon C, et al: A modified AIDA protocol with anthracycline-based consolidation results in high antileukemic efficacy and reduced toxicity in newly diagnosed PML/RARalpha-positive acute promyelocytic leukemia. PETHEMA group. *Blood.* 94:3015-21, 1999

[73] O'Connor OA: Developing new drugs for the treatment of lymphoma. *Eur. J. Haematol.* Suppl:150-8, 2005

[74] Luong QT, O'Kelly J, Braunstein GD, et al: Antitumor activity of suberoylanilide hydroxamic acid against thyroid cancer cell lines in vitro and in vivo. *Clin. Cancer Res.* 12:5570-7, 2006

[75] Yaccoby S, Wezeman MJ, Zangari M, et al: Inhibitory effects of osteoblasts and increased bone formation on myeloma in novel culture systems and a myelomatous mouse model. *Haematologica.* 91:192-9, 2006

[76] Ocker M, Alajati A, Ganslmayer M, et al: The histone-deacetylase inhibitor SAHA potentiates proapoptotic effects of 5-fluorouracil and irinotecan in hepatoma cells. *J. Cancer Res. Clin. Oncol.* 131:385-94, 2005

[77] Hurwitz H, Fehrenbacher L, Novotny W, et al: Bevacizumab plus irinotecan, fluorouracil, and leucovorin for metastatic colorectal cancer. *N. Engl. J. Med.* 350:2335-42, 2004

[78] Sandler A, Gray R, Perry MC, et al: Paclitaxel-carboplatin alone or with bevacizumab for non-small-cell lung cancer. *N. Engl. J. Med.* 355:2542-50, 2006

[79] Wedam SB, Low JA, Yang SX, et al: Antiangiogenic and antitumor effects of bevacizumab in patients with inflammatory and locally advanced breast cancer. *J. Clin. Oncol.* 24:769-77, 2006

[80] Jain RK: Normalization of tumor vasculature: an emerging concept in antiangiogenic therapy. *Science.* 307:58-62, 2005

[81] Calabrese C, Poppleton H, Kocak M, et al: A perivascular niche for brain tumor stem cells. *Cancer Cell.* 11:69-82, 2007

Reviewed by Anne W. Hamburger, Professor of Pathology, University of Maryland, Baltimore, MD, USA.

This work was supported by the Maryland Cancer Research Fund with a grant to AMB.

In: Encyclopedia of Stem Cell Research (2 Volume Set) ISBN: 978-1-61761-835-2
Editor: Alexander L. Greene © 2012 Nova Science Publishers, Inc.

Chapter VI

MESENCHYMAL STEM CELLS IN BONE DISEASES: STATE OF THE ART AND FUTURE PROSPECTS

Gael Y. Rochefort and C. L. Benhamou*
Inserm, CHR Orleans, France

ABSTRACT

Bone remodeling is a physiological process determined by the sequential and coordinated interaction of osteoclasts, osteoblasts and angiogenesis. During bone repair, osteoblastic cells, originated from mesenchymal stem cells (MSCs), are highly regulated to proliferate and to produce an osteogenic matrix, thus forming a new bone. MSCs are multipotential and undifferentiated cells that are present in the adult bone marrow. They serve *in vitro* and *in vivo* as precursors for bone marrow stroma, bone, fat, cartilage, muscle (smooth, cardiac and skeletal) and neural cells. MSCs are usually isolated from adult bone marrow but can also be isolated from several other tissues, such as fetal liver, adult circulating blood, umbilical cord blood, placenta or adipose tissue. In the bone marrow, MSCs give rise to mesenchymal cells residing in the bone (osteogenic, chondrogenic and adipogenic cells) and also support hematopoiesis. Therefore, MSCs regulate both osteogenesis and hematopoiesis, and they are responsible in part for the regenerative capacity of bone tissue. Osteoporosis, resulting of an imbalance between resorption and formation of endosteal and trabecular bone surfaces, is a systemic disorder characterized by a low bone mass and an altered bone quality with a consistent increase in bone fragility and susceptibility to fracture correlated to functional aberrations in MSCs. This chapter highlights current status and progresses in the use of MSCs to treat or attenuate bone diseases, including osteoporosis.

---

* Tel. (+33) 238 744 055; gael.rochefort@gmail.com

I. INTRODUCTION

Stem cells are generally described as clonogenic and undifferentiated cells that are able to self-renew and to differentiate into one or more types of differentiated and committed cells [1-4]. To date, stem cells have been isolated and characterized from tissues of all ages, including embryonic, fetal and adult tissues. Among the collective term of adult (i.e. postnatal) stem cells, mesenchymal stem cells (MSCs) represent a population of multipotential cells which are currently defined by a combination of morphologic, phenotypic, and functional properties, and which are capable of giving rise to at least mesenchymal-derived tissues, including bone, cartilage, fat, tendon and muscle [2, 4-9]. MSCs have been identified into a large number of adult tissues, including the bone marrow where they provide the cellular microenvironment supporting hematopoiesis. As a part of the stromal fraction, MSCs also regulate osteogenesis and are responsible in part, for the regenerative capacity of bone tissue [10].

Since MSCs differentiate into osteogenic cells, they have been used to develop new clinical therapies to treat or attenuate a number of skeletal disorders. Therefore, the purpose of the chapter is to review the literature on the adult MSC biology and their potential in bone engineering and bone disease treatment ensuring the future clinical application success [11-13].

II. MESENCHYMAL STEM CELLS: BIOLOGICAL PROPERTIES AND CHARACTERISTICS

A. MSC Sources

MSC, or progenitor cells with similar features, can be isolated from many different common species, including human, murine and rat origin [4, 14-25]. Furthermore, MSCs can also be extracted from guinea pigs, cats, baboons, sheep, dogs, pigs, cows and horses [26-34].

Usually, MSCs are isolated form the stromal fraction of the bone marrow where they represent only 0.01-0.0001 % of the nucleated cells [18, 19, 35]. In fact, these multipotential stem cells are typically obtained by flushing the marrow out of animal bones with culture medium or from human bone marrow aspirates and transferred into a culture dish. However, MSCs and cells featuring MSC characteristics were also reported in several tissues adult and fetal tissues, including spleen, liver, kidney, pancreas, lung, thymus, smooth muscle, skeletal muscle, aorta, vena cava, brain, dental pulp, deciduous teeth, scalp tissue and hair follicle, periosteum, trabecular bone, adipose tissue, synovium, placenta, amniotic fluid and umbilical cord vein [4, 16-20, 22, 36-54]. Another MSC source of particular importance is provided by blood samples where MSCs can be extracted from umbilical cord blood and cryopreserved cord blood, but also from normal adult and from healthy women during or following pregnancy [14, 35, 48, 53, 55-60].

At last, MSCs can be mobilized into the bloodstream after treatment (chemotherapy, cytokine injection) or physiopathological events and thus can increase the physiological release of stem cells and progenitors from reservoirs, such as the bone marrow, in response to stress signals during injury and inflammation. In fact, MSCs are increased in blood after repeated stimulations with cytokines such as granulocyte colony-stimulating factor (G-CSF) or granulocyte-macrophage colony-stimulating factor (GM-CSF), or recently by several physiopathological circumstances, such as chronic hypoxia, myocardial infarction or encephalopathy [23, 55, 61-65].

B. Hematopoiesis Supportive Capacity

The hematopoietic bone marrow microenvironment can be subdivided into a hematopoietic cell compartment, which is represented by the hematopoietic stem cells and their descendants, and a stromal compartment [35, 66]. This last compartment is composed of osteoblasts and their extra-cellular products, adipocytic cells and several ad-luminal mural stromal cells with smooth muscle characteristics, including in particular fibroblasts, endothelial cells and capillary pericytes. All these stromal compartment cells might derive from MSCs since they are able to differentiate into osteoblasts, adipocytes, vascular smooth muscle-like stroma, and more controversially into endothelial cells [66-73].

The specific role of MSC-derived marrow stromal cells in hematopoiesis and osteogenesis was firstly evidenced by Friedenstein in an historical report where bone-like structures ("ossicles") were formed when marrow stromal cells transplanted under the capsule kidney, and where the donor stroma was colonized by hematopoietic cells deriving from the host [1-3]. Further reports described the donor hematopoietic stem cell engraftment in the host stromal microenvironment during clinical bone marrow transplantation *in vivo*. At last, MSCs were demonstrated to support hematopoiesis *in vitro* for periods longer than 6 months in Dexter cultures and to allow the generation of all blood lineages, including myeloid, lymphoid, and megakaryocytic cells [35, 74].

C. MSC Characteristics

1. Maker Expression

To date, MSCs are not reported to exhibit specific immuno-phenotypic markers. However, MSCs expressed a large variety of makers presented by many other cell types. Thus, MSCs are positive for CD13, CD29, CD44, CD49a, CD49e, CD73 (SH3 and SH4), CD90, CD105 (SH2), CD106, CD166 and HLA ABC but are negative for the hematopoietic and/or endothelial markers CD31, CD34, CD45 and HLA DR [4, 7, 18, 75].

2. Multilineage Differentiation Potential

Adult stem cells including MSCs are able to differentiate into cells of the tissue in which they reside. Thus, MSCs are not only able to differentiate into mesodermal tissues, including osteoblasts, chondroblasts, adipocytes, fibroblasts and skeletal myoblasts [4, 6-9], but they are also able to acquire characteristics of non-mesodermal lineages, such as endothelial cells [76, 77], neural cells [78-80], and cells of the endoderm [76, 81-83], *in vitro* and *in vivo* [84-86].

a) Adipogenic Potential

When cultured in a medium supplemented with insulin, dexamethasone, indomethacin, 3-isobutyl-1-methylxanthine (IBMX) and a peroxisome proliferator-activated receptor γ (PPAR-γ) agonist such as BRL-49653 [87], MSCs are able to differentiate into mature adipocytes. This adipogenic differentiation may be evidenced by the staining of lipid-filled droplets with oil red O, but also the expression of several adipogenic markers [23, 88-90]. In fact, MSCs express small amounts of the crucial transcription factors that promote adipogenesis, such as CCAAT-enhancer-binding protein α (C/EBPα) and PPARγ [91-95].

b) Osteogenic Potential

MSCS can be differentiated into osteogenic cells *in vitro* when cultured in a defined medium supplemented with several exogenous cytokines and growth factors, including various isoforms of bone morphogenic protein (BMP), interleukin-6, growth hormone, leptin, sortilin, and transglutaminase [96-104]. Furthermore, the osteogenic differentiation may also be obtained when using other chemical compounds, such as prostaglandin E_2 (a natural eicosanoid), 1,25-dihydroxyvitamin D3 (the active form of vitamin D3 also known as calcitriol), L-ascorbic acid (vitamin C), dexamethasone (a synthetic steroid), β-glycerol phosphate, the synthetic potent inducer TAK-778, and statins [105-116]. At last, the osteogenic differentiation may also be obtained when MSCs are co-cultured with osteoblasts [108, 116], with osteocytes-derived proteins (bone sialoprotein osteopontin osteonectin osteocalcin and osteocrin) [108, 117-120], or *in vivo* when MSCs are seeded on extracellular matrices made of hydroxyapatite, tricalcium phosphate or poly-L-lactide-co-glycolide [121-124]. When differentiated into osteogenic cells, MSCs express specific osteogenic factors, including RUNX2, MSX2, DLX5, and osterix [125-127], and excrete an extracellular matrix that can be mineralized and specifically stained [23].

c) Chondrogenic Potential

To promote the chondrogenic differentiation of MSCs *in vitro*, MSCs may be cultured in "pellets" after gentle centrifugation [128-132] and with a high-glucose medium supplemented with insulin, transferrin, selenious acid, linoleic acid, ascorbate 2-phosphate, dexamethasone and TGF-β [128, 129]. Then, the chondrogenic differentiation is evidenced by the Safranin O or toluidine blue specific staining of cartilage glycosaminoglycans on formalin-fixed paraffin or resin embedded aggregates, whereas up-regulation of both type II and X collagens may also be confirmed.

d) Myogenic Potential

MSCs can be differentiated *in vitro* into skeletal muscle cells after incubation with various chemical compounds, including 5-azacytidine, basic fibroblast growth factor, forskolin, platelet-derived growth factor, neuregulin, vascular endothelial growth factor, insulin-like growth factor or amphotericin B [20, 25, 133-137]. During the myogenic differentiation process, adjacent MSCs fused and formed multinucleated myotubes [20, 137-140]. MSC-derived myotubes express several myogenic markers, including Pax3, Pax7, Myo-D, myogenin, Myf5 and the myogenic regulatory factor 4, and are able to contract [133, 135, 139, 141-144].

MSCs are also able to differentiate into cardiomyocyte-like cells, after culturing with including 5-azacytidine, amphotericin B or oxytocin [138, 143, 145-151]. The MSC-derived cardiomyocyte-like cells exhibit a myotubes-like structure spontaneously beating and typical sarcomeres, and express several structural and contractile proteins, including myosin heavy chain, beta-actin, desmin, phospholamban, adrenergic and muscarinic receptors, connexin 43, titin, and troponins C, I and T [138, 146-153]. At last, cardiomyocyte-like cells thus obtained display gap junction with a cell-to-cell coupling, but also sinus node–like and ventricular cell–like action potentials [143, 154, 155].

At last, MSCs can differentiate into smooth muscle-like cells when cultured into a Dexter-type medium (basic medium supplemented with fetal calf serum and β-mercaptoethanol), with ascorbic acid or with dimethyl sulfoxide [156-158]. The smooth muscle-like cells thus obtained express various smooth muscle markers (alpha-smooth muscle actin, SM22α, h-caldesmon, h1-calponin). Finally, these cells also exhibit a contraction capacity correlated to their alpha-smooth muscle actin content [144].

3. MSC Therapeutic Potential

Next to their differentiation potential, MSCs display other properties that promote them as good candidates for cell-based therapies.

Firstly, MSCs are generally considered as poorly immunogenic cells, they are of great importance for therapeutic purposes (e.g. hematopoietic stem/progenitor cell engraftment or graft-versus-host disease). In fact, MSCs constitutively express low surface densities of MHC class I molecules and are negative for MHC class II and for co-stimulatory molecules (e.g. CD40, CD80 and CD86), both up-regulated by inflammatory stimuli [159, 160]. Thus, MSCs exert immuno-regulatory activity, such as immuno-suppression by inhibiting T-cell responses both to polyclonal stimuli and to their cognate peptide [161-163].

Secondly, when intravenously injected, donor mesenchymal stem cells have the capacity to domiciliate and survive at long-term. Indeed, donor MSC contribution in recipient bone and BM was estimated in mice and represent 5% of the total cell content 5 months after intravenous injection [164]. Furthermore, MSCs were still detected after 12 weeks in NOD/SCID mice in lungs, kidneys, liver, intestine and brain, in addition to bone, bone marrow and spleen [165] but also after 1 year in baboons after infusion [27].

At last, MSCs, which are easily accessible from healthy human subjects, exhibit a high proliferative potential [4, 164, 166-169] with a self-renewal capacity [170], and they are able to regenerate a target tissue after injury [171, 172]

III. MSC-BASED BONE ENGINEERING

A. Bone Regenerative Capacities

Bones are rigid organs that form part of the skeleton. They provide the mechanical stability to hold up the body and supports muscles and soft organs. They also serve as reservoir for mineral and they harbor the bone marrow that produces red and white blood cells. Bone is a dynamic and highly vascularized tissue that is able to remodel after an injury without scar. In the adult skeleton, bones exhibit a complex architecture and they are arranged either in a porous sponge-like trabecular pattern (cancellous bone) or in a compact pattern (cortical bone) [173].

Bones are composed of cells (osteoblasts, osteocytes and osteoclasts) where osteocytes are embedded in a mineralized matrix composed of collagen, glycoproteins, proteoglycans and sialoproteins. During bone development (modeling) and remodeling, both cells and matrix interact and coordinate in response to stimuli. The high regenerative potential allows bones to heal the majority of fractures under standard conservative or surgical therapy. However, extended bone defects following trauma or cancer resection or non-unions of fractures may require some sophisticated treatment, such as bone grafts or reconstruction using MSCs and biomaterials [174].

B. Matrices and Scaffolds

MSCs can also be differentiated into osteogenic cells *in vivo* by seeding them on non-cellular matrices and scaffolds. Indeed, the team of Goshima was the first to evidence that rat bone marrow mesenchymal cells had an osteogenic potential with new bone deposition when cells were seeded in porous bioceramic scaffolds and implanted *in vivo* into immuno-compromised rodents [175-177]. Then, in 1997 Krebsbach *et al.* demonstrated that marrow stromal fibroblasts (i.e. MSCs) were able to form bone structures when cultured on vehicles containing hydroxyapatite/tricalcium phosphate ceramics and then subcutaneously implanted *in vivo* into NOD/SCID mice [178]. Following these studies, other authors have obtained similar results in different animal models, including syngeneic rats or immuno-deficient mice [176, 178-183].

MSCs seeded on porous hydroxyapatite ceramics were next successfully used to repair critical size animal segmental bone defects, in rabbit, sheep, rat, mice, goat, pig and dog [184-193]. Furthermore, qualitative and quantitative evaluations of the performance of scaffolds seeded with MSCs, using micro-diffraction and X-ray synchrotron radiation computed micro-tomography (micro-CT), reported a positive impact of MSCs on the bone formation kinetics and the scaffold resorption [194-196]. Moreover, some authors also used MSC-seeded scaffolds to create vascularized bone flaps to facilitate the vascularization of the newly formed bone [197, 198]. Then, nonporous, biologically inert materials (ceramics or titanium), and porous, resorbable and osteoconductive biomaterials (hydroxyapatite and tricalcium phosphate) were used as natural or synthetic biomaterial carriers for MSC delivery in human orthopedic applications [122, 123, 199]. At last, the *in vivo* reparation of critical segmental bone defects, but also the reconstruction of phalanx or mandible, was performed in human when using cell-matrix compounds, composed of MSCs seeded on hydroxyapatite/tricalcium phosphate ceramics or poly-L-lactide-co-glycolide [11, 121, 124, 200, 201].

C. Gene Therapy-Coupled Osteogenesis

Next to opportunities offer by MSC injections or by MSC-seeded scaffolds, the stem cell-based therapy may also be coupled to a gene therapy to restore invalid genes or to stimulate bone remodeling in the treatment or the attenuation of bone disorders.

Such a strategy has already been used to transfect some stem cell populations with both viral and non-viral vectors to over-express osteogenic factors that induce bone formation and fracture repair through paracrine and autocrine signal pathways [202-204]. In that purpose, transfected bone marrow-derived, muscle-derived and adipose tissue-derived stem cells have been examined for bone tissue engineering applications [202-204]. Shen *et al.* thus compared the ability of primary muscle-derived cells and muscle-derived stem cells to induce bone formation after *ex vivo* transfection with a retroviral vector expressing human bone morphogenetic protein 4 (BMP4) [203]. Results indicated that all transduced cell populations secreted high levels of BMP4 differentiated toward the osteogenic lineage. Furthermore, this osteogenic potential was more effective with muscle-derived stem cells than with the primary muscle-derived cell populations. At last, when implanted *in vivo* into immunocompetent syngeneic mice, the transfected muscle-derived stem cells secreting high levels of BMP4 were able to produce mineralized bone, persisted for a significantly longer period at the bone forming sites, and triggered a low immunogenic response. All together, these results indicated that muscle-derived stem cells might exhibit several advantages in the improvement of bone healing, with lower immunogenicity and higher capacity for *in vivo* survival [203].

Genetically modified MSCs, over-expressing bone morphogenetic protein 2 and 4 or type I collagen, have also been tested with success to enhance or increase the stem cell capacities for bone tissue engineering or bone remodeling [205-209].

IV. MSC-BASED BONE DISEASE ATTENUATION AND TREATMENT

The MSC-based therapy to treat or attenuate bone diseases started in 1995 with the pioneer experiment of Pereira who demonstrated that culture-expanded bone marrow-derived MSCs can serve as long-lasting precursors for mesenchymal cells in bone, but also in other tissues, such as cartilage and lung [164]. Similarly and few years later, Horwitz and his group reported the ability of MSCs to be transplanted into allogeneic bone marrow without any side effect. Furthermore, this team also demonstrated an osteoblast number increase after infusion of MSCs into children suffering of osteogenesis imperfecta, with formation of new lamellar bone and an increase of the total body mineral content, suggesting the feasibility of the MSC-based therapy to treat bone disorders such as osteogenesis imperfecta [13].

A. Fracture Consolidation

In human, the skeletal bone mass increases until the peak bone mass is reach (between the age of 18 and 30) after which bone mass progressively decreases. Bone remodeling and bone loss, as a function of age, are under the control of bone cells, particularly osteoblasts that regulate bone deposition, and osteoclasts that command bone resorption [210, 211]. Furthermore, maturing people inexorably exhibit aged tissues and decreased capacities of replacing aged tissues, including bone [212]. Thus, the bone loss associated with aging is mainly due both to a bone formation decrease (intrinsic decrease in osteoblast activity) and to an increase in bone resorption (by extrinsic factors such as calcium-vitamin D deficiency). This results in osteopenia or osteoporosis with a higher fracture risk and osteoporosis [213]. Furthermore, the bone repair process may be altered after a fracture [214] or in case of pseudarthrosis [215]. Thus, the osteogenic differentiation potential of MSCs provides great hopes for bone repair in reconstructive surgery to heal fractures in aging people.

The fracture healing process may be assisted by using bone forming osteoprogenitor cells, such as MSCs, coupled with appropriate carriers, including growth factors, matrix and scaffolds. Thus, several carriers have been reported to exhibit a positive impact on bone healing, including guanidine extracted demineralized bone matrix, polymeric or ceramic implants, hydrogel biocompatible scaffolds or bone grafts [184, 216-220]. Bone fracture healing was also improved when using growth factors to initiate the migration, the proliferation and the differentiation of MSCs into osteogenic cells, including human recombinant osteogenic protein-1, or bone morphogenic proteins [218, 219, 221, 222]. At last, local infusion of bone marrow-derived MSCs can enhance fracture healing and furthermore provide an osteogenic microenvironment that favors blood vessels formation [223-226].

B. Osteoporosis

Osteoporosis is the consequence of an imbalance between bone resorption and bone formation, which occurs mainly in post-menopausal women, a situation characterized by a bone resorption increase without adequate compensation in bone formation [227-229]. Osteoporosis is also characterized by a bone strength loss with a bone density and bone mass decrease, and a fracture prevalence increase.

Osteoporosis has been classified into primary and secondary subtypes [230-232]. Primary osteoporosis is an age-associated disease occurring in both sexes, but mainly in post-menopausal women where estrogen homeostasis is altered [233]. On the contrary, secondary osteoporosis is usually caused by factors including adverse effects of glucocorticoid therapy, hyperparathyroidism, anorexia, immobilization, marrow-ablative chemotherapy, diseases of the gastrointestinal or biliary tract and cancer [234-241].

Imbalance between bone resorption and bone formation was also suggested to be linked to functional aberrations in MSC functions including a proliferation decrease, alterations of response to growth and mitogenic factors, a decrease of the osteogenic differentiation capacity with an increased adipogenic differentiation capacity, and a deficient production of type I collagen [242-244]. Thus, several strategies were conducted to reduce this phenomenon and to replace MSCs. Using a senescence-accelerated mouse model, Ichioka and his team were among the first to demonstrate the positive impact of the local (i.e. intra-bone marrow) bone marrow transplantation (containing both mesenchymal and hematopoietic stem cells) in the bone loss treatment [245, 246]. In fact, they demonstrated in the mouse osteoporosis model that allogeneic bone marrow transplantation significantly attenuated the loss of bone mineral density, but also maintained the urinary deoxy-pyridinoline (a biochemical indicator of bone resorption) levels, thus preventing excessive bone resorption associated with osteoporosis. Furthermore, after transplantation, donor MSCs were able to produce interleukin 6, that regulates osteoclastogenesis, and interleukin 11, that inhibits adipogenesis and enhances osteoblastogenesis [247, 248]. Therefore, MSC injection in osteoporotic animals may contribute in maintaining the balance between bone formation and resorption and thus contribute to the reduction of bone loss [245].

Post-menopausal osteoporosis is also the result of increased osteoclast activity, in part induced by increased levels of two cytokines, interleukin-1 (IL-1) and tumor necrosis factor (TNF), both involved in the differentiation of bone marrow precursors into active mature osteoclasts [249], whereas another soluble protein, osteoprotegerin, inhibits osteoclast formation, function, and survival by an action on the RANK-RANKL system [250]. Blocking IL-1 or TNF activity, by administrating an IL-1 receptor agonist or a soluble type I TNF receptor, induced a reduction of bone loss in ovariectomized rodents (an animal model of post-menopausal osteoporosis) [251, 252]. However, both recombinant proteins exhibited a so short half-life that this protein-based therapy would require the use of invasive pumping devices to maintain an adequate drug level allowing a therapeutic effect. Therefore, some researchers explored successfully the adenoviral-based therapy to deliver locally the adequate recombinant protein levels via natural cellular mechanisms. Injections of adenovirus, encoding the IL-1 receptor agonist or osteoprotegerin, resulted in a systemic delivery of the recombinant proteins and thus in protective effect against osteoporosis [250, 253]. Although the recombinant protein expression was only transient, the adenoviral-based therapy may provide new opportunities in the osteoporosis treatment.

At last, studies, associating MSC infusion and bone morphogenetic protein expression, were conducted for the treatment of bone loss associated with osteoporosis. As an example, Zhang et al. reported the positive impact of the intra-femoral infusion of MSCs transfected to over-express the bone morphogenetic protein BMP-4 on the mouse bone mineral constitution. In fact, the bone mineral density was increased by 20.5% at 14 days post-infusion, whereas the total bone density was increased by 10.4% at 56 days post-implantation in comparison with untreated controls [206]. Although engrafted MSCs subsequently declined to undetectable levels into trabecular bone as from 56 days, these reported results evidenced the positive impact of MSC-based therapy to prevent osteoporosis bone loss, and therefore suggested that multiple cycles of MSC infusions may be necessary to allow therapeutic benefits.

C. Osteogenesis Imperfecta

Osteogenesis imperfecta, commonly known as brittle bone disease, is a genetic bone disorder owed to an osteoblast abnormal collagen production caused by mutations in the alpha chains of collagen type I and therefore characterized by osteopenia and bone fragility.

However, type I collagen represents 95% of the bone collagen content and approximately 80% of the total protein composing bones [254]. The type I collagen macromolecule is composed of polymerized collagen polypeptide proa1 and proa2 chains that are encoded by the Col1a1 and Col1a2 genes, respectively [255]. The dominant-negative point mutation characterizing osteogenesis imperfecta induces a collagen triple helix disruption, a polymerization disturbance and therefore causes severe skeletal abnormalities.

Current treatments, used to alleviate the symptoms of the disease, include the employment of orthopedic devices, such as internal rods and external orthotics, and pharmacologic agents, such as bisphosphonates, which prevent osteoclasts resorption [255]. A gene therapy approach to treat the disease was developed, using autologous bone marrow-derived MSCs in human patients suffering from severe osteogenesis imperfecta [205]. After isolation, culture-expanded MSCs were transfected with an adeno-associated virus vector to disrupt the muted collagen gene and allow the wild-type collagen gene to be solely expressed. *In vitro*, around half of the human transfected MSCs had an appropriate gene insertion, a specific mutant allele disruption and thus an effective restoration of the wild type I collagen expression. These successfully transfected MSCs produced collagen fibrils similar to wild type in size, diameter and melting temperatures. When cultured *in vitro* in a hydroxyapatite/tricalcium phosphate matrix and afterwards implanted *in vivo* into immuno-deficient mice, the human donor transfected MSCs were able to differentiate into bone cells, to produce wild type I collagen and to exhibit a mineralized bone matrix [205]. Therefore, even if to date the selection and expansion of individual MSC clones may not be feasible in human clinical situation, this MSC-based gene therapy-coupled approach clearly offers attractive perspectives in the treatment of bone disorders, such as osteogenesis imperfecta.

Conclusion

Since MSCs exhibit an osteogenic differentiation potential when injected *in vivo* or when cultured onto scaffolds, are able to be transfected thus modulating their protein expression pattern and furthermore display an immunogenic tolerance, MSC-based therapy may represent a powerful strategy to restore or attenuate bone-disorders. However, several concerns remain. Firstly, after intravenous injection, MSCs are immediately trapped in the lungs [24, 256], whereas the intra-bone marrow route seems to be more effective [257]. Secondly, the steady state MSC turnover in mesenchymal organs is small (years are for example needed to achieve the complete bone renewal), but this turnover may be dramatically increased in the normal period of growth or after injury [166, 258]. Therefore, the recipient condition is a critical parameter in the MSC homing capacity to allow a significant MSC homing increase [137, 149, 259]. Thirdly, injected MSCs can be detected in a given tissue after long periods; however, this detection does not necessarily mean engraftment, but at least indicate cell survival in tissue [260, 261]. At last, several controversial studies reported that positive effects after MSC infusions might be the results of MSC cell fusion with *in situ* cells [85, 140, 262-265].

In the specific case of bone reconstruction, additional work should be performed to select required factors, to facilitate the MSC perfusion throughout scaffolds and to facilitate the implant connection to the host vascular network. Others studies should also focus on an ideal scaffold, which should be biocompatible. This scaffold should have structural integrity, and act as a stem cell support for the new bone to be generated. A last, this scaffold should exhibit a proper balance between mechanical properties, porous architecture, and degradability while remaining osteoconductive.

REFERENCES

[1] Friedenstein, A.J., U.F. Deriglasova, N.N. Kulagina, A.F. Panasuk, S.F. Rudakowa, E.A. Luria, and I.A. Ruadkow, Precursors for fibroblasts in different populations of hematopoietic cells as detected by the in vitro colony assay method. *Exp. Hematol.*, 1974. 2(2): p. 83-92.

[2] Friedenstein, A.J., A.A. Ivanov-Smolenski, R.K. Chajlakjan, U.F. Gorskaya, A.I. Kuralesova, N.W. Latzinik, and U.W. Gerasimow, Origin of bone marrow stromal mechanocytes in radiochimeras and heterotopic transplants. *Exp. Hematol.*, 1978. 6(5): p. 440-4.

[3] Friedenstein, A.J., S. Piatetzky, II, and K.V. Petrakova, Osteogenesis in transplants of bone marrow cells. *J. Embryol. Exp. Morphol.*, 1966. 16(3): p. 381-90.

[4] Pittenger, M.F., A.M. Mackay, S.C. Beck, R.K. Jaiswal, R. Douglas, J.D. Mosca, M.A. Moorman, D.W. Simonetti, S. Craig, and D.R. Marshak, Multilineage potential of adult human mesenchymal stem cells. *Science*, 1999. 284(5411): p. 143-7.

[5] Latsinik, N.V., F. Gorskaia Iu, A.G. Grosheva, S.P. Domogatskii, and S.A. Kuznetsov, [The stromal colony-forming cell (CFUf) count in the bone marrow of mice and the clonal nature of the fibroblast colonies they form]. *Ontogenez*, 1986. 17(1): p. 27-36.

[6] Fridenshtein, A., [Stromal bone marrow cells and the hematopoietic microenvironment]. *Arkh. Patol.*, 1982. 44(10): p. 3-11.

[7] Haynesworth, S.E., M.A. Baber, and A.I. Caplan, Cell surface antigens on human marrow-derived mesenchymal cells are detected by monoclonal antibodies. *Bone*, 1992. 13(1): p. 69-80.

[8] Gronthos, S. and P.J. Simmons, The biology and application of human bone marrow stromal cell precursors. *J. Hemather.*, 1996. 5(1): p. 15-23.

[9] Prockop, D.J., Marrow stromal cells as stem cells for nonhematopoietic tissues. *Science*, 1997. 276(5309): p. 71-4.

[10] Muraglia, A., R. Cancedda, and R. Quarto, Clonal mesenchymal progenitors from human bone marrow differentiate in vitro according to a hierarchical model. *J. Cell Sci*, 2000. 113 (Pt 7): p. 1161-6.

[11] Quarto, R., M. Mastrogiacomo, R. Cancedda, S.M. Kutepov, V. Mukhachev, A. Lavroukov, E. Kon, and M. Marcacci, Repair of large bone defects with the use of autologous bone marrow stromal cells. *N. Engl. J. Med.*, 2001. 344(5): p. 385-6.

[12] Wakitani, S., K. Imoto, T. Yamamoto, M. Saito, N. Murata, and M. Yoneda, Human autologous culture expanded bone marrow mesenchymal cell transplantation for repair of cartilage defects in osteoarthritic knees. *Osteoarthritis Cartilage,* 2002. 10(3): p. 199-206.

[13] Horwitz, E.M., D.J. Prockop, L.A. Fitzpatrick, W.W. Koo, P.L. Gordon, M. Neel, M. Sussman, P. Orchard, J.C. Marx, R.E. Pyeritz, and M.K. Brenner, Transplantability and therapeutic effects of bone marrow-derived mesenchymal cells in children with osteogenesis imperfecta. *Nat. Med.*, 1999. 5(3): p. 309-13.

[14] Zvaifler, N.J., L. Marinova-Mutafchieva, G. Adams, C.J. Edwards, J. Moss, J.A. Burger, and R.N. Maini, Mesenchymal precursor cells in the blood of normal individuals. *Arthritis Res.*, 2000. 2(6): p. 477-88.

[15] Kuznetsov, S.A., M.H. Mankani, S. Gronthos, K. Satomura, P. Bianco, and P.G. Robey, Circulating skeletal stem cells. *J. Cell Biol.*, 2001. 153(5): p. 1133-40.

[16] Covas, D.T., J.L. Siufi, A.R. Silva, and M.D. Orellana, Isolation and culture of umbilical vein mesenchymal stem cells. *Braz. J. Med. Biol. Res.*, 2003. 36(9): p. 1179-83.

[17] In 't Anker, P.S., S.A. Scherjon, C. Kleijburg-van der Keur, G.M. de Groot-Swings, F.H. Claas, W.E. Fibbe, and H.H. Kanhai, Isolation of mesenchymal stem cells of fetal or maternal origin from human placenta. *Stem Cells*, 2004. 22(7): p. 1338-45.

[18] Zhang, Y., C.D. Li, X.X. Jiang, H.L. Li, P.H. Tang, and N. Mao, Comparison of mesenchymal stem cells from human placenta and bone marrow. *Chin. Med. J.* (Engl), 2004. 117(6): p. 882-7.

[19] Miao, Z., J. Jin, L. Chen, J. Zhu, W. Huang, J. Zhao, H. Qian, and X. Zhang, Isolation of mesenchymal stem cells from human placenta: Comparison with human bone marrow mesenchymal stem cells. *Cell Biol. Int.*, 2006. 30(9): p. 681-7.

[20] Phinney, D.G., G. Kopen, R.L. Isaacson, and D.J. Prockop, Plastic adherent stromal cells from the bone marrow of commonly used strains of inbred mice: variations in yield, growth, and differentiation. *J. Cell Biochem.*, 1999. 72(4): p. 570-85.

[21] Baddoo, M., K. Hill, R. Wilkinson, D. Gaupp, C. Hughes, G.C. Kopen, and D.G. Phinney, Characterization of mesenchymal stem cells isolated from murine bone marrow by negative selection. *J. Cell Biochem.*, 2003. 89(6): p. 1235-49.

[22] Tropel, P., D. Noel, N. Platet, P. Legrand, A.L. Benabid, and F. Berger, Isolation and characterisation of mesenchymal stem cells from adult mouse bone marrow. *Exp. Cell Res*, 2004. 295(2): p. 395-406.

[23] Rochefort, G.Y., B. Delorme, A. Lopez, O. Herault, P. Bonnet, P. Charbord, V. Eder, and J. Domenech, Multipotential mesenchymal stem cells are mobilized into peripheral blood by hypoxia. *Stem Cells*, 2006. 24(10): p. 2202-8.

[24] Rochefort, G.Y., P. Vaudin, N. Bonnet, J.C. Pages, J. Domenech, P. Charbord, and V. Eder, Influence of hypoxia on the domiciliation of mesenchymal stem cells after infusion into rats: possibilities of targeting pulmonary artery remodeling via cells therapies? *Respir Res.*, 2005. 6: p. 125.

[25] Santa Maria, L., C.V. Rojas, and J.J. Minguell, Signals from damaged but not undamaged skeletal muscle induce myogenic differentiation of rat bone-marrow-derived mesenchymal stem cells. *Exp. Cell Res.*, 2004. 300(2): p. 418-26.

[26] Martin, D.R., N.R. Cox, T.L. Hathcock, G.P. Niemeyer, and H.J. Baker, Isolation and characterization of multipotential mesenchymal stem cells from feline bone marrow. *Exp. Hematol.*, 2002. 30(8): p. 879-86.

[27] Devine, S.M., A.M. Bartholomew, N. Mahmud, M. Nelson, S. Patil, W. Hardy, C. Sturgeon, T. Hewett, T. Chung, W. Stock, D. Sher, S. Weissman, K. Ferrer, J. Mosca, R. Deans, A. Moseley, and R. Hoffman, Mesenchymal stem cells are capable of homing to the bone marrow of non-human primates following systemic infusion. *Exp. Hematol.*, 2001. 29(2): p. 244-55.

[28] Airey, J.A., G. Almeida-Porada, E.J. Colletti, C.D. Porada, J. Chamberlain, M. Movsesian, J.L. Sutko, and E.D. Zanjani, Human mesenchymal stem cells form Purkinje fibers in fetal sheep heart. *Circulation,* 2004. 109(11): p. 1401-7.

[29] Silva, G.V., S. Litovsky, J.A. Assad, A.L. Sousa, B.J. Martin, D. Vela, S.C. Coulter, J. Lin, J. Ober, W.K. Vaughn, R.V. Branco, E.M. Oliveira, R. He, Y.J. Geng, J.T. Willerson, and E.C. Perin, Mesenchymal stem cells differentiate into an endothelial phenotype, enhance vascular density, and improve heart function in a canine chronic ischemia model. *Circulation*, 2005. 111(2): p. 150-6.

[30] Moscoso, I., A. Centeno, E. Lopez, J.I. Rodriguez-Barbosa, I. Santamarina, P. Filgueira, M.J. Sanchez, R. Dominguez-Perles, G. Penuelas-Rivas, and N. Domenech, Differentiation "in vitro" of primary and immortalized porcine mesenchymal stem cells into cardiomyocytes for cell transplantation. *Transplant. Proc.*, 2005. 37(1): p. 481-2.

[31] Bosch, P., S.L. Pratt, and S.L. Stice, Isolation, characterization, gene modification, and nuclear reprogramming of porcine mesenchymal stem cells. *Biol. Reprod.*, 2006. 74(1): p. 46-57.

[32] Bosnakovski, D., M. Mizuno, G. Kim, S. Takagi, M. Okumura, and T. Fujinaga, Isolation and multilineage differentiation of bovine bone marrow mesenchymal stem cells. *Cell Tissue Res.*, 2005. 319(2): p. 243-53.

[33] Worster, A.A., A.J. Nixon, B.D. Brower-Toland, and J. Williams, Effect of transforming growth factor beta1 on chondrogenic differentiation of cultured equine mesenchymal stem cells. *Am. J. Vet. Res.*, 2000. 61(9): p. 1003-10.

[34] Ringe, J., T. Haupl, and M. Sittinger, [Mesenchymal stem cells for tissue engineering of bone and cartilage]. *Med. Klin.* (Munich), 2003. 98 Suppl 2: p. 35-40.

[35] Dazzi, F., R. Ramasamy, S. Glennie, S.P. Jones, and I. Roberts, The role of mesenchymal stem cells in haemopoiesis. *Blood Rev.*, 2006. 20(3): p. 161-71.

[36] Howell, J.C., W.H. Lee, P. Morrison, J. Zhong, M.C. Yoder, and E.F. Srour, Pluripotent stem cells identified in multiple murine tissues. *Ann. NY Acad. Sci.*, 2003. 996: p. 158-73.

[37] da Silva Meirelles, L., P.C. Chagastelles, and N.B. Nardi, Mesenchymal stem cells reside in virtually all post-natal organs and tissues. *J. Cell Sci*, 2006. 119(Pt 11): p. 2204-13.

[38] Herrera, M.B., S. Bruno, S. Buttiglieri, C. Tetta, S. Gatti, M.C. Deregibus, B. Bussolati, and G. Camussi, Isolation and Characterization of a Stem Cell Population from Adult Human Liver. *Stem Cells*, 2006.

[39] Seeberger, K.L., J.M. Dufour, A.M. Shapiro, J.R. Lakey, R.V. Rajotte, and G.S. Korbutt, Expansion of mesenchymal stem cells from human pancreatic ductal epithelium. *Lab. Invest.,* 2006. 86(2): p. 141-53.

[40] Yoshimura, H., T. Muneta, A. Nimura, A. Yokoyama, H. Koga, and I. Sekiya, Comparison of rat mesenchymal stem cells derived from bone marrow, synovium, periosteum, adipose tissue, and muscle. *Cell Tissue Res.*, 2006.

[41] Barry, F.P. and J.M. Murphy, Mesenchymal stem cells: clinical applications and biological characterization. *Int. J. Biochem. Cell Biol.*, 2004. 36(4): p. 568-84.

[42] Pierdomenico, L., L. Bonsi, M. Calvitti, D. Rondelli, M. Arpinati, G. Chirumbolo, E. Becchetti, C. Marchionni, F. Alviano, V. Fossati, N. Staffolani, M. Franchina, A. Grossi, and G.P. Bagnara, Multipotent mesenchymal stem cells with immunosuppressive activity can be easily isolated from dental pulp. *Transplantation*, 2005. 80(6): p. 836-42.

[43] Shih, D.T., D.C. Lee, S.C. Chen, R.Y. Tsai, C.T. Huang, C.C. Tsai, E.Y. Shen, and W.T. Chiu, Isolation and characterization of neurogenic mesenchymal stem cells in human scalp tissue. *Stem Cells*, 2005. 23(7): p. 1012-20.

[44] Hoogduijn, M.J., E. Gorjup, and P.G. Genever, Comparative characterization of hair follicle dermal stem cells and bone marrow mesenchymal stem cells. *Stem Cells Dev*, 2006. 15(1): p. 49-60.

[45] Moon, M.H., S.Y. Kim, Y.J. Kim, S.J. Kim, J.B. Lee, Y.C. Bae, S.M. Sung, and J.S. Jung, Human adipose tissue-derived mesenchymal stem cells improve postnatal neovascularization in a mouse model of hindlimb ischemia. *Cell Physiol. Biochem.*, 2006. 17(5-6): p. 279-90.

[46] Dan, Y.Y., K.J. Riehle, C. Lazaro, N. Teoh, J. Haque, J.S. Campbell, and N. Fausto, Isolation of multipotent progenitor cells from human fetal liver capable of differentiating into liver and mesenchymal lineages. *Proc. Natl. Acad. Sci. USA*, 2006. 103(26): p. 9912-7.

[47] In 't Anker, P.S., W.A. Noort, S.A. Scherjon, C. Kleijburg-van der Keur, A.B. Kruisselbrink, R.L. van Bezooijen, W. Beekhuizen, R. Willemze, H.H. Kanhai, and W.E. Fibbe, Mesenchymal stem cells in human second-trimester bone marrow, liver, lung, and spleen exhibit a similar immunophenotype but a heterogeneous multilineage differentiation potential. *Haematologica*, 2003. 88(8): p. 845-52.

[48] Campagnoli, C., I.A. Roberts, S. Kumar, P.R. Bennett, I. Bellantuono, and N.M. Fisk, Identification of mesenchymal stem/progenitor cells in human first-trimester fetal blood, liver, and bone marrow. *Blood*, 2001. 98(8): p. 2396-402.

[49] Rzhaninova, A.A., S.N. Gornostaeva, and D.V. Goldshtein, Isolation and phenotypical characterization of mesenchymal stem cells from human fetal thymus. *Bull Exp. Biol. Med.*, 2005. 139(1): p. 134-40.

[50] Hu, Y., L. Liao, Q. Wang, L. Ma, G. Ma, X. Jiang, and R.C. Zhao, Isolation and identification of mesenchymal stem cells from human fetal pancreas. *J. Lab Clin. Med.*, 2003. 141(5): p. 342-9.

[51] Igura, K., X. Zhang, K. Takahashi, A. Mitsuru, S. Yamaguchi, and T.A. Takashi, Isolation and characterization of mesenchymal progenitor cells from chorionic villi of human placenta. *Cytotherapy*, 2004. 6(6): p. 543-53.

[52] Tsai, M.S., J.L. Lee, Y.J. Chang, and S.M. Hwang, Isolation of human multipotent mesenchymal stem cells from second-trimester amniotic fluid using a novel two-stage culture protocol. *Hum. Reprod.*, 2004. 19(6): p. 1450-6.

[53] Erices, A., P. Conget, and J.J. Minguell, Mesenchymal progenitor cells in human umbilical cord blood. *Br. J. Haematol.,* 2000. 109(1): p. 235-42.

[54] Kim, J.W., S.Y. Kim, S.Y. Park, Y.M. Kim, J.M. Kim, M.H. Lee, and H.M. Ryu, Mesenchymal progenitor cells in the human umbilical cord. *Ann. Hematol.,* 2004. 83(12): p. 733-8.

[55] Villaron, E.M., J. Almeida, N. Lopez-Holgado, M. Alcoceba, L.I. Sanchez-Abarca, F.M. Sanchez-Guijo, M. Alberca, J.A. Perez-Simon, J.F. San Miguel, and M.C. Del Canizo, Mesenchymal stem cells are present in peripheral blood and can engraft after allogeneic hematopoietic stem cell transplantation. *Haematologica,* 2004. 89(12): p. 1421-7.

[56] O'Donoghue, K., M. Choolani, J. Chan, J. de la Fuente, S. Kumar, C. Campagnoli, P.R. Bennett, I.A. Roberts, and N.M. Fisk, Identification of fetal mesenchymal stem cells in maternal blood: implications for non-invasive prenatal diagnosis. *Mol. Hum. Reprod.,* 2003. 9(8): p. 497-502.

[57] O'Donoghue, K., J. Chan, J. de la Fuente, N. Kennea, A. Sandison, J.R. Anderson, I.A. Roberts, and N.M. Fisk, Microchimerism in female bone marrow and bone decades after fetal mesenchymal stem-cell trafficking in pregnancy. *Lancet,* 2004. 364(9429): p. 179-82.

[58] Romanov, Y.A., V.A. Svintsitskaya, and V.N. Smirnov, Searching for alternative sources of postnatal human mesenchymal stem cells: candidate MSC-like cells from umbilical cord. *Stem Cells,* 2003. 21(1): p. 105-10.

[59] Lee, O.K., T.K. Kuo, W.M. Chen, K.D. Lee, S.L. Hsieh, and T.H. Chen, Isolation of multipotent mesenchymal stem cells from umbilical cord blood. *Blood,* 2004. 103(5): p. 1669-75.

[60] Lee, M.W., J. Choi, M.S. Yang, Y.J. Moon, J.S. Park, H.C. Kim, and Y.J. Kim, Mesenchymal stem cells from cryopreserved human umbilical cord blood. *Biochem. Biophys. Res. Commun.,* 2004. 320(1): p. 273-8.

[61] Kassis, I., L. Zangi, R. Rivkin, L. Levdansky, S. Samuel, G. Marx, and R. Gorodetsky, Isolation of mesenchymal stem cells from G-CSF-mobilized human peripheral blood using fibrin microbeads. *Bone Marrow Transplant,* 2006. 37(10): p. 967-76.

[62] Kucia, M., J. Ratajczak, R. Reca, A. Janowska-Wieczorek, and M.Z. Ratajczak, Tissue-specific muscle, neural and liver stem/progenitor cells reside in the bone marrow, respond to an SDF-1 gradient and are mobilized into peripheral blood during stress and tissue injury. *Blood Cells Mol. Dis.,* 2004. 32(1): p. 52-7.

[63] Fernandez, M., V. Simon, G. Herrera, C. Cao, H. Del Favero, and J.J. Minguell, Detection of stromal cells in peripheral blood progenitor cell collections from breast cancer patients. *Bone Marrow Transplant,* 1997. 20(4): p. 265-71.

[64] Zyuz'kov, G.N., N.I. Suslov, A.M. Dygai, V.V. Zhdanov, and E.D. Gol'dberg, Role of stem cells in adaptation to hypoxia and mechanisms of neuroprotective effect of granulocytic colony-stimulating factor. *Bull Exp. Biol. Med.,* 2005. 140(5): p. 606-11.

[65] Kawada, H., J. Fujita, K. Kinjo, Y. Matsuzaki, M. Tsuma, H. Miyatake, Y. Muguruma, K. Tsuboi, Y. Itabashi, Y. Ikeda, S. Ogawa, H. Okano, T. Hotta, K. Ando, and K. Fukuda, Nonhematopoietic mesenchymal stem cells can be mobilized and differentiate into cardiomyocytes after myocardial infarction. *Blood,* 2004. 104(12): p. 3581-7.

[66] Kopp, H.G., S.T. Avecilla, A.T. Hooper, and S. Rafii, The bone marrow vascular niche: home of HSC differentiation and mobilization. *Physiology* (Bethesda), 2005. 20: p. 349-56.

[67] Gupta, P., T.R. Oegema, Jr., J.J. Brazil, A.Z. Dudek, A. Slungaard, and C.M. Verfaillie, Structurally specific heparan sulfates support primitive human hematopoiesis by formation of a multimolecular stem cell niche. *Blood,* 1998. 92(12): p. 4641-51.

[68] Calvi, L.M., G.B. Adams, K.W. Weibrecht, J.M. Weber, D.P. Olson, M.C. Knight, R.P. Martin, E. Schipani, P. Divieti, F.R. Bringhurst, L.A. Milner, H.M. Kronenberg, and D.T. Scadden, Osteoblastic cells regulate the haematopoietic stem cell niche. *Nature,* 2003. 425(6960): p. 841-6.

[69] Shi, S. and S. Gronthos, Perivascular niche of postnatal mesenchymal stem cells in human bone marrow and dental pulp. *J. Bone Miner Res.,* 2003. 18(4): p. 696-704.

[70] Moore, K.A., Recent advances in defining the hematopoietic stem cell niche. *Curr. Opin. Hematol,* 2004. 11(2): p. 107-11.

[71] Arai, F., A. Hirao, and T. Suda, Regulation of hematopoietic stem cells by the niche. *Trends Cardiovasc. Med.,* 2005. 15(2): p. 75-9.

[72] Charbord, P., [The hematopoietic stem cell and the stromal microenvironment]. *Therapie,* 2001. 56(4): p. 383-4.

[73] Chagraoui, J., A. Lepage-Noll, A. Anjo, G. Uzan, and P. Charbord, Fetal liver stroma consists of cells in epithelial-to-mesenchymal transition. *Blood,* 2003. 101(8): p. 2973-82.

[74] Dexter, T.M., T.D. Allen, and L.G. Lajtha, Conditions controlling the proliferation of haemopoietic stem cells in vitro. *J. Cell Physiol.,* 1977. 91(3): p. 335-44.

[75] Barry, F., R. Boynton, M. Murphy, S. Haynesworth, and J. Zaia, The SH-3 and SH-4 antibodies recognize distinct epitopes on CD73 from human mesenchymal stem cells. *Biochem. Biophys. Res. Commun.,* 2001. 289(2): p. 519-24.

[76] Jiang, Y., B.N. Jahagirdar, R.L. Reinhardt, R.E. Schwartz, C.D. Keene, X.R. Ortiz-Gonzalez, M. Reyes, T. Lenvik, T. Lund, M. Blackstad, J. Du, S. Aldrich, A. Lisberg, W.C. Low, D.A. Largaespada, and C.M. Verfaillie, Pluripotency of mesenchymal stem cells derived from adult marrow. *Nature,* 2002. 418(6893): p. 41-9.

[77] Reyes, M., A. Dudek, B. Jahagirdar, L. Koodie, P.H. Marker, and C.M. Verfaillie, Origin of endothelial progenitors in human postnatal bone marrow. *J. Clin. Invest.,* 2002. 109(3): p. 337-46.

[78] Brazelton, T.R., F.M. Rossi, G.I. Keshet, and H.M. Blau, From marrow to brain: expression of neuronal phenotypes in adult mice. *Science,* 2000. 290(5497): p. 1775-9.

[79] Sanchez-Ramos, J., S. Song, F. Cardozo-Pelaez, C. Hazzi, T. Stedeford, A. Willing, T.B. Freeman, S. Saporta, W. Janssen, N. Patel, D.R. Cooper, and P.R. Sanberg, Adult bone marrow stromal cells differentiate into neural cells in vitro. *Exp. Neurol.,* 2000. 164(2): p. 247-56.

[80] Zhao, L.X., J. Zhang, F. Cao, L. Meng, D.M. Wang, Y.H. Li, X. Nan, W.C. Jiao, M. Zheng, X.H. Xu, and X.T. Pei, Modification of the brain-derived neurotrophic factor gene: a portal to transform mesenchymal stem cells into advantageous engineering cells for neuroregeneration and neuroprotection. *Exp. Neurol.,* 2004. 190(2): p. 396-406.

[81] Schwartz, R.E., M. Reyes, L. Koodie, Y. Jiang, M. Blackstad, T. Lund, T. Lenvik, S. Johnson, W.S. Hu, and C.M. Verfaillie, Multipotent adult progenitor cells from bone marrow differentiate into functional hepatocyte-like cells. *J. Clin. Invest.*, 2002. 109(10): p. 1291-302.

[82] Verfaillie, C.M., Adult stem cells: assessing the case for pluripotency. *Trends Cell Biol.*, 2002. 12(11): p. 502-8.

[83] Sata, M., D. Fukuda, K. Tanaka, Y. Kaneda, H. Yashiro, and I. Shirakawa, The role of circulating precursors in vascular repair and lesion formation. *J. Cell Mol. Med.*, 2005. 9(3): p. 557-68.

[84] Liechty, K.W., T.C. MacKenzie, A.F. Shaaban, A. Radu, A.M. Moseley, R. Deans, D.R. Marshak, and A.W. Flake, Human mesenchymal stem cells engraft and demonstrate site-specific differentiation after in utero transplantation in sheep. *Nat. Med.*, 2000. 6(11): p. 1282-6.

[85] Sato, Y., H. Araki, J. Kato, K. Nakamura, Y. Kawano, M. Kobune, T. Sato, K. Miyanishi, T. Takayama, M. Takahashi, R. Takimoto, S. Iyama, T. Matsunaga, S. Ohtani, A. Matsuura, H. Hamada, and Y. Niitsu, Human mesenchymal stem cells xenografted directly to rat liver are differentiated into human hepatocytes without fusion. *Blood*, 2005. 106(2): p. 756-63.

[86] Togel, F., Z. Hu, K. Weiss, J. Isaac, C. Lange, and C. Westenfelder, Administered mesenchymal stem cells protect against ischemic acute renal failure through differentiation-independent mechanisms. *Am. J. Physiol. Renal. Physiol.*, 2005. 289(1): p. F31-42.

[87] Sottile, V., C. Halleux, F. Bassilana, H. Keller, and K. Seuwen, Stem cell characteristics of human trabecular bone-derived cells. *Bone,* 2002. 30(5): p. 699-704.

[88] Scavo, L.M., M. Karas, M. Murray, and D. Leroith, Insulin-like growth factor-I stimulates both cell growth and lipogenesis during differentiation of human mesenchymal stem cells into adipocytes. *J. Clin. Endocrinol. Metab.*, 2004. 89(7): p. 3543-53.

[89] Kim, S.J., H.H. Cho, Y.J. Kim, S.Y. Seo, H.N. Kim, J.B. Lee, J.H. Kim, J.S. Chung, and J.S. Jung, Human adipose stromal cells expanded in human serum promote engraftment of human peripheral blood hematopoietic stem cells in NOD/SCID mice. *Biochem. Biophys. Res. Commun.*, 2005. 329(1): p. 25-31.

[90] Lin, T.M., J.L. Tsai, S.D. Lin, C.S. Lai, and C.C. Chang, Accelerated growth and prolonged lifespan of adipose tissue-derived human mesenchymal stem cells in a medium using reduced calcium and antioxidants. *Stem Cells Dev.*, 2005. 14(1): p. 92-102.

[91] Neubauer, M., C. Fischbach, P. Bauer-Kreisel, E. Lieb, M. Hacker, J. Tessmar, M.B. Schulz, A. Goepferich, and T. Blunk, Basic fibroblast growth factor enhances PPARgamma ligand-induced adipogenesis of mesenchymal stem cells. *FEBS Lett*, 2004. 577(1-2): p. 277-83.

[92] Ogawa, R., H. Mizuno, A. Watanabe, M. Migita, H. Hyakusoku, and T. Shimada, Adipogenic differentiation by adipose-derived stem cells harvested from GFP transgenic mice-including relationship of sex differences. *Biochem. Biophys. Res. Commun.*, 2004. 319(2): p. 511-7.

[93] Pakala, R., P. Kuchulakanti, S.W. Rha, E. Cheneau, R. Baffour, and R. Waksman, Peroxisome proliferator-activated receptor gamma: its role in metabolic syndrome. *Cardiovasc. Radiat Med.*, 2004. 5(2): p. 97-103.

[94] She, H., S. Xiong, S. Hazra, and H. Tsukamoto, Adipogenic transcriptional regulation of hepatic stellate cells. *J. Biol. Chem.*, 2005. 280(6): p. 4959-67.

[95] Tominaga, S., T. Yamaguchi, S. Takahashi, F. Hirose, and T. Osumi, Negative regulation of adipogenesis from human mesenchymal stem cells by Jun N-terminal kinase. *Biochem. Biophys. Res. Commun.*, 2005. 326(2): p. 499-504.

[96] Taguchi, Y., M. Yamamoto, T. Yamate, S.C. Lin, H. Mocharla, P. DeTogni, N. Nakayama, B.F. Boyce, E. Abe, and S.C. Manolagas, Interleukin-6-type cytokines stimulate mesenchymal progenitor differentiation toward the osteoblastic lineage. *Proc. Assoc. Am. Physicians,* 1998. 110(6): p. 559-74.

[97] Thomas, T., F. Gori, S. Khosla, M.D. Jensen, B. Burguera, and B.L. Riggs, Leptin acts on human marrow stromal cells to enhance differentiation to osteoblasts and to inhibit differentiation to adipocytes. *Endocrinology,* 1999. 140(4): p. 1630-8.

[98] Kroger, H., E. Soppi, and N. Loveridge, Growth hormone, osteoblasts, and marrow adipocytes: a case report. *Calcif. Tissue Int.*, 1997. 61(1): p. 33-5.

[99] Maeda, S., T. Nobukuni, K. Shimo-Onoda, K. Hayashi, K. Yone, S. Komiya, and I. Inoue, Sortilin is upregulated during osteoblastic differentiation of mesenchymal stem cells and promotes extracellular matrix mineralization. *J. Cell Physiol.*, 2002. 193(1): p. 73-9.

[100] Ramoshebi, L.N., T.N. Matsaba, J. Teare, L. Renton, J. Patton, and U. Ripamonti, Tissue engineering: TGF-beta superfamily members and delivery systems in bone regeneration. *Expert Rev. Mol. Med.*, 2002. 2002: p. 1-11.

[101] Canalis, E., A.N. Economides, and E. Gazzerro, Bone morphogenetic proteins, their antagonists, and the skeleton. *Endocr. Rev.*, 2003. 24(2): p. 218-35.

[102] Rawadi, G., B. Vayssiere, F. Dunn, R. Baron, and S. Roman-Roman, BMP-2 controls alkaline phosphatase expression and osteoblast mineralization by a Wnt autocrine loop. *J. Bone Miner Res.,* 2003. 18(10): p. 1842-53.

[103] Sykaras, N. and L.A. Opperman, Bone morphogenetic proteins (BMPs): how do they function and what can they offer the clinician? *J. Oral Sci.*, 2003. 45(2): p. 57-73.

[104] Nurminskaya, M., C. Magee, L. Faverman, and T.F. Linsenmayer, Chondrocyte-derived transglutaminase promotes maturation of preosteoblasts in periosteal bone. *Dev. Biol.*, 2003. 263(1): p. 139-52.

[105] Rogers, J.J., H.E. Young, L.R. Adkison, P.A. Lucas, and A.C. Black, Jr., Differentiation factors induce expression of muscle, fat, cartilage, and bone in a clone of mouse pluripotent mesenchymal stem cells. *Am. Surg.,* 1995. 61(3): p. 231-6.

[106] Buttery, L.D., S. Bourne, J.D. Xynos, H. Wood, F.J. Hughes, S.P. Hughes, V. Episkopou, and J.M. Polak, Differentiation of osteoblasts and in vitro bone formation from murine embryonic stem cells. *Tissue Eng,* 2001. 7(1): p. 89-99.

[107] Sottile, V., A. Thomson, and J. McWhir, In vitro osteogenic differentiation of human ES cells. *Cloning Stem Cells,* 2003. 5(2): p. 149-55.

[108] zur Nieden, N.I., G. Kempka, and H.J. Ahr, In vitro differentiation of embryonic stem cells into mineralized osteoblasts. *Differentiation,* 2003. 71(1): p. 18-27.

[109] Notoya, K., H. Nagai, T. Oda, M. Gotoh, T. Hoshino, H. Muranishi, S. Taketomi, T. Sohda, and H. Makino, Enhancement of osteogenesis in vitro and in vivo by a novel osteoblast differentiation promoting compound, TAK-778. *J. Pharmacol. Exp. Ther.*, 1999. 290(3): p. 1054-64.

[110] Rosa, A.L. and M.M. Beloti, TAK-778 enhances osteoblast differentiation of human bone marrow cells. *J. Cell Biochem.*, 2003. 89(6): p. 1148-53.

[111] van Leeuwen, J.P., M. van Driel, G.J. van den Bemd, and H.A. Pols, Vitamin D control of osteoblast function and bone extracellular matrix mineralization. *Crit. Rev. Eukaryot Gene Expr,* 2001. 11(1-3): p. 199-226.

[112] Raisz, L.G., C.C. Pilbeam, and P.M. Fall, Prostaglandins: mechanisms of action and regulation of production in bone. *Osteoporos. Int*, 1993. 3 Suppl 1: p. 136-40.

[113] Weinreb, M., A. Grosskopf, and N. Shir, The anabolic effect of PGE2 in rat bone marrow cultures is mediated via the EP4 receptor subtype. *Am. J. Physiol.*, 1999. 276(2 Pt 1): p. E376-83.

[114] Sugiyama, M., T. Kodama, K. Konishi, K. Abe, S. Asami, and S. Oikawa, Compactin and simvastatin, but not pravastatin, induce bone morphogenetic protein-2 in human osteosarcoma cells. *Biochem. Biophys. Res. Commun.*, 2000. 271(3): p. 688-92.

[115] Ohnaka, K., S. Shimoda, H. Nawata, H. Shimokawa, K. Kaibuchi, Y. Iwamoto, and R. Takayanagi, Pitavastatin enhanced BMP-2 and osteocalcin expression by inhibition of Rho-associated kinase in human osteoblasts. *Biochem. Biophys. Res. Commun.*, 2001. 287(2): p. 337-42.

[116] Phillips, B.W., N. Belmonte, C. Vernochet, G. Ailhaud, and C. Dani, Compactin enhances osteogenesis in murine embryonic stem cells. *Biochem. Biophys. Res. Commun,* 2001. 284(2): p. 478-84.

[117] Bianco, P., L.W. Fisher, M.F. Young, J.D. Termine, and P.G. Robey, Expression of bone sialoprotein (BSP) in developing human tissues. *Calcif. Tissue Int.*, 1991. 49(6): p. 421-6.

[118] Helder, M.N., A.L. Bronckers, and J.H. Woltgens, Dissimilar expression patterns for the extracellular matrix proteins osteopontin (OPN) and collagen type I in dental tissues and alveolar bone of the neonatal rat. *Matrix*, 1993. 13(5): p. 415-25.

[119] Bronckers, A.L., S. Gay, R.D. Finkelman, and W.T. Butler, Developmental appearance of Gla proteins (osteocalcin) and alkaline phosphatase in tooth germs and bones of the rat. *Bone Miner,* 1987. 2(5): p. 361-73.

[120] Thomas, G., P. Moffatt, P. Salois, M.H. Gaumond, R. Gingras, E. Godin, D. Miao, D. Goltzman, and C. Lanctot, Osteocrin, a novel bone-specific secreted protein that modulates the osteoblast phenotype. *J. Biol. Chem.*, 2003. 278(50): p. 50563-71.

[121] Bruder, S.P., A.A. Kurth, M. Shea, W.C. Hayes, N. Jaiswal, and S. Kadiyala, Bone regeneration by implantation of purified, culture-expanded human mesenchymal stem cells. *J. Orthop. Res.*, 1998. 16(2): p. 155-62.

[122] Rose, F.R. and R.O. Oreffo, Bone tissue engineering: hope vs hype. *Biochem. Biophys. Res. Commun.*, 2002. 292(1): p. 1-7.

[123] Vats, A., N.S. Tolley, J.M. Polak, and J.E. Gough, Scaffolds and biomaterials for tissue engineering: a review of clinical applications. *Clin. Otolaryngol. Allied Sci.*, 2003. 28(3): p. 165-72.

[124] El-Amin, S.F., M. Attawia, H.H. Lu, A.K. Shah, R. Chang, N.J. Hickok, R.S. Tuan, and C.T. Laurencin, Integrin expression by human osteoblasts cultured on degradable polymeric materials applicable for tissue engineered bone. *J. Orthop. Res.*, 2002. 20(1): p. 20-8.

[125] Spinella-Jaegle, S., G. Rawadi, S. Kawai, S. Gallea, C. Faucheu, P. Mollat, B. Courtois, B. Bergaud, V. Ramez, A.M. Blanchet, G. Adelmant, R. Baron, and S. Roman-Roman, Sonic hedgehog increases the commitment of pluripotent mesenchymal cells into the osteoblastic lineage and abolishes adipocytic differentiation. *J. Cell Sci.*, 2001. 114(Pt 11): p. 2085-94.

[126] Bennett, C.N., K.A. Longo, W.S. Wright, L.J. Suva, T.F. Lane, K.D. Hankenson, and O.A. MacDougald, Regulation of osteoblastogenesis and bone mass by Wnt10b. *Proc. Natl. Acad. Sci. USA*, 2005. 102(9): p. 3324-9.

[127] Suh, J.M., X. Gao, J. McKay, R. McKay, Z. Salo, and J.M. Graff, Hedgehog signaling plays a conserved role in inhibiting fat formation. *Cell Meta*b., 2006. 3(1): p. 25-34.

[128] Johnstone, B., T.M. Hering, A.I. Caplan, V.M. Goldberg, and J.U. Yoo, In vitro chondrogenesis of bone marrow-derived mesenchymal progenitor cells. *Exp. Cell Res.*, 1998. 238(1): p. 265-72.

[129] Yoo, J.U., T.S. Barthel, K. Nishimura, L. Solchaga, A.I. Caplan, V.M. Goldberg, and B. Johnstone, The chondrogenic potential of human bone-marrow-derived mesenchymal progenitor cells. *J. Bone Joint Surg. Am.*, 1998. 80(12): p. 1745-57.

[130] Kavalkovich, K.W., R.E. Boynton, J.M. Murphy, and F. Barry, Chondrogenic differentiation of human mesenchymal stem cells within an alginate layer culture system. *In Vitro Cell Dev. Biol. Anim.*, 2002. 38(8): p. 457-66.

[131] Lee, J.W., Y.H. Kim, S.H. Kim, S.H. Han, and S.B. Hahn, Chondrogenic differentiation of mesenchymal stem cells and its clinical applications. *Yonsei Med. J.*, 2004. 45 Suppl: p. 41-7.

[132] Yang, I.H., S.H. Kim, Y.H. Kim, H.J. Sun, S.J. Kim, and J.W. Lee, Comparison of phenotypic characterization between "alginate bead" and "pellet" culture systems as chondrogenic differentiation models for human mesenchymal stem cells. *Yonsei Med. J.*, 2004. 45(5): p. 891-900.

[133] Muguruma, Y., M. Reyes, Y. Nakamura, T. Sato, H. Matsuzawa, H. Miyatake, A. Akatsuka, J. Itoh, T. Yahata, K. Ando, S. Kato, and T. Hotta, In vivo and in vitro differentiation of myocytes from human bone marrow-derived multipotent progenitor cells. *Exp. Hematol.*, 2003. 31(12): p. 1323-30.

[134] Dezawa, M., H. Kanno, M. Hoshino, H. Cho, N. Matsumoto, Y. Itokazu, N. Tajima, H. Yamada, H. Sawada, H. Ishikawa, T. Mimura, M. Kitada, Y. Suzuki, and C. Ide, Specific induction of neuronal cells from bone marrow stromal cells and application for autologous transplantation. *J. Clin. Invest.*, 2004. 113(12): p. 1701-10.

[135] Dezawa, M., Insights into autotransplantation: the unexpected discovery of specific induction systems in bone marrow stromal cells. *Cell Mol. Life Sci.*, 2006. 63(23): p. 2764-72.

[136] Dezawa, M., H. Ishikawa, Y. Itokazu, T. Yoshihara, M. Hoshino, S. Takeda, C. Ide, and Y. Nabeshima, Bone marrow stromal cells generate muscle cells and repair muscle degeneration. *Science*, 2005. 309(5732): p. 314-7.

[137] Wu, G.D., J.A. Nolta, Y.S. Jin, M.L. Barr, H. Yu, V.A. Starnes, and D.V. Cramer, Migration of mesenchymal stem cells to heart allografts during chronic rejection. *Transplantation,* 2003. 75(5): p. 679-85.

[138] Toma, C., M.F. Pittenger, K.S. Cahill, B.J. Byrne, and P.D. Kessler, Human mesenchymal stem cells differentiate to a cardiomyocyte phenotype in the adult murine heart. *Circulation,* 2002. 105(1): p. 93-8.

[139] Bhagavati, S. and W. Xu, Isolation and enrichment of skeletal muscle progenitor cells from mouse bone marrow. *Biochem. Biophys. Res. Commun.,* 2004. 318(1): p. 119-24.

[140] Schulze, M., F. Belema-Bedada, A. Technau, and T. Braun, Mesenchymal stem cells are recruited to striated muscle by NFAT/IL-4-mediated cell fusion. *Genes Dev.,* 2005. 19(15): p. 1787-98.

[141] Mizuno, H., P.A. Zuk, M. Zhu, H.P. Lorenz, P. Benhaim, and M.H. Hedrick, Myogenic differentiation by human processed lipoaspirate cells. *Plast Reconstr. Surg.,* 2002. 109(1): p. 199-209; discussion 210-1.

[142] Gang, E.J., S.H. Hong, J.A. Jeong, S.H. Hwang, S.W. Kim, I.H. Yang, C. Ahn, H. Han, and H. Kim, In vitro mesengenic potential of human umbilical cord blood-derived mesenchymal stem cells. *Biochem. Biophys. Res. Commun.,* 2004. 321(1): p. 102-8.

[143] Wakitani, S., T. Saito, and A.I. Caplan, Myogenic cells derived from rat bone marrow mesenchymal stem cells exposed to 5-azacytidine. *Muscle Nerve,* 1995. 18(12): p. 1417-26.

[144] Kinner, B., J.M. Zaleskas, and M. Spector, Regulation of smooth muscle actin expression and contraction in adult human mesenchymal stem cells. *Exp. Cell Res.,* 2002. 278(1): p. 72-83.

[145] Makino, S., K. Fukuda, S. Miyoshi, F. Konishi, H. Kodama, J. Pan, M. Sano, T. Takahashi, S. Hori, H. Abe, J. Hata, A. Umezawa, and S. Ogawa, Cardiomyocytes can be generated from marrow stromal cells in vitro. *J. Clin. Invest.,* 1999. 103(5): p. 697-705.

[146] Bittira, B., J.Q. Kuang, A. Al-Khaldi, D. Shum-Tim, and R.C. Chiu, In vitro preprogramming of marrow stromal cells for myocardial regeneration. *Ann. Thorac. Surg.,* 2002. 74(4): p. 1154-9; discussion 1159-60.

[147] Min, J.Y., Y. Yang, K.L. Converso, L. Liu, Q. Huang, J.P. Morgan, and Y.F. Xiao, Transplantation of embryonic stem cells improves cardiac function in postinfarcted rats. *J. Appl. Physiol.,* 2002. 92(1): p. 288-96.

[148] Cheng, F., P. Zou, H. Yang, Z. Yu, and Z. Zhong, Induced differentiation of human cord blood mesenchymal stem/progenitor cells into cardiomyocyte-like cells in vitro. *J. Huazhong Univ. Sci. Technolog. Med. Sci.,* 2003. 23(2): p. 154-7.

[149] Erices, A.A., C.I. Allers, P.A. Conget, C.V. Rojas, and J.J. Minguell, Human cord blood-derived mesenchymal stem cells home and survive in the marrow of immunodeficient mice after systemic infusion. *Cell Transplant,* 2003. 12(6): p. 555-61.

[150] Fukuda, K., Application of mesenchymal stem cells for the regeneration of cardiomyocyte and its use for cell transplantation therapy. *Hum. Cell,* 2003. 16(3): p. 83-94.

[151] Rangappa, S., J.W. Entwistle, A.S. Wechsler, and J.Y. Kresh, Cardiomyocyte-mediated contact programs human mesenchymal stem cells to express cardiogenic phenotype. *J. Thorac. Cardiovasc. Surg.*, 2003. 126(1): p. 124-32.

[152] Vanelli, P., S. Beltrami, E. Cesana, D. Cicero, A. Zaza, E. Rossi, F. Cicirata, C. Antona, and A. Clivio, Cardiac precursors in human bone marrow and cord blood: in vitro cell cardiogenesis. *Ital. Heart J.*, 2004. 5(5): p. 384-8.

[153] Xu, W., X. Zhang, H. Qian, W. Zhu, X. Sun, J. Hu, H. Zhou, and Y. Chen, Mesenchymal stem cells from adult human bone marrow differentiate into a cardiomyocyte phenotype in vitro. *Exp. Biol. Med.* (Maywood), 2004. 229(7): p. 623-31.

[154] Potapova, I., A. Plotnikov, Z. Lu, P. Danilo, Jr., V. Valiunas, J. Qu, S. Doronin, J. Zuckerman, I.N. Shlapakova, J. Gao, Z. Pan, A.J. Herron, R.B. Robinson, P.R. Brink, M.R. Rosen, and I.S. Cohen, Human mesenchymal stem cells as a gene delivery system to create cardiac pacemakers. *Circ. Res.*, 2004. 94(7): p. 952-9.

[155] Valiunas, V., S. Doronin, L. Valiuniene, I. Potapova, J. Zuckerman, B. Walcott, R.B. Robinson, M.R. Rosen, P.R. Brink, and I.S. Cohen, Human mesenchymal stem cells make cardiac connexins and form functional gap junctions. *J. Physiol.*, 2004. 555(Pt 3): p. 617-26.

[156] Cai, D., R. Marty-Roix, H.P. Hsu, and M. Spector, Lapine and canine bone marrow stromal cells contain smooth muscle actin and contract a collagen-glycosaminoglycan matrix. *Tissue Eng.*, 2001. 7(6): p. 829-41.

[157] Arakawa, E., K. Hasegawa, N. Yanai, M. Obinata, and Y. Matsuda, A mouse bone marrow stromal cell line, TBR-B, shows inducible expression of smooth muscle-specific genes. *FEBS Lett.*, 2000. 481(2): p. 193-6.

[158] Hegner, B., M. Weber, D. Dragun, and E. Schulze-Lohoff, Differential regulation of smooth muscle markers in human bone marrow-derived mesenchymal stem cells. *J. Hypertens*, 2005. 23(6): p. 1191-202.

[159] Tintut, Y., Z. Alfonso, T. Saini, K. Radcliff, K. Watson, K. Bostrom, and L.L. Demer, Multilineage potential of cells from the artery wall. *Circulation*, 2003. 108(20): p. 2505-10.

[160] Eliopoulos, N., J. Stagg, L. Lejeune, S. Pommey, and J. Galipeau, Allogeneic marrow stromal cells are immune rejected by MHC class I- and class II-mismatched recipient mice. *Blood,* 2005. 106(13): p. 4057-65.

[161] Di Nicola, M., C. Carlo-Stella, M. Magni, M. Milanesi, P.D. Longoni, P. Matteucci, S. Grisanti, and A.M. Gianni, Human bone marrow stromal cells suppress T-lymphocyte proliferation induced by cellular or nonspecific mitogenic stimuli. *Blood,* 2002. 99(10): p. 3838-43.

[162] Krampera, M., S. Glennie, J. Dyson, D. Scott, R. Laylor, E. Simpson, and F. Dazzi, Bone marrow mesenchymal stem cells inhibit the response of naive and memory antigen-specific T cells to their cognate peptide. *Blood*, 2003. 101(9): p. 3722-9.

[163] Glennie, S., I. Soeiro, P.J. Dyson, E.W. Lam, and F. Dazzi, Bone marrow mesenchymal stem cells induce division arrest anergy of activated T cells. *Blood*, 2005. 105(7): p. 2821-7.

[164] Pereira, R.F., K.W. Halford, M.D. O'Hara, D.B. Leeper, B.P. Sokolov, M.D. Pollard, O. Bagasra, and D.J. Prockop, Cultured adherent cells from marrow can serve as long-lasting precursor cells for bone, cartilage, and lung in irradiated mice. *Proc. Natl. Acad. Sci. USA,* 1995. 92(11): p. 4857-61.

[165] Bensidhoum, M., A. Chapel, S. Francois, C. Demarquay, C. Mazurier, L. Fouillard, S. Bouchet, J.M. Bertho, P. Gourmelon, J. Aigueperse, P. Charbord, N.C. Gorin, D. Thierry, and M. Lopez, Homing of in vitro expanded Stro-1- or Stro-1+ human mesenchymal stem cells into the NOD/SCID mouse and their role in supporting human CD34 cell engraftment. *Blood,* 2004. 103(9): p. 3313-9.

[166] Bruder, S.P., N. Jaiswal, and S.E. Haynesworth, Growth kinetics, self-renewal, and the osteogenic potential of purified human mesenchymal stem cells during extensive subcultivation and following cryopreservation. *J. Cell Biochem.,* 1997. 64(2): p. 278-94.

[167] Banfi, A., G. Bianchi, R. Notaro, L. Luzzatto, R. Cancedda, and R. Quarto, Replicative aging and gene expression in long-term cultures of human bone marrow stromal cells. *Tissue Eng.,* 2002. 8(6): p. 901-10.

[168] Simmons, P.J., B. Masinovsky, B.M. Longenecker, R. Berenson, B. Torok-Storb, and W.M. Gallatin, Vascular cell adhesion molecule-1 expressed by bone marrow stromal cells mediates the binding of hematopoietic progenitor cells. *Blood,* 1992. 80(2): p. 388-95.

[169] Kawano, S., K. Otsu, S. Shoji, K. Yamagata, and M. Hiraoka, Ca(2+) oscillations regulated by Na(+)-Ca(2+) exchanger and plasma membrane Ca(2+) pump induce fluctuations of membrane currents and potentials in human mesenchymal stem cells. *Cell Calcium.,* 2003. 34(2): p. 145-56.

[170] Bonyadi, M., S.D. Waldman, D. Liu, J.E. Aubin, M.D. Grynpas, and W.L. Stanford, Mesenchymal progenitor self-renewal deficiency leads to age-dependent osteoporosis in Sca-1/Ly-6A null mice. *Proc. Natl. Acad. Sci. USA,* 2003. 100(10): p. 5840-5.

[171] Pereira, R.F., M.D. O'Hara, A.V. Laptev, K.W. Halford, M.D. Pollard, R. Class, D. Simon, K. Livezey, and D.J. Prockop, Marrow stromal cells as a source of progenitor cells for nonhematopoietic tissues in transgenic mice with a phenotype of osteogenesis imperfecta. *Proc. Natl. Acad. Sci. USA,* 1998. 95(3): p. 1142-7.

[172] Horwitz, E.M., D.J. Prockop, P.L. Gordon, W.W. Koo, L.A. Fitzpatrick, M.D. Neel, M.E. McCarville, P.J. Orchard, R.E. Pyeritz, and M.K. Brenner, Clinical responses to bone marrow transplantation in children with severe osteogenesis imperfecta. *Blood,* 2001. 97(5): p. 1227-31.

[173] Aubin, J.E., Bone stem cells. *J. Cell Biochem. Suppl.,* 1998. 30-31: p. 73-82.

[174] Perry, C.R., Bone repair techniques, bone graft, and bone graft substitutes. *Clin. Orthop. Relat. Res.,* 1999(360): p. 71-86.

[175] Goshima, J., V.M. Goldberg, and A.I. Caplan, Osteogenic potential of culture-expanded rat marrow cells as assayed in vivo with porous calcium phosphate ceramic. *Biomaterials,* 1991. 12(2): p. 253-8.

[176] Goshima, J., V.M. Goldberg, and A.I. Caplan, The origin of bone formed in composite grafts of porous calcium phosphate ceramic loaded with marrow cells. *Clin. Orthop. Relat. Res.,* 1991(269): p. 274-83.

[177] Goshima, J., V.M. Goldberg, and A.I. Caplan, The osteogenic potential of culture-expanded rat marrow mesenchymal cells assayed in vivo in calcium phosphate ceramic blocks. *Clin. Orthop. Relat. Res.,* 1991(262): p. 298-311.

[178] Krebsbach, P.H., S.A. Kuznetsov, K. Satomura, R.V. Emmons, D.W. Rowe, and P.G. Robey, Bone formation in vivo: comparison of osteogenesis by transplanted mouse and human marrow stromal fibroblasts. *Transplantation*, 1997. 63(8): p. 1059-69.

[179] Martin, I., A. Muraglia, G. Campanile, R. Cancedda, and R. Quarto, Fibroblast growth factor-2 supports ex vivo expansion and maintenance of osteogenic precursors from human bone marrow. *Endocrinology*, 1997. 138(10): p. 4456-62.

[180] Kadiyala, S., R.G. Young, M.A. Thiede, and S.P. Bruder, Culture expanded canine mesenchymal stem cells possess osteochondrogenic potential in vivo and in vitro. *Cell Transplant,* 1997. 6(2): p. 125-34.

[181] Krebsbach, P.H., S.A. Kuznetsov, P. Bianco, and P.G. Robey, Bone marrow stromal cells: characterization and clinical application. Crit Rev Oral Biol Med, 1999. 10(2): p. 165-81.

[182] Krebsbach, P.H., M.H. Mankani, K. Satomura, S.A. Kuznetsov, and P.G. Robey, Repair of craniotomy defects using bone marrow stromal cells. *Transplantation,* 1998. 66(10): p. 1272-8.

[183] Ohgushi, H., V.M. Goldberg, and A.I. Caplan, Repair of bone defects with marrow cells and porous ceramic. Experiments in rats. *Acta Orthop. Scand.,* 1989. 60(3): p. 334-9.

[184] Kon, E., A. Muraglia, A. Corsi, P. Bianco, M. Marcacci, I. Martin, A. Boyde, I. Ruspantini, P. Chistolini, M. Rocca, R. Giardino, R. Cancedda, and R. Quarto, Autologous bone marrow stromal cells loaded onto porous hydroxyapatite ceramic accelerate bone repair in critical-size defects of sheep long bones. *J. Biomed. Mater. Res.*, 2000. 49(3): p. 328-37.

[185] Petite, H., V. Viateau, W. Bensaid, A. Meunier, C. de Pollak, M. Bourguignon, K. Oudina, L. Sedel, and G. Guillemin, Tissue-engineered bone regeneration. *Nat. Biotechnol.*, 2000. 18(9): p. 959-63.

[186] Chen, F., T. Mao, K. Tao, S. Chen, G. Ding, and X. Gu, Injectable bone. *Br. J. Oral. Maxillofac. Surg.*, 2003. 41(4): p. 240-3.

[187] Chang, S.C., H. Chuang, Y.R. Chen, L.C. Yang, J.K. Chen, S. Mardini, H.Y. Chung, Y.L. Lu, W.C. Ma, and J. Lou, Cranial repair using BMP-2 gene engineered bone marrow stromal cells. *J. Surg. Res.,* 2004. 119(1): p. 85-91.

[188] Schantz, J.T., D.W. Hutmacher, C.X. Lam, M. Brinkmann, K.M. Wong, T.C. Lim, N. Chou, R.E. Guldberg, and S.H. Teoh, Repair of calvarial defects with customised tissue-engineered bone grafts II. Evaluation of cellular efficiency and efficacy in vivo. *Tissue Eng.,* 2003. 9 Suppl 1: p. S127-39.

[189] Dai, K.R., X.L. Xu, T.T. Tang, Z.A. Zhu, C.F. Yu, J.R. Lou, and X.L. Zhang, Repairing of goat tibial bone defects with BMP-2 gene-modified tissue-engineered bone. *Calcif Tissue Int.,* 2005. 77(1): p. 55-61.

[190] Li, Z., Y. Yang, C. Wang, R. Xia, Y. Zhang, Q. Zhao, W. Liao, Y. Wang, and J. Lu, Repair of sheep metatarsus defects by using tissue-engineering technique. *J. Huazhong Univ. Sci. Technolog. Med. Sci.*, 2005. 25(1): p. 62-7.

[191] Meinel, L., R. Fajardo, S. Hofmann, R. Langer, J. Chen, B. Snyder, G. Vunjak-Novakovic, and D. Kaplan, Silk implants for the healing of critical size bone defects. *Bone,* 2005. 37(5): p. 688-98.

[192] Brodke, D., H.A. Pedrozo, T.A. Kapur, M. Attawia, K.H. Kraus, C.E. Holy, S. Kadiyala, and S.P. Bruder, Bone grafts prepared with selective cell retention technology heal canine segmental defects as effectively as autograft. *J. Orthop. Res.*, 2006. 24(5): p. 857-66.

[193] Yoon, E., S. Dhar, D.E. Chun, N.A. Gharibjanian, and G.R. Evans, In Vivo Osteogenic Potential of Human Adipose-Derived Stem Cells/Poly Lactide-Co-Glycolic Acid Constructs for Bone Regeneration in a Rat Critical-Sized Calvarial Defect Model. *Tissue Eng,* 2006.

[194] Mastrogiacomo, M., V.S. Komlev, M. Hausard, F. Peyrin, F. Turquier, S. Casari, A. Cedola, F. Rustichelli, and R. Cancedda, Synchrotron radiation microtomography of bone engineered from bone marrow stromal cells. *Tissue En*g, 2004. 10(11-12): p. 1767-74.

[195] Mastrogiacomo, M., A. Papadimitropoulos, A. Cedola, F. Peyrin, P. Giannoni, S.G. Pearce, M. Alini, C. Giannini, A. Guagliardi, and R. Cancedda, Engineering of bone using bone marrow stromal cells and a silicon-stabilized tricalcium phosphate bioceramic: evidence for a coupling between bone formation and scaffold resorption. *Biomaterials,* 2007. 28(7): p. 1376-84.

[196] Komlev, V.S., F. Peyrin, M. Mastrogiacomo, A. Cedola, A. Papadimitropoulos, F. Rustichelli, and R. Cancedda, Kinetics of in vivo bone deposition by bone marrow stromal cells into porous calcium phosphate scaffolds: an X-ray computed microtomography study. *Tissue Eng,* 2006. 12(12): p. 3449-58.

[197] Casabona, F., I. Martin, A. Muraglia, P. Berrino, P. Santi, R. Cancedda, and R. Quarto, Prefabricated engineered bone flaps: an experimental model of tissue reconstruction in plastic surgery. *Plast Reconstr. Surg.,* 1998. 101(3): p. 577-81.

[198] Mankani, M.H., P.H. Krebsbach, K. Satomura, S.A. Kuznetsov, R. Hoyt, and P.G. Robey, Pedicled bone flap formation using transplanted bone marrow stromal cells. *Arch. Surg.*, 2001. 136(3): p. 263-70.

[199] Cancedda, R., B. Dozin, P. Giannoni, and R. Quarto, Tissue engineering and cell therapy of cartilage and bone. *Matrix Biol.*, 2003. 22(1): p. 81-91.

[200] Vacanti, C.A., L.J. Bonassar, M.P. Vacanti, and J. Shufflebarger, Replacement of an avulsed phalanx with tissue-engineered bone. *N. Engl. J. Med.*, 2001. 344(20): p. 1511-4.

[201] Warnke, P.H., I.N. Springer, J. Wiltfang, Y. Acil, H. Eufinger, M. Wehmoller, P.A. Russo, H. Bolte, E. Sherry, E. Behrens, and H. Terheyden, Growth and transplantation of a custom vascularised bone graft in a man. *Lancet,* 2004. 364(9436): p. 766-70.

[202] Shen, H.C., H. Peng, A. Usas, B. Gearhart, F.H. Fu, and J. Huard, Structural and functional healing of critical-size segmental bone defects by transduced muscle-derived cells expressing BMP4. *J. Gene Med.,* 2004. 6(9): p. 984-91.

[203] Shen, H.C., H. Peng, A. Usas, B. Gearhart, J. Cummins, F.H. Fu, and J. Huard, Ex vivo gene therapy-induced endochondral bone formation: comparison of muscle-derived

stem cells and different subpopulations of primary muscle-derived cells. *Bone*, 2004. 34(6): p. 982-92.

[204] Yang, M., Q.J. Ma, G.T. Dang, K. Ma, P. Chen, and C.Y. Zhou, In vitro and in vivo induction of bone formation based on ex vivo gene therapy using rat adipose-derived adult stem cells expressing BMP-7. *Cytotherapy*, 2005. 7(3): p. 273-81.

[205] Chamberlain, J.R., U. Schwarze, P.R. Wang, R.K. Hirata, K.D. Hankenson, J.M. Pace, R.A. Underwood, K.M. Song, M. Sussman, P.H. Byers, and D.W. Russell, Gene targeting in stem cells from individuals with osteogenesis imperfecta. *Science*, 2004. 303(5661): p. 1198-201.

[206] Zhang, X.S., T.A. Linkhart, S.T. Chen, H. Peng, J.E. Wergedal, G.G. Guttierez, M.H. Sheng, K.H. Lau, and D.J. Baylink, Local ex vivo gene therapy with bone marrow stromal cells expressing human BMP4 promotes endosteal bone formation in mice. *J. Gene Med.*, 2004. 6(1): p. 4-15.

[207] Chen, F., T. Mao, K. Tao, S. Chen, G. Ding, and X. Gu, Bone graft in the shape of human mandibular condyle reconstruction via seeding marrow-derived osteoblasts into porous coral in a nude mice model. *J. Oral Maxillofac. Surg.*, 2002. 60(10): p. 1155-9.

[208] Pelled, G., T. G, H. Aslan, Z. Gazit, and D. Gazit, Mesenchymal stem cells for bone gene therapy and tissue engineering. *Curr. Pharm. Des.*, 2002. 8(21): p. 1917-28.

[209] Xie, C., D. Reynolds, H. Awad, P.T. Rubery, G. Pelled, D. Gazit, R.E. Guldberg, E.M. Schwarz, R.J. O'Keefe, and X. Zhang, Structural bone allograft combined with genetically engineered mesenchymal stem cells as a novel platform for bone tissue engineering. *Tissue Eng.*, 2007. 13(3): p. 435-45.

[210] Ettinger, M.P., Aging bone and osteoporosis: strategies for preventing fractures in the elderly. *Arch. Intern. Med.*, 2003. 163(18): p. 2237-46.

[211] Seeman, E., Invited Review: Pathogenesis of osteoporosis. *J. Appl. Physiol.*, 2003. 95(5): p. 2142-51.

[212] D'Ippolito, G., P.C. Schiller, C. Ricordi, B.A. Roos, and G.A. Howard, Age-related osteogenic potential of mesenchymal stromal stem cells from human vertebral bone marrow. *J. Bone Miner Res.*, 1999. 14(7): p. 1115-22.

[213] Stromsoe, K., Fracture fixation problems in osteoporosis. *Injury,* 2004. 35(2): p. 107-13.

[214] Rozen, N., D. Lewinson, T. Bick, S. Meretyk, and M. Soudry, Role of bone regeneration and turnover modulators in control of fracture. *Crit. Rev. Eukaryot Gene Expr.*, 2007. 17(3): p. 197-213.

[215] Sama, A.A., S.N. Khan, E.R. Myers, R.C. Huang, F.P. Cammisa, Jr., H.S. Sandhu, and J.M. Lane, High-dose alendronate uncouples osteoclast and osteoblast function: a study in a rat spine pseudarthrosis model. *Clin. Orthop. Relat Res.*, 2004(425): p. 135-42.

[216] Langstaff, S., M. Sayer, T.J. Smith, S.M. Pugh, S.A. Hesp, and W.T. Thompson, Resorbable bioceramics based on stabilized calcium phosphates. Part I: rational design, sample preparation and material characterization. *Biomaterials,* 1999. 20(18): p. 1727-41.

[217] Service, R.F., Tissue engineers build new bone. *Science*, 2000. 289(5484): p. 1498-500.

[218] Yamamoto, M., Y. Tabata, and Y. Ikada, Ectopic bone formation induced by biodegradable hydrogels incorporating bone morphogenetic protein. *J. Biomater. Sci. Polym. Ed.*, 1998. 9(5): p. 439-58.

[219] den Boer, F.C., B.W. Wippermann, T.J. Blokhuis, P. Patka, F.C. Bakker, and H.J. Haarman, Healing of segmental bone defects with granular porous hydroxyapatite augmented with recombinant human osteogenic protein-1 or autologous bone marrow. *J. Orthop. Res.*, 2003. 21(3): p. 521-8.

[220] Srouji, S. and E. Livne, Bone marrow stem cells and biological scaffold for bone repair in aging and disease. *Mech. Ageing Dev.*, 2005. 126(2): p. 281-7.

[221] Lieberman, J.R., L.Q. Le, L. Wu, G.A. Finerman, A. Berk, O.N. Witte, and S. Stevenson, Regional gene therapy with a BMP-2-producing murine stromal cell line induces heterotopic and orthotopic bone formation in rodents. *J. Orthop Res.*, 1998. 16(3): p. 330-9.

[222] Chang, S.C., F.C. Wei, H. Chuang, Y.R. Chen, J.K. Chen, K.C. Lee, P.K. Chen, C.L. Tai, and J. Lou, Ex vivo gene therapy in autologous critical-size craniofacial bone regeneration. *Plast Reconstr. Surg.*, 2003. 112(7): p. 1841-50.

[223] Cancedda, R., G. Bianchi, A. Derubeis, and R. Quarto, Cell therapy for bone disease: a review of current status. *Stem Cells*, 2003. 21(5): p. 610-9.

[224] Caplan, A.I. and S.P. Bruder, Mesenchymal stem cells: building blocks for molecular medicine in the 21st century. *Trends Mol. Med.*, 2001. 7(6): p. 259-64.

[225] Gruber, R., B. Kandler, P. Holzmann, M. Vogele-Kadletz, U. Losert, M.B. Fischer, and G. Watzek, Bone marrow stromal cells can provide a local environment that favors migration and formation of tubular structures of endothelial cells. *Tissue Eng.*, 2005. 11(5-6): p. 896-903.

[226] Guillot, P.V., O. Abass, J.H. Bassett, S.J. Shefelbine, G. Bou-Gharios, J. Chan, H. Kurata, G.R. Williams, J. Polak, and N.M. Fisk, Intrauterine transplantation of human fetal mesenchymal stem cells from first trimester blood repairs bone and reduces fractures in osteogenesis imperfecta mice. *Blood*, 2007.

[227] Egermann, M., E. Schneider, C.H. Evans, and A.W. Baltzer, The potential of gene therapy for fracture healing in osteoporosis. *Osteoporos Int.*, 2005. 16 Suppl 2: p. S120-8.

[228] Marie, P., Growth factors and bone formation in osteoporosis: roles for IGF-I and TGF-beta. *Rev. Rhum. Engl. Ed.*, 1997. 64(1): p. 44-53.

[229] Marie, P., F. Debiais, M. Cohen-Solal, and M.C. de Vernejoul, New factors controlling bone remodeling. *Joint Bone Spine*, 2000. 67(3): p. 150-6.

[230] Stein, E. and E. Shane, Secondary osteoporosis. *Endocrinol. Metab. Clin. North Am.*, 2003. 32(1): p. 115-34, vii.

[231] Boling, E.P., Secondary osteoporosis: underlying disease and the risk for glucocorticoid-induced osteoporosis. *Clin. Ther.*, 2004. 26(1): p. 1-14.

[232] Lane, J.M., M.J. Gardner, J.T. Lin, M.C. van der Meulen, and E. Myers, The aging spine: new technologies and therapeutics for the osteoporotic spine. *Eur. Spine J.*, 2003. 12 Suppl 2: p. S147-54.

[233] Stepan, J.J., F. Alenfeld, G. Boivin, J.H. Feyen, and P. Lakatos, Mechanisms of action of antiresorptive therapies of postmenopausal osteoporosis. *Endocr. Regul.*, 2003. 37(4): p. 225-38.

[234] Ohnaka, K., H. Taniguchi, H. Kawate, H. Nawata, and R. Takayanagi, Glucocorticoid enhances the expression of dickkopf-1 in human osteoblasts: novel mechanism of glucocorticoid-induced osteoporosis. *Biochem. Biophys. Res. Commun.*, 2004. 318(1): p. 259-64.

[235] Cormier, C., J.C. Souberbielle, and A. Kahan, Primary hyperparathyroidism and osteoporosis in 2004. *Joint Bone Spine*, 2004. 71(3): p. 183-9.

[236] Misra, M. and A. Klibanski, Anorexia nervosa and osteoporosis. Rev Endocr Metab Disord, 2006. 7(1-2): p. 91-9.

[237] Norimatsu, H., S. Mori, J. Kawanishi, Y. Kaji, and J. Li, Immobilization as the pathogenesis of osteoporosis: experimental and clinical studies. *Osteoporos Int.*, 1997. 7 Suppl 3: p. S57-62.

[238] Dwivedy, I. and S. Ray, Recent developments in the chemotherapy of osteoporosis. *Prog. Drug Res.*, 1995. 45: p. 289-338.

[239] Lichtenstein, G.R., Evaluation of bone mineral density in inflammatory bowel disease: current safety focus. *Am. J. Gastroenterol.*, 2003. 98(12 Suppl): p. S24-30.

[240] Allain, T.J., Prostate cancer, osteoporosis and fracture risk. *Gerontology*, 2006. 52(2): p. 107-10.

[241] Fontanges, E., A. Fontana, and P. Delmas, Osteoporosis and breast cancer. *Joint Bone Spine*, 2004. 71(2): p. 102-10.

[242] Rodriguez, J.P., S. Garat, H. Gajardo, A.M. Pino, and G. Seitz, Abnormal osteogenesis in osteoporotic patients is reflected by altered mesenchymal stem cells dynamics. *J. Cell Biochem.*, 1999. 75(3): p. 414-23.

[243] Rodriguez, J.P., L. Montecinos, S. Rios, P. Reyes, and J. Martinez, Mesenchymal stem cells from osteoporotic patients produce a type I collagen-deficient extracellular matrix favoring adipogenic differentiation. *J. Cell Biochem.*, 2000. 79(4): p. 557-65.

[244] Verma, S., J.H. Rajaratnam, J. Denton, J.A. Hoyland, and R.J. Byers, Adipocytic proportion of bone marrow is inversely related to bone formation in osteoporosis. *J. Clin. Pathol.*, 2002. 55(9): p. 693-8.

[245] Ichioka, N., M. Inaba, T. Kushida, T. Esumi, K. Takahara, K. Inaba, R. Ogawa, H. Iida, and S. Ikehara, Prevention of senile osteoporosis in SAMP6 mice by intrabone marrow injection of allogeneic bone marrow cells. *Stem Cells*, 2002. 20(6): p. 542-51.

[246] Takada, K., M. Inaba, N. Ichioka, Y. Ueda, M. Taira, S. Baba, T. Mizokami, X. Wang, H. Hisha, H. Iida, and S. Ikehara, Treatment of senile osteoporosis in SAMP6 mice by intra-bone marrow injection of allogeneic bone marrow cells. *Stem Cells*, 2006. 24(2): p. 399-405.

[247] Gimble, J.M., F. Wanker, C.S. Wang, H. Bass, X. Wu, K. Kelly, G.D. Yancopoulos, and M.R. Hill, Regulation of bone marrow stromal cell differentiation by cytokines whose receptors share the gp130 protein. *J. Cell Biochem.*, 1994. 54(1): p. 122-33.

[248] Dai, J., D. Lin, J. Zhang, P. Habib, P. Smith, J. Murtha, Z. Fu, Z. Yao, Y. Qi, and E.T. Keller, Chronic alcohol ingestion induces osteoclastogenesis and bone loss through IL-6 in mice. *J. Clin. Invest*, 2000. 106(7): p. 887-95.

[249] Tanaka, Y., S. Nakayamada, and Y. Okada, Osteoblasts and osteoclasts in bone remodeling and inflammation. *Curr. Drug. Targets Inflamm. Allergy*, 2005. 4(3): p. 325-8.

[250] Bolon, B., C. Carter, M. Daris, S. Morony, C. Capparelli, A. Hsieh, M. Mao, P. Kostenuik, C.R. Dunstan, D.L. Lacey, and J.Z. Sheng, Adenoviral delivery of osteoprotegerin ameliorates bone resorption in a mouse ovariectomy model of osteoporosis. *Mol. Ther.*, 2001. 3(2): p. 197-205.

[251] Kimble, R.B., J.L. Vannice, D.C. Bloedow, R.C. Thompson, W. Hopfer, V.T. Kung, C. Brownfield, and R. Pacifici, Interleukin-1 receptor antagonist decreases bone loss and bone resorption in ovariectomized rats. *J. Clin. Invest.*, 1994. 93(5): p. 1959-67.

[252] Kimble, R.B., S. Bain, and R. Pacifici, The functional block of TNF but not of IL-6 prevents bone loss in ovariectomized mice. *J. Bone Miner Res.*, 1997. 12(6): p. 935-41.

[253] Baltzer, A.W., J.D. Whalen, P. Wooley, C. Latterman, L.M. Truchan, P.D. Robbins, and C.H. Evans, Gene therapy for osteoporosis: evaluation in a murine ovariectomy model. *Gene Ther.*, 2001. 8(23): p. 1770-6.

[254] Mante, M., B. Daniels, E. Golden, D. Diefenderfer, G. Reilly, and P.S. Leboy, Attachment of human marrow stromal cells to titanium surfaces. *J. Oral Implantol.*, 2003. 29(2): p. 66-72.

[255] Andrades, J.A., J.A. Santamaria, M.E. Nimni, and J. Becerra, Selection and amplification of a bone marrow cell population and its induction to the chondro-osteogenic lineage by rhOP-1: an in vitro and in vivo study. *Int. J. Dev. Biol.*, 2001. 45(4): p. 689-93.

[256] Gao, J., J.E. Dennis, R.F. Muzic, M. Lundberg, and A.I. Caplan, The dynamic in vivo distribution of bone marrow-derived mesenchymal stem cells after infusion. *Cells Tissues Organs*, 2001. 169(1): p. 12-20.

[257] Mahmud, N., W. Pang, C. Cobbs, P. Alur, J. Borneman, R. Dodds, M. Archambault, S. Devine, J. Turian, A. Bartholomew, P. Vanguri, A. Mackay, R. Young, and R. Hoffman, Studies of the route of administration and role of conditioning with radiation on unrelated allogeneic mismatched mesenchymal stem cell engraftment in a nonhuman primate model. *Exp. Hematol.*, 2004. 32(5): p. 494-501.

[258] Caplan, A.I., Mesenchymal stem cells. *J. Orthop Res.*, 1991. 9(5): p. 641-50.

[259] Francois, S., M. Bensidhoum, M. Mouiseddine, C. Mazurier, B. Allenet, A. Semont, J. Frick, A. Sache, S. Bouchet, D. Thierry, P. Gourmelon, N.C. Gorin, and A. Chapel, Local irradiation not only induces homing of human mesenchymal stem cells at exposed sites but promotes their widespread engraftment to multiple organs: a study of their quantitative distribution after irradiation damage. *Stem Cells*, 2006. 24(4): p. 1020-9.

[260] Bianco, P., M. Riminucci, S. Gronthos, and P.G. Robey, Bone marrow stromal stem cells: nature, biology, and potential applications. *Stem Cells*, 2001. 19(3): p. 180-92.

[261] Javazon, E.H., K.J. Beggs, and A.W. Flake, Mesenchymal stem cells: paradoxes of passaging. *Exp. Hematol.*, 2004. 32(5): p. 414-25.

[262] Alvarez-Dolado, M., R. Pardal, J.M. Garcia-Verdugo, J.R. Fike, H.O. Lee, K. Pfeffer, C. Lois, S.J. Morrison, and A. Alvarez-Buylla, Fusion of bone-marrow-derived cells

with Purkinje neurons, cardiomyocytes and hepatocytes. *Nature*, 2003. 425(6961): p. 968-73.

[263] Goncalves, M.A., A.A. de Vries, M. Holkers, M.J. van de Watering, I. van der Velde, G.P. van Nierop, D. Valerio, and S. Knaan-Shanzer, Human mesenchymal stem cells ectopically expressing full-length dystrophin can complement Duchenne muscular dystrophy myotubes by cell fusion. *Hum. Mol. Genet.*, 2006. 15(2): p. 213-21.

[264] Shi, D., H. Reinecke, C.E. Murry, and B. Torok-Storb, Myogenic fusion of human bone marrow stromal cells, but not hematopoietic cells. *Blood,* 2004. 104(1): p. 290-4.

[265] Spees, J.L., S.D. Olson, J. Ylostalo, P.J. Lynch, J. Smith, A. Perry, A. Peister, M.Y. Wang, and D.J. Prockop, Differentiation, cell fusion, and nuclear fusion during ex vivo repair of epithelium by human adult stem cells from bone marrow stroma. *Proc. Natl. Acad. Sci. USA*, 2003. 100(5): p. 2397-402.

In: Encyclopedia of Stem Cell Research (2 Volume Set) ISBN: 978-1-61761-835-2
Editor: Alexander L. Greene © 2012 Nova Science Publishers, Inc.

Chapter VII

RADIAL GLIA IN THE REPAIR OF CENTRAL NERVOUS SYSTEM INJURY

I. Kulbatski and C. H. Tator

Institute of Medical Science, University of Toronto and Toronto Western Research Institute, University Health Network, Toronto, Ontario, Canada

ABSTRACT

During central nervous system (CNS) development, radial glia function as specialized scaffold cells that guide migrating neurons. Radial glia also proliferate during neurogenesis, give rise to oligodendrocytes and astrocytes, and guide migrating glial precursors. In most cases, radial glia are only present for as long as they function during CNS development, however, some radial glia remain into adulthood. In lower vertebrates such as birds and amphibians in which there is continual neurogenesis into adulthood, radial glia are always present, and may play a role in regeneration. In the adult rat, radial glia emerge following spinal cord injury and likely play a role in neural regeneration. It was recently shown that embryonic rat radial glia transplanted into the injured rat spinal cord formed bridges and promoted functional recovery.

Radial glia comprise the majority of precursors in the ventricular zones in most areas of the CNS, especially in the brain. Radial glia in neonates and radial glia-derived cells in the adult lateral ventricle exhibit neural stem/precursor cell (NSPC) properties, since they generate self-renewing multipotent neurospheres in vitro. We recently showed that NSPCs isolated from the adult rat spinal cord and propagated in vitro, differentiate into large numbers of radial glia, and appear to function as guidance scaffolds. This suggests a recapitulation of their developmental role in vitro. This role may extend to reflect their capacity to act as NSPCs within the adult CNS, and highlights their potential for transplantation therapies.

This chapter focuses on the function of radial glia in the CNS, with particular emphasis on their role as NSPCs, their endogenous response following CNS injury, and the potential of therapies that enhance the endogenous radial glial response or supply an exogenously expanded source of radial glia in the form of a cellular transplant strategy for CNS regeneration.

INTRODUCTION

Regenerative medicine uses the body's endogenous cell populations to replace or repair cells, tissues, and organs, and includes stem cell therapy among its strategies. The application of stem cells for regeneration of the central nervous system (CNS) following trauma and disease is being investigated using various therapeutic paradigms. Among the illnesses that could derive benefit from stem cell therapy are spinal cord injury (SCI), traumatic brain injury (TBI), stroke, and other neurodegenerative conditions like Alzheimer's Disease, Parkinson's Disease and multiple sclerosis. Implementing novel stem cell therapies to enhance repair of the CNS holds great promise for millions of individuals. This chapter will describe the role of radial glia in the developing CNS, their emerging role as neural stem/precursor cells (NSPCs) both during development and following CNS injury, and the potential of radial glial transplantation therapies for CNS regeneration. Strategies to stimulate the endogenous radial glial response to trauma in vivo and/or maximize their potential to repair the injured brain or spinal cord after transplantation will also be addressed.

Current Status of Traumatic Brain and Spinal Cord Injury and Treatment in Humans

TBI is defined as externally inflicted brain trauma, which can impair a person's physical, cognitive, psychological, emotional, and social functioning (McArthur et al. 2004). Epidemiological data shows that in many countries, TBI occurs at a rate of almost 2 million people a year, and almost 100,000 individuals annually suffer a TBI that results in long-term, severe functional deficits (McArthur et al. 2004). The annual rate of acute SCI in most countries is 20-40 per million (Tator 1995). The main causes of both TBI and SCI are motor vehicle crashes, sports and recreation, injuries at work, violence, and falls at home(McArthur et al. 2004; Tator 1995). Each major TBI or complete SCI costs society several million dollars for medical costs and lost earning in addition to the great personal loss sustained by the victims and their families (McArthur et al. 2004; Tator 1995).

Over the years, there have been significant improvements in the acute care of TBI and SCI, including faster emergency care, quicker, safer, and more effective transportation to specialized facilities, and innovations in medical management of acute TBI and SCI (McArthur et al. 2004; Tator 1995). Nevertheless, there are currently no effective long-term clinical therapies to regenerate injured CNS tissue and function (McArthur et al. 2004; Tator 2006). Current treatments focus on physical, cognitive, and behavioral rehabilitation, pharmacotherapy, surgery, environmental manipulation, psychotherapy, education, and assistive technologies.

There is evidence that a secondary injury of the brain or spinal cord occurs after the initial mechanical trauma, and that therapy can interrupt this secondary process and lead to improved recovery. A variety of clinical trials have emerged over the past decade examining the potential of various neuroprotective drugs to improve TBI outcome, but none of the trials that has reached phase III showed a significant improvement in treating clinical TBI, despite the encouraging pre-clinical data (Doppenberg and Bullock 1997; Maas 2001; Maas et al.

2004). Similarly, the trend toward improved neurological recovery in SCI patients in randomized, prospective clinical trials of pharmacotherapy with agents such as methylprednisolone or GM-1 ganglioside supports the concept of a treatable secondary injury (Bracken et al. 1990; Geisler et al. 2001; Tator 2006). Unfortunately, the improvements in these trials were minimal (Tator 2006).

More recently, the focus of pre-clinical studies for CNS repair following TBI and SCI has shifted to the potential of enhancing the endogenous NSPC response and/or supplementing this response with an exogenous source of NSPCs (Kulbatski et al. 2005). Both of these strategies have the potential to substantially improve the acute and long-term management of clinical TBI and SCI.

ROLE OF RADIAL GLIA IN CENTRAL NERVOUS SYSTEM DEVELOPMENT

Radial glia arise from a population of neuroepithelial cells that surround the neural tube (Misson et al. 1991; Schmechel and Rakic 1979; Voigt 1989). Radial glia are mitotically active cells, whose nuclei reside in the ventricular zone (VZ) of the brain, and undergo interkinetic nuclear migration (Misson et al. 1988; Stagaard and Mollgard 1989). The bipolar morphology of radial glia is one of their distinguishing characteristics, and allows these specialized cells to maintain contact of one endfoot on the ventricular surface, with the other radial process contacting the pia (Misson et al. 1991; Schmechel and Rakic 1979; Voigt 1989). During brain development, particularly during the period of neurogenesis, radial glia act as scaffold cells to guide migrating neurons (Gotz and Huttner 2005; Hartfuss et al. 2001; Hatten 1999). Radial glia may also guide migrating glial precursors (Diers-Fenger et al. 2001; O'Rourke et al. 1992). Interestingly, radial glia also exhibit a structural role in brain development by restricting the migration of neurons to particular areas through region specific gene expression, thereby creating a barrier between different regions of the brain (Chapouton et al. 2001). Moreover, radial glia have been shown to release particular factors, such as retinoic acid and sonic hedgehog, that influence the local differentiation of specific neuronal subtypes (Campbell and Gotz 2002; Toresson et al. 1999).

Although the primary role of radial glia has traditionally been defined by their ability to guide migrating neurons, their differentiation into astroyctes following neurogenesis and migration is well documented (Gaiano et al. 2000; Misson et al. 1991; Schmechel and Rakic 1979; Voigt 1989). It has also been shown that radial glia produce neurons (Alvarez-Buylla 1990; Gotz 2003; Halliday and Cepko 1992; Hartfuss et al. 2001; Malatesta et al. 2000; Miyata et al. 2001; Noctor et al. 2001; Weissman et al. 2003). In fact, several studies have shown that radial glia generate the majority of pyramidal neurons in the cerebral cortex (Malatesta et al. 2003; Noctor et al. 2002; Tamamaki et al. 2001).

During early spinal cord development, radial glia span the spinal cord from the ventricular to the pial surface, similar to their orientation in the developing brain (McMahon and McDermott 2002). It is believed that radial glia serve a similar role during spinal cord development as they do during brain development, in that they act as a guidance scaffold for migrating spinal cord neurons (McDermott et al. 2005), after which they differentiate into astrocytes (Barry and McDermott 2005). Additionally, spinal cord radial glia have been shown to differentiate into oligodendrocytes (Aloisi et al. 1992; Choi and Kim 1985; Fogarty et al. 2005; Hirano and Goldman 1988). Overall, however, less is known about the function of radial glia in mammalian spinal cord development compared to the brain.

McMahon and McDermott (2002) performed a careful investigation of radial glia within the developing rat spinal cord, and found that at embryonic day (E)14 the classic radial glial morphology was seen, with the disappearance of full radial processes occurring as development progresses. Radial glia in the spinal cord exhibit extensive interaction with axons, and are thought to play a crucial role during white matter patterning, particularly in regulating axon outgrowth and pathfinding (Brusco et al. 1995). Developing axonal tracts are thought to be ensheathed by radial glia in the developing spinal cord (Brusco et al. 1995), similar to the way in which olfactory ensheathing glia act to guide and support axonal growth in the olfactory system (Chuah and West 2002; Doucette 1995, 1990). The close apposition between radial glia and axons of the corticospinal tract, taken together with electron microscopic evidence of adhesive contact between the axons and radial glia suggest that radial glia offer both physical and trophic support for axonal migration (Joosten and Gribnau 1989; Joosten et al. 1989). Tessier-Lavigne and colleagues showed that radial glia are involved in the chemotropic guidance of developing axons in the adult mammalian CNS (Tessier-Lavigne et al. 1988). For a complete review of the role of radial glia in patterning and boundary formation during spinal cord development see McDermott et al. (2005).

ENDOGENOUS NEURAL STEM/PRECURSOR CELLS IN THE BRAIN AND SPINAL CORD

Developmentally, neural stem cells are highly proliferative cells, giving rise to increasing numbers of stem cells, which progressively undergo lineage restriction, to produce the three terminally differentiated major cell types within the CNS: neurons, astrocytes, and oligodendrocytes (Davis and Temple 1994; Gage 2000). The initial symmetric cell division that occurs in the developing CNS, specifically during the period of neural tube formation, produces more stem cells. As development progresses, symmetric cell division is replaced by asymmetric cell division, and neural precursor cells are produced (Temple 2001). When cultured in vitro, neural stem/precursor cells (NSPCs) form neurospheres, which are free-floating spherical clusters composed of proliferating cells that retain the potential to differentiate into neurons and glia. The term "NSPCs" was devised as a way to avoid the controversial issue of what constitutes true "stemness" (Gage et al. 1995; McKay 1997; Scheffler et al. 1999), in particular within the context of in vitro neurosphere populations. Moreover, "NSPC" is an all-inclusive term that incorporates the complete spectrum of proliferative cells within the CNS that can generate all the nervous system cells.

NSPCs are found in embryonic, fetal, and adult mammalian brain and spinal cord (Gage 2000; McKay 1997; Rietze et al. 2000; Tropepe et al. 2001; van der Kooy and Weiss 2000), and can also be derived from more primitive embryonic stem cells cultured from the blastocyst (Gage 2000; McKay 1997; Rietze et al. 2000; van der Kooy and Weiss 2000). The adult mammalian CNS contains both multipotent and lineage restricted NSPCs (Temple and

Alvarez-Buylla 1999) which are regulated by trophic factors (Craig et al. 1996; Kuhn et al. 1997; Morshead et al. 1994; Tropepe et al. 1997; Weiss et al. 1996). Fischer, Rao, and colleagues are among several groups that have identified neural restricted precursors (NRPs) and glial restricted precursors (GRPs) (Han et al. 2004; Lepore and Fischer 2005; Lepore et al. 2004; Lepore et al. 2006). NRPs and GRPs fall under the broader umbrella of lineage-restricted precursors, and a variety of neuronal and glial precursor subtypes have been identified, including oligodendrocyte precursor cells (OPCs) (Gensert and Goldman 1996; Gregori et al. 2002; Levison and Goldman 1993; Luskin et al. 1993; Miller et al. 2004; Wilson et al. 2003). These cells share the common feature that they are more limited in their differentiation potential than their multipotent stem cell counterparts.

During embryogenesis, the mammalian brain develops from the neuroepithelial-derived neural tube, which consists of a population of multipotential, proliferating NSPCs that are initially localized to the luminal cell layer of the ventricular zone (VZ), and as maturation progresses, are found beneath the VZ in a region called the subventricular zone (SVZ) (Cepko et al. 1990; Davis and Temple 1994; Johe et al. 1996; Temple 2001; Temple and Alvarez-Buylla 1999; Weiss et al. 1996). The adult forebrain retains a mitotically active layer of the primitive SVZ (Doetsch et al. 1999). These cells migrate towards the olfactory bulb, where they subsequently differentiate into neurons (Lois and Alvarez-Buylla 1994). NSPCs can be isolated from the adult brain SVZ (Gritti et al. 1996; Morshead et al. 1994; Reynolds and Weiss 1992; Richards et al. 1992), and the prevailing view identifies the periventricular region of the adult mammalian forebrain as the major stem cell niche in the CNS. In vitro, these SVZ-derived NSPCs can be propagated in long-term cultures in the presence of epidermal growth factor (EGF) and fibroblast growth factor-2 (FGF2) and in the absence of serum, exhibiting the hallmark characteristics of self-renewal and multipotentiality (Gritti et al. 1996; Morshead et al. 1994; Reynolds and Weiss 1992; Richards et al. 1992).

Adrian and Walker (1962) first identified a small population of mitotically active cells surrounding the central canal of the adult rat spinal cord (Adrian and Walker 1962). More recently, Horner and colleagues used BrdU labeling to identify proliferative cells in the adult rat spinal cord, and to study their spatial distribution and differentiation potential. Interestingly, they found highly proliferative cells throughout the entire spinal cord, most notably in the white matter regions, and the majority of these cells co-expressed immature glial markers such as NG2 chondroitin sulphate proteoglycan. These cells were identified as GRPs, since none of them differentiated into neurons, only astrocytes and oligodendrocytes (Horner et al. 2000). Others have also demonstrated the presence of NSPCs in the adult mammalian spinal cord (Horner et al. 2000; Johansson et al. 1999; Kehl et al. 1997; Namiki and Tator 1999; Shihabuddin 2002; Shihabuddin et al. 2000; Shihabuddin et al. 1997; Weiss et al. 1996), and have shown that proliferative cells isolated from the adult rat spinal cord can be propagated in culture and will differentiate into neurons, astrocytes, and oligodendrocytes (Shihabuddin et al. 1997; Weiss et al. 1996). More recently, it has been shown that murine spinal cord NSPCs reside near the central canal since multipotent, self-renewing neurospheres are generated only if the region of the central canal is cultured (Martens et al. 2002; Martens et al. 2000). In contrast, the peripheral regions of the adult rat spinal cord, beyond the region containing the central canal, yield spheres, although these peripheral spheres are composed of

GRPs, since they are limited in their differentiation potential to the glial lineage (Yamamoto et al. 2001).

The precise cellular origin of adult NSPCs in the proliferative regions of the CNS is controversial. One theory identifies NSPCs as ependymal cells (Johansson et al. 1999), while a second theory identifies them as astrocyte-like cells (Doetsch et al. 1999; Laywell et al. 2000). Yet a third theory claims that adult NSPCs originate from radial glia (Hartfuss et al. 2003; Hartfuss et al. 2001; Heins et al. 2002; Malatesta et al. 2003; Malatesta et al. 2000; Merkle et al. 2004; Miyata et al. 2001; Noctor et al. 2001; Noctor et al. 2002; Tamamaki et al. 2001). The remainder of this chapter focuses on studies that demonstrate that radial glia behave as NSPCs during embryogenesis, and give rise to NSPCs in adulthood- reviewed further by others (Bonfanti and Peretto 2007; Malatesta et al. 2007).

Radial Glia as Neural Stem/Precursor Cells

A fascinating body of knowledge has recently begun to emerge, demonstrating that radial glia function as NSPCs in the mammalian CNS (Anthony et al. 2004; Fricker-Gates 2006). Radial glia proliferate during neurogenesis (Misson et al. 1988; Schmechel and Rakic 1979, 1979), and give rise to neurons (Campbell and Gotz 2002; Hartfuss et al. 2001), oligodendrocytes and astrocytes (Choi and Kim 1985; Hirano and Goldman 1988). Their differentiation into astrocytes coincides with the cessation of neurogenesis (Culican et al. 1990; Edwards et al. 1990; Misson et al. 1991; Schmechel and Rakic 1979, 1979; Voigt 1989; Yang et al. 1993).

Historically, radial glia were viewed as glial precursor cells, entirely distinct from the large population of neuronal precursors present during neurogenesis, which had a different morphology and exhibited no glial characteristics. Since the majority of the earlier work in the field demonstrated that radial glia differentiate into astrocytes (Culican et al. 1990; Edwards et al. 1990; Misson et al. 1991; Schmechel and Rakic 1979, 1979; Voigt 1989; Yang et al. 1993), radial glia were often regarded as a specialized subtype of astrocytes. The population of NSPCs in the subventricular zone (SVZ) of the adult mammalian brain generate new neurons that migrate to the olfactory bulb along the rostral migratory stream (RMS) (Alvarez-Buylla and Garcia-Verdugo 2002). Interestingly, these NSPCs have the morphological and ultrastructural characteristics of astrocytes, and express the mature astrocytic marker, glial fibrillary acidic protein (GFAP) (Doetsch et al. 1999; Imura et al. 2003; Laywell et al. 2000). For a review of the relationship between radial glia, astrocytic adult NSPCs and astrocytes see (Ihrie and Alvarez-Buylla 2007). Fiona Doetsch also provides a comprehensive review of the glial identity of neural stem cells, with particular emphasis on the relationships between the neuroepithelial, radial glial and astrocytic lineages (Doetsch 2003).

However, more recently, it has been shown that radial glia comprise the majority of precursors in the ventricular zones in most areas of the CNS, especially in the brain (Hartfuss et al. 2003; Hartfuss et al. 2001; Heins et al. 2002; Malatesta et al. 2003; Malatesta et al. 2000; Miyata et al. 2001; Noctor et al. 2001; Noctor et al. 2002; Tamamaki et al. 2001). Radial glia generate astrocytes and oligodendrocytes (Choi and Kim 1984; Hirano and

Goldman 1988), as well as neurons (Campbell and Gotz 2002; Hartfuss et al. 2001). Furthermore, it was shown that both radial glia in neonates and radial glia-derived cells in the adult lateral ventricle generate self-renewing multipotent neurospheres in vitro (Merkle et al. 2004). Based on this evidence, they concluded that radial glia act as progenitors for a large number of neurons and glia postnatally, as well as giving rise to NSPCs in the adult SVZ that contribute to ongoing neurogenesis into adulthood (Merkle et al. 2004).

This same group proved that adult ependymal cells, which have been previously suggested to function as NSPCs (Johansson et al. 1999), are in fact post-mitotic, and are produced during embryogenesis by radial glia (Malatesta et al. 2003; Spassky et al. 2005). Ependymal cells are ciliated cells that line the central canal of the spinal cord and the ventricular walls of the brain, and are thought to act as a barrier between the cerebrospinal fluid and the underlying parenchyma (Bruni 1998; Bruni and Reddy 1987). In lower vertebrates such as amphibians and lizards, the ependyma in the spinal cord plays a significant role in neuronal regeneration (Dervan and Roberts 2003; Egar and Singer 1972; Nordlander and Singer 1978; Simpson 1968; Simpson and Duffy 1994). In these animals, the ependymal cells of the transected spinal cord rapidly proliferate, migrate and differentiate to regenerate the cord. The proliferating ependymal cells extend long processes to guide the caudally regenerating central axons, and subsequently, these cells differentiate into neurons which send axons rostrally within the regenerated cord (Beattie et al. 1990; Michel and Reier 1979; Simpson and Duffy 1994).

In immature (Bruni and Anderson 1987; Gilmore and Leiting 1980) and adult (Adrian and Walker 1962; Bruni 1998; Horner et al. 2000; Kraus-Ruppert et al. 1975; Rakic and Sidman 1968) mammals, there is proliferative activity in the ependyma of the normal and injured spinal cord (Beattie et al. 1997; Matthews et al. 1979; Takahashi et al. 2003; Vaquero et al. 1981; Wallace et al. 1987). Frisen and others (Frisen et al. 1998; Frisen et al. 1995; Johansson et al. 1999) hypothesized that precursors exist around the central canal and that following SCI these cells undergo rapid proliferation (Johansson et al. 1999; Kojima and Tator 2002; Mothe and Tator 2005; Namiki and Tator 1999; Wallace et al. 1987), and differentiate mainly into astroyctes, which contribute to the formation of the glial scar in situ (Johansson et al. 1999). Electron microscopic (EM) observations have been made by Matthews et al. (1979) who described the relationship between regenerating axons and ependymal cells. Clusters of axons became engulfed by the ependymal cells, and in some instances, mesaxons were formed suggestive of an "attempt to support a regenerative process" (Matthews et al. 1979).

There is evidence that in the mouse brain, radial glia themselves give rise to ependymal cells during embryogenesis and that the ependymal cells do not divide in adulthood (Spassky et al. 2005). Under normal conditions, ependymal cells are not thought to be NSPCs (Chiasson et al. 1999; Johansson et al. 1999; Rietze et al. 2001).

During CNS development, precursor cells have similar biochemical and morphological characteristics. They are bipolar, with long processes and express the same intermediate filaments such as nestin and vimentin. Our laboratory found that adult rat spinal cord neurospheres express high levels of radial glia markers including nestin, RC1, 3CB2 and BLBP (Kulbatski et al. 2007). Our results also suggested that radial glia derived from the adult rat spinal cord function as guidance scaffolds in vitro, which suggests a recapitulation of their developmental role in vitro. This role may extend to reflect their capacity to act as progenitors for neurons and glia within the adult spinal cord, especially in light of the recent study by Merkle et al. (2004). Future lineage tracking studies would be useful to provide a definitive answer.

Our findings corroborate the work of Dromard and colleagues, who found that neurospheres derived from the embryonic and adult CNS are composed predominantly of cells that coexpress the radial glial markers GLAST, RC2, and BLBP and the oligodendrdoglial lineage markers PDGFR-alpha, NG2, and A2B5 (Dromard et al. 2007). These results (Dromard et al. 2007; Kulbatski et al. 2007) suggest that culture conditions can induce phenotypic changes in NSPCs. These were the first studies to demonstrate the radial glial potential for adult rat spinal cord NSPCs, although previous studies demonstrated such potential for human fetal brain NSPCs (Caldwell et al. 2001) and mouse embryonic and adult brain NSPCs (Gregg and Weiss 2003). Interestingly, phenotypic changes that favour the radial glial and/or oligodendroglial lineages may offer advantages for future transplantation trials for CNS repair, by providing a source of radial glia to guide neuronal migration and oligodendrocytes for remyelination of regenerating or spared axons.

RADIAL GLIA, NEURAL STEM/PRECURSORS AND THEIR PROGENY: IDENTIFICATION BY IMMUNOCYTOCHEMISTRY

The identification of radial glia, NSPCs, and their progeny by immunocytochemistry is essential to the understanding of their distribution and differentiation potential in both in vivo and in vitro studies. A wide variety of antigenic markers exist for identifying these various cell types. The identification of mature differentiated CNS cell types is largely based on immunocytochemical staining for neurons, astrocytes, and oligodendrocytes. Since the expression of the various cellular markers progresses in a temporal fashion as cellular differentiation and maturation occur, a particular cell type may co-express more than one marker at any given time. For example, astrocytes express nestin as well as glial-fibrillary acid protein (GFAP). Moreover, since astrocytes and radial glia share a common lineage, many of the radial glial markers such as RC1 and 3CB2 also label astrocytes and related precursor cell types such as NG2 positive glial precursors (Dromard et al. 2007; Edwards et al. 1990; Liu and Rao 2004).

Radial Glia

Among the immunocytochemical markers used to identify radial glia are glutamate transporter (GLAST) (Shibata et al. 1997), 3CB2 (Prada et al. 1995), RC1 (Edwards et al. 1990), RC2 (Misson et al. 1988), brain lipid binding protein (BLBP) (Feng et al. 1994), NG2 (Wu et al. 2005), glial fibrillary acidic protein (GFAP) (Dahl et al. 1985), vimentin (Pixley and de Vellis 1984; Yang et al. 1993), and nestin (Hockfield and McKay 1985). BLBP is an especially useful marker for radial glia since developmentally, radial glia express BLBP during neuronal migration, and BLBP transcription occurs in vitro in the presence of differentiating neurons (Feng et al. 1994; Feng and Heintz 1995). That is, BLBP expression in radial glia is specific to the presence of differentiating and/or migrating neurons.

Neural Stem/Precursor Cells

The intermediate filament protein, nestin, is the hallmark immunocytochemical marker used to identify NSPCs (Lendahl et al. 1990). During spinal cord development, nestin is observed in cells lining the central canal, and is progressively reduced with maturation (Tohyama et al. 1992). However, glial and neural precursor cells, immature and reactive astrocytes, and radial glia also express nestin, to an extent (Kornblum and Geschwind 2001; Lin et al. 1995; Menet et al. 2001). NSPCs are also identified with vimentin (Dahl 1981; Dahl et al. 1981).

Astrocytes

Astrocytes are the most abundant glial cells in the CNS, providing structural support for surrounding neurons, participating in the blood-brain barrier, and releasing a variety of neuronal growth factors (Svendsen 2002). In the adult brain, astrocytes influence neurogenesis by providing cues to undifferentiated cells to produce neuronal progeny, as well as regulating neural synaptic formation (Song et al. 2002; Ullian et al. 2001). The most common immunocytochemical marker for mature astrocytes is GFAP, whereas immature astrocytes are known to express nestin, as well as radial glial markers such as 3CB2 and RC1. The traditional view regarding the role of astrocytes following SCI is that they become reactive and contribute to the glial scar and an inhibitory environment for axonal regeneration (Fawcett 1997; Fawcett and Asher 1999; Matsui and Oohira 2004; Ribotta et al. 2004; Rudge and Silver 1990). However, astrocytes may also serve a variety of important roles such as regulating the immune response and blood-brain barrier, promoting oligodendrocyte remyelination, influencing the localized metabolism of glutamate (thereby reducing glutamate toxicity and secondary injury), and providing trophic support for surviving neurons (Sofroniew 2000).

Oligodendrocytes

As the myelin-forming cells of the CNS, oligodendrocytes play a crucial role in the conduction of the action potential. Myelin is an extension of the oligodendrocyte plasma membrane, and because it is composed of large amounts of lipids, it functions as an electrical insulator (Baumann and Pham-Dinh 2001). Among the markers used to identify oligodendrocytes is the regulator of phenobarbitol-inducible P450 (RIP), which identifies immature and mature non-myelinating oligodendrocytes, as well as mature myelinating oligodendrocytes. Another oligodendrocyte marker is myelin basic protein (MBP), which labels mature myelinating and non-myelinating oligodendrocytes (Baumann and Pham-Dinh

2001). Myelin and myelin-associated proteins, produced by oligodendrocytes, contain molecules that are inhibitory to axonal regeneration (Caroni et al. 1988; Caroni and Schwab 1988; Chen et al. 2000; Fournier et al. 2001; Horner and Gage 2000; McKerracher et al. 1994; Mukhopadhyay et al. 1994; Niederost et al. 1999; Schwab 1996; Schwab and Bartholdi 1996; Schwab and Caroni 1988; Schwab et al. 1993). Nevertheless, there is ample evidence to date that remyelination of surviving axons following SCI offers functional benefits, primarily by increasing axonal conduction and promoting survival of spared axons (Cloutier et al. 2006; Eftekharpour et al. 2007; Faulkner and Keirstead 2005; Karimi-Abdolrezaee et al. 2006; Keirstead 2005; Keirstead and Blakemore 1999; Keirstead et al. 2005; Nistor et al. 2005; Totoiu and Keirstead 2005; Totoiu et al. 2004).

Neurons

Although neurons in the embryonic and adult CNS are classified based on their morphology and function, there are certain markers that are ubiquitous neuronal markers, such as microtubule associated protein-2 (MAP2), beta-III-tubulin (β-IIII tubulin), and neurofilament (Ferreira and Caceres 1992; Geisert and Frankfurter 1989; Huneeus and Davison 1970). There is no evidence to date that replacement of injured neurons after SCI is a viable regenerative strategy in terms of restoration of function. One of the main reasons for this is that the adult CNS is inhibitory to axonal outgrowth, and therefore, transplanted neurons (or NSPCs/NRPs that differentiate into neurons) are unlikely to generate long axons and thus, are unlikely to make the correct connections. However, since it is possible to overcome this inhibition (Huber and Schwab 2000), and fetal neurons are not as sensitive to the adult CNS' inhibitory environment (Clowry et al. 1991; Reier et al. 1992; Reier et al. 1992; Tessler 1991), transplants of neurons or neuronal progeny may prove to be a viable option for enhancing axonal connectivity post-SCI. Replacement neurons may provide an intermediate relay-type synaptic connection for endogenous axons, or may act as a bridge across the injury site. Moreover, transplanted neurons or neuronal progeny may provide trophic support and/or molecules that regulate glial scarring and remyelination.

REGENERATIVE CAPACITY OF ENDOGENOUS RADIAL GLIA FOLLOWING ADULT CENTRAL NERVOUS SYSTEM INJURY

In most cases, radial glia are only present for as long as they function during CNS development, although some radial glia remain into adulthood (Liuzzi and Miller 1987; Schnitzer et al. 1981). In lower vertebrates in which there is continual neurogenesis into adulthood, such as birds and amphibians, radial glia are always present, contributing to neurogenesis, and playing a role in regeneration (Rosen et al. 1994). Widespread and robust neurogenesis occurs in the adult brain of amphibians (Polenov and Chetverukhin 1993), reptiles (Font et al. 2001; Garcia-Verdugo et al. 2002; Lopez-Garcia et al. 1988), fish (Birse et al. 1980; Raymond and Easter 1983; Raymond et al. 1983; Zupanc 1999; Zupanc and Ott 1999), and birds (Alvarez-Buylla 1990; Alvarez-Buylla et al. 1987; Goldman and Nottebohm

1983; Ling et al. 1997; Paton and Nottebohm 1984; Paton et al. 1985). The brain periventricular zones in these species contain a population of adult radial glia-like cells, which undergo mitotic divisions (Lopez-Garcia et al. 1988; Polenov et al. 1972). It is in this same region that adult neurons arise.

Radial glia have also been shown to play a vital role in CNS regeneration following SCI in salamanders and amphibians (Margotta et al. 1991), and cortical injury in reptiles (Font et al. 2001; Molowny et al. 1995). The regenerative capacity of radial glia has also been demonstrated in the adult amphibian telencephalon (Margotta et al. 1992), and the adult lizard hippocampus (Font et al. 2001; Lopez-Garcia et al. 1992). Zupanc and colleagues showed a correlation between the upregulation of somatostatin in radial glia and a profound increase in neurogenesis in the injured teleost fish brain (Zupanc and Clint 2001). This study implicates radial glia as mediators of neuronal regeneration. Similarly, Peterson and colleagues demonstrated that in the injured songbird hippocampus, radial glia are activated to upregulate aromatase, which is believed to stimulate neurogenesis via local estrogen production (Peterson et al. 2004).

It has been shown that following brain injury in the adult mouse, cortical astrocytes adopt a radial morphology, express radial glial markers, and these radial glia support the migration of neurons following injury (Leavitt et al. 1999). In the adult rat, radial glia emerge following SCI (Shibuya et al. 2003) and demyelinating lesions (Talbott et al. 2005), and likely play a role in neuronal regeneration. Most recently, Zhang and colleagues showed that in the adult rat brain, stroke induces proliferation of the ependymal cells of the lateral ventricle, and that these ependymal cells transform into radial glia, based on evidence that they possess the morphology, genotype, and phenotype of radial glia (Zhang et al. 2007). Moreover, the radial glia transformed from ependymal cells may contribute to post-ischemic neurogenesis in the adult brain, similar to their developmental role as a primary source of neurogenesis (Gotz and Barde 2005; Miyata et al. 2001; Noctor et al. 2001). With respect to cellular organization, Zhang et al. (2007) found that in the adult ischemic brain, single radial glial cells were surrounded by neuroblasts (neuronal progenitors), which is comparable to the organization during cortical neurogenesis, where groups of neuroblasts in the ventricular zone surround single radial glial cells (Bittman et al. 1997). Intriguingly, Zhang et al. (2007) demonstrated further that these radial glia also aid neuronal migration following brain ischemia. Taken together, their results strongly suggest a recapitulation of the developmental role of radial glia following brain injury in the adult.

ENHANCING THE ENDOGENOUS RADIAL GLIAL RESPONSE VERSUS TRANSPLANTATION OF RADIAL GLIA FOR CENTRAL NERVOUS SYSTEM REPAIR

It is still unclear whether the endogenous radial glial response to CNS injury in adult mammals can be stimulated to exert the same major beneficial regenerative effects as those in lower vertebrates. Although these cells in the adult mammalian CNS are stimulated to proliferate, differentiate, and guide neuronal migration after injury, it is clear that they are unable to reconstitute the normal cellular architecture of the mammalian CNS. The ineffectiveness of the endogenous response to regenerate the mammalian spinal cord indicates the potential for transplantation therapies using exogenously expanded radial glia. Studies of brain and spinal cord repair by transplanting radial glia in experimental animals have great relevance to patients with CNS injury who may not have sufficient endogenous NSPCs or appropriate endogenous radial glial activation to respond to stimulation by growth factors or pharmacological agents.

Augmentation of the Endogenous Radial Glia Response

The major advantage of augmenting the endogenous radial glial response to CNS injury is that it obviates the need for an external cell source. However, this response to trauma may be too weak and the number of cells too low for augmentation by external cues. Moreover, one of the major obstacles to implementing a therapeutic strategy based on enhancing the endogenous response lies in determining and administering the precise combination of molecular signals, in the appropriate sequence, and in the appropriate location needed to induce proliferation and differentiation of endogenous radial glia. This obstacle is compounded by the limited regional distribution of the endogenous radial glial/NSPC response. This is especially true in the case of TBI, since much of the endogenous response to injury arises from the cells in the subventricular zone and hippocampus.

Nevertheless, much work is being done to understand the basic mechanisms and signalling pathways that control the lineage fate of radial glia. Zheng and Feng (2006) examined the mechanisms that maintain the radial glial scaffold postnatally in the hippocampus of rats. In particular, they found that exogenous and endogenous Neuregulin (a member of the epidermal growth factor family of proteins) promote radial glial proliferation and maintain their morphology and antigenic properties, respectively (Zheng and Feng 2006). This study corroborated the work of Schmid and colleagues who found that Neuregulin signalling regulates the establishment of radial glia and their eventual transformation into astrocytes (Schmid et al. 2003). Furthermore, the Notch signalling pathway, which is known to influence cellular fate during mammalian CNS development, has been shown to influence radial glial formation (Dang et al. 2006; Patten et al. 2006). Maintenance of the radial glial phenotype can be achieved by persistent expression of stabilized beta-catenin (Wrobel et al. 2007), which delays radial glial maturation into intermediate progenitor cells. Conversely, BMP and LIF/CNTF promote radial glia lineage restriction into glial and neuronal restricted precursors (GRPs and NRPs) (Li and Grumet 2007), and chondroitin sulphate glycosaminoglycans have recently been implicated in promoting radial glial differentiation (Sirko et al. 2007).

Taken together, this literature suggests that regulation of the radial glial phenotype can be achieved by a diffusible factor and that the radial glial cell potential is amenable to control by extrinsic and intrinsic factors. As more basic studies yield information about the regulatory mechanisms that guide proliferation and differentiation of radial glia, therapies targeting such pathways may eventually be applied to in vivo experimental models for enhancing the endogenous radial glial response.

Transplantation of Radial Glia

Alternatively, radial glial transplantation therapies aim to restore or preserve neurological function post-injury by introducing a new population of cells that are capable of differentiating and reintegrating into the host tissue in a way that appropriately replaces lost neuronal tissue and function. Among the mechanisms that can account for such regenerative support are the ability of radial glia to proliferate as NSPCs, differentiate into neurons and glia, and guide neuronal and/or axonal elongation. Moreover, NSPCs are known to secrete a variety of growth factors (Lu et al. 2003) that may support myelination, neuroprotection, and regeneration of host tissue. Radial glia, in particular, have been shown to express high levels of IGF-1 immunoreactivity, which may promote neuronal recruitment from the adult songbird subventricular zone (Jiang et al. 1998). Collectively, these features may provide the opportunity for cellular reintegration into the host tissue in a manner that appropriately supports regeneration (Bjorklund and Lindvall 2000; Gates et al. 2000). The possible disadvantages of exogenous cell transplants include limited tissue availability, the need for immunosuppression, the risk of infection, the risk of tumorigenicity due to uncontrolled cellular proliferation, and impaired cell survival.

Radial glia can be isolated from embryonic, fetal, or neonatal CNS tissue (Caldwell et al. 2001; Espinosa-Jeffrey et al. 2002; Gregg and Weiss 2003; McMahon and McDermott 2007; Moreels et al. 2005; Pollard and Conti 2007; van der Pal et al. 1991), induced in culture from embryonic stem cells (Liour and Yu 2003; Pollard and Conti 2007) or adult NSPCs (Gregg and Weiss 2003; Kulbatski et al. 2007), or expanded from radial glia-like cell lines (Hasegawa et al. 2005; Hormigo et al. 2001; Pollard and Conti 2007).

To date, the literature on transplantation of radial glia for repair of CNS injury is minimal. Grumet and colleagues investigated the potential of the radial glia cell line C6-R to support neuronal migration in vivo post-transplantion. This cell line is derived from C6 gliomas and shows distinct characteristics of radial glia in vitro, namely the capacity to guide neuronal migration (Hormigo et al. 2001). Grumet and colleagues transplanted C6-R cells into the normal and injured brain and spinal cord together with embryonic neurons, and found that the radial glia promoted neuronal migration. This study serves as an important proof of principle that radial glial co-transplants may serve an important role in designing future studies of cellular transplants for CNS regeneration. Grumet and colleagues also isolated immortalized radial glial clones from the embryonic rat CNS (clone RG3.6) (Hasegawa et al. 2005). When transplanted into the contused adult rat spinal cord, the RG3.6 cells formed cellular bridges surrounding the lesion site and promoted functional recovery following SCI by protecting against secondary damage and activated macrophage accumulation (Hasegawa et al. 2005). More recently, McMahon and McDermott (2007) examined the developmental potential of embryonic spinal cord radial glia transplanted into the developing brain ventricular system. Their aim was to discern the influence of the local progenitor cell environment on the cell fate of transplanted radial glial progenitors. They found a correlation between the age of the host and the migration and differentiation of transplanted cells, in that the younger the host the farther the transplanted cells migrated and the later they differentiated (McMahon and McDermott 2007).

Our laboratory recently showed that when cultured in vitro, adult rat spinal cord derived NSPCs grown as neurospheres and differentiated as monolayers, exhibit the morphological and immunocytochemical characteristics of radial glia (Kulbatski et al. 2007). One of the hallmark characteristics of neurospheres is that plating them on an adhesive substrate initiates migration of cells out of the neurospheres, followed by their phenotypic differentiation into neurons, oligodendrocytes, and astrocytes. NSPCs migrate from neurospheres via chain migration (Jacques et al. 1998; Lois et al. 1996), and are guided by radial glial scaffolds in differentiating neurospheres from the embryonic rat (Espinosa-Jeffrey et al. 2002), mouse (Gregg and Weiss 2003), and fetal human brain (Caldwell et al. 2001), and mouse embryonic stem cell lines (Liour and Yu 2003). We showed for the first time that adult rat spinal cord neurospheres differentiate abundantly into radial glia, which may act as scaffolds to aid NSPC and/or neuronal migration.

Moreover, we found that dissociated neurospheres do not differentiate into this radial morphology, which provides support for the concept of transplantation of whole neurospheres rather than dissociated cells. Our laboratory recently found improved graft survival and integration into the injured rat spinal cord with whole versus dissociated neurosphere transplants (Mothe et al., submitted January 2007). While this is likely due to the positive influence of the neurosphere microenvironment on cell survival (i.e. cell-cell contact, neurotrophin secretion (Ourednik et al. 2002), the role of radial glia in guiding NSPC migration and axonal regeneration may be crucial, especially in light of the study by Hasegawa et al. (2005) which showed that embryonic rat radial glia transplanted into the injured rat spinal cord formed bridges and promoted functional recovery.

Conclusion

Alvarez-Buylla et al. (2001) proposed a unified hypothesis on the lineage of neural stem cells. They theorized that radial glia provide a link between the presence of NSPCs during brain development and in the adult brain. The persistence into adulthood of specialized astrocytes that retain contact with the ventricular wall is thought to occur via differentiation from radial glia postnatally. A niche is maintained within particular regions of the adult brain, allowing for the development and maintenance of a pool of adult NSPCs (Alvarez-Buylla et al. 2001). Such a theory provides context for the role of radial glia specifically, and glia, in general, in the developing and traumatized CNS. The application of radial glia as therapeutic transplants for CNS repair is still in its infancy. As new data emerges regarding the role of endogenous radial glia in the adult mammalian CNS, new therapies can be conceived and tested. Among such therapies are the co-transplantation of radial glia with other cells types such as NSPCs, and/or pharmacotherapy to augment the endogenous radial glial response to injury. An integrated approach such as this may maximize the innate potential of CNS radial glia to regenerate lost tissue and function following injury, thereby offering hope to millions of individuals living with the effects of CNS injury.

ACKNOWLEDGMENTS

Funding for this work was provided by grants from the Ontario Neurotrauma Foundation, Canadian Paraplegic Association (Ontario Branch), Physician's Services Incorporated, and the Christopher Reeve Paralysis Foundation (C.H. Tator). Personal support was provided by an Ontario Student Opportunity Trust Fund/Vision Sciences Scholarship and Sandra and David Smith Graduate Student Award (I. Kulbatski). We gratefully acknowledge Dr. A. Keating for providing us with the EGFP rats (originally generated by Dr. Kobayashi) for our studies.

REFERENCES

Adrian E, Walker B (1962) Incorporation of Thymidine-H3 by Cells in Normal and Injured Mouse Spinal Cord. *J. Neuropath. Exp. Neurol.* 21:597-609

Aloisi F, Giampaolo A, Russo G, Peschle C, Levi G (1992) Developmental appearance, antigenic profile, and proliferation of glial cells of the human embryonic spinal cord: an immunocytochemical study using dissociated cultured cells. *Glia.* 5:171-181

Alvarez-Buylla A (1990) Commitment and migration of young neurons in the vertebrate brain. *Experientia.* 46:879-882

Alvarez-Buylla A (1990) Mechanism of neurogenesis in adult avian brain. *Experientia.* 46:948-955

Alvarez-Buylla A, Buskirk DR, Nottebohm F (1987) Monoclonal antibody reveals radial glia in adult avian brain. *J. Comp. Neurol.* 264:159-170

Alvarez-Buylla A, Garcia-Verdugo JM (2002) Neurogenesis in adult subventricular zone. *J. Neurosci.* 22:629-634

Alvarez-Buylla A, Garcia-Verdugo JM, Tramontin AD (2001) A unified hypothesis on the lineage of neural stem cells. *Nat. Rev. Neurosci.* 2:287-293

Anthony TE, Klein C, Fishell G, Heintz N (2004) Radial glia serve as neuronal progenitors in all regions of the central nervous system. *Neuron.* 41:881-890

Barry D, McDermott K (2005) Differentiation of radial glia from radial precursor cells and transformation into astrocytes in the developing rat spinal cord. *Glia.* 50:187-197

Baumann N, Pham-Dinh D (2001) Biology of oligodendrocyte and myelin in the mammalian central nervous system. *Physiol. Rev.* 81:871-927

Beattie MS, Bresnahan JC, Komon J, Tovar CA, Van Meter M, Anderson DK, Faden AI, Hsu CY, Noble LJ, Salzman S, Young W (1997) Endogenous repair after spinal cord contusion injuries in the rat. *Exp. Neurol.* 148:453-463.

Beattie MS, Bresnahan JC, Lopate G (1990) Metamorphosis alters the response to spinal cord transection in Xenopus laevis frogs. *J. Neurobiol.* 21:1108-1122

Birse SC, Leonard RB, Coggeshall RE (1980) Neuronal increase in various areas of the nervous system of the guppy, Lebistes. *J. Comp. Neurol.* 194:291-301

Bittman K, Owens DF, Kriegstein AR, LoTurco JJ (1997) Cell coupling and uncoupling in the ventricular zone of developing neocortex. *J. Neurosci.* 17:7037-7044

Bjorklund A, Lindvall O (2000) Cell replacement therapies for central nervous system disorders. *Nat. Neurosci.* 3:537-544

Bonfanti L, Peretto P (2007) Radial glial origin of the adult neural stem cells in the subventricular zone. *Prog. Neurobiol.* 83:24-36

Bracken MB, Shepard MJ, Collins WF, Holford TR, Young W, Baskin DS, Eisenberg HM, Flamm E, Leo-Summers L, Maroon J, et al. (1990) A randomized, controlled trial of methylprednisolone or naloxone in the treatment of acute spinal-cord injury. Results of the Second National Acute Spinal Cord Injury Study. *N. Engl. J. Med.* 322:1405-1411.

Bruni JE (1998) Ependymal development, proliferation, and functions: a review. *Microsc. Res. Tech.* 41:2-13

Bruni JE, Anderson WA (1987) Ependyma of the rat fourth ventricle and central canal: response to injury. *Acta Anat.* (Basel) 128:265-273

Bruni JE, Reddy K (1987) Ependyma of the central canal of the rat spinal cord: a light and transmission electron microscopic study. *J. Anat.* 152:55-70

Brusco A, Gomez LA, Lopez EM, Tagliaferro P, Saavedra JP (1995) Relationship between glial organization and the establishment of nerve tracts in rat spinal cord. *Int. J. Neurosci.* 82:25-31

Caldwell MA, He X, Wilkie N, Pollack S, Marshall G, Wafford KA, Svendsen CN (2001) Growth factors regulate the survival and fate of cells derived from human neurospheres. *Nat. Biotechnol.* 19:475-479.

Caldwell MA, He X, Wilkie N, Pollack S, Marshall G, Wafford KA, Svendsen CN (2001) Growth factors regulate the survival and fate of cells derived from human neurospheres. *Nat. Biotechnol.* 19:475-479

Campbell K, Gotz M (2002) Radial glia: multi-purpose cells for vertebrate brain development. *Trends Neurosci.* 25:235-238

Caroni P, Savio T, Schwab ME (1988) Central nervous system regeneration: oligodendrocytes and myelin as non-permissive substrates for neurite growth. *Prog Brain. Res.* 78:363-370

Caroni P, Schwab ME (1988) Antibody against myelin-associated inhibitor of neurite growth neutralizes nonpermissive substrate properties of CNS white matter. *Neuron.* 1:85-96

Cepko CL, Austin CP, Walsh C, Ryder EF, Halliday A, Fields-Berry S (1990) Studies of cortical development using retrovirus vectors. *Cold Spring Harb. Symp. Quant. Biol.* 55:265-278

Chapouton P, Schuurmans C, Guillemot F, Gotz M (2001) The transcription factor neurogenin 2 restricts cell migration from the cortex to the striatum. *Development.* 128:5149-5159

Chen MS, Huber AB, van der Haar ME, Frank M, Schnell L, Spillmann AA, Christ F, Schwab ME (2000) Nogo-A is a myelin-associated neurite outgrowth inhibitor and an antigen for monoclonal antibody IN-1. *Nature.* 403:434-439

Chiasson BJ, Tropepe V, Morshead CM, van der Kooy D (1999) Adult mammalian forebrain ependymal and subependymal cells demonstrate proliferative potential, but only subependymal cells have neural stem cell characteristics. *J. Neurosci.* 19:4462-4471

Choi BH, Kim RC (1985) Expression of glial fibrillary acidic protein by immature oligodendroglia and its implications. *J. Neuroimmunol.* 8:215-235

Choi BH, Kim RC (1984) Expression of glial fibrillary acidic protein in immature oligodendroglia. *Science.* 223:407-409

Chuah MI, West AK (2002) Cellular and molecular biology of ensheathing cells. *Microsc. Res. Tech.* 58:216-227

Cloutier F, Siegenthaler MM, Nistor G, Keirstead HS (2006) Transplantation of human embryonic stem cell-derived oligodendrocyte progenitors into rat spinal cord injuries does not cause harm. *Regen. Med.* 1:469-479

Clowry G, Sieradzan K, Vrbova G (1991) Transplants of embryonic motoneurones to adult spinal cord: survival and innervation abilities. *Trends Neurosci.* 14:355-357

Craig CG, Tropepe V, Morshead CM, Reynolds BA, Weiss S, van der Kooy D (1996) In vivo growth factor expansion of endogenous subependymal neural precursor cell populations in the adult mouse brain. *J. Neurosci.* 16:2649-2658

Culican SM, Baumrind NL, Yamamoto M, Pearlman AL (1990) Cortical radial glia: identification in tissue culture and evidence for their transformation to astrocytes. *J. Neurosci.* 10:684-692

Dahl D (1981) The vimentin-GFA protein transition in rat neuroglia cytoskeleton occurs at the time of myelination. *J. Neurosci. Res.* 6:741-748

Dahl D, Crosby CJ, Sethi JS, Bignami A (1985) Glial fibrillary acidic (GFA) protein in vertebrates: immunofluorescence and immunoblotting study with monoclonal and polyclonal antibodies. *J. Comp. Neurol.* 239:75-88

Dahl D, Rueger DC, Bignami A, Weber K, Osborn M (1981) Vimentin, the 57 000 molecular weight protein of fibroblast filaments, is the major cytoskeletal component in immature glia. *Eur. J. Cell Biol.* 24:191-196

Dang L, Yoon K, Wang M, Gaiano N (2006) Notch3 signaling promotes radial glial/progenitor character in the mammalian telencephalon. *Dev. Neurosci.* 28:58-69

Davis AA, Temple S (1994) A self-renewing multipotential stem cell in embryonic rat cerebral cortex. *Nature.* 372:263-266

Dervan AG, Roberts BL (2003) Reaction of spinal cord central canal cells to cord transection and their contribution to cord regeneration. *J. Comp. Neurol.* 458:293-306

Diers-Fenger M, Kirchhoff F, Kettenmann H, Levine JM, Trotter J (2001) AN2/NG2 protein-expressing glial progenitor cells in the murine CNS: isolation, differentiation, and association with radial glia. *Glia.* 34:213-228

Doetsch F (2003) The glial identity of neural stem cells. *Nat. Neurosci.* 6:1127-1134

Doetsch F, Caille I, Lim DA, Garcia-Verdugo JM, Alvarez-Buylla A (1999) Subventricular zone astrocytes are neural stem cells in the adult mammalian brain. *Cell.* 97:703-716

Doppenberg EM, Bullock R (1997) Clinical neuro-protection trials in severe traumatic brain injury: lessons from previous studies. *J. Neurotrauma.* 14:71-80

Doucette R (1995) Olfactory ensheathing cells: potential for glial cell transplantation into areas of CNS injury. *Histol. Histopathol.* 10:503-507

Doucette R (1990) Glial influences on axonal growth in the primary olfactory system. *Glia.* 3:433-449

Dromard C, Bartolami S, Deleyrolle L, Takebayashi H, Ripoll C, Simonneau L, Prome S, Puech S, Tran VB, Duperray C, Valmier J, Privat A, Hugnot JP (2007) NG2 and Olig2 expression provides evidence for phenotypic deregulation of cultured central nervous system and peripheral nervous system neural precursor cells. *Stem Cells.* 25:340-353

Edwards MA, Yamamoto M, Caviness VS, Jr. (1990) Organization of radial glia and related cells in the developing murine CNS. An analysis based upon a new monoclonal antibody marker. *Neuroscience.* 36:121-144

Eftekharpour E, Karimi-Abdolrezaee S, Wang J, El Beheiry H, Morshead C, Fehlings MG (2007) Myelination of congenitally dysmyelinated spinal cord axons by adult neural precursor cells results in formation of nodes of Ranvier and improved axonal conduction. *J. Neurosci.* 27:3416-3428

Egar M, Singer M (1972) The role of ependyma in spinal cord regeneration in the urodele, Triturus. *Exp. Neurol.* 37:422-430

Espinosa-Jeffrey A, Becker-Catania SG, Zhao PM, Cole R, Edmond J, de Vellis J (2002) Selective specification of CNS stem cells into oligodendroglial or neuronal cell lineage: cell culture and transplant studies. *J. Neurosci. Res.* 69:810-825

Faulkner J, Keirstead HS (2005) Human embryonic stem cell-derived oligodendrocyte progenitors for the treatment of spinal cord injury. *Transpl. Immunol.* 15:131-142

Fawcett JW (1997) Astrocytic and neuronal factors affecting axon regeneration in the damaged central nervous system. *Cell Tissue Res.* 290:371-377

Fawcett JW, Asher RA (1999) The glial scar and central nervous system repair. *Brain Res. Bull.* 49:377-391.

Feng L, Hatten ME, Heintz N (1994) Brain lipid-binding protein (BLBP): a novel signaling system in the developing mammalian CNS. *Neuron.* 12:895-908

Feng L, Heintz N (1995) Differentiating neurons activate transcription of the brain lipid-binding protein gene in radial glia through a novel regulatory element. *Development.* 121:1719-1730

Ferreira A, Caceres A (1992) Expression of the class III beta-tubulin isotype in developing neurons in culture. *J. Neurosci. Res.* 32:516-529

Fogarty M, Richardson WD, Kessaris N (2005) A subset of oligodendrocytes generated from radial glia in the dorsal spinal cord. *Development.* 132:1951-1959

Font E, Desfilis E, Perez-Canellas MM, Garcia-Verdugo JM (2001) Neurogenesis and neuronal regeneration in the adult reptilian brain. *Brain Behav. Evol.* 58:276-295

Fournier AE, GrandPre T, Strittmatter SM (2001) Identification of a receptor mediating Nogo-66 inhibition of axonal regeneration. *Nature.* 409:341-346

Fricker-Gates RA (2006) Radial glia: a changing role in the central nervous system. *Neuroreport.* 17:1081-1084

Frisen J, Johansson CB, Lothian C, Lendahl U (1998) Central nervous system stem cells in the embryo and adult. *Cell Mol. Life Sci.* 54:935-945

Frisen J, Johansson CB, Torok C, Risling M, Lendahl U (1995) Rapid, widespread, and longlasting induction of nestin contributes to the generation of glial scar tissue after CNS injury. *J. Cell Biol.* 131:453-464

Gage FH (2000) Mammalian neural stem cells. *Science.* 287:1433-1438.

Gage FH, Coates PW, Palmer TD, Kuhn HG, Fisher LJ, Suhonen JO, Peterson DA, Suhr ST, Ray J (1995) Survival and differentiation of adult neuronal progenitor cells transplanted to the adult brain. *Proc. Natl. Acad. Sci. U. S. A.* 92:11879-11883

Gaiano N, Nye JS, Fishell G (2000) Radial glial identity is promoted by Notch1 signaling in the murine forebrain. *Neuron.* 26:395-404

Garcia-Verdugo JM, Ferron S, Flames N, Collado L, Desfilis E, Font E (2002) The proliferative ventricular zone in adult vertebrates: a comparative study using reptiles, birds, and mammals. *Brain Res. Bull.* 57:765-775

Gates MA, Fricker-Gates RA, Macklis JD (2000) Reconstruction of cortical circuitry. *Prog. Brain Res.* 127:115-156

Geisert EE, Jr., Frankfurter A (1989) The neuronal response to injury as visualized by immunostaining of class III beta-tubulin in the rat. *Neurosci. Lett.* 102:137-141

Geisler FH, Coleman WP, Grieco G, Poonian D (2001) The Sygen multicenter acute spinal cord injury study. *Spine.* 26:S87-98

Gensert JM, Goldman JE (1996) In vivo characterization of endogenous proliferating cells in adult rat subcortical white matter. *Glia.* 17:39-51

Gilmore SA, Leiting JE (1980) Changes in the central canal area of immature rats following spinal cord injury. *Brain Res.* 201:185-189

Goldman SA, Nottebohm F (1983) Neuronal production, migration, and differentiation in a vocal control nucleus of the adult female canary brain. *Proc. Natl. Acad. Sci. U. S. A.* 80:2390-2394

Gotz M (2003) Glial cells generate neurons--master control within CNS regions: developmental perspectives on neural stem cells. *Neuroscientist.* 9:379-397

Gotz M, Barde YA (2005) Radial glial cells defined and major intermediates between embryonic stem cells and CNS neurons. *Neuron.* 46:369-372

Gotz M, Huttner WB (2005) The cell biology of neurogenesis. *Nat. Rev. Mol. Cell Biol.* 6:777-788

Gregg C, Weiss S (2003) Generation of functional radial glial cells by embryonic and adult forebrain neural stem cells. *J. Neurosci.* 23:11587-11601

Gregori N, Proschel C, Noble M, Mayer-Proschel M (2002) The tripotential glial-restricted precursor (GRP) cell and glial development in the spinal cord: generation of bipotential oligodendrocyte-type-2 astrocyte progenitor cells and dorsal-ventral differences in GRP cell function. *J. Neurosci.* 22:248-256

Gritti A, Parati EA, Cova L, Frolichsthal P, Galli R, Wanke E, Faravelli L, Morassutti DJ, Roisen F, Nickel DD, Vescovi AL (1996) Multipotential stem cells from the adult mouse brain proliferate and self-renew in response to basic fibroblast growth factor. *J. Neurosci.* 16:1091-1100

Halliday AL, Cepko CL (1992) Generation and migration of cells in the developing striatum. *Neuron.* 9:15-26

Han SS, Liu Y, Tyler-Polsz C, Rao MS, Fischer I (2004) Transplantation of glial-restricted precursor cells into the adult spinal cord: survival, glial-specific differentiation, and preferential migration in white matter. *Glia.* 45:1-16

Hartfuss E, Forster E, Bock HH, Hack MA, Leprince P, Luque JM, Herz J, Frotscher M, Gotz M (2003) Reelin signaling directly affects radial glia morphology and biochemical maturation. *Development.* 130:4597-4609

Hartfuss E, Galli R, Heins N, Gotz M (2001) Characterization of CNS precursor subtypes and radial glia. *Dev. Biol.* 229:15-30

Hasegawa K, Chang YW, Li H, Berlin Y, Ikeda O, Kane-Goldsmith N, Grumet M (2005) Embryonic radial glia bridge spinal cord lesions and promote functional recovery following spinal cord injury. *Exp. Neurol.* 193:394-410

Hatten ME (1999) Central nervous system neuronal migration. *Annu. Rev. Neurosci.* 22:511-539

Heins N, Malatesta P, Cecconi F, Nakafuku M, Tucker KL, Hack MA, Chapouton P, Barde YA, Gotz M (2002) Glial cells generate neurons: the role of the transcription factor Pax6. *Nat. Neurosci.* 5:308-315

Hirano M, Goldman JE (1988) Gliogenesis in rat spinal cord: evidence for origin of astrocytes and oligodendrocytes from radial precursors. *J. Neurosci. Res.* 21:155-167

Hockfield S, McKay RD (1985) Identification of major cell classes in the developing mammalian nervous system. *J. Neurosci.* 5:3310-3328

Hormigo A, McCarthy M, Nothias JM, Hasegawa K, Huang W, Friedlander DR, Fischer I, Fishell G, Grumet M (2001) Radial glial cell line C6-R integrates preferentially in adult white matter and facilitates migration of coimplanted neurons in vivo. *Exp. Neurol.* 168:310-322

Horner PJ, Gage FH (2000) Regenerating the damaged central nervous system. *Nature.* 407:963-970

Horner PJ, Power AE, Kempermann G, Kuhn HG, Palmer TD, Winkler J, Thal LJ, Gage FH (2000) Proliferation and differentiation of progenitor cells throughout the intact adult rat spinal cord. *J. Neurosci.* 20:2218-2228.

Huber AB, Schwab ME (2000) Nogo-A, a potent inhibitor of neurite outgrowth and regeneration. *Biol. Chem.* 381:407-419

Huneeus FC, Davison PF (1970) Fibrillar proteins from squid axons. I. Neurofilament protein. *J. Mol. Biol.* 52:415-428

Ihrie RA, Alvarez-Buylla A (2007) Cells in the astroglial lineage are neural stem cells. *Cell. Tissue Res*

Imura T, Kornblum HI, Sofroniew MV (2003) The predominant neural stem cell isolated from postnatal and adult forebrain but not early embryonic forebrain expresses GFAP. *J. Neurosci.* 23:2824-2832

Jacques TS, Relvas JB, Nishimura S, Pytela R, Edwards GM, Streuli CH, ffrench-Constant C (1998) Neural precursor cell chain migration and division are regulated through different beta1 integrins. *Development.* 125:3167-3177

Jiang J, McMurtry J, Niedzwiecki D, Goldman SA (1998) Insulin-like growth factor-1 is a radial cell-associated neurotrophin that promotes neuronal recruitment from the adult songbird edpendyma/subependyma. *J. Neurobiol.* 36:1-15

Johansson CB, Momma S, Clarke DL, Risling M, Lendahl U, Frisen J (1999) Identification of a neural stem cell in the adult mammalian central nervous system. *Cell.* 96:25-34

Johe KK, Hazel TG, Muller T, Dugich-Djordjevic MM, McKay RD (1996) Single factors direct the differentiation of stem cells from the fetal and adult central nervous system. *Genes Dev.* 10:3129-3140

Joosten EA, Gribnau AA (1989) Astrocytes and guidance of outgrowing corticospinal tract axons in the rat. An immunocytochemical study using anti-vimentin and anti-glial fibrillary acidic protein. *Neuroscience.* 31:439-452

Joosten EA, Gribnau AA, Dederen PJ (1989) Postnatal development of the corticospinal tract in the rat. An ultrastructural anterograde HRP study. *Anat. Embryol.* (Berl) 179:449-456

Karimi-Abdolrezaee S, Eftekharpour E, Wang J, Morshead CM, Fehlings MG (2006) Delayed transplantation of adult neural precursor cells promotes remyelination and functional neurological recovery after spinal cord injury. *J. Neurosci.* 26:3377-3389

Kehl LJ, Fairbanks CA, Laughlin TM, Wilcox GL (1997) Neurogenesis in postnatal rat spinal cord: a study in primary culture. *Science.* 276:586-589

Keirstead HS (2005) Stem cells for the treatment of myelin loss. *Trends Neurosci.* 28:677-683

Keirstead HS, Blakemore WF (1999) The role of oligodendrocytes and oligodendrocyte progenitors in CNS remyelination. *Adv. Exp. Med. Biol.* 468:183-197

Keirstead HS, Nistor G, Bernal G, Totoiu M, Cloutier F, Sharp K, Steward O (2005) Human embryonic stem cell-derived oligodendrocyte progenitor cell transplants remyelinate and restore locomotion after spinal cord injury. *J. Neurosci.* 25:4694-4705

Kojima A, Tator C (2002) Intrathecal administration of Epidermal growth Factor and Fibroblast Growth Factor 2 Promotes Ependymal Proliferation and Functional Recovery after Spinal Cord Injury in Adult Rats. *Journal of Neurotrauma.* 19:223-238

Kornblum HI, Geschwind DH (2001) Molecular markers in CNS stem cell research: hitting a moving target. *Nat. Rev. Neurosci.* 2:843-846

Kraus-Ruppert R, Laissue J, Burki H, Odartchenko N (1975) Kinetic studies on glial, Schwann and capsular cells labelled with [3H] thymidine in cerebrospinal tissue of young mice. *J. Neurol. Sci.* 26:555-563

Kuhn HG, Winkler J, Kempermann G, Thal LJ, Gage FH (1997) Epidermal growth factor and fibroblast growth factor-2 have different effects on neural progenitors in the adult rat brain. *J. Neurosci.* 17:5820-5829

Kulbatski I, Mothe AJ, Keating A, Hakamata Y, Kobayashi E, Tator CH (2007) Oligodendrocytes and radial glia derived from adult rat spinal cord progenitors: morphological and immunocytochemical characterization. *J. Histochem. Cytochem.* 55:209-222

Kulbatski I, Mothe AJ, Nomura H, Tator CH (2005) Endogenous and exogenous CNS derived stem/progenitor cell approaches for neurotrauma. *Curr. Drug Targets.* 6:111-126

Laywell ED, Rakic P, Kukekov VG, Holland EC, Steindler DA (2000) Identification of a multipotent astrocytic stem cell in the immature and adult mouse brain. *Proc. Natl. Acad. Sci. U. S. A.* 97:13883-13888

Leavitt BR, Hernit-Grant CS, Macklis JD (1999) Mature astrocytes transform into transitional radial glia within adult mouse neocortex that supports directed migration of transplanted immature neurons. *Exp. Neurol.* 157:43-57

Lendahl U, Zimmerman LB, McKay RD (1990) CNS stem cells express a new class of intermediate filament protein. *Cell.* 60:585-595

Lepore AC, Fischer I (2005) Lineage-restricted neural precursors survive, migrate, and differentiate following transplantation into the injured adult spinal cord. *Exp. Neurol.* 194:230-242

Lepore AC, Han SS, Tyler-Polsz CJ, Cai J, Rao MS, Fischer I (2004) Differential fate of multipotent and lineage-restricted neural precursors following transplantation into the adult CNS. *Neuron. Glia Biol.* 1:113-126

Lepore AC, Neuhuber B, Connors TM, Han SS, Liu Y, Daniels MP, Rao MS, Fischer I (2006) Long-term fate of neural precursor cells following transplantation into developing and adult CNS. *Neuroscience.* 142:287-304

Levison SW, Goldman JE (1993) Both oligodendrocytes and astrocytes develop from progenitors in the subventricular zone of postnatal rat forebrain. *Neuron.* 10:201-212

Li H, Grumet M (2007) BMP and LIF signaling coordinately regulate lineage restriction of radial glia in the developing forebrain. *Glia.* 55:24-35

Lin RC, Matesic DF, Marvin M, McKay RD, Brustle O (1995) Re-expression of the intermediate filament nestin in reactive astrocytes. *Neurobiol. Dis.* 2:79-85

Ling C, Zuo M, Alvarez-Buylla A, Cheng MF (1997) Neurogenesis in juvenile and adult ring doves. *J. Comp. Neurol.* 379:300-312

Liour SS, Yu RK (2003) Differentiation of radial glia-like cells from embryonic stem cells. *Glia.* 42:109-117

Liu Y, Rao MS (2004) Olig genes are expressed in a heterogeneous population of precursor cells in the developing spinal cord. *Glia.* 45:67-74

Liuzzi FJ, Miller RH (1987) Radially oriented astrocytes in the normal adult rat spinal cord. *Brain Res.* 403:385-388

Lois C, Alvarez-Buylla A (1994) Long-distance neuronal migration in the adult mammalian brain. *Science.* 264:1145-1148

Lois C, Garcia-Verdugo JM, Alvarez-Buylla A (1996) Chain migration of neuronal precursors. *Science.* 271:978-981

Lopez-Garcia C, Molowny A, Garcia-Verdugo JM, Ferrer I (1988) Delayed postnatal neurogenesis in the cerebral cortex of lizards. *Brain Res.* 471:167-174

Lopez-Garcia C, Molowny A, Martinez-Guijarro FJ, Blasco-Ibanez JM, Luis de la Iglesia JA, Bernabeu A, Garcia-Verdugo JM (1992) Lesion and regeneration in the medial cerebral cortex of lizards. *Histol. Histopathol.* 7:725-746

Lu P, Jones LL, Snyder EY, Tuszynski MH (2003) Neural stem cells constitutively secrete neurotrophic factors and promote extensive host axonal growth after spinal cord injury. *Exp. Neurol.* 181:115-129

Luskin MB, Parnavelas JG, Barfield JA (1993) Neurons, astrocytes, and oligodendrocytes of the rat cerebral cortex originate from separate progenitor cells: an ultrastructural analysis of clonally related cells. *J. Neurosci.* 13:1730-1750

Maas AI (2001) Neuroprotective agents in traumatic brain injury. *Expert Opin. Investig. Drugs.* 10:753-767

Maas AI, Marmarou A, Murray GD, Steyerberg EW (2004) Clinical trials in traumatic brain injury: current problems and future solutions. *Acta Neurochir. Suppl.* 89:113-118

Malatesta P, Appolloni I, Calzolari F (2007) Radial glia and neural stem cells. *Cell Tissue Res.*

Malatesta P, Hack MA, Hartfuss E, Kettenmann H, Klinkert W, Kirchhoff F, Gotz M (2003) Neuronal or glial progeny: regional differences in radial glia fate. *Neuron.* 37:751-764

Malatesta P, Hartfuss E, Gotz M (2000) Isolation of radial glial cells by fluorescent-activated cell sorting reveals a neuronal lineage. *Development.* 127:5253-5263

Margotta V, Filoni S, Del Vecchio P (1992) Degenerative and regenerative phenomena in brain heterotopic homoplastic transplants of adult Triturus carnifex (Urodele Amphibians). *J. Hirnforsch.* 33:3-9

Margotta V, Fonti R, Palladini G, Filoni S, Lauro GM (1991) Transient expression of glial-fibrillary acidic protein (GFAP) in the ependyma of the regenerating spinal cord in adult newts. *J. Hirnforsch.* 32:485-490

Martens DJ, Seaberg RM, van der Kooy D (2002) In vivo infusions of exogenous growth factors into the fourth ventricle of the adult mouse brain increase the proliferation of neural progenitors around the fourth ventricle and the central canal of the spinal cord. *Eur. J. Neurosci.* 16:1045-1057

Martens DJ, Tropepe V, van Der Kooy D (2000) Separate proliferation kinetics of fibroblast growth factor-responsive and epidermal growth factor-responsive neural stem cells within the embryonic forebrain germinal zone. *J. Neurosci.* 20:1085-1095

Matsui F, Oohira A (2004) Proteoglycans and injury of the central nervous system. *Congenit. Anom.* (Kyoto) 44:181-188

Matthews MA, St Onge MF, Faciane CL (1979) An electron microscopic analysis of abnormal ependymal cell proliferation and envelopment of sprouting axons following spinal cord transection in the rat. *Acta Neuropathol.* (Berl) 45:27-36

McArthur DL, Chute DJ, Villablanca JP (2004) Moderate and severe traumatic brain injury: epidemiologic, imaging and neuropathologic perspectives. *Brain Pathol.* 14:185-194

McDermott KW, Barry DS, McMahon SS (2005) Role of radial glia in cytogenesis, patterning and boundary formation in the developing spinal cord. *J. Anat.* 207:241-250

McKay R (1997) Stem cells in the central nervous system. *Science.* 276:66-71

McKerracher L, David S, Jackson DL, Kottis V, Dunn RJ, Braun PE (1994) Identification of myelin-associated glycoprotein as a major myelin-derived inhibitor of neurite growth. *Neuron.* 13:805-811

McMahon SS, McDermott KW (2007) Developmental potential of radial glia investigated by transplantation into the developing rat ventricular system in utero. *Exp. Neurol.* 203:128-136

McMahon SS, McDermott KW (2002) Morphology and differentiation of radial glia in the developing rat spinal cord. *J. Comp. Neurol.* 454:263-271

Menet V, Gimenez y Ribotta M, Chauvet N, Drian MJ, Lannoy J, Colucci-Guyon E, Privat A (2001) Inactivation of the glial fibrillary acidic protein gene, but not that of vimentin, improves neuronal survival and neurite growth by modifying adhesion molecule expression. *J. Neurosci.* 21:6147-6158

Merkle FT, Tramontin AD, Garcia-Verdugo JM, Alvarez-Buylla A (2004) Radial glia give rise to adult neural stem cells in the subventricular zone. *Proc. Natl. Acad. Sci. U. S. A.* 101:17528-17532

Michel ME, Reier PJ (1979) Axonal-ependymal associations during early regeneration of the transected spinal cord in Xenopus laevis tadpoles. *J. Neurocytol.* 8:529-548

Miller RH, Dinsio K, Wang R, Geertman R, Maier CE, Hall AK (2004) Patterning of spinal cord oligodendrocyte development by dorsally derived BMP4. *J. Neurosci. Res.* 76:9-19

Misson JP, Austin CP, Takahashi T, Cepko CL, Caviness VS, Jr. (1991) The alignment of migrating neural cells in relation to the murine neopallial radial glial fiber system. *Cereb. Cortex.* 1:221-229

Misson JP, Edwards MA, Yamamoto M, Caviness VS, Jr. (1988) Identification of radial glial cells within the developing murine central nervous system: studies based upon a new immunohistochemical marker. *Brain Res. Dev. Brain Res.* 44:95-108

Misson JP, Edwards MA, Yamamoto M, Caviness VS, Jr. (1988) Mitotic cycling of radial glial cells of the fetal murine cerebral wall: a combined autoradiographic and immunohistochemical study. *Brain Res.* 466:183-190

Miyata T, Kawaguchi A, Okano H, Ogawa M (2001) Asymmetric inheritance of radial glial fibers by cortical neurons. *Neuron.* 31:727-741

Molowny A, Nacher J, Lopez-Garcia C (1995) Reactive neurogenesis during regeneration of the lesioned medial cerebral cortex of lizards. *Neuroscience.* 68:823-836

Moreels M, Vandenabeele F, Deryck L, Lambrichts I (2005) Radial glial cells derived from the neonatal rat spinal cord: morphological and immunocytochemical characterization. *Arch. Histol. Cytol.* 68:361-369

Morshead CM, Reynolds BA, Craig CG, McBurney MW, Staines WA, Morassutti D, Weiss S, van der Kooy D (1994) Neural stem cells in the adult mammalian forebrain: a relatively quiescent subpopulation of subependymal cells. *Neuron.* 13:1071-1082

Mothe AJ, Tator CH (2005) Proliferation, migration, and differentiation of endogenous ependymal region stem/progenitor cells following minimal spinal cord injury in the adult rat. *Neuroscience.* 131:177-187

Mukhopadhyay G, Doherty P, Walsh FS, Crocker PR, Filbin MT (1994) A novel role for myelin-associated glycoprotein as an inhibitor of axonal regeneration. *Neuron.* 13:757-767

Namiki J, Tator CH (1999) Cell proliferation and nestin expression in the ependyma of the adult rat spinal cord after injury. *J. Neuropathol. Exp. Neurol.* 58:489-498.

Niederost BP, Zimmermann DR, Schwab ME, Bandtlow CE (1999) Bovine CNS myelin contains neurite growth-inhibitory activity associated with chondroitin sulfate proteoglycans. *J. Neurosci.* 19:8979-8989

Nistor GI, Totoiu MO, Haque N, Carpenter MK, Keirstead HS (2005) Human embryonic stem cells differentiate into oligodendrocytes in high purity and myelinate after spinal cord transplantation. *Glia.* 49:385-396

Noctor SC, Flint AC, Weissman TA, Dammerman RS, Kriegstein AR (2001) Neurons derived from radial glial cells establish radial units in neocortex. *Nature.* 409:714-720

Noctor SC, Flint AC, Weissman TA, Wong WS, Clinton BK, Kriegstein AR (2002) Dividing precursor cells of the embryonic cortical ventricular zone have morphological and molecular characteristics of radial glia. *J. Neurosci.* 22:3161-3173

Nordlander RH, Singer M (1978) The role of ependyma in regeneration of the spinal cord in the urodele amphibian tail. *J. Comp. Neurol.* 180:349-374

O'Rourke NA, Dailey ME, Smith SJ, McConnell SK (1992) Diverse migratory pathways in the developing cerebral cortex. *Science.* 258:299-302

Ourednik J, Ourednik V, Lynch WP, Schachner M, Snyder EY (2002) Neural stem cells display an inherent mechanism for rescuing dysfunctional neurons. *Nat. Biotechnol.* 20:1103-1110

Paton JA, Nottebohm FN (1984) Neurons generated in the adult brain are recruited into functional circuits. *Science.* 225:1046-1048

Paton JA, O'Loughlin BE, Nottebohm F (1985) Cells born in adult canary forebrain are local interneurons. *J. Neurosci.* 5:3088-3093

Patten BA, Sardi SP, Koirala S, Nakafuku M, Corfas G (2006) Notch1 signaling regulates radial glia differentiation through multiple transcriptional mechanisms. *J. Neurosci.* 26:3102-3108

Peterson RS, Lee DW, Fernando G, Schlinger BA (2004) Radial glia express aromatase in the injured zebra finch brain. *J. Comp. Neurol.* 475:261-269

Pixley SK, de Vellis J (1984) Transition between immature radial glia and mature astrocytes studied with a monoclonal antibody to vimentin. *Brain Res.* 317:201-209

Polenov AL, Chetverukhin VK (1993) Ultrastructural radioautographic analysis of neurogenesis in the hypothalamus of the adult frog, Rana temporaria, with special reference to physiological regeneration of the preoptic nucleus. II. Types of neuronal cells produced. *Cell Tissue Res.* 271:351-362

Polenov AL, Chetverukhin VK, Jakovleva IV (1972) The role of the ependyma of the recessus praeopticus in formation and the physiological regeneration of the nucleus praeopticus in lower vertebrates. *Z. Mikrosk. Anat. Forsch.* 85:513-532

Pollard SM, Conti L (2007) Investigating radial glia in vitro. *Prog. Neurobiol.* 83:53-67

Prada FA, Dorado ME, Quesada A, Prada C, Schwarz U, de la Rosa EJ (1995) Early expression of a novel radial glia antigen in the chick embryo. *Glia.* 15:389-400

Rakic P, Sidman RL (1968) Subcommissural organ and adjacent ependyma: autoradiographic study of their origin in the mouse brain. *Am. J. Anat.* 122:317-335

Raymond PA, Easter SS, Jr. (1983) Postembryonic growth of the optic tectum in goldfish. I. Location of germinal cells and numbers of neurons produced. *J. Neurosci.* 3:1077-1091

Raymond PA, Easter SS, Jr., Burnham JA, Powers MK (1983) Postembryonic growth of the optic tectum in goldfish. II. Modulation of cell proliferation by retinal fiber input. *J. Neurosci.* 3:1092-1099

Reier PJ, Anderson DK, Thompson FJ, Stokes BT (1992) Neural tissue transplantation and CNS trauma: anatomical and functional repair of the injured spinal cord. *J. Neurotrauma.* 9 Suppl 1:S223-248

Reier PJ, Stokes BT, Thompson FJ, Anderson DK (1992) Fetal cell grafts into resection and contusion/compression injuries of the rat and cat spinal cord. *Exp. Neurol.* 115:177-188

Reynolds BA, Weiss S (1992) Generation of neurons and astrocytes from isolated cells of the adult mammalian central nervous system. *Science.* 255:1707-1710

Ribotta MG, Menet V, Privat A (2004) Glial scar and axonal regeneration in the CNS: lessons from GFAP and vimentin transgenic mice. *Acta Neurochir. Suppl.* 89:87-92

Richards LJ, Kilpatrick TJ, Bartlett PF (1992) De novo generation of neuronal cells from the adult mouse brain. *Proc. Natl. Acad. Sci. U. S. A.* 89:8591-8595

Rietze R, Poulin P, Weiss S (2000) Mitotically active cells that generate neurons and astrocytes are present in multiple regions of the adult mouse hippocampus. *J. Comp. Neurol.* 424:397-408

Rietze RL, Valcanis H, Brooker GF, Thomas T, Voss AK, Bartlett PF (2001) Purification of a pluripotent neural stem cell from the adult mouse brain. *Nature.* 412:736-739

Rosen GD, Sherman GF, Galaburda AM (1994) Radial glia in the neocortex of adult rats: effects of neonatal brain injury. *Brain Res. Dev. Brain Res.* 82:127-135

Rudge JS, Silver J (1990) Inhibition of neurite outgrowth on astroglial scars in vitro. *J. Neurosci.* 10:3594-3603

Scheffler B, Horn M, Blumcke I, Laywell ED, Coomes D, Kukekov VG, Steindler DA (1999) Marrow-mindedness: a perspective on neuropoiesis. *Trends Neurosci.* 22:348-357

Schmechel DE, Rakic P (1979) Arrested proliferation of radial glial cells during midgestation in rhesus monkey. *Nature.* 277:303-305

Schmechel DE, Rakic P (1979) A Golgi study of radial glial cells in developing monkey telencephalon: morphogenesis and transformation into astrocytes. *Anat. Embryol.* (Berl) 156:115-152

Schmid RS, McGrath B, Berechid BE, Boyles B, Marchionni M, Sestan N, Anton ES (2003) Neuregulin 1-erbB2 signaling is required for the establishment of radial glia and their transformation into astrocytes in cerebral cortex. *Proc. Natl. Acad. Sci. U. S. A.* 100:4251-4256

Schnitzer J, Franke WW, Schachner M (1981) Immunocytochemical demonstration of vimentin in astrocytes and ependymal cells of developing and adult mouse nervous system. *J. Cell. Biol.* 90:435-447

Schwab ME (1996) Molecules inhibiting neurite growth: a minireview. *Neurochem. Res.* 21:755-761

Schwab ME, Bartholdi D (1996) Degeneration and regeneration of axons in the lesioned spinal cord. *Physiol. Rev.* 76:319-370

Schwab ME, Caroni P (1988) Oligodendrocytes and CNS myelin are nonpermissive substrates for neurite growth and fibroblast spreading in vitro. *J. Neurosci.* 8:2381-2393

Schwab ME, Kapfhammer JP, Bandtlow CE (1993) Inhibitors of neurite growth. *Annu. Rev. Neurosci.* 16:565-595

Shibata T, Yamada K, Watanabe M, Ikenaka K, Wada K, Tanaka K, Inoue Y (1997) Glutamate transporter GLAST is expressed in the radial glia-astrocyte lineage of developing mouse spinal cord. *J. Neurosci.* 17:9212-9219

Shibuya S, Miyamoto O, Itano T, Mori S, Norimatsu H (2003) Temporal progressive antigen expression in radial glia after contusive spinal cord injury in adult rats. *Glia.* 42:172-183

Shihabuddin LS (2002) Adult rodent spinal cord derived neural stem cells. Isolation and characterization. *Methods Mol. Biol.* 198:67-77

Shihabuddin LS, Horner PJ, Ray J, Gage FH (2000) Adult spinal cord stem cells generate neurons after transplantation in the adult dentate gyrus. *J. Neurosci.* 20:8727-8735.

Shihabuddin LS, Ray J, Gage FH (1997) FGF-2 is sufficient to isolate progenitors found in the adult mammalian spinal cord. *Exp. Neurol.* 148:577-586

Simpson SB, Jr. (1968) Morphology of the regenerated spinal cord in the lizard, Anolis carolinensis. *J. Comp. Neurol.* 134:193-210

Simpson SB, Jr., Duffy MT (1994) The lizard spinal cord: a model system for the study of spinal cord injury and repair. *Prog. Brain Res.* 103:229-241

Sirko S, von Holst A, Wizenmann A, Gotz M, Faissner A (2007) Chondroitin sulfate glycosaminoglycans control proliferation, radial glia cell differentiation and neurogenesis in neural stem/progenitor cells. *Development.* 134:2727-2738

Sofroniew MV (2000) Astrocyte failure as a cause of CNS dysfunction. *Mol. Psychiatry.* 5:230-232

Song H, Stevens CF, Gage FH (2002) Astroglia induce neurogenesis from adult neural stem cells. *Nature.* 417:39-44

Spassky N, Merkle FT, Flames N, Tramontin AD, Garcia-Verdugo JM, Alvarez-Buylla A (2005) Adult ependymal cells are postmitotic and are derived from radial glial cells during embryogenesis. *J. Neurosci.* 25:10-18

Stagaard M, Mollgard K (1989) The developing neuroepithelium in human embryonic and fetal brain studied with vimentin-immunocytochemistry. *Anat. Embryol.* (Berl) 180:17-28

Svendsen CN (2002) The amazing astrocyte. *Nature.* 417:29-32

Takahashi M, Arai Y, Kurosawa H, Sueyoshi N, Shirai S (2003) Ependymal cell reactions in spinal cord segments after compression injury in adult rat. *J. Neuropathol. Exp. Neurol.* 62:185-194

Talbott JF, Loy DN, Liu Y, Qiu MS, Bunge MB, Rao MS, Whittemore SR (2005) Endogenous Nkx2.2+/Olig2+ oligodendrocyte precursor cells fail to remyelinate the demyelinated adult rat spinal cord in the absence of astrocytes. *Exp. Neurol.* 192:11-24

Tamamaki N, Nakamura K, Okamoto K, Kaneko T (2001) Radial glia is a progenitor of neocortical neurons in the developing cerebral cortex. *Neurosci. Res.* 41:51-60

Tator C (1995) Epidemiology and General Characteristics of the Spinal Cord Injury Patient. In Benzel E, C.H.Tator, eds. Contemporary Management of Spinal Cord Injury. Park Ridge, Illinois, American Association Of Neurological Surgeons, 9-13

Tator CH (2006) Review of treatment trials in human spinal cord injury: issues, difficulties, and recommendations. *Neurosurgery.* 59:957-982; discussion 982-957

Temple S (2001) The development of neural stem cells. *Nature.* 414:112-117

Temple S, Alvarez-Buylla A (1999) Stem cells in the adult mammalian central nervous system. *Curr. Opin. Neurobiol.* 9:135-141

Tessier-Lavigne M, Placzek M, Lumsden AG, Dodd J, Jessell TM (1988) Chemotropic guidance of developing axons in the mammalian central nervous system. *Nature.* 336:775-778

Tessler A (1991) Intraspinal transplants. *Ann. Neurol.* 29:115-123

Tohyama T, Lee VM, Rorke LB, Marvin M, McKay RD, Trojanowski JQ (1992) Nestin expression in embryonic human neuroepithelium and in human neuroepithelial tumor cells. *Lab. Invest.* 66:303-313

Toresson H, Mata de Urquiza A, Fagerstrom C, Perlmann T, Campbell K (1999) Retinoids are produced by glia in the lateral ganglionic eminence and regulate striatal neuron differentiation. *Development.* 126:1317-1326

Totoiu MO, Keirstead HS (2005) Spinal cord injury is accompanied by chronic progressive demyelination. *J. Comp. Neurol.* 486:373-383

Totoiu MO, Nistor GI, Lane TE, Keirstead HS (2004) Remyelination, axonal sparing, and locomotor recovery following transplantation of glial-committed progenitor cells into the MHV model of multiple sclerosis. *Exp. Neurol.* 187:254-265

Tropepe V, Craig CG, Morshead CM, van der Kooy D (1997) Transforming growth factor-alpha null and senescent mice show decreased neural progenitor cell proliferation in the forebrain subependyma. *J. Neurosci.* 17:7850-7859

Tropepe V, Hitoshi S, Sirard C, Mak TW, Rossant J, van der Kooy D (2001) Direct neural fate specification from embryonic stem cells: a primitive mammalian neural stem cell stage acquired through a default mechanism. *Neuron.* 30:65-78

Ullian EM, Sapperstein SK, Christopherson KS, Barres BA (2001) Control of synapse number by glia. *Science.* 291:657-661

van der Kooy D, Weiss S (2000) Why stem cells? *Science.* 287:1439-1441

van der Pal RH, Klein W, van Golde LM, Lopes-Cardozo M (1991) Developmental profiles of arylsulfatases A and B in rat cerebral cortex and spinal cord. *Biochim. Biophys. Acta.* 1081:315-320

Vaquero J, Ramiro MJ, Oya S, Cabezudo JM (1981) Ependymal reaction after experimental spinal cord injury. *Acta Neurochir.* (Wien) 55:295-302

Voigt T (1989) Development of glial cells in the cerebral wall of ferrets: direct tracing of their transformation from radial glia into astrocytes. *J. Comp. Neurol.* 289:74-88

Wallace MC, Tator CH, Lewis AJ (1987) Chronic regenerative changes in the spinal cord after cord compression injury in rats. *Surg. Neurol.* 27:209-219.

Weiss S, Dunne C, Hewson J, Wohl C, Wheatley M, Peterson AC, Reynolds BA (1996) Multipotent CNS stem cells are present in the adult mammalian spinal cord and ventricular neuroaxis. *J. Neurosci.* 16:7599-7609

Weiss S, Reynolds BA, Vescovi AL, Morshead C, Craig CG, van der Kooy D (1996) Is there a neural stem cell in the mammalian forebrain? *Trends Neurosci.* 19:387-393

Weissman T, Noctor SC, Clinton BK, Honig LS, Kriegstein AR (2003) Neurogenic radial glial cells in reptile, rodent and human: from mitosis to migration. *Cereb Cortex.* 13:550-559

Wilson HC, Onischke C, Raine CS (2003) Human oligodendrocyte precursor cells in vitro: phenotypic analysis and differential response to growth factors. *Glia.* 44:153-165

Wrobel CN, Mutch CA, Swaminathan S, Taketo MM, Chenn A (2007) Persistent expression of stabilized beta-catenin delays maturation of radial glial cells into intermediate progenitors. *Dev. Biol.* 309:285-297

Wu D, Shibuya S, Miyamoto O, Itano T, Yamamoto T (2005) Increase of NG2-positive cells associated with radial glia following traumatic spinal cord injury in adult rats. *J. Neurocytol.* 34:459-469

Yamamoto S, Yamamoto N, Kitamura T, Nakamura K, Nakafuku M (2001) Proliferation of parenchymal neural progenitors in response to injury in the adult rat spinal cord. *Exp. Neurol.* 172:115-127

Yang HY, Lieska N, Shao D, Kriho V, Pappas GD (1993) Immunotyping of radial glia and their glial derivatives during development of the rat spinal cord. *J. Neurocytol.* 22:558-571

Zhang RL, Zhang ZG, Wang Y, LeTourneau Y, Liu XS, Zhang X, Gregg SR, Wang L, Chopp M (2007) Stroke induces ependymal cell transformation into radial glia in the subventricular zone of the adult rodent brain. *J. Cereb. Blood Flow Metab.* 27:1201-1212

Zheng CH, Feng L (2006) Neuregulin regulates the formation of radial glial scaffold in hippocampal dentate gyrus of postnatal rats. *J. Cell Physiol.* 207:530-539

Zupanc GK (1999) Neurogenesis, cell death and regeneration in the adult gymnotiform brain. *J. Exp. Biol.* 202:1435-1446

Zupanc GK, Clint SC (2001) Radial glia-mediated up-regulation of somatostatin in the regenerating adult fish brain. *Neurosci. Lett.* 309:149-152

Zupanc GK, Ott R (1999) Cell proliferation after lesions in the cerebellum of adult teleost fish: time course, origin, and type of new cells produced. *Exp. Neurol.* 160:78-87

In: Encyclopedia of Stem Cell Research (2 Volume Set) ISBN: 978-1-61761-835-2
Editor: Alexander L. Greene © 2012 Nova Science Publishers, Inc.

Chapter VIII

A REVIEW OF CORNEAL EPITHELIAL STEM CELL THERAPY

David Hui-Kang Ma[1,2], *Arvin Chi-Chin Sun*[3,4], *Jui-Yang Lai*[5,6] *and Jan-Kan Chen*[7]

[1]Limbal Stem Cell Laboratory, Department of Ophthalmology,
Chang Gung Memorial Hospital, Taoyuan, Taiwan, ROC
[2]Department of Chinese Medicine, College of Medicine,
Chang Gung University, Taoyuan, Taiwan, ROC
[3]Department of Ophthalmology, Chang Gung
Memorial Hospital, Keelung, Taiwan, ROC
[4]Department of Medicine, College of Medicine,
Chang Gung University, Taoyuan, Taiwan, ROC
[5]Institute of Biochemical and Biomedical Engineering,
Chang Gung University, Taoyuan, Taiwan, ROC
[6]Molecular Medicine Research Center,
Chang Gung University, Taoyuan, Taiwan, ROC
[7]Department of Physiology, College of Medicine,
Chang Gung University, Taoyuan, Taiwan, ROC

ABSTRACT

Owing to the rapid progress in biomedical science and the highly anticipated therapeutic potentials, stem cell-related research has boomed since the beginning of the new millennium. However, in contrast to enormous basic research papers that have been published, clinical applications of stem cells, except hematopoietic stem cell transplantation, are still in infancy. Nevertheless, during the last decade we have witnessed a remarkable success in corneal epithelial stem cell therapy, which merits special attention to what has been found regarding corneal epithelial biology, and what has been reported regarding the therapeutic modalities.

The corneal epithelial stem cells are located in the basal layer of limbus (therefore are called limbal stem cells – LSCs), and are pivotal for the maintenance of corneal transparency and avascularity. In event of LSC deficiency that is caused by burns or autoimmune diseases, conjunctival epithelial cell invasion is accompanied by pannas ingrowth and persistent inflammation. Transplantation of autologous or allogeneic healthy limbal tissue restores corneal epithelium and therefore improves vision.

In recent years, LSC transplantation has evolved to become a successful example of tissue engineering. Corneal, conjunctival, and oral mucosal epithelial cells (as an alternative source of corneal epithelium) can be harvested in small size, cultured and expanded in vitro. Preserved human amniotic membrane (AM) is the natural biomaterial that most widely used as the carrier for cultivated epithelium. It has been well documented that AM preserves epithelial progenitor cells during cultivation, and inhibits corneal inflammation and angiogenesis after transplantation. Fibrin has also been used to transport the cultivated epithelium, but was less reported.

However, either with AM or fibrin, the graft transparency may be affected, and in order to further improve vision, penetrating or lamellar keratoplasty is sometimes needed after epithelial transplantation.

Thermo-responsive culture surface (TRCS) is a newly developed intelligent interface that enables complete detachment of the epithelial sheet upon lowering of temperature without the use of proteolytic enzymes. Because the integrity of basement membrane was maintained, the epithelial sheet graft can attach to the recipient bed readily without the need for laborious suturing procedure, while the graft transparency is optimal. TRCS has been used for cultivated oral mucosal and corneal epithelial cell transplantation, and in near future, it may even facilitate cultivated corneal endothelial cell transplantation, which may eventually solve the problem of global shortage of donor corneas.

INTRODUCTION: A REVIEW OF CORNEAL EPITHELIAL STEM CELL BIOLOGY

The Limbus and Corneal Epithelial Stem Cells

The normal ocular surface is covered by corneal, limbal, and conjunctival epithelial cells that, together with a stable pre-ocular tear film, maintain its integrity. The limbal zone is a transitional area between the cornea and conjunctiva. The corneal epithelium exists in a state of dynamic equilibrium, with the superficial epithelial cells being constantly shed into the tear pool. Terminal differentiation of cells, coupled with cell death by apoptosis, prompts the cell loss via desquamation, a process aided by eyelid blinking.[1] The cells with rapid and continuous turnover shed from the corneal surface are replaced through proliferation of a distinct subpopulation of cells, known as stem cells (SCs).[2]

Evidences for the limbal localization of the corneal epithelial SCs are obtained from different studies. Davanger and Evensen were the first to propose the concept of the limbal location of corneal epithelial SCs.[3] They observed pigmented epithelial migration lines that traveled from the limbus towards the central cornea during the healing phase of eccentric epithelial defects and postulated that the limbal palisades of Vogt are the proliferative reservoir for renewal of corneal epithelial cells.

Thereafter, Schermer et al showed that keratin 3 (K3), a 64-kDa basic keratin, was expressed throughout the entire corneal epithelium as well as the suprabasal limbal epithelium, but neither in the limbal basal epithelium nor in adjacent conjunctiva.[4] Their findings implied that corneal and conjunctival epithelial cells represented two distinct cell lineages, and limbal basal cells were less differentiated than the cells in the central cornea. Together with the well known centripetal migration of corneal epithelial cells, they hypothesized that corneal epithelial SCs were located in the limbal basal epithelium, so called the limbal stem cells (LSCs). They further suggested that corneal basal cells corresponded to transient amplifying cells (TACs) and that corneal suprabasal cells corresponded to post-mitotic cells (PMCs) and terminally differentiated cells (TDCs). Both SCs and TACs are capable of mitosis and remain in contact with the basement membrane. The differentiation of LSCs into TACs accounts for the centripetal migration of cells towards the central cornea. In contrast, PMCs and TDCs are displaced vertically into the suprabasal layers, undergone apoptosis and shed into the tear pool (figure 1). Taken together, these data suggested that cells derived from the limbus are progenitors of the corneal epithelial cells.

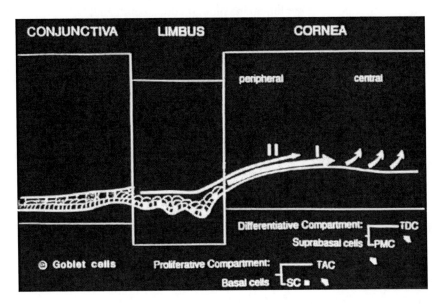

Figure 1. Localization of corneal epithelial stem cells (SCs) in the limbus. The limbal SCs (solid white blocks) are located in the basal layer of limbal epithelial papillae. The progeny of SCs, the transient amplifying cells (TACs) are located in the basal epithelia of limbus as well as in the peripheral cornea. Continuous propagation and migration of TACs toward central cornea gives rise to post-mitotic cells (PMCs) in the suprabasal layer. The PMCs further differentiate into terminally differentiated cells (TDCs) in the superficial layer, which form tight junctions that protect the cornea from environmental insults. Without proliferative ability, the TDCs are constantly shed into the tear film.

Properties of Limbal Stem Cells (LSCs)

By definition, SCs are cells capable of 'unlimited' divisions during the life of the organism, giving rise to progeny that enter a differentiation pathway with subsequent terminal differentiation.[5] Therefore, cells qualified to be SCs must have certain unique characteristics, which include longevity, lack of differentiation, increased potential for error-free proliferation, high capacity of self renewal with a long cell cycle time and a short S-phase duration, and capacity for asymmetric division.[6] In addition, SCs are usually under protection.

The fact that K3-negative cells were found in limbal basal epithelium indicates that these cells are less differentiated compared to corneal epithelial cells.[4] In humans, cells from the limbal area have been demonstrated to possess a greater proliferative potential in culture,[7] which is also a characteristic of SCs. Moreover, the slow-cycling LSCs could be identified by long-term labeling the dividing cells with a DNA precursor such as tritiated thymidine (^{3}H) or 5-bromo-2-deoxyuridine (BrdU).[8,9] This is done because SCs are normally slow-cycling, whereas the TACs are rapidly cycling. Therefore, following a chase period about 4–8 weeks, the TACs lose most of their labels due to dilution resulted from active division, while cells that cycle slowly (i.e. the SCs) retain BrdU labeling. In this way, the SCs can be identified as 'label-retaining cells'.[10] Previous studies have shown that label-retaining cells were found exclusively in the basal layer of the peripheral corneal epithelium in the limbal zone,[9; 11; 12] providing strong support of the limbal location of corneal epithelial SCs.

The self-renewing character of LSCs is evidenced by their ability to undergo asymmetric cell division in the cornea to generate progeny with different proliferative capability. Asymmetric cell division means that one of the daughter cells stays in the stem cell pool to maintain the stem cell population, whereas the other daughter cell, that is, the early TACs, moves out of the pool and divides to give rise to TACs. The TACs then divide further to the more differentiated K3-positive corneal epithelial basal cells. The TACs which move from the limbus to the central cornea become TDCs and are shed into the tear film (figure 1). The LSCs can be induced in response to injury or stimulatory factors and give rise to their progeny, the TACs.

In order to function properly, the LSCs are postulated to be protected in a microenvironmental "niche" that helps the SCs maintain their unique properties.[13] There is a body of evidence supporting the limbal SC "niche" theory, for example:

1. LSCs are located in the heavily pigmented basal layer and, thus, are well protected.[14]
2. The highly undulating epithelial-stromal junction in the limbal palisades of Vogt provides considerable protection from shearing forces.[15] This would be also advantageous for retention of LSCs while facing environmental insults.
3. From immunohistochemical studies, SCs may be more abundant in the superior and inferior limbus compared with the nasal and temporal sectors.[16] (possibly because the nature position of eyelids confers protection.)
4. Melanin deposits in the palisades offer photoprotection from ultraviolet radiation and the subsequent generation of oxygen radicals.

Therefore, LSCs exist in a distinctive environment that not only helps them maintain their unique properties but also protects them from potential insults.

Markers for Limbal Stem Cells

It would tremendously facilitate the study of limbal stem cell (LSC) biology if we could identify and label the SCs with specific markers. Despite a number of biochemical markers have been proposed as potential LSC markers, however, a definitive marker remains elusive and all methods presently used for the identification of LSCs are indirect. Currently available putative molecular markers for LSCs can be classified as differentiation-related markers or stem cell-associated markers (table 1). Members in the category of differentiation-related marker include keratin 3/keratin 12 (K3/K12), connexins, nestin and involucrin. The intracellular keratin pair K3/K12 is not present in the limbal basal region but is found in the central cornea,[4;17] reflecting the fact that limbal cells are more primitive than corneal basal cells. Another example is the gap-junction proteins, connexin 43 (Cx43) and Cx50. Connexins are integral membrane proteins on the cell surface. They have been reported to be absent from the basal layer of the human limbal epithelium, whereas suprabasal limbal cells showed weakly positive membranous staining.[18-20] It has been suggested that the expression of Cx43 represents the differentiation of corneal TACs.[18;20]

Table 1. Expression of putative limbal stem cells markers (differentiation-related and stem cell-associated markers) by human limbal and corneal epithelia

	Limbal epithelium		Corneal epithelium	
	Basal	Suprabasal	Basal	Suprabasal
Differentiation-related markers				
K3/K12	–	++	+++	+++
Connexin 43	–	+++	+	+++
Connexin 50	–	+++	–	+++
Involucrin	–	+++	+	+++
Nestin	–	+++	+	+++
Stem cell-associated markers				
Keratin 19	+++	+	–	–
Vimentin	+++	+	–	–
P63	+++	±	±	–
Integrin $\alpha 9$	+++	±	–	–
ABCG2	+++	±	–	–

–, no expression; ±, very weak expression; +, weak expression; ++, moderate expression; +++, strong expression.

Nestin, a specific marker for neural SC,[21] has been proposed as a potential marker for LSC characteristic of its neuroectodermal origin. However, instead of limbal basal cells, nestin is only expressed in human corneal epithelial cells. Likewise, a cytosolic structural protein, involucrin, is only expressed in superficial epithelial cells in the human cornea and limbus, but not in the basal layer of the limbal epithelium,[19] thus serving as a marker of differentiation.

Stem cell-associated markers are consisted of molecules that are highly expressed in the limbal basal region versus the rest of the ocular surface, such as keratin 19 (K19), vimentin, p63, integrin α9 and ABCG2. For example, K19 and vimentin, a component of cellular intermediate filaments, have been shown to be localized to the basal cells of the human limbal epithelium.[22] Furthermore, limbal epithelial cells co-localized with both proteins have been found to be identical with label-retaining cells.[23] However, a recent study demonstrated that the intensity of K19 staining between limbal and corneal epithelia was not differed significantly.[19] These findings indicated that K19 is not a specific LSC marker. Transcription factor p63, preferentially expressed in the basal layer of the limbus but not in the corneal epithelium of human corneas, was proposed to be a LSC marker.[24] However, subsequent study has demonstrated that p63-positive cells were also observed in the majority of the basal cells in the peripheral and central cornea.[25] Several lines of evidence nowadays are in agreement with the notion that p63-positivity is not specific for LSCs, and that p63-positivity may be representative of cells in a proliferative state, such as TACs.[26-28] Alternatively, it might be that only one isoform (deltaNp63α) of the p63 family functions as LSC marker, as reported by Di Iorio.[29]

Since LSCs reside in a "niche", the interactions between limbal SCs and their matrix undoubtly play a role in maintaining "stemness" of these cells. The cell-cell matrix interactions are predominantly mediated by integrins, a major class of the adhesion molecules, that function as cell surface receptors composed of heterodimers of the α and β subunits.[30] It has been shown that α9 integrin is expressed in a subpopulation of cells in the limbus, but not in the central cornea in mice.[31] In human corneas, integrin α9 was also localized to some limbal basal epithelial cells but not to suprabasal limbal or corneal epithelial cells.[19] Nevertheless, like the other putative markers mentioned above, present data support the notion that α9 integrin is present on subpopulations of early TACs intermixed with the stem cells at the limbus, not exclusively on the SCs themselves.

Recently, a member of the ATP binding cassette (ABC) transporters, ABCG2, has been proposed as a universal SC marker in a variety of tissues.[32;33] Immunolocalization studies demonstrated ABCG2-positive cells in basal layer of the limbal epithelium, but not in the corneal and conjunctival epithelia.[27;34] ABCG2 staining was present in the cell membrane and cytoplasm of these cells. In contrast to most putative SC markers that label the majority of limbal basal cells, ABCG2-positive staining was confined to small clusters of limbal basal cells.[27] Moreover, positive ABCG2 staining was co-localized with an absence of Cx43-staining. Therefore, it seems that at present ABCG2 is the most useful surface marker for the identification and isolation of LSCs.

In summary, although no single marker is available to identify the LSCs to date, the relative expression of these markers in the corneolimbal epithelium allows us to describe a putative SC phenotype. At present, the combination of differentiation-related markers (e.g. K3/K12, Cx43/Cx50, or involucrin) and putative SC-associated markers (e.g. K19, vimentin, integrin α9 or ABCG2) appears to be the best strategy to identify human LSCs.

Limbal Stem Cell Deficiency (LSCD) and Its Management

In addition to serving as an ultimate source in the regeneration of the entire corneal epithelium under both physiological and pathological conditions,[35] limbal epithelial SCs also act as a "barrier" to conjunctival epithelial cells, and normally prevent them from migrating onto the corneal surface.[36] When limbal epithelium is deficient due to any causes, conjunctival epithelium can encroach onto the corneal surface, a process known as 'conjunctivalization' of the cornea. Severe damage to the limbal epithelial cells from injuries like chemical or thermal burns, autoimmune diseases like Stevens-Johnson syndrome (SJS), ocular cicatricial pemphigoid (OCP), contact lens over-wearing, severe microbial infection, multiple surgical procedures, or cryotherapy in the limbal region may lead to loss of the limbal epithelial cells,[36] so called limbal stem cell deficiency (LSCD). Alternatively, LSCD may also be caused by alteration in the microenvironment that supports the LSCs. In addition to rare hereditary diseases like aniridia and keratitis associated with multiple endocrine deficiency, chronic inflammation is the main cause that inhibit LSCs proliferation, and ultimate loss of the LSCs population.[37] A primary reason for understanding the cell biology of corneal epithelial SCs is to find the treatment modalities for LSCD. LSCD is a condition that leads to patient's suffering and loss of vision. Corneal conjunctivalization is the hall mark of LSCD, manifested by chronic inflammation, neovascularization, and goblet cell invasion into the cornea,[38] which may be complicated by persistent epithelial defects, ulceration, and even perforation of the cornea.[35;37;39;40] The cornea may ultimately be healed by fibrosis, however, the vision will be greatly impaired (figure 2).

The most important features to be considered in evaluating patients with LSCD include the degree of LSC loss, the extent of conjunctival disease, and the presence and etiology of ocular surface inflammation. Other important factors are tear film and eyelid abnormalities, keratinization of the ocular surface, laterality of the disease process, health and age of the patient. Careful consideration of all of these factors helps tremendously in tailoring the most suitable method of treatment for each patient.

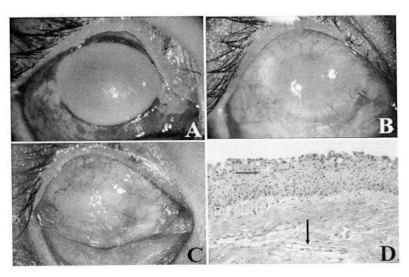

Figure 2. Clinical manifestations of total limbal stem cell deficiency. A 38 years old male suffered from alkaline burn damaging the entire cornea and limbus OD (A). Five months later, prominent blood vessels ingrowth, persistent corneal inflammation and epithelial detect were evident (B). One year after the injury, the cornea was healed by conjunctival epithelium (C), which was confirmed histologically by the presence of goblet cells (red arrow) and blood vessels (black arrow) in the corneal tissue (D).

CORNEAL RECONSTRUCTION BY AUTOLOGOUS LIMBAL TISSUE TRANSPLANTATION

Autologous Limbal Stem Cell Transplantation (LSCT)

The surgical management of severe ocular surface disease has benefited from numerous advances in recent years (for review, see [41]). Thoft was the first to perform autologous conjunctiva transplantation to reconstruct eyes with damaged ocular surface epithelium and superficial vascularization. Although some cases showed successful reepithelialization from the conjunctiva and the vision improved, the result was variable. It is now understood that conjunctival graft not containing LSCs is unable to fully recover the corneal surface.[42]

The first breakthrough came when Kenyon and Tseng reconstituted the entire corneal epithelium of patients with unilateral LSCD using the novel technique of "limbal stem cell transplantation"(LSCT).[43] The operation involved surgical removal of superficial conjunctivalized tissue from the lesion eye, followed by harvesting two free grafts of limbal tissue from the contralateral healthy eye, then transplanted the grafts onto the diseased eye. If only part of the limbus is damaged, limbal tissue can be harvested from the healthy part of the same eye.[44] The procedure resulted in improved visual acuity, rapid re-epithelialization with a smooth and stable corneal surface, healing of persistent epithelial defects, and regression of neovascularization. Impression cytology confirmed the restoration of the corneal epithelial phenotype. This provides further evidence that limbal epithelium contains the SCs requisite for the formation and maintenance of a healthy corneal epithelium. At the same time, it is now becoming apparent that the transplanted limbo-corneal epithelium can secrete several anti-angiogenic and anti-inflammatory factors that inhibit the ingrowth of blood vessels.[45;46]

In patients who suffered from unilateral LSCD, or from bilateral LSCD but affecting different areas of the limbus, the disorder may be treated by conjunctivo-limbal autograft (CLAU) transplantation, and the clinical outcome was promising (figure 3).[47] To handle the residual corneal opacity following removal of the surface pannus, CLAU can be performed simultaneously with penetrating keratoplasty (PKP; transplantation of full-thickness donor cornea)[48] or lamellar keratoplasty (LKP; transplantation of donor cornea devoid of posterior stroma, Descement's membrane, and endothelium).[49] CLAU combined simultaneously or at a later stage with LKP is a more favorable procedure than CLAU combined with PKP in that the risk of allograft rejection is significantly reduced.

However, a serious limitation of transplantation of CLAU is that one or two limbal tissue grafts, spanning two to three clock hours of the limbus, have to be removed from the healthy eyes. As such, the potential complication of iatrogenic LSCD in the donor's eye could be a major concern, because LSCD can occur in rabbits if the central corneal epithelium is sequentially removed from the donor eyes,[50;51] although no report has described such complication in human. Meallet et al reported combined CLAU with amniotic membrane transplantation (AMT) for the management of total LSCD. In this technique the AM was transplanted to the donor site as well as to the recipient cornea followed by fixation of the conjunctivo-limbal grafts. The AM may promote the proliferation of corneal epithelial cells so as to retard fibrovascular ingrowth not only at the donor site but also at the recipient limbal area not covered by conjunctivo-limbal grafts.[52]

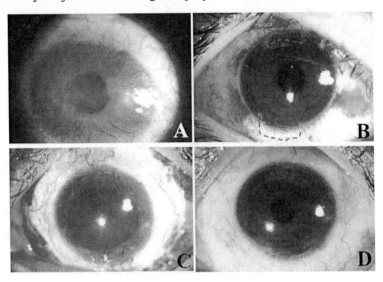

Figure 3. Combined conjunctivo-limbal autografting and amniotic membrane transplantation in a 20 years old male suffered from acid burn OS. Pre-operatively, the cornea was covered by conjunctival epithelium with neovascularization. The visual acuity was only 20/200 (A). Two conjunctivo-limbal grafts 2 o'clock in width were harvest from the right eye (dotted areas; B). One month after transplantation, the grafts were re-vascularized, and positioned above a doughnut-shaped amniotic membrane graft (C). One year after transplantation, the cornea remained clear and was free of blood vessels. The visual acuity improved to 20/20 (D).

Amniotic Membrane Transplantation (AMT)

The amniotic membrane (AM) is the innermost layer of fetal membrane that protects the fetus in the uterus. Histologically, the AM is composed of a single layer of cuboidal epithelium, a thick basement membrane zone, and a gelatinous stroma containing the AM stromal cells. The AM's basement membrane (BM) contains type IV and type VII collagen, laminin-1, -5, heparan sulfate and fibronectin.[53] The AM BM type IV collagen contains subchain $\alpha 2(IV)$, which is also found in the conjunctival BM,[53] and subchain $\alpha 5(IV)$, also found in the corneal BM.[54] The fibronectin and laminin component of AM play an important role in facilitating epithelial cell adhesion. Type I collagen is confined to the AM stroma along with significant amounts of keratan and chondroitin sulfate.[55] As an endogenous BM, AM supports the proliferation,[56] migration,[57;58] adhesion,[59-61] and differentiation of epithelial cells,[62-65] and also prevents epithelial cell apoptosis.[66;67] The AM stroma contains a number of growth factors like EGF, KGF, HGF, bFGF, TGF-α and –β,[68] and NGF.[69] These growth factors provide survival signals for the LSCs in culture. Taken together, these features enable AM to serve as an invaluable natural substrate for ex vivo cultivation of human limbo-corneal epithelial (HLE) cells (so called stromal "niche"). Intact AM as a substrate for cultivating HLE cells exhibit a unique property of keeping the epithelium limbal but not corneal in phenotype, presumably by maintaining more progenitor cells in vitro (discussed later).[70;71]

The AM stroma also contains various anti-angiogenic and anti-inflammatory proteins, and natural protease inhibitors.[72] The production of IL-1 by HLE cells cultivated on AM is down-regulated,[73] while secretion of IL-1ra, the potent endogenous inhibitors of IL-1 increases.[66] Polymorphonuclear neutrophils are induced to undergo apoptosis when in contact with AM stroma.[74] These features explain why AMT may decrease corneal inflammation and melting, and thereby promote reepithelialization. As mentioned above, a chronic inflamed limbal stroma alone is able to cause LSCD, and negatively affect the viability of transplanted limbal tissue,[37] therefore, by exhibiting these anti-inflammatory acitvities AMT may create a non-inflamed stroma that is permissive for the regrowth of LSCs.

Kim et al were the first to demonstrate frozen but not fresh AM was able to reconstruct corneal surface,[75] because following cryopreservation the AM cells are killed and therefore the immunogenicity of the AM is reduced. Clinically, the purpose to perform AMT can be grossly categorized as: 1. promotion of corneal re-epithelialization (sterile or infectious corneal ulcers) 2. conjunctival reconstruction (pterygium and symblepharon) 3. prevention of corneal melting (AM dressing for acute chemical burn; for review, see[76;77]). The necessity to combine AMT with LSCT for corneal reconstruction depends on the severity of LSCD. If the degree of LSCD is only partial (less than one half of the limbus affected), then reconstruct the limbus with AMT alone is most likely to re-establish the limbal barrier,[78] because the progenitor cells from the remaining healthy limbus may migrate to the area limbal covered by AM. However, if the degree of LSCD is extensive, AMT alone is ineffective to prevent conjunctivalization and corneal noevascularization. Under such circumstances, AMT is often performed together with auto- or alloneneic limbal tissue transplantation, in the hope to control stromal inflammation and to promote epithelial outgrowth from the transplanted limbal tissue. The tremendous success of using AM as a substrate and a carrier for ex vivo cultivation of LSCs is discussed later in this chapter.

ALLOGENEIC LIMBAL STEM CELL TRANSPLANTATION (LSCT)

Keratolimbal Allografting (KLAL)

In many incidences, both eyes of a patient are affected, therefore it is impossible to obtain healthy self-limbal tissue. CLAU is not feasible for patients with bilateral LSCD, and under such circumstances either cadaveric[79] or living-related keratolimbal allograft (KLAL)[80] is an alternative treatment. In 1994, Tsai et al. first reported their results of using donor corneas as the source of limbal tissue. Their patients included 16 eyes mainly with thermal or chemical burns, and chronic keratoconjunctivitis. The recipient eye first received superficial lamellar keratectomy to remove fibrovascular pannus, then randomly selected cadaveric limbocorneal graft was transplanted. Oral cyclosporine A was administered immediately for 2.9 months. During the 18.5 months follow-up, vision improved in 13 eyes (81.3%), and rapid (within 1 week) surface healing in 10 eyes (62.5%). This is the first report indicating that limbal allograft transplantation may be able to reconstruct a corneal surface that has suffered from diffuse LSC loss (figure 4).[79] Although the authors reported that no acute graft failure or allograft rejection was identified, over the years it became apparent that the rejection rate in mismatched KLAL is very high. Because much higher number of antigen-presenting Langerhans' cells are present in the limbal area than in the central cornea;[81;82] therefore, limbal grafts are believed to be more susceptible to immunologic rejection. Uncontrolled inflammation due to the underlying disease such as SJS further elicit allograft sensitization and hence rejection.

Signs of allograft rejection include intense sectoral injection, diffuse or perilimbal conjunctival injection, edema, and infiltration of the KLAL grafts, leading to punctate epithelial erosions, epithelial defects, and surface keratinization. Rejected specimens also reveal T-lymphocyte infiltration with strong HLA-DR expression.[83] In a comprehensive review on KLAL technique, Espana et al proposed a step-by-step corneal reconstruction by KLAL.[84] The first strategy is to restore ocular surface defense, such as punctal occlusion for severe dry eye, or blepharoplasty for lid abnormalities. The second strategy is to perform KLAL. Penetrating keratoplasty may be performed at the same time of KLAL, or 3–6 months later. The third strategy is to restore limbal stromal environment. This usually implies to reconstruct the ocular surface with AM. The fourth strategy is to employ effective immunosuppressants, which comprises oral prednisolone, Mycophenolate mophetyl, and Tacrolimus (FK506), an analog to cyclosporin A in action, but a more potent and safer immunosuppressant.[85] Despite the continuous administration of systemic cyclosporin A, the success rate of allogeneic LSCT declines from 75–80% in 1 year[79;85-87] to 50% in 3 years of follow-up.[88-91] Although the length of immunosuppression in KLAL has not been established, it is believed that it should be administered for a prolonged, if not indefinite, period of time.[84]

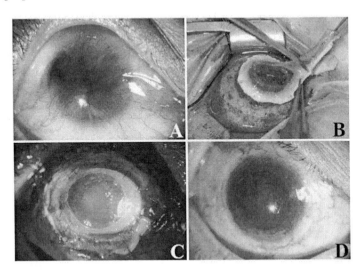

Figure 4. Kerato-limbal allografting combined with amniotic membrane (AM) transplantation in a 45 years old male with acid burn OD. Pre-operatively the vision was only counting fingers (A). During operation, after removing the surface pannas and performing AM transplantation, lamellar dissection on the cadaveric donor limbal tissue was done to obtain the graft (B), which was sutured on top of the doughnut-shaped AM graft. The central part of the AM graft was excised to facilitate light transmission (C). One year after transplantation, under systemic immunosuppression the cornea was clear and quiet, and the best corrected vision was 20/40.

Keratolimbal Allografting Combined with Penetrating Keratoplasty

Although successful allogeneic LSCT regresses corneal neovascularization, residual stromal opacity, if severe, may still interfere with vision. Penetrating keratoplasty (PKP) is sometimes needed for full recovery of vision following LSCT. However, corneal allograft rejection is a main concern when PKP is performed simultaneously with allogeneic LSCT, in that additional antigenic challenge from the limbal tissue may stimulate rejection to the donor cornea even under immunosupression. Tseng et al first reported combined KLAL and PKP in 14 eyes with total LSCD mainly due to chemical burn. During the mean follow-up of 15.4 months, corneal graft rejection occurred in 9 (64%) of the 14 eyes even under systemic cyclosporine A , and 2 eyes were associated with reversible engorgement of limbal vessels, a sign of limbal rejection.[92] Tsubota et al evaluated 70 KLAL transplantations to 43 eyes of 39 patients with severe ocular surface disorders and limbal dysfunction. In 28 eyes, standard PKP was also performed, and systemic cyclosporine A was kept for more than 6 months. A mean of 1163 days after operation, 22 of the 43 eyes (51 %) had corneal epithelialization. Complications of the first transplantation included persistent defects in the corneal epithelium in 26 eyes, ocular hypertension in 16 eyes, and rejection of the corneal graft in 13 of the 28 eyes.[88] Solomon et al. reviewed 53 KLAL with AMT performed in 39 eyes, of which 23 eyes received simultaneous PKP at the time of the first KLAL. Oral cyclosporin A was given continuously. The mean follow-up was 34.0 months. A progressive decrease in the survival of KLAL was noted during more than 5 years of follow-up. The survival of KLAL was 76.9% at 1 year, 47.4% at 3 years, and only 23.7% at 5 years. Performing PKP with KLAL at the same time was associated with a markedly reduced KLAL survival. An overall progressive decline in central corneal graft survival was observed from 47.8% after the first year to 13.7% after 3 years. The survival of PKP was significantly worse in SJS compared with the other causes that after 2 years of follow-up, none of the SJS central grafts survived.[91]

In contrast, Shimazaki et al reported 45 eyes underwent simultaneous KLAL and PKP, and were followed for an averaged 41.8 months. Oral cyclosporine A was given for at least 3 months. Endothelial rejection of the central graft was found in 16 eyes (35.6%), with four eyes showing limbal graft rejection which existed before the episodes.[93] The incidence is compatible with that found in high-risk PKP using systemic cyclosporine A (16.7 to 48.8%).[94-96] The authors attributed the lowered incidence not only to the topical and systemic immunosuppression by cyclosporine A; moreover, it is noteworthy that the number of Langerhans cells in the limbal area decreases during preservation. The authors used donor corneas preserved in Optisol GS for several days; therefore, immunoreactivity may become less than that in fresh tissues. The poor prognosis of corneal transplantation combined with KLAL might be explained in part by the increased exposure of the host immune system to the donor corneal antigens through the recognition and sensitization to limbal allograft antigens when the limbal and corneal graft are originated from the same donor. Furthermore, inflammation generated by KLAL might put the eye susceptible to concomitant PKP sensitization.[84] Most authors now agree that a two-step reconstruction (KLAL followed by PKP at least 3 to 6 months later) is preferred.[97]

Living Related Conjunctivo-limbal Allografting (lrCLAL)

Because rejection rate of allogeneic LSCT is high, and it is impossible to obtain human leukocyte antigen (HLA) phenotype data from most donor corneas; a practical method to obtain HLA-matched tissue is to harvest graft from living related donors. Rao et al first reported the results of limbal allograft transplantation, from HLA-matched and -unmatched related live donors in 8 patients (9 eyes) with severe chemical burns (7 eyes) and SJS (2 eyes). Superior and inferior limbal grafts were obtained from related live HLA-matched (none had more than two mismatches on the HLA A, B, and C loci.) (n = 7) and -unmatched donors (n = 2). Since systemic cyclosporine was not used in any of the recipients, during a mean observation period of 17.2 months, in all the HLA-matched eyes, gradual recurrence of peripheral corneal vascularization occurred, and features of graft rejection developed in three (42.9%) of the 7 eyes. In two HLA-unmatched eyes, transplantation failed to reconstitute the corneal surface. Visual acuity of 20/400 or greater was observed in only two (22.2%) eyes at last follow-up.[80]

Daya et al published a study containing eight recipients (10 eyes) with SJS (3 eyes), ectodermal dysplasia (3 eyes), chemical injury (2 eyes), OCP (1 eye), and atopic keratoconjunctivitis (1 eye). Seven eyes had previously received cadaveric KLAL but failed. Conjunctivo-limbal tissue was harvested from the best matched HLA relative donor. All subjects initially received intravenous methylprednisolone followed by oral prednisolone. Systemic cyclosporine was also administered in all subjects during the follow-up period. After a mean follow-up of 26.2 months, two highly inflamed eyes failed to re-epithelialize. The remainder all survived with restoration of corneal epithelium and reduction of vascularization. Reduced corneal opacification and visual improvement was achieved in seven eyes. Although allograft rejection occurred in two eyes (25%) with SJS and two class I HLA mismatches, both were treated successfully with intensive immunosuppressive therapy for several months. Their result proved that systemic cyclosporine, even at low doses, is useful in ensuring long-term allograft survival.[98]

Santos et al analyzed 10 eyes underwent conjunctivo-limbal autograft (CLAU) and 23 eyes underwent lrCLAL with HLA compatible (N = 10) and non-compatible donors (N = 13). PKP was performed in 16 eyes, and 70% of them simultaneously with KLAL. The overall cumulative survival after a mean follow-up time of 33 months was 80% in the CLAU group and 13% in the lrCLAL recipients. The survival of PKP associated with ocular surface reconstruction observed in this study was 25% after a mean follow-up time of 33 months. Eyes with SJS, dry eye, keratinization, and eyelid abnormalities, and that receiving HLA non-compatible limbal transplants developed graft failure more frequently. Preoperative dry eye was the most important prognostic parameter for surgical outcome. In the study, despite the low incidence of limbal rejection, low-grade inflammation was present in many allogeneic transplant recipient eyes, even in those that were HLA-compatible, and this inflammation, which may represent subclinical rejection, compromised the longevity of the limbal allograft.[99] Similarly, in the report of Gomes et al with purely SJS patients, the result of combined AMT and lrCLAL, even under systemic cyclosporine A was unsatisfactory, with only 20% success rate in 10 patients. A high proportion of post-operative complications, especially infections, seemed to undermine the outcome.[100] Nevertheless, lrCLAL is still preferable to unmatched allograft for reconstructing cornea in SJS patient, especially in young children.[101;102]

Survival of Allogeneic Limbo-corneal Epithelial Cells after Transplantation

Espana et al reported a woman with chemical burn underwent a successful KLAL combined with AMT to reconstruct her cornea. PKP and cataract surgery was performed 6 months later. Immunihistochemical studies on the corneal button revealed that the reconstructed epithelium to be corneal in phenotype in that the expression of keratin 3 (K3), connexin 43, laminin 5 and integrins were identical to those of normal corneal epithelium.[103] However, the article didn't mention whether the corneal epithelium is donor-derived or not. Shimazaki et al were the first to prove the persistence of donor-derived epithelial cells after KLAL. The epithelial cells were obtained in the paracentral cornea, and were subjected to fluorescence in situ hybridization (FISH) using sex chromosome–specific probes and polymerase chain reaction restriction fragment length polymorphism (RFLP) analysis to examine HLA-DPB1 antigens. After the mean follow-up period of 445 days, donor-derived epithelial cells were detected in three of five eyes (60.0%) in the FISH analysis, and in seven of nine eyes (77.8%) in the RFLP analysis. Among these eyes, one and three eyes in the FISH and RFLP analysis, respectively, had both donor- and recipient-derived cells.[104] Using the same technique to analyze epithelial cells obtained upon suture removal, Egarth et al reported that donor-derived epithelial cells were found one year after operation in two out of seven cases following combined limbal and corneal transplantation, and the percentage of donor-derived cells in the two cases was 2.4% and 29%, respectively.[105] Djalilian et al. analyzed DNA microsatellite markers with PCR technique and reported that exclusively nonrecipient cells (presumed to be donor) in corneal buttons up to 3.5 years after KLAL. Long term systemic immunosuppressive therapy was necessary to maintain the outcome.[106] However, Henderson et al found that in no instances were donor-derived cells recovered 3–5 years after KLAL.[107] However, in the eyes without donor-derived cells, it might be the residual LSCs from the recipient that ultimately repopulate the cornea, a mechanism that will be discussed later in this chapter.

CORNEAL RECONSTRUCTION BY CULTIVATED EPITHELIAL STEM CELLS

Transplantation of Ex Vivo Expanded Corneal Epithelial Cells Cultivated on Amniotic Membrane

Because autologous LSCT doesn't cause rejection, the reported long-term results were mostly favorable. However, there is a risk of damaging donor eye with resultant iatrogenic LSCD at the biopsy site. It would be advisable to minimize the size of donor limbal tissue that can generate sufficient progeny to repopulate the corneal surface in event of total LSCD.

As early as in 1975, Rheinwald and Green reported that normal human epidermal keratinocytes can be serially cultivated in the presence of 3T3 cells.[108] Being normal cells, although human diploid keratinocytes have a finite culture lifetime ranged from 20-50 cell generations, this nevertheless inspires other investigators with the notion that the population of keratinocytes can be expanded in vitro, and later be transplanted back to the donor for tissue repair.[109] Techniques described in that article, like the use of trypsin-EDTA to release keratinocyte stem cells from tissue for suspension culture, the use of non-proliferative 3T3 fibroblasts as feeder cells, and the DMEM and F-12- based culture medium formula have all become the gold standards for subsequent keratinocyte research.

The earliest example of cell therapy using cultured keratinocyte stem cells dated back to the 1980s, when it was first demonstrated that human epidermal keratinocytes could be grown in vitro and transplanted back to burn patients to reconstruct a new skin.[110] The relatively easy access to the cornea, the homogeneity of the cells forming the corneal epithelium, and the improvement of cell culture protocols are factors contributing to considerable success in corneal epithelium restoration.[111] In 1997, Pellegrini et al. were the first to report the use of cultivated corneal epithelium to reconstruct corneal surface damaged by severe alkaline burn in two patients.[112] The epithelial cells were cultivated from a 1 mm^2 biopsy sample taken from the limbus of the uninjured eye. The biopsy sample was mechanically and enzymatically disrupted and co-cultured with lethally irradiated 3T3-J2 cells. The grafts were prepared from confluent secondary cultures, mounted on a soft contact lens, then were placed to the recipient site. Keratin 3 positive epithelium in a corneal biopsy taken two years later provided evidence for the persistence of epithelial stem cells in the cornea.

A suitable substrate has been a key issue in cultivated epithelium transplantation in that the substrate should support the growth of the epithelial cells in vitro, and later as a carrier to transfer the cultivated cells to the recipient site. Dispase-separated epithelial sheet is very fragile, and has poor adhesion to contact lens, making the manipulation difficult. Schwab and his colleague worked on collagen gel and collagen shield as carriers, they found that both were unsatisfactory in that the collagen products were very difficult to manipulate and to maintain the integrity. They tended to melt soon after transplantation.[113] By late 1990s, preserved human amniotic membrane (AM) has been widely used for the treatment of ocular surface diseases. The fact that AM transplantation promotes re-epithelialization of the cornea inspired the team to use denuded AM (AM removed of epithelium) as a carrier. Although cell adhesion remained a problem, they found that AM can be a superior carrier. The authors were also the first to report transplanting cultivated related living donor's corneal epithelium. However, the diagnoses for most cases were recurrent pterygia, and therefore the severity of LSCD is only partial, consequently it remained unclear whether the transplanted cells or the host's own cells were responsible for tissue repair.[113;114]

Tsai and co-workers published a different approach to use AM as a carrier.[115] In stead of removing the AM epithelium, the AM was maintained intact. A piece of 1 by 2 mm limbal tissue was harvested from the donor eye, and the limbal epithelial explants were inoculated onto the basement-membrane side of the AM in a 35-mm dish. After two to three weeks, the epithelial cells grew and spread to form a cell layer covering an area 2 to 3 cm in diameter. Interestingly, the AM covered by expanded limbal epithelial cells became much more transparent, due to the matrix metalloproteinases released by the epithelial cells as was reported later.[116] Such grafts were used to reconstruct corneal surface in four patients with partial LSCD, and two patients with total LSCD. Complete re-epithelialization of the corneal surface occurred within two to four days of transplantation in all six eyes. After a mean follow-up period of 15 months, in five of the six eyes (83 percent), the mean visual acuity improved from 20/112 to 20/45. Especially in a case of chemical burn with total LSCD and persistent inflammation, a single surgery resulted in a quiescent corneal surface, and improved the vision from counting fingers to 20/200 after follow-up for 15 months. No patient had recurrent neovascularization or inflammation in the transplanted area during the follow-up period. Tsai's report was the first to show that autologous human limbo-corneal epithelial cells (HLE cells) cultured on AM were able to reconstruct corneal surface with total LSCD (figure 5). Still, like previous and subsequent reports, the ultimate source of epithelium covering the cornea can not be identified.

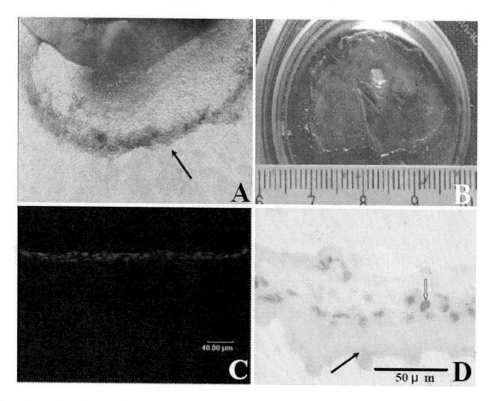

Figure 5. Ex vivo expansion of human limbo-corneal epithelial (HLE) cells on intact amniotic membrane (AM). Epithelial outgrowth from the explant is usually evident (arrow) around one week after cultivation (A). An epithelial sheet 2 to 3 cm in diameter is suitable for transplantation, which is often obtained about 3 weeks following cultivation. Keratin 3 (red) is immunolocalized to the suprabasal but not basal layer of the graft (C). This, together with BrdU label-retaining HLE cells (white arrow) detected in nude mice after xenografting suggest that epithelial progenitor cells can be preserved in vitro on intact AM (D; black arrow: remnant of human AM).

Following Tsai's report, there were several papers reporting modifications of the techniques. Koizumi et al used limbal explants from unmatched donor corneas cultured on denuded AM, and were further cocultured with 3T3 cells.[117] Unlike previous technique, the mitomycin C-inactivated 3T3 cells were place in the lower wells of 6 well culture plate, while the denuded AM carrying the HLE cells was placed in a 25 mm culture insert above. The cultures were submerged in the medium for 2 weeks, after which they were exposed to the air (air-lifting) to promote epithelial stratification for 1 to 2 weeks. In the study, oral prednisolone and cycosporin A were given to prevent allograft rejection, and cyclophosphamide for corneal inflammation. Visual acuity improved in all eyes after surgery, and 10 of the total 13 eyes were restored to good vision (visual acuity improved two or more lines) 6 months after the operation. During the mean follow-up period of 11.2 months, the corneal surfaces were clear, although three eyes experienced epithelial rejection, which was manifested by the sudden onset of corneal epithelial damage with conjunctiva inflammation. For these patients experiencing epithelial rejection and subepithelial opacities, the same group found that the failed epithelial graft and AM can be easily removed, and replaced with a new allograft. Immunosuppressants were given longer than before to prevent postoperative inflammation and allograft rejection. At the end of 12 months' follow-up, all corneas remained clear with improved vision. It is therefore possible to repeat transplantation with newly cultivated epithelium on AM.[118] The pathological finding of the graft removed after allograft rejection revealed the presence of inflammatory cells in the epithelial layer and within the AM. Most of the AM was covered by conjunctival epithelial cells and goblet cells. Only a few areas of cultivated corneal epithelial cells were found.[119]

Shimazaki et al reported the reconstruction of 13 eyes of 13 patients with living related donor's limbal epithelial cells cultivated on AM with explant culture method.[120] The AM was denuded by 10% ammonium for 15 minutes followed by gentle scraping. After the surgery, the epithelium regenerated and covered the ocular surface in eight eyes (61.5%). However, three of the eight eyes developed partial conjunctival invasion, and two eyes later developed epithelial defects. At last examination, corneal epithelialization was achieved in six eyes (46.2%). Five eyes had conjunctivalization, one eye had dermal epithelialization, and one eye was not epithelialized. Although in this article Shimazaki et al did not mention the observation of epithelial rejection, the authors attributed the poorer result to the underlying diseases, mainly SJS and OCP.

There has been no study comparing the effect on corneal inflammation and long-term graft survival by cultivated stem cell transplantation (CSCT) and conventional kerato-limbal allografting (KLAL). Nevertheless, Ang et al reported a patient with SJS and bilateral total LSCD underwent allogeneic CSCT in the right eye, followed by conventional KLAL in the left eye three weeks later. The patient was under immunosuppression with a tapering dose of systemic corticosteroid, cyclosporine, and cyclophosphamide. Complete corneal epithelialization was achieved within 48 hours after CSCT, compared with three weeks after KLAL. Ocular inflammation and tear IL-8 levels decreased more rapidly in the eye with CSCT. Four years after surgery, more severe corneal scarring and opacification were noted in the KLAL eye. The authors thus concluded that CSCT resulted in a better clinical result and vision, with less stromal scarring compared with conventional KLAL.[121] Transplantation of cultivated allogeneic HLE cells has also been demonstrated to dramatically suppress corneal inflammation and promote re-epithelialization and healing in eyes with total LSCD and persistent epithelial defect due to acute SJS.[122]

Phenotype of Cultivated Human Limbo-Corneal Epithelial Cells on Amniotic Membrane

Currently, limbal explant culture or limbal single cell suspension culture on a mitomycin C treated 3T3 fibroblast feeder layer are both used for human corneal epithelial cultivation. Previously, it was unclear which culture method may retain more epithelial progenitor cells in cultures. Kim et al reported that the cell morphology in single cell suspension culture was generally smaller, more compact and uniform, and immunostaining showed a greater number of the small cells expressing putative stem cell markers p63, EGFR, keratin 19 and integrin β1, while more larger cells stained positively for differentiation markers keratin 3, involucrin and connexin 43 in both culture systems. BrdU-label retaining cells were identified in 2.3±0.7% of explant cultures and 3.7±1.5% of single cell cultures chased for 21 days. They concluded that the phenotypes of corneal epithelial cells, ranging from basal cells to superficial differentiated cells, are well maintained in both culture systems, and the suspension culture system seemed to preserve somewhat more progenitor cells in vitro.[123] Nevertheless, animal model has shown that epithelial sheets generated by explant culture technique were able to maintain a stable corneal surface (positive keratin 3 and negative MUC5AC staining) over one year, indicating the preservation of epithelial progenitor cells by that technique.[124]

Shimazaki et al later analyzed their results using either explant culture or cell suspension culture technique combining 3T3 feeder cells and air-lifting to generating transplantable epithelial sheets for 27 patients that had severe chronic cicatricial ocular surface disorders.[125] They found that the treatment is feasible for conjunctivalized corneas with non-immune-mediated disorders. However, eyes with SJS had poor final corneal epithelialization compared with other diseases. Eyes treated with grafts generated by explant culture suffered more severe postoperative complications such as infection, ulceration, and perforation. Epithelial sheets generated by suspension culture technique had better structural integrity, and seemed to be superior to obtain early postoperative epithelialization and to avoid serious postoperative complications (figure 6).

Subsequent penetrating keratoplasty (PKP) poses a challenge to previously transplanted epithelial sheet in that if epithelial stem cells are not present in the cornea, there will be a high risk of persistent epithelial defect of the corneal graft following PKP, with resulting graft melting or infection. Sangwan et al. reported a total of 125 patients treated with cultivated HLE cell transplantation, 15 of them (11 autologous, and 4 allogenic transplantation with adequate immunosuppression) underwent PKP. Fourteen (93%) of the 15 eyes had a successful corneal graft with a stable corneal epithelium. This suggests that the transplanted HLE cells are able to proliferate and repopulate the graft, and stabilize the corneal surface.[126] The corneal buttons removed after PKP from eyes previously transplanted with cultivated HLE cells offer a unique opportunity to examine the phenotype of cultivated cells on AM in vivo.

Comparison between explant and suspension culture method

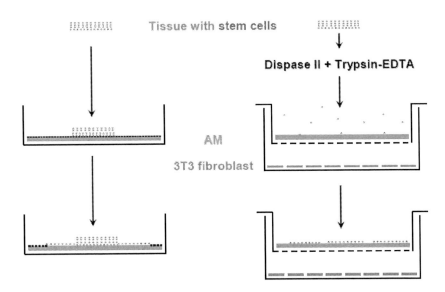

Figure 6. Comparison of explant (left) and suspension culture method (right) for cultivating limbo-corneal epithelial cells on cryo-preserved amniotic membrane (AM). In the explant culture method, one or more pieces of limbal tissue are placed on top of the intact AM. An enlarging epithelial sheet is generated from the explant, with the most actively proliferating cells in the periphery. In the suspension culture method, the epithelial cells are first separated from the limbal tissue by dispase II, then dispersed by trypsin-EDTA treatment. The progenitor cells but not the older cells are preferentially attached to the denuded AM (AM removed of the epithelium). Colonies from individual stem cells may grow and coalesce into a homogenous epithelial sheet. 3T3 feeder cells are often included in the culture system to promote the viability of the epithelial cells.

Using in vitro and animal model, Grueterich and his colleague demonstrated that HLE cells cultivated on intact AM retain a limbal epithelial phenotype characterized by negative keratin 3 and connexin 43 expression, and increased BrdU retention in the basal layer of the epithelium, whereas those on denuded AM (especially further cocultured with 3T3 fibroblasts) differentiate into a corneal phenotype, and were keratin 3 and connexin 43 positive in the basal layer.[71;127;128] The authors also reported a 31-year-old male with a severe acid burn received cultivated autologous HLE cells (limbal explant culture technique on intact AM) to his left eye to replace a failed keratolimbal allograft. Five and a half months later, the patient received a PKP, and immunofluorescence staining of the corneal button revealed that the epithelial phenotype was limbal but not corneal, based on the negative expression of keratin 3 and connexin 43 of the basal epithelium.[129] This is the first evidence suggesting that cultivated HLE progenitor cells may be preserved following transplantation.

Harkin et al. further reported a 75 year old male with a severe alkali burn to his right eye received two cultivated autologous HLE cells on AM followed by a corneal transplantation. HLE cells suspension cultures grown in the presence of 3T3 fibroblasts (submerged, not air-lifting) or on denuded AM displayed positive staining for keratins 14 and 19, and p63, but poor staining for keratin 3. The excised corneal button, on the contrary, stained positively for keratin 3, but not keratin14, keratin 19, or p63. Reactivity to the keratin 3 was greatest in the superficial layers and extended across the width of the excised corneal button. These data suggest that cultivated HLE cells contain predominantly undifferentiated cells with the potential to proliferate, however, after transplantation on denuded AM, the epithelial phenotype resembles normal corneal epithelium, which is compatible with the findings of Grueterich et al.[71;127;128]

Despite the clinical success following transplantation of cultivated HLE cells described above, little evidence support the long-term existence of donor-derived cells in the graft. Daya et al reported transplantation of allogeneic HLE cells in 10 eyes of 10 patients with profound LSCD (3 eyes with ectodermal dysplasia, 3 eyes with SJS, 2 eyes with chemical injury, one eye with thermal injury, and one eye with rosacea blepharoconjuntivitis). The cells were cultured in suspension with 3T3 fibroblasts on plastic dish, and transplanted to the recipient eye using a nonadherent nylon dressing as a vehicle. Nine patients received systemic cyclosporine A immunosuppression, and the DNA genotype was performed in the first 7 case using specimen obtained by surface impression cytology. The mean follow-up period was 28 months, and 7 of 10 eyes had improved parameters of LSCD. However, DNA genotyping revealed the presence of ex vivo cultured donor cell DNA only in 2 eyes (at 2 and 7 months respectively), and repeated examination after 9 months showed no evidence of donor-derived cells. The rest were positive only for host DNA when initially tested between 1 and 7 months postoperatively.[130] Because in Daya's study the long term source of epithelium was exclusively host in origin, this raises the questions regarding the fate of ex vivo expanded stem cells, and more intriguingly, the origin of donor-derived corneal epithelial cells, as in most cases the extent of LSCD was severe. It could be: 1. subtle, chronic allograft rejection, 2. insufficient stem cells included in the graft, or 3. competition with donor derived epithelial cells that outnumber the donor cells in the long run. Recently, it is proposed that the limbal SCs may lie very deep, and are in close contact with mesenchymal (niche) cells.[131] Kawasaki et al reported that clusters of keratin 12 positive cells can be found in bulbar conjunctival epithelium, and the gene expression patterns of these cells were highly similar to that of corneal epithelial cells. This suggests that a small number of the corneal epithelial progenitor cells can reside ectopically in the conjunctival epithelium.[132] Taken together, it is conceivable that even in eyes with very severe LSCD, a small number of LSCs might still be preserved but kept in a dormant state. Transplantation of ex vivo expanded HLE cells especially on AM may exert an anti-angiogenic/anti-inflammatory effect that favors the restoration of the stem cell niche,[133;134] together with the growth factors/anti-apoptotic factors released by the allogeneic HLE cells,[66] these remaining LSCs are revived and are stimulated to proliferate. Although the population of donor cells may decline over the years, as long as there is no further insult such as inflammation, these eyes may ultimately have long-term visual rehabilitation mainly by host's own LSCs.

Transplantation of Ex Vivo Expanded Conjunctival Epithelial Cells Cultivated on Amniotic Membrane

The SCs of conjunctival epithelium are enriched in the forniceal area.[135;136] Although conjunctival SCs are present more diffusely in the ocular surface, they are not immune to various insults like chemical burns or autoimmune diseases. The clinical conjunctival SC deficiency is manifested as symblepharon, ankyloblepharon, and shortening or even obliteration of the fornix. Although not necessarily vision-threatening, conjunctival SC deficiency will almost certainly cause motility restriction of the eye, and is conceivably disfiguring. Transplantation of ex vivo cultivated autologous conjunctival epithelial cells is a feasible way to correct this disorder.

Scuderi et al. were the first to harvest conjunctiva from the healthy eyelid bed of four patients with oculopalpebral diseases. An epithelial sheet was generated and grafted similar to the technique described by Pellegrini et al (suspension culture on 3T3 feeder cells).[112] The biological structure of the cultured epithelium closely matched that of normal conjunctiva and its properties, including clarity, smoothness, and mucus secretion.[137] Following transplantation, the integration of the graft was stable, resulting in great improvement of patient's symptoms and cosmesis.[138]

Ang et al compared the in vitro and in vivo proliferative potential of human conjunctival epithelial cells (HCE) cells cultivated in serum-free media alone (keratinocyte growth media with supplements), serum-free media with a 3T3 feeder layer, and serum-containing media with a 3T3 feeder layer. They found that HCE cells cultivated in the three conditions achieved similar colony-forming efficiencies (CFE), number of population doublings, in vivo growth in athymic mice, and the degree of epithelial stratification. This has important clinical implications, since this culture system avoids the use of animal serum and cells.[139] In addition, the authors also compared the use of human serum (HS) with fetal bovine serum (FBS) and bovine pituitary extract (BPE) for supporting the in vitro and in vivo proliferation of HCE cells. They found that the CFE, BrdU uptake, Goblet cell density, and in vivo epithelial stratification in HS supplemented cultures were comparable to FBS supplemented and BPE supplemented cultures This justifies the use of autologous serum to culture patient's own cells in order to eliminate any animal material from the culture system.[140]

Tan et al reported the use of cultivated conjunctival epithelial sheets for ocular surface reconstruction in seven patients (one extensive conjunctival nevus, three pterygia, two persistent leaking trabeculectomy blebs, and one superior limbic keratoconjunctivitis). HCE cells were harvested from the forniceal conjunctiva two weeks before operation, and were cultivated with explant culture technique on denuded AM under serum-free conditions. After a mean follow-up period of 11.6 months, successful outcome, defined as resolution of the disease, maintenance of conjunctival epithelialization and graft integrity, and absence of significant complications were obtained in all seven patients.[141] Ang et al further investigated the efficacy of cultivated autologous conjunctival epithelial cell transplantation for the treatment of 22 patients with primary pterygia. Excision of the pterygia was followed by reconstruction using a serum-free derived cultivated conjunctival equivalent. The recurrence rate was compared with reconstruction using conventional denuded AM in 18 patients. Although the recurrence rate was similar in both groups (22.7% in the former group and 25.0% in the latter), transplantation of cultivated conjunctival epithelial sheet facilitated early postoperative epithelialization and wound healing, and may aid in preventing serious surgical complications, such as scleral necrosis and secondary infection.[142]

Fibrin Gel as a Natural Scaffold for Cultivation of Human Limbo-Corneal Epithelial Cells

Conventional biomaterials used in tissue engineering like polyglycolic acid (PGA) or PLGA (polylactic and glycolic acid) are not suitable for cultivating HLE cells, because they are neither biodegradable nor soft. In contrast to the tremendous success of AM as a substrate for cultivating HLE cells, only few other biomaterials have been tried clinically. Fibrin gel was first used as a biodegradable scaffold for cultivating chondrocytes[143] or myofibroblasts.[144] In 1994, Kaiser et al reported three patients with deep partial and full skin thickness burns treated with cultured autologous keratinocytes suspended in fibrin glue. In two of these patients the keratinocyte-fibrin matrix was overgrafted with allogeneic, glycerine-preserved split thickness cadaver skin. The non-confluent cells developed into a continuous epithelial layer within 4 days, and histological examination showed a stratified neoepidermis. Clinically the new skin had satisfactory stability and mechanical quality. The fibrin glue matrix seems to give sufficient adherence stability to keratinocytes that are grafted in an actively proliferating state.[145] Later, Pellegrini et al. showed that the relative percentage of holoclones (keratinocyte stem cells) is maintained when epidermal keratinocytes are cultivated on fibrin, and the clonogenic ability, growth rate, and long-term proliferative potential of epidermal keratinocytes are not affected. When fibrin-cultured autografts bearing stem cells are applied on massive full-thickness burns, the "take" of keratinocytes is high, reproducible, and permanent, suggesting that fibrin is a suitable substrate for keratinocyte cultivation and transplantation.[146]

Later, the same group published their results of using fibrin sealant to culture autologous HLE cells in the presence of feeder cells to reconstruct 18 eyes predominantly with total LSCD. They first demonstrated that the clonogenic ability, overall size, morphology and growth rate of HLE cells grown on plastic or on fibrin were identical. Fibrin-cultured epithelial sheet, isolated from a 1-mm^2 limbal biopsy was composed of a well-conserved basal layer formed by cuboidal cells and of several suprabasal layers. Transplantation of fibrin-cultured HLE cells was successful in 14 of 18 patients. Re-epithelialization occurred within the first week. Inflammation and vascularization regressed within the first 3-4 weeks. By the first month, the corneal surface was covered by a transparent, normal-looking epithelium. At 12-27 months follow-up, corneal surfaces were clinically and cytologically stable. However, because of the residual stromal scarring, three patients had a penetrating keratoplasty approximately 1 year later. As expected, the epithelium uniformly expressed keratin 3 but not keratin 19, further demonstrating that fibrin-cultured stem cells have been engrafted and were able to permanently restore the corneal surface.[147] Such fibrin-based scaffold may further be cross-linked to fibronectin by the action of the transglutaminase factor XIII, which may dramatically enhance keratinocyte adhesion, spreading, and migration, thereby contributes to corneal wound healing.[148]

Cultivated Oral Mucosal Epithelial Cells as an Alternative Source of Corneal Epithelium

Allograft rejection is the main cause of failure following transplantation of allogeneic HLE cells, conventional or ex vivo cultivated alike. The success rate is even lower in eyes with autoimmune diseases, especially active SJS.[88-91] Theoretically, systemic immunosuppressant can be tapered one year after uneventful transplantation, but frequently it is hard to differentiate disease-associated corneal inflammation from chronic rejection, making the decision to discontinue immunosuppressant difficult.[84] What is more, patients with systemic diseases such as diabetes, renal failure, or liver cirrhosis are particularly at risk to receive systemic immunosuppressants. Patients at the extreme of age (very young or very old) should also be concerned. Harvesting tissue from living related donors is one way to reduce allograft rejection, however, the recipient still need to be immunosuppressed. These concerns raise the urgency of using alternative autologous keratinocytes for corneal reconstruction.

The use of autologous oral mucosa to reconstruct conunctiva is nothing new. As early as in 1960s there were articles describing reconstructing conjunctival defect with buccal mucosa following burns or removal of tumors.[149-152] The buccal mucosa is routinely used by oculoplastic surgeons to reconstruct conjunctival fornix. However, normal oral mucosa consists of at least 20-30 layers of stratified squamous epithelium, alone with a dense submucosal layer, making it almost impossible to reconstruct the corneal surface with intact oral mucosa. Gipson et al were the first to propose transplantation of oral mucosal epithelium to ocular surface wounds, and that the grafts can be maintained. In their experiments, oral mucosal epithelial sheets were freed from underlying connective tissue and basal lamina by dispase II treatment, and then sutured to abraded or keratectomized rabbit corneas. Even after four months, the grafts maintained some histological characteristics of oral mucosal epithelium.[153]

One intriguing nature of the oral mucosa is that its spinous cell layer shows homogeneous staining for keratin 3, the keratin that was thought to be cornea-specific.[154;155] The expression of keratin 3 by human oral mucosal epithelial (HOME) cells can be further enhanced when HOME cells are culture on AM. This, together with successful short-term result from animal study encourages the clinical use of cultivated autologous HOME cells as a substitute for corneal epithelium.[156;157] Some evidences supported the presence of keratinocyte stem cells in the oral mucosa, that cultivated HOME cells formed colony in vitro, and clonal analysis revealed that holoclone-type (stem cell compartment), meroclone-type (intermediate compartment), and paraclone-type (transient amplifying cell compartment) cells, previously identified in the skin and the ocular surface, were present in HOME cells. Holoclone-type cells showed stronger low-affinity neurotrophin receptor p75 expression at both the mRNA and protein level. p75(+) subset were smaller, did not actively cycle in vivo, and possessed higher in vitro proliferative capacity and clonal growth potential than the p75(-) subset, therefore p75 is suggested to be a potential marker of oral keratinocyte stem/progenitor cells.[158]

In 2004, almost simultaneously two Japanese groups reported their results of cultivated autologous HOME cell transplantation. Nishida et al. reported harvesting 3-by-3-mm specimens of oral mucosal tissue from four patients (one SJS and 3 OCP) with bilateral total LSCD. Epithelial sheets were generated by culturing dispersed HOME cells for two weeks on temperature responsive cell culture surfaces (discussed later) paved with mitomycin C-inactivated 3T3 feeder cells. The presence of keratinocyte progenitor cells in culture was confirmed by colony-forming efficiency in vitro, and positive staining of epithelial stem cell and progenitor cell marker β1 integrin and p63 in basal epithelial cells. The sheet of cultured HOME cells can be separated from the culture surface simply following temperature reduction. After removing conjunctival fibrovascular tissue, the epithelial sheet can be transplanted directly to the corneal surfaces without sutures. After a mean follow-up period of 14 months, all corneal surfaces remained transparent, the vision was significantly improved, and there were no complications.[159] Nakamura et al. also reported their result of transplanting cultivated HOME cells in patients with SJS (three eyes) or chemical burns (three eyes). They were using denuded AM as a carrier in the presence of 3T3 fibroblasts and air-lifting. During the mean follow-up period of 13.8 months, the corneal surface remained stable in all eyes. Although all eyes manifested with mild peripheral neovascularization, the visual acuity was unanimously improved.[160] Later, the authors performed a longer-term assessment of the outcome. There were 15 eyes from 12 patients (including the original 4 cases) mainly with SJS, chemical and thermal injury. The patients were followed up for an averaged 20 months; with the longest follow-up being 34 months. During the follow-up period, all eyes manifested some peripheral corneal neovascularization, and in 10 of 15 eyes (67%) the ocular surface was stable and transparent without any major complications, and the transplanted epithelium survived for at least 34 months. In 10 eyes, postoperative visual acuity was improved by more than 2 lines. However, five eyes, including four with severe SJS, developed small but longstanding epithelial defects; three of them healed spontaneously, and two (13%) required re-operation. The authors suggested that persistent corneal inflammation in SJS may be detrimental to the transplanted epithelium, and short-term, postoperative immunosuppression for reducing postoperative inflammation and control of primary diseases may still be required.[161] Currently, a government-supervised human trial of the technique is under way in our institute. The preliminary results are shown in figures 7 and 8.

Although central corneal clarity is maintained, unlike cultivated HLE cell sheet, following transplantation of cultivated HOME cell sheet, the graft frequently induces mild peripheral neovascularization. To evaluate the angiogenic activity of cultivated HLE and HOME cell sheets, Sekiyama et al examined the expression of angiogenesis-related factors by these cell sheets, which included thrombospondin-1 (TSP-1), pigment epithelium derived factor (PEDF), endostatin, angiostatin, vascular endothelial growth factor (VEGF), Fms-like tyrosine kinase 1 (Flt-1), kinase insert domain receptor (KDR), and basic fibroblast growth factor (bFGF). They found that TSP-1 expression was significantly higher in HLE cell sheet than in HOME cell sheet, while there was no significant difference in the expression of other angiogenic/anti-angiogenic factors. The authors thus concluded that decreased expression of anti-angiogenic factors particularly TSP-1 in HOME cell sheet may be related to the superficial peripheral neovascularization encountered after cultivated HOME cell transplantation.[162]

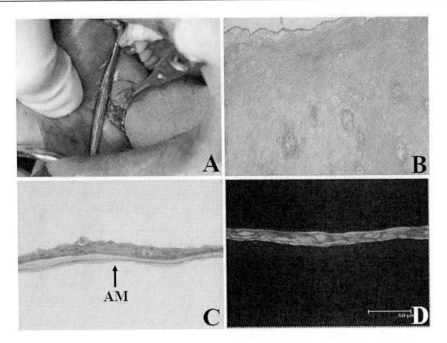

Figure 7. Cultivation of human oral mucosal epithelial (HOME) cells on amniotic membrane (AM). A 6X6 mm biopsy was taken from the buccal mucosa (A). The original oral mucosa (B) is too thick to be transplanted to the cornea. However, following cultivation on denuded AM and coculture with 3T3 feeder cells, the HOME cells were at most 3 to 5 layers thick (C), and were homogenously stained positive for keratin 3 (D; green)

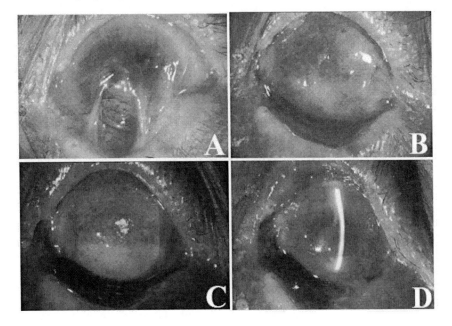

Figure 8. Cultivated autologous oral mucosal epithelial cell transplantation in a 73 years old female with ocular cicatricial pemphigoid. Pre-operatively, the cornea was covered by dense fibrovascular tissue with symblepharon formation. The vision was only hand motion (A). Two months after operation, the transplanted epithelium became stabilized (C, D; fluorescein staining). Eight months after operation, the cornea became more transparent, and the vision improved to 20/2000 (D).

Cataract surgery and lamellar keratoplasty are commonly combined surgical procedures at the time of cultivated HOME cell transplantation in order to further improve vision. However, these procedures are not easy to perform in cases with corneal irregularities and opacities. Inatomi et al introduced simultaneous automated lamellar therapeutic keratoplasty (ALTK) to correct corneal stromal opacity, which is a procedure based on microkeratome-assisted lamellar keratoplasty and provides smooth and sharp stromal excision. This surgical procedure is also very useful to improve intraoperative visibility at the time of cataract surgery in patients with hazy cornea. At the completion of ATLK, the corneal surface is covered with cultivated HOME cells. Such combined corneal and cataract surgery result in dramatic improvement of visual acuity, without the need for further operation.[163]

Regarding the epithelial phenotype of cultivated HOME cells on AM, Inatomi et al. reported that one patient with SJS and one with chemical burn were treated with cultivated HOME cell transplantation, followed about half an year later by a combined penetrating keratoplasty, cataract extraction and intraocular lens implantation. During the mean follow-up period of 22.5 months, the corneal surface remained stable, and the vision was improved in both cases. Histological study demonstrated that the epithelial structure and cell density in the basal cell layer of the corneal buttons were similar to normal stratified corneal epithelium without goblet cells. Keratin 3, but not keratin 12, was expressed by the transplanted HOME cells that was similar to oral mucosal tissue.[164] Nakamura et al. further analyzed corneal buttons obtained from four successful and two failed cases of HOME cell transplantation. In failed grafts, neighboring conjunctival epithelial cells apparently invaded a large portion of the corneal surface, and the epithelial phenotype was mainly keratin 3 negative and Muc5AC (goblet cell-derived mucin) positive; there were also many blood vessels and inflammatory cells in the corneal stroma. In successful grafts, transplanted mucosal epithelial cells survived and had adapted well to the host corneal tissues, and the epithelial phenotype was predominantly keratin 3 positive and Muc5AC negative; there was no infiltration by inflammatory cells, nor was there dissolution of the AM substrate. This study confirmed that in clinically successful eyes, cultivated HOME cells survive on the corneal surface and maintain the ocular surface integrity.[165]

Finally, because there has always been a concern of spreading mad cow disease or other animal-derived diseases when using bovine serum to culture human cells for transplantation, Nakamura et al proposed to use the patient's own serum to replace bovine serum. The BrdU proliferation assay and colony-forming efficiency analysis showed that HOME and HLE cells cultivated with autologous serum-supplemented media showed comparable proliferative capacities compared with bovine serum-supplemented media. The epithelial morphology, expression of tissue-specific keratins and basement membrane assembly were all similar.[166] Having reported the success of transplantating autologous serum-cultivated HLE cells in 9 patients with total LSCD,[167] the authors went on to publish their results of using autologous serum from 10 patients with total LSCD to develop cultivated oral epithelial equivalents. They demonstrated that following transplantation, the ocular surface remained stable, without major complications in all eyes during a mean follow-up of 12.6 months. The visual acuity improved by more than 2 lines in 9 of 10 eyes, with transplanted HOME cells surviving up to 19 months. The successful use of autologous serum in cultivating HOME cells to treat severe ocular surface disease represents an important advance in the pursuit of completely autologous, xenobiotic-free bioengineered ocular equivalents for clinical transplantation.[168]

Thermo-responsive Culture Surface as a Novel Substrate for Stem Cell Transplantation

Corneal epithelial SC transplantation has gained much attention in the past decade. In 1997, Pellegrini et al first reported a clinical application of autologous cultivated corneal epithelium to treat patients with LSCD.[112] Later, several investigators have shown that the biological tissue materials such as AM can be used as a matrix carrier for ex vivo expanded corneal epithelial stem cells as bioengineered ocular surface. Cultivated HLE cell transplantation in conjunction with AM has been proven to be an effective technique for the therapeutic treatment of ocular surface diseases, such as SJS and chemical/thermal burns.[114;115;117] In addition to AM, other carrier substrates such as fibrin gel[147] and chitosan-coated alginate membranes[169] have recently been investigated for their potential use in corneal epithelial regeneration. Although cultivated cell transplantation using carrier substrates can strengthen the tissue-engineered epithelial grafts, the presence of carrier materials postoperatively may decrease optical transparency and pose a risk of inflammatory reaction.[170] To overcome these limitations, Nishida et al recently fabricated bioengineered corneal epithelial cell sheets by using thermo-responsive poly(*N*-isopropylacrylamide) (PNIPAAm)-grafted polystyrene (PS) culture surfaces.[171] In a rabbit model, functional corneal epithelial sheet grafts were successfully transplanted without any carriers.

The cell sheet engineering technique using thermo-responsive culture dishes represents a novel approach for tissue regeneration without artificial scaffolds.[172] Okano and his colleagues have developed thermo-responsive culture surfaces (TRCS) that are created by the covalent grafting of the temperature-sensitive polymer PNIPAAm to ordinary tissue culture dishes.[173] Under normal culture conditions at 37°C, the dish surfaces are relatively hydrophobic and cells attach, spread, and proliferate similarly to on typical tissue culture dishes. However, upon temperature reduction below the polymer's lower critical solution temperature (LCST) of 32°C, the polymer surface becomes hydrophilic and swells, forming a hydration layer between the dish surface and the cultured cells, allowing for spontaneous detachment of the cells from the dish, without the need for enzymatic treatments such as trypsinization. By avoiding proteolytic treatment, critical cell surface proteins such extracellular matrix (ECM), growth factor receptors and cell-cell junction proteins remain intact, and cells can be harvested as intact sheets noninvasively along with their deposited ECM.[170]

A recent report from Nishida's laboratory indicated that the bioengineered cell sheet grafts are feasible for corneal epithelial regeneration.[171] Human or rabbit limbal stem cells were cocultured with mitomycin C-treated 3T3 feeder layers on TRCS at 37°C. After 2 weeks of cultivation, multilayered corneal epithelial cell sheets were harvested from the dishes simply by reducing the temperature to 20°C without the use of proteases. Cell-cell junctions and ECM on the basal side of the sheet, critical to sheet integrity and function, remained intact. Additionally, a viable population of corneal epithelial progenitor cells, close in number to that originally seeded, was found in the sheets. Using a polyvinylidene difluoride (PVDF) membrane, the bioengineered corneal epithelial sheet grafts were transferred to the recipient corneal stroma. Corneal epithelial cell sheet transplantation in a rabbit model demonstrated that the autografts cover the entire cornea and result in a clear and smooth surface. In cases with bilateral total LSCD, the group of Nishida has recently shown that keratinocyte SCs can be isolated from the patient's own oral mucosa and used as an alternative cell source.[159] Interestingly, oral mucosal epithelial cell sheets cultured on temperature-responsive dishes more closely resemble native corneal epithelium than native oral mucosal epithelium. After receiving cell sheet grafts, complete reepithelialization of the corneal surfaces occurred within one week in all four treated eyes. Clinical results have also demonstrated the recovery of visual acuity with corneal transparency maintained for over one year. Additionally, colony-forming assays and immunostaining for p63, β1integrin, and connexin 43 indicated retention of viable stem and/or progenitor cell populations in the bioengineered rabbit oral mucosal epithelial cell sheets. The transplanted rabbit oral mucosal epithelial sheet grafts show phenotypic modulation after transplantation to the denuded corneal stroma.[174] By excluding the use of both scaffolds and carrier substrates, corneal transparency can be maximized. Sutureless transplantation of tissue-engineered cell sheets composed of autologous oral mucosal epithelium hold high promise to reconstruct the ocular surface. The carrier-free cell sheet engineering technique may overcome the drawbacks associated with conventional corneal transplantation surgery, which remains the most common form of treatment for corneal epithelial dysfunction. However, in more than half of cases requiring corneal transplantation, the endothelial cell layer is the only corneal component that requires replacement.[175] Therefore, corneal endothelial reconstruction is an attractive research field in tissue engineering since it is of high clinical importance.

The corneal endothelium is a thin monolayer of cells that form the posterior boundary of the cornea and maintain corneal deturgescence and clarity.[176] Human corneal endothelial cells (HCECs) do not proliferate in vivo, and the number of these cells decreases gradually with aging.[177] Due to the limited regenerative capacity of human corneal endothelium, continued lost of HCECs may cause irreversible corneal edema and loss of vision. In the mid to late 1970s, corneal endothelial transplantation was first attempted by McCulley et al[178] who directly injected a suspension of cultured endothelial cells into rabbit's anterior chamber to repopulate previously damaged corneal endothelium. However, the experiment was only partially successful because only scattered clumps of endothelial cells randomly attached to the recipient cornea and to other ocular tissues such as the iris and lens. In order to overcome the problems associated with injection of isolated cells, several investigators have reported a method to transplant CECs expanded ex vivo on different carrier substrates made of biopolymers such as gelatin,[179] collagen-coated dextran,[180] and collagen,[181] synthetic polymer materials like methyl methacrylate/N-vinyl pyrrolidone copolymers,[182], and biological tissues such as Descemet's membrane[183] and AM[184]. In 1980, Maurice's group prepared a thin gelatin film about 1 μm thick by cross-linking with glutaraldehyde, resulting in a transparent, wrinkle-free, water-permeable substrate which was used to support the growth of cultured CECs.[185] However, such a system would involve the use of cyanoacrylate adhesives, which may result in unstable attachment of the carrier substrate to the recipient corneal stroma. In 1994, Mohay et al. investigated the feasibility of using hydrogel lens as cell carrier device in a feline or rabbit allogeneic transplantation model.[186] They found that the hydrogel device was mechanically stable to allow for easy handling of fragile cell grafts, but the implantation of a foreign body carrier may potentially induce rejection reaction. Recently, the human AM without epithelium has also been applied as a carrier for cultivated HCEC transplantation in a rabbit model.[184] The problems with CEC carrier substrates may include poor graft-host integration, optical interference, risk of foreign body reaction, and disturbance of endothelial cell function because of the presence of carrier materials between the implanted cells and the host tissue.

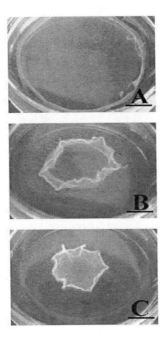

Figure 9. Gross observations of cultured HCEC detachment from thermo-responsive surfaces after incubation at 20°C for 10 min (A), 25 min (B), and 45 min (C). Bars indicate 5 mm.

To overcome these limitations, we have developed the cell sheet engineering technique for the treatment of corneal endothelial deficiency.[187] A novel strategy for corneal endothelial reconstruction using functional biomedical materials is shown in figure 9. By means of plasma chemistry, the polyethylene (PE) surfaces were modified with 1.6 µg/cm^2 of PNIPAAm. Untransformed adult HCECs derived from eye bank corneas were plated on the thermo-responsive PNIPAAm-grafted culture substrates and incubated for 3 weeks at 37°C. When the surrounding temperature was lowered to 20°C, the confluent cultures were harvested as intact cell monolayers. The characteristics of tissue-engineered HCEC sheets are similar to those observed in the donor corneas.[188] Fabrication of bioengineered HCEC sheets from thermo-responsive PNIPAAm-grafted culture dishes[189] or poly(NIPAAm-co-diethyleneglycol methacrylate (DEGMA)) substrates[190] have also been recently reported by other groups. They confirmed proper structure and function of the thermally detached HCEC monolayers. While these findings suggest that transplantable HCEC sheets can feasibly be used as tissue equivalents for replacing compromised endothelium, it is apparent that targeted delivery of cell sheet to the corneal posterior surface is another very important issue. The merits of the technique include that since HCECs from a single donor cornea can be amplified for several folds, and can be cryo-preserved before transplantation, this may not only help to solve the problem of global shortage of donor corneas, and may also make possible the pre-operative matching of donor to reduce transplantation rejection.

Despite constructing a tissue-like architecture, the thermally detached cell sheets were easy to wrinkle and fold during removal.[191] In the field of cell sheet transfer, Shimizu et al have introduced the hydrophilically modified PVDF membranes as a supporter, which enables three-dimensional manipulation of cardiomyocyte sheets into layered constructs.[192] Recently, a doughnut-shaped PVDF supporter has been successfully used for cultured epithelial cell sheet transplantation.[159] However, intraocular grafting is different from ocular surface transplantation, because the anterior chamber is perfused with large amounts of tissue fluid, which may cause unstable attachment of implanted cell sheets to lesion sites. In these cases, it is necessary to provide a temporary supporting structure for enhancing the graft-host integration during and after intraocular delivery of the bioengineered cell monolayer. By avoiding permanent residence of foreign supporting materials in the host, we have utilized the biodegradable and cell-adhesive gelatin discs as a supporter for transportation and surgical handling of well-organized cell sheets.[193] Upon exposure to the aqueous humor, the swelling of gelatin occurred, which allows the attachment and spread of HCEC sheets onto the lesion area of rabbit cornea (figure 10). The gelatins with a negative charge and higher molecular weight may show stable mechanical property, appropriate biodegradability, and acceptable biocompatibility, making these materials interesting candidates for intraocular delivery of thermally detached HCEC sheets.

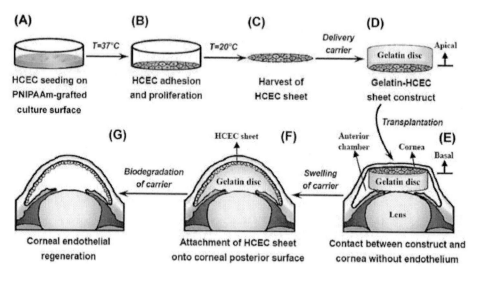

Figure 10. A novel strategy for corneal endothelial reconstruction with a tissue-engineered cell sheet cultivated on thermo-responsive culture dish. Schematic illustrations show the cultivated human corneal endothelial cell (HCEC) sheet is harvested via temperature modulation of a thermo-responsive PNIPAAm-grafted surface (A-C), and is delivered to the posterior surface of cornea (devoid of endothelium) using a bioadhesive gelatin hydrogel disc (D). After swelling (E) and biodegradation (F) of the gelatin carrier, the transplanted HCEC sheet with uniformly proper polarity is attached and integrated onto the denuded cornea to allow regeneration of endothelial monolayer (G).

The advantage of implantation of a gelatin disc may be that it improves the capability of cell sheet integration into host tissue. Since these supporting materials are substantially completely degraded and absorbed in vivo, we believe that this novel cell therapy technique will have a high success rate in treating CEC loss. A long-term (i.e., 6 months) study in a rabbit model strongly suggested that the corneal clarity was restored by implanting the bioengineered HCEC sheets (figure 11) and we have recently confirmed that the cultured HCECs and functional biomedical polymers, PNIPAAm and gelatin, hold high promise for corneal tissue engineering and regeneration.[194] Despite encouraging results from experimental work and clinical trials with regard to the cell sheet-based therapy, more studies are necessary to further evaluate the feasibility of bioengineered cell sheet grafts and functional biomedical polymers before clinical application.

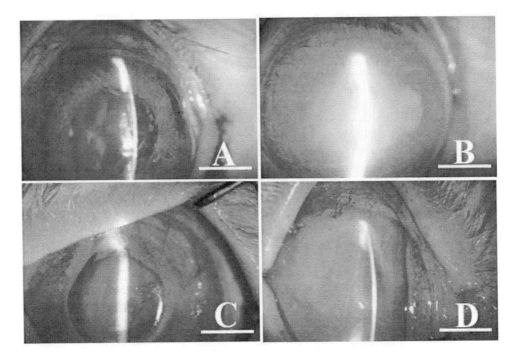

Figure 11. Representative slit-lamp microscopic images revealed that (A) the rabbit corneal endothelium on the Descemet's membrane was mechanically stripped from the cornea. (B) At postoperative 6 months, the corneas in the wounded groups were seriously edematous and cloudy. (C) In the human corneal endothelial cells (HCECs) sheet transplantation groups, gelatin-HCEC sheet construct was inserted into the anterior chamber, and an intact monolayer of HCECs was attached onto the recipient cornea previously denuded of endothelial cells. (D) Corneal opacity and edema were significantly improved at 6 months postoperatively. Scale bars, 5 mm.

CONCLUSION

The rapid progress in the understanding of LSC biology in recent years has enabled clinicians to develop effective therapeutic techniques for corneal epithelial stem cell transplantation. Currently, autologous/allogeneic limbal tissue transplantation combined with amniotic membrane transplantation is the main stream treatment. However, tissue-engineered epithelial sheet transplantation has emerged as a promising technique due to less traumatic to the donor site, faster re-epithelialization, anti-inflammatory and anti-angiogenic effect, and therefore sooner visual recovery. However, more evidences are still needed to document the existence of donor-derived stem cells in the graft after transplantation. On the other hand, cultivating human corneal endothelial cells on thermo-responsive culture surface for transplantation is another promising technology, which highlights the significance of biomaterial surface technology in facilitating stem cell transplantation. It is foreseeable that combining techniques for ex vivo expansion of corneal stem cells (epithelium, stroma, and endothelium) and techniques for fabricating layered cell sheets containing the stem cells may ultimately lead to the creation of genuine biosynthetic cornea.

REFERENCES

[1] Ren H, Wilson G. Apoptosis in the corneal epithelium. *Invest. Ophthalmol. Vis. Sci.* 1996;37:1017-25.
[2] Hall PA, Watt FM. Stem cells: the generation and maintenance of cellular diversity. *Development.* 1989;106:619-33.
[3] Davanger M, Evensen A. Role of the pericorneal papillary structure in renewal of corneal epithelium. *Nature.* 1971;229:560-1.
[4] Schermer A, Galvin S, Sun TT. Differentiation-related expression of a major 64K corneal keratin in vivo and in culture suggests limbal location of corneal epithelial stem cells. *J. Cell Biol.* 1986;103:49-62.
[5] Potten CS, Loeffler M. Stem cells: attributes, cycles, spirals, pitfalls and uncertainties. Lessons for and from the crypt. *Development.* 1990;110:1001-20.
[6] Dua HS, Azuara-Blanco A. Limbal stem cells of the corneal epithelium. *Surv. Ophthalmol.* 2000;44:415-25.
[7] Pellegrini G, Golisano O, Paterna P, et al. Location and clonal analysis of stem cells and their differentiated progeny in the human ocular surface. *J. Cell Biol.* 1999;145:769-82.
[8] Lavker RM, Tseng SC, Sun TT. Corneal epithelial stem cells at the limbus: looking at some old problems from a new angle. *Exp. Eye Res.* 2004;78:433-46.
[9] Cotsarelis G, Cheng SZ, Dong G, et al. Existence of slow-cycling limbal epithelial basal cells that can be preferentially stimulated to proliferate: implications on epithelial stem cells. *Cell.* 1989;57:201-9.
[10] Bickenbach JR. Identification and behavior of label-retaining cells in oral mucosa and skin. *J. Dent. Res.* 1981;60 Spec. No. C:1611-20.
[11] Lavker RM, Wei ZG, Sun TT. Phorbol ester preferentially stimulates mouse fornical conjunctival and limbal epithelial cells to proliferate in vivo. *Invest. Ophthalmol. Vis. Sci.* 1998;39:301-7.
[12] Lehrer MS, Sun TT, Lavker RM. Strategies of epithelial repair: modulation of stem cell and transit amplifying cell proliferation. *J. Cell Sci.* 1998;111 (Pt 19):2867-75.
[13] Schofield R. The stem cell system. *Biomed. Pharmacother.* 1983;37:375-80.
[14] Lavker RM, Dong G, Cheng SZ, et al. Relative proliferative rates of limbal and corneal epithelia. Implications of corneal epithelial migration, circadian rhythm, and

suprabasally located DNA-synthesizing keratinocytes. *Invest. Ophthalmol. Vis. Sci.* 1991;32:1864-75.
[15] Gipson IK. The epithelial basement membrane zone of the limbus. *Eye.* 1989;3 (Pt 2):132-40.
[16] Wiley L, SundarRaj N, Sun TT, Thoft RA. Regional heterogeneity in human corneal and limbal epithelia: an immunohistochemical evaluation. *Invest. Ophthalmol. Vis. Sci.* 1991;32:594-602.
[17] Kurpakus MA, Stock EL, Jones JC. Expression of the 55-kD/64-kD corneal keratins in ocular surface epithelium. *Invest. Ophthalmol. Vis. Sci.* 1990;31:448-56.
[18] Matic M, Petrov IN, Chen S, et al. Stem cells of the corneal epithelium lack connexins and metabolite transfer capacity. *Differentiation.* 1997;61:251-60.
[19] Chen Z, de Paiva CS, Luo L, et al. Characterization of putative stem cell phenotype in human limbal epithelia. *Stem Cells.* 2004;22:355-66.
[20] Wolosin JM, Xiong X, Schutte M, et al. Stem cells and differentiation stages in the limbo-corneal epithelium. *Prog. Retin. Eye Res.* 2000;19:223-55.
[21] Lendahl U, Zimmerman LB, McKay RD. CNS stem cells express a new class of intermediate filament protein. *Cell.* 1990;60:585-95.
[22] Kasper M, Moll R, Stosiek P, Karsten U. Patterns of cytokeratin and vimentin expression in the human eye. *Histochemistry.* 1988;89:369-77.
[23] Kasper M. Patterns of cytokeratins and vimentin in guinea pig and mouse eye tissue: evidence for regional variations in intermediate filament expression in limbal epithelium. *Acta Histochem.* 1992;93:319-32.
[24] Pellegrini G, Dellambra E, Golisano O, et al. p63 identifies keratinocyte stem cells. *Proc. Natl. Acad. Sci. U. S. A.* 2001;98:3156-61.
[25] Dua HS, Joseph A, Shanmuganathan VA, Jones RE. Stem cell differentiation and the effects of deficiency. *Eye.* 2003;17:877-85.
[26] Hsueh YJ, Wang DY, Cheng CC, Chen JK. Age-related expressions of p63 and other keratinocyte stem cell markers in rat cornea. *J. Biomed. Sci.* 2004;11:641-51.
[27] Schlotzer-Schrehardt U, Kruse FE. Identification and characterization of limbal stem cells. *Exp. Eye Res.* 2005;81:247-64.
[28] Wang DY, Hsueh YJ, Yang VC, Chen JK. Propagation and phenotypic preservation of rabbit limbal epithelial cells on amniotic membrane. *Invest. Ophthalmol. Vis. Sci.* 2003;44:4698-704.
[29] Di Iorio E, Barbaro V, Ruzza A, et al. Isoforms of DeltaNp63 and the migration of ocular limbal cells in human corneal regeneration. *Proc. Natl. Acad. Sci. U. S. A.* 2005;102:9523-8.
[30] Hynes RO. Integrins: versatility, modulation, and signaling in cell adhesion. *Cell.* 1992;69:11-25.
[31] Stepp MA, Zhu L, Sheppard D, Cranfill RL. Localized distribution of alpha 9 integrin in the cornea and changes in expression during corneal epithelial cell differentiation. *J. Histochem. Cytochem.* 1995;43:353-62.
[32] Zhou S, Schuetz JD, Bunting KD, et al. The ABC transporter Bcrp1/ABCG2 is expressed in a wide variety of stem cells and is a molecular determinant of the side-population phenotype. *Nat. Med.* 2001;7:1028-34.
[33] Kim M, Turnquist H, Jackson J, et al. The multidrug resistance transporter ABCG2 (breast cancer resistance protein 1) effluxes Hoechst 33342 and is overexpressed in hematopoietic stem cells. *Clin. Cancer Res.* 2002;8:22-8.

[34] de Paiva CS, Chen Z, Corrales RM, et al. ABCG2 transporter identifies a population of clonogenic human limbal epithelial cells. *Stem. Cells.* 2005;23:63-73.
[35] Tseng SC. Regulation and clinical implications of corneal epithelial stem cells. *Mol. Biol. Rep.* 1996;23:47-58.
[36] Tseng SC. Concept and application of limbal stem cells. *Eye.* 1989;3 (Pt 2):141-57.
[37] Tsai RJ, Tseng SC. Effect of stromal inflammation on the outcome of limbal transplantation for corneal surface reconstruction. *Cornea.* 1995;14:439-49.
[38] Huang AJ, Tseng SC. Corneal epithelial wound healing in the absence of limbal epithelium. *Invest. Ophthalmol. Vis. Sci.* 1991;32:96-105.
[39] Puangsricharern V, Tseng SC. Cytologic evidence of corneal diseases with limbal stem cell deficiency. *Ophthalmology.* 1995;102:1476-85.
[40] Tsai RJ, Sun TT, Tseng SC. Comparison of limbal and conjunctival autograft transplantation in corneal surface reconstruction in rabbits. *Ophthalmology.* 1990;97:446-55.
[41] Holland EJ, Schwartz GS. The evolution of epithelial transplantation for severe ocular surface disease and a proposed classification system. *Cornea.* 1996;15:549-56.
[42] Thoft RA. Conjunctival transplantation. *Arch. Ophthalmol.* 1977;95:1425-7.
[43] Kenyon KR, Tseng SC. Limbal autograft transplantation for ocular surface disorders. *Ophthalmology.* 1989;96:709-22.
[44] Nishiwaki-Dantas MC, Dantas PE, Reggi JR. Ipsilateral limbal translocation for treatment of partial limbal deficiency secondary to ocular alkali burn. *Br. J. Ophthalmol.* 2001;85:1031-3.
[45] Ma DH, Chen JK, Zhang F, et al. Regulation of corneal angiogenesis in limbal stem cell deficiency. *Prog. Retin. Eye Res.* 2006;25:563-90.
[46] Ma DH, Tsai RJ, Chu WK, et al. Inhibition of vascular endothelial cell morphogenesis in cultures by limbal epithelial cells. *Invest. Ophthalmol. Vis. Sci.* 1999;40:1822-8.
[47] Basti S, Rao SK. Current status of limbal conjunctival autograft. *Curr. Opin. Ophthalmol.* 2000;11:224-32.
[48] Dua HS, Azuara-Blanco A. Autologous limbal transplantation in patients with nilateral corneal stem cell deficiency. *Br. J. Ophthalmol.* 2000;84:273-8.
[49] Yao YF, Zhang B, Zhou P, Jiang JK. Autologous limbal grafting combined with deep lamellar keratoplasty in unilateral eye with severe chemical or thermal burn at late stage. *Ophthalmology.* 2002;109:2011-7.
[50] Chen JJ, Tseng SC. Corneal epithelial wound healing in partial limbal deficiency. *Investigative Ophthalmology and Visual Science.* 1990;31:1301-14.
[51] Chen JJ, Tseng SC. Abnormal corneal epithelial wound healing in partial-thickness removal of limbal epithelium. *Invest. Ophthalmol. Vis. Sci.* 1991;32:2219-33.
[52] Meallet MA, Espana EM, Grueterich M, et al. Amniotic membrane transplantation with conjunctival limbal autograft for total limbal stem cell deficiency. *Ophthalmology.* 2003;110:1585-92.
[53] Fukuda K, Chikama T, Nakamura M, Nishida T. Differential distribution of subchains of the basement membrane components type IV collagen and laminin among the amniotic membrane, cornea, and conjunctiva. *Cornea.* 1999;18:73-9.
[54] Endo K, Nakamura T, Kawasaki S, Kinoshita S. Human amniotic membrane, like corneal epithelial basement membrane, manifests the alpha5 chain of type IV collagen. *Invest. Ophthalmol. Vis. Sci.* 2004;45:1771-4.
[55] Cooper LJ, Kinoshita S, German M, et al. An investigation into the composition of amniotic membrane used for ocular surface reconstruction. *Cornea.* 2005;24:722-9.

[56] Higa K, Shimmura S, Kato N, et al. Proliferation and differentiation of transplantable rabbit epithelial sheets engineered with or without an amniotic membrane carrier. *Invest. Ophthalmol. Vis. Sci.* 2007;48:597-604.

[57] Sun CC, Cheng CY, Chien CS, et al. Role of matrix metalloproteinase-9 in ex vivo expansion of human limbal epithelial cells cultured on human amniotic membrane. *Invest. Ophthalmol. Vis. Sci.* 2005;46:808-15.

[58] Woo HM, Kim MS, Kweon OK, et al. Effects of amniotic membrane on epithelial wound healing and stromal remodelling after excimer laser keratectomy in rabbit cornea. *Br. J. Ophthalmol.* 2001;85:345-9.

[59] Resch MD, Schlotzer-Schrehardt U, Hofmann-Rummelt C, et al. Adhesion structures of amniotic membranes integrated into human corneas. *Invest. Ophthalmol. Vis. Sci.* 2006;47:1853-61.

[60] Kim MK, Heo JW, Lee JL, et al. Adhesion complex in cultivated limbal epithelium on amniotic membrane after in vivo transplantation. *Curr. Eye Res.* 2005;30:639-46.

[61] Kurpakus-Wheater M. Laminin-5 is a component of preserved amniotic membrane. *Curr. Eye Res.* 2001;22:353-7.

[62] Ohno-Matsui K, Ichinose S, Nakahama K, et al. The effects of amniotic membrane on retinal pigment epithelial cell differentiation. *Mol. Vis.* 2005;11:1-10.

[63] Stanzel BV, Espana EM, Grueterich M, et al. Amniotic membrane maintains the phenotype of rabbit retinal pigment epithelial cells in culture. *Exp. Eye Res.* 2005;80:103-12.

[64] Grueterich M, Espana E, Tseng SC. Connexin 43 expression and proliferation of human limbal epithelium on intact and denuded amniotic membrane. *Invest. Ophthalmol. Vis. Sci.* 2002;43:63-71.

[65] Meller D, Tseng SC. Conjunctival epithelial cell differentiation on amniotic membrane. *Invest. Ophthalmol. Vis. Sci.* 1999;40:878-86.

[66] Sun CC, Su Pang JH, Cheng CY, et al. Interleukin-1 receptor antagonist (IL-1RA) prevents apoptosis in ex vivo expansion of human limbal epithelial cells cultivated on human amniotic membrane. *Stem Cells.* 2006;24:2130-9.

[67] Wang MX, Gray TB, Park WC, et al. Reduction in corneal haze and apoptosis by amniotic membrane matrix in excimer laser photoablation in rabbits. *J. Cataract. Refract. Surg.* 2001;27:310-9.

[68] Koizumi NJ, Inatomi TJ, Sotozono CJ, et al. Growth factor mRNA and protein in preserved human amniotic membrane. *Curr. Eye Res.* 2000;20:173-7.

[69] Touhami A, Grueterich M, Tseng SC. The role of NGF signaling in human limbal epithelium expanded by amniotic membrane culture. *Invest. Ophthalmol. Vis. Sci.* 2002;43:987-94.

[70] Meller D, Pires RT, Tseng SC. Ex vivo preservation and expansion of human limbal epithelial stem cells on amniotic membrane cultures. *Br. J. Ophthalmol.* 2002;86:463-71.

[71] Grueterich M, Tseng SC. Human limbal progenitor cells expanded on intact amniotic membrane ex vivo. *Arch. Ophthalmol.* 2002;120:783-90.

[72] Hao Y, Ma DH, Hwang DG, et al. Identification of antiangiogenic and antiinflammatory proteins in human amniotic membrane. *Cornea.* 2000;19:348-52.

[73] Solomon A, Rosenblatt M, Monroy D, et al. Suppression of interleukin 1alpha and interleukin 1beta in human limbal epithelial cells cultured on the amniotic membrane stromal matrix. *Br. J. Ophthalmol.* 2001;85:444-9.

[74] Shimmura S, Shimazaki J, Ohashi Y, Tsubota K. Antiinflammatory effects of amniotic membrane transplantation in ocular surface disorders. *Cornea.* 2001;20:408-13.

[75] Kim JC, Tseng SC. Transplantation of preserved human amniotic membrane for surface reconstruction in severely damaged rabbit corneas. *Cornea.* 1995;14:473-84.

[76] Gomes JA, Romano A, Santos MS, Dua HS. Amniotic membrane use in ophthalmology. *Curr. Opin. Ophthalmol.* 2005;16:233-40.

[77] Sippel KC, Ma JJ, Foster CS. Amniotic membrane surgery. *Curr. Opin. Ophthalmol.* 2001;12:269-81.

[78] Anderson DF, Ellies P, Pires RT, Tseng SC. Amniotic membrane transplantation for partial limbal stem cell deficiency. *Br. J. Ophthalmol.* 2001;85:567-75.

[79] Tsai RJ, Tseng SC. Human allograft limbal transplantation for corneal surface reconstruction. *Cornea.* 1994;13:389-400.

[80] Rao SK, Rajagopal R, Sitalakshmi G, Padmanabhan P. Limbal allografting from related live donors for corneal surface reconstruction. *Ophthalmology.* 1999;106:822-8.

[81] Holland EJ, DeRuyter DN, Doughman DJ. Langerhans cells in organ-cultured corneas. *Arch. Ophthalmol.* 1987;105:542-5.

[82] Gillette TE, Chandler JW, Greiner JV. Langerhans cells of the ocular surface. *Ophthalmology.* 1982;89:700-11.

[83] Daya SM, Bell RW, Habib NE, et al. Clinical and pathologic findings in human keratolimbal allograft rejection. *Cornea.* 2000;19:443-50.

[84] Espana EM, Di Pascuale M, Grueterich M, et al. Keratolimbal allograft in corneal reconstruction. *Eye.* 2004;18:406-17.

[85] Dua HS, Azuara-Blanco A. Allo-limbal transplantation in patients with limbal stem cell deficiency. *Br. J. Ophthalmol.* 1999;83:414-9.

[86] Reinhard T, Sundmacher R, Spelsberg H, Althaus C. Homologous penetrating central limbo-keratoplasty (HPCLK) in bilateral limbal stem cell insufficiency. *Acta Ophthalmol. Scand.* 1999;77:663-7.

[87] Tan DT, Ficker LA, Buckley RJ. Limbal transplantation. *Ophthalmology.* 1996;103:29-36.

[88] Tsubota K, Toda I, Saito H, et al. Reconstruction of the corneal epithelium by limbal allograft transplantation for severe ocular surface disorders. *Ophthalmology.* 1995;102:1486-96.

[89] Ilari L, Daya SM. Long-term outcomes of keratolimbal allograft for the treatment of severe ocular surface disorders. *Ophthalmology.* 2002;109:1278-84.

[90] Shimazaki J, Shimmura S, Fujishima H, Tsubota K. Association of preoperative tear function with surgical outcome in severe Stevens-Johnson syndrome. *Ophthalmology.* 2000;107:1518-23.

[91] Solomon A, Ellies P, Anderson DF, et al. Long-term outcome of keratolimbal allograft with or without penetrating keratoplasty for total limbal stem cell deficiency. *Ophthalmology.* 2002;109:1159-66.

[92] Tseng SC, Prabhasawat P, Barton K, et al. Amniotic membrane transplantation with or without limbal allografts for corneal surface reconstruction in patients with limbal stem cell deficiency. *Arch. Ophthalmol.* 1998;116:431-41.

[93] Shimazaki J, Maruyama F, Shimmura S, et al. Immunologic rejection of the central graft after limbal allograft transplantation combined with penetrating keratoplasty. *Cornea.* 2001;20:149-52.

[94] Hill JC. Immunosuppression in corneal transplantation. *Eye.* 1995;9 (Pt 2):247-53.

[95] Hill JC. Systemic cyclosporine in high-risk keratoplasty: long-term results. *Eye.* 1995;9 (Pt 4):422-8.
[96] Hill JC. Systemic cyclosporine in high-risk keratoplasty. Short- versus long-term therapy. *Ophthalmology.* 1994;101:128-33.
[97] Holland EJ, Schwartz GS. Epithelial stem-cell transplantation for severe ocular-surface disease. *N. Engl. J. Med.* 1999;340:1752-3.
[98] Daya SM, Ilari FA. Living related conjunctival limbal allograft for the treatment of stem cell deficiency. *Ophthalmology.* 2001;108:126-33.
[99] Santos MS, Gomes JA, Hofling-Lima AL, et al. Survival analysis of conjunctival limbal grafts and amniotic membrane transplantation in eyes with total limbal stem cell deficiency. *Am. J. Ophthalmol.* 2005;140:223-30.
[100] Gomes JA, Santos MS, Ventura AS, et al. Amniotic membrane with living related corneal limbal/conjunctival allograft for ocular surface reconstruction in Stevens-Johnson syndrome. *Arch. Ophthalmol.* 2003;121:1369-74.
[101] Tsubota K, Shimmura S, Shinozaki N, et al. Clinical application of living-related conjunctival-limbal allograft. *Am. J. Ophthalmol.* 2002;133:134-5.
[102] Tsubota K, Shimazaki J. Surgical treatment of children blinded by Stevens-Johnson syndrome. *Am. J. Ophthalmol.* 1999;128:573-81.
[103] Espana EM, Grueterich M, Ti SE, Tseng SC. Phenotypic study of a case receiving a keratolimbal allograft and amniotic membrane for total limbal stem cell deficiency. *Ophthalmology.* 2003;110:481-6.
[104] Shimazaki J, Kaido M, Shinozaki N, et al. Evidence of long-term survival of donor-derived cells after limbal allograft transplantation. *Invest. Ophthalmol. Vis. Sci.* 1999;40:1664-8.
[105] Egarth M, Hellkvist J, Claesson M, et al. Longterm survival of transplanted human corneal epithelial cells and corneal stem cells. *Acta Ophthalmol. Scand.* 2005;83:456-61.
[106] Djalilian AR, Mahesh SP, Koch CA, et al. Survival of donor epithelial cells after limbal stem cell transplantation. *Invest. Ophthalmol. Vis. Sci.* 2005;46:803-7.
[107] Henderson TR, Coster DJ, Williams KA. The long term outcome of limbal allografts: the search for surviving cells. *Br. J. Ophthalmol.* 2001;85:604-9.
[108] Rheinwald JG, Green H. Serial cultivation of strains of human epidermal keratinocytes: the formation of keratinizing colonies from single cells. *Cell.* 1975;6:331-43.
[109] Green H, Kehinde O, Thomas J. Growth of cultured human epidermal cells into multiple epithelia suitable for grafting. *Proc. Natl. Acad. Sci. U. S. A.* 1979;76:5665-8.
[110] Gallico GG, III, O'Connor NE, Compton CC, et al. Permanent coverage of large burn wounds with autologous cultured human epithelium. *N. Engl. J. Med.* 1984;311:448-51.
[111] Pellegrini G, De Luca M, Arsenijevic Y. Towards therapeutic application of ocular stem cells. *Semin. Cell Dev. Biol.* 2007.
[112] Pellegrini G, Traverso CE, Franzi AT, et al. Long-term restoration of damaged corneal surfaces with autologous cultivated corneal epithelium. *Lancet.* 1997;349:990-3.
[113] Schwab IR. Cultured corneal epithelia for ocular surface disease. *Trans. Am. Ophthalmol. Soc.* 1999;97:891-986.
[114] Schwab IR, Reyes M, Isseroff RR. Successful transplantation of bioengineered tissue replacements in patients with ocular surface disease. *Cornea.* 2000;19:421-6.
[115] Tsai RJ, Li LM, Chen JK. Reconstruction of damaged corneas by transplantation of autologous limbal epithelial cells. *N. Engl. J. Med.* 2000;343:86-93.

[116] Li W, He H, Kuo CL, et al. Basement membrane dissolution and reassembly by limbal corneal epithelial cells expanded on amniotic membrane. *Invest. Ophthalmol. Vis. Sci.* 2006;47:2381-9.

[117] Koizumi N, Inatomi T, Suzuki T, et al. Cultivated corneal epithelial stem cell transplantation in ocular surface disorders. *Ophthalmology.* 2001;108:1569-74.

[118] Nakamura T, Koizumi N, Tsuzuki M, et al. Successful regrafting of cultivated corneal epithelium using amniotic membrane as a carrier in severe ocular surface disease. *Cornea.* 2003;22:70-1.

[119] Cooper LJ, Fullwood NJ, Koizumi N, et al. An investigation of removed cultivated epithelial transplants in patients after allocultivated corneal epithelial transplantation. *Cornea.* 2004;23:235-42.

[120] Shimazaki J, Aiba M, Goto E, et al. Transplantation of human limbal epithelium cultivated on amniotic membrane for the treatment of severe ocular surface disorders. *Ophthalmology.* 2002;109:1285-90.

[121] Ang LP, Sotozono C, Koizumi N, et al. A comparison between cultivated and conventional limbal stem cell transplantation for Stevens-Johnson syndrome. *Am. J. Ophthalmol.* 2007;143:178-80.

[122] Koizumi N, Inatomi T, Suzuki T, et al. Cultivated corneal epithelial transplantation for ocular surface reconstruction in acute phase of Stevens-Johnson syndrome. *Arch. Ophthalmol.* 2001;119:298-300.

[123] Kim HS, Jun S, X, de Paiva CS, et al. Phenotypic characterization of human corneal epithelial cells expanded ex vivo from limbal explant and single cell cultures. *Exp. Eye Res.* 2004;79:41-9.

[124] Ti SE, Grueterich M, Espana EM, et al. Correlation of long term phenotypic and clinical outcomes following limbal epithelial transplantation cultivated on amniotic membrane in rabbits. *Br. J. Ophthalmol.* 2004;88:422-7.

[125] Shimazaki J, Higa K, Morito F, et al. Factors influencing outcomes in cultivated limbal epithelial transplantation for chronic cicatricial ocular surface disorders. *Am. J. Ophthalmol.* 2007;143:945-53.

[126] Sangwan VS, Matalia HP, Vemuganti GK, et al. Early results of penetrating keratoplasty after cultivated limbal epithelium transplantation. *Arch. Ophthalmol.* 2005;123:334-40.

[127] Grueterich M, Espana EM, Tseng SC. Ex vivo expansion of limbal epithelial stem cells: amniotic membrane serving as a stem cell niche. *Surv. Ophthalmol.* 2003;48:631-46.

[128] Grueterich M, Espana EM, Tseng SC. Modulation of keratin and connexin expression in limbal epithelium expanded on denuded amniotic membrane with and without a 3T3 fibroblast feeder layer. *Invest. Ophthalmol. Vis. Sci.* 2003;44:4230-6.

[129] Grueterich M, Espana EM, Touhami A, et al. Phenotypic study of a case with successful transplantation of ex vivo expanded human limbal epithelium for unilateral total limbal stem cell deficiency. *Ophthalmology.* 2002;109:1547-52.

[130] Daya SM, Watson A, Sharpe JR, et al. Outcomes and DNA analysis of ex vivo expanded stem cell allograft for ocular surface reconstruction. *Ophthalmology.* 2005;112:470-7.

[131] Li W, Hayashida Y, Chen YT, Tseng SC. Niche regulation of corneal epithelial stem cells at the limbus. *Cell Res.* 2007;17:26-36.

[132] Kawasaki S, Tanioka H, Yamasaki K, et al. Clusters of corneal epithelial cells reside ectopically in human conjunctival epithelium. *Invest. Ophthalmol. Vis. Sci.* 2006;47:1359-67.

[133] Ma DH, Yao JY, Yeh LK, et al. In vitro antiangiogenic activity in ex vivo expanded human limbocorneal epithelial cells cultivated on human amniotic membrane. *Invest. Ophthalmol. Vis. Sci.* 2004;45:2586-95.

[134] Ma DH, Yao JY, Kuo MT, et al. Generation of endostatin by matrix metalloproteinase and cathepsin from human limbocorneal epithelial cells cultivated on amniotic membrane. *Invest. Ophthalmol. Vis. Sci.* 2007;48:644-51.

[135] Wei ZG, Sun TT, Lavker RM. Rabbit conjunctival and corneal epithelial cells belong to two separate lineages. *Invest. Ophthalmol. Vis. Sci.* 1996;37:523-33.

[136] Wei ZG, Cotsarelis G, Sun TT, Lavker RM. Label-retaining cells are preferentially located in fornical epithelium: implications on conjunctival epithelial homeostasis. *Invest. Ophthalmol. Vis. Sci.* 1995;36:236-46.

[137] Alfano C, Chiummariello S, Fioramonti P, et al. Ultrastructural study of autologous cultivated conjunctival epithelium. *Ophthalmic. Surg. Lasers Imaging.* 2006;37:378-82.

[138] Scuderi N, Alfano C, Paolini G, et al. Transplantation of autologous cultivated conjunctival epithelium for the restoration of defects in the ocular surface. *Scand J. Plast. Reconstr. Surg. Hand Surg.* 2002;36:340-8.

[139] Ang LP, Tan DT, Phan TT, et al. The in vitro and in vivo proliferative capacity of serum-free cultivated human conjunctival epithelial cells. *Curr. Eye Res.* 2004;28:307-17.

[140] Ang LP, Tan DT, Seah CJ, Beuerman RW. The use of human serum in supporting the in vitro and in vivo proliferation of human conjunctival epithelial cells. *Br. J. Ophthalmol.* 2005;89:748-52.

[141] Tan DT, Ang LP, Beuerman RW. Reconstruction of the ocular surface by transplantation of a serum-free derived cultivated conjunctival epithelial equivalent. *Transplantation.* 2004;77:1729-34.

[142] Ang LP, Tan DT, Cajucom-Uy H, Beuerman RW. Autologous cultivated conjunctival transplantation for pterygium surgery. *Am. J. Ophthalmol.* 2005;139:611-9.

[143] van Susante JL, Buma P, Schuman L, et al. Resurfacing potential of heterologous chondrocytes suspended in fibrin glue in large full-thickness defects of femoral articular cartilage: an experimental study in the goat. *Biomaterials.* 1999;20:1167-75.

[144] Ye Q, Zund G, Benedikt P, et al. Fibrin gel as a three dimensional matrix in cardiovascular tissue engineering. *Eur. J. Cardiothorac. Surg.* 2000;17:587-91.

[145] Kaiser HW, Stark GB, Kopp J, et al. Cultured autologous keratinocytes in fibrin glue suspension, exclusively and combined with STS-allograft (preliminary clinical and histological report of a new technique). *Burns.* 1994;20:23-9.

[146] Pellegrini G, Ranno R, Stracuzzi G, et al. The control of epidermal stem cells (holoclones) in the treatment of massive full-thickness burns with autologous keratinocytes cultured on fibrin. *Transplantation.* 1999;68:868-79.

[147] Rama P, Bonini S, Lambiase A, et al. Autologous fibrin-cultured limbal stem cells permanently restore the corneal surface of patients with total limbal stem cell deficiency. *Transplantation.* 2001;72:1478-85.

[148] Han B, Schwab IR, Madsen TK, Isseroff RR. A fibrin-based bioengineered ocular surface with human corneal epithelial stem cells. *Cornea.* 2002;21:505-10.

[149] Bauer F, Kincses E. [On girdle-like conjunctival formation from oral mucosa]. *Klin. Monatsbl. Augenheilkd.* 1967;151:28-31.

[150] Boudet C, Philippot M, Boulad L. [Graft of the sclera and oral mucosa in deep conjunctival tumors]. *Bull. Soc. Ophtalmol. Fr.* 1965;65:358-9.

[151] Darabos G, Szabo E. [Transplantation of buccal mucosa into the conjunctiva]. *Acta Morphol. Acad. Sci. Hung.* 1967;15:49-60.
[152] Coscas G, Esta A. [Buccal mucosa grafts]. *Bull. Mem. Soc. Fr. Ophtalmol.* 1968;81:206-14.
[153] Gipson IK, Geggel HS, Spurr-Michaud SJ. Transplant of oral mucosal epithelium to rabbit ocular surface wounds in vivo. *Arch. Ophthalmol.* 1986;104:1529-33.
[154] Collin C, Ouhayoun JP, Grund C, Franke WW. Suprabasal marker proteins distinguishing keratinizing squamous epithelia: cytokeratin 2 polypeptides of oral masticatory epithelium and epidermis are different. *Differentiation.* 1992;51:137-48.
[155] Juhl M, Reibel J, Stoltze K. Immunohistochemical distribution of keratin proteins in clinically healthy human gingival epithelia. *Scand. J. Dent. Res.* 1989;97:159-70.
[156] Nakamura T, Endo K, Cooper LJ, et al. The successful culture and autologous transplantation of rabbit oral mucosal epithelial cells on amniotic membrane. *Invest. Ophthalmol. Vis. Sci.* 2003;44:106-16.
[157] Nakamura T, Kinoshita S. Ocular surface reconstruction using cultivated mucosal epithelial stem cells. *Cornea.* 2003;22:S75-S80.
[158] Nakamura T, Endo K, Kinoshita S. Identification of human oral keratinocyte stem/progenitor cells by neurotrophin receptor p75 and the role of neurotrophin/p75 signaling. *Stem Cells.* 2007;25:628-38.
[159] Nishida K, Yamato M, Hayashida Y, et al. Corneal reconstruction with tissue-engineered cell sheets composed of autologous oral mucosal epithelium. *N. Engl. J. Med.* 2004;351:1187-96.
[160] Nakamura T, Inatomi T, Sotozono C, et al. Transplantation of cultivated autologous oral mucosal epithelial cells in patients with severe ocular surface disorders. *Br. J. Ophthalmol.* 2004;88:1280-4.
[161] Inatomi T, Nakamura T, Koizumi N, et al. Midterm results on ocular surface reconstruction using cultivated autologous oral mucosal epithelial transplantation. *Am. J. Ophthalmol.* 2006;141:267-75.
[162] Sekiyama E, Nakamura T, Kawasaki S, et al. Different expression of angiogenesis-related factors between human cultivated corneal and oral epithelial sheets. *Exp. Eye Res.* 2006;83:741-6.
[163] Inatomi T, Nakamura T, Koizumi N, et al. Current concepts and challenges in ocular surface reconstruction using cultivated mucosal epithelial transplantation. *Cornea.* 2005;24:S32-S38.
[164] Inatomi T, Nakamura T, Kojyo M, et al. Ocular surface reconstruction with combination of cultivated autologous oral mucosal epithelial transplantation and penetrating keratoplasty. *Am. J. Ophthalmol.* 2006;142:757-64.
[165] Nakamura T, Inatomi T, Cooper LJ, et al. Phenotypic investigation of human eyes with transplanted autologous cultivated oral mucosal epithelial sheets for severe ocular surface diseases. *Ophthalmology.* 2007;114:1080-8.
[166] Nakamura T, Ang LP, Rigby H, et al. The use of autologous serum in the development of corneal and oral epithelial equivalents in patients with Stevens-Johnson syndrome. *Invest. Ophthalmol. Vis. Sci.* 2006;47:909-16.
[167] Nakamura T, Inatomi T, Sotozono C, et al. Transplantation of autologous serum-derived cultivated corneal epithelial equivalents for the treatment of severe ocular surface disease. *Ophthalmology.* 2006;113:1765-72.

[168] Ang LP, Nakamura T, Inatomi T, et al. Autologous serum-derived cultivated oral epithelial transplants for severe ocular surface disease. *Arch. Ophthalmol.* 2006;124:1543-51.

[169] Ozturk E, Ergun MA, Ozturk Z, et al. Chitosan-coated alginate membranes for cultivation of limbal epithelial cells to use in the restoration of damaged corneal surfaces. *Int. J. Artif. Organs.* 2006;29:228-38.

[170] Yang J, Yamato M, Kohno C, et al. Cell sheet engineering: recreating tissues without biodegradable scaffolds. *Biomaterials.* 2005;26:6415-22.

[171] Nishida K, Yamato M, Hayashida Y, et al. Functional bioengineered corneal epithelial sheet grafts from corneal stem cells expanded ex vivo on a temperature-responsive cell culture surface. *Transplantation.* 2004;77:379-85.

[172] Yamato M, Utsumi M, Kushida A, et al. Thermo-responsive culture dishes allow the intact harvest of multilayered keratinocyte sheets without dispase by reducing temperature. *Tissue Eng.* 2001;7:473-80.

[173] Kwon OH, Kikuchi A, Yamato M, et al. Rapid cell sheet detachment from poly(N-isopropylacrylamide)-grafted porous cell culture membranes. *J. Biomed. Mater Res.* 2000;50:82-9.

[174] Hayashida Y, Nishida K, Yamato M, et al. Ocular surface reconstruction using autologous rabbit oral mucosal epithelial sheets fabricated ex vivo on a temperature-responsive culture surface. *Invest. Ophthalmol. Vis. Sci.* 2005;46:1632-9.

[175] Ignacio TS, Nguyen TT, Sarayba MA, et al. A technique to harvest Descemet's membrane with viable endothelial cells for selective transplantation. *Am. J. Ophthalmol.* 2005;139:325-30.

[176] Maurice DM. The location of the fluid pump in the cornea. *J. Physiol.* 1972;221:43-54.

[177] Joyce NC. Proliferative capacity of the corneal endothelium. *Prog. Retin. Eye Res.* 2003;22:359-89.

[178] McCulley JP, Maurice DM, Schwartz BD. Corneal endothelial transplantation. *Ophthalmology.* 1980;87:194-201.

[179] Jumblatt MM, Maurice DM, Schwartz BD. A gelatin membrane substrate for the transplantation of tissue cultured cells. *Transplantation.* 1980;29:498-9.

[180] Insler MS, Lopez JG. Microcarrier cell culture of neonatal human corneal endothelium. *Curr. Eye Res.* 1990;9:23-30.

[181] Mimura T, Yamagami S, Yokoo S, et al. Cultured human corneal endothelial cell transplantation with a collagen sheet in a rabbit model. *Invest. Ophthalmol. Vis. Sci.* 2004;45:2992-7.

[182] Mohay J, Lange TM, Soltau JB, et al. Transplantation of corneal endothelial cells using a cell carrier device. *Cornea.* 1994;13:173-82.

[183] Lange TM, Wood TO, McLaughlin BJ. Corneal endothelial cell transplantation using Descemet's membrane as a carrier. *J. Cataract. Refract. Surg.* 1993;19:232-5.

[184] Ishino Y, Sano Y, Nakamura T, et al. Amniotic membrane as a carrier for cultivated human corneal endothelial cell transplantation. *Invest. Ophthalmol. Vis. Sci.* 2004;45:800-6.

[185] Jumblatt MM, Maurice DM, Schwartz BD. A gelatin membrane substrate for the transplantation of tissue cultured cells. *Transplantation.* 1980;29:498-9.

[186] Mohay J, Lange TM, Soltau JB, et al. Transplantation of corneal endothelial cells using a cell carrier device. *Cornea.* 1994;13:173-82.

[187] Hsiue GH, Lai JY, Chen KH, Hsu WM. A novel strategy for corneal endothelial reconstruction with a bioengineered cell sheet. *Transplantation.* 2006;81:473-6.

[188] Lai JY, Chen KH, Hsu WM, et al. Bioengineered human corneal endothelium for transplantation. *Arch. Ophthalmol.* 2006;124:1441-8.

[189] Ide T, Nishida K, Yamato M, et al. Structural characterization of bioengineered human corneal endothelial cell sheets fabricated on temperature-responsive culture dishes. *Biomaterials.* 2006;27:607-14.

[190] Nitschke M, Gramm S, Gotze T, et al. Thermo-responsive poly(NiPAAm-co-DEGMA) substrates for gentle harvest of human corneal endothelial cell sheets. *J. Biomed. Mater Res. A.* 2007;80:1003-10.

[191] Hirose M, Kwon OH, Yamato M, et al. Creation of designed shape cell sheets that are noninvasively harvested and moved onto another surface. *Biomacromolecules.* 2000;1:377-81.

[192] Shimizu T, Yamato M, Isoi Y, et al. Fabrication of pulsatile cardiac tissue grafts using a novel 3-dimensional cell sheet manipulation technique and temperature-responsive cell culture surfaces. *Circ. Res.* 2002;90:e40.

[193] Lai JY, Lu PL, Chen KH, et al. Effect of charge and molecular weight on the functionality of gelatin carriers for corneal endothelial cell therapy. *Biomacromolecules.* 2006;7:1836-44.

[194] Lai JY, Chen KH, Hsiue GH. Tissue-engineered human corneal endothelial cell sheet transplantation in a rabbit model using functional biomaterials. *Transplantation.* 2007;84:1222-32.

Chapter IX

TOWARDS IMAGE-GUIDED STEM CELL THERAPY

Kimberly J. Blackwood, Eric Sabondjian, Donna E. Goldhawk, Michael S. Kovacs, Gerald Wisenberg, Peter Merrifield, Frank S. Prato, Janice M. DeMoor and Robert Z. Stodilka[*]

Imaging Program, Lawson Health Research Institute;
Dept. of Diagnostic Imaging, St. Joseph's Health Care - London;
Dept. of Anatomy and Cell Biology, and Dept. of Medical Biophysics,
University of Western Ontario, Canada

ABSTRACT

Cellular imaging is the non-invasive and repetitive imaging of targeted cells and cellular processes in living organisms. Previously, lack of technology prevented *in vivo* study of cell populations; studies of cellular dynamics relied on "snapshot" images from *ex vivo* histology. With the emergence of cell tracking technologies, it may become possible to study *in vivo* cell distribution, migration, gene expression, differentiation, proliferation, engraftment, and death. Cellular imaging has been used to monitor migration of transplanted cells in therapies for neurodegenerative, cerebral ischemic, cardiac, and oncologic disorders, and to characterize cell migration during the developmental stages of an organism. Many imaging modalities are being evaluated for application to cell tracking and monitoring of regenerative therapy - with no clear leading contender. This article discusses the advantages and disadvantages among leading modalities, including MRI, SPECT, PET, optical, as well as "hybrid" modalities such as SPECT/CT and PET/MRI. We also describe cell labeling strategies such as *ex vivo* labeling with radioactivity (for SPECT), superparamagnetic iron oxide nanoparticles (for

---

[*] CORRESPONDENCE: Robert Z Stodilka, PhD MCCPM; Imaging Program, Lawson Health Research Institute; 268 Grosvenor Street London, Ontario, Canada, N6A 4V2; Stodilka@lawsonimaging.ca

MRI), reporter gene expression, and their associated challenges such as toxicity, contrast dilution, and non-specific uptake. From a clinical perspective, we focus on cardiology applications due to the importance of myocardial regeneration, and finally feature two in-depth examples of cell tracking using imaging: SPECT imaging of radiolabeled cells for monitoring myocardial stem cell therapy, and a magnetosome gene-based contrast agent for cell tracking and molecular imaging with MRI.

Keywords: Cell Tracking, Image-Guided Therapy, MRI, Pet, Spect, Stem Cell

INTRODUCTION

Our title "Towards Image-Guided Stem Cell Therapy" would have been regarded as science fiction ten years ago but by the mid 2000s it seemed to some of us as achievable. It must be realized that cell labeling followed by non-invasive imaging and monitoring have been successful technologies for some 30 years. The removal, labeling and re-injection of red and white blood cells continues to be the business of nuclear medicine for the determination of red blood cell survival and the imaging of infection sites which accumulate white blood cells [Desai *et al.* 1986]. What is new is the need to locate ever smaller numbers of transplanted cells and specifically, for stem cells, to determine cell function as it relates to the purpose of cell transplantation.

In addition there has been a bit of a roller coaster ride with respect to the concept of stem cell therapy. For example, small animal studies initially suggested that myocardial tissue regeneration would be realizable using adult stem cells [Orlic *et al.* 2001] but the original work has been difficult to verify and clinical studies have given mixed results [Meyer *et al.* 2006, Lunde *et al.* 2006, Schächinger *et al.* 2006]. However, we must put things in perspective. In the treatment of a number of forms of bone cancer, autologous adult stem cell therapy has been very successful – albeit often as a therapy of last resort [Nutman *et al* 2007, Ortega *et al* 2003]. Also, although technically not stem cell therapy, we are seeing more and more work on the transplantation of mature adult cells such as the transplantation of islets for the treatment of type 1 diabetes [Sandek 2007]. Such cell therapies, whether of differentiated cells or stem cells, would develop to successful therapies faster if we could monitor non-invasively, the fate of the transplanted cells.

Although most of what is presented in this chapter will be relevant to stem cell therapy in general, we will focus our examples primarily in the area of myocardial stem cell therapy. The reason for this is two-fold: first, myocardial regeneration is extremely important (the World Health Organization estimates heart disease will be the number one cause of disability world wide by 2020) [Boom 2005] and second, because of this, there is an abundance of relevant research. Hence the section on *Clinical Perspectives* introduces the need of regenerative medicine in heart failure and the section on *Diversity of Cell Types for Cellular Cardiomyoplasty* discusses the issues regarding what cells should be transplanted. It is these important questions that need answers before myocardial stem cell therapy can be an effective therapy, and this can be most effectively determined if we have methods of tracking cells non-invasively with respect to their viability and function. In table 1 we present the ideal scenario for autologous myocardial stem cell therapy. It is important to keep in mind that imaging already has a significant established role. First of all, we currently have very good non-invasive imaging methods to diagnose the amount of permanently damaged myocardial tissue. Using modern imaging methods, particularly Magnetic Resonance Imaging (MRI) and Positron Emission Tomography (PET), we can accurately quantitate the amount of permanently damaged tissue and its impact on heart function [Thornhill *et al.* 2006, Saab G *et al.* 2003]. Also, we have excellent imaging tools to guide the harvesting of cells and the *in vivo* transplantation of those cells [Dick *et al.* 2005]. Finally, we have excellent methods to quantitate the final outcome of therapy using those same imaging methods that were used to diagnose the extent of the disease. What we do not have – and critically need – however are non-invasive imaging methods to 1) determine the number of successfully transplanted cells, 2) the viability of those cells and how viability changes with time, 3) the number and types of cells that are differentiating from the stem cells, and finally 4) if those cells are engrafting, meaning if the new tissue is functioning in synchrony with the remaining native tissue.

Table 1. Ideal scenario for autologous image-guided myocardial stem cell therapy

Event	Role of Imaging
Heart Attack and Risk of Heart Failure	Amount of Permanent Damage and Impact on Function
Remove Cells from Patients	Guide Biopsy
Transplant Cells	Guide Transplantation
Validate Transplanted Cell Location	*In vivo* Cellular Location
Cells are Viable?	*In vivo* Cellular Viability
Cells are Differentiating?	Molecular/Cellular Detection
Cells are Engrafting?	Molecular/Cellular Detection
Functional Recovery?	Biochemical and Functional Recovery

Past nuclear medicine experiences with labeling cells *in vitro* prior to re-injection suggest that quantifying the number of transplanted cells and characterizing their viability as a function of time could be achieved with such *in vitro* labeling methods prior to transplantation. This is covered in the section called *Direct Labeling* with application to the myocardium. However methods to measure non-invasively molecular events within the transplanted cells requires the application of molecular biology to medical imaging to develop imaging probes capable of signaling molecular events associated with differentiation and engraftment. Such reporter probes have been available for optical imaging for some time [Miyawaki 2003, Pike *et al.* 2006]. These include those that have evolved from green fluorescent protein (GFP) and firefly luciferase (i.e. bioluminescence imaging).

Although these optical molecular reporter probes have revolutionized cell and very small animal imaging, light scatter and attenuation have limited their application to small samples. What is needed are ways to image the transplanted cells in large animals and humans. In recent years, members of the nuclear medicine community have approached this problem in two ways. First, they have developed a reporter probe/reporter gene system using viral thymidine kinase genes [Jacobs *et al.* 2001]. Figure 1 is a schematic diagram explaining the concept which is further discussed in detail in the section on *Radiochemistry and Probe Development*. This approach has worked well in small animals, where pre-clinical Single

Photon Emission Computed Tomography (SPECT) and PET imaging instruments provide spatial resolution on the order of a millimeter cubed. However, there is difficulty extending the reporter gene/ reporter probe paradigm to large animals (and, by inference, to humans) due to the relatively poor spatial resolution of clinical SPECT and PET instruments. Here, resolution is approximately one centimeter cubed, which corresponds to a thousand-fold increase in volume of tissue, and increase in number of cells per imaging voxel from one million (small animal) to one billion (large animal). Since we typically inject ten million cells, the non-specific uptake of the radioactive reporter probe drastically reduces the contrast-to-noise in images. The other nuclear medicine approach is to introduce into cells to be transplanted the gene that creates the cell membrane-bound sodium/iodide symporter (NIS for sodium [Na], iodine [I] and S [symporter]) [Miyagawa et al. 2005a]. Hence cells successfully transfected would concentrate a radioiodine or a radiotechnitium molecule above that of endogenous non-thyroid cells. However, to date, this method has had limited use.

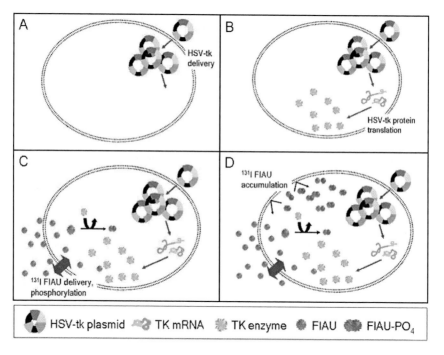

Figure 1. Herpes simplex virus thymidine kinase (HSV-*tk*) transgene expression system for SPECT cellular imaging. A. The HSV-*tk* plasmid is delivered to the cell of interest by various methods. B. HSV-*tk* over-expression produces thymidine kinase (TK) enzyme. C. After intravenous injection of the SPECT imaging probe ^{131}I FIAU ([^{131}I] 5-iodo-1-2-deoxy-2-fluoro-β-D-arabinofuranosyl uracil), the TK enzyme phosphorylates the probe. D. Phosphorylated ^{131}I FIAU is not able to cross the cellular membrane and thus accumulates in the cell. Unphosphorylated ^{131}I FIAU will transiently move into and out of cells not expressing HSV-*tk* thereby contributing to the non specific uptake in these cells. Background ^{131}I FIAU signal will also exist in the extracellular spaces.

The major problem with the nuclear medicine approaches have been the poor spectral resolution and the significant background or non-specific uptake of an externally injected contrast agent (i.e. the radioactive reporter probe). Note that this is also a problem with targeted contrast agents in MRI. There are chemistry approaches that can increase the MRI signal once the target is reached but contrast-to-noise remains a problem [Arbab *et al.* 2003]. What we need is a probe for large animal and future human imaging with spatial resolution similar to MRI (one millimeter cubed) and using a contrast agent with little to no non-specific uptake. MRI has the needed resolution but lacks a reporter gene/reporter probe with no non-specific uptake. In the section *Molecular Imaging Using Genes for Cellular Contrast* we present preliminary data suggesting that such MRI reporter genes may be possible.

Figure 2 shows a modification of figure 1 wherein the concept of an MRI reporter gene without non-specific uptake approach is proposed. In this case the gene that produces *de novo* MRI contrast material is "turned on" (i.e. reports on a cellular molecular event). This approach is described in detail in section *Molecular Imaging Using Genes for Cellular Contrast*.

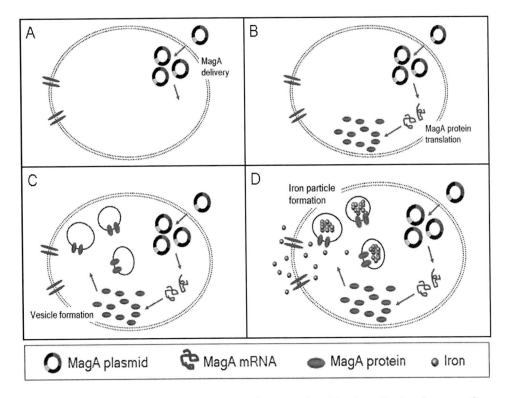

Figure 2. MagA expression system for cellular imaging using iron biomineralization for magnetic resonance (MR) contrast. A. *MagA* transgene is delivered to the cell of interest by various methods. B. *MagA* over-expression results in production of a bacterial iron transport protein. C. MagA is an integral membrane protein, putatively localized to intracellular vesicles. D. Extracellular iron may be stored and biomineralized in MagA-expressing intracellular vesicles. MR signal will only come from dense particles of iron in vesicles therefore non-specific uptake will not be a problem in cells not expressing MagA.

In summary, in this chapter, we identify the imaging technology that still has to be developed to achieve Image Guided Myocardial Stem Cell Therapy. Specifically we need quantitative methods to determine, after cell transplantation, cell number, cell viability and cell function. In the sections that follow we describe the state-of-the-art in achieving those goals and borrow extensively on our experience in myocardial stem cell therapy.

CLINICAL PERSPECTIVES

Myocardial infarction (MI) remains today as a frequent and often life-altering event, despite improvements in treatment to lessen the extent of acute myocardial injury. Subsequent to the acute event, contracting myocardium is gradually replaced, over months, by fibrotic scar. If the extent of permanent injury is large, the clinical syndrome of congestive heart failure will ensue, and the individual's quality and length of life will be accordingly reduced. Unlike some organs, the heart has a very limited capacity to regenerate new functioning myocardium after such an injury. In fact, for decades, it was thought that the adult heart was a terminally differentiated organ with essentially no proliferative capacity. Although several groups have demonstrated the presence of resident cardiac stem cells/progenitor cells, in a number of species including mice, rat, dog, pig, and humans, it is clear that there are either insufficient numbers of these cells or a limited capability to effect significant repair in the clinical setting of moderate to large MIs.

However, recently, there has developed some optimism that either physically transplanted or mobilized marrow-derived stem cells may produce a significant degree of myocardial repair which may lead to potentially important improvements in clinically measurable endpoints, such as heart failure. Seven years ago, based on studies in mice, it was reported that the extent of myocardial fibrosis could be significantly reduced through the transplantation of marrow-derived cells and subsequent differentiation into cardiomyocytes [Orlic et al 2001]. This created an explosion of interest, and some skepticism, regarding the field of myocardial regeneration. The subsequent years have seen investigations into a variety of related areas including 1) the optimum cell population, source, and numbers of cells required, 2) routes of cell delivery, and 3) understanding the mechanisms of repair. As with any new proposed treatment, there is often an initial surge of enthusiasm that the "holy grail" for the condition has been found, followed by tempering of that initial enthusiasm with the realities that the treatment may either not work, or not to the extent originally predicted. This would appear to be the current status of myocardial regenerative therapy.

On review of the currently available data, from both animal and limited clinical trials, we can state that 1) the benefit produced by marrow-derived transplantation is mediated not by transdifferentiation of the transplanted cells [Murry et al. 2004], but rather by a paracrine effect where the transplanted cells produce a local increase in vasculogenesis, lessen the degree of evolving myocardial fibrosis, and perhaps stimulate the production of new cardiomyocytes [Niagara et al. 2007, Gnecchi et al. 2005], 2) a relatively small number of cells remain resident at the transplanted site following intracoronary injection [Kang et al. 2006]; although the numbers of cells is higher with direct injection techniques, there appears to be relatively rapid clearance of these cells, particularly in our own experience, when these cells are injected on the day of infarction [Kong et al. 2005], 3) the optimum cell population still remains as an unresolved issue. Investigators have proposed the use of bone marrow (mesenchymal) stromal cells (BMSCs), bone marrow monocytes (BMMCs), endothelial progenitor cells which can be isolated from either marrow or peripheral blood, cells of embryonic origin, or skeletal muscle satellite cells (SMSCs). All have their strong proponents and detractors.

Few studies to date have taken the disciplined approach that is generally applied currently to the assessment of newly developed pharmacological interventions, where the burden of proof is high to establish the efficacy of treatment. Most initial clinical trials were designed to assess safety rather than efficacy, and suggested a moderate improvement in global or regional cardiac function using this surrogate endpoint. However a recent randomized trial, the BOOST study, although demonstrating an improvement in magnetic resonance measured ejection fraction at 6 months following intracoronary injection, showed no effect at 18 months [Meyer et al. 2006]. As well, the ASTAMI study, in 100 patients, demonstrated no improvement in either left ventricular ejection fraction, or infarct size at 6 months [Lunde et a.l 2006], although the REPAIR-AMI trial, in 200 patients, suggested a small improvement in ejection fraction [Schächinger et al. 2006]. There are many explanations for the divergent findings observed in both animal and clinical trial results, including the baseline severity of left ventricular dysfunction, the timing of cell delivery, the route of cell injection, and the method of cell isolation, and the quality and purity of the cells.

For myocardial regenerative therapy to advance to the next level, that of being an established proven technique that holds real promise for the treatment of the post MI patient, it will be imperative to establish that the treatment produces meaningful benefit in important clinical endpoints, and to correlate the dose of treatment (cell-type and numbers) with measurable treatment effect, thus defining a dose response curve. This approach would be similar to the one used for the evaluation of pharmacological therapies in phase IV clinical trials. In this case, the clinical endpoints would be not just an improvement in the surrogate endpoint of ejection fraction, which can occur spontaneously in many patients following MI, but a reduction in the incidence of clinical heart failure and an improvement in survival in comparison to placebo treated controls in randomized trials. The latter will require long-term studies over several years with large numbers of patients.

However, in the short term, towards the important goal of establishing dose-response curves, imaging can play a vital role in addressing the challenges of "proving" that this therapy works. The labeling of cells prior to their transplantation will help us in assessing the kinetics of cell engraftment and clearance from injection sites. By using tailored genetic approaches, we may be able to ascertain with greater accuracy the mechanisms by which myocardial repair is generated, such as whether the conversion or differentiation of the transplanted cells plays any meaningful role. By coupling techniques to track the cells with those that will evaluate changes in myocardial cell fibrosis, we may be able to truly establish dose response curves. MRI has proven to be a valuable tool to allow the serial assessment of the extent of myocardial injury in both animal models and clinically [Pereira et al. 1999, Thornhill et al. 2006]. We have used MRI to assess the relative changes in infarct size that occur over the course of the first 12 weeks following a 3 hour left anterior descending coronary artery occlusion followed by reperfusion in a canine model (figure 3).

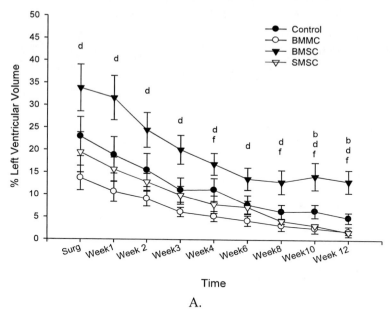

A.

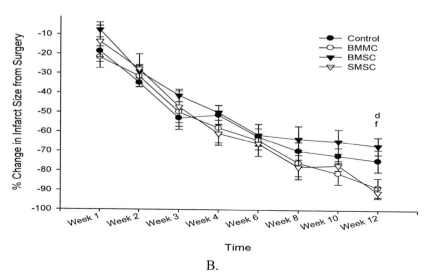

B.

a=Control different from BMMC, b=Control different from BMSC,
c=Control different from SMSC, d= BMMC different from BMSC,
e=BMMC different from SMSC, f=BMSC different from SMSC.

Figure 3. Changes that occurred in the degree of signal enhancement after direct injection of either undifferentiated bone marrow monocytes (BMMCs), bone marrow stromal cells (BMSCs), skeletal muscle satellite cells (SMSCs), or saline (control) injections. Despite the significant differences in baseline infarct size between treatment groups (A), all groups had a comparable degree of relative infarct shrinkage compared to the day of infarction, for the first 6 weeks (B). Subsequently, the curves began to diverge, with a modest treatment effect observed in the bone marrow monocyte and skeletal muscle satellite cell treated groups (i.e. a decrease in the size of the infarct).

The next few years will hopefully witness the resolution of many of the issues and questions that still exist. We remain cautiously optimistic that stem cell treatment will play an important role for the treatment of the post MI patient, and potentially those with chronic conditions leading to extensive myocardial fibrosis.

DIVERSITY OF CELL TYPES USED FOR CELLULAR CARDIOMYOPLASTY

During MI, loss of blood supply to cardiac tissue results in hypoxia, death of cardiomyocytes and their replacement by an inert scar. One approach for limiting and/or reversing the damage caused by MI is the transplantation of cardiogenic cells to the site of injury – an approach known as cellular cardiomyoplasty. The ideal cell type for such studies would be 1) simple to harvest, 2) easy to grow *in vitro*, 3) resistant to hypoxia, 4) able to differentiate into cardiomyocytes which become electrically coupled to resident cells, 5) histocompatable with the host, and 6) have little or no potential for forming tumours. While a number of different cell types have been used for cardiomyoplasty, there is currently no one cell type which fulfills all these requirements.

In animal models, cardiogenic cell lines (such as the mouse AT-1 line) have been isolated which differentiate into cardiomyocytes *in vitro*. When these cells were injected into damaged myocardium in a mouse model for MI, they differentiated into cardiomyocytes which became electrically coupled to resident cardiomyocytes [Koh *et al.* 1993]. While human cardiogenic cell lines have not yet been identified, attempts are being made to isolate such cell lines for therapeutic purposes. Primary cultures of cardiomyocytes have been isolated from fetal hearts of several species and used for cellular cardiomyoplasty of damaged hearts [Koh *et al.* 1995], but these cells are difficult to expand *in vitro*. Although a population of cardiomyogenic precursor cells have been isolated from fetal rodents and human hearts which can be enriched and expanded *in vitro* [Laugwitz *et al.* 2005], these cells are not retained in adult hearts and the ethical problems associated with harvesting fetal hearts on a larger scale limits the therapeutic potential of these cells.

A more promising approach to cellular cardiomyoplasty involves the use of multipotential stem cells to repair damaged myocardium. By definition, stem cells have the ability to self-renew and to differentiate into multiple cell types. Practically, stem cells can be characterized as embryonic stem (ES) cells or adult stem cells, based on their developmental origins. ES cells, derived from the inner cell mass of blastocysts, tend to have a broader developmental potential than adult stem cells, but also have a greater potential for forming tumors. Because of these qualities, the hope is that large numbers of human stem cells can be obtained *in vitro* which will differentiate exclusively into cardiomyocytes in response to local cues following injection into damaged myocardium. There are numerous reports of successful rodent ES cell engraftment into rodent hearts and progress is being made with human ES cells transplanted into rodent hearts [LaFlamme *et al.*2007]. To date, the therapeutic use of human ES cells in clinical trials to treat myocardial infarct has not been attempted. Adult stem cells (often referred to as mesenchymal stem cell or multipotential adult precursor cells), with the characteristics described above, have been identified in most adult tissues of mice and men, including brain, adipose tissue, endothelial lining of vessels, blood, skeletal muscle, heart, testes, skin and bone marrow [Sohn et al. 2007]. Of these tissues, SMSCs and bone marrow stem cells have been investigated most intensely.

SMSCs were the first adult stem cell type used for cardiomyoplasty in animal models [Chiu et al 1995], and while there was initially some hope that they would transdifferentiate into cardiomyocytes, it is now known that SMSCs injected into damaged hearts differentiate into skeletal muscle fibers which do not become electrically coupled (via gap junctions) to resident cardiomyocytes [Reinecke et al. 2002]. While there is growing evidence that cardiomyoplasty using SMSCs improves cardiac function, this may be due to their ability to promote neovascularization of heart muscle via a paracrine mechanism [Oshima et al. 2005]. Orlic et al. [2001] first suggested that bone marrow stem cells transdifferentiated into cardiomyocytes when injected into infarcted mouse myocardium. The transplanted cells expressed cardiac-specific troponin I and myosin heavy chain, but these studies could not be repeated by others [Murry et al. 2004] and it is now believed that Orlic's original observations were flawed, since immunofluorescence analysis is somewhat subjective and because bone marrow stem cells can fuse with adult cardiomyocytes and adopt their phenotype. Several studies have reported improved cardiac function following cardiomyoplasty with bone marrow stem cells and there is good evidence that this may result from paracrine signaling from transplanted cells which secrete multiple proangiogenic cytokines, including vascular endothelial growth factor, hepatocyte growth factor, granulocyte factor and granulocyte–macrophage colony-stimulating factor [Uemura et al. 2006]. Recently, bone marrow stem cells have been genetically engineered to over-express these factors, and shown to increase neovascularization and improve cardiac function following cellular cardiomyoplasty [Matsumoto et al. 2005].

In light of the successful use of SMSCs and bone marrow stem cells in animal models, phase 1 clinical trials have been carried out using both cell types. Menasché and colleagues [2001] were the first to perform a clinical study using transplanted autologous SMSCs into a patient while undergoing concomitant coronary artery bypass grafting. They followed the patient over eight months and determined that within five months, there was evidence of improved contraction in the patient's heart. Around the same time, a controlled clinical study by Strauer and colleagues [2002] was published using bone marrow stem cells for cardiovascular therapy. The BMMCs were injected into 10 patients by an intracoronary method while the patients underwent percutaneous transluminal coronary angioplasty (PCI). The control group, also consisting of 10 patients, was given only standard PCI therapy. Over a three month period, improvements in the experimental group were seen over the control in decreased infarct size and increased ejection fraction of the left ventricle. Recently, clinical trials (MAGIC, TOPCARE-AMI, and BOOST) were designed that focused on injecting bone marrow-derived stem cells via intracoronary means. All three groups reported subsequent improvements in cardiac output in patients after six month observations. However, by 18 months, the BOOST trial showed that the increase in ventricular ejection fraction was not sustained compared to control patients, raising concerns about the long-term potential for this type of therapy [Meyer et al. 2006]. This controversy and the increased number of clinical trials currently underway has created a great demand for molecular imaging techniques to study cell survival, differentiation and functional integration non-invasively, in real time over an extended period.

IMAGING TECHNOLOGIES

The imaging modalities receiving the most attention for cell tracking applications are MRI, SPECT, PET and Optical Imaging. Efforts are underway to develop, for each modality, cell tracking technologies using direct labeling methods as well as reporter-gene approaches.

Magnetic Resonance Imaging

MRI can provide anatomical images with millimeter resolution. Thus MRI can place signals from labeled cells into context by allowing the cell locations to be superimposed onto images of underlying anatomy. In this sense, MRI is unique as a stand-alone modality, whereas SPECT and PET require hybridization, often with X-ray Computed Tomography (CT), to facilitate this context.

Detection of labeled cells is dependent on the relaxivity of the contrast agent, the cell labeling efficiency, the number of implanted cells, and the characteristics of the magnetic field. The most common contrast agents for MRI are gadolinium-based, however these agents suffer from poor detectability. More recently, contrast agents based on superparamagnetic iron oxide (SPIO) particles are coming to the forefront for MRI-based cell tracking. The iron oxide particles consist of a crystalline iron oxide core, often coated with dextran or starch, and have a hydrodynamic diameter of approximately 30 nm. Although labeled cells can be localized with exquisite millimeter accuracy and precision, micromolar concentrations of SPIO are required, thus the detection threshold is currently around 10^5 cells [Bengel et al 2005] in stationary organs using conventional MRI scanners without sequence modification. SPIO particles have among the shortest T2/T2* relaxivities known, making them easy to detect. However, their short relaxivities also result in negative contrast, making quantification extremely difficult. Detection of labeled cells can be improved substantially in some situations with specialized hardware. For example, detection of few or even single SPIO-labeled cells suspended in gelatin has been achieved using magnetic resonance microscopy, albeit with highly-customized gradient coils [Foster-Garneau et al 2003]. Although the majority of MRI cell tracking strategies involve direct-labeling, recent work is demonstrating potential for gene-based imaging using magnetite-producing transgenes, discussed elsewhere in this chapter.

Unlike radionuclides, MRI contrast agents are non-radioactive, making them more suitable for labeling radiosensitive cells, and potentially allowing directly labeled cells to be tracked for longer periods of time. A particular concern with MRI is that many patients with implantable devices such as pacemakers and defibrillators will likely be candidates for stem cell clinical trials, and these devices are contraindications to MRI scanning.

Single Photon Emission Computed Tomography

Nuclear medicine has been used since the mid-1970's to track in humans autologous leukocytes directly labeled with ^{111}In (Indium) radiotracers [Thakur et al. 1977]. More recently, SPECT has been used to track directly labeled cells in porcine and murine models of MI for as long as 14 days [Aicher et al. 2003, Chin et al. 2003].

SPECT is inherently multi-spectral, allowing it to image multiple radionuclides simultaneously. For example, one study has shown simultaneous cell tracking (^{111}In-radiolabeled cardiomyoblasts) in the heart and imaging of myocardial perfusion (using ^{99m}Tc-sestamibi) [Zhou et al. 2005]. Our site has built upon this work by demonstrating, in a canine model, triple radionuclide imaging, where the third parameter measured is reporter gene expression using ^{131}I-FIAU (2'-fluoro-2'-deoxy-5-[124I]iodo-1-β-D-arabino-furanosyluracil) [Stodilka et al. 2006]. Multi-parameter imaging places additional demands on hardware and increases the complexity of obtaining quantitative images. However, it does provide perfect registration which is especially important in situations involving extensive non-specific uptake such as reporter probe imaging. Recently, interest in SPECT is renewing due to its hybridization with X-ray CT. SPECT/CT, like MRI, can then visualize labeled cells in the context of underlying anatomy. SPECT is not nearly as sensitive as PET; although a recent study using a phantom suggests that approximately 10,000 directly labeled cells could be imaged by SPECT in approximately 16 minutes using standard clinical equipment [Jin et al. 2005].

Positron Emission Tomography

PET has two great strengths for cell tracking: an unbeatable sensitivity ranging in the picomolar (10^{-11} – 10^{-12} mol/l) [Zhou et al. 2006] and an ability to label a multitude of biologically-relevant molecules via the positron emitting radionuclides ^{11}C, ^{13}N, and ^{18}F. Cardiac transgene expression was first demonstrated in PET using the reporter gene / reporter probe paradigm: herpes simplex virus type 1 thymidine kinase (HSV1-*tk*) and the reporter probe FIAU [Bengel et al. 2003].

PET produces higher resolution clinical images than SPECT, although PET cannot discriminate between different radionuclides and so cannot simultaneously image multiple parameters. The primary limitations to PET are its expense and the short half-lives of its positron emitting radionuclides. PET radionuclides are made in medical cyclotrons, which although becoming more common, can generally only be maintained by large institutions due to high costs. Short half lives of radiotracers (<2 hours) limits PET to tracking directly-labeled cells for time scales on the order of hours. Further, only reporter probes with fast binding kinetics can be used – although faster binding kinetics often goes hand-in-hand with higher levels of non-specific uptake.

Like SPECT, PET enables the visualization of contrast agent distributions. The distribution of underlying anatomy cannot be observed directly, although it can be inferred in the presence of extensive non-specific uptake. Like SPECT, PET is benefitting tremendously from hybridization, both with X-ray CT (to form PET/CT) [Beyer et al. 2000], and more recently hybrid PET/MRI platforms are being explored [Gilbert et al. 2006]. Although costly for the time being, such hybridization promises to deliver the best of each modality.

Optical Imaging

Optical imaging has allowed substantial progress in cell tracking in small animals via fluorescence and bioluminescence. Bioluminescence imaging relies on light emitted when the enzyme luciferase is exposed to the luciferin substrate, which it oxidizes. Photon emissions are then often detected by a charge-coupled device (CCD) camera. Like all reporter gene expression imaging methods, an important drawback to bioluminescence imaging is the requirement of stable expression of non-human genes, and injection of high concentrations of substrates which may have pharmacologic or immunogenic responses. Fluorescence imaging uses exogenous fluorophores as contrast agents that can directly label cells. Of these, the near-infrared fluorophores have the greatest clinical potential, since they can be detected up to approximately 10 mm in tissue [Ntziachristos et al. 2003] – although these depths would limit optical imaging to near-surface applications such as intra-operative tracking of transplanted cells. In optical imaging, frequencies typically used (400-1000 nm) are highly absorbed and scattered by tissue, thus making small animal imaging the primary application of this modality. For the present, optical imaging is not tomographic.

RADIOCHEMISTRY AND PROBE DEVELOPMENT

There are two main families of reporter probes that have been developed to image HSV1-*tk* expression for use in cell tracking using SPECT and PET imaging. Both evolved from antiviral drugs which were known to be incorporated into DNA by the promiscuous viral thymidine kinases such as HSV1-*tk*, but incorporated at much lower rates by mammalian thymidine kinases.

Pyrimidine nucleosides labeled with radioiodine (e.g. FIAU) have been shown to be the superior imaging agents for the wild type HSV1-*tk* variant [Tjuvajev et al. 2002]. With iodine labeling, FIAU can be used for SPECT (^{123}I, ^{131}I) imaging [Vaidyanathan et al. 1998] or PET imaging (^{124}I) [Tjuvajev et al.1998]. FIAU was developed to improve the stability of the earlier generation pyrimidine nucleoside imaging agent IUdR (figure 4). The resistance of enzymatic cleavage at the N-glycosidic bond by nucleoside phosphorylases [Conti et al.1995] was greatly improved by introduction of a fluorine at C2 of the arabinose sugar ring [Watanabe et al. 1979].

With PET increasingly becoming the imaging modality of choice, there have also been efforts to develop a 2nd class of reporter probes. Utilizing fluorine-substituted analogues of the acycloguanosine antiviral drug ganciclovir such as [^{18}F]FHBG and [^{18}F]FHPG (figure 5), the expression of the mutant gene HSV1-*sr39tk* has been imaged using PET [Gambhir et al. 2000]. With their two hour half-life, ^{18}F-labeled probes allow repetitive imaging of subjects compared to ^{124}I PET probes or $^{123/131}$I SPECT probes. However, FHBG has been shown to be a poorer imaging agent of the stably transfected HSV1-*tk* variant than FIAU [Tjuvajev *et al.* 2002, Min *et al.* 2003].

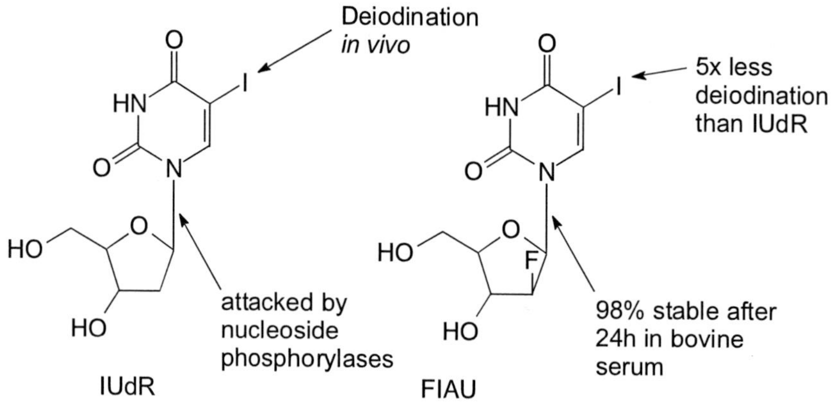

Figure 4. Pyrimidine Nucleosides used in imaging HSV1-*tk* Expression.

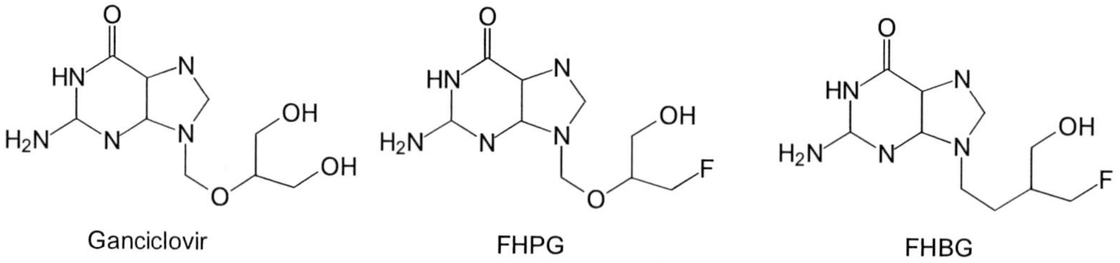

Figure 5. Acyloguanosine Nucleosides used in imaging HSV1-sr39*tk* Expression.

Another approach has been to attempt the synthesis of [^{18}F]FIAU for imaging HSV1-*tk* with a short-lived PET probe [Mangner *et al* 2003]. For routine use, it is desirable to have a probe and a synthetic route to produce it in high yield, with reliability and consistency, and by the simplest route possible in terms of the number of synthetic and purification steps. Unfortunately, although the radiochemical yields are reasonable, the synthesis of [^{18}F]FIAU and other derivatives require a complicated multi-step sequence and a synthesis time of 3 hours.

To make synthesis of an [^{18}F]FIAU derivative more suitable for simple two-step radiolabeling and preparation on an automated synthesis unit (ASU), another approach has been to prepare a new probe [^{18}F]FFEAU (figure 6) [Balantoni *et al.* 2005]. Although reported in low yield, two different precursors were labeled with ^{18}F in only two synthetic steps.

Probe development for the imaging of gene expression has become relatively stabilized. The future is in extending this technology towards being more suitable for clinical use. For routine clinical acceptance, it is most advantageous to use a short-lived probe for performing PET, either FHBG or one of the newer FIAU probes labeled with ^{18}F. Ideally, the probe should be obtainable in a reliably high radiochemical yield in relatively few synthetic steps utilizing an ASU. The probe should be easy to purify and obtain in high radiochemical purity with no chemical impurities, and as an apyrogenic and sterile injectable.

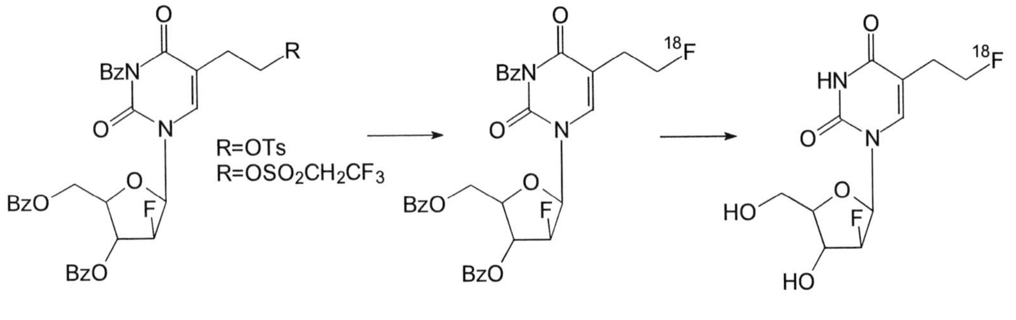

Figure 6. [^{18}F]FFEAU.

A recent development of great promise is the application of the sodium iodide symporter (NIS) to reporter probe imaging. NIS is an intrinsic transmembrane glycoprotein expressed naturally in the thyroid gland where it enables follicular cells to accumulate the iodide anion 20-40 times over plasmid concentration levels. [Miyagawa et al. 2005a] NIS has been cloned from both rat (*NIS*) and human (*hNIS*) genes and have both been shown to be functional *in vitro*. Cells expressing NIS are capable of accumulating radioiodine, e.g. ^{123}I (SPECT), ^{124}I (PET), ^{131}I (SPECT) and ^{99m}TcO$_4^-$ (SPECT), and therefore can be imaged with great ease as the imaging agents are readily available without the need for specialized radiochemistry personnel and equipment.

A comparison between NIS (^{124}I), HSV1-*tk* ([^{124}I]FIAU) and HSV1-*sr39tk* ([^{18}F]FHBG) has demonstrated the utility of NIS in rat cardiac PET studies [Miyagawa et al. 2005b]. Compared to controls, the maximum cardiac uptake of ^{124}I was 6.88-fold higher in cardiac cells transfected with the *hNIS* gene at 30-40 min post injection. The efflux rate of ^{124}I was mild and was measured to be 22.3% thereafter to 120 min post injection. In contrast, both [^{124}I]FIAU (1.34-fold) and [^{18}F]FHBG (4.15-fold) had lower uptake compared to the control animals. In addition, [^{124}I]FIAU was rapidly excreted from the heart but there was no appreciable excretion of [^{18}F]FHBG. NIS shows great promise as a next generation reporter gene.

In our group, we have been developing a method to track transplanted BMSCs in the canine heart to repetitively image transplanted cell viability and function *in vivo* with dual isotope SPECT [Stodilka et al. 2006]. Simultaneous acquisition of ^{111}In and ^{131}I gamma rays is a practical way to image the functional capacity of transplanted cells using *a priori* information provided by ^{111}In. In these studies, HSV1-*tk* transfected BMSCs were co-labeled with ^{111}In-tropolone and [^{131}I]FIAU, and subsequently imaged with SPECT to generate time-activity curves out to 48 hours. (figure 7) Although initial [^{131}I]FIAU efflux was demonstrated out to about 10 hours, it slowed down thereafter to give a mean biological half-life of 20.6 hours. The longer biological half life of 4.5 days for ^{111}In is strongly indicative that the transplanted cells are alive and that the [^{131}I]FIAU excretion is not largely due to cell death.

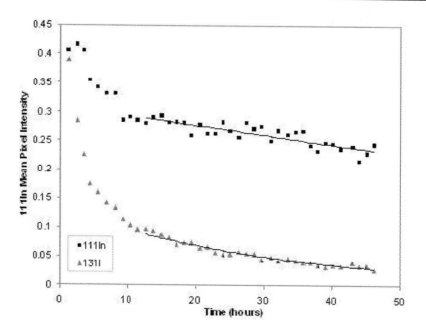

Figure 7. Spect time activity curves showing efflux of ^{131}I and ^{111}In from dual labeled canine BMSCs expressing HSV-*tk* after transplantation in canine myocardium. Curves were fit to a mono-exponential curve and the biological half-life was calculated for each radiolabel. Biological half-lives for [^{131}I]FIAU and ^{111}In were 20.6 hours and 4.5 days, respectively.

MOLECULAR IMAGING USING GENES FOR CELLULAR CONTRAST

Adapting molecular cloning strategies for use with non-invasive imaging modalities entails selection of expression vectors to suit the detection system. For example, firefly luciferase constructs have been exploited in optical imaging [Pike *et al.* 2006]; viral thymidine kinase vectors have been used for imaging with radiolabels [Jacobs *et al* 2001]; and fusion protein constructs have been used to combine imaging modalities [Jacobs *et al.* 1999, Ray *et al* 2007]. While gene expression systems broaden the possibilities for targeted, long-term cell tracking, each imaging technique nevertheless has its advantages and limitations. Factors such as depth of penetration in tissue, substrate delivery, longevity of the label and tissue resolution affect the choice of expression vector and imaging modality. In the case of MRI, which provides excellent tissue resolution and depth of penetration, cellular detail is not readily obtained. Gene expression systems that impart magnetic properties to cells are under development [Gilad *et al.* 2007, Weissleder *et al.* 2000]. This section will discuss challenges in molecular MRI and advances in vector design for generating cellular contrast.

Non-invasive mapping of cellular or subcellular events in living organisms relies on intracellular contrast agents, many of which are based on SPIO particles. These magnetite crystals consist of a mixture of ferrous and ferric oxides. For MRI contrast, these particles must be as small as possible and yet retain permanent magnetic properties [Bulte *et al.* 1994].

Numerous companies have developed nanosphere and microsphere SPIO particles that are biologically compatible, using a variety of materials to coat the magnetite, including protein, phospholipids, polysaccharide, dextran [Arbab et al. 2003] and silane polymer shells that may or may not include target-specific antibodies. However, they are not useful for long-term studies in which labelled cells divide and the SPIO contrast agent becomes diluted. In addition, SPIO particles alone cannot provide information on cellular and molecular function. For these reasons, gene expression systems are needed to couple protein expression with the formation of suitable contrast agents.

Overexpression of the iron binding protein, ferritin, produced detectable contrast in C6 glioma cells analyzed by MRI at 4.7T [Cohen et al. 2005]. This same GFP and heavy chain ferritin construct was subsequently been used to examine the inducible expression of intracellular contrast in transgenic mice [Cohen et al. 2007]. Others have used modified ferritin subunits to enhance iron loading in lung adenocarcinoma cells [Genove et al. 2005]. In this report, cellular contrast from bound, superparamagnetic ferrihydrite was recorded by MRI at 11.7T. Mobilization of unbound iron was also increased, as reflected by upregulation of transferrin receptor levels. The latter gene has been modified for overexpression by removal of 3' untranslated region sequences that bear iron-responsive and mRNA destabilizing elements [Weissleder et al. 2000, Casey et al. 1989]. Another endogenous contrast agent is the magnetosome, a membrane-bound structure produced by magnetotactic bacteria and containing magnetite [Bazylinski and Frankel 2004, Lang et al 2007, Matsunaga et al. 2007]. Due to their size specificity and distinctive crystal morphology, magnetosomes are an ideal *in vivo* imaging contrast agent. However, the full complement of genes responsible for magnetosome synthesis in bacteria is still under investigation [Lang et al. 2007, Komeili et al. 2006, Schüler 2004], and the entire magnetosome structure has not yet been reproduced in foreign cells.

Adapting the process of iron biomineralization for use in reporter gene expression is complicated by the number of genes involved and the complex nature of iron homeostasis. In mammalian cells, iron accumulation is regulated by ferritin, transferrin and transferrin receptor [Beutler 2004]; and modifications in these genes have demonstrated that iron uptake and retention may be manipulated to enhance intracellular contrast [Deans et al. 2006]. In a model of magnetosome assembly, magnetite is synthesized within a specialized compartment equipped to import iron and sequester the nascent crystal [Matsunaga et al. 2004]. Hence, the magnetosome may provide the cell with superparamagnetic iron while protecting it from cytotoxicity in much the same way as the lysosome sequesters proteases for specific purposes.

Toward further development of reporter genes for MRI, we are transfecting mammalian cells with select magnetosome genes, to impart magnetosome-like character to the host cell for the purpose of enhancing intracellular contrast. This research is predicated on reports that higher vertebrates and mammals form magnetite and, in some species, geomagnetic field sensing abilities have been attributed to it [Kirschvink 1989, Moatamed and Johnson 1986]. There is also evidence that magnetite is synthesized in human and rat brains [Dunn et al 1995, Kirschvink et al. 1992], and is increased in some neurodegenerative diseases [Collingwood and Dobson 2006]. An iron regulated gene, *magA*, which encodes a membrane-bound, iron-transport protein involved in magnetite synthesis has been identified in *Magnetospirillum* species of bacteria [Bazylinski and Frankel 2004, Matsunaga et al. 1992, Nakamura et al.

1995]. We are using MagA expression to improve cellular contrast in mammalian cells and facilitate cell tracking by MRI. Our results show an increase in cellular contrast after stable expression of GFP-MagA fusion protein in a population of neuroblastoma cells (figure 8). Correlation of negative and positive contrast images indicates that signal voids are attributed to fluid-filled species, such as cells. The lack of signal in spin echo measurements confirms that disturbances in the magnetic field are not due to air pockets in the matrix. In serial planes, MagA expression allows detection of cells in adjacent layers, resolving cellular detail from a mixed population of cells (figure 9). These findings suggest that MagA-derived contrast has potential for MRI of small clusters of cells, if not individual cells.

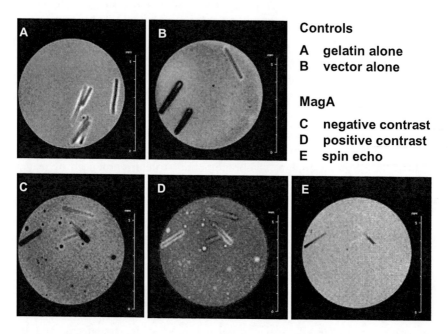

Figure 8. Molecular MRI of MagA Expression in Mouse Neuroblastoma Cells. MagA was expressed in N2A cells from pEGFP-C3 and cultured under selection to obtain a population of stably-expressing clones. Medium was supplemented with 250 µM ferric nitrate for 7 days prior to mounting cells in gelatin/phosphate buffered saline pH 7.4 and imaging by MRI at 11T. Panels A and B are negative contrast images showing an axial cross section through the gelatin phantom and gelatin containing 10^6 cells expressing vector alone, respectively. The plane of focus is marked by human hair. Panels C-E show negative contrast, positive contrast and spin echo images of a single, axial cross section through gelatin containing 10^6 MagA-expressing cells.

The *in vivo* tracking of cells, including progenitors that may differentiate into mature cells with highly specific functions, is a valuable research and clinical tool. The potential of iron binding or transport proteins to augment intracellular contrast for non-invasive MRI of cellular and molecular detail, represents a major advance in molecular imaging and will complement SPIO methodology. Genetically engineering cells to produce or upregulate synthesis of iron biominerals confers magnetic properties to the cell, subject to regulation by specific promoter activity, and provides reporter gene expression for MRI to follow migration, proliferation, differentiation and apoptosis of transfected cells. Development of this technology is expected to expand the application of MRI to all types of cells and therapeutic treatments.

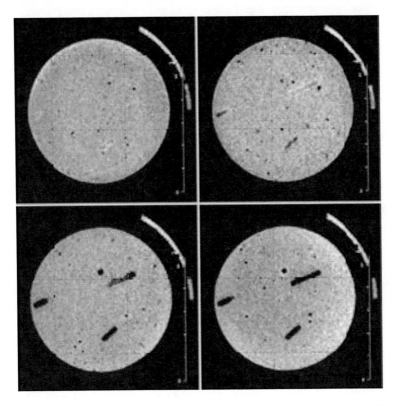

Figure 9. MagA Expression in Adjacent Focal Planes. N2A cells were prepared as described above. MRI at 11T was performed on adjacent, axial cross sections through gelatin containing 10^6 MagA-expressing cells. Panels A-D are serial, negative contrast images, moving into the plane of focus marked by human hair. Slice thickness is 60 μm.

DIRECT LABELING USING RADIONUCLIDES

Clinical nuclear medicine imaging primarily makes use of SPECT and PET and acquires functional information based on tracer amounts of radioisotopes. Due to the high specific activity of injected radioisotopes, SPECT and PET can detect relatively low amounts of contrast agent, compared to MRI for example, detecting radiotracer material in the picomolar to nanomolar range [Sharma et al. 2002]. With that said, radioisotopes have been used extensively in cellular tracking to monitor homing and biodistribution by first directly labeling the cells of interest *in vitro* [Bindslev et al. 2006]. However, quantitative cellular tracking would be ideal to allow the determination of transplanted cell number and survival at any given location in the body. Accomplishing this is not trivial using radioisotope imaging for a number of reasons, as described by Fragioni and Hajjar [2004]. Firstly, increasing the amount of radioactive label per cell will improve cell detectability by SPECT and PET; however care must be taken to avoid radiotoxicity. Secondly, radiolabel leakage from viable cells and the non-specific uptake of radiolabel from dead or leaking cells into surrounding tissue precludes quantitative imaging. Thirdly, quantitatively imaging viable cells must ensure that any radiolabel found within the extravascular and extracellular spaces, due to cell death or leakage, must be promptly removed. Lastly, accurately assessing cell number *in vivo* based on non-specific radiotracers can be difficult as the radiolabel per cell decreases with respect to the number of divisions a cell undergoes [Frangioni and Hajjar 2004].

Our group has addressed some of these concerns using ^{111}In-tropolone and SPECT in canine myocardium. ^{111}In-tropolone can readily and non-specifically label any kind of cell and allows serial, dynamic imaging due to a relatively long half-life of 2.82 days [Kraitchman *et al.* 2005]. Previous work has shown that tropolone surrounds the ^{111}In nuclei facilitating diffusion across the cellular membrane into the cytosol, where proteins competitively bind the radiolabel [Dewanjee *et al.* 1981]. More importantly, it has been widely used clinically to image leukocyte distribution in inflammation, dendritic cell migration, transplanted hepatocyte biodistribution, and stem cell trafficking [Bindslev *et al.* 2006].

We have been interested in quantitatively assessing transplanted bone marrow cell viability using ^{111}In-tropolone and clinical SPECT in a large animal model of acute MI. As previously mentioned, one of the key concerns in quantitatively imaging transplanted cell viability is determining what happens to the radiolabel once the cell dies and how long its associated radiolabel takes to clear the site of injection. We focused our attention our characterizing clearance *in vivo* of ^{111}In labeled cellular debris (i.e. cytosolic proteins) from the site of cell transplantation and how this time dependent clearance affected the signal from viable cells once transplanted in canine myocardium. To address the ^{111}In clearance characteristics due to instantaneous cell death of transplanted cells *in vivo*, ^{111}In labeled cells were lysed *in vitro* followed by direct epicardial injection *in vivo* within normal and infarcted canine myocardium. ^{111}In time activity curves (TAC) were determined from continuous SPECT imaging following injection. TAC analysis revealed a double component clearance with a fast initial phase followed by a slower secondary phase [Blackwood *et al.* 2007a]. Experiments in our laboratory indicated that the initial phase might be due to injectate loss through the needle track. Therefore, only the secondary phase was considered to be the true clearance of radiolabeled debris, which we named the Debris Impulse Response Function (DIRF).

While DIRF describes the lower limit with which cell viability can be estimated, an upper limit is described by the ^{111}In clearance from cells that do not die. This was also determined *in vivo* and ultimately established how stable the ^{111}In radiolabel was in viable cells. Although ^{111}In has been shown to be stable with minimal leakage *in vitro* [Ballinger and Gnanasegaran 2005], initial radiolabel efflux has been shown followed by stabilization *in vivo* [Tran *et al.* 2006]. To understand ^{111}In radiolabel leakage *in vivo*, we took a different approach by labeling endogenous myocardial tissue *in situ* with ^{111}In-tropolone with the assumption that any ^{111}In loss would represent ^{111}In leakage only and not ^{111}In released from dead cells as cardiomyocytes are post-mitotic. We were able to show that ^{111}In was relatively stable in viable cells and had a biological half-life that was ~25 times longer than from dead cells. With this work, we have been able to identify a time window within which the viability of labeled cells can be accurately determined [Blackwood *et al.* 2007b]. As such, when viable labeled cells are transplanted into the myocardium the combination of cell death and survival demonstrate ^{111}In clearance kinetics that fall within this window. Figure 10 shows the differences in ^{111}In clearance from dead cells, cells that do not die, and transplanted viable cells. While this suggests that discriminating between cell death and viability is possible, it also highlights the importance of understanding the effects of DIRF for imaging viable transplanted cells *in vivo*.

One of the current challenges for cell therapy in the myocardium is that of cell survival following transplantation [Zhang *et al.* 2001]. In this sense, the concept of DIRF can be applied to most current forms of quantitative cellular imaging using clinically available tracking agents. Quantitative cellular imaging using targeted (e.g. reporter probe accumulation) or non-specific contrast agents will require some information on how the contrast agent associated with dead cells is removed from the region of interest particularly if the signal is still present following cell death. We anticipate that the kinetics of DIRF will also vary with respect to the organ of interest and perhaps the cell of interest depending on how the contrast agent is sequestered within the cell to be tracked. Within the myocardium itself, we can likely expect that changes in blood flow (normal vs. chronically occluded vs. reperfused myocardium) will also affect DIRF kinetics depending on where cells are transplanted.

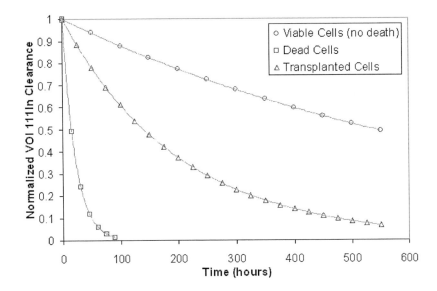

Figure 10. *In vivo* clearance kinetics (slow phase) of ^{111}In from cardiomyocytes labeled in situ (○), viable BMSCs injected into canine myocardium (△), and one DIRF curve from labeled BMSCs lysed *in vitro* and injected into canine myocardium (□).

CONCLUSION

In conclusion, in this chapter we have identified the technology that still needs to be developed to achieve Imaging Guided Myocardial Stem Cell Therapy. We suggest that the quantitative methods needed to determine the number of cells successfully transplanted and their viability with time can be achieved using in vitro labeling prior to transplantation. There are two front runners: a) labeling with iron particles and then imaging with MRI and b) labeling with radioactive compounds and then imaging with SPECT or PET. Although MRI has superior resolution, it is the sensitivity and the ability to quantify by correcting for released label that may give the nuclear medicine methods the advantage. However, the quantitative methods needed to determine function and molecular events within the cells are much less developed. When considering large animals and humans the nuclear medicine methods suffer from poor spatial resolution and the significant background or non-specific uptake of the externally injected contrast agent. These issues with nuclear medicine make it difficult to quantify the measured results and follow the cells for long periods of time. One solution may arise from the recent advancements made using MagA as a reporter gene for MRI, which has the potential to reduce non-specific uptake and thus improve the contrast-to-noise in MRI images. Improving quantitative methods to image viability, function and engraftment of transplanted cells will accelerate discovery and optimize methods of therapy.

ACKNOWLEDGMENTS

The authors thank Yves Bureau, Caroline Culshaw, Savita Dhanvantari, Lela Dorrington, Yuan Jin, Jim Koropatnick, Claude Lemaire, Benoit Lewden, Andrea Mitchell, Jane Sykes, Alex Thomas, Terry Thompson, and Glenn Wells for numerous discussions and scientific insights – many of which helped with the preparation of this chapter.

This work was supported by grants from the Canadian Institutes of Health Research, the Natural Sciences and Engineering Research Council, the Canadian Foundation for Innovation, the Heart and Stroke Foundation of Canada, Cancer Care Ontario (distributed through the Cancer Imaging Network of Ontario), the Ontario Research and Development Challenge Fund (distributed through the Behavioral Research and Imaging Network) and Multi Magnetics Inc.

REFERENCES

Aicher A, Brenner W, Zuayra M, Badorff C, Massoudi S, Assmus B, et al. Assessment of the tissue distribution of transplanted human endothelial progenitor cells by radioactive labeling. *Circulation*. 2003;107(16):2134-9.

Arbab A, Bashaw L, Miller BR, Jordan E, Bulte J, Frank J. Intracytoplasmic tagging of cells with ferumoxides and transfection agent for cellular magnetic resonance imaging after cell transplantation: methods and techniques. *Transplantation*. 2003;76(7):1123-30.

Balatoni JA, Doubrovin M, Ageyeva L, Pillarsetty N, Finn RD, Gelovani JG, et al. Imaging herpes viral thymidine kinase-1 reporter gene expression with a new ^{18}F-labeled probe: 2'fluoro-2'deoxy-5-[^{18}F]fluoroethyl-1-β-D-arabinofuranosyl uracil. *Nucl. Med. Biol.* 2005;32(8):811-9.

Ballinger, JR, Gnanasegaran G. Radiolabelled leukocytes for imaging inflammation: how radiochemistry affects clinical use. *Q. J. Nucl. Med. Mol. Imaging*. 2005: 49(4):308-18.

Bazylinski D, Frankel R. Magnetosome formation in prokaryotes. *Nat. Rev. Microbiol.* 2004;2(3):217-30.

Bengel FM, Anton M, Richter T, Simoes MV, Haubner R, Henke J, et al. Noninvasive imaging of transgene expression by use of positron emission tomography in a pig model of myocardial gene transfer. *Circulation.* 2003;108(17):2127-33.

Bengel FM, Schachinger V, Dimmeler S. Cell-based therapies and imaging in cardiology. *Eur. J. Nucl. Med. Mol. Imaging.* 2005;32 Suppl 2:S404-16.

Beutler E. "Pumping" iron: the proteins. *Science.* 2004;306(5704):2051-3.

Beyer T, Townsend DW, Brun T, Kinahan PE, Charron M, Roddy R, et al. A combined PET/CT scanner for clinical oncology. *J. Nucl. Med.* 2000;41(8):1369-79.

Bindslev L, Haack-Sørensen M, Bisgaard K, Kragh L, Mortensen S, Hesse B, et al. Labeling of human mesenchymal stem cells with indium-111 for SPECT imaging: effect on cell proliferation and differentiation. *Eur. J. Nucl. Med. Mol. Imaging.* 2006;33(10):1171-7.

Blackwood KJ, Lewden B, Stodilka RZ, Prato FS 2007a Mathematical modeling to quantify transplanted cell survival in canine myocardium in vivo. *Joint Molecular Imaging Conference Abstract Book ,* 271. 9-8-2007

Blackwood KJ, Lewden B, Stodilka RZ, Sykes J, Jin Y, Kong H et al 2007b In vivo SPECT imaging of cell viability after transplantation in the canine heart. *Joint Molecular Imaging Conference Abstract Book ,* 389. 9-8-2007

Bloom BR. Public health in transition. *Scientific American.* 2005 Sept;293(3):92-99.

Bulte J, Douglas T, Mann S, Frankel R, Moskowitz B, Brooks R, et al. Magnetoferritin. Biomineralization as a novel molecular approach in the design of iron-oxide-based magnetic resonance contrast agents. *Invest. Radiol.* 1994;29 Suppl 2:S214-S6.

Casey J, Koellert D, Ramin V, Klausner R, Harford J. Iron regulation of transferrin receptor mRNA levels requires iron-responsive elements and a rapid turnover determinant in the 3' untranslated region of the mRNA. *EMBO J.* 1989;8(12):3693-9.

Chin BB, NakamotoY, Bulte JWM, Pittenger MF, Wahl R, Kraitchman DL. ^{111}In oxine labelled mesenchymal stem cell SPECT after intravenous administration in myocardial infarction. *Nucl. Med. Commun.* 2003;24(11):1149-54.

Chiu RC, Zibaitis A, Kao RL. Cellular cardiomyoplasty: myocardial regeneration with satellite cell implantation. *Ann. Thorac. Surg.* 1995;60(1):12-18.

Cohen B, Dafni H, Meir G, Harmelin A, Neeman M. Ferritin as an endogenous MRI reporter for noninvasive imaging of gene expression in C6 glioma tumors. *Neoplasia.* 2005;7(2):109-17.

Cohen B, Ziv K, Plaks V, Israely T, Kalchenko V, Harmelin A, et al. MRI detection of transcriptional regulation of gene expression in transgenic mice. *Nat. Med.* 2007;13(4):498-503.

Collingwood J, Dobson J. Mapping and characterization of iron compounds in Alzheimer's tissue. *J. Alzheimer's Dis. 2006*;10(2-3):215-22.

Conti PS, Alauddin MM, Fissekis, JR, Schmall B, Watanabe KA. Synthesis of 2'-fluoro-5-[^{11}C]methyl-1-β-D-arabinofuranosyluracil ([^{11}C]-FMAU: A potential nucleoside analog for *in vivo* study of cellular proliferation with PET. *Nuc. Med. Biol.* 1995;22(6):783-9.

Deans A, Wadghiri Y, Bernas L, Yu X, Rutt B, Turnbull D. Cellular MRI contrast via coexpression of transferrin receptor and ferritin. *Magn. Reson. Med.* 2006;56(1):51-9.

Desai AG, Thakur ML. Radiolabeled blood cells: techniques and applications. *Crit. Rev. Clin. Lab. Sci.* 1986;24(2):95-122.

Dewanjee MK, Rao SA, Didisheim P. Indium-111 tropolone, a new high-affinity platelet label: preparation and evaluation of labeling parameters. *J. Nucl. Med.* 1981;22(11):981-7.

Dick AJ, Lederman RJ. MRI-guided myocardial cell therapy. *Int. J. Cardiovasc. Intervent.* 2005;7(4):165-70.

Dunn J, Fuller M, Zoeger J, Dobson J, Heller F, Hammann J, *et al*. Magnetic material in the human hippocampus. *Brain Res. Bull.* 1995;36(2):149-53.

Foster-Gareau P, Heyn C, Alejski A, Rutt BK. Imaging single mammalian cells with a 1.5 T clinical MRI scanner. *Magn. Reson. Med.* 2003;49(5):968-71.

Frangioni JV, Hajjar RJ. *In vivo* tracking of stem cells for clinical trials in cardiovascular disease. *Circulation.* 2004;110(21):3378-83.

Gambhir SS, Bauer E, Black ME, Liang Q, Kokoris MS, Barrio JR, *et al*. A mutant herpes simplex virus type 1 thymidine kinase reporter gene shows improved sensitivity for imaging reporter gene expression with positron emission tomography. *Proc. Natl. Acad. Sci. USA.* 2000;97(6):2785-90.

Genove G, DeMarco U, Xu H, Goins W, Ahrens E. A new transgene reporter for *in vivo* magnetic resonance imaging. *Nat. Med.* 2005;11(4):450-4.

Gilad A, Winnard P, van Zijl P, Bulte J. Developing MR reporter genes: promises and pitfalls. *NMR Biomed.* 2007;20(3):275-90.

Gilbert KM, Handler WB, Scholl TJ, Odegaard JW, Chronik BA. Design of field-cycled magnetic resonance systems for small animal imaging. *Phys. Med. Biol.* 2006;51(11):2825-41.

Gnecchi M, He H, Liang OD, Melo LG, Morello F, Mu H, *et al*. Paracrine action accounts for marked protection of ischemic heart by Akt-modified mesenchymal stem cells. *Nat. Med.* 2005;11(4):367-8.

Heyn C, Ronald JA, Ramadan SS, Snir JA, Barry AM, MacKenzie LT, *et al*. In vivo MRI of cancer cell fate at the single-cell level in a mouse model of breast cancer metastasis to the brain. *Magn. Reson. Med.* 2006;56(5):1001-10.

Jacobs A, Dubrovin M, Hewett J, Sena-Esteves M, Tan C, Slack M, *et al*. Functional coexpression of HSV-1 thymidine kinase and green fluorescent protein: implications for noninvasive imaging of transgene expression. *Neoplasia.* 1999;1(2):154-61.

Jacobs A, Voges J, Reszka R, Lercher M, Gossmann A, Kracht L, *et al*. Positron-emission tomography of vector-mediated gene expression in gene therapy for gliomas. *Lancet.* 2001;358(9283):727-9.

Jin Y, Kong H, Stodilka RZ, Wells RG, Zabel P, Merrifield PA, *et al*. Determining the minimum number of detectable cardiac transplanted ^{111}In-tropolone- labelled bone-marrow-derived mesenchymal cells by *SPECT Phys. Med. Biol.* 2005;50(19):4445-55.

Kang WJ, Kang HJ, Kim HS, Chung JK, Lee MC, Lee DS. Tissue distribution of 18F-FDG-labeled peripheral hematopoietic stem cells after intracoronary administration in patients with myocardial infarction. *J. Nucl. Med.* 2006;47(8):1295-301.

Kirschvink J. Magnetite biomineralization and geomagnetic sensitivity in higher animals: an update and recommendations for future study. *Bioelectromagnetics.* 1989;10(3):239-59.

Kirschvink J, Kobayashi-Kirschvink A, Woodford B. Magnetite biomineralization in the human brain. *Proc. Nat. Acad. Sci. USA.* 1992;89(16):7683-7.

Koh GY, Soonpaa MH, Klug MG Field LJ. Long-term survival of AT-1 cardiomyocyte grafts in syngeneic myocardium. *Am. J. Physiol.* 1993;264(5 Pt 2):H1727-33.

Koh GY, Soonpaa MH, Klug MG, Pride HP, Cooper BJ, Zipes DP, *et al*. Stable fetal cardiomyocyte grafts in the hearts of dystrophic mice and dogs. *J. Clin. Invest.* 1995;96(4):2034-42.

Komeili A, Li Z, Newman D, Jensen G. Magnetosomes are cell membrane invaginations organized by the actin-like protein MamK. *Science.* 2006;311(5758):242-5.

Kong H, Blackwood KJ, Stodilka RZ, Wells RG, Wisenberg G, Merrifield P, et al. 111In-Tropolone labeling of canine bone marrow mesenchymal cells: in vitro viability and washout kinetics. The Society of Nuclear Medicine 52nd Annual Meeting; June 18-22, 2005; Toronto, Ontario.

Kraitchman DL, Tatsumi M, Gilson WD, Ishimori T, Kedziorek D, Walczak P, et al. Dynamic imaging of allogeneic mesenchymal stem cells trafficking to myocardial infarction. *Circulation.* 2005;112(10):1451-61.

LaFlamme MA, Chen KY, Naumova AV, Muskheli V, Fugate JA, Dupras SK, et al. Cardiomyocytes derived from human embryonic stem cells in pro-survival factors enhance function of infarcted rat hearts. *Nat. Biotechnol.* 2007;25(9):1015-1024.

Lang C, Schüler D, Faivre D. Synthesis of magnetite nanoparticles for bio- and nanotechnology: genetic engineering and biomimetics of bacterial magnetosomes. *Macromolec. Biosci.* 2007;7(2):144-51.

Laugwitz KL, Moretti A, Lam J, Gruber P, Chen Y, Woodard S, et al. Postnatal isl1+ cardioblasts enter fully differentiated cardiomyocyte lineages. *Nature.* 2005;433(7026):647-53.

Lunde K, Solheim S, Aakhus S, Arnesen H, Abdelnoor M, Egeland T, et al. Intracoronary injection of mononuclear bone marrow cells in acute myocardial infarction. *N. Eng. J. Med.* 2006;355(12):1199-209.

Mangner TJ, Klecker RW, Anderson L, Shields AF. Synthesis of 2'-deoxy-2'-[^{18}F]fluoro-β-D-arabinofuranosyl nucleosides, [^{18}F]FAU, [^{18}F]FMAU, [^{18}F]FBAU and [^{18}F]FIAU, as potential PET agents for imaging cellular proliferation. *Nucl. Med. Biol.* 2003;30(3):215-24.

Matsumoto R, Omura,T, Yoshiyama M, Hayashi T, Inamoto S, Koh KR, et al. Vascular endothelial growth factor–expressing mesenchymal stem cell transplantation for the treatment of acute myocardial infarction. *Arterioscler. Thromb. Vasc. Biol.* 2005;25(6):1168-73.

Matsunaga T, Nakamura C, Burgess J, Sode K. Gene transfer in magnetic bacteria: transposon mutagenesis and cloning of genomic DNA fragments required for magnetosome synthesis. *J. Bacteriol.* 1992;174(9):2748-53.

Matsunaga T, Sakaguchi T, Okamura Y. Molecular and biotechnological aspects of bacterial magnetite. In: Baeuerlein E, editor. Biomineralization: progress in biology, molecular biology and application. Weinheim: Wiley-VCH; 2004. p. 91-106.

Matsunaga T, Suzuki T, Tanaka M, Arakaki A. Molecular analysis of magnetotactic bacteria and development of functional bacterial magnetic particles for nano-biotechnology. *Trends Biotech.* 2007;25(4):182-8.

Menasché P, Hagège AA, Scorsin M, Pouzet B, Desnos M, Duboc D, et al. Myoblast transplantation for heart failure. *Lancet.* 2001;357(9252):279-80.

Meyer GP, Wollert KC, Lotz J, Steffens J, Lippolt P, Fichtner S, et al. Intracoronary bone marrow cell transfer after myocardial infarction: eighteen months' follow-up data from the randomized, controlled BOOST (Bone marrow transfer to enhance ST-elevation infarct regeneration) trial. *Circulation.* 2006;113(10):1287-94.

Min JJ, Iyer M, Gambhir SS. Comparison of [(18)F]FHBG and [14C]FIAU for imaging of HSV1-*tk* reporter gene expression: adenoviral infection vs stable transfection. *Eur. J. Nucl. Med. Mol. Imaging.* 2003;30(11):1547-60.

Miyagawa M, Beyer M, Wagner B, Anton M, Spitzweg C, Gansbacher B, et al. Cardiac reporter gene imaging using the human sodium/iodide symporter gene. *Cardiovasc. Res.* 2005a;65(1):195-202

Miyagawa M, Anton M, Wagner B, Haubner R, Souvatzoglou M, Gansbacher B et al. Non-invasive imaging of cardiac transgene expression with PET: comparison of the human sodium/iodide symporter gene and HSV1-*tk* as the reporter gene. *Eur. J. Nucl. Med. Mol. Imaging.* 2005b;32(9):1108-14.

Miyawaki A. Fluorescence imaging of physiological activity in complex systems using GFP-based probes. *Curr. Opin. Neurobiol.* 2003 Oct;13(5):591-6.

Moatamed F, Johnson F. Identification and significance of magnetite in human tissues. *Arch. Pathol. Lab. Med.* 1986;110(7):618-21.

Murry CE, Soonpaa MH, Reinecke H, Nakajima H, Nakajima HO, Rubart M, et al. Haematopoietic stem cells do not transdifferentiate into cardiac myocytes in myocardial infarcts. *Nature.* 2004;428(6983):664-8.

Nakamura C, Burgess J, Sode K, Matsunaga T. An iron-regulated gene, *magA*, encoding an iron transport protein of *Magnetospirillum* sp. strain AMB-1. *J. Biol. Chem.* 1995;270(47):28392-6.

Niagara MI, Haider HK, Jiang S, Ashraf M. Pharmacologically preconditioned skeletal myoblasts are resistant to oxidative stress and promote angiomyogenesis via release of paracrine factors in the infarcted heart. *Circ. Res.* 2007;100(4):545-55.

Ntziachristos V, Bremer C, Weissleder R. Fluorescence imaging with near-infrared light: new technological advances that enable *in vivo* molecular imaging. *Eur. Radiol.* 2003;13(1):195-208.

Nutman A, Postovsky S, Zaidman I, Elhasid R, Vlodavsky E, Kreiss Y et al. Primary intraspinal primitive neuroectodermal tumor treated with autologous stem cell transplantation: case report and review of literature. *Pediatr. Hematol. Oncol.* 2007 Jan-Feb;24(1):53-61.

Orlic D, Kajstura J, Chimenti S, Jakoniuk I, Anderson SM, Li B, et al. Bone marrow cells regenerate infarcted myocardium. *Nature.* 2001;410(6829):701-5.

Ortega JJ, Diaz de Heredia C, Olive T, Bastida P, Llort A, Armadans L, et al. Allogeneic and autologous bone marrow transplantation after consolidation therapy in high-risk acute myeloid leukemia in children. Towards a risk-oriented therapy. *Haematologica.* 2003 Mar;88(3):290-9.

Oshima H, Payne TR, Urish KL, Sakai T, Ling Y, Gharaibeh B, et al. Differential myocardial infarct repair with muscle stem cells compared to myoblasts. *Mol. Ther.* 2005;12(6):1130-41.

Pereira RS, Prato FS, Sykes J, Wisenberg G. Assessment of myocardial viability using MRI during a constant infusion of Gd-DTPA: further studies at early and late periods of reperfusion. *Mag. Reson. Med.* 1999;42(1):60-8.

Pike L, Petravicz J, Wang S. Bioluminescence imaging after HSV amplicon vector delivery into brain. *J. Gene Med.* 2006;8(7):804-13.

Ray P, Tsien R, Gambhir S. Construction and validation of improved triple fusion reporter gene vectors for molecular imaging of living subjects. *Cancer Res.* 2007;67(7):3085-93.

Reinecke H, Poppa V, Murry CE. Skeletal muscle stem cells do not transdifferentiate into cardiomyocytes after cardiac grafting. *J. Mol. Cell Cardiol.* 2002;34(2):241-249.

Saab G, DeKemp RA, Ukkonen H, Ruddy TD, Germano G, Beanlands RS. Gated fluorine 18 fluorodeoxyglucose positron emission tomography: determination of global and regional left ventricular function and myocardial tissue characterization. *J. Nucl. Cardiol.* 2003 May-Jun;10(3):297-303.

Sandek F. Transplantation in the treatment of diabetes. *Vnitr. Lek.* 2007 Jul-Aug;53(7-8):859-64.

Schächinger V, Erbs S, Elsässer A, Haberbosch W, Hambrecht R, Hölschermann H, et al. REPAIR-AMI Investigators. Intracoronary bone marrow-derived progenitor cells in acute myocardial infarction. *N. Eng. J. Med.* 2006;355(12):1210-21.

Schüler D. Molecular analysis of a subcellular compartment: the magnetosome membrane in *Magnetospirillum gryphiswaldense*. *Arch. Microbiol.* 2004;181(1):1-7.

Sharma V, Luker GD, Piwnica-Worms D. Molecular imaging of gene expression and protein function *in vivo* with PET and SPECT. *J. Magn. Reson. Imaging.* 2002;16(4):336-51.

Sohn RL, Jain M, Liao R. Adult stem cells and heart regeneration. *Expert. Rev. Cardiovasc. Ther.* 2007;5(3):507-17.

Stodilka RZ, Blackwood KJ, Kong H, Prato FS Method for Quantitative Cell Tracking using SPECT for the Evaluation of Myocardial Stem Cell Therapy. *Nucl. Med. Commun.* 2006 27 807-813

Strauer BE, Brehm, M, Zeus T, Köstering M, Hernandez A, Sorg RV, et al. Repair of infarcted myocardium by autologous intracoronary mononuclear bone marrow cell transplantation in humans. *Circulation.* 2002;106(15):1913-8.

Thakur ML, Lavender JP, Arnot RN, Silverster DJ, Segal AW 1977 Indium–111-labelled autologous leukocytes in man. *J. Nucl. Med.* 18 1014-1021

Thornhill RE, Prato FS, Wisenberg G, White JA, Nowell J, Sauer A. Feasibility of the single-bolus strategy for measuring the partition coefficient of Gd-DTPA in patients with myocardial infarction: independence of image delay time and maturity of scar. *Magn. Reson. Med.* 2006;55(4):780-9.

Tran N, Li Y, Maskali F, Antunes L, Maureira P, Laurens MH et al. Short-term heart retention and distribution of intramyocardial delivered mesenchymal cells within necrotic or intact myocardium. *Cell Transplant.* 2006; 15(4):351-358.

Tjuvajev JG, Avril N, Oku T, Sasajima T, Miyagawa T, Joshi R, et al. Imaging herpes virus thymidine kinase gene transfer and expression by positron emission tomography. *Cancer Res.* 1998;58(19):4333-41.

Tjuvajev JG, Doubrovin M, Akhurst T, Cai S, Balatoni J, Alauddin MM, et al. Comparison of radiolabeled nucleoside probes (FIAU, FHBG, FHPG) for PET imaging of HSV-*tk* gene expression. *J. Nucl. Med.* 2002;43(8):1072-83.

Uemura R, Xu M, Ahmad N, Ashraf M. Bone marrow stem cells prevent left ventricular remodeling of ischemic heart through paracrine signaling. *Circ. Res.* 2006;98(11):1414-21.

Vaidyanathan G, Zalutsky MR, Preparation of 5-[^{131}I]Iodo- and 5-[^{211}At]astato-1-(2-deoxy-2-fluoro--β-D-arabinofuranosyl) uracil by a halodestannylation reaction. *Nucl. Med. Biol.* 1998;25(5):487-96.

Watanabe KA, Reichman U, Hirota K, Lopez C, Fox JJ. Nucleosides. 110. Synthesis and antiherpes virus activity of some 2'-fluoro-2'-deoxyarabinofuranosylpyrimidine nucleosides. *J. Med. Chem.* 1979;22(1):21-4.

Weissleder R, Moore A, Mahmood U, Bhorade R, Benveniste H, Chiocca E, et al. In vivo magnetic resonance imaging of transgene expression. *Nat. Med.* 2000;6(3):351-5.

Wu JC, Chen IY, Sundaresan G, Min JJ, De A, Qiao JH, et al. Molecular imaging of cardiac cell transplantation in living animals using optical bioluminescence and positron emission tomography. *Circulation.* 2003;108(11):1302-5.

Zhang M, Methot D, Poppa V, Fujio Y, Walsh K, Murry CE. Cardiomyocyte grafting for cardiac repair: graft cell death and anti-death strategies. *J. Mol. Cell Cardiol.* 2001;33(5):907-21.

Zhou R, Acton PD, Ferrari VA. Imaging stem cells implanted in infarcted myocardium. *J. Am. Coll. Cardiol.* 2006;48(10):2094-106.

Zhou R, Thomas DH, Qiao H, Bal HS, Choi SR, Alavi A, *et al. In vivo* detection of stem cells grafted in infarcted rat myocardium. *J. Nucl. Med.* 2005;46(5):816-22.

In: Encyclopedia of Stem Cell Research (2 Volume Set) ISBN: 978-1-61761-835-2
Editor: Alexander L. Greene © 2012 Nova Science Publishers, Inc.

Chapter X

HUMAN POST-NATAL STEM CELLS IN ORGANS PRODUCED BY TISSUE ENGINEERING FOR CLINICAL APPLICATIONS

Lucie Germain, Danielle Larouche,
François A. Auger and Julie Fradette[*]

LOEX Laboratory, Centre de recherche,
Hôpital du Saint-Sacrement du CHAUQ, Quebec, Quebec, G1S 4L8,
and Départements de Chirurgie, d'Oto-rhino-laryngologie et ophtalmologie,
Université Laval, Quebec, Quebec, Canada

ABSTRACT

This chapter will focus on the clinical applications of post-natal stem cells. Massive tissue loss frequently requires grafting for proper healing. Considering that there is a shortage of organ donors, the expansion of cells in vitro and the reconstruction of tissues or organs constitute a very valuable alternative solution. The first clinical application of such tissues has been the autologous culture of epidermal cells for the treatment of burn patients, and will be presented herein. Since the cutaneous epithelium forms squames that are lost, it is continuously renewed every 28 days and its long-term regeneration depends on stem cells. The importance of preserving stem cells during in vitro expansion and after grafting will thus be discussed. Clinical applications of cultured cells from other tissues, such as limbal stem cells for corneal epithelium (surface of the eye) replacement, will also be reviewed. Finally, the development of new promising technologies and methods taking advantage of other sources of stem cells that could be isolated after birth from tissues such as adipose depots will also be presented.

---

[*] Corresponding author: Dr. Julie Fradette, Laboratoire d'Organogénèse Expérimentale, Hôpital du Saint-Sacrement du CHAUQ, 1050 Chemin Sainte-Foy, Québec, Québec, Canada, G1S 4L8. Telephone: (418) 682-7995 or 7663. Fax: (418) 682-8000. Email: julie.fradette@chg.ulaval.ca ; www.loex.qc.ca

INTRODUCTION

Progress in tissue engineering offers hope for patients suffering from tissue loss. Organ transplantation or tissue grafting are classical treatments for the replacement of damaged organs or severe tissue destruction. However, this procedure is limited by tissue/organ availability. For example, in the case of burn patients, the amount of skin loss may limit the availability of donor sites from which autologous skin can be harvested for grafting. In the case of allogeneic organ transplantation, the waiting list is long, indicating a severe shortage of organ donors [1]. Moreover, for some organs such as the cornea, the lack of suitable organ is expected to markedly increase in the future. Indeed, the treatment of corneas with laser surgery, an increasingly popular approach for correcting eye disorders, changes the optical properties of the corneas that then become unsuitable for transplantation to a receiver [2].

Tissue engineering is an innovative field that includes various approaches based on the utilisation of biomaterials, extracellular matrix components and cells to produce substitutes for the replacement of wounded or diseased tissues. The presence of living cells is clearly advantageous when a tissue substitute is required to replace a large defect or injury. Thus, such substitutes can integrate in a biologically active fashion into the surrounding tissues. Furthermore, the self-healing properties of these reconstructed organs should be preserved as has been shown in the use of cultured autologous epidermis [3-9].

Several considerations must be taken into account for the development of alternatives to the transplantation of allogeneic organs through tissue engineering. Autologous tissue is evidently a preferable transplant material because of the unavoidable rejection reaction problem associated with allogeneic grafts that consequently necessitate lifelong immunosuppressive treatment.

The choice of the cell source is very important since the quality of the tissue substitute will be a reflection of the quality of the cells used for its reconstitution. The ideal cell source should provide cells with extensive proliferation potential (self-renewal capacity) and appropriate differentiation abilities (able to give rise to the targeted differentiated progeny) in order to ensure the repair, regeneration and functionality of the tissue substitutes after grafting. Interestingly, these are typical properties of stem cells.

Although embryonic stem cells have been hailed as an alternative cell source in the future, there are practical and ethical obstacles to their use in the various clinical applications presented in this chapter. Tissue substitutes comprise both stem cells and their differentiated progeny. Thus, the advantages of multipotency of embryonic stem cells may become a limitation since the induction of differentiation must be perfectly controlled in order to avoid ectopic tissue formation such as teratomas or bone material in the heart with ensuing catastrophic complications [10, 11]. The rejection problem is another challenge that must be overcome. Indeed, the functionality of the living substitute often resides in differentiated cells. Although embryonic stem cells do not present histocompatibility antigens, their differentiated progeny, necessary for tissue functionality, do express them [10, 11].

In contrast, post-natal stem cells may have a more restricted potential of differentiation thus being able to generate a few lineages or perhaps only one. However, this lower lineage plasticity becomes an advantage when stem cells are isolated from a biopsy of the tissue targeted for reconstruction since it is easier to control their differentiation pathway towards the desired cell type. Interestingly, multipotent stem cells can also be isolated from some post-natal tissues. As such, these cells represent a good autologous cellular pool to produce a variety of tissues especially when there are obvious difficulties or no possibility of harvesting stem cells from the diseased tissue.

The present chapter will focus on the development of living tissue substitutes for permanent tissue replacement. Skin and corneal epithelial cells will serve as examples of cultured stem cells used in the treatment of large wound defects. Whether it is necessary to purify stem cells will also be discussed. Moreover, promising results from the study of multipotent post-natal stem cells isolated from adipose tissue will be presented.

HUMAN EPIDERMAL AUTOLOGOUS GRAFTS PRODUCED FROM SKIN EPITHELIAL CELL CULTURES CONTAINING POST-NATAL STEM CELLS

Cultured epidermal autografts (CEA) have been used for the treatment of burn patients in several countries. Although this approach provides only the epidermis, the superficial layer of the skin (figure 1Aa), it proved to be life-saving for many patients [3, 4, 12-20] especially those who have insufficient donor sites to use the classical therapeutic approach that requires the harvesting of such spared sites. Thus, the possibility of producing thousands of square centimetres from the small (1-5 cm^2) initial biopsy (figure 1Ba) was a significant breakthrough into this demanding clinical arena [8]. The thin cultured epidermis (figure 1Bd) matures after transplantation into a full-thickness epidermis (figure 1Be). The wounds are then efficiently and permanently covered with a self-regenerating living tissue. Moreover, these grafts can repair themselves if they are wounded [4]. The differentiated stratum corneum that forms after in vivo grafting then ensures the reappearance of many skin functions such as protection against desiccation and mechanical damage. The use of autologous cultures prevents the problems associated with rejection that would develop with allogeneic cells since keratinocytes are immunogenic [21, 22].

In the skin, stem cells have been localized in the basal layer of the epidermis [23] (for review see Watt et al. (2006) [24]). Keratinocytes differentiate as they move towards the outer surface of the epithelium. In hairy anatomic sites, the bulge region of the hair follicles is particularly enriched in stem cells [25-31]. The figure 1Aa,b presents schematic representations of the localisation of stem cells in hairy and glabrous skin. Thus, it is advantageous to isolate cells especially from these portions of the epithelium in order to maximize the number of stem cells harvested. In the initial cell culture method, human skin was digested with trypsin [32]. The addition of a skin digestion step with thermolysin has the advantage of removing the dermis while harvesting hair follicles and epidermis including a complete basal cell layer that are then digested with trypsin [33, 34].

Human skin epithelial cells can be grown in culture in the presence of a feeder layer of irradiated fibroblasts and medium supplemented with various additives (including serum, EGF, insulin, cholera toxin) that prolong lifespan and increase the growth rate of keratinocyte cultures in vitro [32, 35]. Keratinocytes can be subcultured for several passages using this method. The feeder layer favours the clonal growth of keratinocytes, and its influence on transcription factors will be discussed below.

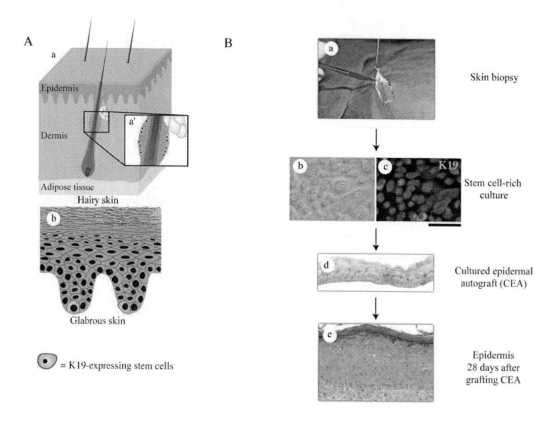

Figure 1. (A) Schematic representation of hairy (a) and glabrous (b) skin showing the localisation of K19-expressing stem cells (green). (a') High magnification of boxed area in (a) showing the bulge region of the hair follicle. (B) Summary of the production of epidermal sheets used for the treatment of burn patients. A small (1-5 cm^2) biopsy is excised from the patient (a) and epithelial cells are extracted by an enzymatic treatment. Epithelial cells are seeded on fibroblast feeder layers in culture flasks, they form colonies in culture as shown by phase contrast microscopy (b) and Hoechst staining of the nuclei (c). After amplification by subculturing, epithelial cells are detached from the culture flasks without breaking cell-cell links to form cultured epidermal autograft (CEA)(d). After grafting, the thin CEA matures into full-thickness epidermis (e). Bar: 100 µm.

In culture, it has been observed that skin epithelial cells form colonies that are several layers thick. Notably, proliferative cells are located at the edge of the colonies, in the basal layer where they attach to the plastic substrate [36]. Differentiated cells can detach from the plastic substrate, then leave the basal layer to form the suprabasal layers in which cells are bound to their neighbours by desmosomes [37, 38]. The high concentration of calcium in the culture medium sustains cell differentiation and allows the formation of these desmosomes [37-39]. Therefore, such epidermal cultures contain a combination of cells with various differentiation levels.

In vitro, individual keratinocytes form three distinct types of colonies named holoclones, meroclones and paraclones [40]. Holoclones present a high proliferative capacity in the absence of terminal differentiation. They contain uniformly small keratinocytes that form large colonies (figure 2A,C). Paraclones, which are small colonies, characteristically present large cells (figure 2B,D). These keratinocytes stopped proliferating after a few divisions and underwent differentiation. Meroclones contain a mixture of keratinocytes with various proliferation/differentiation potential and are considered an intermediate stage between holoclones and paraclones. The extensive proliferation potential of keratinocytes forming holoclones is reminiscent of stem cells.

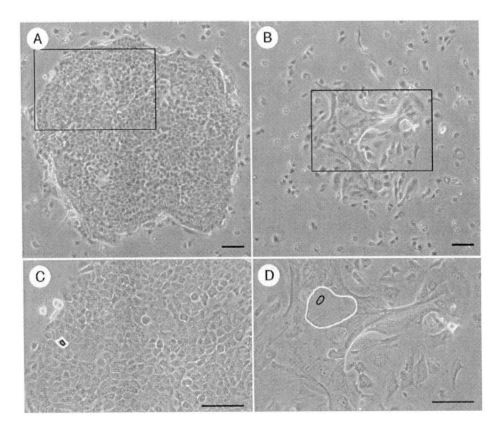

Figure 2. Phase contrast micrographs of a holoclone (A) and a paraclone (B). (C and D) high magnification of boxed area in A and B, respectively. One cell have been delineated using a white line in C and D. Note that holoclone (A, C) contains uniformly small keratinocytes with a high nucleus (black line in C) to cytoplasm (white line in C) ratio typical of less differentiated cells, while paraclone (B, D) contains differentiated keratinocytes with a small nucleus (black line in D) to cytoplasm (white line in D) ratio. Bars: 100 μm.

The identification of keratin 19 (K19), a structural protein present in the cytoplasm of stem cells but absent from the other keratinocytes of the cutaneous epithelium, allowed us to better characterize stem cells in situ and in vitro [26, 41]. The observed increase in the percentage of K19-positive cells during the first passages of skin epithelial cell cultures indicates that stem cells do proliferate under these culture conditions [26]. A greater percentage of K19-expressing stem cells was observed in skin from children compared to adults. The number of holoclones is also greater in cultures established from young compared to older subjects (Germain et al., unpublished results and [42, 43]). Moreover, the amount of epithelium that can be produced from a small biopsy (1 to 4 cm^2) is much larger for a child (1 x 10^{32} cells that could cover 10^{17} km^2) compared to an adult (a few square meters). However, it is worth mentioning that such a surface area is sufficient to treat an adult patient.

In general, it is difficult to track stem cells in vivo after transplantation, therefore the long-term survival and proliferation of transplanted CEA and their epithelial stem cells is difficult to assess directly. Usually, very few biopsies can be performed, obviously to spare the newly epithelialized region from a potentially deleterious additional trauma. Despite these difficulties, a direct demonstration of the survival of stem cells after CEA grafting in vivo was published by Mavilio et al. [44]. They took advantage of the transplantation of genetically-modified epithelial stem cells to follow their fate months after their transfer on a patient suffering from epidermolysis bullosa. This successful direct assessment of stem cell survival and other clinical evidence support the long-term regeneration of the newly formed epithelium and thus indicates the persistence of stem cells during the first passages in culture as well as after grafting CEA. Indeed, cultured epithelium forms normal epidermis that survives for years after grafting on patients [3]. However, the complete regeneration of the underlying dermis is a very long process [45].

More complex skin substitutes comprising both the dermis and the epidermis are currently under development by our and other teams. The addition of a living dermal substitute to the construct should facilitate recovery of the properties associated with the dermis such as elasticity and mechanical resistance and decrease scar retraction in vivo. Different approaches have been developed such as cells seeded in collagen gels, natural or synthetic scaffolds [5, 6, 8, 46-56]. Alternatively, skin substitutes can be produced from autologous cells only, without biomaterials, using culture methods promoting the secretion and organization of a dense extracellular matrix as in our self-assembly approach [56-59]. These skin substitutes have many histological characteristics that are close to those of normal human skin (figure 3A).

Various skin substitutes have been used to treat chronic wounds such as venous or diabetic ulcers [17, 55, 60-70], but very few were reported as permanent skin replacement for third degree burns [71]. One challenge is that the time of production of these living bi-layered substitutes is longer than for the production of CEA. However, the delay will probably be shortened as technology progresses, as it was the case for CEA for which the production time of 28 days for the initial graft, decreased to 12 days.

Promising results were obtained following animal transplantation of such bi-layered human skin substitutes on full-thickness surgical wounds for a 1 to 6-month period [58, 72-76]. In addition to providing a permanent coverage with an histologically normal and adequately differentiated epithelium, mechanical properties associated with the dermal component were also imparted to the transplant site by such complete dermal\epidermal cultured grafts. Moreover, these substitutes are easier to manipulate since they are more resistant than the relatively fragile CEA. The improved mechanical properties after grafting were attributed to the well-developed dermo-epidermal junction (figure 3Ab) as well as the ultrastructural aspect of the dermal components [58, 73]. Indeed, complex collagen and elastin fiber networks are observed [58, 73, 77].

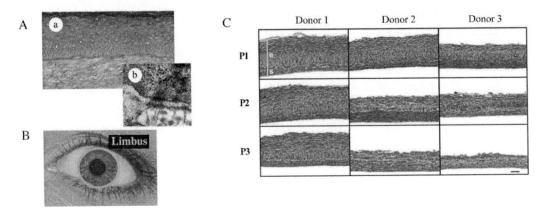

Figure 3. (A) Skin reconstructed by the self-assembly approach. (a) Masson's trichrome staining. (b) Transmission electron microscopy observation showing the basement membrane with an hemidesmosome. Note the formation of a differentiated epidermis with all layers including the stratum corneum, and the presence of a complete basement membrane with lamina lucida, lamina densa and hemidesmosomes. (B) Human eye. The corneal stem cells are located in the limbus area (labeled in green). (C) Histological cross sections of reconstructed cornea produced in vitro with epithelial cells from three different donors after passage 1 (P1), passage 2 (P2) and passage 3 (P3). Note that the quality of the reconstructed tissues differs according to the cells used. Bar = 100 μm (C). Taken from Gaudreault et al. (2003) [78] with permission.

In the case of chronic wounds, the substitutes used for treatment are not necessarily intended to fully integrate into the wound in a fashion similar to autologous full-thickness skin grafts. Therefore, the presence of epithelial stem cells may not be essential because of the short-term survival of this biological dressing. These substitutes favour and enhance the healing process attributed to the migration of the autologous keratinocytes surrounding the wound. Then, it follows that such a temporary coverage does not necessitate the use of autologous tissue [70]. Multiple applications of allogeneic cultured epithelium may be required if large defects are treated.

HUMAN CORNEAL GRAFTS PRODUCED FROM EPITHELIAL CELL POPULATIONS CONTAINING POST-NATAL LIMBAL STEM CELLS

The corneal epithelium localized at the surface of the eye is also a continuously renewing tissue although less differentiated than the epidermis. It must remain very transparent to ascribe adequate optical properties for good eyesight. The maintenance of the homeostasis in the cornea is achieved through a balance between proliferation and differentiation. In contrast to skin, stem cells are not uniformly distributed along the entire corneal surface. Actually, the central cornea is devoid of stem cells, and only contains relatively differentiated cells expressing the K3/K12 keratins [79-82]. Stem cells are restricted to the periphery of the cornea [83] at the junction with the conjunctiva in the region named the limbus (figure 3B).

The epithelium is thicker in the limbus, comprising 10 cell layers compared to the 4-6 cell layers of the central cornea.

The method allowing clonal growth and extensive expansion of skin keratinocytes by co-culturing them with irradiated fibroblasts is also adequate for the culture of corneal epithelial cells [84, 85]. Human epithelial cells isolated after a dispase digestion from the central corneal or the limbus have been compared in culture. Limbal cells can be subcultured for several passages (seven passages, 25 to 35 population doublings) [86, 87]. In contrast, cells from the central cornea have a shorter lifetime in culture as they can barely be subcultured (2 or 3 passages at the most). Thus, the proliferative potential of cells isolated from different portions of the ocular epithelium varies in culture. The longer lifespan of cells isolated from the limbus is consistent with the preservation of stem cells in vitro under these culture conditions. Our observations [86] are similar to those published by others [84, 88].

The type of colonies formed in culture is also different according to the anatomic origin of the cells [88]. Cells isolated from the central cornea form paraclones (small colonies containing large cells with a low nucleus to cytoplasm ratio, indicating that they are differentiated cells) which is consistent with their low proliferative potential [40]. In contrast, limbal cells produce holoclones. Large colonies are constituted of small cells that possess a high nucleus to cytoplasm ratio typical of less differentiated cells [40].

The limbus that contains stem cells is of a relatively small size. As such, the initial biopsy represents a particular challenge, since it must be quite small. This prompted studies into the minimal biopsy size necessary to initiate successful cell culture. Indeed, one clinical application for these cultures is the treatment of stem cell deficiency, following chemical burns. Typically, one eye is affected and the other may also be partially affected. Thus, the limbal biopsy sampling must be of a minor size to limit as much as possible the potential risk of causing total limbal stem cell deficiency in the healthy portion of the eye affected by partial stem cell deficiency. In keeping with these clinical limitations, our team and others have shown that limbal epithelial cells can be successfully isolated and cultured from a 1 to 3 mm^2 human limbal biopsy [84, 89-91].

With such a small size biopsy, the concentration of stem cells in the initial tissue biopsy should then be maximized. The limbus is not a homogeneous tissue and its morphological characteristics vary with the anatomic localisation. Cells harvested from the four quadrants have distinct growth potential. Higher colony forming efficiency within the limbus is attributed to cells from the superior and inferior quadrants compared to cells from nasal or temporal limbus [88, 92]. These results indicate that it would probably be better to harvest biopsies from these very sites.

Since stem cells are expected to be present in a protected area, the preferential localisation of stem cells in the superior and inferior quadrants is logical considering the protection provided by eyelids against most environmental and mechanical injuries.

The successful treatment of limbal stem cell deficiency using ex vivo cultured limbal epithelial stem cells was first reported by Pellegrini [89]. Since then, several groups have cultured limbal cells in vitro for the treatment of limbal stem cell deficiency (for review see Shortt (2007) [93]). Several culture methods were concurrently reported [89, 94-97]. A better preservation of the precious stem cells was attributed to the use of substrates such as fibrin or amniotic membrane [88, 90, 98].

When limbal stem cell deficiency is total, an adequate amount of autologous or allogeneic limbal stem cells must be transplanted if a stable corneal epithelial phenotype is to be regained [93]. However, the survival of the allogeneic cells after grafting may be limited to 7 to 9 months since allogeneic DNA was not identified at a later post-transplantation time as reported in nine patients. DNA genotyping was performed on epithelial cells harvested by impression cytology after grafting allogeneic cultures. The corresponding DNA genotype of donor cells was only identified in two patients after two and seven months [99]. Autologous grafting is clearly desirable since it avoids the risk of immune rejection. The best alternative cell source in cases when use of autologous limbal epithelial cells is not possible remains to be determined (for review see Shortt (2007) [93]).

As discussed previously for the cutaneous CEA, it is difficult but not impossible to follow the fate of limbal stem cells in vitro and after grafting. The efficiency of limbal cells to form colonies (cfe assay) indicates that stem cells are present in these cultures [89, 90, 100]. Other characteristics such as the absence of K3/K12 in the basal layer of cultured substitutes is evidence, but not proof, of the presence of stem cells. The published successful treatment of stem cell deficiency is another circumstantial indication of the presence of stem cells. Several clinical parameters can be assessed before and after the treatment with cultured cells: the presence of a stable, transparent corneal epithelium, the resolution of persistent epithelial defects and regression of corneal vascularization. However, one must take into account the fact that the extent of the initial stem cell deficiency could obviously influence the outcome. Thus, if this deficiency was not total, the culture may act as a specialized dressing that then essentially helps the remaining host stem cells survive.

The regeneration of a normal corneal epithelium, the absence of Goblet cells and the expected K3 expression pattern have been shown on biopsies obtained from two patients, 19 and 24 months after grafting [89]. The study of impression cytology after grafting is a non-invasive mean to assess the success of corneal regeneration. In these harvested cells, the expression of K3 and K12 is indicative of an appropriate corneal phenotype [90].

PRACTICAL CONSIDERATIONS IN THE PRODUCTION OF CULTURED SUBSTITUTES FOR GRAFTING

The advantage of the feeder layer on the production of colonies from single cells has been clearly demonstrated [32, 40]. It is very difficult if not impossible to initiate and expand epithelial cell cultures from a small normal human skin or limbus biopsy without a feeder layer. The feeder cells produce growth factors and deposit extracellular matrix that promote epithelial growth. The presence of irradiated fibroblasts also limits the outgrowth of human fibroblasts that may have been isolated with the epithelial cells, likely by a mechanism of contact inhibition. These fibroblast feeder layers also possess anti-apoptotic activity [101]. In vivo, stem cells occupy specific positions or "niches" in the basal layer of the epithelium. It is possible that the feeder layer plays a similar role in vitro. However, the exact mechanism of action of these accompanying cells still remains to be clarified.

Cell proliferation and differentiation is dependent on specific gene expression. The transcription of these genes is modulated either positively or negatively by nuclear transcription factors. In order to evaluate whether the feeder layer had an effect on transcription factors [102], newborn and adult human skin keratinocytes were serially passaged until senescence in the presence or absence of irradiated fibroblasts. The lifespan extension of keratinocytes cultured with irradiated fibroblasts was associated with the stabilization of the DNA binding properties of Sp1 without altering its transcription. In the absence of feeder layer, keratinocyte expression of Sp1 rapidly diminishes and the lifetime of the culture is much shorter (figure 4). In addition, the observation of the higher proportion of keratin 10-expressing keratinocytes in the absence of feeder layer (table 1) indicated that this condition induces more differentiation. Since Sp1/Sp3 regulates the transcription of a high number of genes, the alteration of such a fundamental transcription factor is a remarkable mean for the cell to influence its proliferation/differentiation. Thus, these results suggest that the interaction between the feeder layer and keratinocytes delays their terminal differentiation by preventing alterations in the expression of transcription factors, such as Sp1 and Sp3 [102].

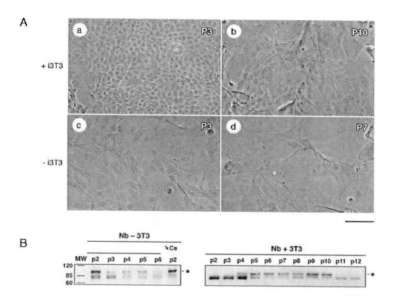

Figure 4. (A) Phase contrast micrographs of newborn skin keratinocytes grown either with i3T3 (a, b) or without i3T3 (c,d) at passage 3 (a, c), 10 (b) and 7 (d). Bar: 100 µm. (B) Western blot analyses of the nuclear proteins from newborn (Nb) skin keratinocytes grown either with (+3T3) or without (-3T3) i3T3 and harvested at different passages (P2-P12) using polyclonal antibodies raised against Sp1 (Santa Cruz Biotechnology, Inc.) ↓ Ca: Keratinocytes grown in low calcium medium. The position of a variant of Sp1 with a low electrophoretic mobility in gel is indicated (*). The position of the molecular weight markers (120-, 85-, 60-kDa) is provided. Note that expression of Sp1 is altered by cell passages in culture, but the loss of Sp1 is delayed when keratinocytes are cultivated with i3T3. Taken from Masson-Gadais et al. (2006) [102] with permission.

In the cornea, the lifespan of human limbal epithelial cells cultured from post-mortem human eye varies with the donors as does their morphological aspect in culture. Some cultures present a higher proportion of differentiated cells at early passages (figure 5). This has an impact on the ability of these cultures to differentiate and stratify after seeding on a reconstructed stroma in bi-layered corneal substitutes (figure 3C). This variation has been correlated with changes in the expression of the transcription factors of the Sp1 family [78]. Therefore, the expression of Sp1/Sp3 might represent a good predictor for selecting human limbal epithelial cell cultures that are most likely to proliferate, stratify and differentiate properly when used for the production of reconstructed corneal substitutes.

Table 1. Percentage of keratin 10-positive cells as a function of the passage of human skin keratinocytes in the presence or absence of irradiated fibroblast (i3T3)

Passage (P)	P3		P5		P7		P9	
	%±SD	(n)	%±SD	(n)	%±SD	(n)	%±SD	(n)
+ i3T3	9±2	(10)	10±3	(10)	18§±4	(10)	39§±4	(5)
− i3T3	21*±6	(6)	36*§±8	(5)	41*±2	(5)	NA	

* : Statistically significant difference with keratinocytes at the same passage co-cultured with i3T3. $P<0.005$
§ : Statistically significant difference with keratinocytes at the preceding passage of the same culture condition (-i3T3 or +i3T3). $P<0.05$
NA: skin keratinocytes are already senescent after P7, therefore no analysis could be performed at P9.

One of the advantages of using post-natal stem cells harvested from healthy portions of the same organ needing reconstruction is that no purification step of the stem cell population is then necessary. Indeed, the two examples reported here for epithelial cells cultured from skin and cornea show that the expected differentiation pathways do occur in the epithelial cells cultured in vitro. Although, epithelial cells exhibiting various differentiation status, from stem cells to terminally differentiated cells (holoclones to paraclones) coexist in the culture, their differentiation pathway is normal. Skin or cornea of normal histological appearance can be produced as substitutes in vitro or after grafting in vivo. This, in combination with the absence of aberrant differentiation pathways, then renders stem cell purification unnecessary for these tissues.

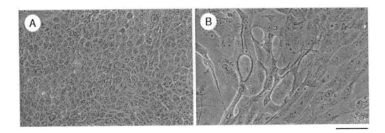

Figure 5. Phase contrast micrographs of human corneal epithelial cell cultures from two different donors at the same passage (P3). (A) Colony containing less differentiated cells. (B) Colony containing differentiated cells. Bar = 100 µm (A,B).

Stem cells are crucial for the long-term survival of the tissue/organ after transplantation because of their essential role in tissue turnover and regeneration. Thus, it is worth studying the preservation of stem cells under the chosen culture conditions. The various components of the culture reagents (serum, growth factors, trypsin, etc.) should be tested. In addition, quality control is necessary in each and every laboratory and for each tissue-engineered construct. The preservation of stem cells may vary in different substitutes. For example, there is an upward migration of keratin 19-positive cells in skin equivalent produced by the collagen gel model indicating that stem cells are lost during the maturation stage [103]. They migrate to the stratum corneum where they will desquamate. In contrast, keratin 19-positive cells are present in the basal layer of the epithelium of tissue-engineered skin produced by the self-assembly approach even after 21 days of culture at the air-liquid interface indicating that stem cells are preserved in their expected position. This difference between these two skin substitutes is attributed to the presence of a well-structured basement membrane under the epithelium in the latter substitute (figure 3Ab) in contrast to the collagen gel model [103] and thus demonstrates the crucial importance of the stromal compartment.

POST-NATAL STEM CELLS FROM THE MESENCHYME: CELLULAR THERAPIES AND TISSUE ENGINEERING STRATEGIES

The mesenchymal portion of many tissues is gaining attention as a source of multipotent stem cells for regenerative processes, including tissue engineering for organ reconstruction. Bone marrow mesenchymal stem cells have been widely studied and are a reference in the field of adult stem cells [104-107]. Recently, mesenchymal stem cell populations from tissues such as placenta [108], umbilical cord matrix [109, 110], dermis [111, 112] and adipose tissue [113, 114] have been described and characterized. Adipose tissue, or subcutaneous fat (figure 1Aa), will be presented here as a very promising new source of human post-natal cells for regenerative therapies as well as an important target organ for soft tissue reconstruction.

Since 2001, human adipose tissue has raised great interest in the research community. This tissue, once described as a passive storage site for triglycerides, has revealed itself to be not only an active secretory organ [115] but also a prevalent and accessible tissue harbouring a subpopulation of multipotent stem cells [113, 114]. When adipose tissue from individuals of normal body mass index (BMI) is harvested and its stroma digested with collagenase, the non-adipocyte stromal cells can be cultured and amplified as adherent cells in vitro. Among these stromal cells, a subpopulation of human adipose-derived stem cells (ASCs) can be induced to differentiate specifically into various cell types including adipocytes, osteoblasts, myocytes, chondrocytes [113], as well as cells displaying neuronal [116] or epithelial (hepatocytes) [117, 118] characteristics.

The cell surface phenotype of cultured ASCs is very similar, although not identical, to the immunophenotype of bone marrow-derived stem cells. These two populations express common stromal markers such as CD73 and CD105 (endoglin) but lack expression of the haematopoietic marker CD45 and of the endothelial marker CD31 [114, 119-121]. While combinations of surface markers have been described to help enrich freshly isolated ASCs [122, 123], no unique single marker allows localisation of ASCs in situ or their identification among cultured adipose-derived stromal cells. At the transcriptome level, recent studies also relate a high correlation between human adipose and bone marrow stem cell populations analyzed by microarrays [120, 124-126]. The major advantages of using stem cells extracted from adipose tissue in regenerative medicine include the availability of large amounts of tissue harvested by standard lipoaspiration procedures, and the high proportion of cells able to differentiate into multiple lineages. Indeed, adipose tissue can supply a very high number of stem cells. Interestingly, 2% of stromal cells exhibit stem cell characteristics in comparison with only 0.002 % for bone marrow stem cells [127]. This translates into a higher yield of high-quality autologous cells available for clinical applications, therefore reducing the need of extensive in vitro amplification before implantation or tissue reconstruction.

ASCs are presently the focus of intense research efforts, and the non-profit organization IFATS (International Federation for Adipose Therapeutics and Science) is actively promoting research investigating their potential for tissue repair of many organs. Two main trends have emerged among the various regenerative medicine strategies using ASCs being currently tested: cellular therapy and the reconstruction of tissue-engineered organs. The hypothesis supporting the use of ASCs as cellular entities mediating therapeutic repair in different organs mostly relies on their paracrine effects. ASCs secretion of a variety of bioactive molecules including pro-angiogenic factors would stimulate endogenous repair mechanisms when injected at injured sites. The local implantation of ASCs could also stimulate the recruitment of endogenous stem cells to this site where their differentiation into the appropriate lineage would be promoted by specific cues from the microenvironment. These proposed mechanisms of action gathered from the work of many investigators are discussed in [126].

Despite their recent history compared to cells from bone marrow, which have widely proven their value in clinical applications for haematological pathologies, cardiovascular diseases and recovery after chemotherapy for cancer patients (reviewed in Giordano (2007) [128]), ASCs are already used in a few ongoing clinical trials. These human studies are mainly taking place in Asia and in Europe for the moment. They assess the potential benefit of ASCs as cell-based therapies for a range of therapeutic applications including fistula's repair (Spain, Germany, United Kingdom), breast augmentation (Japan [129]), and cardiovascular repair with trials such as The PRECISE study for chronic myocardial ischemia (Spain) and The APPOLO trial for treatment of heart attacks (Netherlands, Spain) (www.clinicaltrials.gov).

The use of mesenchymal stem cells (MSCs) including adipose-derived stem cells is also very frequent in orthopaedic research. MSCs are either utilized alone or in combination with lattices and scaffolds for promising cartilage and bone repair/formation [130, 131]. As mentioned previously, in presence of larger defects, in vitro tissue engineering strategies are needed to achieve repair of the injured site. ASCs are then used as building blocks in combination with a large number of different matrices and biomaterials. Among the numerous tissues that could be reconstructed from multipotent ASCs, adipose tissue itself is an important organ highly in demand [132]! Soft-tissue loss can be caused by trauma, tumour resection, extensive deep burns, and congenital or acquired anomalies. The demand for soft tissue substitutes in reconstructive and plastic surgery is continually increasing since most current fat autograft techniques fail to produce long-term satisfactory replacement [133]. This is due in part to the fragility of adipose tissue and the lack of appropriate vascularization after grafting [134, 135]. Tissue engineering strategies are very promising as an alternative therapeutic approach to address the low predictability of successful autologous fat transplantation.

Pioneering work in establishing the basis of in vitro adipose tissue engineering was made using mouse embryonic 3T3-L1 cell lines [136, 137] or primary cells extracted from animal fat depots [138, 139]. A variety of natural or synthetic polymer scaffolds have also been tested in combination with adipocyte precursor cells derived from human bone marrow [140-143] or human fat itself in order to produce adipose substitutes. More specifically, different in vitro strategies for adipose tissue engineering based on the use of adipose-derived stem/stromal cells (ASCs) of human origin are highlighted in table 2. The variety of scaffolding elements that have been examined for adipose reconstruction (from synthetic polymers to collagen microbeads, decellularized placenta matrix or endogenously produced human matrix) is a reflection of the particular needs of adipocyte precursors for optimal attachment, viability and when applicable, pore size optimization of the biomaterial to accommodate lipid accumulation in adipocytes as differentiation proceeds. Moreover, adipose substitutes should be easy to manipulate but also soft and flexible in order to avoid discomfort after implantation. Limitations related to the use of synthetic biomaterials often resided in pore size, cell distribution within the polymers and stiffness of the matrices. Modelling such a specialized conjunctive tissue is a challenge and despite recent advances, tissue-engineered adipose substitutes have not made it into the clinical realm yet, thus indicating the need to optimize the current models or to innovate with novel strategies for engineering this peculiar type of tissue.

Table 2. In vitro tissue engineering strategies for reconstruction of adipose tissue from human ASCs

Authors	Year	Scaffold
Mauney et al. [144]	2007	Comparison of silk fibroin, collagen, and poly-lactic acid (PLA) scaffolds
Rubin et al. [145]	2007	Collagenous microbeads
Flynn et al. [146]	2007	Decellularized human placenta and crosslinked hyaluronan (XLHA)
Vermette et al. [147]	2007	Self-assembled human extracellular matrix components
Hong et al. [148]	2006	Gelatin sponges (Gelform)
Cho et al. [149]	2006	Fibrin gels containing preadipocytes cultured in adipogenic-inducing conditions with or without bFGF
Hemmrich et al. [150]	2006	Nonwoven co-poly(ester amide) based on ε-caprolactam, adipic acid and 1,4-butanediol
Hableib et al. [151]	2003	Hyaluronic-acid based scaffolds
Kimura et al. [152]	2003	Collagen sponges with human preadipocytes and gelatin microspheres containing bFGF
Von Heimburg et al. [153, 154]	2001	Collagen sponges
Kral et al. [155]	1999	Polytetrafluoroethylene (PTFE)

Among new technologies being developed (table 2), a trend is seen towards the choice of scaffolding elements of more natural origins. As an example, we recently described the production of a human adipose substitute using a cell-based tissue engineering approach adapted from the self-assembly approach described earlier in this chapter for vascular, cutaneous and corneal reconstruction [56, 57, 59, 78, 156]. The stimulation of adipose-derived stromal cells with ascorbic acid and serum in vitro leads to the secretion and organization of their own extracellular matrix (ECM) components. When we concomitantly differentiated these ASC cultures with a classic adipogenic cocktail including the inducers IBMX and rosiglitazone, adipose sheets were produced, and then superposed to reconstruct thicker adipose substitutes [147]. The human reconstructed adipose tissues displayed histological (figure 6A-D) as well as scanning electron microscopic features (figure 6E) representative of native adult human tissue (figure 6F). Importantly, these substitutes were functional, as defined by triglycerides biosynthesis, adipokine secretion (leptin, adiponectin) and beta-adrenergic mediated lipolysis in vitro [147]. This ability to influence surrounding cells and respond to signals from their environment will likely favour engraftment as well as appropriate remodelling and integration of the adipose substitutes after implantation. In addition, using this adapted self-assembly approach has the obvious benefit of avoiding the need for exogenous or synthetic biomaterials. These substitutes featured functional adipocytes embedded into a natural scaffold produced by stromal cells endogenous to human adipose tissue itself, recreating a proper physiological environment without chemical alterations or potential scaffold-related immunogenicity/inflammation.

Adipose tissue does not possess a high cellular turnover rate such as skin or cornea. In fact, radioactive tracer studies have suggested that the turnover rate for cells within adipose tissue does range between 6 to 15 months in humans [157]. However, adipose tissue presents a remarkable ability to undergo important volume changes during short periods of time. Relatively small increase in volume are usually accommodated by adipocyte hypertrophy, but more important metabolic changes will result in the production of new adipocytes from precursors, an expansion usually paralleled by remodelling of adipose vasculature [158]. How adipose stem cells give rise to preadipocytes in vivo is not as well understood as the steps inducing preadipocytes to differentiate into lipid-filled adipocytes, and many fundamental questions remain concerning the origin of the stem cell population found in adipose depots. Likewise, whether mesenchymal stem cells are preserved into tissue-engineered substitutes produced from adipose-derived stem cells and what degree of plasticity they could then retain will have to be investigated, in particular in relationship with the scaffolding components used to produce such substitute. But it can be hypothesized that reconstructed tissues containing functional differentiated cells embedded into a stroma closely related to their endogenous microenvironnement would lead to a better vascularisation and integration with the surrounding host tissues after grafting, good volume retention and appropriate remodelling in the long-term. Subcutaneous adipose tissue definitely represents an interesting source of autologous multipotent stem cells for use in tissue engineering applications or cell-based therapies for a large number of conditions in addition to soft-tissue reconstruction. Moreover, by integrating the specific knowledge acquired from studies of stem cells from both the epithelial and mesenchymal compartments, new substitutes with superior long-term gain of function will certainly be developed in the future.

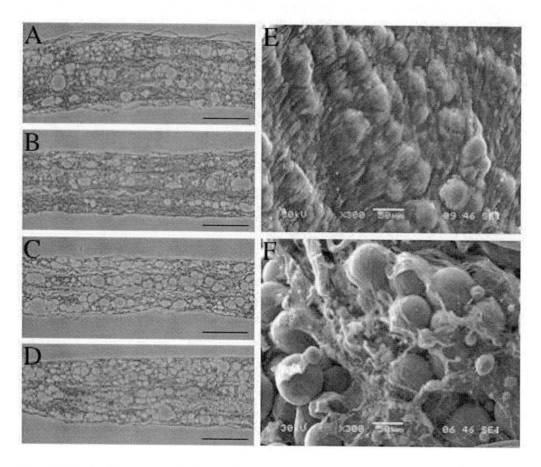

Figure 6. Human adipose tissues in vitro-engineered using an adapted self-assembly approach. (A-D) Histological cross-sections after Masson's trichrome staining of reconstructed tissues produced by superposing three self-assembled adipose sheets. Lipid-filled adipocytes are embedded into a rich human extracellular matrix (collagen in blue) after a total of 35 days in culture. (A-B) Reconstructed adipose tissue produced using stromal cells extracted, cryopreserved and expanded from a lipoaspirate of a 36 year-old donor, while (C-D) is from a 35 year-old donor. These examples are representative of the intrinsic abilities of stromal/stem cells to differentiate into adipocytes under proper induction on one hand, and to secrete and organize extracellular matrix components after ascorbic acid supplementation on the other hand. These potentials can slightly vary between cell populations extracted from different individuals (A-B versus C-D) and can be partly modulated by modifying culture conditions. The appearance of reconstructed adipose tissues (E) is very similar to the aspect of native human fat (F) when viewed by scanning electron microscopy. A higher content of extracellular matrix is seen for reconstructed tissues compared to human fat. While not impacting on the functionality of the substitutes, this results in the production of reconstructed tissues easier to manipulate, with a lower risk of damaging fragile adipocytes. Bar = 100 μm (A-D), 50 μm (E-F).

CONCLUSION

In conclusion, stem cells are present in nearly all post-natal tissues. They have been isolated and cultured from several organs [104-107, 109-114, 159, 160]. This opens the possibility of growing autologous substitutes for the treatment of extensive tissue loss without having to deal with the problems of organ rejection. We gave examples of the usefulness and potency of epithelial stem cells from skin and cornea for the regeneration of their respective epithelium. Thus, although these ectodermal stem cells may already be committed towards a specific lineage and possess a more restricted plasticity, their efficiency for the regeneration of organs on a long-term basis is quite appropriate. In fact, these stem cells may be much better candidates for such a task since they naturally differentiate into the cell lineage desired for a good engraftment. Indeed, even though specific culture conditions are necessary to preserve these stem cells in vitro such as a feeder layer, thereafter differentiation occurs naturally and transdifferentiation does not occur. The clinical application of these cultured substitutes has a significant impact on patient healthcare especially for those with large wounds or defects. More complex substitutes are now in development in which a stroma is added to the epithelium. These tissue-engineered grafts should improve the clinical outcomes since they will also allow the replacement of the mesenchymal compartment. This technology also presents some limitations associated with the amount of time as well as the highly qualified personnal necessary to reconstruct autologous substitutes by tissue engineering. Finally, recently described sources of mesenchymal stem cells such as adipose tissue will likely have a significant impact on therapeutic applications in regenerative medicine. The higher frequency of multipotent stem cells in such abundant and accessible depots as adipose tissue is a key factor driving the development of both cell-based therapies and tissue engineering approaches to treat affected organs or mitigate the consequences of pathological conditions such as cardiovascular diseases, cartilage and bone loss and soft-tissue atrophy.

ACKNOWLEDGMENTS

We are grateful to the members of the LOEX. This work was supported by the Canadian Institutes of Health Research (CIHR), the 'Réseau de Recherche en Santé de la Vision' from the 'Fonds de la Recherche en Santé du Québec' (FRSQ) and the 'Fondation des hôpitaux Enfant-Jésus et Saint-Sacrement' et 'Fondation des Pompiers du Québec pour les Grands Brûlés'. LG is the holder of the Canadian Research Chair on Stem Cell and Tissue Engineering from the CIHR. JF is Scholar from the FRSQ.

REFERENCES

[1] Port, FK; Merion, RM; Goodrich, NP; Wolfe, RA. (2006) Recent trends and results for organ donation and transplantation in the United States, 2005. *Am J Transplant.* 6: 1095-1100.

[2] Armour, RL; Ousley, PJ; Wall, J; Hoar, K; Stoeger, C; Terry, MA. (2007) Endothelial keratoplasty using donor tissue not suitable for full-thickness penetrating keratoplasty. *Cornea*. 26: 515-519.

[3] Gallico, GG, 3rd; O'Connor, NE; Compton, CC; Kehinde, O; Green, H. (1984) Permanent coverage of large burn wounds with autologous cultured human epithelium. *N Engl J Med*. 311: 448-451.

[4] Carver, N & Leigh, IM. (1991) Keratinocyte grafts and skin equivalents. *Int J Dermatol*. 30: 540-551.

[5] Langer, R & Vacanti, JP. (1993) Tissue engineering. *Science*. 260: 920-926.

[6] Damour, O; Gueugniaud, PY; Berthin-Maghit, M; Rousselle, P; Berthod, F; Sahuc, F; Collombel, C. (1994) A dermal substrate made of collagen--GAG--chitosan for deep burn coverage: first clinical uses. *Clin Mater*. 15: 273-276.

[7] Berthod, F & Damour, O. (1997) In vitro reconstructed skin models for wound coverage in deep burns. *Br J Dermatol*. 136: 809-816.

[8] Auger, FA; Berthod, F; Moulin, V; Pouliot, R; Germain, L. (2004) Tissue-engineered skin substitutes: from in vitro constructs to in vivo applications. *Biotechnol Appl Biochem*. 39: 263-275.

[9] Auger, FA & Germain, L. (2004) Tissue Engineering. In: GE Wnek & GL Bowlin (eds.), *Encyclopedia of Biomaterials and Biomedical Engineering*. New York: Marcel Dekker; 1477-1483.

[10] Swijnenburg, RJ; Tanaka, M; Vogel, H; Baker, J; Kofidis, T; Gunawan, F; Lebl, DR; Caffarelli, AD; de Bruin, JL; Fedoseyeva, EV; Robbins, RC. (2005) Embryonic stem cell immunogenicity increases upon differentiation after transplantation into ischemic myocardium. *Circulation*. 112: I166-172.

[11] Nussbaum, J; Minami, E; Laflamme, MA; Virag, JA; Ware, CB; Masino, A; Muskheli, V; Pabon, L; Reinecke, H; Murry, CE. (2007) Transplantation of undifferentiated murine embryonic stem cells in the heart: teratoma formation and immune response. *Faseb J*. 21: 1345-1357.

[12] Cuono, C; Langdon, R; McGuire, J. (1986) Use of cultured epidermal autografts and dermal allografts as skin replacement after burn injury. *Lancet*. 1: 1123-1124.

[13] Eldad, A; Burt, A; Clarke, JA; Gusterson, B. (1987) Cultured epithelium as a skin substitute. *Burns Incl Therm Inj*. 13: 173-180.

[14] Auger, FA. (1988) The role of cultured autologous human epithelium in large burn wound treatment. *Transplantation/Implantation Today*. 5: 21-24.

[15] Green, H & Barrandon, Y. (1988) Cultured epidermal cells and their use in the generation of epidermis. *News Physiol Sci*. 3: 53-56.

[16] Kumagai, N; Nishina, H; Tanabe, H; Hosaka, T; Ishida, H; Ogino, Y. (1988) Clinical application of autologous cultured epithelia for the treatment of burn wounds and burn scars. *Plast Reconstr Surg*. 82: 99-110.

[17] Teepe, RG; Kreis, RW; Koebrugge, EJ; Kempenaar, JA; Vloemans, AF; Hermans, RP; Boxma, H; Dokter, J; Hermans, J; Ponec, M; et al. (1990) The use of cultured autologous epidermis in the treatment of extensive burn wounds. *J Trauma*. 30: 269-275.

[18] Damour, O; Braye, F; Foyattier, J-L; Fabreguette, A; Rousselle, P; Vissac, S; Petit, P. (1997) Culture autologous epidermis for massive burns wounds: 15 years of practice. In: M Rouabhia (ed.), *Skin substitute production by tissue engineering: clinical and fundamental applications*. Austin, TX, USA: Landes Bioscience; 47-74.

[19] Pellegrini, G; Bondanza, S; Guerra, L; De Luca, M. (1998) Cultivation of human keratinocyte stem cells: current and future clinical applications. *Med Biol Eng Comput.* 36: 778-790.
[20] Pellegrini, G; Ranno, R; Stracuzzi, G; Bondanza, S; Guerra, L; Zambruno, G; Micali, G; De Luca, M. (1999) The control of epidermal stem cells (holoclones) in the treatment of massive full-thickness burns with autologous keratinocytes cultured on fibrin. *Transplantation.* 68: 868-879.
[21] Rouabhia, M; Germain, L; Bergeron, J; Auger, FA. (1995) Allogeneic-syngeneic cultured epithelia. A successful therapeutic option for skin regeneration. *Transplantation.* 59: 1229-1235.
[22] Rouabhia, M. (1996) Permanent skin replacement using chimeric epithelial cultured sheets comprising xenogeneic and syngeneic keratinocytes. *Transplantation.* 61: 1290-1300.
[23] Lavker, RM & Sun, TT. (1982) Heterogeneity in epidermal basal keratinocytes: morphological and functional correlations. *Science.* 215: 1239-1241.
[24] Watt, FM; Lo Celso, C; Silva-Vargas, V. (2006) Epidermal stem cells: an update. *Curr Opin Genet Dev.* 16: 518-524.
[25] Cotsarelis, G; Sun, T-T; Lavker, RM. (1990) Label retaining cells reside in the bulge area of pilosebacous unit: Implication for follicular stem cells, hair cycle and skin carcinogenesis. *Cell.* 61: 1329-1337.
[26] Michel, M; Torok, N; Godbout, MJ; Lussier, M; Gaudreau, P; Royal, A; Germain, L. (1996) Keratin 19 as a biochemical marker of skin stem cells in vivo and in vitro: keratin 19 expressing cells are differentially localized in function of anatomic sites, and their number varies with donor age and culture stage. *J Cell Sci.* 109 (Pt 5): 1017-1028.
[27] Taylor, G; Lehrer, MS; Jensen, PJ; Sun, TT; Lavker, RM. (2000) Involvement of follicular stem cells in forming not only the follicle but also the epidermis. *Cell.* 102: 451-461.
[28] Oshima, H; Rochat, A; Kedzia, C; Kobayashi, K; Barrandon, Y. (2001) Morphogenesis and renewal of hair follicles from adult multipotent stem cells. *Cell.* 104: 233-245.
[29] Blanpain, C; Lowry, WE; Geoghegan, A; Polak, L; Fuchs, E. (2004) Self-renewal, multipotency, and the existence of two cell populations within an epithelial stem cell niche. *Cell.* 118: 635-648.
[30] Morris, RJ; Liu, Y; Marles, L; Yang, Z; Trempus, C; Li, S; Lin, JS; Sawicki, JA; Cotsarelis, G. (2004) Capturing and profiling adult hair follicle stem cells. *Nat Biotechnol.* 22: 411-417.
[31] Tumbar, T; Guasch, G; Greco, V; Blanpain, C; Lowry, WE; Rendl, M; Fuchs, E. (2004) Defining the epithelial stem cell niche in skin. *Science.* 303: 359-363.
[32] Rheinwald, JG & Green, H. (1975) Serial cultivation of strains of human epidermal keratinocytes: the formation of keratinizing colonies from single cells. *Cell.* 6: 331-343.
[33] Germain, L; Rouabhia, M; Guignard, R; Carrier, L; Bouvard, V; Auger, FA. (1993) Improvement of human keratinocyte isolation and culture using thermolysin. *Burns.* 19: 99-104.
[34] Germain, L; Michel, M; Fradette, J; Xu, W; Godbout, M-J; Li, H. (1997) Skin stem cell identification and culture: a potential tool for rapid epidermal sheet production and grafting. In: M Rouabhia (ed.), *Skin substitute production by tissue engineering: clinical and fundamental applications.* Austin, Tx, USA: Landes Bioscience; 177-210.
[35] Green, H; Kehinde, O; Thomas, J. (1979) Growth of cultured human epidermal cells into multiple epithelia suitable for grafting. *Proc Natl Acad Sci U S A.* 76: 5665-5668.

[36] Barrandon, Y & Green, H. (1987) Cell migration is essential for sustained growth of keratinocyte colonies: the roles of transforming growth factor-alpha and epidermal growth factor. *Cell.* 50: 1131-1137.

[37] Holbrook, KA & Hennings, H. (1983) Phenotypic expression of epidermal cells in vitro: a review. *J Invest Dermatol.* 81: 11s-24s.

[38] Watt, FM. (1983) Involucrin and other markers of keratinocyte terminal differentiation. *J Invest Dermatol.* 81: 100s-103s.

[39] Yuspa, SH; Hennings, H; Tucker, RW; Jaken, S; Kilkenny, AE; Roop, DR. (1988) Signal transduction for proliferation and differentiation in keratinocytes. *Ann N Y Acad Sci.* 548: 191-196.

[40] Barrandon, Y & Green, H. (1987) Three clonal types of keratinocyte with different capacities for multiplication. *Proc Natl Acad Sci U S A.* 84: 2302-2306.

[41] Fradette, J; Germain, L; Seshaiah, P; Coulombe, PA. (1998) The type I keratin 19 possesses distinct and context-dependent assembly properties. *J Biol Chem.* 273: 35176-35184.

[42] Barrandon, Y & Green, H. (1985) Cell size as a determinant of the clone-forming ability of human keratinocytes. *Proc Natl Acad Sci U S A.* 82: 5390-5394.

[43] De Luca, M; Pellegrini, G; Green, H. (2006) Regeneration of squamous epithelia from stem cells of cultured grafts. *Regen Med.* 1: 45-57.

[44] Mavilio, F; Pellegrini, G; Ferrari, S; Di Nunzio, F; Di Iorio, E; Recchia, A; Maruggi, G; Ferrari, G; Provasi, E; Bonini, C; Capurro, S; Conti, A; Magnoni, C; Giannetti, A; De Luca, M. (2006) Correction of junctional epidermolysis bullosa by transplantation of genetically modified epidermal stem cells. *Nat Med.* 12: 1397-1402.

[45] Compton, CC; Gill, JM; Bradford, DA; Regauer, S; Gallico, GG; O'Connor, NE. (1989) Skin regenerated from cultured epithelial autografts on full-thickness burn wounds from 6 days to 5 years after grafting. A light, electron microscopic and immunohistochemical study. *Lab Invest.* 60: 600-612.

[46] Bell, E; Ivarsson, B; Merrill, C. (1979) Production of a tissue-like structure by contraction of collagen lattices by human fibroblasts of different proliferative potential in vitro. *Proc Natl Acad Sci U S A.* 76: 1274-1278.

[47] Bell, E; Ehrlich, HP; Buttle, DJ; Nakatsuji, T. (1981) Living tissue formed in vitro and accepted as skin-equivalent tissue of full thickness. *Science.* 211: 1052-1054.

[48] Burke, JF; Yannas, IV; Quinby, WC, Jr.; Bondoc, CC; Jung, WK. (1981) Successful use of a physiologically acceptable artificial skin in the treatment of extensive burn injury. *Ann Surg.* 194: 413-428.

[49] Yannas, IV; Burke, JF; Orgill, DP; Skrabut, EM. (1982) Wound tissue can utilize a polymeric template to synthesize a functional extension of skin. *Science.* 215: 174-176.

[50] Boyce, ST & Hansbrough, JF. (1988) Biologic attachment, growth, and differentiation of cultured human epidermal keratinocytes on a graftable collagen and chondroitin-6-sulfate substrate. *Surgery.* 103: 421-431.

[51] Yannas, IV; Lee, E; Orgill, DP; Skrabut, EM; Murphy, GF. (1989) Synthesis and characterization of a model extracellular matrix that induces partial regeneration of adult mammalian skin. *Proc Natl Acad Sci U S A.* 86: 933-937.

[52] Berthod, F; Hayek, D; Damour, O; Collombel, C. (1993) Collagen synthesis by fibroblasts cultured within a collagen sponge. *Biomaterials.* 14: 749-754.

[53] Boyce, ST; Greenhalgh, DG; Kagan, RJ; Housinger, T; Sorrell, JM; Childress, CP; Rieman, M; Warden, GD. (1993) Skin anatomy and antigen expression after burn

wound closure with composite grafts of cultured skin cells and biopolymers. *Plast Reconstr Surg.* 91: 632-641.

[54] Hansbrough, JF; Morgan, JL; Greenleaf, GE; Bartel, R. (1993) Composite grafts of human keratinocytes grown on a polyglactin mesh-cultured fibroblast dermal substitute function as a bilayer skin replacement in full-thickness wounds on athymic mice. *J Burn Care Rehabil.* 14: 485-494.

[55] Mansbridge, J; Liu, K; Patch, R; Symons, K; Pinney, E. (1998) Three-dimensional fibroblast culture implant for the treatment of diabetic foot ulcers: metabolic activity and therapeutic range. *Tissue Eng.* 4: 403-414.

[56] Auger, FA; Rémy-Zolghadri, M; Grenier, G; Germain, L. (2000) The self-assembly approach for organ reconstruction by tissue engineering. e-biomed: a *Journal of Regenerative Medicine.* 1: 75-86.

[57] Michel, M; L'Heureux, N; Pouliot, R; Xu, W; Auger, FA; Germain, L. (1999) Characterization of a new tissue-engineered human skin equivalent with hair. *In Vitro Cell Dev Biol Anim.* 35: 318-326.

[58] Pouliot, R; Larouche, D; Auger, FA; Juhasz, J; Xu, W; Li, H; Germain, L. (2002) Reconstructed human skin produced in vitro and grafted on athymic mice. *Transplantation.* 73: 1751-1757.

[59] Larouche, D; Paquet, C; Fradette, J; Carrier, P; Auger, FA; Germain, L. (In press) Regeneration of skin and cornea by tissue engineering. In: J Audet & WL Stanford (eds.), *Stem cells in regenerative medicine for the methods in molecular medicine series.* Totowa, NJ, USA: Humana Press

[60] Leigh, IM; Purkis, PE; Navsaria, HA; Phillips, TJ. (1987) Treatment of chronic venous ulcers with sheets of cultured allogenic keratinocytes. *Br J Dermatol.* 117: 591-597.

[61] Phillips, TJ; Kehinde, O; Green, H; Gilchrest, BA. (1989) Treatment of skin ulcers with cultured epidermal allografts. *J Am Acad Dermatol.* 21: 191-199.

[62] Beele, H; Naeyaert, JM; Goeteyn, M; De Mil, M; Kint, A. (1991) Repeated cultured epidermal allografts in the treatment of chronic leg ulcers of various origins. *Dermatologica.* 183: 31-35.

[63] Sabolinski, ML; Alvarez, O; Auletta, M; Mulder, G; Parenteau, NL. (1996) Cultured skin as a 'smart material' for healing wounds: experience in venous ulcers. *Biomaterials.* 17: 311-320.

[64] Naughton, G; Mansbridge, J; Gentzkow, G. (1997) A metabolically active human dermal replacement for the treatment of diabetic foot ulcers. *Artif Organs.* 21: 1203-1210.

[65] Falanga, V. (1998) Apligraf treatment of venous ulcers and other chronic wounds. *J Dermatol.* 25: 812-817.

[66] Sibbald, RG. (1998) Apligraf living skin equivalent for healing venous and chronic wounds. *J Cutan Med Surg. 3 Suppl 1*: S1-24-28.

[67] Bogensberger, G; Eaglstein, WH; Kirsner, RS. (2000) Chronic leg ulcers in a patient with combined arterial and venous disease successfully treated with a human skin equivalent: a case report. *Wounds.* 12: 118-121.

[68] Veves, A; Falanga, V; Armstrong, DG; Sabolinski, ML. (2001) Graftskin, a human skin equivalent, is effective in the management of noninfected neuropathic diabetic foot ulcers: a prospective randomized multicenter clinical trial. *Diabetes Care.* 24: 290-295.

[69] Brem, H; Young, J; Tomic-Canic, M; Isaacs, C; Ehrlich, HP. (2003) Clinical efficacy and mechanism of bilayered living human skin equivalent (HSE) in treatment of diabetic foot ulcers. *Surg Technol Int.* 11: 23-31.

[70] Amini-Adle, M; Auxenfants, C; Allombert-Blaise, C; Deroo-Berger, MC; Ly, A; Jullien, D; Faure, M; Damour, O; Claudy, A. (2007) Rapid healing of long-lasting sickle cell leg ulcer treated with allogeneic keratinocytes. *J Eur Acad Dermatol Venereol.* 21: 707-708.

[71] Boyce, ST; Kagan, RJ; Greenhalgh, DG; Warner, P; Yakuboff, KP; Palmieri, T; Warden, GD. (2006) Cultured skin substitutes reduce requirements for harvesting of skin autograft for closure of excised, full-thickness burns. *J Trauma.* 60: 821-829.

[72] Vicanova, J; Ponec, M; Weerheim, A; Swope, V; Westbrook, M; Harriger, D; Boyce, S. (1997) Epidermal lipid metabolism of cultured skin substitutes during healing of full-thickness wounds in athymic mice. *Wound Repair Regen.* 5: 329-338.

[73] Berthod, F; Germain, L; Li, H; Xu, W; Damour, O; Auger, FA. (2001) Collagen fibril network and elastic system remodeling in a reconstructed skin transplanted on nude mice. *Matrix Biol.* 20: 463-473.

[74] Braye, FM; Stefani, A; Venet, E; Pieptu, D; Tissot, E; Damour, O. (2001) Grafting of large pieces of human reconstructed skin in a porcine model. *Br J Plast Surg.* 54: 532-538.

[75] Supp, DM; Wilson-Landy, K; Boyce, ST. (2002) Human dermal microvascular endothelial cells form vascular analogs in cultured skin substitutes after grafting to athymic mice. *Faseb J.* 16: 797-804.

[76] Tremblay, PL; Hudon, V; Berthod, F; Germain, L; Auger, FA. (2005) Inosculation of tissue-engineered capillaries with the host's vasculature in a reconstructed skin transplanted on mice. *Am J Transplant.* 5: 1002-1010.

[77] Duplan-Perrat, F; Damour, O; Montrocher, C; Peyrol, S; Grenier, G; Jacob, MP; Braye, F. (2000) Keratinocytes influence the maturation and organization of the elastin network in a skin equivalent. *J Invest Dermatol.* 114: 365-370.

[78] Gaudreault, M; Carrier, P; Larouche, K; Leclerc, S; Giasson, M; Germain, L; Guerin, SL. (2003) Influence of sp1/sp3 expression on corneal epithelial cells proliferation and differentiation properties in reconstructed tissues. *Invest Ophthalmol Vis Sci.* 44: 1447-1457.

[79] Liu, JJ; Kao, WW; Wilson, SE. (1999) Corneal epithelium-specific mouse keratin K12 promoter. *Exp Eye Res.* 68: 295-301.

[80] Moll, R; Franke, WW; Schiller, DL; Geiger, B; Krepler, R. (1982) The catalog of human cytokeratins: patterns of expression in normal epithelia, tumors and cultured cells. *Cell.* 31: 11-24.

[81] Schermer, A; Galvin, S; Sun, TT. (1986) Differentiation-related expression of a major 64K corneal keratin in vivo and in culture suggests limbal location of corneal epithelial stem cells. *J Cell Biol.* 103: 49-62.

[82] Kivela, T & Uusitalo, M. (1998) Structure, development and function of cytoskeletal elements in non-neuronal cells of the human eye. *Prog Retin Eye Res.* 17: 385-428.

[83] Cotsarelis, G; Cheng, SZ; Dong, G; Sun, TT; Lavker, RM. (1989) Existence of slow-cycling limbal epithelial basal cells that can be preferentially stimulated to proliferate: implications on epithelial stem cells. *Cell.* 57: 201-209.

[84] Lindberg, K; Brown, ME; Chaves, HV; Kenyon, KR; Rheinwald, JG. (1993) In vitro propagation of human ocular surface epithelial cells for transplantation. *Invest Ophthalmol Vis Sci.* 34: 2672-2679.

[85] Germain, L; Auger, FA; Grandbois, E; Guignard, R; Giasson, M; Boisjoly, H; Guerin, SL. (1999) Reconstructed human cornea produced in vitro by tissue engineering. *Pathobiology.* 67: 140-147.

[86] Germain, L; Carrier, P; Auger, FA; Salesse, C; Guerin, SL. (2000) Can we produce a human corneal equivalent by tissue engineering? *Prog Retin Eye Res.* 19: 497-527.
[87] Deschambeault, A; Carrier, P; Talbot, M; Germain, L. (2003) In vivo characterization of human limbal epithelial cells isolated from the four quadrants. *ARVO Meeting Abstracts.* 44: 1357.
[88] Pellegrini, G; Golisano, O; Paterna, P; Lambiase, A; Bonini, S; Rama, P; De Luca, M. (1999) Location and clonal analysis of stem cells and their differentiated progeny in the human ocular surface. *J Cell Biol.* 145: 769-782.
[89] Pellegrini, G; Traverso, CE; Franzi, AT; Zingirian, M; Cancedda, R; De Luca, M. (1997) Long-term restoration of damaged corneal surfaces with autologous cultivated corneal epithelium. *Lancet.* 349: 990-993.
[90] Rama, P; Bonini, S; Lambiase, A; Golisano, O; Paterna, P; De Luca, M; Pellegrini, G. (2001) Autologous fibrin-cultured limbal stem cells permanently restore the corneal surface of patients with total limbal stem cell deficiency. *Transplantation.* 72: 1478-1485.
[91] Talbot, M; Carrier, P; Giasson, CJ; Deschambeault, A; Guerin, SL; Auger, FA; Bazin, R; Germain, L. (2006) Autologous transplantation of rabbit limbal epithelia cultured on fibrin gels for ocular surface reconstruction. *Mol Vis.* 12: 65-75.
[92] Deschambeault, A; Carrier, P; Talbot, M; Guérin, SL; Auger, FA; Germain, L. (2002) Regional variation in the localization of limbal stem cells. *Invest Ophthalmol Vis Sci.* 43: E-Abstract 1621.
[93] Shortt, AJ; Secker, GA; Notara, MD; Limb, GA; Khaw, PT; Tuft, SJ; Daniels, JT. (2007) Transplantation of ex vivo cultured limbal epithelial stem cells: a review of techniques and clinical results. *Surv Ophthalmol.* 52: 483-502.
[94] Schwab, IR. (1999) Cultured corneal epithelia for ocular surface disease. *Trans Am Ophthalmol Soc.* 97: 891-986.
[95] Tsai, RJ; Li, LM; Chen, JK. (2000) Reconstruction of damaged corneas by transplantation of autologous limbal epithelial cells. *N Engl J Med.* 343: 86-93.
[96] Nakamura, T; Inatomi, T; Sotozono, C; Koizumi, N; Kinoshita, S. (2004) Successful primary culture and autologous transplantation of corneal limbal epithelial cells from minimal biopsy for unilateral severe ocular surface disease. *Acta Ophthalmol Scand.* 82: 468-471.
[97] Sangwan, VS; Murthy, SI; Vemuganti, GK; Bansal, AK; Gangopadhyay, N; Rao, GN. (2005) Cultivated corneal epithelial transplantation for severe ocular surface disease in vernal keratoconjunctivitis. *Cornea.* 24: 426-430.
[98] Meller, D; Pires, RT; Tseng, SC. (2002) Ex vivo preservation and expansion of human limbal epithelial stem cells on amniotic membrane cultures. *Br J Ophthalmol.* 86: 463-471.
[99] Daya, SM; Watson, A; Sharpe, JR; Giledi, O; Rowe, A; Martin, R; James, SE. (2005) Outcomes and DNA analysis of ex vivo expanded stem cell allograft for ocular surface reconstruction. *Ophthalmology.* 112: 470-477.
[100] Schwab, IR; Reyes, M; Isseroff, RR. (2000) Successful transplantation of bioengineered tissue replacements in patients with ocular surface disease. *Cornea.* 19: 421-426.
[101] Tseng, SC; Kruse, FE; Merritt, J; Li, DQ. (1996) Comparison between serum-free and fibroblast-cocultured single-cell clonal culture systems: evidence showing that epithelial anti-apoptotic activity is present in 3T3 fibroblast-conditioned media. *Curr Eye Res.* 15: 973-984.

[102] Masson-Gadais, B; Fugere, C; Paquet, C; Leclerc, S; Lefort, NR; Germain, L; Guerin, SL. (2006) The feeder layer-mediated extended lifetime of cultured human skin keratinocytes is associated with altered levels of the transcription factors Sp1 and Sp3. *J Cell Physiol*. 206: 831-842.

[103] Michel, M; L'Heureux, N; Auger, FA; Germain, L. (1997) From newborn to adult: phenotypic and functional properties of skin equivalent and human skin as a function of donor age. *J Cell Physiol*. 171: 179-189.

[104] Caplan, AI. (1991) Mesenchymal stem cells. *J Orthop Res*. 9: 641-650.

[105] Prockop, DJ. (1997) Marrow stromal cells as stem cells for nonhematopoietic tissues. *Science*. 276: 71-74.

[106] Pittenger, MF; Mackay, AM; Beck, SC; Jaiswal, RK; Douglas, R; Mosca, JD; Moorman, MA; Simonetti, DW; Craig, S; Marshak, DR. (1999) Multilineage potential of adult human mesenchymal stem cells. *Science*. 284: 143-147.

[107] Jiang, Y; Jahagirdar, BN; Reinhardt, RL; Schwartz, RE; Keene, CD; Ortiz-Gonzalez, XR; Reyes, M; Lenvik, T; Lund, T; Blackstad, M; Du, J; Aldrich, S; Lisberg, A; Low, WC; Largaespada, DA; Verfaillie, CM. (2002) Pluripotency of mesenchymal stem cells derived from adult marrow. *Nature*. 418: 41-49.

[108] Li, CD; Zhang, WY; Li, HL; Jiang, XX; Zhang, Y; Tang, P; Mao, N. (2005) *Isolation and Identification of a Multilineage Potential Mesenchymal Cell from Human Placenta. Placenta*. [epub ahead of print]

[109] Wang, HS; Hung, SC; Peng, ST; Huang, CC; Wei, HM; Guo, YJ; Fu, YS; Lai, MC; Chen, CC. (2004) Mesenchymal stem cells in the Wharton's jelly of the human umbilical cord. *Stem Cells*. 22: 1330-1337.

[110] Sarugaser, R; Lickorish, D; Baksh, D; Hosseini, MM; Davies, JE. (2005) Human umbilical cord perivascular (HUCPV) cells: a source of mesenchymal progenitors. *Stem Cells*. 23: 220-229.

[111] Toma, JG; McKenzie, IA; Bagli, D; Miller, FD. (2005) Isolation and characterization of multipotent skin-derived precursors from human skin. *Stem Cells*. 23: 727-737.

[112] Gingras, M; Champigny, MF; Berthod, F. (2007) Differentiation of human adult skin-derived neuronal precursors into mature neurons. *J Cell Physiol*. 210: 498-506.

[113] Zuk, PA; Zhu, M; Mizuno, H; Huang, J; Futrell, JW; Katz, AJ; Benhaim, P; Lorenz, HP; Hedrick, MH. (2001) Multilineage cells from human adipose tissue: implications for cell-based therapies. *Tissue Eng*. 7: 211-228.

[114] Zuk, PA; Zhu, M; Ashjian, P; De Ugarte, DA; Huang, JI; Mizuno, H; Alfonso, ZC; Fraser, JK; Benhaim, P; Hedrick, MH. (2002) Human adipose tissue is a source of multipotent stem cells. *Mol Biol Cell*. 13: 4279-4295.

[115] Ailhaud, G. (2006) Adipose tissue as a secretory organ: from adipogenesis to the metabolic syndrome. *C R Biol*. 329: 570-577; discussion 653-575.

[116] Safford, KM; Hicok, KC; Safford, SD; Halvorsen, YD; Wilkison, WO; Gimble, JM; Rice, HE. (2002) Neurogenic differentiation of murine and human adipose-derived stromal cells. *Biochem Biophys Res Commun*. 294: 371-379.

[117] Seo, MJ; Suh, SY; Bae, YC; Jung, JS. (2005) Differentiation of human adipose stromal cells into hepatic lineage in vitro and in vivo. *Biochem Biophys Res Commun*. 328: 258-264.

[118] Talens-Visconti, R; Bonora, A; Jover, R; Mirabet, V; Carbonell, F; Castell, JV; Gomez-Lechon, MJ. (2007) Human mesenchymal stem cells from adipose tissue: Differentiation into hepatic lineage. *Toxicol In Vitro*. 21: 324-329.

[119] Katz, AJ; Tholpady, A; Tholpady, SS; Shang, H; Ogle, RC. (2005) Cell surface and transcriptional characterization of human adipose-derived adherent stromal (hADAS) cells. *Stem Cells*. 23: 412-423.

[120] Wagner, W; Wein, F; Seckinger, A; Frankhauser, M; Wirkner, U; Krause, U; Blake, J; Schwager, C; Eckstein, V; Ansorge, W; Ho, AD. (2005) Comparative characteristics of mesenchymal stem cells from human bone marrow, adipose tissue, and umbilical cord blood. *Exp Hematol*. 33: 1402-1416.

[121] Kern, S; Eichler, H; Stoeve, J; Kluter, H; Bieback, K. (2006) Comparative analysis of mesenchymal stem cells from bone marrow, umbilical cord blood, or adipose tissue. *Stem Cells*. 24: 1294-1301.

[122] Miranville, A; Heeschen, C; Sengenes, C; Curat, CA; Busse, R; Bouloumie, A. (2004) Improvement of postnatal neovascularization by human adipose tissue-derived stem cells. *Circulation*. 110: 349-355.

[123] Sengenes, C; Lolmede, K; Zakaroff-Girard, A; Busse, R; Bouloumie, A. (2005) Preadipocytes in the human subcutaneous adipose tissue display distinct features from the adult mesenchymal and hematopoietic stem cells. *J Cell Physiol*. 205: 114-122.

[124] Lee, RH; Kim, B; Choi, I; Kim, H; Choi, HS; Suh, K; Bae, YC; Jung, JS. (2004) Characterization and expression analysis of mesenchymal stem cells from human bone marrow and adipose tissue. *Cell Physiol Biochem*. 14: 311-324.

[125] Liu, TM; Martina, M; Hutmacher, DW; Hui, JH; Lee, EH; Lim, B. (2007) Identification of common pathways mediating differentiation of bone marrow- and adipose tissue-derived human mesenchymal stem cells into three mesenchymal lineages. *Stem Cells*. 25: 750-760.

[126] Gimble, JM; Katz, AJ; Bunnell, BA. (2007) Adipose-derived stem cells for regenerative medicine. *Circ Res*. 100: 1249-1260.

[127] Strem, BM & Hedrick, MH. (2005) The growing importance of fat in regenerative medicine. *Trends Biotechnol*. 23: 64-66.

[128] Giordano, A; Galderisi, U; Marino, IR. (2007) From the laboratory bench to the patient's bedside: an update on clinical trials with mesenchymal stem cells. *J Cell Physiol*. 211: 27-35.

[129] Yoshimura, K; Sato, K; Aoi, N; Kurita, M; Hirohi, T; Harii, K. (2008) Cell-Assisted Lipotransfer for Cosmetic Breast Augmentation: Supportive Use of Adipose-Derived Stem/Stromal Cells. *Aesthetic Plast Surg*. 32: 48-45.

[130] Guilak, F; Awad, HA; Fermor, B; Leddy, HA; Gimble, JM. (2004) Adipose-derived adult stem cells for cartilage tissue engineering. *Biorheology*. 41: 389-399.

[131] Kimelman, N; Pelled, G; Helm, GA; Huard, J; Schwarz, EM; Gazit, D. (2007) Review: gene- and stem cell-based therapeutics for bone regeneration and repair. *Tissue Eng*. 13: 1135-1150.

[132] Gomillion, CT & Burg, KJ. (2006) Stem cells and adipose tissue engineering. *Biomaterials*. 27: 6052-6063.

[133] Patrick, CW, Jr. (2001) Tissue engineering strategies for adipose tissue repair. *Anat Rec*. 263: 361-366.

[134] Billings, E, Jr. & May, JW, Jr. (1989) Historical review and present status of free fat graft autotransplantation in plastic and reconstructive surgery. *Plast Reconstr Surg*. 83: 368-381.

[135] Rohrich, RJ; Sorokin, ES; Brown, SA. (2004) In search of improved fat transfer viability: a quantitative analysis of the role of centrifugation and harvest site. *Plast Reconstr Surg*. 113: 391-395; discussion 396-397.

[136] Fischbach, C; Spruss, T; Weiser, B; Neubauer, M; Becker, C; Hacker, M; Gopferich, A; Blunk, T. (2004) Generation of mature fat pads in vitro and in vivo utilizing 3-D long-term culture of 3T3-L1 preadipocytes. *Exp Cell Res.* 300: 54-64.

[137] Fischbach, C; Seufert, J; Staiger, H; Hacker, M; Neubauer, M; Gopferich, A; Blunk, T. (2004) Three-dimensional in vitro model of adipogenesis: comparison of culture conditions. *Tissue Eng.* 10: 215-229.

[138] Patrick, CW, Jr.; Chauvin, PB; Hobley, J; Reece, GP. (1999) Preadipocyte seeded PLGA scaffolds for adipose tissue engineering. *Tissue Eng.* 5: 139-151.

[139] Patrick, CW, Jr.; Zheng, B; Johnston, C; Reece, GP. (2002) Long-term implantation of preadipocyte-seeded PLGA scaffolds. *Tissue Eng.* 8: 283-293.

[140] Alhadlaq, A; Tang, M; Mao, JJ. (2005) Engineered adipose tissue from human mesenchymal stem cells maintains predefined shape and dimension: implications in soft tissue augmentation and reconstruction. *Tissue Eng.* 11: 556-566.

[141] Hong, L; Peptan, I; Clark, P; Mao, JJ. (2005) Ex vivo adipose tissue engineering by human marrow stromal cell seeded gelatin sponge. *Ann Biomed Eng.* 33: 511-517.

[142] Neubauer, M; Hacker, M; Bauer-Kreisel, P; Weiser, B; Fischbach, C; Schulz, MB; Goepferich, A; Blunk, T. (2005) Adipose tissue engineering based on mesenchymal stem cells and basic fibroblast growth factor in vitro. *Tissue Eng.* 11: 1840-1851.

[143] Stosich, MS & Mao, JJ. (2007) Adipose tissue engineering from human adult stem cells: clinical implications in plastic and reconstructive surgery. *Plast Reconstr Surg.* 119: 71-83; discussion 84-75.

[144] Mauney, JR; Nguyen, T; Gillen, K; Kirker-Head, C; Gimble, JM; Kaplan, DL. (2007) Engineering adipose-like tissue in vitro and in vivo utilizing human bone marrow and adipose-derived mesenchymal stem cells with silk fibroin 3D scaffolds. *Biomaterials.* 28: 5280-5290.

[145] Rubin, JP; Bennett, JM; Doctor, JS; Tebbets, BM; Marra, KG. (2007) Collagenous microbeads as a scaffold for tissue engineering with adipose-derived stem cells. *Plast Reconstr Surg.* 120: 414-424.

[146] Flynn, L; Prestwich, GD; Semple, JL; Woodhouse, KA. (2007) Adipose tissue engineering with naturally derived scaffolds and adipose-derived stem cells. *Biomaterials.* 28: 3834-3842.

[147] Vermette, M; Trottier, V; Menard, V; Saint-Pierre, L; Roy, A; Fradette, J. (2007) Production of a new tissue-engineered adipose substitute from human adipose-derived stromal cells. *Biomaterials.* 28: 2850-2860.

[148] Hong, L; Peptan, IA; Colpan, A; Daw, JL. (2006) Adipose tissue engineering by human adipose-derived stromal cells. *Cells Tissues Organs.* 183: 133-140.

[149] Cho, SW; Kim, I; Kim, SH; Rhie, JW; Choi, CY; Kim, BS. (2006) Enhancement of adipose tissue formation by implantation of adipogenic-differentiated preadipocytes. *Biochem Biophys Res Commun.* 345: 588-594.

[150] Hemmrich, K; Meersch, M; Wiesemann, U; Salber, J; Klee, D; Gries, T; Pallua, N. (2006) Polyesteramide-derived nonwovens as innovative degradable matrices support preadipocyte adhesion, proliferation, and differentiation. *Tissue Eng.* 12: 3557-3565.

[151] Halbleib, M; Skurk, T; de Luca, C; von Heimburg, D; Hauner, H. (2003) Tissue engineering of white adipose tissue using hyaluronic acid-based scaffolds. I: in vitro differentiation of human adipocyte precursor cells on scaffolds. *Biomaterials.* 24: 3125-3132.

[152] Kimura, Y; Ozeki, M; Inamoto, T; Tabata, Y. (2003) Adipose tissue engineering based on human preadipocytes combined with gelatin microspheres containing basic fibroblast growth factor. *Biomaterials*. 24: 2513-2521.

[153] von Heimburg, D; Zachariah, S; Heschel, I; Kuhling, H; Schoof, H; Hafemann, B; Pallua, N. (2001) Human preadipocytes seeded on freeze-dried collagen scaffolds investigated in vitro and in vivo. *Biomaterials*. 22: 429-438.

[154] von Heimburg, D; Zachariah, S; Low, A; Pallua, N. (2001) Influence of different biodegradable carriers on the in vivo behavior of human adipose precursor cells. *Plast Reconstr Surg*. 108: 411-420; discussion 421-412.

[155] Kral, JG & Crandall, DL. (1999) Development of a human adipocyte synthetic polymer scaffold. *Plast Reconstr Surg*. 104: 1732-1738.

[156] L'Heureux, N; Paquet, S; Labbe, R; Germain, L; Auger, FA. (1998) A completely biological tissue-engineered human blood vessel. *Faseb J*. 12: 47-56.

[157] Strawford, A; Antelo, F; Christiansen, M; Hellerstein, MK. (2004) Adipose tissue triglyceride turnover, de novo lipogenesis, and cell proliferation in humans measured with 2H2O. *Am J Physiol Endocrinol Metab*. 286: E577-588.

[158] Rupnick, MA; Panigrahy, D; Zhang, CY; Dallabrida, SM; Lowell, BB; Langer, R; Folkman, MJ. (2002) Adipose tissue mass can be regulated through the vasculature. *Proc Natl Acad Sci U S A*. 99: 10730-10735.

[159] Atala, A. (2006) Recent developments in tissue engineering and regenerative medicine. *Curr Opin Pediatr*. 18: 167-171.

[160] Schmelzer, E; Zhang, L; Bruce, A; Wauthier, E; Ludlow, J; Yao, HL; Moss, N; Melhem, A; McClelland, R; Turner, W; Kulik, M; Sherwood, S; Tallheden, T; Cheng, N; Furth, ME; Reid, LM. (2007) Human hepatic stem cells from fetal and postnatal donors. *J Exp Med*. 204: 1973-1987.

In: Encyclopedia of Stem Cell Research (2 Volume Set)   ISBN: 978-1-61761-835-2
Editor: Alexander L. Greene   © 2012 Nova Science Publishers, Inc.

Chapter XI

CELL DIFFERENTIATION: THERAPEUTICAL CHALLENGES IN DIABETES

Enrique Roche, Nestor Vicente-Salar,
Maribel Arribas and Beatriz Paredes
Instituto de Bioingenieria, Universidad Miguel Hernandez, Alicante, Spain

ABSTRACT

Stem cells, derived from either embryonic or adult tissues, are considered to be potential sources of insulin-secreting cells to be transplanted into type 1 and advanced stages of type 2 diabetic patients. Many laboratories have considered this possibility, resulting in a large amount of published protocols, with a wide degree of complexity among them. Our group was the first to report that it was possible to obtain insulin-secreting cells from mouse embryonic stem cells, proving the feasibility of this new challenge. The same observation was immediately reported using human embryonic stem cells. However, the resulting cell product was not properly characterised, affecting the reproducibility of the protocol by other groups. A more elaborated protocol was developed by Lumelsky and co-workers, demonstrating that neuroectodermal cells could be an alternative source for insulin-producing cells. However, the resulting cells of this protocol produced low amounts of the hormone. This aimed other groups to perform key changes in order to improve the insulin content of the resulting cells. Recently, Baetge's group has published a new protocol based on the knowledge accumulated in pancreatic development. In this protocol, human embryonic stem cells were differentiated into islet-like structures through a five step protocol, emulating the key steps during embryonic development of the endocrine pancreas. The final cell product, however, seemed to be in an immature state, thus further improvement is required. Despite this drawback, the protocol represents the culmination of work performed by different groups and offers new research challenges for the investigators in this exciting field. Concerning adult stem cells, the possibility of identifying pancreatic precursors or of reprogramming extrapancreatic derived cells are key possibilities that may circumvent the problems that appear when using embryonic stem cells, such as immune rejection and tumour formation.

INTRODUCTION

Insulin injection is the only effective palliative method to normalize high circulating glucose levels in diabetic subjects. This forces the patients to maintain a tight control of their lifestyle, including balanced diets, proper exercise, precise pharmacological intervention and motivation. Before the discovery of insulin by Frederick Banting, Herbert Best and Richard McLeod in Toronto in the year 1922, this disease resulted fatal for the patients. Their findings allowed the patients to survive, and diabetes passed on to become a chronic disease. Ever since this discovery, many laboratories around the world search for a cure, however, understanding diabetes is not an easy task, and as a result of this complexity there is still no definitive cure for the disease.

Although pharmacological agents and insulin formulations have reached a high degree of specificity, the correct control of blood glucose has not been achieved. The poor control of glycaemia in diabetic patients is related with the development of secondary complications, such as neuropathy, nephropathy, retinopathy and cardiovascular disorders that impair the quality of life of affected patients [1]. Over recent years, key advances have been made in islet transplantation [2], although this strategy still faces many problems such as graft immune-compatibility, side effects of immunosuppressors in β-cell viability, adjustment of the correct number of islets, implant survival and finally scarcity of the biomaterial [3-6]. Therefore, alternative sources of β-cell surrogates need to be investigated to offer new therapeutic alternatives.

In this sense, generation of viable, functional and customized β-cells could be theoretically achieved from embryonic (ESCs) or adult stem cells (ASCs) (figure 1). This is possible because stem cells bear two key properties: self-renewal by symmetric divisions and differentiation to diverse cell fates by asymmetric divisions [7]. In addition, these cells can be cultured in vitro, allowing the study of these cells and facilitating gene manipulation in order to solve problems related with tumour formation, immune rejection or functional reprogramming [8]. Embryonic stem cells are obtained from the inner cell mass of in vitro developing blastocysts. To maintain human embryonic stem cells in culture, they have to be cultured on feeder layers of embryonic inactivated fibroblasts [7, 8]. These fibroblasts supposedly secrete to the medium specific factors that maintain the cells undifferentiated and at the same time favour cell divisions through Wnt, BMP (Bone Morphogenetic Protein)/TGF-β1 (Transforming Growth Factor-β1), activin and IGF-1 (Insulin-like Growth Factor-1) pathways, among others [9]. Usually, ESCs display slow division kinetics, however, progenitors are formed very quickly in vitro, displaying lower degree of plasticity and constrained commitment to particular cell fates [10]. These precursor cells tend to accumulate chromosomal aberrations and very often are reluctant to the agents used in the differentiation protocols, maintaining a tumourigenic potential [11]. In this context, it should be interesting to search for factors that maintain the plasticity of the stem cell population over precursors, avoiding their neuroectodermal commitment [12]. In addition, ESCs present an additional problem of immunocompatibility that severely limits their clinical applications [3]. Nevertheless, ESCs are a good testing material in order to check the efficiency of extracellular factors and culture conditions that could be instrumental in specific protocols.

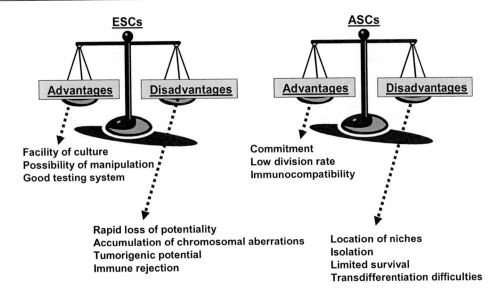

Figure 1. Advantages and disadvantages of embryonic and adult stem cells to use in Cell Therapy protocols.

Conversely to ESCs, ASCs do not pose problems related with immune rejection (provided that donor and recipient is the same person) and apparently under normal circumstances display homeostatic division rates. This usually occurs when ASCs are maintained in their natural niches, where the cells receive the appropriate signals to cover regular tissue turnover or exceptional tissue repopulation in cases of severe aggression [13, 14]. ASCs from different tissues, such as liver, intestine and bone marrow have shown their potential to produce insulin-secreting cells [15-19]. However, the mechanisms underlying such differentiation processes remain largely unidentified. As of yet, it is still unknown whether bone marrow stem cells are capable of transdifferentiating into insulin-producing cells during pancreas repopulation or if they enhance β-cell regeneration [16, 17]. In this context, it is not clear which transcription factor is more instrumental in reprogramming liver cells to insulin-producing cells [18, 19]. The exact identification of candidate cells in the different tissues by cell surface markers and the identification of specific niches for differentiation will be new scientific challenges in a near future.

Despite the large amount of research being performed on the subject, the location and identification of pancreatic stem cells, which would represent a key discovery in diabetes cell therapy, is currently unknown. Ducts (of pancreatic or hepatic origin) seem to bear a precursor population that can be manipulated in vitro to obtain insulin-producing cells [20, 21]. However, the results have been modest and need further improvements. On the other hand, the presence of precursors associated with islet structures have also been proposed, although the phenotypic characterization and the in vivo differentiating mechanism are still elusive matters [22]. Bioengineered mesenchymal stem cells from pancreatic or extrapancreatic tissues could represent alternative sources to obtain insulin-secreting cells, however the in vitro differentiation protocols are still poorly developed. Mesenchymal stem cells seem to be a heterogeneous population and thus identification and isolation of cell clones capable of differentiating to insulin-secreting cells is still unknown [23]. Pancreatic exocrine cells represent another source for insulin-positive cells, although several authors claim the opposite [24, 25]. Finally, it seems that β cells can rely on their auto-replicative capacity, although they are poorly operative in diabetes, where the tax of death overpasses the replication capacity of mature β-cells [26, 27].

Although there is still much work to do, somewhat efficient several protocols are currently available, suggesting that research is walking in a good direction and is a matter of time before a consistent protocol is found. This Chapter will try to resume the key work that has been performed in this field, recapitulating the key reports that have presented substantial features in ESCs and ASCs.

IT IS POSSIBLE TO WALK FROM AN EMBRYONIC STEM CELL TO AN INSULIN-POSITIVE CELL

Our laboratory was the first to report that it was possible to obtain insulin-secreting cells from undifferentiated mouse ESCs [28]. This was a key paper, as it established the main proof of principle in this field. Transfecting mouse ESCs with a neomycin-selection cassette under the control of the insulin gene promoter, we were capable of selecting insulin-positive cells from the rest of the cells [29]. In addition, the paper introduced some key determinants that were instrumental in the in vitro differentiation process, which have been successfully used by others [30-33]. Specifically, we proposed the use of nicotinamide during the final maturation step and the lowering of extracellular glucose concentrations in the culture medium. In addition, we also recommended the formation of three-dimensional structures that mimicked the islet cell cluster.

Although this was a pioneering report in the field, the protocol left several unsolved questions. One of them concerned the reproducibility of the protocol. Spontaneous expression of insulin can be easily obtained [34], although its concentration at different cell passages was not totally reproducible. At that time, we did not have a convincing explanation for this, but our current research indicated that, as it has been observed in neuronal stem cells [35], totipotent ESCs coexist in culture within a population of precursors. These precursors display division kinetics faster than the differentiated stem cells, leading to an accumulation of this population over several passages. We have observed that this precursor population tends to differentiate in vitro mainly to an ectodermal fate, mostly due to the fact that commitment to this embryonic layer does not require complex signals and is a default pathway [36]. Neuroectodermal tissues also express the insulin gene, in particular insulin II in mice. Thus, our selection system results in the isolation of a diverse population of insulin-positive cells, deriving from the neuroectoderm, primitive endoderm and definitive endoderm.

Therefore, in the mouse model, the expression of insulin II could alert about the presence of insulin-positive cells of ectodermal origin (cells derived from primitive endoderm can also express the insulin II gene) [37]. Insulin I is the marker of mouse insulin-positive cells derived from definitive endoderm (the embryonic layer from which β-cell derives). It is true that in this original work, the contribution of ectodermal and endodermal layers to the final insulin-positive population was not assessed [28]. Experience in our laboratory indicates that insulin-positive cells in this report [28] could represent a mixed population from different origins in which, and according to insulin II expression, non-endodermal precursors are the primary contributors. Over passages, this population increases, leading to insulin II-positive cells [10].

Our report showed that transplantation of insulin-producing cells in the spleen of streptozotocin-induced diabetic mice could restore their glycaemia levels. However, our group, which has been corroborated by other investigators, has seen that the spleen is not the ideal location to study the evolution of an implant. Subsequent reports have implanted biomaterials in the renal capsule, which seems to be a more adequate location [31, 33, 38]. This strategy allows the following of any likely in vivo maturation processes by simple nefrectomy, providing at the same time evidence of possible pancreas regeneration, which sometimes occurs when using chemically-induced diabetic models.

The third key point concerns the possibility of teratoma formation after implantation. We have identified cells escaping from the differentiation processes and remaining undifferentiated during the entire protocol. The tracing of these cells and subsequent characterization presented chromosomal aberrations, an altered pattern of oncogene expression, and a high degree of BrdU incorporation [11, 39]. Teratoma formation in transplanted animals was observed after 3 months of post-implantation, differing from other publications in which the implant was only present for 15 days [11, 38].

A similar strategy has been used with human ESCs. However, the real origin of the insulin-positive cells (ectoderm, primitive or definitive endoderm) was not addressed, while the functional analysis of insulin release in response to glucose concentrations was not sufficiently conclusive to demonstrate the presence of a regulated secretion process [40]. Despite these drawbacks, the report presented for the first time that it was also possible to walk from human ESCs to insulin-producing cells, as we have previously demonstrated with mouse ESCs.

Since key transcription factors in endocrine pancreas development are also expressed in ESCs, an alternative strategy is to isolate pure populations of such precursors and apply different maturation strategies. This approach has been afforded by Leon-Quinto et al [38], using a selection cassette under the control of the Nkx6.1 promoter. This transcription factor belongs to the NK homeobox family of proteins. During endocrine pancreas development, Nkx6.1 expression is restricted exclusively to β-cell precursors [41]. Again, the main problem to face concerns the observation that the expression of many of the transcription factors involved in islet development are also expressed in neuroectodermal-derived cells [42], questioning, therefore, the real origin of the obtained cells. In any case, and by using this strategy, this report described reproducible amounts of intracellular insulin, although they were still very low to envisage a therapeutic purpose. An interesting finding of this report was the description that anti-Shh (Sonic hedgehog) was very effective in inducing insulin gene expression. In fact, Shh inhibition in vivo is a key event in order to induce the transcription factor Pdx-1 and subsequently commence pancreas development [43]. This finding indicates that the information raised from embryonic development could be instrumental in bioengineering protocols [44]. In this context, it has been demonstrated that Shh inhibition by cyclopamine administration is a key step in differentiation protocols to obtain insulin-secretory cells [45]. In other words, improving our knowledge in understanding embryonic pancreas development subsequently supports the advancement in the tissue engineering field.

NEUROECTODERM DERIVATIVES FROM EMBRYONIC STEM CELLS REPRESENTS AN ALTERNATIVE SOURCE FOR INSULIN-PRODUCING CELLS

Islet cells and certain neurons share many features, including the expression of several transcription factors, as well as proteins of the secretory pathway and enzymes of the glucose sensing machinery [46]. Insulin is expressed in both systems, despite the different embryonic origin [37]. Surprisingly nestin, which is a protein of intermediate filaments found in neural precursors, was also detected in pancreatic progenitors [22]. These findings resulted in a research group to consider a strategy based in the differentiation of a nestin-rich cell population from ESCs that subsequently is committed to express insulin [30].

However, the protocol displayed several limitations that were derived from an incomplete interpretation of the above mentioned arguments. Indeed, neuroectoderm-derived hypothalamic neurons are capable of sensing extracellular glucose and to express and secrete insulin [46]. However, the processing of the hormone is not completed, yielding mainly pro-insulin, which exerts different biological actions than pancreatic insulin [47]. In addition, the amount of biosynthesized pro-insulin was very low to envisage future clinical applications, remaining far from what is found in adult pancreatic β-cells. Furthermore, nestin does not seem to be the marker of pancreatic precursors, but rather of vimentin-positive mesenchymal cells, stellate cells and vascular endothelial cells [48-50].

Aside from these constraints, the designed protocol [30] yielded low but reproducible amounts of the hormone, representing a positive aspect not reported before [28]. This should imply that specific modifications could substantially increase the intracellular insulin biosynthesis. Unfortunately, coaxial and directional manipulations have not advanced significantly in this direction [31-33]. Furthermore, the real origin of the insulin detected inside the cells by immunocytochemistry could be in fact the insulin that was present in the culture medium (ITSFn medium used in this protocol contains insulin) and caught by the cells when they enter apoptosis [51].

However, in positive terms, this group of strategies clearly indicates that neuroectoderm could be a candidate source of insulin-positive cells. Insulin II is the major form of insulin expressed in these protocols when using mouse ESCs [37]. Humans have only one insulin gene, which is also expressed in certain cells of the nervous system [47]. Compared to definitive endoderm, from which pancreatic β-cells are derived, neuroectoderm is relatively easy to obtain in vitro using bioengineering protocols. We can hypothesize that with well-directed manipulations, it could be possible to obtain insulin-secreting cells producing sufficient insulin to envisage transplantation trials. To this end, it is important to centre research in specific aspects, including hormone production and processing, as well as regulation of the gene expression.

Mimicking Pancreas Organogenesis Is a Key Approach to Produce In Vitro Insulin-Secreting Cells from Embryonic Stem Cells

Aside from the neural pathway [30], insulin-producing cells can be obtained by replicating in vitro the pancreatic developmental pathway. The spontaneous expression of specific transcription factors involved in pancreas development during ESC cultures has encouraged some groups to hypothesize that some steps of islet development could be reproduced in vitro [52, 53]. These spontaneous differentiation programmes were triggered in ESCs when they were transferred from adherent monolayers to bacteriological Petri dishes. Under these culture suspension conditions, ESCs associate forming heterogeneous cell aggregates called embryoid bodies (EBs). The activation of differentiation programmes is confirmed by the expression of typical markers of the three embryonic layers: primitive and definitive endoderm, ectoderm and mesoderm [54]. How this differentiation pattern is achieved is not well known. It is believed that gradients established between the outside and the inside of the EB are instrumental in nutrient, oxygen and growth factor distribution, thereby affecting cell differentiation. Cell-to-cell interactions, as well as paracrine and biophysical determinants seem to also be instrumental during this process.

However, the rationale behind this assumption is doubtful, since it has not been rigorously demonstrated that ESCs can follow specific developmental steps in vitro when forming EB structures. First, some of the so-called β-cell specific transcription factors are not so specific, being expressed in other cell types, such as the ectoderm [42]. Therefore, the detection of a transcription factor by RT-PCR in EBs is not a guarantee that a specific differentiation programme is operating in the cells. The time sequence when these transcription factors are expressed in EBs is variable and, very often, not coincident with the onset observed during pancreatic embryogenesis [53]. In addition, EBs obtained from ESC monolayers are heterogeneous, and display a large variety of morphologies [54]. The most conciliatory explanation is that there is no general differentiation pattern when EBs are formed from ESC monolayers. It seems that each particular EB structure follows its own gene expression pattern, activated and modulated by unknown determinants. It is a rare event for any given EB to spontaneously follow the steps of pancreatic development.

This chaotic patterning in EBs could be circumvented by coaxial and/or directional strategies, thereby committing EBs to desired cell fates. Although this seems to be an obvious approach, a 100% commitment to a specific cell lineage is difficult to achieve. First of all, ESC monolayers contain precursors that very easily differentiate to ectoderm derivatives, thus conditioning the lineages present in EB structures. In addition, it is technically difficult in coaxial strategies to facilitate an equal access of medium determinants to all cells placed inside the EB. Therefore, the total commitment to definitive endoderm, which is the germ layer from which the endocrine pancreas derives, using EBs is difficult to reach. In the best of the cases, EB structures can be modestly enriched in particular cell types that express definitive endoderm markers and progress to pancreatic fates [55, 56]. On the other hand, directional strategies require the transfection of ESCs with inducible transgenes coding for key transcription factors involved in pancreas development [55, 56]. Again, the expression of these transcription factors in other tissues could constrain the application of this approach.

A recent report [57] circumvents this and other problems through the use of a differentiation strategy that recapitulates in vitro pancreas ontogeny in ESC monolayer cultures, obtaining β-cell-like surrogates. The cells were submitted to specific compounds in 5 differentiation steps. In each step, the expression of endocrine pancreas-specific genes and proteins were analyzed (figure 2). A key point in this protocol was the enrichment of the human ESC monolayers in definitive endoderm precursors. As a result, 80% of the culture were definitive endoderm-derived cells [58], compared to the 2.7% seen in the previous method, where EBs were used [59].

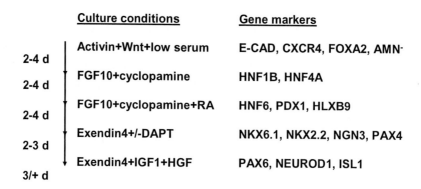

Figure 2. Scheme of the protocol developed by Baetge's group to obtain insulin-producing cells from ESCs. Abbreviations used: HGF, Hepatic Growth Factor; RA, Retinoic Acid.

One of the main obstacles addressed in this protocol concerns the distinction between definitive and primitive endoderm. Both lineages perform very similar functions during embryonic development and thus share many markers, including insulin (insulin II in mice) [60]. Therefore, the use of a combination of various markers to establish lineage association has been the proper criterion adopted for the identification of definitive endoderm precursors [57, 61].

During mouse embryonic gastrulation, the primitive streak recruits cells from specific regions of the epiblast, where they undergo the epithelial-to-mesenchymal transition, giving rise to mesoderm and definitive endoderm [62-64]. This common origin within the primitive streak supports the idea that both lineages arise from an original progenitor called the mesendoderm. This concept, when applied in vitro, has resulted in human and mouse ESCs to differentiate towards definitive endoderm derivatives. In this context, selection of brachyury-positive cells gave rise to definitive endoderm fates [55], although brachyury gene expression is not exclusively restricted to mesoderm, being also expressed in visceral endoderm [65].

Yasunaga and coworkers reported that it was possible to isolate mouse cells committed to definitive endoderm through the use of specific selection strategies and culture conditions [61]. Based on the expression of Gsc (goosecoid) and Sox17/CD25, they established a mesendoderm precursor line. Gsc is a mesoderm marker, while Sox17/CD25 is a well-known marker of definitive and visceral endoderm. Therefore, cell lines $Gsc^-/Sox17^+$ are committed to visceral endoderm, whereas $Gsc^+/Sox17^+$ are mesendoderm precursors. In addition, primitive endoderm commitment can also be validated by the positive expression of amnionless, which seems to be exclusively present in primitive endoderm [57, 61, 66] (figure 3).

	Gsc	Sox17	Bry	Ecad	Cxcr4	Foxa2	Amn
Mesoderm	+	-	+	-	-	-	-
Primitive endoderm	-	+	+	+	+	+	+
Definitive endoderm	-	+	-	+	+	+	-
Mesendoderm	+	+	+	+	+	+	-

Figure 3. Useful combination of gene markers to discriminate definitive endoderm from primitive endoderm and mesoderm.

Specific conditions are required to guide the progenitors towards definitive endoderm, which include serum deprivation, a cell density lower than 10^5 cells/mL, and the addition of Nodal, a TGFβ family member. Alternatively, activin A is capable of binding to Nodal receptors and subsequently mimic the same intracellular signalling events [61, 64, 67]. The limitation of serum seems to restrain the action of specific factors, such as IGF, which support ESC self-renewal [61, 68, 69], favouring at the same time specific imprinted gene expression profiles [70]. In addition, inhibitors of the PI3K pathway, such as LY294002, seem to mimic low foetal calf serum/serum replacement culture conditions [67].

Specific culture conditions are subsequently required to drive the cells from definitive endoderm towards endocrine pancreatic cells. In this sense, endoderm-derived organs follow particular patterns which can be mimicked by adding specific factors to the culture medium. For instance, BMP-4 seems to be required for in vitro hepatic differentiation [71], however it does not play a key role in endocrine pancreas differentiation [45, 57]. Several extracellular factors that have been used to obtain insulin-producing cells are FGFs (Fibroblast Growth Factors), the Shh-inhibitor cyclopamine, retinoic acid and the GLP-1 (Glucagon-Like Peptide-1) analog exendin-4 [45]. Although these factors have been used in several protocols with human and mouse ESCs [38, 72-78], their results have varied greatly. Thus, the efficiency of these factors is directly related to their concentration and exposition time. From all these data, it can be deduced, first, that the efficiency of the afore-mentioned compounds is enhanced when cells are committed to definitive endoderm, and second, that the timing and concentration of incubation for each compound is critical in order to obtain the proper cell fate, since inappropriate timing can give rise to different lineages [72]. Therefore, this can explain why some compounds such as retinoic acid or cyclopamine have modest or even no effect in some protocols going through EB formation. In EBs, definitive endoderm seems to arise very late, as indicated by glucagon gene expression. This explains why, for example, retinoic acid and cyclopamine did not produce any effect when added during the first day of EB formation [53]. Also, it has been proven that low concentrations of serum is instrumental in inducing definitive endoderm in monolayer culture [45], meanwhile high serum concentration is required in some protocols going through EB formation [73].

One remaining question is to know whether the classical approach via EB formation allows spontaneous commitment towards definitive endoderm lineages or if the addition of specific factors is necessary for this end. It is clear that the use of monolayers [45] allows the direct access of extracellular factors to the cells, improving the reproducibility of the protocols. However, it is difficult to control all the microenvironmental determinants during EB formation due to its heterogeneity [54, 79], yielding different amounts of insulin-producing cells between the different protocols. The advantage of using EBs vs monolayers during differentiation processes is the presence of different cell types, such as those derived from the ectoderm, mesoderm and primitive endoderm that could produce key factors and thereby mimic certain steps of pancreatic development. Nevertheless, this point remains to be fully demonstrated inside EB structures. The presence of glucagon mRNA in spontaneous differentiation protocols could suggest that EBs may give rise to definitive endoderm derivatives after long periods of culture [54]. However, it must be considered that some differentiation pathways could be blocked at the EB level. This could be related to the observation that Shh is produced by EBs, repressing any likely endocrine pancreas differentiation. In fact, it has been shown that Shh inhibition can improve the yield of insulin-producing cells [80, 81].

Baetge's report has supposed a hallmark in diabetes cell therapy, and at the same time has shown that there is still much information unknown concerning the pancreatic developmental biology in mouse and humans, as well as the difficulty to transfer this knowledge to the culture plate. For example, the differentiation protocol presents a duration of approximately 15 days to go from totipotent ESCs to pancreatic endocrine immature cells, whereas in vivo this process is around 4 times longer. One explanation could be that under these artificial conditions in the culture dish, the differentiation may be strongly favoured over proliferation or enlargement processes which are typical in mammalian organogenesis. Although the resulting cells possessed high insulin concentrations, close to those found in mature β-cells, the hormone is predominantly expressed as proinsulin. In addition, the cells responded to multiple secretagogues; however they had a low response to extracellular glucose. Furthermore, some cell clusters were co-expressing insulin and glucagon or insulin and somatostatin, indicating an immature phenotype. In this context, the expression of MAFA transcription factors is required to obtain mature β-cells [82], which have not been considered in this protocol [45]. An important point to indicate is that this protocol is specific for definitive endoderm precursors. The application to neuroectoderm or primitive endoderm does not produce the same results [45].

All these results indicate that the cells obtained by Baetge's protocol present an immature phenotype that requires further maturation steps in order to obtain functional insulin-secreting cells. Thus, the search for new determinants could complete and improve this in vitro differentiation protocol [45]. The characterization of the microenvironment or niche in which the pancreas develops could help in finding instrumental determinants to culminate this differentiation process. In this rationale, when human ESCs were cotransplanted with mouse foetal dorsal pancreas, they expressed processed insulin as well as many transcription factors found in β-cells during embryonic development [83]. Therefore, analytical approaches can be applied to develop pancreas environments in order to find key factors that could be transferred to an in vitro system. It can be hypothesized that this niche should contain a mixture of key molecules derived from the same endocrine pancreas, as well from surrounding tissues. Cell-to-cell interactions have to also be taken in account. Complexity increases if we consider that this niche is subject to dynamic processes in which concentration, composition and time of action of the different determinants is changing according to particular patterns specified by orchestrated developmental programmes [84].

In this context, certain groups have searched for factors released by adult and developing pancreas (pancreatic buds) that could act as autocrine factors, inducing self-renewal and/or differentiation [85, 86]. Although the idea seems interesting in theory, it needs to be sustained by consistent proof and solid experiments. At present, the first study [86] addressing this point presents such a poor design that all subsequent conclusions were completely useless for bioengineering protocols. First of all, this study does not report whether the insulin gene that is expressed corresponds to insulin I or II. The correct processing of the hormone was obviated as well. Furthermore, it did not address if the cells were initially committed to definitive endoderm. The functional tests did not give any useful information. In addition, the resulting cells released 20% of the insulin content when stimulated with glucose, showing a very rare and unusual secretion pattern. Finally, and taken in account the large amounts of BrdU (Br-deoxyuridine) incorporated into the cells, it can be concluded that the final cell line was closest to a tumoural rather than a therapeutic cell fate.

PANCREATIC STEM CELLS AND THE POSSIBILITY TO OBTAIN ADULT B-CELLS

Since it is quite obvious that human beings are not born with all the battery of islet cells necessary for the duration of their lives, it is logical to assume that the endocrine pancreas turnover must occur during normal life. However, this process is not as evident as in other endoderm-derived organs, such as the liver. Therefore, a very active area of research is searching for the source from which β-cell arises in vivo and the molecular mechanisms that operate. The main goal in the context of Regenerative Medicine applied to diabetes should be the in vitro expansion of islets in order to obtain sufficient amounts to rescue the patient from the disease when they are re-implanted (figure 4). At best, the accumulated knowledge should give key information in order to design pharmacological agents that could stimulate in vivo, and specifically β-cell turnover, complementing the action of drugs designed to improve β-cell function. Currently several agents, such as exendin, a pharmacological product derived from GLP-1, β-cellulin, nicotinamide, gastrin, EGF-1 (Epidermal Growth factor-1), thyroid hormone, among others, have shown promising results in β-cell regeneration in diabetes [87].

The β-cell mass in a healthy organism is maintained by several processes that include neogenesis from pancreatic stem cells and the replication of pre-existing β-cells. In pathological situations where insulin production is deficient, β-cell function adapts through hypertrophy (increased cell size). Replication is also enhanced, however it usually fails if the damage persists, favouring death over proliferation/hypertrophy. The location of candidate niches for pancreatic stem cell location (ducts, islets, acini) and the characteristics of the cellular progenitors (epithelium, mesenchyme, exocrine tissue, β-cells) remain reluctant questions at present [88].

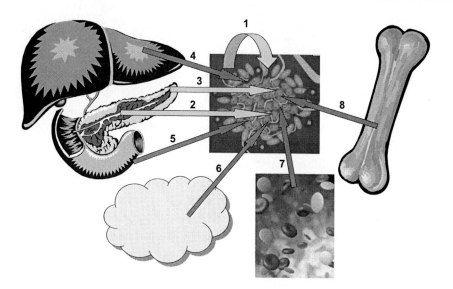

Figure 4. Locations containing candidate ASCs that could contribute to derive insulin-producing cells. 1) β-cell self renewal 2) Pancreatic ducts 3) Pancreatic acini 4) Liver 5) Intestine 6) Adipose tissue 7) Peripheral blood and 8) Bone marrow.

The self-replicating capacity of pancreatic β-cells, but not the existence of precursors, has been demonstrated by convincing cell-tracing experiments [89]. In any case, the best proliferation records are displayed by embryonic β-cells (10% of β-cell mass/day) compared to adult β-cells (4% of β-cell mass/day in rodents and less than 1% in humans). Most likely, the β-cell self-renewal could be the operating mechanism in normal pancreas turnover, which declines with age in humans and rodents (less than 0.1% of β-cell mass/day). Many determinants can alter the β-cell cycle [88]. However, the pancreas is capable of displaying some degree of plasticity towards specific physiological (pregnancy) and pathological situations (obesity, insulin resistance, diabetes), thereby increasing its turnover rate through self-replication, neogenesis and hypertrophy [41]. Nevertheless, when the damage strongly favours β-cell death (autoimmune attack, apoptosis) and disrupts repair and turnover, insulin levels drop and the nutrients remain in circulation with no insulin-mediated access to target tissues, leading to overt diabetes [27].

Concerning islet/β-cell neogenesis, the observation of islet budding from pancreatic ducts has suggested the existence of islet precursors in this tissue. The identification of the epithelial cell capable of differentiating towards insulin-positive cells remains elusive. This candidate cell has received several names, such as CHIBs (Cultivated Human Islet Buds) [20], IPSCs (Islet Pluripotent Stem Cells) [21], NIPs (Nestin-positive Islet-derived Progenitors, also found associated with islets) [22] and NEPEC (Non-Endocrine Pancreatic Epithelial Precursor) [91]. Certain gene markers, such as CK19 or nestin, have been ascribed to these precursor cells. However, none of these studies could establish the molecular determinants that direct the differentiation process in these cells, as well as the insulin-biosynthetic and secretory capacity. On the other hand, duct epithelium can be easily purified from the rest of the pancreatic cell types such as islets and exocrine tissue [20]. This could favour subsequent bioengineering, thereby offering a new potential application of human ductal tissue obtained from cadaveric pancreata. Several agents could favour islet neogenesis from the ducts, such as INGAP (Islet Neogenesis-Associated Protein) peptide or all-trans retinoic acid, although the mechanism through which these molecules are operating has not been fully characterized [44, 92]. In this context, it is well-known that during pancreatic development, duct-like cells can give rise to islet cells and all express the homeobox transcription factor PDX-1. Complete ablation of PDX-1 expression leads to pancreatic agenesis [93]. Also, it has been shown that this transcription factor is present in ductal precursors after acute necrotizing pancreatitis as well as after IFNγ (interferon-γ)-induced immune damage [94, 95].

Concerning islet studies, several reports also claim the existence of progenitors inside or associated to islet structures, such as the afore-mentioned NIPs, which were isolated from rat and human islets. These progenitors display proliferative activity and express endocrine and exocrine pancreatic markers as well as hepatic genes [22]. In this system as well as in the ductal system, nestin has been described as a β-cell precursor marker. However, this has been recently questioned due to its widespread expression in pancreas, including a specific subpopulation of mesenchymal cells, as well as in pancreatic stellate cells, exocrine precursors and vascular endothelial cells [48, 96, 97]. In addition, insulin-positive cells derived from nestin$^+$/Pdx-1$^-$-ESCs indicate that this lineage is different from the pancreas [98].

Aside from their location, the pathways from which new β-cells appear are unknown. The proposed mechanism, called the epithelial-to-mesenchymal-to-epithelial transition, implies the dedifferentiation of islets cells to mesenchymal cells in order to re-differentiate again into islets [99, 100]. However, whether this mechanism, that has been described only in vitro, occurs in vivo is a debated question [101-105]. Alternatively, exocrine acinar cells could provide progenitors capable of differentiating into insulin-secreting cells [24], although this is again a matter of debate [25].

At present, the studies previously cited prove that the endocrine pancreatic tissue exhibits a low turnover activity operating under normal conditions [106, 107], but at the same time possesses a certain plasticity managed by still poorly-characterized precursors cells [108]. This pancreatic stem cell population does not seem to have an obvious niche in the organ, and more likely it is spread throughout the pancreatic structure (duct, islet, acini, mesenchyme), representing a heterogeneous population and responding to a wide variety of stimuli. The better identification of endocrine pancreas precursors and signals that favour pancreas regeneration could allow the design of pharmacological agents to restore endocrine pancreatic mass lost in diabetic pathology.

EXTRAPANCREATIC STEM CELLS AND THE POSSIBILITY TO OBTAIN INSULIN-SECRETING CELLS

The possibility of ectopic expression of insulin gene in several non-pancreatic tissues opens alternative options to circumvent the problems posed by pancreas bioengineering [109] (figure 4). In this context, bone marrow represents the most studied ASC population in the organism, displaying a wide plasticity and offering the possibility of obtaining insulin-secreting cells. However, the reports concerning this possibility have been contradictory in some instances. The experiment designed by Ianus et al reported that bone marrow stem cells contribute modestly (1.7-3%) to transdifferentiate into insulin-positive cells [16]. However, other reports failed to reproduce these results [110, 111]. In any case, many questions remain concerning the signals that promote mobilization from bone marrow to pancreas, the requirement of a pancreatic lesion and the mechanisms operating when bone marrow stem cells migrate into the pancreatic tissue [112-114].

A possible explanation is that bone marrow harbours a heterogeneous population of cell precursors, such as hematopoietic, endothelial, mesenchymal, etc, which are capable of responding to a large variety of stimuli and thereby deriving towards different cell fates that could favour insulin production through different mechanisms. In this context, endothelial progenitor cells can indirectly favour islet regeneration through new vasculature formation [17], although in all cases the contribution of these precursors is modest and fusion events cannot be discarded. Mesenchymal cells also form part of the bone marrow stem cell repertoire. They are located in the stroma, displaying the ability to differentiate into mesoderm-derived tissues, such as bone, cartilage and adipoblasts. In vitro experiments have shown that bone marrow mesenchymal stem cells display the ability, either by coaxed culture conditions or by transfection with β-cell specific DNA constructs, to differentiate into pancreatic precursors [115-118]. Nevertheless, this is not always reproducible; indicating that precise phenotyping of this heterogeneous population is required. In this sense, bone marrow-derived CD29+/CD44+/CD106+ mesenchymal cells can differentiate to insulin-positive cells, while CD14+/CD34+/CD45+ cannot [119]. Interestingly, mesenchymal stem cells from adipose tissue present many phenotypic similarities with bone marrow mesenchymal cells. The culture of these adipose-derived cells in the presence of bFGF (basic Fibroblast Growth Factor) and high glucose concentration induced islet gene expression [120]. Altogether, these reports indicate an interesting plasticity for either bone marrow or adipose-derived mesenchymal cells, which deserves more attention.

Similarly, a precise phenotypic characterization can be extended to other populations of stem cells. For instance, it has been described that circulating monocytes could be coaxed to express insulin [121]. However, the progenitor population has not been characterized in detail, explaining the impossibility of reproducing these results by others. Recently, a human stem cell population derived from peripheral blood has been discovered. This population displays positive expression of Oct-4, Nanog and the hematopietic markers CD9, CD45 and CD117, and is negative for CD34 as well as for markers of the monocyte and lymphocyte lineages [122]. A possible interpretation to these contradictory results is that the monocyte population isolated in the first report [121] contained progenitor cells, but was not properly characterized.

Conversely to pancreas, liver displays a robust self-renewing capacity due to the existence of a hepatic stem cell population. On the other hand, and as it has been seen in the pancreas, this organ derives from the upper foregut definitive endoderm. In this sense, it has been described that oval hepatic stem cells are capable of differentiating into insulin-positive cells, hepatocytes and bile duct epithelium [123, 124]. A hepatic mesenchymal cell population has been isolated, displaying the expression of CD29, CD73, CD44, CD90, nestin and vimentin markers. This population possesses the ability to differentiate into pancreatic endocrine fates [125]. On the other hand, human foetal hepatic stem cells overexpressing Pdx-1 can be transdifferentiated to β-like-cells, synthesizing and secreting insulin in a glucose-dependent manner [126]. Adult human and mouse hepatic cells overexpressing Pdx-1 can ectopically activate insulin genes both in vitro and in vivo [18, 109, 127]. One should be aware, however, that the use of Pdx-1 expression vectors could induce the differentiation of pancreatic exocrine tissue, causing hepatic destruction. This has been circumvented by the overexpression of other specific transcription factors of pancreatic endocrine lineage, such as NeuroD combined with betacellulin, thereby avoiding tissue destruction [19]. Finally, it is interesting to mention that insulin-positive cells have been found in mouse bile ducts, deriving from the liver during embryogenesis [128].

Finally, endocrine cells of the intestinal epithelium could be good candidates for reparative medicine in diabetes with minimal bioengineering. First, these cells can be easily transfected to display ectopic insulin expression. Second, endocrine intestinal cells share many functional characteristics with β-cells, such as the nutrient-sensor machinery that includes the glucose transporter GLUT-2 and glucokinase (the first enzyme of the glycolytic pathway) [129, 130]. However, other cell functions, such as regulated insulin processing and secretion, need to be improved.

Altogether, bone marrow, mesenchymal, liver and gut cells open new avenues for autologous cell therapy in diabetes. To delve inside the molecular mechanisms involved in the differentiation processes is essential to design consistent protocols.

CONCLUSION

The use of ESCs and ASCs in the treatment of diabetes requires substantial improvements before finding a clinical application. In vitro culture conditions have to be assessed in order to establish a reproducible protocol. It is necessary as well to delve inside pancreas ontogeny and physiology in order to transfer knowledge from in vivo to in vitro niches. Immune rejection and tumour formation are serious problems that can hamper the development of future therapeutic trials in humans. Finally, the mechanisms that allow insulin gene expression in extrapancreatic tissues need to be further investigated. In conclusion, the objective is to obtain a cell that produces sufficient amounts of processed insulin and is capable of secreting it in response to several secretagogues (mainly glucose) in a regulated manner. In addition, this cell has to be capable of surviving in an appropriate body niche and without neither giving rise to tumours nor to induce immune rejection.

REFERENCES

[1] DeFronzo, RA; Ferrannini, E; Keen, H; Zimmet, P. International textbook of diabetes mellitus, 3th ed. Chichester (UK): John Wiley and Sons; 2004.

[2] Shapiro, AM; Lakey, JR; Ryan, EA; Korbutt, GS; Toth, E; Warnock, GL; Kneteman, NM; Rajotte, RV. Islet transplantation in seven patients with type 1 diabetes mellitus using a glucocorticoid-free immunosuppressive regimen. *New England Journal of Medicine*, 2000, 343, 230-238.

[3] Roche, E; Reig, JA; Campos, A; Paredes, B; Isaac, JR; Lim, S; Calne, RY; Soria, B. Insulin-secreting cells derived from stem cells: Clinical perspectives, hypes and hopes. *Transplant Immunology*, 2005, 15, 113-129.

[4] Ryan, EA; Paty, BW; Senior, PA; Bigam, D; Alfadhli, E; Kneteman, NM; Lakey, JR; Shapiro, AM. Five-year follow-up after clinical islet transplantation. *Diabetes*. 2005, 54, 2060-2069.

[5] Hermann, M; Margreiter, R; Hengster, P. Molecular and cellular key players in human islet transplantation. *Journal of Cellular and Molecular Medicine*. 2007, 11, 398-415.

[6] Laybutt, DR; Hawkins, YC; Lock, J; Lebet, J; Sharma, A; Bonner-Weir, S; Weir, GC. Influence of diabetes on the loss of β-cell differentiation after islet transplantation in rats. *Diabetologia*, 2007, 50, 2117-2125.

[7] Smith AG. Embryo-derived stem cells: of mice and men. *Annual Review of Cellular and Developmental Biology*, 2001, 17, 435-462.

[8] Smith AG. Culture and differentiation of embryonic stem cells. *Journal of Tissue Culture Methods*, 1991, 13, 89-94.

[9] Prowse, AB; McQuade, LR; Bryant, KJ; Marcal, H; Gray, PP. Identification of potential pluripotency determinants for human embryonic stem cells following proteomic analysis of human and mouse fibroblast conditioned media. *Journal of Proteome Research*, 2007, 6, 3796-3807.

[10] Roche, E; Sepulcre, P; Reig, JA; Santana, A; Soria, B. Ectodermal commitment of insulin-producing cells derived from mouse embryonic stem cells. *FASEB Journal*, 2005, 19, 1341-1343.

[11] Ensenat-Waser, R; Santana, A; Vicente-Salar, N; Cigudosa, JC; Roche, E; Soria, B; Reig, JA. Isolation and characterization of residual undifferentiated mouse embryonic stem cells from embryoid body cultures by fluorescence tracking. *In Vitro Cellular and Developmental Biology-Animal*, 2006, 42, 115-123.

[12] Pumiglia, K; Temple, S. PEDF: bridging neurovascular interactions in the stem cell niche. *Nature Neuroscience*, 2006, 9, 299-300.

[13] Watt, FM; Hogan, BL. Out of eden: stem cells and their niches. *Science*, 2000, 287, 1427-1430.

[14] Barrilleaux, B; Phinney, DG; Prockop, DJ; O'Connor, KC. Ex vivo engineering of living tissues with adult stem cells. *Tissue Engineering*, 2006, 12, 3007-3019.

[15] Fellous, TG; Guppy, NJ; Brittan, M; Alison, MR. Cellular pathways to β-cell replacement. *Diabetes/Metabolism Research and Reviews*, 2007, 23, 87-99.

[16] Ianus, A; Holz, GG; Theise, ND; Hussain, MA. In vivo derivation of glucose-competent pancreatic endocrine cells from bone marrow without evidence of cell fusion. *Journal of Clinical Investigation*, 2003, 111: 843-850.

[17] Hess, D; Li, L; Martin, M; Sakano, S; Hill, D; Strutt, B; Thyssen, S; Gray, DA; Bhatia, M. Bone marrow-derived stem cells initiate pancreatic regeneration. *Nature Biotechnology*, 2003, 21, 763-770.

[18] Ferber, S; Halkin, A; Cohen, H; Ber, I; Einav, Y; Goldberg, I; Barshack, I; Seijffers, R; Kopolovic, J; Kaiser, N; Karasik, A. Pancreatic and duodenal homeobox gene 1 induces expression of insulin genes in liver and ameliorates streptozotocin-induced hyperglycemia. *Nature Medicine*. 2000, 6, 568-572.

[19] Kojima, H; Fujimiya, M; Matsumura, K; Younan, P; Imaeda, H; Maeda, M; Chan, L. NeuroD-betacellulin gene therapy induces islet neogenesis in the liver and reverses diabetes in mice. *Nature Medicine*, 2003, 9, 596-603.

[20] Bonner-Weir, S; Taneja, M; Weir, GC; Tatarkiewicz, K; Song, K-H; Sharma, A; O'Neil, JJ. In vitro cultivation of human islets from expanded ductal tissue. *Proceedings of the National Academy of Sciences of USA*, 2000, 97, 7999-8004.

[21] Ramiya, VK; Maraist, M; Arfors, KE; Schatz, DA; Peck, AB; Cornelius, JG. Reversal of insulin-dependent diabetes using islets generated in vitro from pancreatic stem cells. *Nature Medicine*, 2000, 6, 278-282.

[22] Zulewski, H; Abraham, EJ; Gerlach, MJ; Daniel, PB; Moritzs, W; Müller, B; Vallejo, M; Thomas, MK; Habener, JF. Multipotential nestin-positive stem cells isolated from adult pancreatic islets differentiate ex vivo into pancreatic endocrine, exocrine and hepatic phenotypes. *Diabetes*, 2001, 50, 521-533.

[23] Zulewski, H. Stem cells with potential to generate insulin-producing cells in man. *Swiss Medical Weekly*, 2006, 136: 647-654.

[24] Minami, K; Okuno, M; Miyawaki, K; Okumachi, A; Ishizaki, K; Oyama, K; Kawaguchi, M; Ishizuka, N; Iwanaga, T; Seino, S. Lineage tracing and characterization of insulin-secreting cells generated from adult pancreatic acinar cells. *Proccedings of the National Academy of Sciences of USA*, 2005, 102, 15116-15121.

[25] Desai, BM; Oliver-Krasinski, J; De Leon, DD; Fazard, C; Hong, N; Leach, SD; Stoffers, DA. Preexisting pancreatic acinar cells contribute to acinar cell, but not islet beta cell regeneration. *Journal of Clinical Investigation*, 2007, 117, 971-977.

[26] Dor, Y; Brown, J; Martínez, OI; Melton, DA. Adult pancreatic β-cells are formed by self-duplication rather than stem-cell differentiation. *Nature*, 2004, 429, 41-46.

[27] Kodama, S; Kuhtreiber, W; Fujimura, S; Dale, EA; Faustman, DL. Islet regeneration during the reversal of autoimmune diabetes in NOD mice. *Science*, 2003, 302, 1223-1227.

[28] Soria, B; Roche, E; Bernat, G; León-Quinto, T; Reig, JA; Martínez, F. Insulin-secreting cells derived from embryonic stem cells normalize glycemia in streptozotocin-induced diabetic mice. *Diabetes*, 2000, 49, 157-162.

[29] Roche, E; Burcin, MM; Esser, S; Rüdiger, M; Soria, B. The use of gating technology in bioengineering insulin-secreting cells from embryonic stem cells. *Cytotechnology*, 2003, 41, 145-151.

[30] Lumelsky, N; Blondel, O; Laeng, P; Velasco, I; Ravin, R; McKay, R. Differentiation of embryonic stem cells to insulin-secreting structures similar to pancreatic islets. *Science*, 2001, 292, 1389-1394.

[31] Hori, Y; Rulifson, IC; Tsai, BC; Heit, JJ; Cahoy, JD; Kim, SK. Growth inhibitors promote differentiation of insulin-producing tissue from embryonic stem cells. *Proccedings of the National Academy of Sciences of USA*, 2002, 99, 16105-16110.

[32] Moritoh, Y; Yamato, E; Yasui, Y; Miyazaki, S; Miyazaki, J. Analysis of insulin-producing cells during in vitro differentiation from feeder-free embryonic stem cells. *Diabetes*, 2003, 52, 1163-1168.

[33] Blyszczuk, P; Czyz, J; Kania, G; Wagner, M; Roll, U; St-Onge, L; Wobus, A. Expression of Pax4 in embryonic stem cells promotes differentiation of nestin-positive

progenitor and insulin-producing cells. *Proccedings of the National Academy of Sciences of USA*, 2003, 100, 998-1003.

[34] Soria, B; Skoudy, A; Martín, F. From stem cells to beta cells: new strategies in cell therapy of diabetes mellitus. *Diabetologia*, 2001, 44, 407-415.

[35] Ramirez-Castillejo, C; Sanchez-Sanchez, F; Andreu-Agullo, C; Ferron, SR; Aroca-Aguilar, JD; Sanchez, P; Mira, H; Escribano, J; Farinas, I. Pigment epithelium-derived factor is a niche signal for neural stem cell renewal. *Nature Neuroscience*, 2006, 9, 331-339.

[36] Ying, Q-L ; Stavridis, M; Griffiths, D; Li, M ; Smith, A. Conversion of embryonic stem cells into neuroectodermal precursorsin adherent monoculture. *Nature Biotechnology*, 2003, 21, 183-186.

[37] Kojima, H; Fujimiya, M; Terashima, T; Kimura, H; Chan, L. Extrapancreatic proinsulin/insulin-expressing cells in diabetes mellitus: Is history repeating itself? *Endocrine Journal*, 2006, 53, 715-722.

[38] Leon-Quinto, T; Jones, J; Skoudy, A; Burcin, M; Soria, B. In vitro directed differentiation of mouse embryonic stem cells into insulin-producing cells. *Diabetologia*, 2004, 48, 1095-1104.

[39] Santana, A; Enseñat-Waser, R; Arribas, MI; Reig, JA; Roche, E. Insulin-producing cells derived from stem cells: recent progress and future directions. *Journal of Cellular and Molecular Medicine*, 10, 4, 866-883.

[40] Assady, S; Maor, G; Amit, M; Itskovitz-Eldor, J; Skorecki, KL; Tzukerman, M. Insulin production by human embryonic stem cells. *Diabetes*, 2001, 50, 1691-1697.

[41] Murtaugh, LC. Pancreas and beta-cell development: from the actual to the possible. *Development*, 2007, 134, 427-438.

[42] Chakrabarti, SK; Mirmira, RG. Transcription factors direct the development and function of pancreatic β cells. *TRENDS in Endocrinology and Metabolism*, 2003, 14, 78-84.

[43] Kim, SK; Hebrok, M. Intercellular signals regulating pancreas development and function. *Genes and Development*, 2001, 15, 111-127.

[44] Roche, E; Jones, J; Arribas, MI; Leon-Quinto, T; Soria, B. Role of small bioorganic molecules in stem cell differentiation to insulin-producing cells. *Bioorganic and Medicinal Chemistry*, 2006, 14, 6466-6474.

[45] D'Amour, KA; Bang, AG; Eliazer, S; Kelly, OG; Agulnick, AD; Smart, NG; Moorman, MA; Kroon, E; Carpenter, MK; Baetge, EE. Production of pancreatic hormone-expressing endocrine cells from human embryonic stem cells. *Nature Biotechnology*, 2006, 24, 1392-1401.

[46] Schuit, FC; Huypens, P; Heimberg, H; Pipeleers, DG. Glucose sensing in pancreatic beta-cells: a model for the study of other glucose-regulated cells in gut, pancreas, and hypothalamus. *Diabetes,* 2001, 50, 1-11.

[47] Hernandez-Sanchez, C; Mansilla, A; de la Rosa, EJ; de Pablo, F. Proinsulin in development: new roles for an ancient prohormone. *Diabetologia*, 2006, 49, 1142-1150.

[48] Street, CN; Lakey, JR; Seeberger, K, Helms, L; Rajotte, RV; Shapiro, AM; Korbutt, GS. Heterogeneous expression of nestin in human pancreatic tissue precludes its use as an islet precursor marker. *Journal of Endocrinology*, 2004, 180, 213-225.

[49] Treutelaar, MK; Skidmore, JM; Dias-Leme, CL; Hara M; Zhang, L; Simeone, D; Martin, DM; Burant, CF. Nestin-lineage cells contribute to the microvasculature but not endocrine cells of the islet. *Diabetes*, 2003, 52, 2503-2512.

[50] Humphrey, RK; Bucay, N; Beattie, GM; Lopez, A; Messam, CA; Cirulli, V; Hayek, A. Characterization and isolation of promoter-defined nestin-positive cells from the human fetal pancreas. *Diabetes*, 2003, 52, 2519-2525.

[51] Rajagopal, J; Anderson, WJ; Kume, S; Martínez, OI; Melton, DA. Insulin staining of ES cell progeny from insulin uptake. *Science*, 2003, 299, 363.

[52] Kahan, BW; Jacobson, LM; Hullett, DA; Ochoada, JM; Oberley, TD; Lang, KM; Odorico, JS. Pancreatic precursors and differentiated islet cell types from murine embryonic stem cells. An in vitro model to study islet differentiation. *Diabetes*, 2003, 52, 2016-2024.

[53] Skoudy, A; Rovira, M; Savatier, P; Martin, F; Leon-Quinto, T; Soria, B; Real, FX. Transforming growth factor (TGF)β, fibroblast growth factor (FGF) and retinoid signaling pathways promote pancreatic exocrine gene expression in mouse embryonic stem cells. *Biochemical Journal*, 2004, 379, 749-756.

[54] Ensenat-Waser, R; Santana, A; Paredes, B; Zenke, M; Reig, JA; Roche, E. Embryonic stem cell processing in obtaining insulin-producing cells: A technical review. *Cell Preservation Technology*, 2006, 4, 278-289.

[55] Kubo, A; Shinozaki, K; Shannon, JM; Kouskoff, V; Kennedy, M; Woo, S; Fehling, HJ; Keller, G. Development of definitive endoderm from embryonic stem cells in culture. *Development*, 2004, 131, 1651-1662.

[56] Vincent, R; Treff, N; Budde, M; Kastenberg, Z; Odorico, J. Generation and characterization of novel tetracycline-inducible pancreatic transcription factor-expressing murine embryonic stem cell lines. *Stem Cells Development*, 2006, 15, 953-962.

[57] D'Amour, KA; Agulnick, AD; Eliazer, S; Kelly, OG; Kroon, E; Baetge, EE. Efficient differentiation of human embryonic stem cells to definitive endoderm. *Nature Biotechnology*, 2005, 23, 1534-1541.

[58] Madsen OD, Serup P. Towards cell therapy for diabetes. *Nature Biotechnology*, 2006, 24, 1481-1483.

[59] Ku, HT; Zhang, N; Kubo, A; O'Connor, R; Mao, M; Keller, G; Bromberg, JS. Committing embryonic stem cells to early endocrine pancreas in vitro. *Stem Cells*, 2004, 22, 1205-1217.

[60] Milne, HM; Burns, CJ; Kitsou-Mylona, I; Luther, MJ; Minger, SL; Persaud, SJ; Jones, PM. Generation of insulin-expressing cells from mouse embryonic stem cells. *Biochemical and Biophysical Research Communications*, 2005, 328, 399-403.

[61] Yasunaga, M; Tada, S; Torikai-Nishikawa, S; Nakano, Y; Okada, M; Jakt, LM; Nishikawa, S; Chiba, T; Era, T; Nishikawa, S-I. Induction and monitoring of definitive and visceral endoderm differentiation of mouse ES cells. *Nature Biotechnology*, 2005, 23, 1542-1550.

[62] Shook, D; Keller, R. Mechanisms, mechanics and function of epithelial-mesenchymal transitions in early development. *Mechanisms of Development*, 2003, 120, 1351-1383.

[63] Yamanaka, Y; Ralston, A; Stephenson, RO; Rossant, J. Cell and molecular regulation of the mouse blastocyst. *Developmental Dynamics*, 2006, 235, 2301-2314.

[64] Gadue, P; Huber, TL; Paddison, PJ; Keller, GM. Wnt and TGF-β signaling are required for the induction of an in vitro model of primitive streak formation using embryonic stem cells. *Proceedings of the National Academy of Sciences of USA*, 2006, 103, 16806-16811.

[65] Inman, KE; Downs, KM. Localization of brachyury (T) in embryonic and extraembryonic tissues during mouse gastrulation. *Gene Expression Patterns*, 2006, 6, 783-793.

[66] Tada, S; Era, T; Furusawa, C; Sakurai, H; Nishikawa, S; Kinoshita, M; Nakao, K; Chiba, T; Nishikawa, S-I. Characterization of mesendoderm: a diverging point of the definitive endoderm and mesoderm in embryonic stem cell differentiation culture. *Development*, 2005, 132, 4363-4374.

[67] McLean, AB; D'Amour, KA; Jones, KL; Krishnamoorthy, M; Kulik, MJ; Reynolds, DM; Sheppard, AM; Liu, H; Xu, Y; Baetge, EE; Dalton, S. Activin A efficiently specifies definitive endoderm from human embryonic stem cells only when phosphatidylinositol 3-kinase signaling is suppressed. *Stem Cells*, 2007, 25, 29-38.

[68] Wang, L; Schulz, TC; Sherrer, ES; Dauphin, DS; Shin, S; Nelson, AM; Ware, CB; Zhan, M; Song, CZ; Chen, X; Brimble, SN; McLean, A; Galeano, MJ; Uhl, EW; D'Amour, KA; Chesnut, JD; Rao, MS; Balu, CA; Robins, AJ. Self-renewal of human embryonic stem cells requires insulin-like growth factor-1 receptor and ERBB2 receptor signaling. *Blood*, 2007, doi: 10.1182/blood-2007-03-082586.

[69] Nguyen, TT; Sheppard, AM; Kaye, PL; Noakes, PG. IGF-1 and insulin activate mitogen-activated protein kinase via the type 1 IGF receptor in mouse embryonic stem cells. *Reproduction*, 2007, 134, 41-49.

[70] Baqir, S; Smith, LC. Growth restricted in vitro culture conditions alter the imprinted gene expression patterns of mouse embryonic stem cells. *Cloning and Stem Cells*, 2003, 5, 199-212.

[71] Gouon-Evans, V; Boussemart, L; Gadue, P; Nierhoff, D; Koehler; CI; Kubo, A; Shafritz, DA; Keller, G. BMP-4 is required for hepatic specification of mouse embryonic stem cell-derived definitive endoderm. *Nature Biotechnology*, 2006, 24, 1402-1411.

[72] McKiernan, E; O'Driscoll, L; Kasper, M; Barron, N; O'Sullivan, F; Clynes, M. Directed differentiation of mouse embryonic stem cells into pancreatic-like or neuronal- and glial-like phenotypes. *Tissue Engineering*, 2007, 13, 2419-2430.

[73] Shim, JH; Kim, SE; Woo, DH; Kim, SK; Oh, CH; McKay, R; Kim, JH. Directed differentiation of human embryonic stem cells towards a pancreatic cell fate. *Diabetologia*, 2007, 50, 1228-1238.

[74] Phillips, BW; Hentze, H; Rust, WL; Chen, QP; Chipperfield, H; Tan, EK; Abraham, S; Sadasivam, A; Soong, PL; Wang, ST; Lim, R; Sun, W; Colman, A; Dunn, NR. Directed differentiation of human embryonic stem cells into the pancreatic endocrine lineage. *Stem Cells and Development*, 2007, 16, 561-578.

[75] Jiang, J; Au, M; Lu, K; Eshpeter, A; Korbutt, G; Fisk, G; Majumdar, AS. Generation of insulin-producing islet-like clusters form human embryonic stem cells. *Stem Cells*, 2007, 25, 1940-1953.

[76] Jiang, W; Shi, Y; Zhao, D; Chen, S; Yong, J; Zhang, J; Qing, T; Sun, X; Zhang, P; Ding, M; Li, D; Deng, H. In vitro derivation of functional insulin-producing cells from human embryonic stem cells. *Cell Research*, 2007, 17, 333-344.

[77] Nakanishi, M; Hamazaki, TS; Komazaki, S; Okochi, H; Asashima, M. Pancreatic tissue formation from murine embryonic stem cells in vitro. *Differentiation*, 2007, 75, 1-11.

[78] Bai, I; Meredith, G; Tuch, BE. Glucagon-like peptide-1 enhances production of insulin in insulin-producing cells derived from mouse embryonic stem cells. *Journal of Endocrinology*, 2005, 186, 343-352.

[79] Schroeder, IS; Rolletschek, A; Blyszczuk, P; Kania, G; Wobus, AM. Differentiation of mouse embryonic stem cells to insulin-producing cells. *Nature Protocols*, 2006, 1, 495-507.

[80] Mfopou, JK; De Groote, V; Xu, X; Heimberg, H; Bouwens, L. Sonic hedgehog and other soluble factors from differentiating embryoid bodies inhibit pancreas development. *Stem Cells*, 2007, 25, 1156-1165.

[81] Mfopou, JK; Bouwens, L. Hedgehog signals in pancreatic differentiation from embryonic stem cells: revisiting the neglected. *Differentiation*, 2007, doi: 10.1111/j.1432-0436.2007.00191.x.

[82] Wang, H; Brun, T; Kataoka, K; Sharma, AJ; Wollheim, CB. MAFA controls genes implicated in insulin biosynthesis and secretion. *Diabetologia*, 2007, 50, 348-358.

[83] Brolén, GKC; Heins, N; Edsbagge, J; Semb, H. Signals from the embryonic mouse pancreas induce differentiation of human embryonic stem cells into insulin-producing β-cell-like cells. *Diabetes*, 54, 2005, 2867-2874.

[84] Rivas-Carrillo, JD; Okitsu, T; Tanaka, N; Kobayashi, N. Pancreas development and beta-cell differentiation of embryonic stem cells. *Current Medicinal Chemistry*, 2007, 14, 1573-1578.

[85] Takeshita, F; Kodama, M; Yamamoto, H; Ikarashi, Y; Ueda, S; Teratani, T; Yamamoto, Y; Tamatani, T; Kanegasaki, S; Ochiya, T; Quinn, G. Streptozotocin-induced partial beta cell depletion in nude mice without hyperglycemia induces pancreatic morphogenesis in transplanted embryonic stem cells. *Diabeteologia*, 2006, 49, 2948-2958.

[86] Vaca, P; Martin, F; Vegara-Meseguer, JM; Rovira, JM; Berna, G; Soria, B. Induction of differentiation of embryonic stem cells into insulin secreting cells by fetal soluble factors. *Stem Cells*, 2006, 24, 258-265.

[87] Banerjee, M; Kanitkar, M; Bhonde, RR. Approaches towards endogenous pancreatic regeneration. *The Review of Diabetic Studies*, 2005, 2, 165-176.

[88] Ackermann, AM; Gannon, M. Molecular regulation of pancreatic β-cell mass development, maintenance, and expansion. *Journal of Molecular Endocrinology*, 2007, 38, 193-206.

[89] Dor, Y; Brown, J; Martínez, OI; Melton, DA. Adult pancreatic β-cells are formed by self-duplication rather than stem-cell differentiation. *Nature*, 2004, 429, 41-46.

[90] Atkinson, MA; Rhodes, CJ. Pancreatic regeneration in type I diabetes: dreams on a deserted islet? *Diabetologia*, 2005, 48, 2200-2202.

[91] Hao, E; Tyrberg, B; Itkin-Ansari, P; Lakey, JR; Geron, I; Monosov, EZ; Barcova, M; Mercola, M; Levine, F. Beta-cell differentiation from nonendocrine epithelial cells of the adult human pancreas. *Nature Medicine*, 2006, 12, 310-316.

[92] Rafaeloff, R; Pittenger, GL; Barlow, SW; Qin, XF; Yan, B; Rosenberg, L; Duguid, WP; Vinik, AI. Cloning and sequencing of the pancreatic islet neogenesis associated protein (INGAP) gene and its expression in islet neogenesis in hamsters. *Journal of Clinical Investigation*, 1997, 99, 2100-2109.

[93] Kaneto, H; Miyatsuka, T; Shiraiwa, T; Yamamoto, K; Kato, K; Fujitani, Y; Matsuoka; TA. Crucial role of PDX-1 in pancreas development, beta-cell differentiation, and induction of surrogate beta-cells. *Current Medicinal Chemistry*, 2007, 14, 1745-1752.

[94] Taguchi, M; Yamaguchi, T; Otsuki, M. Induction of PDX-1-positive cells in the main duct during regeneration after acute necrotizing pancreatitis in rats. *Journal of Pathology*, 2002, 197, 638-646.

[95] Kritzik, MR; Jones, E; Chen, Z; Krakowski, M; Krahl, T; Good, A; Wright, C; Fox, H; Sarvetnick, N. PDX-1 and Msx-2 expression in the regenerating and developing pancreas. *Journal of Endocrinology*, 1999, 163, 523-530.

[96] Bonner-Weir, S; Sharma, A. pancreatic stem cells. *Journal of Pathology*, 2002, 197, 519-526.

[97] Ishiwata, T; Kudo, M; Onda M; Fujii, T; Teduka, K; Suzuki, T; Korc, M; Naito, Z. Defined localization of nestin-expressing cells in L-arginine-induced acute pancreatitis. *Pancreas*, 2006, 32, 360-368.

[98] Takayama, I; Miyazaki, S; Tashiro, F; Fujikura, J; Miyazaki, J; Yamato, E. Pdx-1 independent differentiation of mouse embryonic stem cells into insulin-expressing cells. *Diabetes Research and Clinical Practice*, 2007, doi: 10.1016/j.diabres.2007.08.013.

[99] Gershengorn, MC; Hardikar, AA; Hardikar, A; Wei, C; Geras-Raaka, E; Marcus-Samuels, B; Raaka, BM. Epithelial-to-mesenchymal transition generates proliferative human islet precursor cells. *Science*, 2004, 306, 2261-2264.

[100] Davani, B; Ikonomou, L; Raaka, BM; Geras-Raaka, E; Morton, RA; Marcus-Samuels, B; Gershengorn, MC. Human islet-derived precursor cells are mesenchymal stromal cells that differentiate and mature to hormone-expressing cells in vivo. *Stem Cells*, 2007, doi: 0: 2007-0323v1.

[101] Atouf, F; Park, CH; Pechhold, K; Ta, M; Choi, Y; Lumeelsky, NL. No evidence for mouse pancreatic beta-cell epithelial-mesenchymal transition in vitro. *Diabetes*, 2007, 56, 699-702.

[102] Chase, LG; Ulloa-Montoya, F; Kidder, BL; Verfaille, CM. Islet-derived fibroblast-like cells are not derived via epithelial-mesenchymal transition from Pdx-1 or insulin-positive cells. *Diabetes*, 2007, 56, 3-7.

[103] Eberhardt, M; Salmon, P; von Mach, MA; Hengstler, JG; Brulport, M; Linscheid, P; Seboek, D; Oberholzer, J; Barbero, A; Martin, I; Müller, B; Trono, D; Zulewski, H. Multipotential nestin and Isl-1 positive mesenchymal stem cells isolated from human pancreatic islets. *Biochemical and Biophyical Research Communications*, 2006, 345, 1167-1176.

[104] Weinberg, N; Ouziel-Yahalom, L; Knoller, S; Efrat, S; Dor, Y. Lineage tracing evidence for in vitro dedifferentiation but rare proliferation of mouse pancreatic beta-cells. *Diabetes*, 2007, 56, 1299-1304.

[105] D'Alessandro, JS; Lu, K; Fung, BP; Colman, A; Clarke, DL. Rapid and efficient in vitro generation of pancreatic islet progenitor cells from nonendocrine epithelial cells in the adult human pancreas. *Stem Cells and Development*, 2007, 16, 75-89.

[106] Teta, M; Rankin MM; Long, SY; Stein, GM; Kushner, JA. Growth and regeneration of adult beta-cells does not involve specialized progenitors. *Developmental Cell*, 2007, 12, 817-826.

[107] Kayali, AG; Flores, LE; Lopez, AD; Kutlu, B; Baetge, E; Kitamura, R; Hao, E; Beattie, GM; Hayek, A. Limited capacity of human adult islets expanded in vitro to redifferentiate into insulin-producing beta-cells. *Diabetes*, 2007, 56, 703-708.

[108] Tiemann, K; Panienka, R; Kloppel, G. Expression of transcription factors and precursor cell markers during regeneration of beta-cells in pancreata of rats treated with streptozotocin. *Virchows Archives*, 2007, 450, 261-266.

[109] Efrat, S. Prospects for gene therapy of insulin-dependent diabetes mellitus. *Diabetologia*, 1998, 41, 1401-1409.

[110] Choi, JB; Uchino, H; Azuma, K; Iwashita, N; Tanaka, Y; Mochizuki, H; Migita, M; Shimada, T; Kawamori, R; Watada, H. Little evidence of transdifferentiation of bone marrow-derived cells into pancreatic beta cells. *Diabetologia*, 2003, 46, 1366-1374.

[111] Lechner, A; Yang, Y-Q; Blacken, RA; Wang, L; Nolan, AL; Habener, JF. No evidence for significant transdifferentiation of bone marrow into pancreatic β-cells in vivo. *Diabetes*, 2004, 53, 616-623.

[112] Hasegawa, Y; Ogihara, T; Yamada, T; Ishigaki, Y; Imai, J; Uno, K; Gao, J; Kaneko, K; Ishihara, H; Sasano, H; Nakauchi, H; Oka, Y; Katagiri, H. Bone marrow (BM) transplantation promotes beta-cell regeneration after acute injury through BM cell mobilization. *Endocrinology*, 2007, 148, 2006-2015.

[113] Butler, AE; Huang, A; Rao, PN; Bhushan, A; Hogan, WJ; Rizza, RA; Butler, PC. Hematopoietic stem cells derived from adult donors are not a source of pancreatic beta-cells in adult nondiabetic humans. *Diabetes*, 2007, 56, 1810-1816.

[114] Lavazais, E; Pogu, S; Sai, P; Martignat, L. Cytokine mobilization of bone marrow cells and pancreatic lesion do not improve streptozotocin-induced diabetes in mice by transdifefrentiation of bone marrow cells into insulin-producing cells. *Diabetes Metabolism*, 2007, 33, 68-78.

[115] D'Ippolito, G; Diabira, S; Howard, GA; Menei, P; Roos, BA; Schiller, PC. Marrow-isolated adult multilineage inducible (MIAMI) cells, a unique population of postnatal young and old human cells with extensive expansion and differentiation potential. *Journal of Cellular Science*, 2004, 117, 2971-2981.

[116] Tayaramma, T; Ma, B; Rohde, M; Mayer, H. Chromatin-remodeling factors allow differentiation of bone marrow cells into insulin-producing cells. *Stem Cells*, 2006, 24, 2858-2867.

[117] Moriscot, C; De Fraipont, F; Richard, M-J; Marchand, M; Svatier, P; Bosco, D; Favrot, M; Benhamou, P-Y. Human bone marrow mesenchymal stem cells can express insulin and key transcription factors of the endocrine pancreas developmental pathway upon

genetic and/or microenvironmental manipulation in vitro. *Stem Cells*, 2005, 23, 594-604.

[118] Karnieli, O; Izhar-Prato, Y; Bulvik, S; Efrat, S. Generation of insulin-producing cells from human bone marrow mesenchymal stem cells by genetic manipulation. *Stem Cells*, 2007, doi: 0: 2007-0164v1.

[119] Yu, S; Li, C; Xin-guo, H; wei-kai, H; Jian-jun, D; Lei, S; Kuan-xiao, T; Bin, W; Jun, S; Hui, L; Ke-xin, W. Differentiation of bone marrow-derived mesenchymal stem cells from diabetic patients into insulin-producing cells in vitro. *Chinese Medical Journal*, 2007, 120, 771-776.

[120] Timper, K; Seboek, D; Eberhardt, M; Linscheid, P; Christ-Crain, M; Keller, U; Muller, B; Zulewski, H. Human adipose tissue-derived mesenchymal stem cells differentiate into insulin, somatostatin, and glucagon expressing cells. *Biochemical and Biophysical Research Communications*, 2006, 341, 1135-1140.

[121] Ruhnke, M; Ungefroren, H; Nussler, A; Martin, F; Brulport, M; Schorman, W; Hengstler, JG; Klapper, W; Ulrichs, K; Hutchinson, JA; Soria, B; Parwaresch, RM; Heeckt, P; Kremer, B; Fändrich, F. Differentiation of in vitro-modified human peripheral blood monocytes into hepatocyte-like and pancreatic islet-like cells. *Gastroenterology*, 2005, 128, 1774-1786.

[122] Zhao, Y; Huang, Z; Lazzarini, P; Wang, Y; Di, A; Chen, M. A unique human blood-derived cell population displays high potencial for producing insulin. *Biochemical and Biophysical Research Communications*, 2007, 360, 205-211.

[123] Yang, L; Li, S; Hatch, H; Ahrens, K; Cornelius, JG; Petersen, BE; Peck, AB. In vitro trans-differentiation of adult hepatic stem cells into pancreatic endocrine hormone-producing cells. *Proceedings of the National Academy of Sciences of USA*, 2002, 99, 8078-8083.

[124] Kim, S; Shin, JS; Kim, HJ; Fisher, RC; Lee, MJ; Kim, CW. Streptozotocin-induced diabetes can be reversed by hepatic oval cell activation through hepatic transdifferentiation and pancreatic islet regeneration. *Laboratory Investigation*, 2007, 87, 702-712.

[125] Herrera, MB; Bruno, S; Buttiglieri, S; Tetta, C; Gatti, S; Deregibus, MC; Bussolati, B; Camussi, G. Isolation and characterization of a stem cell population from adult human liver. *Stem Cells*, 2006, 24, 2840-2850.

[126] Zalzman, M; Gupta, S; Giri, RK; Berkovich, I; Sappal, BS; Karnieli, O; Zern, MA; Fleischer, N; Efrat, S. Reversal of hyperglycemia in mice by using human expandable insulin-producing cells differentiated from fetal liver progenitor cells. *Proceedings of the National Academy of Sciences of USA*, 2003, 100, 7253-7258.

[127] Shternhall-Ron, K; Quintana, FJ; Perl, S; Meivar-Levy, I; Barshack, I; Cohen, IR; Ferber, S. Ectopic PDX-1 expression in liver ameliorates type 1 diabetes. *Journal of Autoimmunity*, 2007, 28, 134-142.

[128] Dutton, JR; Chillingworth, NL; Eberhard, D; Brannon, CR; Hornsey, MA; Tosh, D; Slack, JM. Beta cells occur naturally in extrahepatic bile ducts of mice. *Journal of Cell Science*, 2007, 120, 239-245.

[129] Kojima, H; Nakamura, T; Fujita, Y; Kishi, A; Fujimiya, M; Yamada, S; Kudo, M; Nishio, Y; Maegawa, H; Haneda, M; Yasuda, H; Kojima, I; Seno, M; Wong, NC;

Kikkawa, R; Kashiwagi, A. Combined expression of pancreatic duodenal homeobox 1 and islet factor 1 induces immature enterocytes to produce insulin. *Diabetes*, 2002, 51, 1398-1408.

[130] Han, J; Lee, HH; Kwon, H; Shin, S; Yoon, JW; Jun, HS. Engineered enteroendocrine cells secrete insulin in response to glucose and reverse hyperglycemia in diabetic mice. *Molecular Therapy*, 2007, 15, 1195-1202.

Chapter XII

MESENCHYMAL STEM CELL BASED THERAPY IN LIVER DISEASE

I. Aurich[1], M. Sgodda[2] and H. Aurich[2]
[1]Martin Luther University Halle-Wittenberg NBL3
Research Group NWG6, Department of Medicine, Germany
[2]Martin Luther University Halle-Wittenberg,
First Department of Internal Medicine, Germany

ABSTRACT

The use of primary human hepatocytes for cell therapy of liver diseases is limited because of the restricted availability of marginal donor organs. Hence, novel cell sources are required to gain hepatocytes of adequate quality and quantity for clinical use. Due to the plasticity and potential to proliferate, stem cells isolated from various origins may be an alternative source to generate functional hepatocytes suitable for clinical use. Within the last decade, different protocols have been published to investigate the potential of adult stem cells to differentiate into hepatocyte-like cells. In contrast, protocols using embryonic stem cells (ESC) still struggle with the problem of tumorigenicity, and major ethical concerns restrict the applicability of human embryonic stem cells. Hence, research focused on adult hematopoietic (HSC) and mesenchymal stem cells (MSC). Regarding availability, in vitro proliferation, cultivation and differentiation, MSC are usually prefered over HSC. The specific surface expression pattern (CD34, CD45, CD105) is clearly different in the two types of stem cells. After expansion of MSC in vitro, the differentiation into hepatocyte-like cells proceeds with treatment applying specific growth factors and supplements. The level of hepatogenic differentiation is indicated by the loss of progenitor cell markers (CX43, CK7, CK19, alpha fetoprotein) and the increase in expression of hepatogenic markers (CK18, CX32, HepPar I, CD26, CYP) as well as hepatocyte-specific functions (urea synthesis, detoxification, albumin expression, storage of polyhydrocarbons). Different animal models have been used to investigate the integration and repopulation of transplanted MSC into injured livers. The hepatogenic differentiated MSC results in an improved integration into the liver parenchyma. After transplantation into regenerating mouse livers, MSC continue to express hepatocyte-specific functions. Besides others, the detection of human serum albumin in the mouse serum and the activation of liver specific promoters indicate a functionality of transplanted human stem cell-derived hepatocytes in the host mouse liver. Thus it is expected that MSC may become a useful source for hepatocyte regeneration in liver-cell therapy.

INTRODUCTION

Every year millions of people die due to end-stage liver diseases despite major advances in the fields of immunology and transplantation. Liver diseases are caused by autoimmune reactions [1], malignant transformation [2], infection agents [3], genetic defects [4], or secondary effects [5]. Liver transplantation is the only effective way that significantly improves the prognosis of patients with end-stage hepatic insufficiency. However, liver replacement is an extremely aggressive form of treatment and requires life-long immunosuppression. Furthermore, the growing disparity between available donor organs and the large number of patients waiting for transplantations gave rise to develop alternative therapies. Recent studies suggest that liver cell transplantation may be a promising option for the treatment of liver failure. However, the numbers of livers available for hepatocyte isolation are limited as are for whole organ transplantation [6]. Residual segments from liver transplants and organs not suitable for transplantation are the usual source of isolated hepatocytes. Fatty livers do not yield liver cells of good quality nor is the number of cells usually sufficient for transplantation [7]. Cryopreserved isolated hepatocytes from multiple donors would increase the number of available cells. However, liver cells after cryopreservation have been shown to engraft worse than freshly isolated hepatocytes [8] and additionally their viability following cryopreservation is poor [9].

Hepatocyte transplantation very rarely resulted in a significant therapeutic outcome in human clinical trials caused by the difficulty to expand hepatocytes *in vitro* and their insufficient numbers to achieve measurable biological effects. Additionally, cultivated primary hepatocytes tend towards dedifferentiation resulting in a short life-span and the rapid loss of liver-specific functions although the methods of their long-term cultivation have been improved in order to delay the rapid loss of the initial hepatic functions [10, 11]. Nevertheless, only hepatocytes immortalized by gene transfer are capable of long-term growth and correcting metabolic defects and thus counteracting liver failure [7, 12, 13].

Because of the difficulties reviewed above the regenerative medicine may be a promising approach for the development of stem-cell-based cell and gene therapy to recreate liver functions [14].

The multipotential differentiation capacity of stem cells, their simple isolation, culture and especially the possibility to expand them *in vitro* make these cells attractive for cell and gene therapy in clinical applications.

Stem cells are cells from embryonic, fetal, or adult origin which under certain conditions have the ability to proliferate themselves for long periods or, in the case of adult stem cells, throughout the life span of the organism.

Stem cells are distinguished from other cell types by the ability to divide for indefinite periods (self replication). Due to the conditions of culture, stem cells are able to differentiate into many different cell types. They have the potency to develop into various mature cells with the respective characteristic shapes and specialized functions.

EMBRYONIC STEM CELLS

The embryonic stem cells (ESC) can self-replicate and are pluripotent – they can give rise to cells derived from all three embryonic germ layers – mesoderm, endoderm, and ectoderm. ESC can be isolated from the inner cell mass of blastocysts. The first study on the isolation of ESC from human blastocytes was published in 1994 [15]. Afterwards, techniques for isolating and culturing human ESC have been refined [16, 17]. The ability to isolate human ESC from blastocysts and retain them in culture highly depends on the integrity, development state, and condition of the blastocyst from which they are isolated. In general, blastocysts with a large and distinct inner cell mass in most cases result in highly efficient stem cell culture. Once the inner cell mass is received from either mice or human blastocysts, the techniques for culturing ESC are similar. The cells are plated in culture dishes containing growth medium which is supplemented with fetal bovine serum (FBS) on feeder cell layers (mouse or human fibroblasts) that had been irradiated to prevent their replication. After the cell mass had been divided and formed clumps, peripher cells were dissociated and replated in the same culture conditions. Much work was done to demonstrate the pluripotency of isolated ESC. Thus, mouse ESC injected subcutaneously in genetically identical or immunodeficient mice develop into teratomas. These tumors contain cell types from all three germ layers (epithelial cells, muscle cells, bone or neural tissue cells) and form typical gut-like structures. Embryonic stem cells can proliferate indefinitely, a characteristic they do not share with adult stem cells.

Thus one of the current advantages regarding the use of these cells for clinical applications is their unlimited ability to proliferate *in vitro*. Studies indicate the possibility to cultivate human ESC for more than one year in serum free medium on feeder cells. Furthermore they are able to generate a wide range of cell types through directed differentiation. A striking disadvantage of the use of ESC for cell therapy in humans is the tendency of undifferentiated cells to form teratomas. The tumor formations have been demonstrated to be avoided by removing any undifferentiated cells prior to transplantation.

However, the isolation of ESC destroys the early embryo at an early stage; for this reason, stem cell research requires profound ethical guidelines. The use of human embryos for research on ESC is broadly discussed on the ethical and political agenda in many countries. Despite the potential benefit of using human ESC for therapies, their use remains highly controversial. For this reason, there is increasing interest in discovering alternative, non-embryonic sources of stem cells.

ADULT STEM CELLS

Adult stem cells are promising candidates for tissue regeneration and their usage overcomes the obstacles of embryonic stem cells, such as ethical concerns and risks of rejection. In the adult stage, stem cells have been considered to be completely determined in their development depending on the tissue in which they grow. This rather view has been revised during the last few years. It has been found that stem cells apart from characteristics of the tissue in which they reside, may also give rise to get nonrelated properties [18, 19]. In this context hematopoietic stem cells which generally produce blood cells have additionally been shown to differentiate into hepatic oval cells [20]. Mesenchymal stem cells generally characterized to differentiate into many cells of the mesenchymal phenotype can be processed to non-mesenchymal cells like neural cells [21]. During development, growth and repair the adult organism apparently has the ability to recruit progenitor cells from other tissues. In case of muscle repair mesenchymal stem cells migrate into skeletal muscles [22].

Adult stem cells are undifferentiated cells in differentiated tissues. They renew themselves, and become specialized to yield all of the cell types of the tissue from which it originated. Adult stem cells are capable of making identical copies of themselves for the lifetime of the organism. Typically, adult stem cells generate one or several intermediate cell types, the so called precursor or progenitor cells, before they achieve their final state of full differentiation. The primary functions of adult stem cells are to maintain the steady state functioning of their undifferentiated forms, in part to replace cells in damaged or diseased tissues.

HEMATOPOIETIC STEM CELLS

The most widely studied adult stem cells are hematopoietic stem cells (HSC) sustaining the formation of the blood and the cellular immune systems. Compared to adult stem cells from other tissues, HSC are easier to obtain, as they can either be recovered directly out of the bone marrow or stimulated to move into the peripheral blood stream by the application of certain cytokines, where they can be easily collected. The main reason making it difficult to purify stem cells is that they are extremely rare. Only 1 in every 10,000 to 15,000 estimated bone marrow cells is thought to be a stem cell. In blood stream the proportion changes to only about 1 in 100,000 blood cells. Like bone marrow, umbilical cord blood is another source enriched of hematopoietic stem cells. The HSC from umbilical cord blood are usually regarded as neonatal stem cells since their degree of maturity is lower than of those stem cells found in the bone marrow of adults or children. The advantages of using stem cells from cord blood as a source are their non-invasive isolation and their abundance in cord blood. HSC are potentially immortal by renewing themselves, migrate out of the bone marrow into the circulating blood, undergo apoptosis, and can differentiate to a variety of cells.

Many groups have reported on the genomic plasticity of HSC enabling them to switch between hematopoietic and non-hematopoietic lineages which make these cells attractive for cellular therapeutic applications. In this context several studies have demonstrated that marrow-derived cells can differentiate into skeletal muscle cells [22-24], into brain cells [25-28], into kidney and lung cells [29-31] as well as into liver cells [20, 32-34]

Because HSC in cell culture look and behave like ordinary white blood cells it is difficult to identify them by means of morphology. Their identification highly depends on the expression of cell-surface markers which have been identified to HSC.

MESENCHYMAL STEM CELLS

The focus of using stem cells in cell therapy has currently shifted to mesenchymal stem cells.

Mesenchymal stem cells (MSC) were first described by Friedenstein *et al.* in 1976 as clonal, plastic-adherent cells being a source of the osteoblastic, adipogenic and chondrogenic cell lines [35]. Mesenchymal stem cells are characterized by dividing without limits and exhibit a high degree of plasticity. Beside from bone marrow [36], they have been isolated from normal blood [37], umbilical cord blood [38], placenta [39, 40], scalp tissue [41], amniotic fluid [42], fetal tissues (43), and adipose tissue [44, 45]. Regarding ethical matters the use of adult stem cells is favourable over fetal stem cells or embryonic stem cells. All these MSC can differentiate *in vitro* into multiple types of lineages such as chondrogenic, osteogenic, adipogenic [36], myogenic [22], neurogenic [46], and hepatogenic [47-50] cells depending on the microenvironment in which they reside.

There is one apparent advantage in using MSC for cell therapy: they can easily be harvested from various tissues. In addition to long-term self renewal capability, MSC possess a versatile differentiation potential and a vast expansion capacity. They are characterized by a stable population doubling and low levels of senescence.

The traditional bone marrow puncture of more than a few millilitres may be painful and requires a general or spinal anaesthesia. Only a small percentage (0.01 to 0.001%) of the total number of isolated mononuclear cells from bone marrow has been shown to be MSC [36]. Thus, autologous bone marrow isolation has clear limitations.

Alternatively adipose tissue is an attractive source of multipotent human MSC. They are under local anesthesia obtainable in large quantities, with minimal discomfort. Adipose tissue-derived stem cells are considered as the multipotent fraction of fibroblast-like adherent cells, which, after isolation of the adipose stromal vascular fraction, attach to plastic culture dishes [35, 51]. Recent, studies have demonstrated that adipose-derived stem cells are similar regarding proliferation and differentiation to bone marrow-derived stem cells. Although they are more heterogeneous [52], they reveal a similar antigen marker profile [53-56], and have a similar differentiation potential [53, 57-62].

ISOLATION OF MSC

As mentioned above, MSC are found in the peripheral blood, umbilical cord blood, bone-marrow, subcutaneous, and peritoneal fat tissue. The techniques to isolate the MSC differ even as MSC were isolated from the same origin. The different published protocols of MSC isolation result in a homogenous population as well as in higher yield of MSC.

For the first step of MSC isolation from blood cell suspension like peripheral, umbilical cord blood stem cells or bone marrow it is necessary to prevent coagulation by adding citrate buffer [63] or heparin [64] to the aspirate. In order to increase the yield of MSC isolated from fat tissue or the yield of umbilical cord blood stem cells the tissue must be disintegrated by a collagenase typ I digestion [45, 52, 61, 65-67]. The digestion of the minced tissue is done in a 0,075% collagenase type 1 solution for 30 min at 37 °C and stopped by adding 4 % FBS. To remove cell debris and undigested material the suspension is filtered through a 100-140 μm nylon mesh [52, 61, 65].

The single cell suspensions received from umbilical cord blood, peripheral blood, bone marrow or fat tissue are further treated by one to three washing steps to remove undesirable material like heparin, citrate, fat cells, and FBS. Furthermore the cells are concentrated and can be applied for further steps.

To separate the MSC from other cells, the suspension is loaded onto a density gradient usually Percoll with 1.047 – 1.077 g/ml and centrifuged for 20-30 min at 300 – 500 x g [36, 63-65, 68-71]. The resulting interphase of mononuclear cells contains the MSC among other mononuclear cells. To further enrich MSC it is possible to remove contaminating cells by negative immunodepletion with antibodies against antigens not expressed on the surface of MSC but on mature blood cells like CD3, CD14, CD38 [68, 71]. Alternatively or in addition it is possible to isolate MSC by positive immunodepletion with antibodies against antigens only expressed on these cells like the CD105 antigen [69].

The last step of the isolation procedure is the selection of the MSC by plastic adherence on culture dishes. The long-term plastic adherence separates the MSC from non-adherent cells like lymphocytes and hard to handle cells like HSC. This leads to a homogeneous MSC population after removing the non-adherent cells by several washing steps (Figure 1). The choice of the expansion media is a critical step for a successful MSC culture. The composition of a suitable medium shows many variations according different authors. Several components are well described and necessary for successful MSC culture. Most of the media consist of the commercial available media Dulbeccos Modified Eagle Medium (DMEM) with high glucose (HG) [57, 70, 72] or a mixture of 60 % DMEM with low glucose (LG) and 40 % of the even commercial available media MCDB-201 (61, 63, 65, 73). A critical point seems to be the composition of the supplements to be added to the media. Essential supplements are apparently ascorbic acid 2-phosphat, dexamethasone, FBS at 10-15 % final concentration [57, 61, 63, 65, 73], transferrin and linolenic acid [57, 63, 65]. Some supplements like Insulin-Transferrin-Sodium Selenit (ITS) or epidermal growth factor (EGF) were used in expansion media [61] or in differentiation media [63, 65].

Cells attached on the plastic surface show a fibroblast like morphology during their proliferation and form colonies (Figure 2). These colony forming units (CFU-F) were first described in 1976 by Friedenstein *et al* [35] as clonogenic fibroblast precursor cells and about 20 years later termed "mesenchymal stem cell" [74]. After an expansion time of about 5-7 days leading to a maximal confluence of 50 % MSC have to be passaged and analysed for their stem cell character by fluorescence activated cell sorting (FACS), gene array, or proteomics. Furthermore it is necessary to split the MSC culture after 5-7 days to prevent them from spontaneous differentiation and to retain their stem cell potential. In different studies the spontaneous differentiation of MSC into different lineages are described [75-77]. The time point of the loss of stem cell character and the start of differentiation is a progressive junction depending on the confluence and/or the time period for which the cells have been cultured according to the lineage and the origin of the stem cells.

However, it is no problem to cryopreserve the MSC in FBS supplemented with 10 % dimethylsulfoxide (DMSO) in liquid nitrogen for further applications.

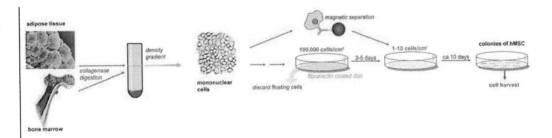

Figure 1. Isolation of human MSC from bone marrow or adipose tissue. Cells were selected by density gradient centrifugation, magnetic sorting and plastic adherence.

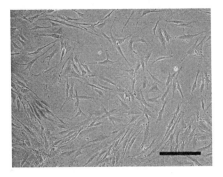

Figure 2. Fibroblast-like morphology of mesenchymal stem cells isolated from human bone marrow 2 days after isolation (bar = 50 μm).

FACS Isolation and Characterisation of MSC

During the expansion phase, the isolated MSC are just selected by the adhesion on polystyrene plastic culture dishes optionally coated with fibronectin. A special importance is the composition of the culture media for maintenance of the cells for maintaining their morphology as fibroblast like cells. Therefore it is necessary to determine the character of MSC regarding their cell surface molecules or their gene expression pattern after the expansion. Protein arrays or gene chip analyses of MSC are time- and costs-consuming procedures. Furthermore it takes a lot of the isolated cells, which does not comfort these analyses any value with respect to differentiation and transplantation studies. The FACS technique is a common method to analyze isolated and cultured cell populations for their cell surface expressed antigen. A lot of proteins which are expressed in MSC have been identified and many of them have been used for the characterisation of MSC populations with respect to the commercial availability of appropriate antibodies. However, no single specific MSC marker has been identified. While MSC express a large number of adhesions molecules, extracellular matrix proteins, cytokines, and growth factor receptors, they express a wide spectrum of antigens also characteristic for other cell types. These are CD13 (aminopeptidase N), CD29 (integrin beta 1), CD44 (HCAM), CD71 (TFR = transferrin receptor), CD73 (nucleotidase, ecto 5), CD90 (Thy1), CD105 (endoglin) and CD166 (ALCAM) which are widely expressed in many tissues or cells of the lymphatic system in addition to their expression in mesenchymal and hematopoietic stem cells. MSC do not express CD14 (monocyte differentiation antigen), CD34 (hematopoietic progenitor cell antigen), CD38 (ADP ribosyl cyclase), CD45 (leukocyte common antigen), and CD117 (c-kit). These antigens are often described as markers to differ between the MSC and HSC/ESC on the other hand (Figure 3).

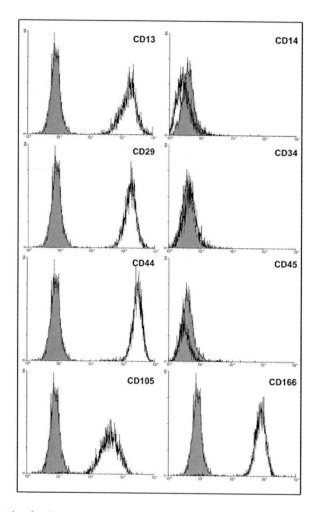

Figure 3. FACS analysis of 5 days cultivated human mesenchymal stem cells isolated from adipose tissue. 5000 cells were used to analyse the CD surface antigen expression. The antigen pattern confirms to these of undifferentiated mesenchymal stem cells. Analyses were performed using direct PE or FITC conjugated antibodies. An internal IgG isotyp control was used to detect unspecific bindings (grey area).

Since there has not been discovered a distinct marker for MSC, the expression profile of different antigens is the only way to characterize the MSC population. According to markers did or did not express by HSC and other mononuclear cells to the marker profile of MSC leads to the identification of the population.

Table 1 shows relevant antigens which are strongly, weakly or not expressed in MSC. The attribution concerning the degree of expression of some markers varies between different authors, because of different cultivation media, various ages of the donors or prolonged stem cell cultures and different antibodies used.

Table 1.

CD	Expression	Author	CD	Expression	Author
13	++	[45, 63, 67, 78-82]	3	--	[67, 82]
29	++	[36, 53, 61, 63, 67, 80-84]	4	--	[53, 67, 82]
44	++	[36, 45, 53, 61, 63, 67, 79-82, 84, 85]	11a	--	[53, 82]
49a	++	[82]	11b	--	[53, 63, 80, 84, 86]
49b	++	[53, 82]	11c	--	[53, 67]
49c	++	[82]	14	--	[45, 52, 61, 63, 67, 81, 82, 84]
49d	++	[45, 53, 67, 81]	15	--	[67, 82]
49e	++	[53, 80-82]	18	--	[53, 82, 84]
49f	++	[82]	21	--	[82]
51	++	[36, 53, 79, 81, 82]	31	--	[45, 52, 53, 67, 82]
54	++	[(67, 81, 82)]	34	--	[45, 52, 61, 63, 81, 82, 84]
71	++	[36, 45, 82]	36	--	[81, 82, 84]
73	++	[52, 82, 84]	38	--	[67, 82]
90	++	[36, 45, 53, 61, 67, 78-80, 82-84, 86]	45	--	[45, 52, 61, 63, 67, 78, 80-82, 84-86]
102	++	[82]	49d	--	[45, 81, 82]
105	++	[45, 52, 61, 63, 67, 78, 82, 83, 85]	49d	+/-	[53, 67]
106	++	[36, 45, 53, 63, 67, 81, 82, 84]	62e	+/-	[45, 53, 82]
120a	++	[36, 82]	62p	+/-	[53, 67]
120b	++	[82]	62l	+/-	[53, 82]
123	++	[82]	80	+/-	[52, 82]
124	++	[82]	82	+/-	[52, 82)
126	++	[36, 82]	117	+/-	[53, 82]
127	++	[82]	133	+/-	[53, 81, 82]
166	++	[52, 63, 82]	HLA-DR	+/-	[53, 61, 63, 80, 81, 83, 87]
140	++	[53, 82]			
HLA-ABC	++	[53, 80-82]			

However, after the determination of the cell population by their surface antigen pattern, it is necessary to expand the cells in a way that does not affect the stem cell characteristics and to avoid any influences on the differentiation of the MSC.

DIFFERENTIATION OF MSC

The differentiation from stem cells to a cell lineage includes the requirement to imitate the natural process in a way which does not alter the cells but keeps them in an undifferentiated state. During the liver development the embryonic anterior-ventral domain of the foregut endoderm and the dorsal domain of the endoderm form buds which fuse and finally create the liver [88]. The two hepatic epithelial cell lineages of the liver, hepatocytes and biliary cells [89], develop during the 4th week of development from a non-embryonic hepatoblast lineage. In the same time the anterior-ventral and the dorsal domain of the endoderm create buds for the lung, thyroid gland and pancreas. The mechanism of this differentiation process and the formation of organs is not completely understood and to imitate this highly complex cell communication leads to many investigations regarding cell signalling and the genetic network of cell proliferation. In the adult liver there is an intra-organ stem cell compartment located in the smallest, most proximal branches of the biliary tree, the canals of Hering. There progenitors named 'oval cells' can be mobilized if they are required within the liver organ. These cells proliferate and differentiate into hepatocytes in case of liver injury. In addition they can be activated at the earliest stages of carcinogenesis induced by chemicals [90]. The knowledge of these stem cell-like liver cells introduced a new period of investigating liver regeneration which currently is focused mainly on these liver-derived stem cells. Not surprisingly, the differentiation of stem cells is a hard discussed field with even as much protocols as different opinions.

As mentioned above confluence and the choice of the media used for isolation procedures and expansion of MSC is a critical point. The most frequently used media, DMEM and the mixture of DMEM and MCDB-201, induces the differentiation of MSC even in the expansion phase. As shown by Lee *et al.* [52] in microarray analysis MSC derived from fat tissue which had been expanded in these different cell media exhibited a different gene expression pattern of 183 genes. Especially the osteoblast specific factor 2 (OSF-2) involved in skeletal development was significantly higher expressed if cultured in DMEM/MCDB-201 than in DMEM alone. The variable gene expression in expanding MSC has been confirmed by other groups. Some of the mentioned genes are known to be expressed only during the embryonic development and in self-renewing tissues which indicates the multipotency of MSC. These genes have been used to indicate the stem cell character of a selected cell population. Katz *et al.* [53] have shown, that only 7 of 172 evaluated genes were not transcribed in MSC derived from adipose tissue. The highest transcription levels have been recorded for the above mentioned flowcytometrically determined markers endoglin (CD105), the integrins $\alpha 5$ (CD49e), integrin $\alpha 11$ and $\beta 1$ (CD29), for FGF 2, 6, and 7, for FGF receptor 3, neurophilin-1,; TGF-β receptors 2 and 3, osteonectin, osteopontin, fibronectin-1, VEGF-D, TNF-α; and matrix metalloprotease 2 (gelatinase A). It has been reported [91] that MSC express inductors of transcription such as OCT-4/POU5F1 the assumed main candidate for the control over the early development. The task of the transcription regulator NANOG, which is involved in inner cell mass and embryonic stem cell, is to prevent them from differentiation towards extraembryonic endoderm and trophetoderm lineages. The same regulatory work has to be fulfilled by Sox-2, which forms ternary complexes with OCT-1 or OCT-3 and acts as a transcriptional activator of FGF-4. Other proteins like the gap junction protein CX43 or the cytokeratins 7 and 19 are markers for the early development and thus are used to define undifferentiated stem cell genotypes [63, 65]. Moreover, MSC also show a high expression rate of the chemokine receptors CCR1, CCR2, CCR4, CCR6, CCR7, CCR8, CCR9, CCR10, XCR, CXCR1, CXCR2, CXCR3, CXCR4, CXCR5, and CXCR6 (92). These receptors are also expressed on different types of leukocytes suggesting a prominent role of MCS in the immune response. In this context *in vitro* studies have demonstrated the immunosuppressive effect of MSC [69, 72, 93, 94].

In conclusion, the expression of specific proteins which have been detected in MSC like chemokine receptors, metalloproteases, adhesion molecules, gap junction proteins as well as regulatory transcriptional proteins are responsible for their differentiation. These proteins show a clear shift during the expansion phase depending on the choice of culture media and the state of confluence.

This cultivation-depend modification of isolated MSC lead to the question whether these cells have the same features as those in their natural habitat niches where they have been isolated from. However, even if the expression of certain genes changes during the expansion phase, it must be postulated that these cells do not have lost their capacity to differentiate at least into three different cell lineages. In addition, the wide spread expression of markers specific for multipotent cells emphasises the multipotency of MSC as well.

For differentiation MSC have to grow up till a cell to cell contact is reached which is about 70-100 % confluence. This confluence is essential for cell communication via gap junction [63, 65, 95-97]. To initiate the differentiation, some protocols use 1µM-20µM 5-azacytidine (5-Aza) [63, 65, 97, 98] which inhibits DNA methyltransferase. This results in a partial or complete demethylation of the DNA allowing transcription factors to bind to the DNA. The use of 5-Aza is discussed controversially as demethylation is known to increase the potential of carcinoma cells to develop towards more invasive cell lines, associated with the induction of various matrix metalloproteases [99]. Otherwise, the binding of transcription factors to DNA reactivate tumor suppressor genes [100]. Furthermore 5-Aza is used as a therapeutic in leukemia [101]. The effect of 5-Aza to primary cell lines such as MSC has not yet been investigated in detail, but the demethylation of DNA is indeed a very invasive step in cell development under *in vitro* conditions.

After the initiation of the differentiation, the expansion media are replaced by certain differentiation media as an essential step of further efficient cell differentiation (Figure 4). Depending on the composition of differentiation media, MSC can differentiate into adipogenic, chondrogenic, osteogenic, neurogenic, and hepatogenic cell lineages [36, 45, 61, 63, 65, 67, 70, 73, 77, 78, 96, 102-104). The numbers of protocols and media compositions used for hepatogenic differentiation are as different as the protocols for expansion media are. According to the culture conditions of primary hepatocytes which are well established the differentiation media are adapted to the hepatocyte culture media. These consist of DMEM supplemented with insulin, dexamethasone, nicotinamide, albumin, galactose, glutamine, ornithine, proline transferrin, gentamycin, EGF, hepatocyte growth factor (HGF), and trace elements like copper and zinc [105].

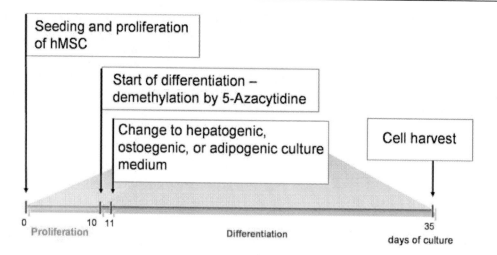

Figure 4. Differentiation of mesenchymal stem cells are performed in specific media after a ten days proliferation phase until 95 % cell confluence is reached.

In the intact liver, hepatocytes do not respond to growth factors like EGF and HGF. They first must be primed to enter the cell cycle and to respond to these growth factors. In the cell culture EGF and HGF are stimulators for DNA replication in hepatocytes [106, 107]. The basal medium of hepatogenic differentiation is DMEM supplemented with 2-10 % FBS [63, 65, 97, 108, 109], 10-40 ng/ml EGF and HGF 10-150 ng/ml alone or in combination with EGF [63, 65, 78, 95-98, 108, 110, 111]. Other groups use acidic fibroblast growth factor (aFGF) or 10-20 ng/ml basic fibroblast growth factor (bFGF) in combination with or without HGF and EGF [97, 98, 108, 110, 111]. The use of dexamethasone has often been described [63, 65, 96, 102, 108, 111] as well as the addition of ITS, insulin and gentamycin [63, 65, 102, 111]. The MSC to be differentiated are treated with these supplements by changing the media after sufficient confluence has been reached.

Two different protocols for differentiation with one-step or two-step instructions have been described. In case of the two-step protocol the first step medium do not contain growth factors. These are added in the second step of differentiation. The addition of 5-Aza is optional [78, 96]. Interestingly, some protocols use the expansion media supplements transferrin or linoelic acid also for the differentiation procedure, but this results even in a proper differentiation [78, 102].

The time point at which MSC are differentiated into the hepatic lineage is not clear because there are different indications to determine the differentiation status of stem cells. Hepatocytes are able to produce urea, to store glycogen, to produce albumin, and to detoxicate via cytochrome P450. Furthermore there is a multiple liver specific gene expression profile for hepatocytes containing the expression of dipeptidylpeptidase IV (CD26), the expression of cytochromes P450 proteins (Cyp1A1, Cyp3A4, Cyp7A1), transferrin, gap junction protein CX32, gluconeogenic PCK1, hepatic nuclear factor (HNF) 1-4α, or cytokeratin 18. The identification of these proteins is often used to verify the successful differentiation process [63, 65, 78, 95, 96, 98, 102, 108, 110]. However, there is no exactly defined time point when the expression begins indicating that differentiation is an insidious process. Some of these markers like glycogen storage, urea production, the expression of albumin, alpha fetoprotein, cytokeratin 18 and PCK1 can be observed after 2-3 weeks of differentiation [63, 65, 78, 95-97, 110]. During the same time the expression of progenitor markers decreases or disappears [Thy1 (CD90), CX43, cytokeratin 7 and 19)] [63, 65, 78]. After 4-6 weeks of differentiation the expression of the later markers of hepatogenic differentiation like HNF4, tyrosine aminotransferase or members of the cytochrome family Cyp1A1, Cyp3A4 and Cyp7A1 increases [63, 65, 96, 102]. The indicators for a successful hepatogenic differentiation have been investigated carefully and are thus well known. There is no question that it is possible to isolate, expand and differentiate MSC into different lineages, but there is only a poor understanding which signalling pathways play a more or less important role. Many signalling pathways contributing to the cell to cell communication in the context of embryonic development are known. However, the investigations to bring them together for an understanding of differentiation process are still missing.

SIGNALLING PATHWAYS IN STEM CELL DIFFERENTIATION

Some interesting pathways involved in differentiation are currently in the focus of research. The Wnt pathway plays an important role in the embryonic development, cancer, self-renewal, liver fibrosis, and differentiation [112]. There are 19 Wnt and 10 Frizzled genes known whereas 11 Wnts and 9 Frizzleds have been shown to be expressed in the adult mouse liver [112]. Furthermore it is known that Wnt5a is expressed in the mouse liver as well as in the human bone marrow by HSC and MSC. There is even an expression of Wnt3a but the origin of its expression has not yet been identified [113]. Another important pathway responsible for cell-cell communication is the Notch pathway, which involves gene regulatory mechanisms controlling multiple cell differentiation processes during embryonic and adult growth. The Notch pathway cross talks with the Wnt pathway in several ways (TGF-b/BMP, Hh and RTK/Ras pathway, all cell to fate determinants) [114]. A key role in the Wnt pathway is beta-catenin, a main downstream effector of the canonical Wnt pathway. In its normal state beta-catenin is targeted for phosphorylation (not at tyrosin residues 654 and 670) via glycogen synthetase kinase 3 beta (GSK3ß) and degradation or alternatively it is associated with e-cadherin and the actin portion of the cytoskeleton at the membrane necessary for cell-cell adhesion. In the liver, beta-catenin is associated with the HGF receptor (c-met), the tyrosine phosphatase domain of c-met which can phosphorylate beta-catenin, finally leading to a nucleus transfer [112]. The unphosphorylated (or tyrosin 654/670 phosphorylated) form of beta-catenin targets genes in combination with Lef/TCF [1,3,4] of the canonical Wnt pathway such as c-myc, cyclin D1-3, Lef itself or Imp. All of these genes are involved in cell proliferation or mRNA stabilization. In MSC differentiate hepatogenically a translocation of beta-catenin is observed which underlined the importance of the Wnt pathway for further investigations. Cellular beta-catenin is stabilized by activation of the Wnt cascade and afterwards translocated into the nucleus at day 7 of the differentiation. Hence it co-activates transcription factors of the TCF/Lef family. After an additional week of differentiation beta-catenin shifts from the nucleus back to the membrane and into the cytosolic pool [97]. Taken together the role of the Wnt pathway with its major downstream effector beta-catenin is involved in embryogenesis, regeneration and cancer. The observation of the beta-catenin translocation during the differentiation process may focus the attention on differentiation and ongoing transplantation of MSC in the context of Wnt pathway signal transduction and its downstream/cross-talk effectors. A better understanding how stem cells (re)-program the status of proliferation and differentiation into a stable, not carcinogenically transformed somatic cell is the goal of further stem cell research. Without this knowledge, a clinical approach remains doubtful because of the risk of cancer.

USE OF MESENCHYMAL STEM CELLS IN LIVER CELL THERAPY

It is one of the ambitions aims of the regenerative medicine to development a stem-cell-based cell and gene therapy for serve liver diseases. Because of the plasticity of stem cells, their multipotency to form differentiated liver cells and thus to generate liver tissue they are the favourable candidates for a cellular transplantation. A cellular therapy may be indicated in three groups of liver diseases: (i) Fulminant hepatic failure caused by viral hepatitis or acetaminophene toxicity in such cases if orthotopic liver organ transplantation is not urgent. (ii) Chronic liver diseases leading to fibrosis until end-stage cirrhosis. (iii) Metabolic diseases originated by inherited genetic defects of one or more hepatic enzymes.

Before stem cells can be used for cell therapy, evidence indicating a potentially successful stem cell integration into a recipient's liver as a consequence of disease correction is required. Several reports have specified the effective transplantation of stem cells isolated from various origins into injured livers. In this context animal models have been developed in which stem cells from different sources were used for syngenic [65, 115-117], allogenic [118] and xenogenic [48, 63, 119] transplantations.

SYNGENIC TRANSPLANTATION

Using a syngenic transplantation model in BALB/c mice Fang *et al.* [115] have evaluated the effect of fetal liver kinase 1^+ (Flk1$^+$) MSC from murine bone marrow (BM) on a carbon tetrachloride (CCl_4) induced fibrosis model. In this study the fibrosis index and donor-cell engraftment were assessed 2 and 5 weeks after CCL_4 treatment. Livers from mice transplanted with Flk^{1+} MSC significantly suppressed fibrosis development immediately after exposure to CCl_4, however no significant suppression in the degree of liver fibrosis was observed in mice receiving Flk1$^+$ MSC one week after CCl_4 exposure in contrast to the exposure for 2 and 5 weeks, respectively. The integration of transplanted cells into recipient livers was verified by in situ hybridisation, PCR analyses and immunohistochemical stainings of expressed albumin. Other groups used dipeptidyl peptidase IV (DPPIV) deficient Fisher 344 rats. Popp *et al.* [116] transplanted BM-derived MSC from wild-type F344 rats into DPPIV deficient syngenic rats. Liver damage was induced by injection of CCL_4 or allyl alcohol (AA) with or without retrorsine pretreatment. As a result hepatocyte chimerism in the recipient livers was observed but MSC did not differentiate into hepatocytes *in vivo* when transplanted under retrosine treatment. Sgodda *et al.* [65] also used the Fisher 344 rat-model for transplantation of undifferentiated MSC *vs.* hepatogenically predifferentiated MSC which have been derived from Fisher 344 rat peritoneal adipose tissue. Undifferentiated stem cells and stem cells (CD26+/+) which had been hepatogenically predifferentiated were transplanted by an intraportal infusion into the livers of CD26 deficient (CD26-/-) animals. Formerly these cells had been lentivirally infected *in vitro* by the GFP-gene under the control of phosphoenolpyruvate carboxykinase1 (PCK1) or ubiquitin (Ub) gene promoter, respectively (Figure 5).

In this model 10 weeks after transplantation of MSC generated from predifferentiated rat adipose tissue, clusters of CD26-positive cells were detected by histochemical staining in the parenchymal host liver. Only these cell clusters were shown to express GFP induced by both the PCK1 and the ubiquitin promoter. In contrast to the clusters of CD26+/+ cells [65], only single cells were detected in the host liver if cells had been transplanted without prior hepatogenic differentiation (Figure 6). Oyagi *et al.* [117] investigated the therapeutic effect of BM-derived MSC which had been treated *in vitro* with HGF transplanted into CCl_4-toxicated rats. In that study cells isolated from BM of wildtype Fisher 344 rats were cultured for two weeks in the presence or absence of HGF labelled with a PKH fluorescent marker (Sigma-Aldrich) and transplanted by injection (3×10^6 cells per rat) into the CCl_4 treated host rats. Blood samples were collected 4 weeks after transplantation and analyzed for albumin production and transaminase levels. Furthermore the amount of fibrosis was determined by histology.

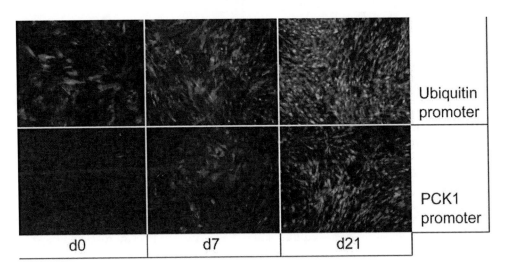

Figure 5. Expression of transgenic green fluorescent protein (GFP) under the control of the human phosphoenolpyruvate carboxykinase 1 (hPCK1) and ubiquitin (Ub) promoter in bone marrow derived hMSC after lentiviral infection. The rising hPCK1-GFP expression indicates the increase of liver specific functions of hMSC during hepatogenic differentiation. (200x magn., 2 sec. exp.).

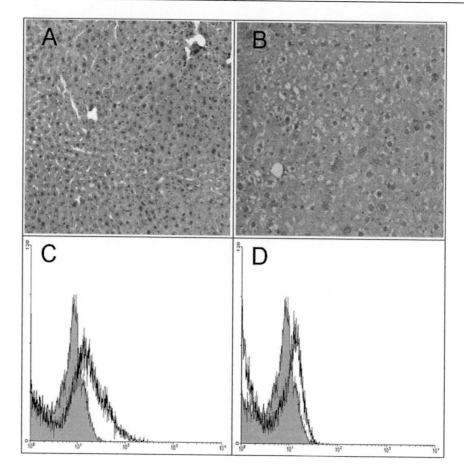

Figure 6. Integration of *in vitro* hepatogenic predifferentiated (A) and undifferentiated (B) rat adipose tissue derived mesenchymal stem cells (rAT-MSC) into the recipients' liver. The transplanted Fisher CD26+/+ rAT-MSC were stably infected with a GFP transgene under the control of the PCK1 (PCK-GFP) gene promoter by lentiviral gene transfer. Undifferentiated or 14 days hepatogenic predifferentiated rAT-MSC was infused intraportally into the liver of Fisher CD26-/- rats. After 10 weeks the livers were analysed by immunohistochemical staining against GFP (A and B). In a second experiment the rAT-MSC were transplanted into the host livers. The livers were disintegrated by collagenase digestion. The resulting cell suspension containing the transplanted CD26 positive cells were identified by FACS analyses.

The BM derived MSC which had been transplanted into liver-injured rats restored their serum albumin levels and suppressed transaminase activity and liver fibrosis significantly. In contrast, these effects were not observed when the BM MSC had been cultured without HGF.

ALLOGENIC TRANSPLANTATION

Using an allogenic model Zhao *et al.* [118] MSC isolated from bone marrow of male Fisher 344 rats were intravenously infused into female Wistar rats which had been treated with CCl_4 or dimethylnitrosamine (DMN). Four to six weeks after the MSC infusion livers were removed and assessed by immunohistochemistry and PCR technique. Transplanted MSC (3×10^6 per rat) reduced the mortality rates in CCl_4 treated rats by 10% and in DMN-induced rats by 50-70%. Furthermore a decrease in collagen and alpha-smooth muscle actin deposition in the recipients' livers by 50-60% was observed in comparison to control rats which had not been infused with MSC. In addition a significant decreasement of the fibrosis index was observed.

XENOGENIC TRANSPLANTATION

Several xenograft models were published in the last few years describing transplantation of human stem cells into animals. Chamberlain and coworkers. [119] reported an efficient regeneration of human hepatocytes after the intrahepatic infusion of human clonal MSC into fetal sheeps. The aim of their investigations was to show whether the human MSC could differentiate and expand into human hepatocytes in the fetal sheep milieu by intrahepatic injection without malignant transformation. The second aim was to investigate whether the route of administration influenced the levels of donor-derived hepatocytes and their pattern of distribution inside the recipient's liver parenchyma. For direct comparison human MSC were transplanted intraperitoneally (IP) or intrahepatically (IH) into fetal sheeps. The livers were monitored 56 – 70 days after transplantation by immunohistochemical analyses, enzyme-linked immunosorbent assays and flowcytometric studies. The intrahepatic injection of MSC was demonstrated to be more reliable and efficient than the IP procedure resulting in 12.5 % +/- 3.5 % (human hepatocytes +/- SD) versus 2.6 % +/- 0.4 % after IP application. The animals which had received an MSC intrahepatically exhibited a widespread distribution of stem cell-derived hepatocytes inside the liver parenchyma. In contrast the intraperitoneal injection resulted mainly in a periportal distribution of transplanted MSC producing higher amounts of albumin (4 +/- 0.48 ng/ml) compared to sheeps transplanted intrahepatically (1.2 +/- 0.8 ng/ml).

Aurich *et al.* (63) investigated the functional integration of human BM-derived MSC in murine livers. MSC were differentiated for 14 days *in vitro*. The cells expressed hepatocyte-specific markers (CK18, Cx32, transferrin, albumin, CYP3A4, CD26, PCK1), stored glycogen, synthesised urea and expressed the hepatocyte-specific HepPar1 gene. These predifferentiated cells were intrasplenically transplanted into immunodeficient Pfp/Rag2-/- mice (1×10^6 cells/mouse). To provide growth advantage of predifferentiated MSC over host hepatocytes, mice were pretreated with propranolol, a ß-receptor antagonist, 48 hours before transplantation followed by a partial hepatectomy. After twelve weeks murine livers were removed and the expression of hepatocyte-specific proteins was assessed by immunohistochemical analyses. Serial sections were analysed to detect human HepPar1, PCK1, Cx32, albumin and glycogen deposition which indicated the functional activity of the transplanted hepatogenic predifferentiated BM-MSC.

Using a Sprague Dawley rat model Sato *et al.* (48) showed that human MSC directly xenografted into rat livers were able to differentiate into human hepatocytes. Rat livers were damaged with AA and human MSC (approximately 1×10^6 cells per rat) were directly injected into the left lateral lobe by intrahepatic injection. Two weeks after transplantation cell clusters positive for human albumin were detectable, which increased during the first four but decreased after 8 weeks. Correspondingly human albumin was detectable in the rat sera by ELISA (1.2 +/- 0.4 ng/ml) at day 14. The concentration increased to 1.8 +/- 0.6 ng/ml until day 28 but decreased to 0.6 +/- 0.4 ng/ml at day 56. During the same time period the expression of CK18 increased whereas the CK19 expression decreased continuously.

PREFERENCE OF MESENCHYMAL STEM CELLS IN HUMAN LIVER CELL THERAPY

Because of their simple availability, plasticity and their high proliferation capacity as well as their potential handling without any ethical controversy, MSC are preferred to embryonic or fetal stem cells in human research. Using various animal models it was demonstrated by many researchers [120, 121] that the pluripotency of ESC allows the differentiation into nearly all cell types including hepatocytes. However, ethical standards strongly restrict investigations using human ESC.

HSC show similar characteristics to MSC regarding their ability of differentiation [122-124] but exhibit disadvantages concerning the culture conditions and proliferation properties. Thus, it may be difficult to get sufficient cell numbers for transplantation applications. Masson *et al.* [125] presented in their review article data on transplantations using HSC in syngenic and xenogenic models. There studies on syngenic transplantations are mentioned which were characterised by a hepatic repopulation of approximately 30 – 50 % after 6 month [33] but in most investigations only by a rate of 0.1 – 2 % (125). Xenogenic transplantations yielded to a marginal hepatic repopulation of about 1%.

Moreover the engraftment and functionality of transplanted human hepatic progenitor cells was reported [126, 127]. For these experiments cells were isolated from human fetal livers. This source, however, appears to be problematical in terms of sufficient availability and of ethical aspect.

TREATMENT OF STEM CELLS BEFORE TRANSPLANTATION

Using different experimental models the cited reports have provided evidence that the transplantation, integration and differentiation of donor-derived stem cells into a hepatogenic lineage is generally possible. However, the predominantly marginal rates of repopulation raise questions concerning therapeutical applications. Thereby the integration of functional hepatic differentiated stem cells particularly in the context of xenografting was detectable only at a minor extent. Concludingly human MSC should be at the focus of investigations. In this context a pretreatment leading to the predifferentiation of MSC before transplantation should yield to better results. In many studies undifferentiated stem cells were used for transplantations subjected to a multitude of passages (up to 30 times) in order to receive an increased cell number [115, 118]. In other reports the stem cells were *in vitro* predifferentiated in the presence of HGF [117] or HGF and EGF in common added to a hepatocyte-specific growth medium [63, 65]. This seems to increase the cell number of hepatocyte-differentiated donor-derived stem cells and to be advantages for their functionality in the recipient liver in contrast to undifferentiated cells. In recent studies hAT-MSC were differentiated *in vitro* before intraspleenic transplantation into immunodeficient mice which were treated using propranolol and by one third hepatectomy.

In these experiments the repopulation predominantly in the periportal area was verify (63). Single cells were detectable after transplantation of undifferentiated cells up to large clusters when AT-hMSC were used which had been predifferentiated *in vitro* with HGF, EGF in hepatocyte-specific medium for 14 days (Figure 6). The differentiation was initiated by treating the undifferentiated stem cells (AT-hMSC) with the demethylating agent 5-Aza for 24 hours at a confluence of 90 – 100 %. The use of 5-Aza in MSC cultures leads to a distinct initialization and a better reproducibility of hepatogenic differentiation compared to MSC cultured without 5-Aza (unpublished data).

Extent clusters of *in vitro* predifferentiated rat adipose-derived mesenchymal stem cells (rAT-MSC) used in syngenic rat transplantation-model were observed in further studies of our group (unpublished data) confirming the major integration of hepatogenically differentiated AT-hMSC in xenogenic transplantations [63].

The findings demonstrating an advantage in the integration of predifferentiated MSC in syngenic and especially in autologous transplantation models provide evidence that the use of MSC isolated from adipose tissue and their autologies transplantation may be an attractive way to a successful cell therapy.

THE ROLE OF MICROENVIRONMENT

Biological systems strongly interact with their environment. In this context the microenvironment of MSC transplanted into liver parenchyma exerts an important influence on their hepatogenic differentiation and their effective repopulation. Several publications addressing this aspect were reviewed by Shafritz and Dabeva [128]. In order to reach a sufficient liver repopulation and regeneration by transplanted cells they need a proliferation advantage in the recipient liver. In animal models livers were treated with propranolol, monocrotalin, or retrorsine before partial hepatectomy to impede the proliferation of residual host hepatocytes. Chronical liver disease like fibrosis were imitated by the treatment of animals with CCl_4 or allyl alcohol [48, 115-118]. Afterwards an additional acute liver damage caused by hepatectomy or irradiation was set to enforce the capability for regeneration by the transplanted donor stem cells. To investigate the difference between the regenerative capacity of transplanted stem cells and the self regeneration mediated by damaged liver cells of the recipients' livers is extremely difficult. Only xenogenic and transgenic models provide a possibility by the detection of species specific or transgenic markers for these analyses. The detection of xenogenically different hepatic markers by immunohistochemical stainings among the recipients' liver cells as well as the detection of donor-specific e.g. human albumin in animal serum provide the most common evidence for successful cell integration. However, the level of integrated donor-derived cells (e.g. hepatocytes, stem cells) which are successfully integrated into the recipients' liver strongly depends on the animal model and the kind of liver damage [129, 130].

ROUTE OF ADMINISTRATION

The optimal way for stem cell applications is currently under discussion. Intrahepatic transplantations (IH) result in a widespread distribution of engrafted cells throughout the whole liver parenchyma, whereas the intraperitoneal injection (IP) mainly leads to the periportal distribution of transplanted cells [119]. This periportal settling pattern of transplanted cells occurred analogously after intraspleenic transplantation (IS) [63]. Intrahepatic administration generally results in higher integration rates, whereas the level of human albumin detected in animal serum was higher after the intraperitoneal than after intrahepatic administration of the cells. It may be concluded that a combined transplantation procedure is the most efficient way necessary for a successful repopulation of the liver.

IMMUNOGENICITY

Many publications deal with the transplantation of adult stem cells into adult recipients. In these studies the outcome is observed 4-12 weeks after transplantation. A decrease in functional parameters of transplanted cells was detectable which was in accordance with a decreasing number of integrated cells up to their complete loss (48). Based on comparative investigations of transplantations dealing with human hepatocytes or predifferentiated BM-hMSC an initial high level of human albumin was detected after the transplantation of human hepatocytes in murine serum which decreased within 8 weeks after transplantation. In contrast after the transplantation of predifferentiated BM-hMSC no human albumin was detected initially whereas an increasing level was recorded after 8 weeks. This data suggest a combined transplantation of human hepatocytes and hMSC because of the antidromic functional development. This is especially interesting with respect to the hypoimmunogenicity and immunosuppressive capacities of MSC [93, 94, 131-134]. In contrast to hepatocytes which are apparently immunogenic in host organism MSC from bone marrow and adipose tissue have been shown to bear immunosuppressive features. They modulate the functions of host dendritic cell and T cell and promote the induction of suppressor and/or regulatory T cells. Furthermore they induce the anergy in T cells by immunomodulatory down-regulating factors like interleukin-10, transforming growth factor-ß, prostaglandin E2 and hepatocyte growth factor. In addition, MSC express the enzyme indoleamine-2,3-dioxygenase leading to a tryptophan-depleted micromilieu that promotes immunosuppression. According to the study of Fibbe *et al.* [135], MSC are not intrinsically immunoprivileged but are capable to induce memory T cell responses which follow the *in vivo* injection into immunocompetent hosts. After cotransplantation into recipients that have received sublethal irradation, allogenic MSC can still induce an alloresponse that may result in graft rejection. This suggests that the immunogenicity of allogenic MSC is not fully prevented by a non-myeloablative regime. MSC have already been and are currently used in clinical applications especially for treatment of therapy-resistant graft-versus-host disease (GVHD) [72, 136, 137].

FUSION

Fusions of donor and recipient cells as well as transdifferentiation of HSC are critcally dicussed. Several groups [123, 138-140] described the fusion of donor stem cells and hepatocytes of the recipients. In the livers of recipient animals, nuclei were identified which were positive for both the genomic human and the recipient animal DNA. Furthermore animal hepatocytes were demonstrated to additionally express human donor specific genes.

No cell fusions were detected after MSC cell transplantations using immunohistochemical or *in situ* hybridisation techniques [48, 63, 122, 124, 141, 142] The phenomenon of cell fusion caused by HSC but not by MSC is currently not understood.

CONCLUSION

Present studies about MSC deal with sources, *in vitro* culture conditions and differentiation protocols of stem cells. Additional important aspects are the dosage of cells for transplantation, their optimal administration route and the microenvironment. MSC represent the best source for cell therapy of the known alternatives in the field of liver regeneration. They represent an autologous source of cells and are easy to isolate. Furthermore they show an extensive expansion rate *in vitro* as well as a broad differentiation potential *in vitro* and *in vivo*. Advantageously they also have a certain immunosuppressive capability.

Further investigations are required to guarantee that stem cell transplantation is a reliable application for therapeutical approaches of liver diseases. In addition to the successful autologous transplantation model the use of xenografts has so far resulted only in a marginal repopulation of injured livers in long-term studies. Only a few of the established animal models are available to study human stem cell transplantations and, thus, may be useful in the cell therapy of human liver diseases, However, all models taken together show promising approaches to use transplanted stem cells for an efficient hepatic regeneration Therefore, additional clinical models with clear clinical relevance are urgently needed to investigate the biological effects of stem cells in human recipients and to understand the complexity of liver regeneration. Especially a better understanding of the mechanisms modulating the development and function of MSC in the physiological context of liver injury is strongly required.

REFERENCES

[1] Strassburg CP, Vogel A, Manns MP. Autoimmunity and hepatitis C. *Autoimmun. Rev.* 2003;2:322-331.

[2] Zhu AX. Hepatocellular carcinoma: are we making progress? *Cancer Invest* 2003;21:418-428.
[3] Soemohardjo S. New options in the treatment of chronic hepatitis. *Adv. Exp. Med. Biol.* 2003;531:191-198.
[4] Ballas CB, Zielske SP, Gerson SL. Adult bone marrow stem cells for cell and gene therapies: implications for greater use. *J. Cell Biochem. Suppl.* 2002;38:20-28.
[5] Gill RQ, Sterling RK. Acute liver failure. *J. Clin. Gastroenterol.* 2001;33:191-198.
[6] Gomez-Lechon MJ, Donato T, Ponsoda X, Castell JV. Human hepatic cell cultures: in vitro and in vivo drug metabolism. *Altern. Lab Anim.* 2003;31:257-265.
[7] Fox IJ, Chowdhury JR. Hepatocyte transplantation. *Am. J. Transplant.* 2004;4 Suppl 6:7-13.
[8] David P, Alexandre E, Audet M, Chenard-Neu MP, Wolf P, Jaeck D, Azimzadeh A, et al. Engraftment and albumin production of intrasplenically transplanted rat hepatocytes (Sprague-Dawley), freshly isolated versus cryopreserved, into Nagase analbuminemic rats (NAR). *Cell Transplant* 2001;10:67-80.
[9] Muller P, Aurich H, Wenkel R, Schaffner I, Wolff I, Walldorf J, Fleig WE, et al. Serum-free cryopreservation of porcine hepatocytes. *Cell Tissue Res.* 2004;317:45-56.
[10] Runge D, Michalopoulos GK, Strom SC, Runge DM. Recent advances in human hepatocyte culture systems. *Biochem. Biophys. Res. Commun.* 2000;274:1-3.
[11] Schneider C, Aurich H, Wenkel R, Christ B. Propagation and functional characterization of serum-free cultured porcine hepatocytes for downstream applications. *Cell Tissue Res.* 2006;323:433-442.
[12] Nakamura J, Okamoto T, Schumacher IK, Tabei I, Chowdhury NR, Chowdhury JR, Fox IJ. Treatment of surgically induced acute liver failure by transplantation of conditionally immortalized hepatocytes. *Transplantation* 1997;63:1541-1547.
[13] Cai J, Ito M, Nagata H, Westerman KA, Lafleur D, Chowdhury JR, Leboulch P, et al. Treatment of liver failure in rats with end-stage cirrhosis by transplantation of immortalized hepatocytes. *Hepatology* 2002;36:386-394.
[14] Weissman IL. Translating stem and progenitor cell biology to the clinic: barriers and opportunities. *Science* 2000;287:1442-1446.
[15] Bongso A, Fong CY, Ng SC, Ratnam S. Isolation and culture of inner cell mass cells from human blastocysts. *Hum. Reprod.* 1994;9:2110-2117.
[16] Reubinoff BE, Pera MF, Fong CY, Trounson A, Bongso A. Embryonic stem cell lines from human blastocysts: somatic differentiation in vitro. *Nat. Biotechnol.* 2000;18:399-404.
[17] Thomson JA, Itskovitz-Eldor J, Shapiro SS, Waknitz MA, Swiergiel JJ, Marshall VS, Jones JM. Embryonic stem cell lines derived from human blastocysts. *Science* 1998;282:1145-1147.
[18] Muraca M, Gerunda G, Neri D, Vilei MT, Granato A, Feltracco P, Meroni M, et al. Hepatocyte transplantation as a treatment for glycogen storage disease type 1a. *Lancet* 2002;359:317-318.
[19] Fox IJ, Chowdhury JR, Kaufman SS, Goertzen TC, Chowdhury NR, Warkentin PI, Dorko K, et al. Treatment of the Crigler-Najjar syndrome type I with hepatocyte transplantation. *N. Engl. J. Med.* 1998;338:1422-1426.

[20] Petersen BE, Bowen WC, Patrene KD, Mars WM, Sullivan AK, Murase N, Boggs SS, et al. Bone marrow as a potential source of hepatic oval cells. *Science* 1999;284:1168-1170.

[21] Kopen GC, Prockop DJ, Phinney DG. Marrow stromal cells migrate throughout forebrain and cerebellum, and they differentiate into astrocytes after injection into neonatal mouse brains. *Proc. Natl. Acad. Sci. USA* 1999;96:10711-10716.

[22] Ferrari G, Cusella-De Angelis G, Coletta M, Paolucci E, Stornaiuolo A, Cossu G, Mavilio F. Muscle regeneration by bone marrow-derived myogenic progenitors. *Science* 1998;279:1528-1530.

[23] Gussoni E, Soneoka Y, Strickland CD, Buzney EA, Khan MK, Flint AF, Kunkel LM, et al. Dystrophin expression in the mdx mouse restored by stem cell transplantation. *Nature* 1999;401:390-394.

[24] Palermo AT, Labarge MA, Doyonnas R, Pomerantz J, Blau HM. Bone marrow contribution to skeletal muscle: a physiological response to stress. *Dev. Biol.* 2005;279:336-344.

[25] Eglitis MA, Mezey E. Hematopoietic cells differentiate into both microglia and macroglia in the brains of adult mice. Proc Natl Acad Sci U S A 1997;94:4080-4085.

[26] Brazelton TR, Rossi FM, Keshet GI, Blau HM. From marrow to brain: expression of neuronal phenotypes in adult mice. *Science* 2000;290:1775-1779.

[27] Mezey E, Chandross KJ, Harta G, Maki RA, McKercher SR. Turning blood into brain: cells bearing neuronal antigens generated in vivo from bone marrow. *Science* 2000;290:1779-1782.

[28] Zeng Z, Yuan X, Liu G, Zeng X, Ng H, Chen H, Jiang T, et al. Manipulation of proliferation and differentiation of human bone marrow-derived neural stem cells in vitro and in vivo. *J. Neurosci. Res.* 2007;85:310-320.

[29] Poulsom R, Forbes SJ, Hodivala-Dilke K, Ryan E, Wyles S, Navaratnarasah S, Jeffery R, et al. Bone marrow contributes to renal parenchymal turnover and regeneration. *J. Pathol.* 2001;195:229-235.

[30] Imasawa T, Utsunomiya Y, Kawamura T, Zhong Y, Nagasawa R, Okabe M, Maruyama N, et al. The potential of bone marrow-derived cells to differentiate to glomerular mesangial cells. *J. Am. Soc. Nephrol.* 2001;12:1401-1409.

[31] van Haaften T, Thebaud B. Adult bone marrow-derived stem cells for the lung: implications for pediatric lung diseases. *Pediatr. Res.* 2006;59:94R-99R.

[32] Theise ND, Nimmakayalu M, Gardner R, Illei PB, Morgan G, Teperman L, Henegariu O, et al. Liver from bone marrow in humans. *Hepatology* 2000;32:11-16.

[33] Lagasse E, Connors H, Al-Dhalimy M, Reitsma M, Dohse M, Osborne L, Wang X, et al. Purified hematopoietic stem cells can differentiate into hepatocytes in vivo. *Nat. Med.* 2000;6:1229-1234.

[34] Zhan Y, Wang Y, Wei L, Chen H, Cong X, Fei R, Gao Y, et al. Differentiation of hematopoietic stem cells into hepatocytes in liver fibrosis in rats. *Transplant. Proc.* 2006;38:3082-3085.

[35] Friedenstein AJ, Gorskaja JF, Kulagina NN. Fibroblast precursors in normal and irradiated mouse hematopoietic organs. *Exp. Hematol.* 1976;4:267-274.

[36] Pittenger MF, Mackay AM, Beck SC, Jaiswal RK, Douglas R, Mosca JD, Moorman MA, et al. Multilineage potential of adult human mesenchymal stem cells. *Science* 1999;284:143-147.

[37] Zvaifler NJ, Marinova-Mutafchieva L, Adams G, Edwards CJ, Moss J, Burger JA, Maini RN. Mesenchymal precursor cells in the blood of normal individuals. *Arthritis Res* 2000;2:477-488.

[38] Bieback K, Kern S, Kluter H, Eichler H. Critical parameters for the isolation of mesenchymal stem cells from umbilical cord blood. *Stem Cells* 2004;22:625-634.

[39] In 't Anker PS, Scherjon SA, Kleijburg-van der Keur C, de Groot-Swings GM, Claas FH, Fibbe WE, Kanhai HH. Isolation of mesenchymal stem cells of fetal or maternal origin from human placenta. *Stem Cells* 2004;22:1338-1345.

[40] Igura K, Zhang X, Takahashi K, Mitsuru A, Yamaguchi S, Takashi TA. Isolation and characterization of mesenchymal progenitor cells from chorionic villi of human placenta. *Cytotherapy* 2004;6:543-553.

[41] Shih DT, Lee DC, Chen SC, Tsai RY, Huang CT, Tsai CC, Shen EY, et al. Isolation and characterization of neurogenic mesenchymal stem cells in human scalp tissue. *Stem Cells* 2005;23:1012-1020.

[42] Tsai MS, Lee JL, Chang YJ, Hwang SM. Isolation of human multipotent mesenchymal stem cells from second-trimester amniotic fluid using a novel two-stage culture protocol. *Hum. Reprod.* 2004;19:1450-1456.

[43] Campagnoli C, Roberts IA, Kumar S, Bennett PR, Bellantuono I, Fisk NM. Identification of mesenchymal stem/progenitor cells in human first-trimester fetal blood, liver, and bone marrow. *Blood* 2001;98:2396-2402.

[44] Zuk PA, Zhu M, Mizuno H, Huang J, Futrell JW, Katz AJ, Benhaim P, et al. Multilineage cells from human adipose tissue: implications for cell-based therapies. *Tissue Eng* 2001;7:211-228.

[45] Zuk PA, Zhu M, Ashjian P, De Ugarte DA, Huang JI, Mizuno H, Alfonso ZC, et al. Human adipose tissue is a source of multipotent stem cells. *Mol. Biol. Cell* 2002;13:4279-4295.

[46] Sanchez-Ramos J, Song S, Cardozo-Pelaez F, Hazzi C, Stedeford T, Willing A, Freeman TB, et al. Adult bone marrow stromal cells differentiate into neural cells in vitro. *Exp. Neurol.* 2000;164:247-256.

[47] Schwartz RE, Reyes M, Koodie L, Jiang Y, Blackstad M, Lund T, Lenvik T, et al. Multipotent adult progenitor cells from bone marrow differentiate into functional hepatocyte-like cells. *J. Clin. Invest* 2002;109:1291-1302.

[48] Sato Y, Araki H, Kato J, Nakamura K, Kawano Y, Kobune M, Sato T, et al. Human mesenchymal stem cells xenografted directly to rat liver are differentiated into human hepatocytes without fusion. *Blood* 2005;106:756-763.

[49] Ong SY, Dai H, Leong KW. Inducing hepatic differentiation of human mesenchymal stem cells in pellet culture. *Biomaterials* 2006;27:4087-4097.

[50] Hong SH, Gang EJ, Jeong JA, Ahn C, Hwang SH, Yang IH, Park HK, et al. In vitro differentiation of human umbilical cord blood-derived mesenchymal stem cells into hepatocyte-like cells. *Biochem. Biophys. Res. Commun.* 2005;330:1153-1161.

[51] Castro-Malaspina H, Gay RE, Resnick G, Kapoor N, Meyers P, Chiarieri D, McKenzie S, et al. Characterization of human bone marrow fibroblast colony-forming cells (CFU-F) and their progeny. *Blood* 1980;56:289-301.

[52] Lee RH, Kim B, Choi I, Kim H, Choi HS, Suh K, Bae YC, et al. Characterization and expression analysis of mesenchymal stem cells from human bone marrow and adipose tissue. *Cell Physiol. Biochem.* 2004;14:311-324.

[53] Katz AJ, Tholpady A, Tholpady SS, Shang H, Ogle RC. Cell surface and transcriptional characterization of human adipose-derived adherent stromal (hADAS) cells. *Stem Cells* 2005;23:412-423.

[54] Wagner W, Wein F, Seckinger A, Frankhauser M, Wirkner U, Krause U, Blake J, et al. Comparative characteristics of mesenchymal stem cells from human bone marrow, adipose tissue, and umbilical cord blood. *Exp. Hematol.* 2005;33:1402-1416.

[55] Gronthos S, Franklin DM, Leddy HA, Robey PG, Storms RW, Gimble JM. Surface protein characterization of human adipose tissue-derived stromal cells. *J. Cell Physiol.* 2001;189:54-63.

[56] Kern S, Eichler H, Stoeve J, Kluter H, Bieback K. Comparative analysis of mesenchymal stem cells from bone marrow, umbilical cord blood, or adipose tissue. *Stem Cells* 2006;24:1294-1301.

[57] Dicker A, Le Blanc K, Astrom G, van Harmelen V, Gotherstrom C, Blomqvist L, Arner P, et al. Functional studies of mesenchymal stem cells derived from adult human adipose tissue. *Exp. Cell Res.* 2005;308:283-290.

[58] Im GI, Shin YW, Lee KB. Do adipose tissue-derived mesenchymal stem cells have the same osteogenic and chondrogenic potential as bone marrow-derived cells? *Osteoarthritis Cartilage* 2005;13:845-853.

[59] Safford KM, Hicok KC, Safford SD, Halvorsen YD, Wilkison WO, Gimble JM, Rice HE. Neurogenic differentiation of murine and human adipose-derived stromal cells. *Biochem. Biophys. Res. Commun.* 2002;294:371-379.

[60] Cao Y, Sun Z, Liao L, Meng Y, Han Q, Zhao RC. Human adipose tissue-derived stem cells differentiate into endothelial cells in vitro and improve postnatal neovascularization in vivo. *Biochem. Biophys. Res. Commun.* 2005;332:370-379.

[61] Seo MJ, Suh SY, Bae YC, Jung JS. Differentiation of human adipose stromal cells into hepatic lineage in vitro and in vivo. *Biochem. Biophys. Res. Commun.* 2005;328:258-264.

[62] De Ugarte DA, Morizono K, Elbarbary A, Alfonso Z, Zuk PA, Zhu M, Dragoo JL, et al. Comparison of multi-lineage cells from human adipose tissue and bone marrow. *Cells Tissues Organs* 2003;174:101-109.

[63] Aurich I, Mueller LP, Aurich H, Luetzkendorf J, Tisljar K, Dollinger MM, Schormann W, et al. Functional integration of hepatocytes derived from human mesenchymal stem cells into mouse livers. *Gut* 2007;56:405-415.

[64] Erices A, Conget P, Minguell JJ. Mesenchymal progenitor cells in human umbilical cord blood. *Br. J. Haematol.* 2000;109:235-242.

[65] Sgodda M, Aurich H, Kleist S, Aurich I, Konig S, Dollinger MM, Fleig WE, et al. Hepatocyte differentiation of mesenchymal stem cells from rat peritoneal adipose tissue in vitro and in vivo. *Exp. Cell Res.* 2007;313:2875-2886.

[66] Covas DT, Siufi JL, Silva AR, Orellana MD. Isolation and culture of umbilical vein mesenchymal stem cells. *Braz. J. Med. Biol. Res.* 2003;36:1179-1183.

[67] De Ugarte DA, Alfonso Z, Zuk PA, Elbarbary A, Zhu M, Ashjian P, Benhaim P, et al. Differential expression of stem cell mobilization-associated molecules on multi-lineage cells from adipose tissue and bone marrow. *Immunol. Lett* 2003;89:267-270.

[68] Lee OK, Kuo TK, Chen WM, Lee KD, Hsieh SL, Chen TH. Isolation of multipotent mesenchymal stem cells from umbilical cord blood. *Blood* 2004;103:1669-1675.

[69] Groh ME, Maitra B, Szekely E, Koc ON. Human mesenchymal stem cells require monocyte-mediated activation to suppress alloreactive T cells. *Exp. Hematol.* 2005;33:928-934.

[70] Barry FP, Murphy JM. Mesenchymal stem cells: clinical applications and biological characterization. *Int. J. Biochem. Cell Biol.* 2004;36:568-584.

[71] Antonitsis P, Ioannidou-Papagiannaki E, Kaidoglou A, Papakonstantinou C. In vitro cardiomyogenic differentiation of adult human bone marrow mesenchymal stem cells. The role of 5-azacytidine. *Interact. Cardiovasc. Thorac Surg.* 2007;6:593-597.

[72] Beyth S, Borovsky Z, Mevorach D, Liebergall M, Gazit Z, Aslan H, Galun E, et al. Human mesenchymal stem cells alter antigen-presenting cell maturation and induce T-cell unresponsiveness. *Blood* 2005;105:2214-2219.

[73] Jiang Y, Jahagirdar BN, Reinhardt RL, Schwartz RE, Keene CD, Ortiz-Gonzalez XR, Reyes M, et al. Pluripotency of mesenchymal stem cells derived from adult marrow. *Nature* 2002;418:41-49.

[74] Caplan AI. Osteogenesis imperfecta, rehabilitation medicine, fundamental research and mesenchymal stem cells. *Connect. Tissue Res.* 1995;31:S9-14.

[75] Tseng PY, Chen CJ, Sheu CC, Yu CW, Huang YS. Spontaneous differentiation of adult rat marrow stromal cells in a long-term culture. *J. Vet. Med. Sci.* 2007;69:95-102.

[76] Bosnakovski D, Mizuno M, Kim G, Takagi S, Okumur M, Fujinag T. Gene expression profile of bovine bone marrow mesenchymal stem cell during spontaneous chondrogenic differentiation in pellet culture system. *Jpn J. Vet. Res.* 2006;53:127-139.

[77] Naruse K, Urabe K, Mukaida T, Ueno T, Migishima F, Oikawa A, Mikuni-Takagaki Y, et al. Spontaneous differentiation of mesenchymal stem cells obtained from fetal rat circulation. *Bone* 2004;35:850-858.

[78] Talens-Visconti R, Bonora A, Jover R, Mirabet V, Carbonell F, Castell JV, Gomez-Lechon MJ. Hepatogenic differentiation of human mesenchymal stem cells from adipose tissue in comparison with bone marrow mesenchymal stem cells. *World J. Gastroenterol.* 2006;12:5834-5845.

[79] Silva WA, Jr., Covas DT, Panepucci RA, Proto-Siqueira R, Siufi JL, Zanette DL, Santos AR, et al. The profile of gene expression of human marrow mesenchymal stem cells. *Stem Cells* 2003;21:661-669.

[80] Aust L, Devlin B, Foster SJ, Halvorsen YD, Hicok K, du Laney T, Sen A, et al. Yield of human adipose-derived adult stem cells from liposuction aspirates. *Cytotherapy* 2004;6:7-14.

[81] Panepucci RA, Siufi JL, Silva WA, Jr., Proto-Siqueira R, Neder L, Orellana M, Rocha V, et al. Comparison of gene expression of umbilical cord vein and bone marrow-derived mesenchymal stem cells. *Stem Cells* 2004;22:1263-1278.

[82] Pittenger MF, Martin BJ. Mesenchymal stem cells and their potential as cardiac therapeutics. *Circ. Res.* 2004;95:9-20.

[83] Lee MW, Choi J, Yang MS, Moon YJ, Park JS, Kim HC, Kim YJ. Mesenchymal stem cells from cryopreserved human umbilical cord blood. *Biochem. Biophys. Res. Commun.* 2004;320:273-278.

[84] Parekkadan B, Sethu P, Van Poll D, Yarmush ML, Toner M. Osmotic Selection of Human Mesenchymal Stem/Progenitor Cells from Umbilical Cord Blood. *Tissue Eng* 2007.

[85] Jager M, Krauspe R. Antigen expression of cord blood derived stem cells under osteogenic stimulation in vitro. *Cell Biol. Int.* 2007;31:950-957.

[86] Yoshimura H, Muneta T, Nimura A, Yokoyama A, Koga H, Sekiya I. Comparison of rat mesenchymal stem cells derived from bone marrow, synovium, periosteum, adipose tissue, and muscle. *Cell Tissue Res.* 2007;327:449-462.

[87] Ishii M, Koike C, Igarashi A, Yamanaka K, Pan H, Higashi Y, Kawaguchi H, et al. Molecular markers distinguish bone marrow mesenchymal stem cells from fibroblasts. *Biochem. Biophys. Res. Commun.* 2005;332:297-303.

[88] Zaret KS. Hepatocyte differentiation: from the endoderm and beyond. *Curr. Opin. Genet. Dev.* 2001;11:568-574.

[89] Wilson JW, Groat CS, Leduc EH. Histogenesis of the Liver. *Ann. NY Acad. Sci.* 1963;111:8-24.

[90] Farber E. Similarities in the sequence of early histological changes induced in the liver of the rat by ethionine, 2-acetylamino-fluorene, and 3'-methyl-4-dimethyl-aminoazobenzene. *Cancer Res.* 1956;16:142-148.

[91] Gonzalez R, Maki CB, Pacchiarotti J, Csontos S, Pham JK, Slepko N, Patel A, et al. Pluripotent marker expression and differentiation of human second trimester Mesenchymal Stem Cells. *Biochem. Biophys. Res. Commun.* 2007;362:491-497.

[92] Ringe J, Strassburg S, Neumann K, Endres M, Notter M, Burmester GR, Kaps C, et al. Towards in situ tissue repair: human mesenchymal stem cells express chemokine receptors CXCR1, CXCR2 and CCR2, and migrate upon stimulation with CXCL8 but not CCL2. *J. Cell Biochem.* 2007;101:135-146.

[93] Di Nicola M, Carlo-Stella C, Magni M, Milanesi M, Longoni PD, Matteucci P, Grisanti S, et al. Human bone marrow stromal cells suppress T-lymphocyte proliferation induced by cellular or nonspecific mitogenic stimuli. *Blood* 2002;99:3838-3843.

[94] Krampera M, Glennie S, Dyson J, Scott D, Laylor R, Simpson E, Dazzi F. Bone marrow mesenchymal stem cells inhibit the response of naive and memory antigen-specific T cells to their cognate peptide. *Blood* 2003;101:3722-3729.

[95] Kang XQ, Zang WJ, Bao LJ, Li DL, Song TS, Xu XL, Yu XJ. Fibroblast growth factor-4 and hepatocyte growth factor induce differentiation of human umbilical cord blood-derived mesenchymal stem cells into hepatocytes. *World J. Gastroenterol.* 2005;11:7461-7465.

[96] Lee KD, Kuo TK, Whang-Peng J, Chung YF, Lin CT, Chou SH, Chen JR, et al. In vitro hepatic differentiation of human mesenchymal stem cells. *Hepatology* 2004;40:1275-1284.

[97] Yoshida Y, Shimomura T, Sakabe T, Ishii K, Gonda K, Matsuoka S, Watanabe Y, et al. A role of Wnt/{beta}-catenin signals in hepatic fate specification of human umbilical cord blood-derived mesenchymal stem cells. *Am. J. Physiol. Gastrointest Liver Physiol.* 2007.

[98] Shimomura T, Yoshida Y, Sakabe T, Ishii K, Gonda K, Murai R, Takubo K, et al. Hepatic differentiation of human bone marrow-derived UE7T-13 cells: Effects of cytokines and CCN family gene expression. *Hepatol. Res.* 2007.

[99] Sato N, Maehara N, Su GH, Goggins M. Effects of 5-aza-2'-deoxycytidine on matrix metalloproteinase expression and pancreatic cancer cell invasiveness. *J. Natl. Cancer Inst* 2003;95:327-330.

[100] Kusaba H, Nakayama M, Harada T, Nomoto M, Kohno K, Kuwano M, Wada M. Association of 5' CpG demethylation and altered chromatin structure in the promoter region with transcriptional activation of the multidrug resistance 1 gene in human cancer cells. *Eur. J. Biochem.* 1999;262:924-932.

[101] Leone G, Voso MT, Teofili L, Lubbert M. Inhibitors of DNA methylation in the treatment of hematological malignancies and MDS. *Clin. Immunol.* 2003;109:89-102.

[102] Banas A, Teratani T, Yamamoto Y, Tokuhara M, Takeshita F, Quinn G, Okochi H, et al. Adipose tissue-derived mesenchymal stem cells as a source of human hepatocytes. *Hepatology* 2007;46:219-228.

[103] Lange C, Bruns H, Kluth D, Zander AR, Fiegel HC. Hepatocytic differentiation of mesenchymal stem cells in cocultures with fetal liver cells. *World J. Gastroenterol* 2006;12:2394-2397.

[104] Okumoto K, Saito T, Haga H, Hattori E, Ishii R, Karasawa T, Suzuki A, et al. Characteristics of rat bone marrow cells differentiated into a liver cell lineage and dynamics of the transplanted cells in the injured liver. *J. Gastroenterol.* 2006;41:62-69.

[105] Runge DM, Runge D, Dorko K, Pisarov LA, Leckel K, Kostrubsky VE, Thomas D, et al. Epidermal growth factor- and hepatocyte growth factor-receptor activity in serum-free cultures of human hepatocytes. *J. Hepatol.* 1999;30:265-274.

[106] Webber EM, Godowski PJ, Fausto N. In vivo response of hepatocytes to growth factors requires an initial priming stimulus. *Hepatology* 1994;19:489-497.

[107] Webber EM, Bruix J, Pierce RH, Fausto N. Tumor necrosis factor primes hepatocytes for DNA replication in the rat. *Hepatology* 1998;28:1226-1234.

[108] Shu SN, Wei L, Wang JH, Zhan YT, Chen HS, Wang Y. Hepatic differentiation capability of rat bone marrow-derived mesenchymal stem cells and hematopoietic stem cells. *World J. Gastroenterol* 2004;10:2818-2822.

[109] Hunter MP, Wilson CM, Jiang X, Cong R, Vasavada H, Kaestner KH, Bogue CW. The homeobox gene Hhex is essential for proper hepatoblast differentiation and bile duct morphogenesis. *Dev. Biol.* 2007;308:355-367.

[110] Qihao Z, Xigu C, Guanghui C, Weiwei Z. Spheroid formation and differentiation into hepatocyte-like cells of rat mesenchymal stem cell induced by co-culture with liver cells. *DNA Cell Biol.* 2007;26:497-503.

[111] Snykers S, Vanhaecke T, De Becker A, Papeleu P, Vinken M, Van Riet I, Rogiers V. Chromatin remodeling agent trichostatin A: a key-factor in the hepatic differentiation of

human mesenchymal stem cells derived of adult bone marrow. *BMC Dev. Biol.* 2007;7:24.

[112] Thompson MD, Monga SP. WNT/beta-catenin signaling in liver health and disease. *Hepatology* 2007;45:1298-1305.

[113] Baksh D, Tuan RS. Canonical and non-canonical Wnts differentially affect the development potential of primary isolate of human bone marrow mesenchymal stem cells. *J. Cell Physiol.* 2007;212:817-826.

[114] Carlson ME, Conboy IM. Regulating the Notch pathway in embryonic, adult and old stem cells. *Curr. Opin. Pharmacol.* 2007;7:303-309.

[115] Fang B, Shi M, Liao L, Yang S, Liu Y, Zhao RC. Systemic infusion of FLK1(+) mesenchymal stem cells ameliorate carbon tetrachloride-induced liver fibrosis in mice. *Transplantation* 2004;78:83-88.

[116] Popp FC, Slowik P, Eggenhofer E, Renner P, Lang SA, Stoeltzing O, Geissler EK, et al. No contribution of multipotent mesenchymal stromal cells to liver regeneration in a rat model of prolonged hepatic injury. *Stem Cells* 2007;25:639-645.

[117] Oyagi S, Hirose M, Kojima M, Okuyama M, Kawase M, Nakamura T, Ohgushi H, et al. Therapeutic effect of transplanting HGF-treated bone marrow mesenchymal cells into CCl4-injured rats. *J. Hepatol.* 2006;44:742-748.

[118] Zhao DC, Lei JX, Chen R, Yu WH, Zhang XM, Li SN, Xiang P. Bone marrow-derived mesenchymal stem cells protect against experimental liver fibrosis in rats. *World J. Gastroenterol.* 2005;11:3431-3440.

[119] Chamberlain J, Yamagami T, Colletti E, Theise ND, Desai J, Frias A, Pixley J, et al. Efficient generation of human hepatocytes by the intrahepatic delivery of clonal human mesenchymal stem cells in fetal sheep. *Hepatology* 2007.

[120] Ishii T, Yasuchika K, Fujii H, Hoppo T, Baba S, Naito M, Machimoto T, et al. In vitro differentiation and maturation of mouse embryonic stem cells into hepatocytes. *Exp. Cell Res.* 2005;309:68-77.

[121] Kumashiro Y, Asahina K, Ozeki R, Shimizu-Saito K, Tanaka Y, Kida Y, Inoue K, et al. Enrichment of hepatocytes differentiated from mouse embryonic stem cells as a transplantable source. *Transplantation* 2005;79:550-557.

[122] Almeida-Porada G, Porada CD, Chamberlain J, Torabi A, Zanjani ED. Formation of human hepatocytes by human hematopoietic stem cells in sheep. *Blood* 2004;104:2582-2590.

[123] Fujino H, Hiramatsu H, Tsuchiya A, Niwa A, Noma H, Shiota M, Umeda K, et al. Human cord blood CD34+ cells develop into hepatocytes in the livers of NOD/SCID/{gamma}cnull mice through cell fusion. *Faseb J.* 2007.

[124] Jang YY, Collector MI, Baylin SB, Diehl AM, Sharkis SJ. Hematopoietic stem cells convert into liver cells within days without fusion. *Nat. Cell Biol.* 2004;6:532-539.

[125] Masson S, Harrison DJ, Plevris JN, Newsome PN. Potential of hematopoietic stem cell therapy in hepatology: a critical review. *Stem Cells* 2004;22:897-907.

[126] Schmelzer E, Zhang L, Bruce A, Wauthier E, Ludlow J, Yao HL, Moss N, et al. Human hepatic stem cells from fetal and postnatal donors. *J. Exp. Med.* 2007;204:1973-1987.

[127] Dan YY, Riehle KJ, Lazaro C, Teoh N, Haque J, Campbell JS, Fausto N. Isolation of multipotent progenitor cells from human fetal liver capable of differentiating into liver and mesenchymal lineages. *Proc. Natl. Acad. Sci. USA* 2006;103:9912-9917.

[128] Shafritz DA, Dabeva MD. Liver stem cells and model systems for liver repopulation. *J. Hepatol.* 2002;36:552-564.

[129] Almeida-Porada G, El Shabrawy D, Porada C, Zanjani ED. Differentiative potential of human metanephric mesenchymal cells. *Exp. Hematol.* 2002;30:1454-1462.

[130] Gregory CA, Ylostalo J, Prockop DJ. Adult bone marrow stem/progenitor cells (MSCs) are preconditioned by microenvironmental "niches" in culture: a two-stage hypothesis for regulation of MSC fate. *Sci. STKE* 2005;2005:pe37.

[131] Uccelli A, Moretta L, Pistoia V. Immunoregulatory function of mesenchymal stem cells. *Eur. J. Immunol.* 2006;36:2566-2573.

[132] Nauta AJ, Fibbe WE. Immunomodulatory properties of mesenchymal stromal cells. *Blood* 2007.

[133] Puissant B, Barreau C, Bourin P, Clavel C, Corre J, Bousquet C, Taureau C, et al. Immunomodulatory effect of human adipose tissue-derived adult stem cells: comparison with bone marrow mesenchymal stem cells. *Br. J. Haematol.* 2005;129:118-129.

[134] Barry FP, Murphy JM, English K, Mahon BP. Immunogenicity of adult mesenchymal stem cells: lessons from the fetal allograft. *Stem Cells Dev.* 2005;14:252-265.

[135] Fibbe WE, Nauta AJ, Roelofs H. Modulation of immune responses by mesenchymal stem cells. *Ann. NY Acad. Sci.* 2007;1106:272-278.

[136] Ringden O, Uzunel M, Rasmusson I, Remberger M, Sundberg B, Lonnies H, Marschall HU, et al. Mesenchymal stem cells for treatment of therapy-resistant graft-versus-host disease. *Transplantation* 2006;81:1390-1397.

[137] Le Blanc K, Rasmusson I, Sundberg B, Gotherstrom C, Hassan M, Uzunel M, Ringden O. Treatment of severe acute graft-versus-host disease with third party haploidentical mesenchymal stem cells. *Lancet* 2004;363:1439-1441.

[138] Vassilopoulos G, Wang PR, Russell DW. Transplanted bone marrow regenerates liver by cell fusion. *Nature* 2003;422:901-904.

[139] Wang X, Willenbring H, Akkari Y, Torimaru Y, Foster M, Al-Dhalimy M, Lagasse E, et al. Cell fusion is the principal source of bone-marrow-derived hepatocytes. *Nature* 2003;422:897-901.

[140] Alvarez-Dolado M, Pardal R, Garcia-Verdugo JM, Fike JR, Lee HO, Pfeffer K, Lois C, et al. Fusion of bone-marrow-derived cells with Purkinje neurons, cardiomyocytes and hepatocytes. *Nature* 2003;425:968-973.

[141] Harris RG, Herzog EL, Bruscia EM, Grove JE, Van Arnam JS, Krause DS. Lack of a fusion requirement for development of bone marrow-derived epithelia. *Science* 2004;305:90-93.

[142] Heo J, Factor VM, Uren T, Takahama Y, Lee JS, Major M, Feinstone SM, et al. Hepatic precursors derived from murine embryonic stem cells contribute to regeneration of injured liver. *Hepatology* 2006;44:1478-1486.

In: Encyclopedia of Stem Cell Research (2 Volume Set) ISBN: 978-1-61761-835-2
Editor: Alexander L. Greene © 2012 Nova Science Publishers, Inc.

Chapter XIII

RECENT ADVANCEMENTS TOWARDS THE DERIVATION OF IMMUNE-COMPATIBLE PATIENT-SPECIFIC HUMAN PLURIPOTENT STEM CELL LINES

Micha Drukker[*]

Institute for Stem Cell Biology and Regenerative Medicine, Beckman Center,
Stanford, CA, US

ABSTRACT

The derivation of human embryonic stem cell lines from blastocyst stage embryos, first achieved almost a decade ago, demonstrated the potential to prepare virtually unlimited numbers of therapeutically beneficial cells *in vitro*. Assuming that large-scale production of differentiated cells is attainable, it is imperative to develop strategies to prevent immune responses towards the grafted cells following transplantation. This paper presents recent advances in the production of pluripotent cell lines using three emerging techniques: somatic cell nuclear transfer into enucleated oocytes and zygotes, parthenogenetic activation of unfertilized oocytes and induction of pluripotency in somatic cells. These techniques have a remarkable potential for generation of patient-specific pluripotent cells that would be tolerated by the immune system.

Keywords: Human embryonic stem cells (hESCs); Immunogenicity; Parthenogenesis; Somatic cell nuclear transfer (SCNT); Induction of pluripotent stem (iPS) cells.

---

[*] Micha Drukker: dmicha@stanford.edu

INTRODUCTION

Human embryonic stem cells (hESCs) have the capacity perpetuate themselves indefinitely in culture conditions while maintaining the potential to differentiate to all cell types of the body upon induction [1, 2]. These cells offer a considerable therapeutic advantage over the lineage-committed adult stem cell types such as hematopoietic stem cells (HSCs) and neuronal stem cells, since they may serve as virtually an infinite source for all cell lineages. Therefore, the isolation of hESCs has lead to numerous studies that aim to isolate beneficial cells for therapeutics [1]. The goal now remains to develop methodologies for harnessing the potential of hESCs in tissue replacement, repair, maintenance, and/or enhancement of function.

As a first step towards this goal, multiple laboratories have developed an array of differentiation protocols to derive specialized cell types, such as neuronal cells, cardiomyocytes, endothelial cells, hematopoietic precursors and hepatocytes (reviewed in [3]). Yet, other aspects of cellular therapeutics should be addressed before successful therapeutic application of hESC-derived cells is possible. For example, differentiation protocols need to improve to the point that homogenous preparations of particular cell types can be produced without any remaining undifferentiated (and potentially teratogenic) cells. In addition, derivation, propagation and differentiation of hESCs should be carried out in animal product-free culture conditions to prevent cross-specie contaminations. Finally, implanted cells must successfully integrate into the patient's tissue without prompting immune responses towards the graft. This review summarizes the current knowledge about the immune properties of hESCs and their differentiated derivatives (for detailed review see [4]) followed by an discussion of novel strategies that could potentially generate histocompatible patient-specific hESC lines.

IMMUNOGENICITY OF HUMAN EMBRYONIC STEM CELLS AND DIFFERENTIATED CELLS

The two arms of the immune system, innate and adaptive, can interact with transplanted allogeneic cells (from genetically non-identical individual) leading to their rejection. Clearly, the major assaults on allogeneic tissues are mediated either directly through the action of cytotoxic T cells or by alloantibodies that are produced by alloreactive B cells against graft-derived antigens (reviewed in [5]). Class I and II MHC proteins (MHC-I and MHC-II, respectively), which are encoded by a highly variable set of human leukocyte antigens (HLA), lie at the heart of these acute allogeneic responses (reviewed in [6]). Following transplantation, foreign MHC molecules, which are expressed on grafted cells, can interact with the recipient's T cells leading to their sensitization and maturation into cytotoxic T cells that attack the transplant (direct recognition) [7]. In addition, host professional antigen presenting cells can processes foreign MHC molecules and present them to host T and B cells leading to alloantibodies secretion by B cells (indirect recognition) [6]. When alloantibodies enter circulation, they bind to transplanted cells and target them for destruction by phagocytosis and the complement system.

To evaluate whether hESCs and their derivatives could potentially induce allogeneic responses, the expression of MHC molecules on these cells was tested in a number of studies [8, 9]. It was found that undifferentiated hESCs express low levels of MHC-I proteins and that differentiation and application of interferons (IFNs) induces 100-fold increase to somatic levels. In contrast, MHC-II proteins seem to be absent under all tested conditions probably due to minimal differentiation towards hematopoietic fate (MHC-II expression is largely restricted to this lineage). Furthermore, together with colleagues, we tested the immunogenicity of hESCs *in vitro* by incubating the cells with pre-stimulated human T cells. We found that following MHC-I induction by IFNs kT cells specifically recognize and lyse hESCs. In contrast, human T-cell response against differentiated hESCs in mice was very weak most probably due to low expression of co-stimulatory signals (CD80 and CD86) that are necessary for T activation [10]. These data indicate that hESCs express sufficient levels of MHC-I molecules to elicit rejection by primed cytotoxic T cells, but have a reduced potential to stimulate T cells.

Another line of immune defense that can potentially reject foreign grafts is natural killer (NK) cells. Theses are cytotoxic lymphocytes that lyse cells based on the balance between stimulating and inhibiting signals that are provided by target cells. It is possible that low expression of MHC-I in hESCs and their derivatives could result in their targeting by NK cells since these molecules serve as ligands for NK-cell inhibitory receptors [11]. When we examined the NK-cell response towards hESCs *in vitro*, we found that irrespective of MHC expression NK cells do not readily lyse hESCs [9]. Additional studies are required to determine whether hESCs are sensitive to NK-mediated rejection *in vivo*, and whether NK cells might pose a significant obstacle to hESC therapeutics. At least in one case, it has been shown that hematopoietic progenies of mouse ES are rejected by NK cells *in vivo* [12].

Based on the existing data regarding antigenicity and immunogenicity of hESCs, a complex picture of their immunological status can be drawn. Differentiation to specialized somatic cell types is likely to induce moderate levels of MHC-I expression and in the case of hematopoietic differentiation MHC-II and co-stimulatory molecules will also be expressed [13-15]. Thus, T-cell mediated immune responses are likely to be directed at differentiated hESCs, and in the case of hematopoietic transplantation this reaction may be even more severe. Also, alloantibodies and NK cells may play a role in graft rejection. Therefore, these immune factors must be considered when designing strategies for preventing rejection of hESC-derived transplants.

STRATEGIES FOR IMMUNE PROTECTION OF DIFFERENTIATED HUMAN EMBRYONIC STEM CELLS

Excluding immunosuppression, currently five major approaches may be used to diminish or abolish the immune response against transplanted hESCs (i-iv were reviewed in [4, 16]). These options include: *i)* transplantation of differentiated therapeutic cells to natural environments that restrict immune responses (immune-privileged sites), such as the brain and testis. *ii*) Generation of large hESC line banks will allow matching MHC haplotypes between patients and cell lines. *iii*) Genetic manipulation of the genes that encode for MHC antigens and other immune modulators in hESC. *iv*) Induction of hematopoietic chimerism – a state that allows acceptance of allografts from the donor cell line that is used for hematopoietic stem cell transplantation. *v*) Generation of genetically identical hESC lines specifically for each patient. The latter approach would alleviate most immunological considerations, but until very recently seemed improbable due to technical and ethical issues. This view is changing now as several seminal advancements made within the last two years have indicated that tailored derivations of patient specific syngeneic (genetically close or identical) hESC lines could be done in the near future. I will discuss these developments hereafter (summarized in table 1).

Table 1. Proposed pathways for derivation of patient specific hESC lines

Method	Cell sources		Gender specificity	Immunological considerations for transplantation	Demonstrated in:	
					Mouse	Human
Parthenogenesis	Metaphase II oocytes [19]		Yes, female	Preferentially, MHC heterozygous cells should be used	+	+
Somatic cell nuclear transfer	Oocytes [28]	+ Somatic nucleus	No	Mitochondrial mHAgs might induce immune responses	+	-
	Zygotes [30]					
Fusion with hESCs	Fibroblasts [34]		No	Should be used only as diploid cells	+	+
			No			
Induced pluripotency	Embryonic and adult fibroblasts [36-41]		No	Unknown	+	+

PARTHENOGENETICALLY ACTIVATED OOCYTES GIVE RISE TO SYNGENEIC ES CELL LINES

Parthenogenesis is the process of embryonic development without male fertilization. Mammals do not reproduce by parthenogenesis, but for many species activation of arrested metaphase oocytes by chemical regents can lead to development into diploid blastocyst stage embryos. Protocols for ESC-derivation from pseudo-zygotes were developed for mouse [17], macaque monkey [18] and recently human embryos by Revazova et al., [19]. Quite strikingly, this study showed that about half of the human oocytes that were chemically activated (23 of

46 embryos) progressed to the blastocyst stage, and of these, six parthenogenetic ESC (pESCs) lines were successfully produced. In mice and presumably also in humans, parthenogenetic embryos do not develop past the early limb bud stage as embryonic development require expression from the two parental genomes [20]. Still, the differentiation capacity of mouse, macaque monkey and human pESCs is striking; for example, mouse pESCs differentiate *in vitro* and contribute to multiple tissues in chimeric mice. When transplantation compatibility of these cells was tested, it was found that differentiated pESC lines engrafted only in MHC matched animals, meaning that they are histocompatible with the nucleus donor [21]. Similarly, human pESCs (phESCs) form embryoid bodies (EBs) in culture and teratomas that include cell types of the three embryonic germ layers, however, their immunological properties are yet to be determined [19].

The extent of homozygosity in parthenogenetic cells depends on oocyte activation stage, metaphase-I or metaphase-II and on recombination events. Activation of metaphase-I arrested oocytes (before first polar body extrusion) gives rise to pESC lines that are identical to the donor as they contain the two maternal chromosome homologs. However, it is unlikely that these cells would be used for therapeutics since experiments in mice showed that they were tetraploid or aneuploid. Metaphase-II arrested mouse and human oocytes (before second polar body extrusion) give rise to pESC lines containing duplicated hemizygote genome and have normal karyotype [17]. Therefore, the latter may be clinically applicable.

Although phESC lines are histocompatible with the oocyte donor, NK cells may actually respond against the cells if they lack one set of MHC genes. This phenomenon is thought to be relevant mainly to rejection of bone marrow by NK cells following transplantation (reviewed in [22]) and therefore should be examined carefully prior clinical application. It seems that all metaphase-II derived phESC lines that were reported by Revazova et al., contained full heterozygosity in the MHC region [19]. This means that during oocyte development, recombination occurred between the centromere and the MHC region on chromosome 6 homologs, and the resulting recombinant sister chromatids contain the whole MHC milieu. Therefore, NK-cell response against differentiated phESCs that retain heterozygosity seems unlikely.

It should be noted that phESCs were probably also derived in experiments carried out by Hwang's group in South Korea. Although the team reported the derivation of "cloned" embryo-derived hESCs they could not provide definitive proof to show that the cell lines were not result of parthenogenesis. Recently, Kim et al., found that the most of the genes in pESCs are heterozygous, but close to the centromere the gene copies show predominant homozygosity [23]. In contrast, nuclear transfer-derived ESCs (ntESCs) contain heterozygosity throughout the genome. Analysis of a hESC line that was claimed to be derived from a cloned embryo [24] showed that the cells contain extensive homozygosity in the MHC loci indicating that this cell line is actually parthenote [23].

PhESC lines that carry only one set of MHC genes (when recombination does not occur) could potentially prove beneficial not only for the oocyte donor but also for genetically related individuals. For example, there is a 50% chance that a cell line that is derived for a patient will be histocompatible to any of her children. Moreover, if a sizable depository of MHC homozygous phESC lines that carry MHC alleles that are common in the population were to be generated, it may serve as a hESC MHC matching bank [25]. In summary, if it would be possible to produce phESC lines as effectively as reported, such cells may become a major source of therapeutic histocompatible cell lines for fertile women, genetically related individuals and the general public. It is important to note that the extent of the NK-cell response against such transplants remains unclear and must be further examined. Immune responses against minor histocompatibility antigens and mitochondrial antigens may jeopardize grafted cells from genetically non-identical hESC lines (discussed below). It is likely that additional factors such as the tissue in question, the transplantation site and the extent of donor-derived vasculature would also influence transplantation outcomes.

DERIVATION OF EMBRYONIC STEM CELLS FROM SOMATIC CELL NUCLEAR TRANSFERRED OOCYTES AND ZYGOTES

The seminal experiment of producing live sheep from oocytes that had their nucleus replaced by somatic nucleus (somatic cell nuclear transfer - SCNT) proved for the first time that the genetic information in the somatic mammalian nucleus could be reprogrammed to the embryonic state [26]. Since then, this technique has been successfully translated to other species, including mouse, rabbit, cat, pig, cow and goat (reviewed in [27]). Cloned mouse embryos can give rise to ESC lines with a relatively high success rate [28]. Since the nucleus donor and the ESC line are genetically identical, except for mitochondrial antigens (discussed below), it has been suggested that differentiated tissues derived from human reprogrammed cell lines would not be rejected by the immune system of the donor.

Currently, there is still no proof for isolation of ntESCs from cloned humans oocytes and previous publications that described the derivation of such lines have been retracted [29, 24]. Nevertheless, these studies were probably the first to report derivation of hESCs from parthenogenetic embryos. If SCNT into human oocytes and the generation of histocompatible ESC lines could be achieved, a significant obstacle lies in acquiring the large numbers of oocytes that would be necessary for the clinical application of this technique. A novel approach that may alleviate this issue utilizes mitotically arrested zygotes to reprogram injected mitotic somatic nuclei, following chromosome removal [30]. After release from mitotic arrest, ~20% of the mouse cloned embryos developed to the blastocyst stage, and of these, ~5% developed to full term following transfer to pseudopregnant recipients (no live births were recorded). Cloned blastocysts could give rise to ESC lines that were shown to contribute extensively to chimeric embryos following injection into recipient blastocysts. The authors went on to prove that murine aneuploid zygotes (containing more than 2 polar bodies) could also serve as recipients to chromosome transfer following zygotic chromosome removal. This means that abnormal human embryos containing more than two nuclei and are therefore discarded following in vitro fertilization (about 5% of the embryos), could potentially be used to generate patient specific hESC lines. Still, it is important to note that SCNT into human oocytes or zygotes was not demonstrated to date.

One final immunological issue not addressed by derivation of hESC lines through SCNT is the potential immune response directed towards mitochondrial histocompatibility antigens. It is known that in mouse and rats certain amino acid substitutions in mitochondrial proteins can lead to generation of specific alloreactive cytotoxic T cells [31]. Therefore, it is possible that certain mitochondrial protein polymorphisms might become antigenic and initiate immune responses following transplantation of differentiated hESCs that were generated following SCNT. But, the small number of encoded proteins in mitochondria and the relatively small number of mitochondrial single nucleotide polymorphisms (~170), suggests that the risk of immune response towards donor-derived mitochondrial antigens would be considerably smaller than mismatched genomes. In accordance, it has been shown in cows that transplantation of organs derived from cloned embryos to the adult nuclear donor did not lead to immune response even though they express different mitochondrial haplotypes [32].

REPROGRAMMING OF SOMATIC CELLS BY FUSION WITH EMBRYONIC STEM CELLS

Similarly to the reprogramming effects of oocytes and zygotes, ESCs also have the capacity to reprogram somatic nucleus to the ESC-state. Since ESCs are small and have a high nucleus-to-cytoplasm ratio, reprogramming by SCNT into these cells is technically challenging and has not been reported to date. Still, fusion of somatic cells with ESC partners has a similar reprogramming effect on the somatic nucleus leading to reactivation of embryonic genes [33]. This concept has been proven recently for human somatic cells fused with hESCs in two studies that used foreskin fibroblasts and hESC-derived myeloid progenitors as fusion partners [34, 35]. In both cases, the resulting hybrid cell lines could gave rise to EBs in vitro and teratomas in vivo. Therefore, fusion of patient's somatic cells with hESCs could potentially circumvent the need for oocytes or embryos as vehicles to reprogram somatic cells to the ESC-stage.

Still, it seems unlikely that tetraploid hybrid cells would be considered suitable as therapeutic reagents due to their genomic instability. Moreover, such cell lines contain 4 copies of the MHC region and therefore, MHC matching is improbable. It is possible that in the future technical advancements will allow elimination of the ESC chromosomes before or after cell fusion. Alternatively, enucleated hESCs may preserve the capacity to reprogram the somatic genome. If these techniques will be developed, issues such as the extent of somatic reprogramming and full differentiation capacity of hESC/somatic cell fusions will have to be investigated further.

REPROGRAMMING SOMATIC CELLS BY DEFINED FACTORS

Successful experiments showing nuclear reprogramming by SCNT and by fusion of somatic cells with ESCs have led to the realization that oocytes, early zygotes and ESCs contain reprogramming factors. Successful reprogramming by fusion is of particular importance in trying to isolate these factors since measurements of gene expression can be carried out reliably in ESCs but not in oocytes and zygotes. Using this rationale, Shinya Yamanaka and colleagues have recently examined the ability of 24 genes that are preferentially expressed in mouse ESCs to reprogram somatic cells [36]. Introduction of the genes was carried out by retroviral transduction and then selection of cells that obtained the pluripotent state was carried out by a knock-in of drug resistance cassette into a gene that is specifically expressed in ES cells. They found that co-transfecting all the 24 factors into murine fetal fibroblasts could induce pluripotent state and colonies that had ESC morphology and expressed pluripotency markers were formed. They went on to determine which of 24 factors are necessary for the process and found that the four transcription factors that are critical for induction of pluripotent stem (iPS) cells are Oct3/4, Klf4, Sox2 and c-Myc. The authors also showed that iPS cells can differentiate into EBs, teratomas and contribute to all cell lineages including germline by generating adult chimeras [37].

During the past year, additional two independent laboratories have confirmed these results [38, 39] and very recently Yamanaka [40] and Thomson [41] groups showed that induction of pluripotency is also applicable to human cells. Yamanaka's group used the same four factors to induce pluripotency in human cells whereas Thomson group used Nanog and Lin28 instead of Klf4 and c-Myc. Furthermore, Yamanaka's group showed that iPS colonies could be isolated just by morphological criteria without the use of gene selection [40]. This elegant investigation showed for the first time that pluripotency can be induced using a relatively simple method of over-expressing transcription factors in somatic cells. From the immunological perspective, iPS cells would be fully compatible with the donor since there is no addition of genetic information to the cells.

Since induction of pluripotency by transcription factors is a very recent development it is still undetermined whether introduction of transgenes expressing Oct3/4, c-Myc and Klf4 is safe for clinical use. For example, as a result of c-Myc reactivation, tumors were found in about a fourth of the F1 offspring that were born to iPS cell injected chimeras [37]. Therefore, strategies to induce pluripotency without stable integration of oncogenes and retroviruses must be developed. If these issues can be met, iPS cells will be generated per patient needs and it is very likely that they will become the primary source of differentiated cells.

CONCLUSION

The extent to which hESC-derived tissues will be used for therapeutics depends first and foremost on the capacity to develop differentiation protocols and methods for isolation of therapeutically relevant cells free from hazardous undifferentiated cells. Once that is successfully achieved, the immunological response represents the next obstacle that will strongly influence transplantation outcomes and hence the feasibility of such treatments. Our current knowledge indicates that following differentiation, hESCs express MHC-I and possibly MHC-II molecules and therefore might be rejected by adaptive immune responses. Circumventing this hurdle depends on the capacity to either actively prevent the immune response, for example by genetic manipulation of the MHC genes, or by the generation and use of patient specific hESC lines. Until very recently, it seemed that generating patient specific hESC lines would be possible only by SCNT into donated oocytes but the scarcity of donated oocytes, as well ethical issues regarding their obtainment and use, represent considerable obstacles for implementation of this technique.

Outlined in the review, several new key developments may now enable derivation of patient specific "tailor made" hESC lines. Parthenogenetic hESC lines that have the full donor MHC repertoire may be derived, but still their derivation and use is likely to be practical only for fertile women. In contrast, SCNT into genetically abnormal zygotes may be used to produce genetically identical hESC lines for virtually any nucleus donor (although mitochondrial antigens may still vary). It seems that the ethical and religious considerations using these two options would be minimal since parthenogenetic embryos cannot fully develop and abnormal zygotes are routinely discarded. Perhaps the most significant breakthrough, however, is the demonstration that human pluripotent stem cells can be induced in somatic cells by the introduction of four pluripotency-inducing genes. Adaptation of this technique for derivation of transplantation-safe patient-specific human pluripotent cell lines would bypass significant technical, as well as ethical issues that are associated with oocyte and zygote usage [42]. Relevant to all these derivation pathways, is the fact that *in vitro* differentiated hESCs might have somewhat modified expression signature of immunological antigens and other molecules that participate in immune responses. Hence, analysis of their immune properties will need to be further pursued prior to clinical use.

ACKNOWLEDGMENTS

I would like to thank Mr. C. Tang and Drs. T. Serwold, R. Ardehali and Y. Mayshar for critical reading of the manuscript. M.D. is supported by a Human Frontier Science Program postdoctoral fellowship.

REFERENCES

[1] Thomson, J. A. Itskovitz-Eldor, J. Shapiro, S. S. Waknitz, M. A. Swiergiel, J. J. Marshall, V. S. and Jones, J. M. (1998). Embryonic stem cell lines derived from human blastocysts. *Science, 282,* 1145-1147.

[2] Reubinoff, B. E. Pera, M. F. Fong, C. Y. Trounson, A. and Bongso, A. (2000). Embryonic stem cell lines from human blastocysts: somatic differentiation in vitro. *Nat. Biotechnol., 18,* 399-404.

[3] Hyslop, L. A. Armstrong, L. Stojkovic, M. and Lako, M. (2005). Human embryonic stem cells: biology and clinical implications. *Expert Rev. Mol. Med, 7,* 1-21.

[4] Drukker, M. and Benvenisty, N. (2004). The immunogenicity of human embryonic stem-derived cells. *Trends. Biotechnol., 22,* 136-141.

[5] Rogers, N. J. and Lechler, R. I. (2001). Allorecognition. *Am. J. Transplant., 1,* 97-102.

[6] Lechler, R. I. Sykes, M. Thomson, A. W. and Turka, L. A. (2005). Organ transplantation--how much of the promise has been realized? *Nat. Med, 11,* 605-613.

[7] Suchin, E. J. Langmuir, P. B. Palmer, E. Sayegh, M. H. Wells, A. D. and Turka, L. A. (2001). Quantifying the frequency of alloreactive T cells in vivo: new answers to an old question. *J. Immunol, 166,* 973-981.

[8] Draper, J. S. Pigott, C. Thomson, J. A. and Andrews, P. W. (2002). Surface antigens of human embryonic stem cells: changes upon differentiation in culture. *J. Anat., 200,* 249-258.

[9] Drukker, M. Katz, G. Urbach, A. Schuldiner, M. Markel, G. Itskovitz-Eldor, J. Reubinoff, B. Mandelboim, O. and Benvenisty, N. (2002). Characterization of the expression of MHC proteins in human embryonic stem cells. *Proc. Natl. Acad. Sci. U. S. A., 99,* 9864-9869.

[10] Drukker, M. Katchman, H. Katz, G. Even-Tov Friedman, S. Shezen, E. Hornstein, E. Mandelboim, O. Reisner, Y. and Benvenisty, N. (2006). Human embryonic stem cells and their differentiated derivatives are less susceptible to immune rejection than adult cells. *Stem Cells, 24,* 221-229.

[11] Raulet, D. H. (2006). Missing self recognition and self tolerance of natural killer (NK) cells. *Semin. Immunol, 18,* 145-150.

[12] Rideout, W. M., 3rd Hochedlinger, K. Kyba, M. Daley, G. Q. and Jaenisch, R. (2002). Correction of a genetic defect by nuclear transplantation and combined cell and gene therapy. *Cell, 109,* 17-27.

[13] Anderson, J. S. Bandi, S. Kaufman, D. S. and Akkina, R. (2006). Derivation of normal macrophages from human embryonic stem (hES) cells for applications in HIV gene therapy. *Retrovirology, 3,* 24.

[14] Kaufman, D. S. Hanson, E. T. Lewis, R. L. Auerbach, R. and Thomson, J. A. (2001). Hematopoietic colony-forming cells derived from human embryonic stem cells. *Proc. Natl. Acad. Sci. U. S. A., 98,* 10716-10721.

[15] Slukvin, II Vodyanik, M. A. Thomson, J. A. Gumenyuk, M. E. and Choi, K. D. (2006). Directed differentiation of human embryonic stem cells into functional dendritic cells through the myeloid pathway. *J. Immunol, 176,* 2924-2932.

[16] Bradley, J. A. Bolton, E. M. and Pedersen, R. A. (2002). Stem cell medicine encounters the immune system. *Nat. Rev. Immunol, 2,* 859-871.

[17] Allen, N. D. Barton, S. C. Hilton, K. Norris, M. L. and Surani, M. A. (1994). A functional analysis of imprinting in parthenogenetic embryonic stem cells. *Development, 120,* 1473-1482.

[18] Cibelli, J. B. Grant, K. A. Chapman, K. B. Cunniff, K. Worst, T. Green, H. L. Walker, S. J. Gutin, P. H. Vilner, L. Tabar, V. Dominko, T. Kane, J. Wettstein, P. J. Lanza, R. P. Studer, L. Vrana, K. E. and West, M. D. (2002). Parthenogenetic stem cells in nonhuman primates. *Science, 295,* 819.

[19] Revazova, E. S. Turovets, N. A. Kochetkova, O. D. Kindarova, L. B. Kuzmichev, L. N. Janus, J. D. and Pryzhkova, M. V. (2007). Patient-Specific Stem Cell Lines Derived from Human Parthenogenetic Blastocysts. *Cloning Stem Cells.*

[20] Kaufman, M. H. Barton, S. C. and Surani, M. A. (1977). Normal postimplantation development of mouse parthenogenetic embryos to the forelimb bud stage. *Nature, 265,* 53-55.

[21] Kim, K. Lerou, P. Yabuuchi, A. Lengerke, C. Ng, K. West, J. Kirby, A. Daly, M. J. and Daley, G. Q. (2007). Histocompatible embryonic stem cells by parthenogenesis. *Science, 315,* 482-486.

[22] Hoglund, P. Sundback, J. Olsson-Alheim, M. Y. Johansson, M. Salcedo, M. Ohlen, C. Ljunggren, H. G. Sentman, C. L. and Karre, K. (1997). Host MHC class I gene control of NK-cell specificity in the mouse. *Immunol. Rev, 155,* 11-28.

[23] Kim, K. Ng, K. Rugg-Gunn, P., G. Shieh, J. Kirak, O. Jaenisch, R. Wakayama, T. Moore, M., A. Pedersen, R., A. and Daley, G., Q. (2007). Recombination Signatures Distinguish Embryonic Stem Cells Derived by Parthenogenesis and Somatic Cell Nuclear Transfer. *Cell Stem Cell, 1,* 1-7.

[24] Hwang, W. S. Ryu, Y. J. Park, J. H. Park, E. S. Lee, E. G. Koo, J. M. Chun, H. Y. Lee, B. C. Kang, S. K. Kim, S. J. Ahn, C. Hwang, J. H. Park, K. Y. Cibelli, J. B. and Moon, S. Y. (2004). Evidence of a Pluripotent Human Embryonic Stem Cell Line Derived from a Cloned Blastocyst. *Science.*

[25] Taylor, C. J. Bolton, E. M. Pocock, S. Sharples, L. D. Pedersen, R. A. and Bradley, J. A. (2005). Banking on human embryonic stem cells: estimating the number of donor cell lines needed for HLA matching. *Lancet, 366,* 2019-2025.

[26] Campbell, K. H. McWhir, J. Ritchie, W. A. and Wilmut, I. (1996). Sheep cloned by nuclear transfer from a cultured cell line. *Nature, 380,* 64-66.

[27] Gurdon, J. B. and Byrne, J. A. (2003). The first half-century of nuclear transplantation. *Proc. Natl. Acad. Sci. U. S. A, 100,* 8048-8052.

[28] Hochedlinger, K. and Jaenisch, R. (2003). Nuclear transplantation, embryonic stem cells, and the potential for cell therapy. *N. Engl. J. Med, 349,* 275-286.

[29] Hwang, W. S. Roh, S. I. Lee, B. C. Kang, S. K. Kwon, D. K. Kim, S. Kim, S. J. Park, S. W. Kwon, H. S. Lee, C. K. Lee, J. B. Kim, J. M. Ahn, C. Paek, S. H. Chang, S. S. Koo, J. J. Yoon, H. S. Hwang, J. H. Hwang, Y. Y. Park, Y. S. Oh, S. K. Kim, H. S. Park, J. H. Moon, S. Y. and Schatten, G. (2005). Patient-specific embryonic stem cells derived from human SCNT blastocysts. *Science, 308,* 1777-1783.

[30] Egli, D. Rosains, J. Birkhoff, G. and Eggan, K. (2007). Developmental reprogramming after chromosome transfer into mitotic mouse zygotes. *Nature, 447,* 679-685.

[31] Loveland, B. Wang, C. R. Yonekawa, H. Hermel, E. and Lindahl, K. F. (1990). Maternally transmitted histocompatibility antigen of mice: a hydrophobic peptide of a mitochondrially encoded protein. *Cell, 60,* 971-980.

[32] Lanza, R. P. Chung, H. Y. Yoo, J. J. Wettstein, P. J. Blackwell, C. Borson, N. Hofmeister, E. Schuch, G. Soker, S. Moraes, C. T. West, M. D. and Atala, A. (2002). Generation of histocompatible tissues using nuclear transplantation. *Nat. Biotechnol, 20,* 689-696.

[33] Tada, M. Takahama, Y. Abe, K. Nakatsuji, N. and Tada, T. (2001). Nuclear reprogramming of somatic cells by in vitro hybridization with ES cells. *Curr. Biol, 11,* 1553-1558.

[34] Cowan, C. A. Atienza, J. Melton, D. A. and Eggan, K. (2005). Nuclear reprogramming of somatic cells after fusion with human embryonic stem cells. *Science, 309,* 1369-1373.

[35] Yu, J. Vodyanik, M. A. He, P. Slukvin, II and Thomson, J. A. (2006). Human embryonic stem cells reprogram myeloid precursors following cell-cell fusion. *Stem Cells, 24,* 168-176.

[36] Takahashi, K. and Yamanaka, S. (2006). Induction of pluripotent stem cells from mouse embryonic and adult fibroblast cultures by defined factors. *Cell, 126,* 663-676.

[37] Okita, K. Ichisaka, T. and Yamanaka, S. (2007). Generation of germline-competent induced pluripotent stem cells. *Nature, 448,* 313-317.

[38] Maherali, N. Sridharan, R. Xie, W. Utikal, J. Eminli, S. Arnold, K. Stadtfeld, M. Yachechko, R. Tchieu, J. Jaenisch, R. Plath, K. and Hochedlinger, K. (2007). Directly Reprogrammed Fibroblasts Show Global Epigenetic Remodeling and Widespread Tissue Contribution. *Cell Stem Cell, 1,* 55-70.

[39] Wernig, M. Meissner, A. Foreman, R. Brambrink, T. Ku, M. Hochedlinger, K. Bernstein, B. E. and Jaenisch, R. (2007). In vitro reprogramming of fibroblasts into a pluripotent ES-cell-like state. *Nature, 448,* 318-324.

[40] Takahashi, K. Tanabe, K. Ohnuki, M. Narita, M. Ichisaka, T. Tomoda, K. and Yamanaka, S. (2007). Induction of pluripotent stem cells from adult human fibroblasts by defined factors. *Cell, 131,* 861-872.

[41] Yu, J. Vodyanik, M. A. Smuga-Otto, K. Antosiewicz-Bourget, J. Frane, J. L. Tian, S. Nie, J. Jonsdottir, G. A. Ruotti, V. Stewart, R. Slukvin, II and Thomson, J. A. (2007). Induced Pluripotent Stem Cell Lines Derived from Human Somatic Cells. *Science*.

[42] Green, R. M. (2007). Can we develop ethically universal embryonic stem-cell lines? *Nat. Rev. Genet, 8,* 480-485.

In: Encyclopedia of Stem Cell Research (2 Volume Set)
Editor: Alexander L. Greene

ISBN: 978-1-61761-835-2
© 2012 Nova Science Publishers, Inc.

Chapter XIV

OXIDATIVE DAMAGE IN AGE-RELATED NEURODEGENERATIVE DISEASES AND INTERVENTIONS

H. Fai Poon[*] *and Sara C. Doore*
Roskamp Institute, Sarasota, FL, US

ABSTRACT

Aging, a universal process of all organisms, is defined as a functional decline of systems, to which the dysregulation of the redox signaling pathway contributes. The brain is not excluded from the aging process, and the aged brain is more susceptible to neurodegenerative diseases than the young one. Much research is being conducted to examine the variables involved in age-related neurodegeneration, as well as its interventions. One potential method of treatment may incorporate stem cells, which could provide a renewed resource for aged neurons or aberrant genes and/or proteins in the degenerated brain. Here, we will examine the biological processes that are affected by the dysregualtion of the redox signaling pathway in age-related degenerative central nervous systems. Furthermore, we will discuss how stem cell research and other treatments could provide potential intervention for these biological processes.

INTRODUCTION

With an increasing percentage of the population growing older, there will probably be corresponding concern with the processes of aging. Specifically, diseases involving neurodegeneration, such as Alzheimer's disease (AD) and Parkinson's disease (PD) are particularly difficult to cope with for patients and their family members alike. It was

---

[*] Address correspondence to: Dr. H. Fai Poon, Roskamp Institute, 2040 Whitfield Ave., Sarasota, FL 34243; Tel: 941 752 2949; Fax: 941 752 2948; e-mail: fpoon@rfdn.org

demonstrated that excessive oxidative stress may contribute to the manifestation of these diseases by modifying and/or damaging components of the cell (Poon et al. 2005a). Particular interest in treatments to alleviate this type of damage and ease the effects of neurodegeneration has turned to stem cell therapy, which would provide a renewed source for neurogenesis. However, components of this type of therapy are still being discussed regarding necessity and ease and efficiency of treatments. Also of importance, and a question to keep in mind, is whether or not treatments derived from stem cells may prevent against future oxidative damage.

One of the prevailing possibilities regarding stem cell treatment includes the grafting of these cells onto damaged tissue, which entails selecting suitable precursor cells for donation, expanding cultures *in vitro*, and injecting the cells into proximal areas of the damage. An alternative method involves the induction of native neuronal stem cells to differentiate and proliferate via the use of exogenously-applied growth factors. It may also be possible to use both types of treatment simultaneously, though this method has not been quite so fully explored (reference). Each method will be discussed relevant to neurodegenerative-diseased brain, as well as the efficiency and factors involved in the longevity of these treatments. Considering the highly oxidative environment of the diseased brain, it is also necessary to examine the ability for transplanted or newly differentiated neural precursor cells/neural stem cells (NPCs/NSCs) to survive once applied. Regarding this, new research regarding the potential of stem cells to possess oxidative resistant mechanisms will be presented.

OXIDATIVE MODIFICATION AND NEURODEGENERATION

Modifications Caused by Reactive Oxygen Species

The most significant source of oxidants in animals is mitochondrial damage and decay, specifically pertaining to injury of complexes in the electron transport chain (Poon et al. 2004). These oxidants, specifically reactive oxygen species (ROS) such as superoxide ($O_2^{\bullet -}$), hydroxyl (HO•), and hypochlorous acid (HOCl), are ultimately derived when O_2 comes into contact with an unpaired electron, and their generation can be exacerbated by the presence of metal ions and/or hydrogen peroxide (H_2O_2), which itself is often considered a ROS as well. Hydrogen peroxide is formed by superoxide dismutases, a group of enzymes which catalyze the reaction of $2O_2^{\bullet -} + 2H+$ into $2H_2O_2 + O_2$ (Poon et al. 2004a).

The toxicity of these ROS molecules lies in the unpaired electron, which is highly reactive and leads to a series of propagation reactions, where electrons are "stolen" from other molecules to make the initiator possess an even number once again, but which simultaneously causes the victim molecule to be radical instead.

Oxidative modification can occur in lipids and proteins, and both affect the rate of brain aging. Regarding lipids specifically, polyunsaturated fatty acids are particularly susceptible to ROS, and propagation reactions ultimately terminate to form aldehydes, such as 4-hydroxyl-2-nonenal (HNE), malondialdehyde (MDA), and acrolein, which bind to certain amino acids of proteins and therefore inhibits their proper function. ROS can also directly attack the proteins themselves, on either the peptide-linked backbones, resulting in either cross-linking or peptide-bond cleavage, or the attack can occur on the amino acid side-chains, resulting in modification of the chemical properties. Oxidative modification contributes to neurodegeneration directly by modifying protein function, whether disabling it partially or inhibiting it completely. Moreover, dysregulation of the redox state of proteins cal also lead to systematic dysfunction (Poon et al. 2005a).

The levels of oxidative modification of lipids and proteins can both be quantified by measuring levels of HNE, MDA, and acrolein, or by measuring levels of carbonyl and 3-nitrotyrosine (3NT), respectively.

Proteins Susceptible to Oxidative Modification

It is possible to determine which specific proteins are modified by measuring the levels of modification in certain samples and then identifying the proteins of interest by mass spectrometry. A previous study by Sultana et al. (2006) has indicated a number of proteins that show oxidative modification in Alzheimer's disease specifically, including the functional groups of ROS regulation, protein folding and degradation, metabolism, pH balance, and cytoskeleton/transport, discussed in detail below.

One protein involved in ROS regulation is peroxiredoxin 2 (Prdx2), an antioxidative enzyme that responds to lipid peroxidation (Poon et al. 2005). This protein has been shown to have increased oxidation in senescence-accelerated prone (SAMP8) mice, a previously-discussed murine model of accelerated aging (Poon et al. 2004b). Human studies have also shown a correlation between deficiency in Prdx2 and cognitive deficiency.

Regarding protein folding and degradation, two proteins known to be oxidatively modified include Pin1, a chaperone and putative cell cycle regulator, and UCHL-1, involved in ubiquitination/de-ubiquitination of proteins (Sultana et al. 2006). When oxidized, Pin1 shows a decrease in protein level, and UCHL-1 shows a decrease in protein activity (Sultana et al. 2006). There also appears to be some correspondence between these proteins and neurofibrillary tangles (NFT) known to develop in AD brains (Kurt et al. 2003). Pin1 has been shown to co-localize with and restore the function of tau, which is hyperphosphorylated in AD and a suspected component of NFTs. Decreased activity of UCHL-1 may also be involved in protein aggregate formation, as dysfunctional protein degradation can cause the conglomeration and aggregation of misfolded proteins. Heat shock protein 86 (hsp86), another chaperone protein, was also oxidatively modified, but no direct correspondence to NFT or protein aggregation has been established.

There are several metabolic proteins shown to be oxidized in AD, including lactate dehydrogenase 2 (LDH-2), creatine kinase, aldolase 3 (brain-specific), TPI, PGMI, and α-enolase (Poon et al. 2005b; Sultana et al. 2006). The oxidation of these proteins all result in lower protein levels, activity, or expression, except for enolase, which shows increased protein levels (Sultana et al. 2006). Another oxidized enzyme in AD, carbonic anhydrase (CAII) is also important in maintaining balanced pH by catalyzing the conversion of CO_2 to HCO_3^-. The reasons underlying why these specific enzymes are targeted still remain to be identified.

The cytoskeleton-associated proteins dihydropyrimidinase-related protein 2 (DRP-2), coronin 1a (coro1a), and γ-SNAP, also appear to be oxidized along with decreased expression or activity (Poon et al. 2005; Sultana et al. 2006). DRP-2 is also involved in neuronal growth cone collapse and axonal growth, and the phosphorylated form of this protein has previously been found in NFTs (Sultana et al. 2006). Coro1a is a cytoskeleton-associated protein that possibly plays roles in endocytosis, specifically in endosome-to-lysosome transport. γ-SNAP is a vesicular transport protein, important for maintaining synaptic integrity and transduction of signal.

These proteins, though only a small representation of the proteome, nonetheless indicate that oxidative modification occurs in the AD brain, and implies that these types of modifications may provide beneficial targets for potential therapeutics.

INTERVENTION OF NEURODEGENERATION BY STEM CELLS

Feasibility of Stem Cells Replacing Damaged Proteins and Cells

Unfortunately, un-damaging previously-synthesized proteins is not a possibility for treatment of neurodegeneration, as such a treatment would require intense specificity and also would possess high variability. Therefore, attention has been turned to replacement therapy, with a focus on stem cells in particular. In the brain, these cells are typically known as either NPCs or NSCs, and they would represent a brand new resource for restoring neuronal function. If these cells could be incorporated and differentiated *in vivo* in a neurodegenerating brain, the hope is that they could resume function of the diseased cells, thereby decreasing (or hopefully reversing) the effects of neurodegeneration. Considering the number of people with diseases such as Alzheimer's, Parkinson's, and amyotrophic lateral sclerosis (to name a few), or those who have experienced traumatic brain injury, this type of treatment could vastly improve the quality of life and restore normal functioning.

Necessity of Stem Cell Grafting and Possibility of Native NPC Induction

Supposing that NPCs may restore some function taken by neurodegeneration, there still remains a question of how, exactly, these stem cells would be placed in the right area, and how they would be regulated to proliferate and/or differentiate. Surgical grafting of stem cells has provided one method of proper placement of NPCs. Although previously thought not to exist in the adult brain, there has been recent evidence showing that NPCs persist throughout adulthood, though they are significantly fewer in number than those present earlier in life (Eriksson et al. 1998). Even in AD brains, NPCs still exist, though they are even fewer than those in normal adult brains (Lovell et al. 2006). This type of treatment is worth considering, with several points to discuss.

Efficiency of Stem Cell Grafting Procedures and Longevity of Grafted Cells

One issue regarding the grafting of stem cells into afflicted brains pertains to the efficiency of the treatment, specifically regarding how long NPCs can remain viable in the brain after introduction. Fortunately, the grafting procedure itself seems relatively simple, as NPCs will automatically migrate to sites of lesion and damage upon introduction (which can be done via injection at sites in proximity to the damage) (Zhang et al. 2007). It also appears that NPCs are able to survive and differentiate in new host tissues, especially if those tissues were previously damaged rather than normal, as shown by immunohistochemical staining (Zhang et al. 2007). However, even if relatively simple, treatment may still prove to be ineffective if the cells cannot live long after application, or if grafting has to be done repeatedly after short periods of time, as this would prove time-consuming and expensive. Indeed, this seemed to be a problem for Zhang et al. (2007), as they noted that a relatively small percentage of cells differentiated into an array of fully-functional neurons. Overall conclusions of successful neuronal differentiation are difficult at this time, as results are quite mixed, with some studies resulting in successful dopaminergic neurons, capable of neurotransmission (Wang et al. 2006; Hattiangady et al. 2007; Sun et al. 2007) and others resulting in only a small percentage of dopaminergic neurons (Horiguchi et al. 2004; Zhang et al. 2007), or in poor integration of stem cells in general (Keene et al. 2007).

It is possible that the number of cells that differentiate into functioning neurons due to the origins of the NPCs. Although stem cells, by definition, are able to differentiate into multiple types of cells, some are more apt to differentiate into specific cell types. Horiguchi et al. (2004) showed that differentiated stem cells do show regional specificities retained by NPCs. Specifically, rostral-derived NPCs proliferate more quickly, though caudal-derived NPCs are more likely to result in tyrosine hydroxylase (TH)-positive neurons, indicative of dopaminergic neurons.

Recently, a method of cell sorting devised by Pruszak et al. (2007) provides a way to identify and isolate immature embryonic stem cells (ES), NPCs, and differentiated neurons. Furthermore, the authors transplanted the differentiated neurons into rodent brains and found that the cells could survive *in vivo* (Pruszak et al. 2007). However, the longevity of these neurons, and whether or not they could restore some memory function was not explored.

The Role of Growth Factors in Stem Cell Differentiation and Proliferation

If transplanting stem cells of foreign origin is not efficient for long-term therapy, then alternatives to induce native stem cells to differentiate and replace damaged neurons can be applied. In the adult brain, there are specific areas in which neurogenesis occurs, namely the subventricular zone (SVZ) and the subgranular zone (SGZ) of the hippocampus (Leker and McKay 2004; Grote et al. 2007). One particular intrigue of working with native stem cells is the fact that application of exogenous stem cells must come from an immortalized cell line, which must be selected carefully before large-scale expansion, whereas induction of native stem cells potentially requires much less time and energy (Leker and McKay 2004; Zhu et al. 2005). Examining the genes and proteins expressed shortly after differentiation of NPCs to neurons, astrocytes, and oligodendrocytes has yielded a large list of data (Salim et al. 2007), but the most focus has been on a few select growth factors involved in regulation of neurogenesis. These growth factors are primarily brain-derived neurotrophic factor (BDNF), epidermal growth factor (EGF), basic fibroblast growth factor (bFGF), insulin-like growth factor (IGF-1), and vascular endothelial growth factor (VEGF) (Chen et al. 2007; Grote et al. 2007; Yu et al. 2007). Deciphering how these growth factors regulate NPC proliferation and differentiation could ultimately lead to a more indirect type of stem cell therapy as well. However, this is quite an ambitious task, and studies are still being performed regarding the roles these growth factors possess (Chen et al. 2007), especially in abnormal situations such as diseased or injured brains. For example, it was discovered that patients with AD have higher levels of VEGF in their serum and in brains, examined post-mortem (Kalaria et al. 1998). Another example is brought up by Williams (2007) in that AD is a generalized disease, and thus FGF, a more general growth factor than NGF, may be more appropriate to focus on for treatments, provided there are no generalized side effects as well.

Some studies have already examined the treatment of injured brains by introducing adeno-associated virus (AAV)-mediated delivery of BDNF (Henry et al. 2007), as well as glial cell line-derived neurotrophic factor (GDNF) and even the tyrosine hydroxylase (TH) enzyme (Wang et al. 2002; Wang et al. 2006). This type of treatment seemed to produce good results, in that progenitor cells were recruited to sites of injury and differentiated as normal (Henry et al. 2007). The differentiated cells also formed functional neurons along with glial cells, which persisted throughout the study of 84 days post-AAV injection *in vivo* (Henry et al. 2007). Furthermore, behavioral studies demonstrated that AAV-GDNF-injected mice improved to near-normal levels of functioning 20 weeks after treatment.

Another interesting method of increasing the longevity and/or functioning of endogenous stem cells is transplantation of astrocytes rather than growth factors or stem cells themselves. One study has shown that transplanted astrocytes continually secrete factors such as bFGF, enhancing the lifespan of progenitor cells, though this effect did not extend to rate or ability to differentiate (Jordan et al. 2007).

The Possibility of Simultaneous Treatments: Growth Factors in Addition to Grafts

The notion of using astrocytes rather than their secreted growth factors alone is particularly interesting and brings up the possibility of treatment with both exogenous stem cells *and* growth factors (or other helpful cells, such as astrocytes) to extend the life of the cells and ensure that they differentiate and proliferate sufficiently.

Similarly, there is also the possibility of using stem cells themselves as delivery vehicles for genes encoding certain neuroprotective or antioxidative proteins. Since stem cells are able to migrate to sites of damage without intervention, they may be able to provide both a source of new cells and a source of their own growth factors (Kabos et al. 2003). The potential of using stem cells to deliver antioxidants is supported by the study where they were able to show that NSCs engineered to express neurotrophin-3 (NT3), a differentiation-inducing compound, were able to migrate to sites of injury and successfully express NT3 at those sites

(Park et al. 2006). NSCs also apparently are able to produce and secrete GDNF and NGF inherently, promoting survival of neighboring injured neurons as well (Llado et al. 2004).

Potential for Stem Cells to Resist Oxidative Stress

This possibility of neuroprotective effects from stem cell therapies is particularly exciting. It would be particularly beneficial if therapy involving NPC grafting could provide not only a chance for neurogeneration, but if those NPCs were less likely to become similarly damaged in the process. One study involving NPCs illustrated that these cells actually exhibit increased expression of antioxidative proteins and maintained mitochondrial function after treatment with 3-nitroproprionic acid (3NP) (Madhavan et al. 2006). Compared to controls, stem cells underwent upregulation of uncoupling protein 2 (UCP2), glutathione peroxidase (GPX), and superoxide dismutase II (SODII) after exposure to 3NP, recovering within five days of treatment. Other studies have found similar oxidative resistance capacities in adipose-derived stem cells (Kim et al. 2007), circulating precursor cells (Dernbach et al. 2004), endothelial progenitor cells (He et al. 2004), and hepatic stellate cells (Novo et al. 2006) (table 1). This would make sense considering the multipotent capacity of each individual cell and potential for mutation amplification. The ability to resist such toxic oxidative stress specifically in the brain indicates increased resistance to oxidative stressors, such as the amyloid-beta protein involved in AD.

However, one study also adds another factor to these findings of increased oxidative resistance, stating that stem cells are actually highly sensitive to oxidative stress and exhibit increased levels of cell death after exposure when compared to differentiated cells (Yin et al. 2006). This proteomic analysis in smooth muscle progenitors acknowledges that stem cells possess superior antioxidant defense mechanisms in the cytoplasm but brings up the point that they also have much higher levels of mitochondrial ROS production, effectively counteracting those defenses (Yin et al. 2006).

To resolve this discontinuity, it would be helpful to perform additional microarray and proteomic studies on neural precursor cells, and more specifically to examine the levels of ROS-mediated genes and proteins in the mitochondria versus the cytoplasm. Although it seems that some sort of increased resistance to ROS is present in all stem cells, whether or not it is actually efficient (or canceled out by increased ROS production of the mitochondria) may need further extrapolation. In addition to examining solely the amount of antioxidants and oxidative stress-related genes and proteins, there should be some studies regarding the extent of lipid peroxidation and protein modification in NPCs versus "old" post-mitotic neural cells, possibly at different stages in the differentiation process. These types of studies may help us understand the true extent of oxidative resistance and whether or not transplanted cells would be able to persist in an oxidative environment, such as the AD brain.

Table 1. A list of upregulated genes and proteins pertaining to oxidative stress in precursor cells compared to post-mitotic cells

Name	Level	Function	Location Found	Reference
Uncoupling protein 2; UCP2	Protein	Mitochondrial uncoupling protein (CNS); suppresses free radical production	Neurons	Andrews et al. 2005; Madhavan et al. 2006
Catalase	mRNA, protein		Blood	Dernbach et al. 2004
Glutathione peroxidase (GPX)	mRNA, protein	Peroxidase; reduction of free radicals	Muscle; neurons	Dernbach et al. 2004; McLean et al. 2005; Lee et al. 2006; Madhavan et al. 2006
Cytosolic superoxide dismutase (CuZnSOD; SOD-I)	mRNA, protein	Catalyzes formation of hydrogen peroxide from superoxide	Endothelial; neurons; muscle	He et al. 2004; Faiz et al. 2006; Yin et al. 2006
Mitochondrial superoxide dismutase (MnSOD; SOD-II)	mRNA, protein	Catalyzes formation of hydrogen peroxide from superoxide	Endothelial; neurons; muscle	Dernbach et al. 2004; He et al. 2004; Madhavan et al. 2006; Yin et al. 2006
Nurr1		Nuclear receptor required for midbrain dopaminergic neuron development	Neurons	Sousa et al. 2007
Heat shock proteins (Hsp, various)	Protein	Chaperones	Muscle	Yin et al. 2006; Salim et al. 2007
Peroxiredoxin 1 (PRDX1; cytosolic)	Protein	Reduces peroxides produced during metabolism to water and alcohol	Muscle	Yin et al. 2006
Peroxiredoxin 2 (PRDX2; cytosolic)	Protein	Reduces peroxides produced during metabolism to water and alcohol	Muscle	Yin et al. 2006
Peroxiredoxin 6 (PRDX6; cytosolic)	Protein	Reduces peroxides produced during metabolism to water and alcohol	Muscle	Yin et al. 2006
Proline dehydrogenase (oxidase)	mRNA	Reduces proline; found in mitochondrial matrix	Blood	Dernbach et al. 2004
Succinate dehydrogenase	mRNA	Involved in transferring electrons from succinate to ubiquinone (coenzyme Q); electron transport chain of mitochondria	Blood	Dernbach et al. 2004
Name	Level	Function	Location Found	Reference

Monoamine oxidase A	mRNA	Oxidizes biogenic and xenobiotic amines, e.g. 5-hydroxytryptamine, norepinephrine, and epinephrine	Blood	Dernbach et al. 2004
NAD(P)H menadione oxidoreductase 1 (Nmo1)	mRNA	Involved in detoxification pathways (by conjugation reactions of hydroquinons)	Blood	Dernbach et al. 2004
Biliverdin IV beta reductase 1	mRNA	Electron transfer from reduced pyridine nucleotides; antioxidant; possible iron metabolism regulation	Blood	Dernbach et al. 2004
Carbonyl reductase 1	mRNA	Reduces carbonyls to corresponding alcohols	Blood	Dernbach et al. 2004
P450 reductase	mRNA	Electron transporter from NADP to cytochrome P450	Blood	Dernbach et al. 2004
Epoxide hydrolase 1	mRNA	Hydrolyzes certain epoxides to become more water-soluble and less reactive	Blood	Dernbach et al. 2004
Acyl coenzyme A oxidase	mRNA	Catalyzes desaturation of long chain acyl-CoAs; produces H_2O_2	Blood	Dernbach et al. 2004
Aldose reductase	mRNA	Reduces carbonyls to corresponding alcohols	Blood	Dernbach et al. 2004
Aldehyde reductase	mRNA	Reduces aldehydes to their corresponding alcohols	Blood	Dernbach et al. 2004

CONCLUSION

The potential of stem cell therapy as a treatment for neurodegenerative disease has undergone much research and scrutiny, but the implications seem promising. Particularly if there is further evidence regarding the superior resistance of NPCs to oxidative stress, this type of therapy may prove extremely helpful in alleviating the symptoms of neurodegeneration in Alzheimer's disease and Parkinson's disease, among others.

REFERENCES

Andrews ZB, Horvath B, Barnstable CJ, Elseworth J, Yang L, Beal MF, Roth RH, Matthews RT, Horvath TL. (2005) Uncoupling protein-2 is critical for nigral dopamine cell survival in a mouse model of Parkinson's disease. *J. Neurosci.* 25(1): 184-191.

Chen K, Henry RA, Hughes SM, Connor B. (2007) Creating a neurogenic environment: The role of BDNF and FGF2. *Mol. Cell. Neurosci.* 36: 108-120.

Eriksson PS, Perfilieva E, Bjork-Eriksson T, Alborn AM, Nordborg C, Peterson DA, Gage FH. (1998) Neurogenesis in the adult human hippocampus. *Nat. Med.* 54(3): 390-401.

Faiz M, Acarin L, Peluffo H, Villapol S, Castellano B, Gonzalez B. (2006) Antioxidant Cu/Zn SOD: expression in postnatal brain progenitor cells. *Neurosci Lett.* 401(1-2): 71-76.

Grote HE, Hannan AJ. (2007) Regulators of adult neurogenesis in the healthy and diseased brain. *Clin. Exp. Pharmacol. Physiol.* 34: 533-545.

Hattiangady B, Shuai B, Cai J, Coksaygan T, Rao MS, Shetty AK. (2007) Increased dentate neurogenesis after grafting of glial restricted progenitors or neural stem cells in the aging hippocampus. *Stem Cells.* 25(8): 2104-2117.

He T, Peterson TE, Holmuhamedov EL, Terzic A, Caplice NM, Oberley LW, Katusic ZS. (2006) Human endothelial progenitor cells tolerate oxidative stress due to intrinsically high expression of manganese superoxide dismutase. *Artherioscler. Thromb. Vasc. Biol.* 24(11): 2021-2027.

Henry RA, Hughes SM, Connor B. (2007) AAV-mediated delivery of BDNF augments neurogenesis in the normal and quinolinic acid-lesioned adult rat brain. *Eur. J. Neurosci.* 25: 3513-3525.

Horiguchi S, Takahashi J, Kishi Y, Morizane A, Okamoto Y, Koyanagi M, Tsuji M, Tashiro K, Honjo T, Fujii S, Hashimoto N. (2004) Neural precursor cells derived from human embryonic brain retain regional specificity. *J. Neurosci. Res.* 75: 817-824.

Jordan PM, Cain LD, Wu P. (2007) Astrocytes enhance long-term survival of cholinergic neurons differentiated from human fetal neural stem cells. *J. Neurosci. Res.*

Kabos P, Ehtesham M, Black KL, Yu JS. (2003) Neural stem cells as delivery vehicles. *Expert Opin. Biol. Ther.* 3(5): 759-770.

Kalaria RN, Cohen DL, Premkumar DR, Nag S, LaManna JC, Lust WD. (1998) Vascular endothelial growth factor in Alzheimer's disease and experimental cerebral ischemia. *Brain Res. Mol. Brain Res.* 62: 101–105.

Keene CD, Sonnen JA, Swanson PD, Kopyov O, Leverenz JB, Bird TD, Montine TJ. (2007) Neural transplantation in Huntington disease: long-term grafts in two patients. *Neurology.* 68(24): 2093-2098.

Kim WS, Park BS, Kim HK, Park JS, Kim KJ, Choi JS, Chung SJ, Kim DD, Sung JH. (2007) Evidence supporting antioxidant action of adipose-derived stem cells: Protection of human dermal fibroblasts from oxidative stress. *J. Dermatol. Sci.*

Kurt MA, Davies DC, Kidd M, Duff K, Howlett DR. (2003) Hyperphosphorylated tau and paired helical filament-like structures in the brains of mice carrying mutant amyloid precursor protein and mutant presenilin-1 transgenes. *Neurobiol. Dis.* 14(1): 89-97.

Leker RR, McKay RD. (2004) Using endogenous neural stem cells to enhance recovery from ischemic brain injury. *Curr. Neurovasc. Res.* 1(5): 421-427.

Lladó J, Haenggeli C, Maragakis NJ, Snyder EY, Rothstein JD. (2004) Neural stem cells protect against glutamate-induced excitotoxicity and promote survival of injured motor neurons through the secretion of neurotrophic factors. *Mol. Cell Neurosci.* 27(3): 322-331.

Lovell MA, Geiger H, Van Zant GE, Lynn BC, Markesbery WR. (2006) Isolation of neural precursor cells from Alzheimer's disease and aged control postmortem brain. *Neurobiol. Aging.* 27: 909-917.

Madhavan L, Ourednik V, Ourednik J. (2006) Increased "vigilance" of antioxidant mechanisms in neural stem cells potentiates their capability to resist oxidative stress. *Stem Cells.* 24(9): 2110-2119.

McLean CW, Mirochnitchenko O, Claus CP, Noble-Haeusslein LJ, Ferriero DM. (2005) Overexpression of glutathione peroxidase protects immature murine neurons from oxidative stress. *Dev. Neurosci.* 27(2-5): 169-175.

Novo E, Marra F, Zamara E, Valfre di Bonzo L, Monitillo L, Cannito S, Petrai I, Mazzocca A, Bonacchi A, De Franco RS, Colombatto S, Autelli R, Pinzani M, Parola M. (2006) Overexpression of Bcl-2 by activated human hepatic stellate cells: resistance to apoptosis as a mechanism of progressive hepatic fibrogenesis in humans. *Gut.* 55(8): 1174-1182.

Park KI, Himes BT, Stieg PE, Tessler A, Fischer I, Snyder EY. (2006) Neural stem cells may be uniquely suited for combined gene therapy and cell replacement: Evidence from engraftment of Neurotrophin-3-expressing stem cells in hypoxic-ischemic brain injury. *Exp. Neurol.* 199(1): 179-190.

Poon HF, Calabrese V, Scapagnini, Butterfield DA. (2004a) Free radicals and brain aging. *Clin. Geriatric Med.* 20(2): 329-359.

Poon HF, Castegna A, Farr SA, Thongboonkerd V, Lynn BC, Banks WA, Morley JE, Klein JB, Butterfield DA. (2004b) Quantitative proteomics analysis of specific protein expression and oxidative modification in aged senescence-accelerated-prone 8 mice brain. *Neuroscience.* 126(4): 915-926.

Poon HF, Frasier M, Shreve N, Calabrese V, Wolozin B, Butterfield DA. (2005a) Mitochondrial associated metabolic proteins are selectively oxidized in A30P alpha-synuclein transgenic mice – a model of familiar Parkinson's disease. *Neurobiol. Dis.* 18(3): 492-498.

Poon HF, Farr SA, Thongboonkerd V, Lynn BC, Banks WA, Morley JE, Klein JB, Butterfield DA. (2005b) Proteomic analysis of specific brain proteins in aged SAMP8 mice treated with alpha-lipoic acid: implications for aging and age-related neurodegerative disorders. *Neurochem Int.* 138(1): 8-16.

Pruszak J, Sonntag KC, Aung MH, Sanchez-Pernaute R, Isacson O. (2007) Markers and methods for cell sorting of human embryonic stem cell-derived neural cell populations. *Stem Cells.* 25(9): 2257-2268.

Sousa KM, Mira H, Hall AC, Jansson-Sjoestrand L, Kusakabe M, Arenas E. (2007) Microarray analyses support a role for Nurr1 in resistance to oxidative stress and neuronal differentiation in neural stem cells. *Stem Cells.* 25(2): 511-519.

Sultana R, Boyd-Kimball D, Poon HF, Cai J, Pierce WM, Klein JB, Merchant M, Markesbery WR, Butterfield DA. (2006) Redox proteomics identification of oxidized proteins in Alzheimer's disease hippocampus and cerebellum: An approach to understand pathological and biochemical alterations in AD. *Neurobiol. Aging.* 27: 1564-1576.

Sun J, Gao Q, Miller K, Wang X, Wang J, Liu W, Bao L, Zhang J, Zhang L, Poon WS, Gao Y. (2007) Dopaminergic differentiation of grafted GFP transgenic neuroepithelial stem cells in the brain of a rat model of Parkinson's disease. *Neurosci. Lett.* 420(1): 23-28.

Wang L, Muramatsu S, Lu Y, Ikeguchi K, Fujimoto K, Okada T, Mizukami H, Hanazono Y, Kume A, Urano F, Ichinose H, Nagatsu T, Nakano I, Ozawa K. (2002) Delayed delivery of AAV-GDNF prevents nigral neurodegeneration and promotes functional recovery in a rat model of Parkinson's disease. *Gene Ther.* 9(6): 381-389.

Wang Q, Matsumoto Y, Shindo T, Miyake K, Shindo A, Kawanishi M, Kawai N, Tamiya T, Nagao S. (2006) Neural stem cells transplantation in cortex in a mouse model of Alzheimer's disease. *J. Med. Invest.* 53: 61-69.

Williams BJ, Eriksdotter-Jonhagen M, Granholm AC. (2007) Nerve growth factor in treatment and pathogenesis of Alzheimer's disease. *Prog. Neurobiol.* 80: 114-128.

Yin X, Mayr M, Xiao Q, Wang W, Xu Q. (2006) Proteomic analysis reveals higher demand for antioxidant protection in embryonic stem cell-derived smooth muscle cells. *Proteomics.* 6: 6437-6446.

Yu Y, Gu S, Huang H, Wen T. (2007) Combination of bFGF, heparin and laminin induce the generation of dopaminergic neurons from rat neural stem cells both in vitro and in vivo. *J. Neuro. Sci.* 255: 81-86.

Zhang X, Jin G, Titan M, Qin J, Huang Z. (2007) The denervated hippocampus provides proper microenvironment for the survival and differentiation of neural progenitors. *Neurosci Lett.* 414(2): 115-20.

Zhu J, Wu X, Zhang HL. (2005) Adult neural stem cell therapy: expansion in vitro, tracking in vivo and clinical transplantation. *Curr. Drug Targets.* 6(1): 97-110.

In: Encyclopedia of Stem Cell Research (2 Volume Set) ISBN: 978-1-61761-835-2
Editor: Alexander L. Greene © 2012 Nova Science Publishers, Inc.

Chapter XV

THE ACTIVATION OF ADULT ENDOGENOUS NEURAL STEM CELLS BY NEURODEGENERATIVE PROCESS WITHIN THE STRIATUM IN AN ANIMAL MODEL OF HUNTINGTON'S DISEASE

Yvona Mazurová[*1], *Emil Rudolf*[2], *Ivana Gunčová*[1] *and Ivan Látr*[3]

[1]Department of Histology and Embryology, Charles University in Prague, Faculty of Medicine in Hradec Králové, Czech Republic
[2]Department of Medical Biology and Genetics, Charles University in Prague, Faculty of Medicine in Hradec Králové, Czech Republic
[3]Neurosurgery Clinic, Faculty Hospital, Hradec Králové, Czech Republic

ABSTRACT

Studies, carried out in the last decade, have demonstrated a continuous postnatal neurogenesis in the subependymal zone (SEZ) of lateral brain ventricles in the normal adult brain. However, some morphological and functional relationships, especially under pathological conditions, remain unclear. Crucial for endogenous neural stem cells (NSCs) is believed a specialized microenvironment – neurogenic niche. The glial nature of adult NSCs is already well documented, indicating that SEZ stem/niche cells are GFAP-positive astrocytes. But some other properties and relationships remain to be investigated.

The neurodegenerative process within the striatum, a hallmark of Huntington's disease (HD), represents severe damage of the brain parenchyma. In an animal model of HD, induced by intrastriatal injection of quolinic acid (QA), neurodegenerative process

---

[*] Address for correspondence: Assoc. Prof. Yvona Mazurová, M.D., Ph.D.; Department of Histology and Embryology; Charles University in Prague; Faculty of Medicine in Hradec Králové; Šimkova 870, P.O. Box 38; 500 38 Hradec Králové; Czech Republic; e-mail: mazurova@lfhk.cuni.cz ; phone: +420 49 5816 440; fax: +420 49 5816 376

initiates immediate intensive cell proliferation, resulting in characteristic enlargement of the SEZ. For that reason, we were interested in a reaction of the neurogenic niche in the SEZ at 7 days after the QA lesion. The reaction of the SEZ changed over time. Therefore a protracted reaction of the SEZ in the ongoing neurodegenerative process within the striatum was observed after 6 months.

We have described the compartmentalization of the SEZ: (1) In the R-SEZ, i.e. in a rostral part of anterior horn of lateral brain ventricles (AP 1.4-1.5 from bregma), related to the rostral migratory stream and olfactory bulb, the generation of new neuronal cell typically prevails, whereas (2) in the more posterior region (AP 1.1-1.2 from bregma), the lateral part of the SEZ (L-SEZ) opposite the degenerated striatum was characteristic by proliferation of both types of cells, with neuronal and mainly with astrocytic properties. Accompanied angiogenesis was also obvious as an integral morphological and functional component of activated SEZ.

Our results show some new morphological features, particularly a wide plasticity of endogenous astrocyte-like stem/niche cells in immediate response to an extensive pathological process in the adult brain but also their inability to become mature neurons in the region of L-SEZ. Our further findings document that astrocyte-like cells in the adult SEZ, during their extensive proliferation, retain some features of embryonic stem cells, including the reexpression of vimentin intermediate filaments which contributes to the suggestion that these astrocyte-like cells are derivatives of radial glia. On the other hand, their following differentiation is limited by the microenvironment of the adult neurogenic niche.

INTRODUCTION

Multipotent neural stem cells play a key role in the development of the nervous system. The new concept of their existence also in the adult brain was first suggested by Joseph Altman in 1962. He supposed that non-differentiated precursors for generation of new neurons in adult brain might be ependymal cells [1]. The evidence for the existence, proliferation and differentiation of adult stem cells in secondary germinal/neurogenic regions, the SEZ of the lateral brain ventricles and the subgranular zone (SGZ) in the dentate gyrus of the hippocampus, in mammals, including primates [e.g. 29, 62] and human [e.g. 19, 28, 31, 65, 74] but also in lower vertebrates is now widely accepted [reviewed e.g. 13, 18, 36, 72]. Multipotent (embryonic/fetal) NSCs undergo self-renewal, and subsequently can enter the quiescent state [55] or die [8, 54, 75] or mature into adult NSCs. In the adult rodent brain, endogenous NSCs in the SEZ in response to the different cues divide to generate neural progenitors (NPCs). NPCs divide to give origin to committed neuronal precursors – neuroblasts which mostly migrate via the rostral migratory stream (RMS) to the olfactory bulb (OB), where they differentiate into two types of interneurons, granule and periglomerular [4, 24, 41, 42, 44, 71]. It is now widely accepted that adult NSCs have the identity of the glial cells [1, 3, 16, 22, 27, 66, 72].

Self-renewal and multilineage differentiation are two generic attributes of stem cells which are also expressed by the cells in the adult SEZ, either *in vitro* or *in vivo*. However, these adult stem cells also possess attributes of differentiated mature glial cells – particularly they contain typical thick bundles of intermediate filaments composed of glial fibrillary acidic protein (GFAP) [e.g. 66]. For these reasons, the term astrocyte-like cells starts to be commonly used for glial cells of the adult SEZ [49]. Crucial for endogenous NSCs proliferation and differentiation *in vivo* is a pocket-like specialized microenvironment – a niche, in which these cells reside [e.g. 15, 21, 45, 56, 72]. A niche is formed by neurogenic cells, specific local signals and morphogens of embryonic character that determine its neurogenic behavior also in adulthood [15, 57]. Three basic types of cells are described in the SEZ niche: (1) slowly dividing astrocytes (B cells) with properties of multipotent NSCs, (2) putative precursors (C cells) and (3) rapidly dividing fate-specific neuroblasts (A cells) migrating in chains to OB. Both, type A and type C cells are apposed to the type B astrocytes [e.g. 5, 6, 15, 72].

Despite missing basal lamina of ependymal cells (they are of only epitheloid character), a specialized basal lamina contacts all SEZ cell types and may play an important role in cell tethering, ligand binding and regulation [51, 52]. Moreover, vessels also represent a very important component of neurogenic niche [6, 15, 43, 61].

Ependymal cells, a single covering layer of columnar cells with cilia in all brain ventricles, are important regulators in the SEZ and promoters of neurogenic niche even though they are not stem cells as was previously suggested [1, 28]. They produce noggin, an antagonist of bone morphogenic proteins (BMPs), which inhibits neurogenesis and this way promotes glial differentiation [5, 35].

A very detailed description is available for the structure and partly also the possible function of adult SEZ and neurogenic niche under the physiological conditions. NSCs are believed to divide very slowly, more slowly than other types of adult stem cells [e.g. 12, 37, 55, 57, 72]. This fact invokes the question of how endogenous adult NSCs respond to brain damage. Increased proliferation of NSCs and NPCs has been observed in relation to different experimentally induced pathological conditions, e.g. in relation to the mechanical injury of the forebrain – aspiration cavity, cut or stab wound [e.g. 73], focal cerebral ischemia - stroke model [e.g. 7, 32, 33], chemical or inflammatory demyelination [58] and partly also to the degenerative process in the striatum as a model of HD [24, 39, 47, 49, 68]. On the other hand, the development of reaction of the adult SEZ in response to protracted neurodegenerative process within the striatum remains to be clearly demonstrated.

MATERIAL AND METHODS

Experimental Design

Adult male Wistar rats (220–230 g of body weight at the beginning of the experiment) were used. All procedures were performed in accordance with the directive of the EEC (86/609/EEC) and the use of animals in present experiments was reviewed and approved by the Animal Ethical Committee of Charles University in Prague, Faculty of Medicine in Hradec Králové.

In total, 14 rats divided in 2 equal groups were assigned to this experiment – 3 rats with quolinic acid (QA) lesion, 2 sham-lesioned and 2 intact control animals per group. For detailed description of surgical procedure and processing of histological material see Mazurova et al [50].

Quolinic acid (Sigma-Aldrich, CR; 120 nmol, i.e. 20 µg/ 2 µl PBS) was stereotaxically injected to the right hemisphere of 6 animals at the following coordinates: A: 1.5, L: 2.2, V: 5.0 and 4.5 (A = anterior to bregma, L = lateral from midline, V = ventral from dura); toothbar at the 0 level. QA was applied in two sites (1 µl per each site) from one injection tract. Similarly, in 4 sham-lesioned rats 0.1 M PBS (2 µl) was applied in the same site. Rats in the group I were sacrificed at 1 week and in the group II at 6 months after the surgery, including age-matched controls. Two i.p. injections of BrdU (120 mg/kg) were applied 15 and 3 hours before animals' sacrifice to distinguish especially the rapidly dividing cell in the SEZ.

Histology and Immunohistochemistry

Rats were killed (in deep anesthesia) by transcardial perfusion of 4% neutral formaldehyde. Blocks of transversely cut brains (through the both hemispheres) were postfixed for 3 days in the same fixative solution and embedded in paraffin. Numbered serial coronal sections (90 serial sections from one brain) were stained with haematoxylin and eosin (each 15th section) and in selected series (related to the R-SEZ and L-SEZ), the immunohistochemical detection of different antibodies was made.

The following sequence of monoclonal primary antibodies was used: anti-BrdU (monoclonal - Dako, Czech Republic; dilution 1:100; polyclonal - ABCAM, UK; dilution 1:50); anti-GFAP (monoclonal - Sigma-Aldrich, Czech Republic; dilution 1:400; polyclonal - Dako, Czech Republic; dilution 1:400), anti-vimentin (monoclonal - Sigma-Aldrich, Czech Republic; dilution 1:40; polyclonal - Chemicon, Czech Republic; dilution 1:20), anti-S 100β (monoclonal - Sigma-Aldrich, Czech Republic; dilution 1:1000; polyclonal - Dako, Czech Republic; dilution 1:300), anti-nestin (DSHB, USA; dilution 1:4) , anti-NCAM (DSHB, USA; dilution 1:4), anti-DCX (polyclonal - Chemicon, Czech Republic; dilution 1:3000), anti-MAP2 (monoclonal - Sigma-Aldrich, Czech Republic; dilution 1:500; polyclonal - Chemicon, Czech Republic; dilution 1:700), anti-ß-III-tubulin (EXBIO, Czech Republic; dilution 1:20), anti-NeuN (Chemicon, Czech Republic; dilution 1:50)

In brief, deparaffinized and rehydrated sections were incubated in water solution of H_2O_2 (dilution 5:1) for 20 min to reduce endogenous peroxidase activity. The pretreatment in microwave 3x5 min at 800 W in the sodium citrate buffer (pH 6.0) and washing in 0.01 M PBS was made. Incubation with mostly monoclonal primary antibodies (see above) was performed overnight at 4°C. Sections were then washed and incubated with appropriate biotinilated secondary antibody for 45 min. at a room temperature, and subsequently with a streptavidin conjugate of peroxidase (DAKO, Czech Republic) also for 45 min. Visualization of bound antibody was performed using DAB (Sigma-Aldrich, Czech Republic) and hydrogen peroxide. Sections were counterstained with 0.1% methyl green.

The sequential technique for immunofluorescent double-labeling of antibodies (always monoclonal antibody in combination with a polyclonal antibody) was used. Avidin or secondary antibody were labeled with either Cy-3 (red) or Alexa 488 (green) and nuclei were counterstained with 4′,6–diamidino-2-phenylindole – DAPI (blue). The following combinations of antibodies were used for double-labeling method (the first-mentioned is a monoclonal antibody, the second is a polyclonal antibody): anti-BrdU + anti-GFAP, anti-nestin + anti-BrdU, anti-NCAM + anti-BrdU, anti-BrdU + anti-DCX, anti-β-III-tubulin + anti-BrdU, anti-BrdU + anti-MAP2, anti-nestin + anti-vimentin, anti-nestin + anti-GFAP, anti-vimentin + anti-GFAP, anti-NeuN + anti-GFAP.

All findings obtained by immunofluorescent detection (double-labeling) were confirmed by a single antibody detection using PAP immunohistochemistry on parallel paraffin sections.

Photomicrographs were made with Cybernetics software version 4.51 (Laboratory Imaging, Prague, Czech Republic) or Lucia G/F software version 4.82 (Laboratory Imaging, Prague, Czech Republic).

RESULTS

Huntington's Disease – The Neurodegenerative Process in the Striatum

The neurodegenerative process in the striatum represents the most characteristic morphological feature in both HD patients and an animal model of HD. Significant for this process is a development of partial necrosis only, i.e. the near complete loss of neurons with preservation of the majority of glial cells (figures 2 a, b). Despite intensive subsequent development of reparative gliosis (a proliferation of reactive astrocytes), the degeneration of striatal neurons followed by the reduction (rarefaction) of the neuropil is such an extensive process that the severe striatal atrophy occurs. The shrinkage of the striatum is accompanied by conspicuous compensatory dilatation of lateral brain ventricles (figures 1 a, b).

Unlike the HD patients, the development of all mentioned processes is very fast in animal brain after the instillation of the neurotoxic acid which, on the other hand, is very useful mechanism for research purposes. Neurodegenerative changes induced by the intrastriatal injection of the QA are well developed after 6 – 7 days and then the process slows down. We have found [50] that at about 1 month, the QA lesion is essentially developed and the following progression of neurodegenerative process within the striatum is comparable with continual deterioration of the state in HD patients. For that reason, we were interested in a reaction of the SEZ 1 week after the application of the QA (immediate reaction) in comparison with the state after 6 months (protracted reaction).

The SEZ in Adult Intact (Normal) Brain

In embryonic period, the primary proliferative zone in developing forbrain is the ventricular zone (VZ) which lines large lateral ventricles. A secondary proliferative region, the subventricular zone (SVZ), develops as a prominent thickening beneath VZ in the region on lateral (LGE) and medial ganglionic eminences. The VZ finally transforms into a terminally differentiated ependymal layer, a lining of brain ventricles. In adult mammalian telencephalon, proliferative subependymal zone is adjacent to the ependymal layer of the lateral walls of the lateral brain ventricles (this region probably derives from LGE). The adult SEZ retains the capacity for self-renewal and can generate both neurons and glia. The SEZ is most prominent in the lateral wall of the lateral brain ventricles, particularly in their dorsal part, where it continues via the rostrocaudal extension, which copies the ventral surface of corpus callosum, rostrally and by the restricted pathway, the rostral migratory stream, to the olfactory bulb.

When using serial coronal sections, it becomes obvious that structure, and in anterior part also thickness of the SEZ, change in antero-posterior direction.

In order to examine the impact of the striatal neurodegenerative process on the adult neurogenesis, the dorsal (upper) part of the SEZ in lateral wall of lateral ventricle was studied. We selected a region closer to the aSEZ and RMS (at approx. level AP 1.4-1.5 from bregma) – the rostral compartment of the SEZ (R-SEZ), and a part of the SEZ adjacent to the striatum (at approx. level AP 1.1-1.2 from bregma) – the lateral compartment of the SEZ (L-SEZ). Surprisingly, we did not note any essential difference between both studied compartments in normal adult brain in relation to the detection of all used antibodies. The only noted difference was in a thickness of the SEZ in the mentioned compartments - the L-SEZ was slightly thicker than the R-SEZ.

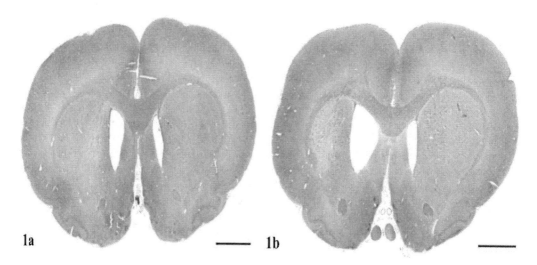

Figure 1. The degeneration of striatal neurons results in a striatal atrophy accompanied by compensatory dilatation of the lateral brain ventricle in a damaged hemisphere (left) which is already well visible at 1 week after neurotoxic (QA) lesion (a); b - the development of neurodegenerative process continues and the dilatation of lateral ventricle becomes very conspicuous in 6-month surviving animals. H&E. Bar: a, b – 1.5 mm.

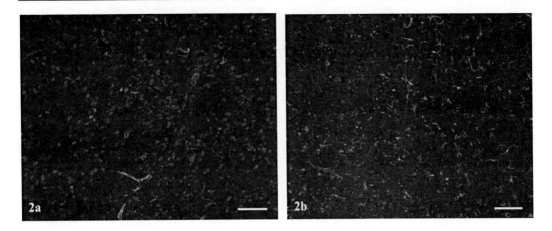

Figure 2. a – The accumulation of the large number of neurons (red – marked by anti-NeuN) and only scattered expression of GFAP (green) by fine protoplasmic astrocytes are typical features of normal striatum. b - The near complete loss of neurons only (the partial necrosis) which are partly replaced by intensive proliferation of GFAP-positive reactive (fibrous) astrocytes is a hallmark of both HD and neurotoxic lesion in an animal model of HD. (Most of blue nuclei stained with DAPI belong to the glial cells, the other to phagocytes at 1 week after the QA lesion.); Anti-NeuN + anti-GFAP (+ DAPI – only in fig. b). Bar: a, b – 100 μm.

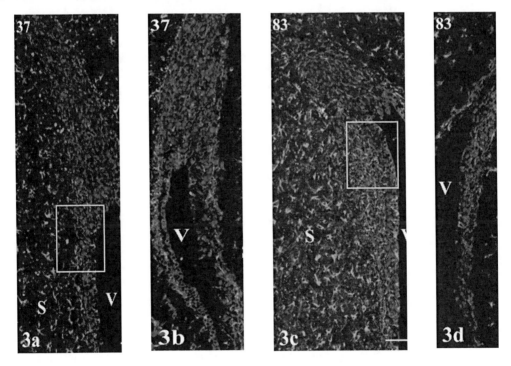

Figure 3. (Continued).

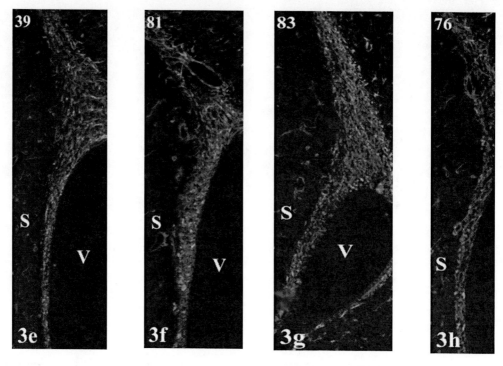

Figure 3. Coronal sections of the hemisphere, where the neurodegenerative process develops in the striatum at 1 week (a – d) or at 6 months (e, f) after unilateral QA lesion, and for comparison, of intact control brain at 1 week (g) and at 6 months (h) of experiment. Differences in reaction of the neurogenic region in the R-SEZ (a, b, e – AP approx. -1.5 from bregma) and the L-SEZ compartments (c, d, f, g, h – AP approx. -1.2 from bregma), as well as the comparison of reaction of the SEZ in lesioned (a, c) and contralateral non-lesioned hemisphere (b, d) are shown. Very intensive proliferation of rapidly dividing BrdU$^+$ cells is characteristic for both (a) the R-SEZ but especially for its dorsolateral extension (related to the RMS) and (b) the L-SEZ. In the L-SEZ compartment, the most significant is its thickening based mainly on the multiplication of GFAP$^+$ astrocyte-like cells. Reactive astrogliosis is apparent in the striatum (S) opposite the L-SEZ region. V – the lateral brain ventricle. Boxed areas represent evaluated parts of the R-SEZ and the L-SEZ compartments. The reaction of the SEZ to the neurodegenerative process within the striatum is diminished at 6 months after lesion; the structure of the R-SEZ (e) essentially does not differ compared with intact brain of age-matched control (h), however, the enlargement and increased proliferation are still conspicuous in the L-SEZ (f). Number in left upper corner represents the number of serial section. Anti-BrdU + anti-GFAP (+ DAPI – only in figs. b, e). Bar: a-h – 100 μm.

The Neurodegenerative Process within the Striatum Affects Neurogenesis in the Adult SEZ

Our previous findings [47, 48] have confirmed that the intensity of reaction of the SEZ (i.e. the proliferation and differentiation of NSCs) depends on the extent and severity of the brain pathology. Since the neurodegenerative process represents both the extensive and also intensive damage of the striatum, striking immediate reaction of the adult SEZ is typical. Unlike in normal adult rat brain (figures 3g, h), a distinct enlargement of the SEZ in a dorsal part of the lateral wall of lateral brain ventricles is based on upregulated proliferation of both, the special type of GFAP-positive astrocytes (the NSCs/niche cells) and the precursors/

neuroblasts in characteristic clusters (figures 3a, c). We have observed that the reaction of the SEZ differs in the amount of proliferating cells but partly also in characteristic of newly generated cells in both compartments, the R-SEZ (figures 3a, b) and the L-SEZ (figures 3c, d). Considering that the process of degeneration in the striatum continues only slowly, the intensity of reaction of neurogenic niche within the adult SEZ decreases in a course of time. However, the number of proliferating cells remains steadily increased in the L-SEZ of the damaged hemisphere (figure 3f) in comparison with the R-SEZ (figure 3e) but especially with contralateral non-lesioned side and age-matched controls (figure 3h). Therefore, the reaction of the R-SEZ and L-SEZ compartments in activated SEZ was assessed in relation to the changes characteristic for 1-week and 6-month period of the development of neurodegenerative process within the striatum.

Intensive development of neurodegenerative process within the striatum influences proliferation also in the SEZ of contralateral undamaged hemisphere in both compartments, but particularly in the L-SEZ (figures 3b, c).

In sham-lesioned rats, only slightly increased proliferation was found in the L-SEZ, less in the R-SEZ, one week after the surgery. No difference was noted in the structure of the SEZ in sham-lesioned 6-month surviving animals in comparison with age-matched controls.

Activated SEZ – The Immediate Reaction of Neurogenic Niche (7 Days after QA Lesion)

Cell proliferation was detected by BrdU labeling. Since only 2 injections of BrdU were applied shortly (15 and 3 hours) before killing of animals, the nuclei of rapidly dividing precursors were labeled predominantly. On the other hand, not all newly generated cells were detected during this short period. The presence of cells with different level of expression of BrdU (figures 4a, b, 9) confirmed subsequent very rapid divisions of these cells, which were likely either neuronal precursors, or transit-amplifying cells of glial phenotype. BrdU-positive nuclei of proliferating cells formed typical large clusters, which participate in enlargement of activated SEZ in both observed compartments (figures 3a-d). In the R-SEZ, a large number of $BrdU^+$ nuclei densely packed in clusters filled the whole width of the SEZ (figures 3a, 4a). Similarly in the L-SEZ, clusters of $BrdU^+$ nuclei rapidly increased in size and formed 2-3 new rows within the SEZ (figures 3b, 4b, 9), in comparison with only 1–2 layers of small clusters in intact brains of control animals (figures 3g, 4c). The largest and most numerous clusters, composed of many $BrdU^+$ cells but also of cells with nuclei counterstained with DAPI only, were located just beneath the ependymal layer (figures 3a, c, 4a, b, 9). The size of these clusters rapidly decreased and their cells became more loosely arranged in the middle and outer layers of enlarged L-SEZ (figures 3c, 4b, 9).

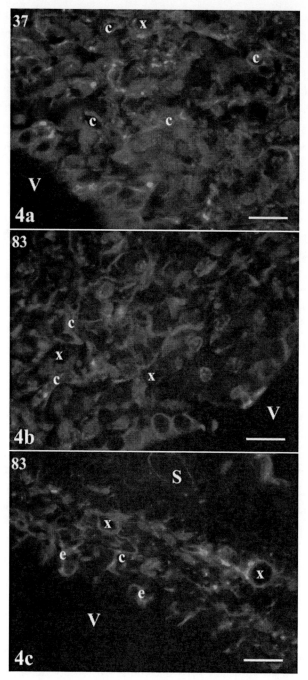

Fig. 4: Details of boxed areas from fig. 3a (**a**) and fig. 3c (**b**) show the typical arrangement of enlarged clusters of rapidly dividing BrdU$^+$ cells in the R-SEZ (**a**) and the L-SEZ (**b**) in comparison with the structure of the L-SEZ in control brain (**c**). Different level of the intensity of BrdU-expression confirms the rapid repeated division of some cells. The scaffolding meshwork formed of GFAP$^+$ astrocyte-like cells includes also enlarged network of vessels (x), particularly of capillaries (c) which wall is marked by GFAP$^+$ vascular end-feet of astrocyte-like cells. Ependymal cells which line the wall of lateral ventricle (V) are also labeled with GFAP. Anti-BrdU + anti-GFAP (+ DAPI – only in fig. a). Bar: a-c – 20 µm.

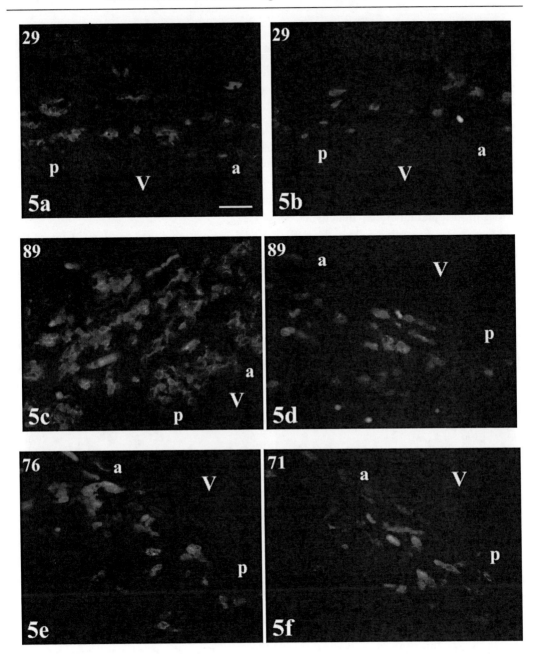

Figure 5. Most of newly generated (BrdU$^+$) cells (red nuclei) are of neuronal identity because of colabeling with the NCAM (green). The most intensive coexpression of BrdU and NCAM is in the L-SEZ region at 1 week after the QA lesion (c) and then in the R-SEZ (a) of the same animal; increased proliferation is also observed in the L-SEZ (d) but not in the R-SEZ (b) of contralateral undamaged side. On the other hand, the partial dissociation of BrdU and NCAM expression is typical for protracted reaction of the L-SEZ (e) and also for its age-matched control (f). The reason is, that a part of formerly BrdU$^+$ cells underwent several mitotic divisions, therefore lost BrdU labeling (which was half by each division) and became postmitotic neuroblasts (only NCAM$^+$). Comparable situation, but with smaller number of cells, is in L-SEZ of age-matched control (f). V - lateral ventricle; a–p - antero–posterior direction. Anti-NCAM + anti-BrdU. Bar: a-f – 20 μm.

A phenotype of BrdU⁺ Cells

The majority of newly generated cells with BrdU$^+$ nuclei in both regions expressed also NCAM, a typical marker of immature neuronal cells – neuroblasts (figures 5a-d). Conspicuous expression of NCAM was in the whole width of enlarged L-SEZ (figure 5a) in contrast to intact SEZ, where only few NCAM$^+$ cells were present (figure 5b). On the other hand, only slight increase in number of newly generated immature neuronal cells was found in a region of the R-SEZ (figure 5c) compared with controls (figure 5d). Most of NCAM-expressing cells can be also marked with β-III-tubulin, less with MAP-2ab but always reveal only a weak positivity for these two markers in comparison with strong positivity of mature neurons in surrounding brain parenchyma.

Most of BrdU-positive cells in the R-SEZ (and especially in dorsolateral extension of the SEZ) expressed also doublecortin (DCX), a marker of migrating neuroblasts (figure 6a); markedly lower expression of DCX was in the L-SEZ (figure 6b) but always higher in comparison with control brains.

On the other hand, some cells with BrdU$^+$ nuclei were of roughly of stellate shape (with only short processes) with conspicuous expression of nestin in their cytoplasm *(see the following)*. Rather larger number of these cells was in the L-SEZ region. The mentioned characteristic contributed to the assumption that these cells were proliferating transit-amplifying cells.

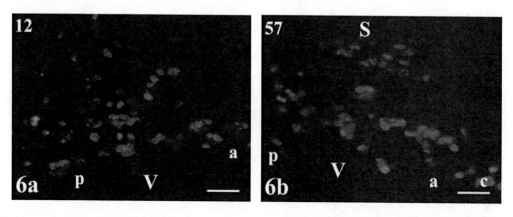

Figure 6. a - In the R-SEZ, BrdU$^+$ (red) cells are less numerous compared with L-SEZ but almost all of them coexpress DCX (green) and alone DCX-labeled cells are also frequent, which confirms that they are neuroblasts continually migrating via the RMS to OB. b – On the other hand, newly generated BrdU$^+$ cells in clusters prevail in early-activated L-SEZ and although most of them coexpress also DCX the number of DCX$^+$cells is markedly lower in this region. V - lateral ventricle; a–p - antero–posterior direction. Anti-DCX + anti-BrdU. Bar: a, b – 20 μm.

Reaction of Neural Stem/Niche Cells and Progenitor Cells

Nestin, principally used as a marker of NSCs and NPCs, was expressed in the whole activated SEZ, primarily in the L-SEZ; a slight to moderate labeling was typical for most of ependymal cells (figures 7a, c). The number and distribution of nestin-expressing cells was always closely related to clusters of immature (mostly BrdU$^+$) cells, which was characteristic for both compartments. Accordingly, increased expression of nestin, related only to the clusters of neuronal cells, was also found in the SEZ of contralateral undamaged hemisphere (figures 7b, d), unlike only scattered labeling in control brains. Typical extensive and prominent meshwork of nestin-positive cells was in the L-SEZ (figures 7b, 8) in relation to the clusters of immature, in majority neuronal cells, which here occupied 3 or more layers (unlike 1-2 layers of clusters in the R-SEZ – figure 7a). The distribution of nestin within the cytoplasm copies the shape of cells, which enables to see a thin rim around large nuclei of the cells packed in clusters but also short thick extensions running between or aside clustered cells – these cells might be supposed the transit-amplifying precursors (figure 8). Few cells belonging to the clusters underneath the ependyma extend long, also nestin-positive process inbetween the ependymal cells to reach the ventricular lumen (figure 8*)*. (If these extensions coexpress two or all three intermediate filaments they evidently carry a vessel – *see the following*.)

The number of nestin$^+$ cells was markedly smaller in the R-SEZ (figure 7a) and only a mild increase of nestin expression occurred in cell clumps in the SEZ of contralateral non-lesioned hemisphere (figure 7b). These differences in a number of nestin-expressing cells well document significant activation of neurogenic niche in the L-SEZ in response to the neurodegenerative process developing in the striatum. The intensive expression of nestin in intimate contact with clusters of closely packed immature cells (both BrdU$^+$ and stained only with DAPI) argues for extensive proliferation of transit-amplifying precursors (C cells) supporting the migratory neuroblasts (A cells) in response to the damage of the brain parenchyma.

(Nestin is also very useful marker of newly formed/sprouted vessels which are very important and therefore numerous in enlarged activated SEZ - *see the following*).

Cells of Astrocytic Phenotype

To characterize morphology and spatial distribution of cells with astrocytic properties, the detection of cytoskeletal intermediate filaments (IFs) vimentin and GFAP was carried out. The extensive labeling for vimentin, a marker of reactive astrocytes, but also of radial glia and ependymal cells, was found in the activated SEZ of the damaged brain hemisphere. All vimentin-positive cells were of astrocytic phenotype (i.e. of stellate shape with branched processes) but their cytoplasmic processes were softer, compared with those of GFAP$^+$ cells (figures 10a-d). They formed both a fine scaffold network for proliferating (BrdU$^+$) and other cells in clusters (figure 9), and more densely arranged scaffolding in nearly whole enlarged SEZ with maximum in a middle layer which subsequently disappeared in the outer layer (figures 10a-d). Unlike the distribution of nestin expression, we did not notice substantial differences between the R-SEZ and the L-SEZ in relation to the detection of vimentin (and also GFAP). Furthermore, a distinct labeling for vimentin was also throughout the SEZ, and especially in the ependymal cells, in control brains (figure 10e). It is necessary to note that also endothelial and smooth muscle cells within the wall of vessels are vimentin-positive.

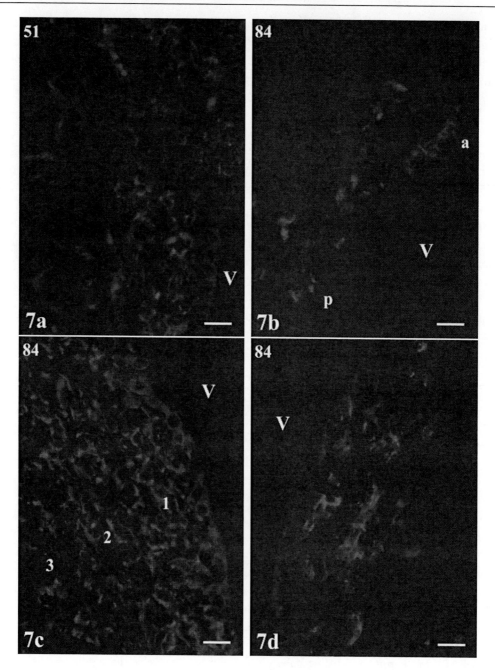

Figure 7. One week after QA lesion. Network-like arrangement of nestin-positive cells is typical for both compartments (a, c) of early-activated SEZ and also for contralateral L-SEZ (d); but only focal and of lesser extent nestin-positivity, related exclusively to the clustered cells, is observed in the L-SEZ of age-matched controls (b). Stellate-shaped nestin$^+$ cells are likely transit-amplifying cells which are most numerous in the L-SEZ compartment (c). They surround single neuronal cells within the clusters (zone 1) but also form a dense network in the middle layer of the SEZ (zone 2) and their number decreases in the outer layer of the SEZ (zone 3). V - lateral ventricle; a–p - antero–posterior direction. Anti-nestin. Bar: a-d – 20 μm.

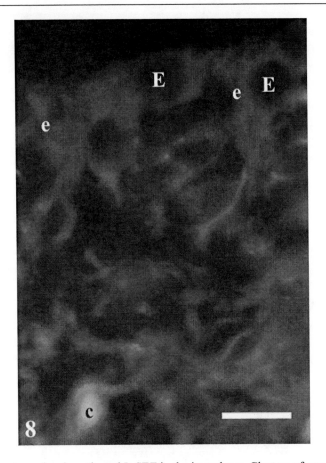

Figure 8. Detailed structure of early-activated L-SEZ in the inner layer. Clusters of mostly neuronal cells as well as single cells (blue nuclei) are surrounded by nestin$^+$ cells (red) of glial phenotype. Many capillaries (C) also express nestin which confirms that they are newly developed. Ependymal cells (E) are mostly vimentin$^+$ (green). The coexpression of nestin and vimentin is sometimes also found in cellular processes (e) which extend from inner layer of probably transit-amplifying cells between ependymal cells to reach a ventrical lumen. Anti-nestin + anti-vimentin. Bar: 5 μm.

The expression of GFAP is considered to be the most characteristic morphological feature of the NSCs/niche astrocyte-like cells within neurogenic regions in both developing and adult brains under the normal as well as pathological conditions (figures 3a-d, g, h, 4a-c). The scaffolding formed of GFAP-positive cells (figure 10c) was also more robust in comparison with that detected by vimentin (figure 10b), and filled in entirely the whole thickness in both observed compartments of activated and intact SEZ. Compared with the arrangement of vimentin-expressing cells/processes, the GFAP-positive processes of astrocyte-like cells entered the clusters of immature cells rarely and they were always only very fine (figure 10d). On the other hand, typical thick GFAP$^+$ processes circled all clusters of densely packed cells, which was most prominent in relation to the largest clusters located underneath the ependyma (figures 4a, b, 10a-d). Scattered thicker and long GFAP$^+$ astrocytic processes (sometimes coepressing vimentin) entered the ependymal layer and reached the lumen of the lateral ventricle (figure 10d).

The coexpression of all detected IFs. Since all the above-described cytoskeletal filaments and proteins were detected in the network-forming cell processes, we tried to investigate their interrelationship by the use of immunofluoresce double-labeling methods. Surprisingly, the coexpression of either nestin and vimentin, or nestin and GFAP, or vimentin and GFAP was of quite small extent not only in both compartments of activated SEZ and in contralateral hemisphere, but also in the SEZ of control brain. In the R-SEZ, this coexpression was of less extent compared with the L-SEZ compartment. Briefly, two almost independent scaffolding networks, one composed of vimentin-positive astrocyte-like cells, and the second formed of the GFAP-positive astrocyte-like cells coexisted in the activated L-SEZ (figures 10a-d).

The only prominent coexpression of all three IFs was in vascular end-feet anchored on the wall of vessels throughout the SEZ in all observed cases. A very fine colocalization was detected in scaffolding of the clusters of neuronal cells, and only rarely in fine network around these clusters. Prominent coexpression was present in "septa" formed of thick processes of GFAP-positive astrocytes. In both these mentioned cases, the overlay of signals resulted from the presence of vessels (figure 10d). Slightly exceptional was the detection of nestin in relation to the wall of vessels, where nestin is expressed not only by astrocytic end-feet on outer surface of vessels but also by endothelium in newly formed sprouted vessels (figure 8).

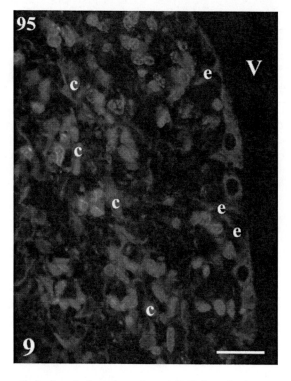

Figure 9. Astrocyte-like cells in the whole early-activated SEZ (here in the L-SEZ) form intensely vimentin-positive (green) scaffolding network. BrdU$^+$ cells are packed in clusters, which size decreases outward. Numerous capillaries (C) represent the integral part of activated neurogenic niche. Also here, the vimentin$^+$ processes (e) of astrocyte-like cells extend between ependymal cells. Anti-BrdU + anti-vimentin + DAPI. Bar: 20 μm.

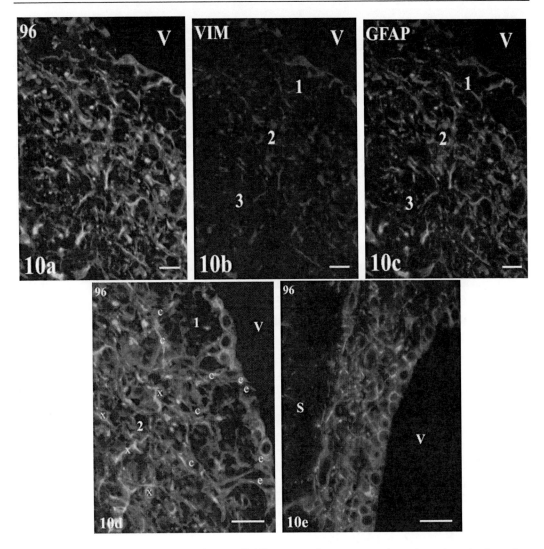

Figure 10. a,d - Two almost independent scaffolding networks are present in early-activated enlarged SEZ, especially in the L-SEZ. b - Finer network is formed of vimentin$^+$ cells; c – denser, coarser network is of GFAP$^+$ astrocyte-like cells. The differences in character and arrangement in all 3 layers of the L-SEZ (1-3) of both networks are well visible on figures (b) and (c). d – Detail of figure (a) shows that the scaffolding for clusters of neuronal cells is formed mainly of vimentin$^+$ (red) cells, and also that the colocalisation of both IFs is mostly only in relation to vascular end-feet of astrocytic cells on the wall of vessels (X), especially capillaries (C). Fine processes (e) of astrocyte-like cells extending between ependymal cells are labeled for one or both IFs. e – In the intact brain, the L-SEZ reveals larger coexpression of vimentin and GFAP, essentially throughout the whole width of the SEZ. However, also here the most intensive coexpression of both IFs is in vascular end-feet. V - lateral ventricle; S – striatum. Anti-vimentin + anti-GFAP (+ DAPI – only in fig. e). Bar: a–e - 20 μm.

The glio-vascular unit represents the specialized relationship of astrocyte end-feet to the wall of vessels in the CNS, including the formation of perivascular limiting membrane and its close relationship to the blood-brain barrier. Blood vessels, and particularly capillaries, represent an inherent very important component of the neurogenic niche. Therefore, it was not any surprise that the enlargement of activated SEZ (especially of the L-SEZ) was accompanied by the augmentation of vascular network, most likely by sprouting of existing vessels (figures 4a, b). As was mentioned before, a very suitable marker of these newly formed vessels was nestin (figure 8), expressed by many vessels in the entire L-SEZ, and in lesser extent in the R-SEZ. Consequently, the vessels within the SEZ were detected according to the astrocyte end-feet for which the coexpression of two or sometime all three IFs is typical. Moreover, the endothelium and also smooth muscle cells in medium-sized and larger vessels are usually marked also by vimentin (figure 10d).

The ependymal cells line in a simple layer all brain cavities in epitheloid arrangement (i.e. devoid of their own basal lamina). They express very intensely vimentin (figures 9, 10b) and a bit less GFAP in all observed groups of animals (figures 3a-h, 4a-c). The vimentin expression is so intensive that mostly lays over the GFAP labeling, if the double-staining method is used (figures 10a, d). Interestingly, the intensity of nestin expression reflected the intensity of the SEZ activation, it means that conspicuous labeling for nestin revealed ependymal cells in the L-SEZ compartment (figure 7c), moderate to slight level of expression was in ependyma of the R-SEZ region but also of L-SEZ compartment in the hemisphere conralateral to the degenerated striatum (figures 7a, d) and in the intact brain, the ependymal cells essentially did not express nestin at all (figure 7b).

Activated SEZ – The Protracted Reaction of Neurogenic Niche (6 Months after QA Lesion)

Even though the degeneration of striatal neurons and neuropil continues slowly and shrinkage of the striatum with compensatory enlargement of lateral brain ventricles progresses (figures 1b, 3e, f), the intensity of reaction of neurogenic niche decreases in a course of time (figures 3e, f).

The intensity of proliferation of rapidly dividing BrdU-positive precursors decreased, however, the number of $BrdU^+$ cells remained steadily increased in the damaged hemisphere (especially in the L-SEZ) in comparison with contralateral non-lesioned side and age-matched controls (figures 3e, f, h). Consequently, large clusters of $BrdU^+$ nuclei underneath the ependymal layer, a hallmark of immediate reaction of the SEZ to the striatal damage, were only few, smaller and exclusively within the L-SEZ at 6 months after the QA lesion (figure 3f). Since the thickness of activated L-SEZ decreased in time, the clusters of neuronal cells were not more typically arranged in layers but they became spread throughout the thinner L-SEZ, and except those few of larger size, all other clusters were quite small (figures 3e, f).

The location of nestin (figure 11a) as well as NCAM expression (figures 5e, 11b) were in close relation to the clusters of neuronal cells like in previously described stage. However, the extent of detection was markedly lower (especially of the nestin) because of substantial reduction of clusters of neuronal cells in both number and size. Nestin expression in particular became typically focal, unlike a network-like arrangement in L-SEZ during the immediate reaction (compare figures 11a and 7c). Reduced extent of NCAM expression is likely caused by maturation of a part of neuroblasts within clusters.

Differences in relation to the vimentin and GFAP expression and coexpression also occurred (figures 12a-c, 3e, f). Despite a typical network-like arrangement of astrocytic cells detected by either vimentin or GFAP, both those scaffolding networks became finer, more loosely arranged and especially of lesser extent in relation to reduced width of the L-SEZ (figures 12a-c). The arrangement of glial cells network (expressing both vimentin and GFAP) was not such precisely defined as formerly. Also the scaffolding for clusters of neuroblasts was formed preferentially by vimentin$^+$ extensions of the glial cells but in a very fine, reduced form only (figure 12b). Quite prominent expression of vimentin persisted in the wall of larger vessels (because of its expression also by endothelial and smooth muscle cells – figures 12a, b).

On the other hand, the coexpression of both IFs was rather more extensive in 6-month survivors, where it spread almost throughout the L-SEZ (compare figures 12a and 10d). This phenomenon might be related to the slow maturation of some astrocyte-like cells. Concurrently, the most conspicuous coexpression of vimentin and GFAP was again in vascular end-feet of astrocyte-like cells (figure 12a).

Vessels, which originated during a prompt and extensive enlargement of the L-SEZ (partly also in the R-SEZ) in the first studied stage of the reaction to the neurodegenerative process (figures 4a, b), became more mature after 6 months which is indicated mainly by increased number of the smooth muscle cells (vimentin-positive) and therefore also increased thickness of their wall is typical. Because of reduced width of activated L-SEZ, vascular network also becomes more densely arranged. The coexpression of vimentin and GFAP in vascular astrocytic end-feet was constantly present. However, the expression of nestin within the wall of vessels (by both the endothelium and the end-feet) was not found. This documented the fact that vessels, originated/sprouted in early stage of SEZ activation, consequently became mature and that essentially no new vessels were formed in later stages of the L-SEZ reaction.

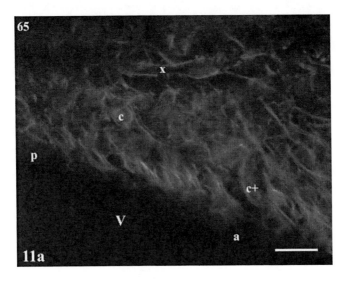

Figure 11. (Continued).

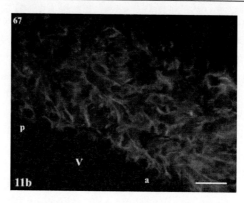

Figure 11. The most characteristic for activated L-SEZ in animals surviving 6 months after the QA lesion is that proliferative activity slows down and therefore the width of the SEZ becomes thinner in comparison with the L-SEZ in 1-week survivors. a – The expression of nestin is subtle, only in connection to the cells in clusters. The vessels (X), mostly capillaries are numerous also in this case. Rarely, the nestin-expressing, e.g. newly formed capillary (C+) can be found underneath the ependyma. b – Surprisingly, NCAM is expressed by some cells of clusters only. The reason is likely the maturation of most of neuronal cells in clusters. a, b - The GFAP$^+$ astrocyte-like cells (green) form typical scaffolding network but of lesser extent. V - lateral ventricle; a–p - antero–posterior direction. a - anti-nestin + anti-GFAP + DAPI, b - anti-NCAM + anti-GFAP + DAPI. Bar: a, b - 20 μm.

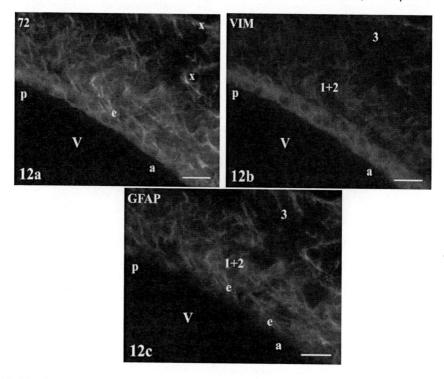

Figure 12. The characteristic arrangement of both vimentin$^+$ (b) and GFAP$^+$ (c) scaffolding network in the L-SEZ of 6-month survivors after the QA lesion. A smaller thickness of the L-SEZ results in reduction (1+2) of 3 layers, described in the L-SEZ of 1 week surviving rats, into 2 layers only. a – Unlike in the early activated L-SEZ, rather larger extent of coexpression of both main IFs is characteristic for this stage, which might be also related to the maturation of some astrocyte-like cells. V - lateral ventricle; a–p - antero–posterior direction. Anti-vimentin + anti-GFAP + DAPI. Bar: a–c - 20 μm.

The Characteristic of Activated Neurogenic Niche in Temporal Study

In enlarged L-SEZ, activated by developing neurodegenerative process within the striatum, we have found a very rapid immediate increase in proliferation of both neuronal precursors and especially glial cells. Considering the design of our experiment, essentially the proliferation of rapidly dividing cells was documented by the expression of BrdU. The BrdU-positive nuclei were always found within densely packed clusters of cells. The coexpression of BrdU and NCAM in most of these cells showed their neuronal identity. Also nestin was intensely expressed in these clusters of cells throughout the enlarged L-SEZ, and in lesser extent in the R-SEZ. Nestin-expressing cells largely revealed short, wider processes of irregular shape which resembled the morphology of the immature astrocyte-like glial cells. Nestin-positive cells appeared to form scaffolding for clustered neuronal cells but further studies are needed to verify whether they are directly the activated proliferating stem/niche cell or only rapidly dividing transit-amplifying cells. The number of these cells decreased in time, and in reaction to 6-month-lasting neurodegenerative process in the striatum, expression of nestin was less extensive, particularly due to lower number of clusters of neural precursors.

The expression of vimentin throughout nearly whole width of both activated and intact SEZ supports the suggestion that astrocyte-like NSCs/niche cells are modified radial glia. Moreover, vimentin-positive stellate-shaped cells (which did not coexpress GFAP) typically formed the scaffolding network for clusters of neuronal precursors. Concurrently, a massive expression of vimentin might also document activation of these astrocyte-like cells (which is in agreement with high expression of vimentin in reactive astrocytes within the brain parenchyma).

In early-activated L-SEZ, two almost independent scaffolding networks were found - one formed of vimentin- and the second of the GFAP-positive astrocyte-like cells. The network formed of vimentin$^+$ cells was more delicate, particularly in the region underneath the ependyma, and did not cover the entire width of the SEZ, in comparison with coarser network of GFAP$^+$ cells which extended up to the boundary with the surrounding brain parenchyma. In animals surviving 6 months after the QA lesion, these two networks were less pronounced as separately arranged also because the L-SEZ subsequently became thinner. On the other hand, the overlay of vimentin and GFAP expression was more frequent in this case, without conspicuous difference between the L-SEZ and R-SEZ.

The coexpression of vimentin and GFAP, although quite frequent in enlarged L-SEZ in comparison with the R-SEZ, was essentially located only in vascular end-feet marking the wall of numerous (in majority newly formed) small to larger vessels. Surprisingly, rather more pronounced overlay of both networks (not only as vascular end-feet) was present in the SEZ at 6 months after the QA lesion. It is likely that some of these activated astrocyte-like cells undergo slow maturation but most of them persist in immature form (resembling their common origin with radial glia cells) for a long time, if not permanently.

Indeed, a very intensive vasculogenesis represents another important integral component of activated neurogenic niche in the SEZ. Certainly, there are several reasons of this phenomenon but one of them is probably most relevant – not only the enlargement of vascular (particularly capillary) network but also increased number and activation of astrocyte end-feet (visualized by their intensive labeling especially with nestin and vimentin), i.e. the formation of glio-vascular unit, is related to increased metabolic needs of highly active SEZ enlarged in response to the neurodegenerative process within the striatum.

DISCUSSION

The adult neurogenesis in animal forebrain has been widely studied especially during last two decades. Vast majority of these studies, however, investigate the structure of the SEZ in the brain of young adult animals under physiological conditions to describe proliferating neuronal precursors. These precursors tangentially migrate within the wall of lateral ventricles and then via the RMS to OB, where they differentiate into interneurons [e.g. 2, 4, 9, 10, 14, 34, 40, 41, 42, 46, 69]. An astrocytic morphology including ultrastructure was confirmed for adult neural stem cell in animal brain [3, 11, 16, 22, 27, 66, 72] as well as in human brain [e.g. 23, 59, 65].

Two types of rapidly dividing cells were identified within the SEZ: the migratory fate-specific neuroblasts (A-cells) and transit-amplifying precursors of glial character (C-cells). Both these types of cells are supposed to derive from NSCs with characteristic of GFAP-positive astrocytes (B-cells). NSC in the SEZ is always defined as a (very) slowly proliferating cell with the ability to self-renew [e.g. 12, 37, 55, 57, 72]. Growing body of evidence suggests developmental relationship of SVZ neural stem cells to the radial glia [e.g. 37, 72]. It is obvious that during the histogenesis of embryonic CNS, the neuroepithelial stem cells give rise to the radial glial stem cells [30, 53, 64] from which the astrocytic stem cells but also neurons of cortical plate are derived. Both the radial glia and NSCs reveal same properties (self-renewal and asymmetric division, production of both neuronal and glial cells). However, the radial glial cells disappear in the perinatal period. It is now supposed that radial glial cells transform into the subpopulation of astrocyte-like cells within the SEZ (and also in the SGZ of hippocampus) [3, 25, 72]. Vimentin is mostly mentioned as a typical marker of radial glial cells [64, 66].

In the SEZ, activated in response to developing neurodegenerative process within the striatum of adult rat brain, we have observed intensive labeling for vimentin within extended scaffolding network of glial cell. Furthermore, two essentially independent scaffolding networks have been found particularly in the L-SEZ: one formed of GFAP-positive astrocyte-like cells and the second of vimentin-positive astrocytic cells. Surprisingly, in relation to protracted reaction of the SEZ (i.e. at 6 months after the QA lesion), the increased coexpression of vimentin and GFAP was typical. It might be a sign of two subtypes of NSCs existing rather independently in the adult SEZ: The first type of astrocyte-like cells detected by GFAP, and the second type (vimentin-positive) are likely the derivates of radial glial cells, with which they share the "stemness". This property might be enhanced by the damage of the brain when they start to proliferate. If the damage is chronic, as in the case of the neurodegenerative process, long-lasting subsequent differentiation of some these astrocyte-like cells occurs. Our findings are also consistent with results of *in vitro* experiments [37] showing that only a small fraction of GFAP-positive cells (type B) can form multipotent neurospheres, so that only a subtype of these astrocytic cells can serve as stem cells.

Simultaneously, the stem cells of neurogenic niche are also suggested niche cells [e.g. 15, 20]. Niche is the primary environment where the stem cell acquires information about whether or not to divide and what types of progeny to generate [45, 70]. The high plasticity of NSCs in neurogenic niche during prenatal period starts to change in time of the birth and then rapidly decreases [e.g. 38, 63]. Our study provides evidence that massive loss of striatal neurons caused by neurodegenerative process launches immediate intensive response of adult neurogenic niche within the SEZ of lateral brain ventricles. The enhanced proliferation of both neuronal precursors as well as glial cells appear very early marked by intensive (and in the L-SEZ also extensive) expression of nestin. It is likely that intensely nestin-positive cells densely packed in clusters are both the neuroblasts and transit-amplifying precursor cells (in both observed compartments). On the other hand, processes characteristic for astrocyte-like cells forming a network among the clusters but particularly in the middle layer of enlarged L-SEZ also express nestin despite its rather lower intensity. Surprisingly, the coexpression of nestin and vimentin was essentially not found in relation to this network. Thus it remains to be investigated, which type of cells is responsible for such intensive proliferation to cause a very rapid conspicuous enlargement of activated SEZ represented by a dense network of GFAP-positive astrocyte-like cells. (Thickening of the SEZ is already found at 1 day after QA lesion – unpublished data).

Even though the compartmentalization is most characteristic for activated SEZ (also in long-term surviving animals), it is present also in the normal intact SEZ. The intriguing possibly rises that the compartmentalization of the SEZ has a relationship to the special function (not fully known yet) of each part of the SEZ [26, 67].

Decreased intensity of proliferation during 6 months of the development of neurodegenerative process in the striatum is related to both, rapidly dividing precursors whose clusters decrease in size and number, and astrocyte-like cells whose networks also become reduced and cease to express nestin. On the other hand, increased coexpression of vimentin and GFAP likely documents slow subsequent maturation of some newly generated astrocyte-like cell.

Considering our current knowledge of the function of astrocytes [e.g. 17, 22, 27, 60] the need for extensive study of astrocyte-like cells role, which play in the SEZ (particularly in the L-SEZ) under physiological and pathological conditions, is highlighted. These cells cannot be considered only neural stem cells but likely they also act as mature astrocytes – probably with specific modifications related to their dual role in neurogenic niche.

CONCLUSION

The immediate response of the L-SEZ is much more intensive compared with R-SEZ. This compartmentalization of activated SEZ probably corresponds to the role which each of mentioned parts plays in adult neurogenesis. The R-SEZ, which is closely related to the neurogenesis for OB, is less involved in response to severe chronic striatal damage, the neurodegenerative process. On the other hand, it would be possible that signals coming from striatum do not promote neurogenesis within the L-SEZ in adequate extent and therefore the gliogenesis here prevails. The intensity of cell proliferation and differentiation either of neuroblasts or glial cells is markedly lower in 6-month survivors but always higher in comparison with contralateral non-lesioned side, sham-operated rats or intact age-matched controls. Typical changes were also noted in the structure of neurogenic niche. Two quite independent scaffolding networks formed of vimentin-positive- and GFAP-positive astrocyte-like cells were described as a characteristic feature of immediate reaction of the SEZ (especially of the L-SEZ). Interestingly, these two formerly individual signals frequently overlap in the SEZ of long-term (6 months) surviving animals. Based on these observations, the hypothesis of the existence of two subtypes of NSCs in the SEZ with selective response to signals activating the neurogenic niche may be proposed. It is also likely that the intensive expression of vimentin is the proof of both the activation of astrocytic cells and developmental relationship between SEZ neural stem cells and radial glial cells. All mentioned features of astrocyte-like stem cells of adult SEZ indicate that these cells retain some characteristics of embryonic stem cells/radial glial cells but their proliferation and differentiation are limited by the microenvironment of adult neurogenic niche. Although the intensity of cellular response of the SEZ to the neurotoxic lesion of the striatum decreases during the time, the characteristic changes in a structure of neurogenic niche have been found during whole studied period.

Our observations also underscore the complexity of activation of neurogenic niche in response to different macro- and microenvironmental cues. Therefore, we must first increase our understanding of regulatory mechanisms of adult neurogenesis and gliogenesis to be able to utilize this potential for therapeutic use.

Acknowledgments

The authors thank M. Hetešová, J. Pipková, H. Hollerová and Z. Komárková for technical assistance. The nestin (clone Rat-401) and NCAM (clone 5B8) were obtained from the Developmental Studies Hybridoma Bank, University of Iowa, IA, USA.

Work was supported by the Research project (MSM0021620820) of the Ministry of Education of the Czech Republic.

References

[1] Altman, J. Autoradiographic study of degenerative and regenerative proliferation of neuroglia cells with tritiated thymidine. *Exp. Neurol.* 1962, 5, 302-318.
[2] Alvarez-Buylla, A; Temple, S. Stem cells in the developing and adult nervous system. *J. Neurobiol.* 1998, 36(2), 105-110.
[3] Alvarez-Buylla, A; García-Verdugo, JM; Tramontin, AD. A unified hypothesis on the lineage of neural stem cells. *Nat. Rev. Neurosci.* 2001, 2(4), 287-293.
[4] Alvarez-Buylla, A; Garcia-Verdugo, JM. Neurogenesis in adult subventricular zone. *J. Neurosci.* 2002a, 22(3), 629-634.
[5] Alvarez-Buylla, A; Seri, B; Doetsch, F. Identification of neural stem cells in the adult vertebrate brain. *Brain Res. Bull.* 2002b, 57(6), 751-758.

[6] Alvarez-Buylla, A; Lim, DA. For the long run: maintaining germinal niches in the adult brain. *Neuron.* 2004, 41(5), 683-686.

[7] Arvidsson, A; Collin, T; Kirik, D; Kokaia, Z; Lindvall, O. Neuronal replacement from endogenous precursors in the adult brain after stroke. *Nat. Med.* 2002, 8(9), 963-970.

[8] Biebl, M; Cooper, CM; Winkler, J; Kuhn, HG. Analysis of neurogenesis and programmed cell death reveals a self-renewing capacity in the adult rat brain. *Neurosci. Lett.* 2000, 291(1), 17-20.

[9] Doetsch, F; Alvarez-Buylla, A. Network of tangential pathways for neuronal migration in adult mammalian brain. *Proc. Natl. Acad. Sci. U.S.A.* 1996, 93, 14895–14900.

[10] Doetsch, F; Garcia-Verdugo, JM; Alvarez-Buylla, A. Cellular composition and three-dimensional organization of the subventricular germinal zone in the adult mammalian brain. *J. Neurosci.* 1997, 17, 5046–5061.

[11] Doetsch, F; Caillé, I; Lim, DA; García-Verdugo, JM; Alvarez-Buylla, A. Subventricular zone astrocytes are neural stem cells in the adult mammalian brain. *Cell.* 1999a, 97(6), 703-716.

[12] Doetsch, F; García-Verdugo, JM; Alvarez-Buylla, A. Regeneration of a germinal layer in the adult mammalian brain. *Proc. Natl. Acad. Sci. U. S. A.* 1999b, 96(20), 11619-11624.

[13] Doetsch, F; Scharff, C. Challenges for brain repair: insights from adult neurogenesis in birds and mammals. *Brain Behav. Evol.* 2001, 58(5), 306-322.

[14] Doetsch, F; Petreanu, L; Caille, I; Garcia-Verdugo, JM; Alvarez-Buylla, A. EGF converts transit-amplifying neurogenic precursors in the adult brain into multipotent stem cells. *Neuron.* 2002, 36, 1021–1034.

[15] Doetsch, F. A niche for adult neural stem cells. *Curr. Opin. Genet. Dev.* 2003a, (5), 543-550.

[16] Doetsch, F. The glial identity of neural stem cells. *Nat. Neurosci.* 2003b, 6(11), 1127-1134.

[17] Emsley, JG; Arlotta, P; Macklis, JD. Star-cross'd neurons: astroglial effects on neural repair in the adult mammalian CNS. *Trends Neurosci.* 2004, 27(5), 238-240.

[18] Emsley, JG; Mitchell, BD; Kempermann, G; Macklis, JD. Adult neurogenesis and repair of the adult CNS with neural progenitors, precursors and stem cells. *Progress Neurobiol.* 2005, 75, 321-341.

[19] Eriksson, PS; Perfilieva, E; Björk-Eriksson, T; Alborn, AM; Nordborg, C; Peterson, DA; Gage, FH. Neurogenesis in the adult human hippocampus. *Nat. Med.* 1998, 4(11), 1313-1317.

[20] Fuchs, E; Tumbar, T; Guasch, G. Socializing with the neighbors: stem cells and their niche. *Cell.* 2004, 116(6), 769-778.

[21] Gage, FH. Neurogenesis in the adult brain. *J. Neurosci.* 2002, 22, 612–613.

[22] Goldman, S. Glia as neural progenitor cells. *Trends Neurosci.* 2003, 26(11), 590-596.

[23] Goldman, SA. Neural progenitor cells of the adult human brain. In: Rao MS. Neural development and stem cells. New Jersey: Humana Press Inc; 2006; 267-297.

[24] Gordon, RJ; Tattersfield, AS; Vazey, EM; Kells, AP; McGregor, AL; Hughes, SM; Connor, B. Temporal profile of subventricular zone progenitor cell migration following quinolinic acid-induced striatal cell loss. *Neuroscience.* 2007, 146(4), 1704-1718.

[25] Götz, M; Steindler, D. To be glial or not-how glial are the precursors of neurons in development and adulthood? *Glia.* 2003, 43(1), 1-3.

[26] Guillemot, F; Parras, C. Adult neurogenesis: a tale of two precursors. *Nat. Neurosci.* 2005, 8(7), 846-848.

[27] Horner, PJ; Palmer, TD. New roles for astrocytes: the nightlife of an 'astrocyte'. La vida loca! *Trends Neurosci.* 2003, 26(11), 597-603.

[28] Johansson, CB; Svensson, M; Wallstedt, L; Janson, AM; Frisen, J. Neural stem cells in the adult human brain. *Exp. Cell Res.* 1999, 253, 733–736.

[29] Kornack, DR; Rakic, P. Cell proliferation without neurogenesis in adult primate neocortex. *Science.* 2001, 294, 2127–2130.

[30] Kriegstein, AR; Götz, M. Radial glia diversity: A matter of cell fate. *Glia.* 2003, 43, 37-43.

[31] Kukekov, VG; Laywell, ED; Suslov, O; Davies, K; Scheffler, B; Thomas, LB; O'Brien, TF; Kusakabe, M; Steindler, DA. Multipotent stem/progenitor cells with similar properties arise from two neurogenic regions of adult human brain. *Exp. Neurol.* 1999, 156(2), 333-344.

[32] Lie, DC; Song, H; Colamarino, SA; Ming, GL; Gage, FH. Neurogenesis in the adult brain: new strategies for central nervous system diseases. *Annu. Rev. Pharmacol. Toxicol.* 2004, 44, 399–421.

[33] Lichtenwalner, RJ; Parent, JM. Adult neurogenesis and the ischemic forebrain. *J. Cereb. Blood Flow Metab.* 2006, 26(1), 1-20.

[34] Lim, DA; Alvarez-Buylla, A. Interaction between astrocytes and adult subventricular zone precursors stimulates neurogenesis. *Proc. Natl. Acad. Sci. U.S.A.* 1999, 96, 7526–7531.

[35] Lim, DA; Tramontin, AD; Trevejo, JM; Herrera, GD; Garcia-Verdugo, JM; Alvarez-Buylla, A. Noggin antagonizes BMP signaling to create a niche for adult neurogenesis. *Neuron.* 2000, 28, 713–726.

[36] Lim, DA; Suárez-Fariñas, M; Naef, F; Hacker, CR; Menn, B; Takebayashi, H; Magnasco, M; Patil, N; Alvarez-Buylla, A. In vivo transcriptional profile analysis reveals RNA splicing and chromatin remodeling as prominent processes for adult neurogenesis. *Mol. Cell Neurosci.* 2006a, 31(1), 131-148.

[37] Lim DA, Alvarez-Buylla A. Neural stem cells in the adult brain. In: Rao MS. *Neural development and stem cells.* New Jersey: Humana Press Inc; 2006b; 29-47.

[38] Lledo, PM; Saghatelyan, A. Integrating new neurons into the adult olfactory bulb: joining the network, life-death decisions, and the effects of sensory experience. *Trends Neurosci.* 2005, 28(5), 248-254.

[39] Lindvall, O; Kokaia, Z; Martinez-Serrano, A. Stem cell therapy for human neurodegenerative disorders-how to make it work. *Nat. Med.* 2004, 10 (Suppl.), S42–S50.

[40] Lois, C; Alvarez-Buylla, A. Proliferating subventricular zone cells in the adult mammalian forebrain can differentiate into neurons and glia. *Proc. Natl. Acad. Sci. U.S.A.* 1993, 90, 2074–2077.

[41] Lois, C; Alvarez-Buylla, A. Long-distance neuronal migration in the adult mammalian brain. *Science.* 1994, 264(5162), 1145-1148.

[42] Lois, C; García-Verdugo, JM; Alvarez-Buylla, A. Chain migration of neuronal precursors. *Science.* 1996, 271(5251), 978-781.

[43] Louissaint, Ajr; Rao, S; Leventhal, C; Goldman, SA. Coordinated interaction of neurogenesis and angiogenesis in the adult songbird brain. *Neuron.* 2002, 34, 945–960.

[44] Luskin, MB. Restricted proliferation and migration of postnatally generated neurons derived from the forebrain subventricular zone. *Neuron.* 1993, 11(1), 173-89.

[45] Ma, DK; Ming, GL; Song, H. Glial influences on neural stem cell development: cellular niches for adult neurogenesis. *Curr. Opin. Neurobiol.* 2005, *15(5), 514-520.*

[46] Marshall, CA; Suzuki, SO; Goldman, JE. Gliogenic and neurogenic progenitors of the subventricular zone: who are they, where did they come from, and where are they going? *Glia.* 2003, 43(1), 52-61.

[47] Mazurová, Y; Valoušková, V; Österreicher, J. The reaction of subependymal layer of the lateral brain ventricles to the striatal ibotenic acid lesion in long-term study. *Acta Histochem.* 2002, 104(4), 375-379.

[48] Mazurová, Y; Látr, I; Österreicher, J; Cerman, J. Proliferation and differentiation of neural stem cells in the subependymal layer of lateral brain ventricles in a reaction to neurodegenerative process in the striatum. *(in Czech) Acta Med. (Suppl),* 2004, 47(2), 63-70.

[49] Mazurová, Y; Rudolf, E; Látr, I; Osterreicher, J. Proliferation and differentiation of adult endogenous neural stem cells in response to neurodegenerative process within the striatum. *Neurodegener. Dis.* 2006a, 3(1-2), 12-18.

[50] Mazurová, Y; Látr, I; Österreicher, J; Gunčová, I. Progressive reparative gliosis in aged hosts and interferences with neural grafts in an animal model of Huntington's disease. *Cell Mol. Neurobiol.* 2006b, 26(7-8), 1423-1441.

[51] Mercier, F; Kitasako, JT; Hatton, GI. Anatomy of the brain neurogenic zones revisited: fractones and the fibroblast/macrophage network. *J. Comp. Neurol.* 2002, 451(2), 170-188.

[52] Mercier, F; Kitasako, JT; Hatton, GI. Fractones and other basal laminae in the hypothalamus. *J. Comp. Neurol.* 2003, 455(3), 324-340.

[53] Morest, DK; Silver, J. Precursors of neurons, neuroglia, and ependymal cells in the CNS: what are they? Where are they from? How do they get where they are going? *Glia.* 2003, 43(1), 6-18.

[54] Morshead, CM; van der Kooy, D. Postmitotic death is the fate of constitutively proliferating cells in the subependymal layer of the adult mouse brain. *J. Neurosci.* 1992, 12(1), 249-256.

[55] Morshead, CM; Reynolds, BA; Craig, CG; McBurney, MW; Staines, WA; Morassutti, D; Weiss, S; van der Kooy, D. Neural stem cells in the adult mammalian forebrain: a relatively quiescent subpopulation of subependymal cells. *Neuron.* 1994, 13(5), 1071-1082.

[56] Morshead, CM; van der Kooy. D. A new 'spin' on neural stem cells? *Curr. Opin. Neurobiol.* 2001, 11(1), 59-65.

[57] Morshead, CM; van der Kooy, D. Disguising adult neural stem cells. *Curr. Opin. Neurobiol.* 2004, 14(1), 125-131.

[58] Nait-Oumesmar, B; Decker, L; Lachapelle, F; Avellana-Adalid, V; Bachelin, C; Van Evercooren, AB. Progenitor cells of the adult mouse subventricular zone proliferate, migrate and differentiate into oligodendrocytes after demyelination. *Eur. J. Neurosci.* 1999, 11(12), 4357-4366.

[59] Nunes, MC; Roy, NS; Keyoung, HM; Goodman, RR; McKhann, G 2nd; Jiang, L; Kang, J; Nedergaard, M; Goldman, SA. Identification and isolation of multipotential neural progenitor cells from the subcortical white matter of the adult human brain. *Nat. Med.* 2003, 9(4), 439-447.

[60] Okano, H; Sakaguchi, M; Ohki, K; Suzuki, N; Sawamoto, K. Regeneration of the central nervous system using endogenous repair mechanisms. *J. Neurochem.* 2007, 102(5), 1459-1465.

[61] Palmer, TD; Willhoite, RA; Gage, FH. Vascular niche for adult hippocampal neurogenesis. *J. Comp. Neurol.* 2000, 425, 479–494.

[62] Pencea, V; Bingaman, KD; Freedman, LJ; Luskin, MB. Neurogenesis in the subventricular zone and rostral migratory stream of the neonatal and adult primate forebrain. *Exp. Neurol.* 2001, 172, 1–16.

[63] Peretto, P; Giachino, C; Aimar, P; Fasolo, A; Bonfanti, L. Chain formation and glial tube assembly in the shift from neonatal to adult subventricular zone of the rodent forebrain. *J. Comp. Neurol.* 2005, 487(4), 407-427.

[64] Rakic, P. Exclusive radial glial cells: historical and evolutionary perspective. *Glia.* 2003, 43, 19-32.

[65] Sanai, N; Tramontin, AD; Quiñones-Hinojosa, A; Barbaro, NM; Gupta, N; Kunwar, S; Lawton, MT; McDermott, MW; Parsa, AT; Manuel-García Verdugo, J; Berger, MS; Alvarez-Buylla, A. Unique astrocyte ribbon in adult human brain contains neural stem cells but lacks chain migration. *Nature.* 2004, 427(6976), 740-744.

[66] Steindler, DA; Leywell, ED. Astrocytes as stem cells: nomenclature, phenotype, and translation. *Glia.* 2003, 43(1), 62-69.

[67] Suzuki, SO; Goldman, JE. Multiple cell populations in the early postnatal subventricular zone take distinct migratory pathways: a dynamic study of glial and neuronal progenitor migration. *J. Neurosci.* 2003, 23(10), 4240-4250.

[68] Tattersfield, AS; Croon, RJ; Liu, YW; Kells, AP; Faull, RLM; Connor, B. Neurogenesis in the striatum of the quinolinic acid lesion model of Huntington's disease. *Neuroscience.* 2004, 127(2), 319-332.

[69] Temple, S; Alvarez-Buylla, A. Stem cells in the adult mammalian central nervous system. *Curr. Opin. Neurobiol.* 1999, 9(1), 135-141.

[70] Temple, S. Defining neural stem cells and their role in normal development of the nervous system. In: Rao MS. *Neural development and stem cells.* New Jersey: Humana Press Inc; 2006; 1-28

[71] Thomas, LB; Gates, MA; Steindler, DA. Young neurons from the adult subependymal zone proliferate and migrate along an astrocyte, extracellular matrix-rich pathway. *Glia.* 1996, 17, 1–14.

[72] Watts, C; McConkey, H; Anderson, L; Caldwell, M. Anatomical perspectives on adult neural stem cells. *J. Anat.* 2005, 207, 197-208.

[73] Weinstein, DE; Burrola, P; Kilpatrick, TJ. Increased proliferation of precursor cells in the adult rat brain after targeted lesioning. *Brain Res.* 1996, 743, 11-16.

[74] Westerlund, U; Moe, MC; Varghese, M; Berg-Johnsen, J; Ohlsson, M; Langmoen, IA; Svensson, M. Stem cells from the adult human brain develop into functional neurons in culture. *Exp. Cell Res.* 2003, 289(2), 378-383.

[75] Young, D; Lawlor, PA; Leone, P; Dragunow, M; During, MJ. Environmental enrichment inhibits spontaneous apoptosis, prevents seizures and is neuroprotective. *Nat. Med.* 1999, 5(4), 448-53

In: Encyclopedia of Stem Cell Research (2 Volume Set)
Editor: Alexander L. Greene

ISBN: 978-1-61761-835-2
© 2012 Nova Science Publishers, Inc.

Chapter XVI

CORNEAL EPITHELIAL STEM CELLS: A BIOLOGICAL AND CLINICAL APPROACH

Maria Notara[*] *and Julie T. Daniels*
Cells for Sight Transplantation and Research Programme;
Ocular Repair and Regeneration Biology Unit,
Institute of Ophthalmology,
London, UK

1. INTRODUCTION

The clinical use of stem cells is a promising alternative treatment of life threatening and dehabilitating conditions such as leukaemia, diabetes, heart disease and spinal cord injury. The ethical and scientific debates regarding the appropriate stem cell source e.g. embryonic versus adult, autologous versus allogeneic etc are ongoing. In this review, we will describe limbal epithelial stem cells (LESC), a population of cells believed to be residing in the vascularised corneoscleral junction (i.e. the limbus) which are responsible for the maintenance and repair of the corneal epithelium. Partial or total depletion of the LESC population can have devastating effects including vision impairment, pain and ultimately blindness. LESCs are already successfully used clinically to treat blinding conditions of the cornea such as chemical burns, Stevens Johnson syndrome or aniridia. The function, properties and cytokine signalling of the LESC-corneal stroma as well as the potentials in exploiting their therapeutic uses will be discussed.

---

[*] Corresponding author: E:mail: m.notara@ucl.ac.uk; Tel: 020 7608 6996; Fax: 020 7608 6887

2. The Cornea

Our window to the world is provided by the cornea on the front surface of the eye. The integrity and functionality of the outer most corneal epithelium is essential for vision. A population of limbal epithelial stem cells (LESC) are responsible for maintaining the epithelium throughout life by providing a constant supply of daughter cells which replenish those constantly lost from the ocular surface during normal wear and tear and following injury. LESC deficiency leads to corneal opacification, inflammation, vascularisation and discomfort [1] [2]. Cultured LESC delivery is one of several examples of successful an adult stem cell therapy used in patients. The clinical precedence for use of stem cell therapy and the accessibility of a transparent stem cell niche make the cornea a unique model for the study of adult stem cells in physiological conditions as well as in disease.

3. The Limbus and the Limbal Epithelial Stem Cells (LESC)

The Limbal Stem Cell Niche Concept

The limbus, or corneoscleral junction, measures 1.5-2 mm in width and is the point at which the cornea becomes continuous with the sclera (figure 1)

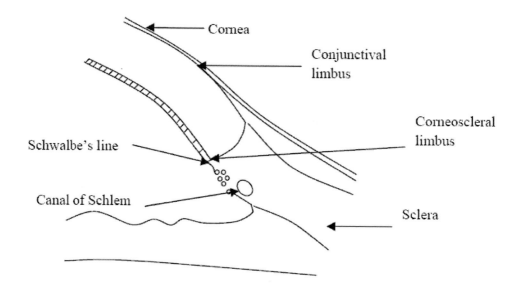

Figure 1. The corneoscleral limbus and associated structures.

LESC are believed to reside in the basal layer of the limbal area, at the vascularised junction between the corneal and conjunctival epithelium.

Davanger and Evensen in 1971 were the first to suggest that the corneal epithelium is maintained and renewed by a cell population residing in the limbus [3]. In the last 35 years, more evidence indicating that the corneal stem cells reside in the limbal region has been presented. For instance, limbal epithelial basal cells can retain tritiated thymidine for prolonged periods thus suggesting that they have long cell cycle [4]. Limbal basal cells have been shown to have higher proliferative potential in vitro than central and paracentral corneal epithelial cells [5]. Finally, wounding or surgical removal of the limbus in a rabbit model, has shown to cause delayed healing and conjunctivalisation of the corneal surface [6, 7].

Limbal Anatomy and Structure

Within the limbus, the LESC are thought to reside in a stem cell niche, which preserves them in their undifferentiated status (figure 2). This stem cell niche has been identified as the palisades of Vogt, which are thrown into folds in the sub-epithelial connective tissue. These structures are believed to provide a protective environment for the LESC. Putative stem cells have been observed at the bottom of the epithelial papillae forming the limbal palisades of Vogt [8]. This irregular intersection between the limbal epithelium and stroma protects the cells from potentially damaging shear stress, while the neighbouring blood vessels supply a source of nutrients for the resident cells [9].

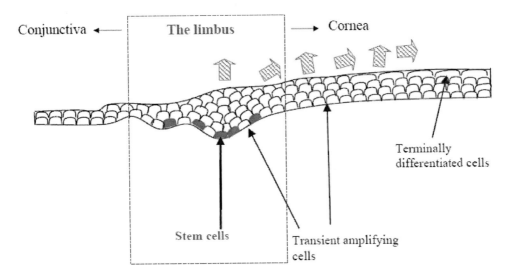

Figure 2. The limbal epithelial stem cells (normally situated in the basal layers of the limbus) give rise to transient amplifying cells which migrate towards the anterior layers of the corneal area eventually forming the terminally differentiated epithelium.

Dua et al. (2005) identified a novel anatomical structure extending from the palisades of Vogt which the authors put forward as a putative LESC stem cell niche, the Limbal Epithelial Crypt (LEC). CK14 staining showed that all the cells in this LEC were epithelial in nature, and the expression of ABCG2, one of proposed putative LESC markers, suggested that the cells within these crypts may be stem cells although no functional evidence was presented [10]. In a recent follow-up study, the same research group further studied the frequency and distribution of LEC, investigated the immunophenotype of the cells within the LEC and studied their ultra structural features with focus to the size, morphology, intercellular connections and basal attachments. Cells within the crypt were shown to express cytokeratins CK32 and CK19 as well as CD 34, vimentin, p63 and connexin 43 whereas they did not express the proliferation marker Ki67, indicating slow cell cycle. Moreover, these cells had a high nuclear to cytoplasmic ratio and were adherent to the underlying basement membrane by multiple cytoplasmic projections. These data suggested that LEC contain a unique sub-population of cells expressing several characteristics that are consistent with it representing a putative LESC niche [11].

Our group has recently identified two distinct candidate LESC niche structures namely limbal crypts and focal stromal projections. These two structures could also be imaged in-vivo in healthy human individuals. Biopsies targeted to limbal regions rich in our proposed LESC niche structures yielded significantly higher numbers of LESCs in culture suggesting that targeted biopsy of adult stem cell niches can improve stem cell yield and may prove to be essential for the successful development of novel adult stem cell therapies [12].

The cornea possesses two unique characteristics that make it ideally suited as a model system for studying adult stem cells and their niche in humans. Firstly, LESCs are found at the corneal limbus (the peripheral extent of the cornea) and are anatomically segregated from their transient amplifying cell progeny which migrate centrally to cover the paracentral and central cornea [13]. Secondly, it is optically transparent tissue and therefore non-invasive imaging of LESCs in humans is possible.

It has been shown in histological tissue sections that LESCs are discretely located in the basal layer of the corneal limbal epithelium, at the junction between the transparent cornea and the opaque sclera [14-16]. However, the total number and distribution of LESCs is unknown. The limbal palisades of Vogt have been proposed as the site of the LESC niche [17]. Photomicrographic, angiographic and histological studies have demonstrated the fibrovascular nature of the palisades and the presence of "ridges of thickened epithelium" in the interpalisade zone [18, 19].

The evidence that LESC reside within the corneal limbus is strong. It is therefore presumed that the corneal limbus constitutes a specialized adult stem cell niche. There is some functional evidence to support this.

4. THE ROLE OF THE LIMBAL STEM CELL NICHE MICROENVIRONMENT IN MAINTAINING LIMBAL EPITHELIAL STEM CELLS

Adult stem cells (SC) have intrinsic characteristics that define their function, phenotype and behaviour, but they also highly depend on specialized environmental locations in the tissue, or niches, to keep them in an undifferentiated state, control their proliferation and guide the commitment of their progeny to defined cell phenotypes. Understanding of the mechanisms that govern these SC-niche interactions is essential to the comprehension of normal SC function and homeostasis. It is also essential to the aim of developing adult SC therapies.

Some characteristics of other adult SC niches such as in the gut, skin and bone marrow have already been investigated [20-22]. Studies on a wide variety of SC niches have identified at least three main mechanisms by which environmental factors regulate SC behaviour.

Secreted factors such as the bone morphogenic protein (bmp) / transforming growth factor β (TGFβ) superfamily and the Wnt families of proteins have been shown to regulate SC proliferation and fate in a variety of species and tissues [20, 22]. For instance haematopoietic stem cell niche can be induced via autocrine secretion of angiopoietin-1 [23].

Moreover, cell-cell interactions mediated by integral membrane proteins such Notch and its ligand Delta, as well as JAK-STAT (Janus Kinase - Signal Transducer and Activator of Transcription) and its ligand Unpaired (Upd) [20, 22] play a significant role in SC maintenance and regulation in both invertebrate and vertebrate organisms.

The third mechanism by which the niche environment may control SC behaviour is through cell-extracellular matrix interactions. Adhesion of cells to the extracellular matrix is mediated by several classes of receptor, the best characterised of which is the integrin family. The role of integrins in regulating SC has been best characterised in the skin where it has been shown that epidermal SC express high levels of β1-integrins [24], that high levels of β1-integrin expression is required for maintenance of epidermal SC [25] and that β1-integrins regulate the differentiation of keratinocytes and other cell types through mitogen-activated protein kinase (MAPK) signalling [25-27]. The ligands for the integrin family of receptors are extracellular matrix molecules (ECM). In the gut ECM composition has been shown to be important in determining the distribution of epithelial SC [28] and ECM/β1-integrin interactions have been shown to play a significant role in neural SC maintenance [29]. Another interesting aspect of integrin mediated regulation of differentiation and proliferation is their functional co-operation with growth factors [30-32].

Extracellular matrix (ECM) composition is thought to be an important component of the LESC niche as it has been shown that the basement membrane composition of the limbus differs significantly from that of the cornea [33-35].

In terms of ECM composition, except from the laminins 1 and 5, the limbal stroma also contains laminin α2β2 chains which are not present in the central cornea area. Also, α1, α2 and α5 type chains of collagen type I are present in the limbal basement membrane whereas α3 and α5 chains are in the corneal part [36, 37].

Espana et al demonstrated by using an ex-vivo rabbit cornea model that the limbal stroma modulates epithelial differentiation, proliferation and apoptosis in the direction favouring stemness, whereas the corneal stroma promotes differentiation [38]. Other than this data, the key structural and functional mechanisms that operate in the limbal niche remain unknown. It is hoped that elucidation of these mechanisms will greatly improve our ability to grow and manipulate LESC for therapeutic purposes.

The use of *ex-vivo* cultured LESCs to treat corneal LSCD in humans was first described by Pellegrini et al in 1997 [39]. Since then, further reports of the use of this technology to treat patients have been published [40-54]. In addition, further studies have reported the transplantation of *ex-vivo* cultured autologous oral mucosal epithelial cells to treat LSCD [44, 55-57]. In all of these studies the ex-vivo expansion of stem cells required the use of a surrogate niche. These were either human amniotic membrane (HAM) [42, 44, 45, 49, 50, 53,

54, 58, 59] or growth arrested 3T3 fibroblast feeder cells [39, 40, 43, 46, 51]. Amniotic membrane has been widely used as a substrate and carrier on which to culture limbal epithelial cells for transplantation. It has been shown that limbal epithelial cells cultured in this way maintain a SC like phenotype [41]. The mechanisms by which this is mediated remain elusive; however, it has been proposed that the basement membrane composition as well as the growth factor content of amniotic membrane have a major function [41, 60]. 3T3 fibroblasts are primitive cells that are isolated from mouse embryos. They have a high proliferative capacity and have been used extensively used in the culture of epithelial stem cells especially in skin and cornea [13, 61, 62]. Induction of 3T3 growth arrest, by irradiation or by treatment with mitomycin C -a DNA cross-linking reagent that halts DNA replication- stimulates the production of the growth factors and matrix constituents that promote epithelial cell duplication and metabolism [61]. Both amniotic membrane and growth arrested 3T3 fibroblasts slow down the differentiation of corneal epithelial cells in vitro, which therefore allows the expansion of the population of LESCs [13, 60].

The clinical outcomes of ex-vivo cultured limbal stem cell therapy suggests that the treatment can successfully restore a functioning corneal epithelium in a previously stem cell deficient cornea. A key question, which remains unanswered, is whether this is due to the survival of transplanted cells or to the recovery of any residual autologous LESC. Whichever is the case, the presence of a functioning niche or the establishment of a new niche is likely to be essential to the long term success of this procedure. This and the other issues discussed above pose interesting questions and are exciting areas for future research.

5. IDENTIFICATION OF LESC: PUTATIVE STEM CELL MARKERS

There is currently no single marker that can be used to definitively identify a LESC. However there are stem cell associated markers that can be used in combination with the absence of differentiation markers to identify putative LESC.

p63

The transcription factor p63 was proposed as a LESC marker by Pellegrini et al. in 2001 [63]. p63 is structurally similar to the tumour suppressor protein p53 [64], and is involved in morphogenesis [65]. p63 knockout mice ($p63^{-/-}$) have major defects in their epithelial development and lack stratified epithelium [66]. This suggests that p63 may be involved in maintaining the stem cell population [66]. Pellegrini et al. (2001) showed that p63 is expressed in the nuclei of human limbal epithelial basal cells but not in TA cells on the surface of the cornea. However, several groups have since found that p63 is also expressed by most of the basal cells in the central human cornea [67, 68]. Therefore although p63 is useful for identifying putative LESC, it is not deemed specific enough to be a definitive marker for these cells.

The alpha isoform of p63 (ΔNp63α) has been shown to be more specific for LESCs than other isoforms of this transcription factor [69]. Holoclones derived from the limbus express high levels of p63α, meroclones express low levels, and paraclones exhibit no expression. Expression of p63α varies depending on the state of the corneal tissue post mortem and this may explain the discrepancy in p63 staining previously found between different research groups. Defects or abrasions on the central cornea, often caused by incomplete closure of the eyelids after death, can result in the cornea becoming 'activated'. In these activated corneas p63α expressing cells from the limbus migrate towards the central cornea and are found in the basal layer. ΔNp beta and gamma isoforms of p63 appear in the suprabasal layers of the cornea and limbus in response to this wounding and therefore indicate more differentiated cells [69].

ABCG2

The ATP binding cassette transporter protein ABCG2 has been proposed as a possible LESC marker [70], and has been proposed as a universal marker for stem cells [71]. Zhou et al. (2001) have found that ABCG2 is expressed in stem cells from bone marrow and skeletal muscle, and also embryonic stem cells. ABCG2 is also known as the breast cancer resistance protein 1 (BCRP1) [71], and mediates drug resistance [72]. ABCG2 expression is responsible for the efflux of many different anticancer drugs from a stem cell, and also its ability to exclude Hoechst 33342 dye [71]. ABCG2 has been found to be expressed in some of the limbal basal cell population but not in corneal epithelial cells thus suggesting that it is a possible marker for LESC [70, 73].

Other Markers

Other putative limbal stem cell associated markers include vimentin, integrin α9 [8] and cytokeratin 19 [74, 75]. Differentiation markers which can be used to identify which cells are not limbal stem cells include involucrin, connexin 43, and the cytokeratins K3 and K12 [8, 73].

In Vitro Limbal Epithelial Stem Cell Characterisation Using Putative Stem Cell Markers

Given the clinical application of limbal epithelial stem cell transplantation after in vitro expansion, it has become imperative to characterise LESC in terms of differentiation in *in vitro* conditions. The putative LESC markers discussed above have only recently started been used *in vitro*.

In a recent detailed investigation, Vascotto and Griffith have examined a broad selection of growth factor receptors and markers correlating their expression in vivo (basal or superficial limbal/conjunctival epithelium and scattered cells within the substantia propria of the bulbar conjunctiva) and in culture. The study demonstrated the direct relation of the in vivo with the in vitro phenotype, covering all the important growth factors and markers of interest in the cornea area such as EGF, ABCG2 and ΔNP63α [76]

ABCG2 has recently started being used as a putative stem cell marker of cultured limbal epithelial cells. De Paiva et al, first mentioned that in primary cultured human limbal epithelial cells, the ABCG2 antibody mainly stained the membranes of clusters of small cells, and minimal or no staining was observed in the large cells. ABCG2− cells accounted for 10.62 ± 4.04% [77]. The same group, in a recent publication, correlated the size of limbal epithelial cells with expression levels of ABCG2 and P63a quantified by real-time PCR. The expression of stem cell–associated markers, ABCG2 and ΔNp63α mRNA, were highest in the population that contained the smallest sized cells with decreasing levels in populations with higher cell size. The lowest mRNA levels were found in the cell population that contained the largest sized cells. On the other hand, mRNA for the differentiation markers involucrin, K12, and K3 were detected at the lowest levels in the population with the smallest cells with increasing expression in the intermediate-sized population and at the highest levels in the population with the biggest cells [78].

6. METHODS FOR THE PURIFICATION OF LIMBAL EPITHELIAL STEM CELL POPULATION IN VITRO

Side Population (SP) Cells

The cells which have the ability to efflux Hoechst 33342 dye are known as the 'side population' (SP) and represent a population enriched for stem cells. SP cells have been found in human limbal epithelium but not in the peripheral and central corneal epithelium, thus indicating that Hoechst dye can be used to partially distinguish and purify LESC [70, 79]. SP cells make up 0.3-0.4% of the limbal epithelial cell population and have been found to have stem cell-like properties such as quiescent state, positive expression of putative stem cell markers e.g. ABCG2, and negative expression of markers for differentiated corneal epithelial cells [70, 79].

Rapid Adhesion to Collagen IV

Collagen IV can be used to partially purify limbal epithelial cells with stem cell like properties [80]. This selectivity is based on the interaction of type β_1 integrins expressed on the surface of putative LESC with collagen IV. β_1 integrin intensity of expression has therefore been proposed as a marker for putative stem cells [80, 81]. Li et al. (2005) demonstrated that cells from the limbal region which adhere to collagen IV within 20 minutes have greater stem cell properties than cells that adhere to collagen IV more slowly. Cells that do not adhere to collagen IV within 2 hours were termed "non-adherent", and those that adhered between 20 minutes and 2 hours were classed as slowly adherent cells (Figure 3).

Rapidly adherent cells were found to have higher proliferative capacity, greater colony forming efficiency, expressed higher levels of integrin β_1, p63 and ABCG2 putative stem cell markers, and retained 5-fold the level of BrdU label retained by non-adherent cells. This population of rapidly adherent cells also did not express the differentiation markers involucrin and cytokeratin 12. It was calculated that 10% of the cells isolated from the limbal region rapidly adhered to collagen IV. This method of enrichment by attachment to collagen IV was based on a method developed by Jones and Watt (1993) for putative epidermal keratinocyte stem cells selection [82].

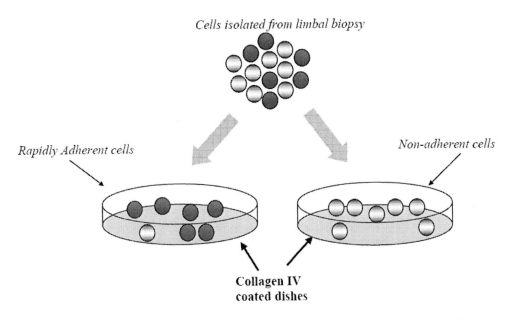

Figure 3. Use of collagen IV to partially purify LESC. Cells which adhere to collagen IV within 20 minutes exhibit stem cell-like phenotype to a greater extent than cells that adhere more slowly.

7. CLINICAL PRACTICE

Limbal Epithelial Stem Cell Failure

LESC deficiency can result from primary aetiologies such as the heritable genetic disorder, aniridia [83] [84]. More commonly LESC deficiency occurs as a result of acquired factors including thermal or chemical injury, Stevens Johnson Syndrome, contact lens wear and multiple surgeries [85] [86] [87] [88] [89]. The outcome is persistent epithelial breakdown, superficial corneal vascularization, chronic discomfort and impaired vision caused by the migration of neighbouring conjunctival epithelial cells and blood vessels onto the corneal surface [90] [91]. LESC deficiency may be partial or total [92]. Partial LESC deficiency can occur in a specific region of limbus leaving an intact population of LESCs in other areas. This results in sectoral ingrowth of conjunctival epithelium in areas of LESC deficiency [87]. In total LESC deficiency there is dysfunction or destruction of the entire LESC population resulting in conjunctivalization of the entire cornea [87].

Limbal Epithelial Stem Cell Therapy Techniques for Graft Preparation

Principally, two different culture types namely the explant system and the single cell suspension system, have been used to produce epithelial sheets containing LESC for delivery to the eye. During explant culture human amniotic membrane is often used as both a substrate and carrier for cultured LESCs. Limbal biopsy tissue is allowed to adhere to the amnion prior to being submerged in culture medium which stimulates the limbal epithelial cells to migrate out of the biopsy and proliferate on the amnion [93] [94] [95] [96] [97] [98] [99]. Once a confluent epithelial sheet has been formed, air lifting is often introduced to promote stratification of multi-layered epithelium. The method of amniotic membrane preparation may have an effect on the phenotype of the cultured limbal epithelial cells (LECs). Grueterich *et al* showed that culturing LECs on amnion with an intact amniotic epithelium may result in a more stem cell like phenotype than de-epithelialised (denuded) amnion [100]. In the authors experience, the use of amniotic membrane does present some disadvantages including unpredictable biological variability between donor tissues, often restricted tissue availability and the inherent semi-opaque nature if the membrane obstructs post-operative visual clarity until the tissue is remodeled (a process that depending on the patient can occur over a period of few days to several months).

The single cell suspension culture system requires first separating the epithelial cells from the stroma using dispase and then dissociating the epithelial cells from one another using trypsin prior to seeding [101] [102] [103] [104] either straight onto amniotic membrane or onto a plastic tissue culture dish containing a feeder layer of growth arrested 3T3 fibroblasts if more extensive *in vitro* cell expansion is desired. The cultures can be incubated for up to three weeks. When a confluent epithelial sheet is formed, it can be transferred to the ocular surface using either a contact lens [101] [102], collagen shield, [102] or fibrin gel [105]. Usually, the suspensions of single limbal epithelial cells seeded onto amniotic membrane are co-cultured with a layer of growth arrested 3T3 fibroblasts in the bottom of the dish.

CONCLUSION

Future Prospects

Although cultured LESC have already been used to repair damaged corneas in patients, the mechanisms by which this occurs are yet to be defined. At the moment it is not clear whether the cultured LESC integrate into the host limbus thus replacing the stem cells that have been previously lost or damaged, or if application of the graft triggers existing previously damaged or non-competent stem cells to resume wound healing.

The definition of a specific marker for LESC would assist to a great extent the isolation and identification of these cells. Also the study and understanding of the LESC niche and how it controls stem cell maintenance and differentiation could facilitate LESC to be preserved for longer in *in vitro* culture systems.

In conclusion, the properties of the corneal tissue provide a unique opportunity to study in detail an adult stem cell population in its natural microenvironment. Recent advances in imaging methods are already providing further information about the structure and functionality of the LESC niche. In combination with the future development of safe and enduring labels for use in animal and human subjects, corneal models can make possible non-invasive experimentation and long-term observation of resident and transplanted stem cells. This can help address important questions concerning physiological LESC functionality and also make therapeutic methods more efficient.

REFERENCES

[1] Daniels JT; Dart JKG; Tuft S and Khaw PT. Corneal stem cells in review. *Wound Rep. Regener.* 2001 9(6), 483-494

[2] Daniels JT; Harris A and Mason C. Corneal epithelial stem cells in health and disease. *Stem Cell Rev.* 2007 *In press*

[3] Davanger M, and Evensen, A. Role of the Pericorneal Papillary Structure in Renewal of Corneal Epithelium. *Nature.* 1971 229 560-561

[4] Cotsarelis G; Cheng, S.Z.; Dong, G.; Sun, T.T. and Lavker, R.M. Existence of slow-cycling limbal epithelial basal cells that can be preferentially stimulated to prliferate: implications on epithelial stem cells. *Cell.* 1989 57 201-209

[5] Pellegrini G, Golisano, O., Paterna, P., Lambiase, A., Bonini, S., Rama, P. and De Luca, M. Location and clonal analysis of stem cells and their differentiated progeny in the human ocular surface. *J. Cell Biol.* 1999 145(4), 769-82

[6] Chen JJ and Tseng SC. Abnormal corneal epithelial wound healing in partial-thickness removal of limbal epithelium. *Invest. Ophthalmol. Vis. Sci.* 1991 32(8), 2219-2233

[7] Huang AJ and Tseng SC. Corneal epithelial wound healing in the absence of limbal epithelium. *Invest. Ophthalmol. Vis. Sci.* 1991 32(1), 96-105

[8] Schlotzer-Schrehardt U and Kruse FE. Identification and characterization of limbal stem cells. *Exp. Eye Res.* 2005 81 247-264

[9] Boulton M and Albon J. Stem cells in the eye. *Int. J. Biochem. Cell Biol.* 2004 36(4), 643-657

[10] Dua HS, Shanmuganathan, V.A., Powell-Richards, A.O., Tighe, P.J and Joseph, A. Limbal epithelial crypts: a novel anatomical structure and a putative limbal stem cell niche. *Br. J. Ophthalmol.* 2005 89(5), 529-32

[11] Shanmuganathan VA; Foster T; Kulkarni BB *et al.* Morphological characteristics of the limbal epithelial crypt. *British Journal of Ophthalmology.* 2007 91(4), 514-519

[12] Shortt AJ; Secker GA; Munro PM*et al.* Characterization of the limbal epithelial stem cell niche: Novel imaging techniques permit in-vivo observation and targeted biopsy of limbal epithelial stem cells. *Stem Cells %R 10.1634/stemcells.2006-0580.* 2007 2006-0580

[13] Pellegrini G; Golisano O; Paterna P*et al.* Location and clonal analysis of stem cells and their differentiated progeny in the human ocular surface. *J.Cell Biol.* 1999 145(4), 769-782

[14] Chen Z; de Paiva CS; Luo L*et al.* Characterization of putative stem cell phenotype in human limbal epithelia. *Stem Cells.* 2004 22(3), 355-366

[15] Cotsarelis G; Cheng SZ; Dong G; Sun TT and Lavker RM. Existence of slow-cycling limbal epithelial basal cells that can be preferentially stimulated to proliferate: implications on epithelial stem cells. *Cell.* 1989 57(2), 201-209

[16] Schermer A; Galvin S and Sun TT. Differentiation-related expression of a major 64K corneal keratin in vivo and in culture suggests limbal location of corneal epithelial stem cells. *J.Cell Biol.* 1986 103(1), 49-62

[17] Davanger M and Evensen A. Role of the pericorneal papillary structure in renewal of corneal epithelium. *Nature.* 1971 229(5286), 560-561

[18] Goldberg MF and Bron AJ. Limbal palisades of Vogt. *Trans.Am.Ophthalmol.Soc.* 1982 80 155-171

[19] Townsend WM. The limbal palisades of Vogt. *Trans.Am.Ophthalmol.Soc.* 1991 89 721-756

[20] Fuchs E; Tumbar T and Guasch G. Socializing with the neighbors: stem cells and their niche. *Cell.* 2004 116(6), 769-778

[21] Spradling A; Drummond-Barbosa D and Kai T. Stem cells find their niche. *Nature.* 2001 414(6859), 98-104

[22] Watt FM and Hogan BL. Out of Eden: stem cells and their niches. *Science.* 2000 287(5457), 1427-1430

[23] Takakura N; Huang XL; Naruse T *et al.* Critical role of the TIE2 endothelial cell receptor in the development of definitive hematopoiesis. *Immunity.* 1998 9(5), 677-686

[24] Jensen UB; Lowell S and Watt FM. The spatial relationship between stem cells and their progeny in the basal layer of human epidermis: a new view based on whole-mount labelling and lineage analysis. *Development.* 1999 126(11), 2409-2418

[25] Zhu AJ; Haase I and Watt FM. Signaling via beta1 integrins and mitogen-activated protein kinase determines human epidermal stem cell fate in vitro. *Proc.Natl.Acad.Sci.U.S.A.* 1999 96(12), 6728-6733

[26] Jones PH; Harper S and Watt FM. Stem cell patterning and fate in human epidermis. *Cell.* 1995 80(1), 83-93

[27] Jones PH and Watt FM. Separation of human epidermal stem cells from transit amplifying cells on the basis of differences in integrin function and expression. *Cell.* 1993 73(4), 713-724

[28] Kedinger M; Lefebvre O; Duluc I; Freund JN and Simon-Assmann P. Cellular and molecular partners involved in gut morphogenesis and differentiation. *Philos.Trans.R.Soc.Lond B Biol.Sci.* 1998 353(1370), 847-856

[29] Campos LS; Leone DP; Relvas JB *et al.* Beta1 integrins activate a MAPK signalling pathway in neural stem cells that contributes to their maintenance. *Development.* 2004 131(14), 3433-3444

[30] Giancotti FG and Ruoslahti E. Integrin signaling. *Science.* 1999 285(5430), 1028-1032

[31] Miyamoto S; Teramoto H; Gutkind JS and Yamada KM. Integrins can collaborate with growth factors for phosphorylation of receptor tyrosine kinases and MAP kinase activation: roles of integrin aggregation and occupancy of receptors. *J.Cell Biol.* 1996 135(6 Pt 1), 1633-1642

[32] Wang F; Weaver VM; Petersen OW *et al.* Reciprocal interactions between beta1-integrin and epidermal growth factor receptor in three-dimensional basement membrane breast cultures: a different perspective in epithelial biology. *Proc.Natl.Acad.Sci.U.S.A.* 1998 95(25), 14821-14826

[33] Fukuda K; Chikama T; Nakamura M and Nishida T. Differential distribution of subchains of the basement membrane components type IV collagen and laminin among the amniotic membrane, cornea, and conjunctiva. *Cornea.* 1999 18(1), 73-79

[34] Kolega J; Manabe M and Sun TT. Basement membrane heterogeneity and variation in corneal epithelial differentiation. *Differentiation.* 1989 42(1), 54-63

[35] Ljubimov AV; Burgeson RE; Butkowski RJ *et al.* Human corneal basement membrane heterogeneity: topographical differences in the expression of type IV collagen and laminin isoforms. *Lab Invest.* 1995 72(4), 461-473
[36] Tuori A; Uusitalo H; Burgeson RE; Terttunen J and Virtanen I. The immunohistochemical composition of the human corneal basement membrane. *Cornea.* 1996 15(3), 286-294
[37] Ljubimov AV; Burgeson RE; Butkowski RJ *et al.* Human Corneal Basement-Membrane Heterogeneity - Topographical Differences in the Expression of Type-Iv Collagen and Laminin Isoforms. *Laboratory Investigation.* 1995 72(4), 461-473
[38] Espana EM; Kawakita T; Romano A *et al.* Stromal niche controls the plasticity of limbal and corneal epithelial differentiation in a rabbit model of recombined tissue. *Invest Ophthalmol.Vis.Sci.* 2003 44(12), 5130-5135
[39] Pellegrini G; Traverso CE; Franzi AT *et al.* Long-term restoration of damaged corneal surfaces with autologous cultivated corneal epithelium. *Lancet.* 1997 349(9057), 990-993
[40] Daya SM; Watson A; Sharpe JR *et al.* Outcomes and DNA analysis of ex vivo expanded stem cell allograft for ocular surface reconstruction. *Ophthalmology.* 2005 112(3), 470-477
[41] Grueterich M; Espana E and Tseng SC. Connexin 43 expression and proliferation of human limbal epithelium on intact and denuded amniotic membrane. *Invest. Ophthalmol. Vis. Sci.* 2002 43(1), 63-71
[42] Koizumi N; Inatomi T; Suzuki T; Sotozono C and Kinoshita S. Cultivated corneal epithelial transplantation for ocular surface reconstruction in acute phase of Stevens-Johnson syndrome. *Arch.Ophthalmol.* 2001 119(2), 298-300
[43] Nakamura T; Inatomi T; Sotozono C *et al.* Transplantation of autologous serum-derived cultivated corneal epithelial equivalents for the treatment of severe ocular surface disease. *Ophthalmology.* 2006 113(10), 1765-1772
[44] Nakamura T; Inatomi T; Sotozono C; Koizumi N and Kinoshita S. Successful primary culture and autologous transplantation of corneal limbal epithelial cells from minimal biopsy for unilateral severe ocular surface disease. *Acta Ophthalmol.Scand.* 2004 82(4), 468-471
[45] Nakamura T; Koizumi N; Tsuzuki M *et al.* Successful regrafting of cultivated corneal epithelium using amniotic membrane as a carrier in severe ocular surface disease. *Cornea.* 2003 22(1), 70-71
[46] Rama P; Bonini S; Lambiase A *et al.* Autologous fibrin-cultured limbal stem cells permanently restore the corneal surface of patients with total limbal stem cell deficiency. *Transplantation.* 2001 72(9), 1478-1485
[47] Sangwan VS; Matalia HP; Vemuganti GK *et al.* Clinical outcome of autologous cultivated limbal epithelium transplantation. *Indian J.Ophthalmol.* 2006 54(1), 29-34
[48] Sangwan VS; Murthy SI; Vemuganti GK *et al.* Cultivated corneal epithelial transplantation for severe ocular surface disease in vernal keratoconjunctivitis. *Cornea.* 2005 24(4), 426-430
[49] Sangwan VS; Vemuganti GK; Iftekhar G; Bansal AK and Rao GN. Use of autologous cultured limbal and conjunctival epithelium in a patient with severe bilateral ocular surface disease induced by acid injury: a case report of unique application. *Cornea.* 2003 22(5), 478-481

[50] Sangwan VS; Vemuganti GK; Singh S and Balasubramanian D. Successful reconstruction of damaged ocular outer surface in humans using limbal and conjuctival stem cell culture methods. *Biosci.Rep.* 2003 23(4), 169-174

[51] Schwab IR. Cultured corneal epithelia for ocular surface disease. *Trans.Am.Ophthalmol.Soc.* 1999 97 891-986

[52] Schwab IR; Reyes M and Isseroff RR. Successful transplantation of bioengineered tissue replacements in patients with ocular surface disease. *Cornea.* 2000 19(4), 421-426

[53] Shimazaki J; Aiba M; Goto E*et al.* Transplantation of human limbal epithelium cultivated on amniotic membrane for the treatment of severe ocular surface disorders. *Ophthalmology.* 2002 109(7), 1285-1290

[54] Tsai RJ; Li LM and Chen JK. Reconstruction of damaged corneas by transplantation of autologous limbal epithelial cells. *N.Engl.J.Med.* 2000 343(2), 86-93

[55] Inatomi T; Nakamura T; Koizumi N*et al.* Midterm results on ocular surface reconstruction using cultivated autologous oral mucosal epithelial transplantation. *Am.J.Ophthalmol.* 2006 141(2), 267-275

[56] Inatomi T; Nakamura T; Kojyo M*et al.* Ocular Surface Reconstruction With Combination of Cultivated Autologous Oral Mucosal Epithelial Transplantation and Penetrating Keratoplasty. *Am.J.Ophthalmol.* 2006 Paper in Press

[57] Nishida K; Yamato M; Hayashida Y*et al.* Corneal reconstruction with tissue-engineered cell sheets composed of autologous oral mucosal epithelium. *N.Engl.J.Med.* 2004 351(12), 1187-1196

[58] Grueterich M; Espana EM; Touhami A; Ti SE and Tseng SC. Phenotypic study of a case with successful transplantation of ex vivo expanded human limbal epithelium for unilateral total limbal stem cell deficiency. *Ophthalmology.* 2002 109(8), 1547-1552

[59] Koizumi N; Inatomi T; Suzuki T; Sotozono C and Kinoshita S. Cultivated corneal epithelial stem cell transplantation in ocular surface disorders. *Ophthalmology.* 2001 108(9), 1569-1574

[60] Grueterich M; Espana EM and Tseng SC. Ex vivo expansion of limbal epithelial stem cells: amniotic membrane serving as a stem cell niche. *Surv.Ophthalmol.* 2003 48(6), 631-646

[61] Freshney RI; *Culture of animal cells: a manual of basic techniques.* 2000, New York: John Wiley and Sons Inc.

[62] Rheinwald JG and Green H. Serial cultivation of strains of human epidermal keratinocytes: the formation of keratinizing colonies from single cells. *Cell.* 1975 6(3), 331-343

[63] Pellegrini G, Dellambra, E., Golisano, O., Martinelli, E., Fantozzi, I., Bondanza, S., Ponzin, D., McKeon, F. and De Luca, M. p63 identifies keratinocyte stem cells. *Proc. Natl. Acad. Sci. USA.* 2001 98(6), 3156-3161

[64] Lohrum MAE, and Vousden, K.H. Regulation and function of the p53-related proteins: same family, different rules. *Trends Cell Biol.* 2000 10(5), 197-202

[65] Mills AA, Zheng, B., Wang, X.J., Vogel, H., Roop, D.R., and Bradley, A. p63 is a p53 homologue required for limb and epidermal morphogenesis. *Nature.* 1999 398(6729), 708-713

[66] Yang A; Schweitzer R; Sun D*et al.* p63 is essential for regenerative proliferation in limb, craniofacial and epithelial development. *Nature.* 1999 398(6729), 714-718

[67] Dua HS, Joseph, A., Shanmuganathan, V.A. and Jones, R.E. Stem cell differentiation and the effects of deficiency. *Eye.* 2003 17(8), 877-885

[68] Chee KYH, Kicic, A. and Wiffen, S.J. Limbal stem cells: the search for a marker. *Clin. Experiment. Ophthalmol.* 2006 34(1), 64-73
[69] Di Iorio E; Barbaro V; Ruzza A*et al.* Isoforms of {Delta}Np63 and the migration of ocular limbal cells in human corneal regeneration. *Proceedings of the National Academy of Sciences of the United States of America.* 2005 102(27), 9523-9528
[70] Watanabe K, Nishida, K., Yamato, M., Umemoto, T., Sumide, T., Yamamoto, K., Maeda, N., Watanabe, H., Okano, T. and Tano, Y. Human limbal epithelium contains side population cells expressing the ATP-binding cassette transporter ABCG2. *FEBS Lett.* 2004 565 6-20
[71] Zhou S, Schuetz, J.D., Bunting, K.D., Colapietro, A.M., Sampath, J., Morris, J.J., Lagutina, I., Grosveld, G.C., Osawa, M., Nakauchi, H. and Sorrentino B.P. The ABC transporter Bcrp1/ABCG2 is expressed in a wide variety of stem cells and is a molecular determinant of the side-population phenotype. *Nat. Med.* 2001 7(9), 1028-34
[72] Doyle LA, and Ross, D.D. Multidrug resistance mediated by the breast cancer resistance protein BCRP (ABCG2). *Oncogene.* 2003 22(47), 7340-7358
[73] Chen Z, De Paiva, C.S., Luo, L., Kretzer, F.L., Pflugfelder, S.C. and Li, D.Q. Characterization of Putative Stem Cell Phenotype in Human Limbal Epithelial Stem Cells. *Stem Cells.* 2004 22 355-366
[74] Kasper M. Patterns of Cytokeratins and Vimentin in Guinea-Pig and Mouse Eye Tissue - Evidence for Regional Variations in Intermediate Filament Expression in Limbal Epithelium. *Acta Histochemica.* 1992 93(1), 319-332
[75] Harkin DG; Barnard Z; Gillies P; Ainscough SL and Apel AJG. Analysis of p63 and cytokeratin expression in a cultivated limbal autograft used in the treatment of limbal stem cell deficiency. *British Journal of Ophthalmology.* 2004 88(9), 1154-1158
[76] Vascotto SG and Griffith M. Localization of candidate stem and progenitor cell markers within the human cornea, limbus, and bulbar conjunctiva in vivo and in cell culture. *Anatomical Record Part a-Discoveries in Molecular Cellular and Evolutionary Biology.* 2006 288A(8), 921-931
[77] De Paiva CS; Chen Z; Corrales RM; Pflugfelder SC and Li DQ. ABCG2 transporter identifies a population of clonogenic human limbal epithelial cells. *Stem Cells.* 2005 23(1), 63-73
[78] De Paiva CS; Pflugfelder SC and Li DQ. Cell size correlates with phenotype and proliferative capacity in human corneal epithelial cells. *Stem Cells.* 2006 24(2), 368-375
[79] Umemoto T, Yamato, M., Nishida, K., Yang, J., Tano, Y. and Okano, T. Limbal epithelial side-population cells have stem cell-like properties, including quiescent state. *Stem Cells.* 2006 24(1), 86-94
[80] Li DQ, Chen, Z., Song, X.J., de Paiva, C.S., Kim, H.S. and Pflugfelder, S.C. Partial enrichment of a population of human limbal epithelial cells with putative stem cell properties based on collagen type IV adhesiveness. *Exp. Eye Res.* 2005 80(4), 581-590
[81] van Rossum MM, Schalkwijk, J., van de Kerkhof, P.C. and van Erp, P.E. Immunofluorescent surface labelling, flow sorting and culturing of putative epidermal stem cells derived from small skin punch biopsies. *J. Immunol. Methods.* 2002 267(2), 109-17
[82] Jones P and Watt F. Separation of human epidermal stem cells from transit amplifying cells on the basis of differences in integrin function and expression. *Cell.* 1993 73(4), 713-724

[83] Holland EJ; Djalilian AR and Schwartz GS. Management of aniridic keratopathy with keratolimbal allograft: a limbal stem cell transplantation technique. *Ophthalmology.* 2003 110(1), 125-130

[84] Nishida K; Kinoshita S; Ohashi Y; Kuwayama Y and Yamamoto S. Ocular surface abnormalities in aniridia. *Am. J. Ophthalmol.* 1995 120(3), 368-375

[85] Clinch TE; Goins KM and Cobo LM. Treatment of contact lens-related ocular surface disorders with autologous conjunctival transplantation. *Ophthalmology.* 1992 99 634-638

[86] Holland EJ. Epithelial transplantation for severe ocular surface disease. *Trans. Am. Ophthalmol. Soc.* 1996 94 677-743

[87] Holland EJ and Schwartz GS. The evolution of epithelial transplantation for severe ocular surface disease and a proposed classification system. *Cornea.* 1996 15 549-556

[88] Dua HS; Saini JS; Azuara-Blanco A and Gupta P. Limbal stem cell deficiency: concept, aetiology, clinical presentation, diagnosis and management. *Indian J. Ophthalmol.* 2000 48(83-92),

[89] Gomes JA; Santos MS; Ventura AS*et al.* Amniotic membrane with living related corneal limbal/conjunctival allograft for ocular surface reconstruction in Stevens-Johnson syndrome. *Arch. Ophthalmol.* 2003 121 1369-1374

[90] Huang AJ and Tseng SC. Corneal epithelial wound healing in the absence of limbal epithelium. *Invest. Ophthalmol. Vis. Sci.* 1991 32 96-105

[91] Puangsricharern V and Tseng SC. Cytologic evidence of corneal diseases with limbal stem cell deficiency. *Ophthalmology.* 1995 102(10), 1476-1485

[92] Dua HS and Azuara-Blanco A. Limbal stem cells of the corneal epithelium. *Surv. Ophthalmol.* 2000 44(5), 415-425

[93] Tsai RJ-F; Li L-M and Chen J-K. Reconstruction of damaged corneas by transplantation of autologous limbal epithelial cells. *New Engl. J. Med.* 2000 343 86-93

[94] Koizumi N; Inatomi T; Suzuki K; Sotozono C and Kinoshita S. Cultivated corneal epithelial stem cell transplantation in ocular surface disorders. *Ophthalmology.* 2001 108 1569-1574

[95] Koizumi N; Inatomi T; Suzuki T; Sotozono C and Kinoshita S. Cultivated corneal epithelial transplantation for ocular surface reconstruction in acute phase of Stevens-Johnson syndrome. *Arch. Ophthalmol.* 2001 119 298-300

[96] Grueterich M; Espana EM; Touhami A; Ti SE and Tseng SC. Phenotypic study of a case with successful transplantation of ex vivo expanded human limbal epithelium for unilateral total limbal stem cell deficiency. *Ophthalmology.* 2002 109(8), 1547-1552

[97] Shimazaki J; Aiba M; Goto E*et al.* Transplantation of human limbal epithelium cultivated on amniotic membrane for the treatment of severe ocular surface disorders. *Ophthalmology.* 2002 109 1285-1290

[98] Nakamura M; Inatomi T; Sotozono C; Koizumi N and Kinoshita S. Successful primary culture and autologous transplantation of corneal limbal epithelial cells from minimal biopsy for unilateral severe ocular surface disorder. *Acta Opthalmol Scand.* 2004 82 468-471

[99] Sangwan VS; Matalia HP; Vemuganti GK*et al.* Clinical outcome of autologous cultivated limbal epithelium transplantation. *Indian J. Ophthalmol.* 2006 54 29-34

[100] Grueterich M; Espana EM and Tseng SC. Connexin 43 expression and proliferation of human limbal epithelium on intact and denuded amniotic membrane. *Invest. Ophthalmol. Vis. Sci.* 2002 43 63-71

[101] Pellegrini G; Traverso CE; Franzi AT*et al*. Long-term restoration of damaged corneal surfaces with autologous cultivated human epithelium. *The Lancet*. 1997 349 990-993
[102] Schwab IR. Cultured corneal epithelia for ocular surface disease. *Trans. Am. Ophthalmol. Soc.* 1999 97 891-986
[103] Daya SM; Watson A; Sharoe JR*et al*. Outcomes and DNA analysis of ex vivo expanded stem cell allograft for ocular surface reconstruction. *Ophthalmology*. 2005 112(3), 470-477
[104] Nakamura M; Inatomi T; Sotozono C *et al*. Transplantation of autologous serum-derived cultivated corneal epithelial equivalents for the treatment of severe ocular surface disease. *Ophthalmology*. 2006 113 1756-1772
[105] Rama P; Bonini S; Lambiase A*et al*. Autologous fibrin-cultured limbal stem cells permanently restore the corneal surface of patients with total limbal stem cell deficiency. *Transplantation*. 2001 72(9), 1478-1485

In: Encyclopedia of Stem Cell Research (2 Volume Set) ISBN: 978-1-61761-835-2
Editor: Alexander L. Greene © 2012 Nova Science Publishers, Inc.

Chapter XVII

IMMUNOLOGICAL RESPONSES OF CD34$^+$ STEM CELLS TO BACTERIAL PRODUCTS

Jung Mogg Kim[*]

Department of Microbiology, Hanyang University College of Medicine,
Seoul, South Korea

ABSTRACT

Since umbilical cord blood contains a significantly higher number of CD34$^+$ stem cells than adult peripheral blood, umbilical cord blood is proposed as an ideal alternative to bone marrow and peripheral blood for the hematopoietic stem cell transplantation. However, the sepsis induced by bacterial infection has known to be one of the complications after cord blood transplantation. Therefore, it is important to evaluate immunological responses of CD34$^+$ stem cells to bacterial infection. We found that CD34$^+$ cells and their cultured cells infected with *Escherichia coli* induced expression of proinflammatory cytokines, such as IL-1α, IL-6, IL-8, and TNF-α, via NF-κB pathway. Expression of the proinflammatory cytokines was mainly generated from granulocytes-macrophage lineages. CD34$^+$ cells may recognize the molecular patterns associated with pathogens and subsequently initiate the transcription of inflammatory genes. These molecular patterns may be specifically conserved components of microbes such as CpG DNA. Exposure of the cells to synthetic oligodeoxynucleotides containing unmethylated CpG motifs (CpG ODN) resulted in a time- and dose-dependent increase of IL-8 expression and activation of phosphorylated mitogen-activated protein kinase (MAPK) such as ERK1/2 and p38. In addition, CpG ODN stimulated AP-1, but not NF-κB signals. Moreover, inhibition of MAPK reduced the IL-8 production, while inhibition of NF-κB did not affect the IL-8 expression increased by CpG ODN. Blocking Toll-like receptor 9 (TLR9) in CD34$^+$ cells decreased CpG ODN-induced up-regulation of IL-8, indicating that CpG DNA, acting on TLR9, activates CD34$^+$ cells to express IL-8 through MAPK-

---

[*] Corresponding author: Jung Mogg Kim, M.D.; Department of Microbiology, Hanyang University College of Medicine; 17 Haengdang-dong, Sungdong-gu, Seoul 133-791, South Korea; Tel: +82-2-2220-0645; Fax: +82-2-2282-0645; E-mail: jungmogg@hanyang.ac.kr

dependent and NF-κB-independent pathways, although whole Gram-negative *E. coli* can activate NF-κB and up-regulate IL-8 in CD34+ cells. Moreover, co-stimulation with lipopolysaccharide and CpG synergistically up-regulates IL-8 in $CD34^+$ cells. Results obtained from our studies may have important implications in host defense and gene therapy strategies. In particular, a new role of CpG DNA and $CD34^+$ cells in systemic bacterial infection is possible. Furthermore, attention should be paid to distinguish the therapeutic gene-mediated biological effect from the CpG-mediated nonspecific effect.

INTRODUCTION

Primitive hematopoietic stem cells (HSCs) are pluripotent cells with the capacity to give rise to all lineages of blood cells. During commitment, progenitor cells are composed mainly of cells with the potential for differentiation into 1 or 2 lineages. The HSCs express CD34 molecules in their surfaces and are pluripotent with the capacity to differentiate into erythrocytes, granulocytes, monocytes, megakaryocytes, and lymphocytes [1]. The numbers of $CD34^+$ stem cells are significantly higher in umbilical cord blood than in adult peripheral blood [2]. Especially, the numbers of colony forming unit-granulocyte-macrophages are much higher in umbilical cord blood than in peripheral blood [3]. Therefore, umbilical cord blood has been proposed as an ideal alternative to bone marrow and peripheral blood for hematopoietic stem cell transplantation. However, the sepsis induced by bacterial infection has known to be one of the complications after cord blood transplantation. For example, early transplant-related mortality after cord blood transplantation is close to 50%, mainly due to infectious complications such as bacteremia [4]. Human HSCs are relatively resistant to infection by bacteria, compared with viral infection [5,6]. However, a report demonstrated that the sepsis induced by *Escherichia coli* infection has been considered as the one of the complications upon transplantation treatment [7].

Proinflammatory cytokines, including tumor necrosis factor (TNF)-α, interleukin (IL)-1, IL-6 and IL-8, are synthesized and secreted by numerous cell types and tissues in response to pathogenic infection [8,9]. TNF-α, IL-1α, and IL-6 are involved in the induction of acute phase proteins, generation of fever, and shock. This phenomenon is known to be observed during the sepsis. In addition, many neutrophils are found in the blood in septic patients. The migration and activation of neutrophils are induced by chemokine IL-8. [10,11]. In this regard, cytokine-induced inflammatory responses are highly characteristic of the septic insult produced by gram-negative bacterial infection. Considering the cytokine-induced inflammatory responses in sepsis, there is a possibility that proinflammatory cytokines may be expressed in $CD34^+$ cells or their cultured cells when bacterial infection occurs during the period of cord blood transplantation.

E. COLI INFECTION UP-REGULATES EXPRESSION OF IL-1α, IL-6, IL-8, AND TNF-α IN THE CD34$^+$ CELLS OR THEIR CULTURED CELLS

IL-1α, IL-6, IL-8, MCP-1, and TNF-α are proinflammatory cytokines that are involved in the inflammatory process [12]. We assessed gene expression of these cytokines in CD34$^+$ cells following *E. coli* infection. CD34$^+$ cells constitutively expressed low levels of IL-1α, IL-6, IL-8, and TNF-α mRNA expression, but the expression of these proinflammatory cytokines increased after *E. coli* infection (figure 1). In addition, up-regulated proinflammatory cytokine mRNA expression such as IL-1α, IL-6, IL-8, and TNF-α were also noted in *E. coli*-infected cultured cells derived from CD34$^+$ (day 7 and 14). Quantification of mRNA using synthetic standard RNA showed that IL-1α, IL-6, IL-8 and TNF-α mRNA expression by *E. coli* infection was 2 to 19 times greater than by control in CD34$^+$ cells [13]. The release of proinflammatory cytokines can contribute to the inflammatory cell infiltration that accompanies bacteremia. In addition, cytokines IL-1, IL-6 and TNF-α are known to be importantly involved in the systemic inflammatory process such as shock, fever, and production of acute phase proteins and antibodies [12,14]. IL-8 is also known to be a chemoattractant and activator for neutrophils [15]. Our results showed that these cytokines were up-regulated in CD34$^+$ cells infected with *E. coli*. Notably, the kinetics of IL-8 mRNA expression was delayed relative to the other cytokines. Therefore, there is a possibility that cytokines released from the cells during infection may mediate the IL-8 response to *E. coli* infection.

To differentiate CD34$^+$ cells in vitro, the CD34$^+$ cells (1 x 10^5 /ml) were seeded at DMEM with 10% heat-inactivated fetal bovine serum (FBS) containing FLT3 ligand (FL, 50 ng/ml), thrombopoietin (TPO, 10 ng/ml), and stem cell factor (SCF, 50 ng/ml) in 35 mm dishes at 37°C in a humidified atmosphere of 5% CO$_2$ in air. Every 3-4 days, a half of the culture volume was removed from the wells to be replaced with fresh medium and growth factors. At various intervals, the cells were harvested (figure 2) [16]. Viability of the cells was assessed using the trypan blue exclusion assay. Under this culture condition, CD34$^+$ fraction was decreased to 21-30% at day 7, and was only 5-6% at day 14, as assessed by FACS analyses. When 1 x 10^5 isolated CD34$^+$ cells were incubated with FL+TPO+SCF at day 0, the viable cells were increased to (1.6 ± 0.7) x 10^7 cells after 7 days culture and (8.6 ± 1.5) x 10^8 cells after 14 days culture (mean ± SD of five separate experiments). The percentage of living cells was 96.2 ± 2.6% (day 7) and 86.8 ± 3.6% (day 14) of total cells (mean ± SD of five separate experiments). The cultured cells derived from CD34$^+$ stem cells increased the numbers of proinflammatory cytokine mRNA transcripts in response to *E. coli* infection (figure 3). However, mRNA expression of MCP-1, RANTES, and eotaxin was not significantly increased in *E. coli*-infected CD34$^+$ cells (day 0) and their cultured cells (day 7 and 14) [13].

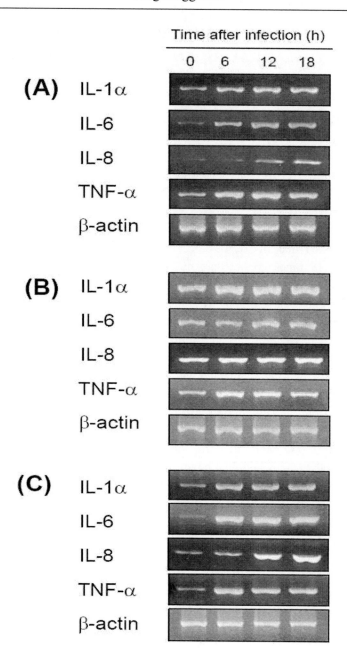

Figure 1. RT-PCR analysis of proinflammatory cytokine mRNA in *E. coli*-infected CD34[+] cells and their cultured cells. The cells (1×10^6) in the 6-well tissue culture plate were infected with *E. coli* for the indicated hours. The ratio of *E. coli* to the cells was adjusted to 10:1. The expression of mRNA for each cytokine and β-actin was assessed by RT-PCR using specific primers. The data are a representative data in more than five separate experiments. (A), freshly isolated CD34[+] hematopoietic stem cells; (B) or (C), the cultured cells which were obtained from CD34+ stem cells incubated with FL + TPO + SCF for 7 days or 14 days, respectively. [13]

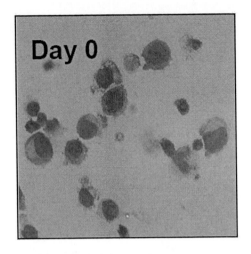 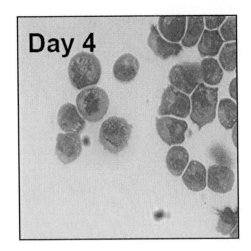
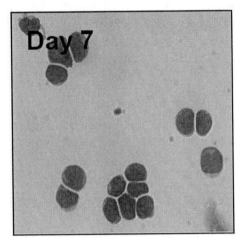 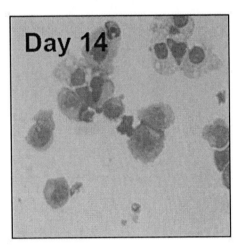

Figure 2. Morphological changes in CD34$^+$ cord blood cells during short-term culture in the presence of FL/TPO/SCF. Wright-Giemsa staining was performed to evaluate the morphology of cells at each time-point. Cells displayed condensed nuclei and decreased nuclear/cytoplasm ratio, even at 4 days after culture, suggesting differentiation into committed cells. [16]

To determine whether increased cytokine mRNA levels were accompanied by increased protein secretion, we measured the amount of cytokine proteins in culture supernatants. The secretions of each cytokine were paralleled by each mRNA expression (figure 4). For example, the cultured cells derived from CD34$^+$ (day 14) infected with *E. coli* produced 3.6-fold higher amounts of IL-1α compared with uninfected controls. However, MCP-1 production in infected and uninfected cells remained relatively constant (~ 18.5 ng/ml). These data suggest that the increased proinflammatory cytokine secretion in response to *E. coli* infection may be due in large part to pretranslational events.

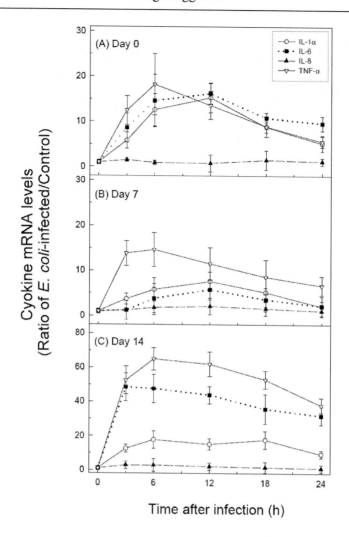

Figure 3. Proinflammatory cytokine mRNA expression in *E. coli*-infected cultured cells derived from CD34+ stem cells. CD34$^+$ stem cells (purity > 98%, 1 x 10^5 cells) were incubated with FLT3 ligand (50 ng/ml) + thrombopoietin (10 ng/ml) + stem cell factor (50 ng/ml) for 7 days or 14 days. Every 3-4 days, a half of the culture volume was removed from the wells to be replaced with fresh medium and growth factors. The cultured cells (1 x 10^6 cells) in 6-well plates were incubated with *E. coli* for the indicated hours. The ratio of *E. coli* to the cultured cells was adjusted to 10:1. For quantification of the expressed transcripts, total RNA was reverse-transcribed using an oligo(dT) primer and synthetic internal RNA standards, and amplified by PCR. [13]

To isolate CFU-GM, BFU-E (burst-forming unit-erythroid), and CFU-GEMM (colony forming unit-granulocyte, erythrocyte, macrophage, megakaryocyte), CD34$^+$ cells were cultured in complete MethoCult^{TM} medium (1% methylcellulose in DMEM, 30% FBS, 1% bovine serum albumin, 3 U/ml erythropoietin, 10^{-4} M 2-mercaptoenthanol, 2 mM L-glutamine, 50 ng/ml stem cell factor, 10 ng/ml GM-CSF, 10 ng/ml IL-3). After 14 days of CD34$^+$ cell culture in the complete MethoCult^{TM} medium, fractions of CFU-GM, BFU-E, and CFU-GEMM were 68%, 29% and 3%, respectively (mean value of three separate experiments). Under the optical inverted microscopy, CFU-GM or BFU-E was collected. To test subpopulation of the cultured cells derived from CD34$^+$ involved in the induction of proinflammatory cytokines in response to *E. coli* infection, the proinflammatory cytokine expression levels were compared between CFU-GM and BFU-E. As shown in figure 5, up-regulation of the proinflammatory cytokines by *E. coli* infection was mainly attributed to CFU-GM in the cultured cells derived from $CD34^+$ [13]. These results indicate that expression of the proinflammatory cytokines was mainly generated from granulocytes-macrophage lineages.

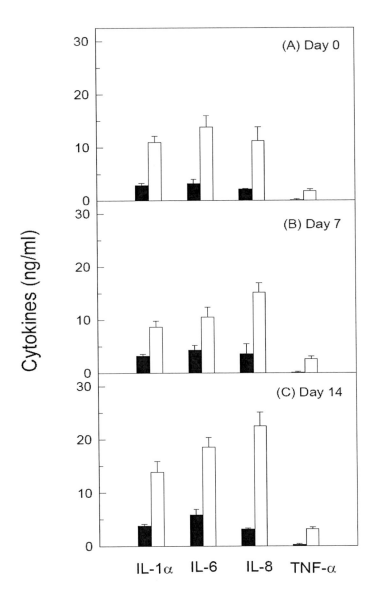

Figure 4. Proinflammatory cytokine secretion by $CD34^+$ cells or their cultured cells infected with *E. coli*. $CD34^+$ cells (day 0, A) or their cultured cells [day 7 (B) and 14 (C)] in 6-well plates were incubated with *E. coli* for 18 h and protein levels of each cytokine were determined by ELISA. Data are the mean ± SEM of seven separate experiments. White bar, *E. coli*-infected; Black bar, non-infected controls. [13]

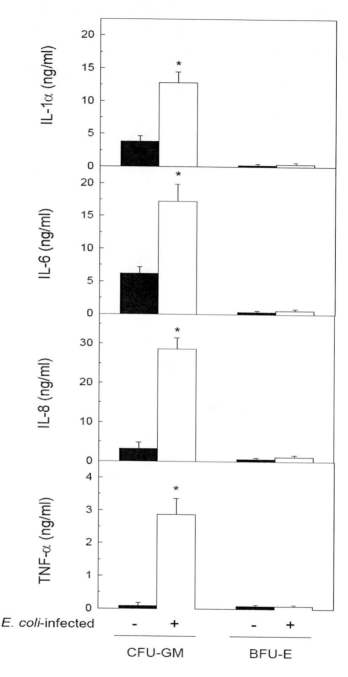

Figure 5. Secretion of proinflammatory cytokines from CFU-GM or BFU-E in response to *E. coli* infection. CFU-GM or BFU-E was isolated from the cultured cells derived from CD34$^+$ cells. The freshly isolated CD34+ cells were cultured in complete MethoCult^{TM} medium for 14 days. Isolated CFU-GM or BFU-E (1 x 10^4) was incubated with *E. coli* (1 x 10^5 CFU) for 18 h and protein levels of each cytokine were determined by ELISA. Data are the mean ± SEM of five separate experiments. Asterisks indicate statistical significance with $P < 0.05$ in comparison with the control. [13]

E. COLI INFECTION INDUCES P50 HOMODIMERIC NF-κB ACTIVATION AND IκBα DEGRADATION IN CD34+ CELLS AND THEIR CULTURED CELLS

Many of the genes that are activated after bacterial infection are target genes of the transcription nuclear factor-kappa B (NF-κB) [17-21]. NF-κB is a dimeric transcription factor composed of homodimers or heterodimers of Rel protein, of which there are five family members in mammalian cells [i.e., RelA (p65), c-Rel, Rel B, NF-κB1 (p50), and NF-κB2 (p52)] [22-24]. NF-κB dimers are held in the cytoplasm in an inactive state by inhibitory proteins, the IκBs. Stimulation of cells with cytokine or bacterial infection activates a signaling cascade that culminates in the phosphorylation of IκBs [18,20]. IκB kinase (IKK) is known to directly phosphorylate IκB, which then undergoes ubiquitin-mediated proteolysis, thereby releasing NF-κB dimers to translocate to the nucleus. The IKK complex contains three subunits: the catalytic subunits, IKK-α and IKK-β, and a regulatory subunit, IKK-γ (also known as NEMO, NF-κB essential modulator) [25,26]. While IKK-α and IKK-β are essential for IκB phosphorylation, IKK-γ forms a tetrameric scaffold that can assemble two kinase dimers to facilitate trans-autophosphorylation [27].

To determine whether *E. coli* activates NF-κB in human CD34+ cells and their cultured cells, DNA binding studies were performed using cell extracts after infection of the cultured cells derived from CD34+ cells (day 14) with *E. coli* [13]. Following infection, these cells increased DNA binding activity of NF-κB, as shown by EMSA (figure 6A). In addition, degradation of IκBα was observed in *E. coli*-infected the cultured cells derived from CD34+, as determined by immunoblot analysis. Notably, an IκBα signal completely disappeared at 1 hr after infection, but then continuously recovered. Similar results were obtained in CD34+ cells (day 0) (figure 6B).

To identify the specific NF-κB subunits that comprise the NF-κB signal detected by EMSAs in *E. coli*-infected CD34+ cells or their cultured cells, supershift assay was performed. Specific antibodies to p50, p52, p65, c-Rel, and Rel B were used for these experiments. Supershift studies demonstrated that the antibody to p50 shifted the entire signal. However, anti-p52, anti-p65, anti-c-Rel, or anti-Rel B antibodies did not shift the NF-κB signals (figure 6C and D). These results suggest that NF-κB activation by *E. coli* infection may be predominantly mediated by homodimers of p50.

Distinct expression profiles for each of the five mammalian NF-κB/Rel members have been observed in developing tissues and organs. Thus, p50/p65 heterodimers are readily activated in most cell types while, in contrast, c-Rel complexes (e.g. p50/c-Rel heterodimers and c-Rel homodimers) are found predominantly in cells of hematopoietic lineage [28]. NF-κB/Rel is known not to affect the potency of hematopoietic stem cells to differentiate into common lymphoid and common myeloid cells. Nevertheless, p50/p65 is crucial for lymphopoiesis, whereas p65/c-Rel is complementary for myeloid development [28]. Our supershift studies showed that *E. coli* infection induced p50/p50 homodimers in CD34+ cells and their cultured cells. Until now, there is little understanding of the induction of p50/p50 homodimers in CD34+ cells and their cultured cells. A recent study reported that p50/p65 was required for proper development of myeloid dendritic cells [29]. However, loss of p50/c-Rel or c-Rel alone did not perturb dendritic cell development, but rather affected the maturation and survival of dendritic cells [29,30]. These findings suggest that p50 is involved in dendritic cell development. Considering that CFU-GM was mainly involved in the proinflammatory cytokine expression in *E. coli*-infected cultured cells derived from CD34$^+$, the activation of p50/p50 homodimer may be due to myeloid lineages of CD34$^+$ stem cells. Further study of the NF-κB subunits in the stage of myeloid development from CD34$^+$ cells seems to be quite necessary.

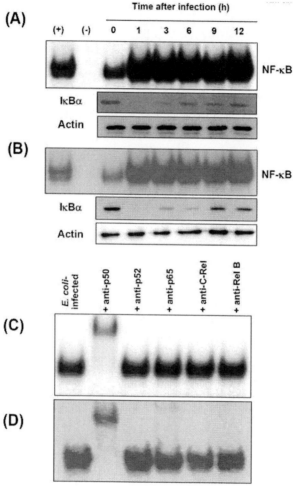

Figure 6. NF-κB activation and IκBα degradation in the CD34$^+$ cells or their cultured cells infected with *E. coli*. (A) The cultured cells (day 14) were incubated with *E. coli*. The ratio of *E. coli* to the cells was adjusted to 10:1. NF-κB DNA binding activity was assessed by EMSA at the indicated times. Immunoblots for concurrent IκBα and actin under the same condition are provided beneath each EMSA time point. The results are representative of five repeated experiments. (+) represents a positive control whereby the cultured cells derived from CD34$^+$ were treated with TNF-α (20 ng/ml) for 3 h. (-) represents negative control. (B) Similar results of NF-κB activation and IκBα degradation were observed in the CD34$^+$ stem cells (day 0). (C) Activation of specific NF-κB subunits in the cultured cells (C, day 14) infected with *E. coli*. Supershift assays were performed using antibodies to p50, p52, p65, c-Rel, and Rel B. The antibody to p50 shifts the entire NF-κB signals. Anti-p52, p65, c-Rel and Rel B did not show the shifts. The results are representative of three repeated experiments. (D) Similar results of supershift assay were obtained from the CD34$^+$ cells (day 0). [13]

INHIBITION OF NF-κB ACTIVITY DOWN-REGULATES THE PROINFLAMMATORY CYTOKINE EXPRESSION IN CD34$^+$ CELLS INFECTED WITH *E. COLI*

Based on that *E. coli* infection activates the NF-κB signals in the CD34$^+$ cells or their cultured cells, we next determined whether the increased proinflammatory cytokine expression after *E. coli* infection was associated with NF-κB pathways. Addition of calphain-1 inhibitor to *E. coli*-infected cultured cells derived from CD34$^+$ cells (day 14) significantly decreased the proinflammatory cytokine secretion [13].

One of the major pathways of NF-κB activation involves the phosphorylation of IκBα, which is in turn followed by IκB degradation and the subsequent migration of NF-κB dimers from the cytoplasm to the nucleus [22,23]. We assayed expression of proinflammatory cytokines in CD34$^+$ cells with suppressed NF-κB activity, which had been transfected with the retrovirus-IκBα-AA [13]. To confirm that the transfection with retrovirus-IκBα-AA was related to a decrease in an NF-κB signal, EMSA were performed. Activation of NF-κB signals was inhibited in the cultured cells derived from CD34$^+$ (day 14) transfected with retrovirus-IκBα-AA (figure 7A). Consistent with this, mRNA expression of IL-1, IL-6, IL-8, and TNF-α in response to *E. coli* infection was also decreased in NF-κB-suppressed cultured cells derived from CD34$^+$ (figure 7B).

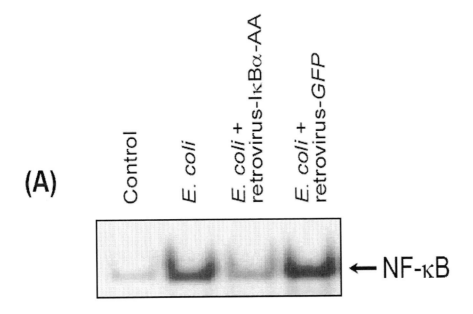

Figure 7. (Continued).

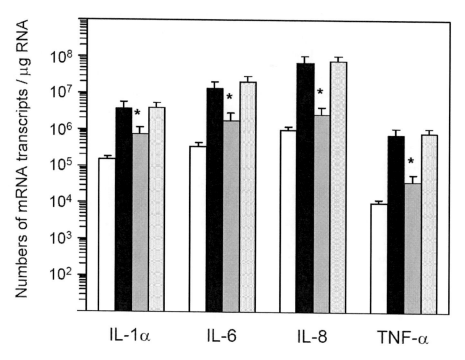

Figure 7. Proinflammatory cytokine expression in *E. coli*-infected cultured cells transfected with retrovirus containing the IκBα super-repressor. (A) The cultured cells (day 14) were transfected with either retrovirus containing IκBα super-repressor (retrovirus-IκBα-AA) or control virus, (retrovirus-*GFP*). At 48 h after transfection, the cells were incubated with *E. coli* for 3 h. NF-κB binding activity was assayed by EMSA. The results are representative of three repeated experiments. (B) Transfected cultured cells (1×10^8 cells) were incubated with *E. coli* (1×10^9 CFU) for 18 h. For quantification of the expressed transcripts, total RNA was reverse-transcribed using an oligo(dT) primer and synthetic internal RNA standards, and amplified by PCR. Data are presented as numbers of mRNA transcripts/μg of total RNA (mean ± SD, n=5). Asterisks indicate statistical significance with $P < 0.05$ in comparison with control virus-transfected cells infected with *E. coli*. □, control; ■, *E. coli*-infected; ▨, *E. coli*-infected cells transfected with retrovirus-IκBα-AA; ▨, *E. coli*-infected cells transfected with control virus (retrovirus-*GFP*). [13]

E. COLI INFECTION INCREASES PHOSPHORYLATED IKK SIGNALS IN THE CULTURED CELLS DERIVED FROM CD34$^+$

Major pathways for NF-κB activation are involved in the activation of IKK, which is followed by IκB degradation [23]. In this study, we found that *E. coli* infection increased signals of the phosphorylated IKKα/β in the cultured cells derived from CD34$^+$ (day 14) (figure 8A). These cultured cells were obtained from CD34$^+$ cells incubated with FL + TPO + SCF for 14 days. In order to study whether the activation of IKK was one of the major pathways that culminated in the expression of proinflammatory cytokines following *E. coli* infection, cultured cells derived from CD34$^+$ (day 14) were treated with an NBD peptide which can block the association of NEMO with the IKK complex [31]. Secretion of the proinflammatory cytokines was inhibited by treatment with an NBD peptide, but not by treatment with mutant type of NBD peptide. Similar results were obtained from the CD34$^+$ cells (day 0) infected with *E. coli*. To confirm that *E. coli*-induced IKK activation was directly associated with reporter gene activation, luciferase assay were also performed. Addition of NBD peptide decreased the activation of IL-8 reporter genes in the cultured cells infected with *E. coli* (figure 8B) [13]. These cultured cells were obtained from CD34$^+$ cells incubated with FL + TPO + SCF for day 14. These results demonstrate that the activation of IKK are involved as crucial steps for NF-κB activation in CD34$^+$ cells or their cultured cells following infection with whole *E. coli* bacterial cells.

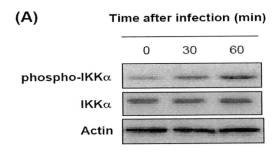

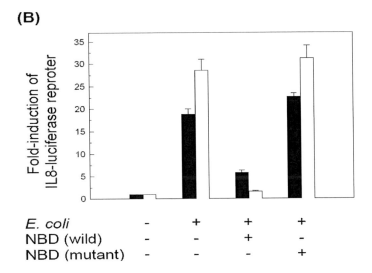

Figure 8. Phosphorylation of IKK and IL-8 reporter gene activation in *E. coli*-infected cultured cells derived from CD34$^+$. (A) The cultured cells (day 14) were incubated with *E. coli* for the indicated times. The ratio of *E. coli* to the cells was adjusted to 10:1. Phosphorylation and protein expression of IKKα and actin were assessed by immunoblot. (B) The cultured cells (day 14) were transfected with pIL-8-luciferase transcriptional reporters. 48 h later, the transfected cells were incubated with *E. coli* (black bar) or TNF-α (20 ng/ml, open bar) for 6 h. Data are expressed as the mean fold induction ± SEM in luciferase activity relative to non-stimulated controls (n=5). [13]

CpG DNA Induces IL-8 Expression in Human CD34+ Cells

In the previous report, we demonstrated that *E. coli* provokes the expression of several proinflammatory cytokines, including IL-8, in CD34+ cells [13]. This suggests that CD34+ cells can recognize the molecular patterns associated with pathogens and subsequently initiate the transcription of inflammatory genes. These molecular patterns may be specifically conserved components of microbes, such as lipopolysaccharide (LPS) from Gram-negative bacteria, CpG DNA, and flagellin [32-34]. Among these specifically conserved components of microbes, unmethylated 5'-CpG-3' dinucleotides with certain flanking bases have been suggested to be responsible for the immunogenicity of bacterial DNA [35]. Synthetic oligodeoxynucleotides (ODN), containing this CpG motif (CpG ODN) [36], have been shown to have immunostimulatory effects similar to those of bacterial DNA [35].

As shown in figure 9, CpG ODN-induced increases of IL-8 mRNA in CD34+ cells were dose-dependent and followed a characteristic time course. However, β-actin mRNA levels in stimulated and unstimulated cells remained relatively constant throughout the same period (~ 6×10^6 transcripts/μg RNA). To determine whether increased IL-8 mRNA levels were accompanied by increased secretion of IL-8 protein, we measured the amount of IL-8 proteins in culture supernatants. The increase of IL-8 mRNA expression was associated with an increase of IL-8 secretion 24 h post-stimulation (control, 0.8 ± 0.3 ng/ml; CpG, 9.8 ± 1.1 ng/ml; mean ± SEM, n=5) [37].

We next determined whether *E. coli* plasmid DNA might be effective in inducing IL-8 expression. Thus, CD34+ cells were treated with plasmid DNA (20 μg/ml), and IL-8 expression was examined 12 h later by quantitative RT-PCR. *E. coli* plasmid DNA also up-regulated IL-8 mRNA expression in CD34+ cells (control, 3.6×10^5; *E. coli* DNA, 5.7×10^7; mean numbers of IL-8 mRNA transcripts/μg RNA, n=5). In this experiment, LPS levels in *E. coli* plasmid DNA was < 0.03 EU/ml [37].

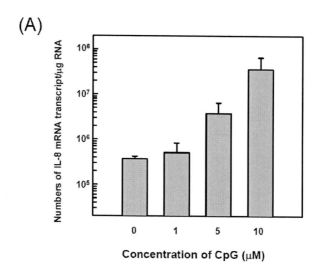

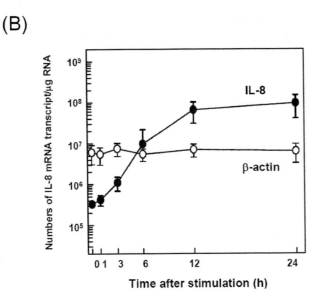

Figure 9. CpG ODN-induced increases of IL-8 expression in CD34$^+$ cells. (A) After treatment of CD34$^+$ cells with various doses of CpG ODN, expression of IL-8 mRNA was analyzed by quantitative RT-PCR. (B) IL-8 mRNA expression in CD34$^+$ cells at different times following treatment with CpG ODN (10 μM). Data are presented as numbers of mRNA transcripts/μg of total RNA (mean ± SD, n=5). [37]

IL-8 Expression through TLR9 within CD34$^+$ Cells in Response to CpG DNA Stimulation

Unlike LPS, which is recognized by Toll-like receptor (TLR) 4, CpG DNA is recognized by TLR9 [38-40]. The signaling of these two receptors, however, shares similar downstream pathways, including activation of mitogen-activated protein kinases (MAPKs) and IKK complex [41,42]. Several studies have shown that CpG DNA has strong stimulatory effects on lymphocytes [35,43-46]. These stimulatory effects include triggering B cell proliferation, resistance to apoptosis, release of IL-6 and IL-12, natural killer cell secretion of interferon (IFN)-γ, increased lytic activity, and monocyte/macrophage secretion of IFN-α/β, IL-6, IL-12, GM-CSF, chemokines, and TNF-α. Since there is no report regarding TLR9 and CpG DNA-induced signaling in CD34$^+$ cells, we investigated the role of TLR9 activation along with the intracellular signaling pathways triggered by CpG DNA in CD34$^+$ cells.

RT-PCR analysis of RNA from CD34$^+$ cells revealed constitutive expression of TLR9 transcripts, and stimulation of CD34$^+$ cells with CpG ODN did not change the TLR9 mRNA expression (figure 10). Subsequent nucleotide sequence analyses of the RT-PCR product from CD34$^+$ cells revealed 100% identity with the published human TLR9 cDNA sequence, confirming that the primers used in this study amplified the correct sequences [37]. This result is provided an evidence for the first time that CD34$^+$ cells constitutively express TLR9 mRNA.

Internalization and endosomal maturation have been shown to be required for CpG DNA to activate TLR9 signaling in immune cells [47,48]. As shown in figure 11, chloroquine, which effectively blocks endosomal maturation [47], significantly inhibited the CpG ODN-induced increase of IL-8 production in CD34$^+$ cells, indicating similar ODN-mediated signaling between CD34$^+$ cells and immune cells.

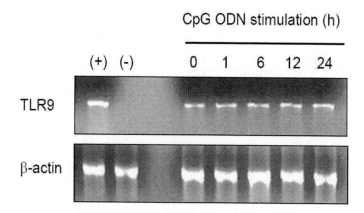

Figure 10. TLR9 mRNA expression in CD34$^+$ cells, revealed by RT-PCR analysis. The cells (1 x 10^6) in the 6-well tissue culture plate were treated with CpG ODN (10 μM) for the indicated periods. The expression of mRNA for TLR9 and β-actin was assessed by RT-PCR using specific primers. (+) and (-) represent positive and negative controls, respectively. Shown in the figure are the representative data of 3 separate experiments. [37]

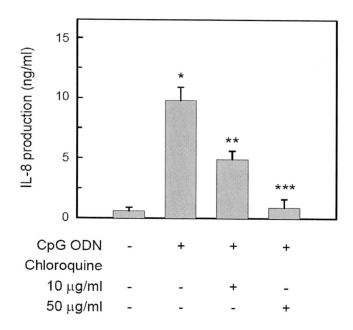

Figure 11. Activation of CD34$^+$ cells by CpG ODN is dependent on endosomal maturation. CD34$^+$ cells were treated with chloroquine (10 μg/ml or 50 μg/ml) for 30 min, followed by CpG ODN treatment (10 μM) for 24 h. IL-8 production was determined by ELISA analysis (mean ± SEM, n = 5; *$P < 0.05$ compared with control, **$P < 0.05$ compared with group treated CpG ODN only, ***$P < 0.01$ compared with group treated CpG ODN only). [37]

CPG DNA ACTIVATES AP-1 SIGNALS IN CD34$^+$ CELLS

MAPKs comprise an important group of serine- and threonine-signaling kinases that transduce a variety of extracellular stimuli through a cascade of protein phosphorylation, leading to the activation of transcription factors. There are three groups of MAPK family members: (i) p46 and p54 c-Jun NH$_2$-terminal kinase (JNK) or stress-activated protein kinase with multiple subisoforms, (ii) p38 MAPK with a, b, g, and d isoforms, and (iii) p42 and p44 extracellular signal-regulated kinase (ERK). All of these signaling cascades have been implicated in controlling the transcription of chemokine IL-8 and have been shown to regulate activator protein-1 (AP-1) activity [49]. Thus, MAPKs can phosphorylate the transcription factor Elk-1, a member of the complex family, which binds the serum response element motif in the c-Fos promoter, thereby inducing c-Fos transcription [50]. In contrast, c-Jun is regulated both transcriptionally and post-transcriptionally, and its transcription is up-regulated by activated MAPK [52]. Subsequently, c-Jun can increase its own transcription by binding to the TRE motif in its promoter. Novel cFos synthesis leads to the formation of Jun/Fos heterodimers, which have a 10-fold higher DNA binding affinity than Jun/Jun homodimers, resulting in increased AP-1 activity [53]. Therefore, AP-1 activation is known to induce the expression of IL-8 in response to stimulation with bacterial products [49,52]. To determine whether CpG DNA could activate AP-1 signals in CD34$^+$ cells, AP-1-DNA binding studies were performed by EMSA using nuclear extracts after stimulation of CD34$^+$ cells with CpG ODN. As shown in figure 12A, stimulation of these cells with CpG ODN increased the binding activity. The specificity of AP-1 signals was confirmed by competition assay: The addition of AP-1 oligomer to nuclear extracts after stimulation of CD34$^+$ cells with CpG ODN for 2 h was shown to suppress the AP-1 signal, however, the addition of AP-1 mutant oligomer or NF-κB oligomer did not change the signals (figure 12B). In contrast to AP-1 signals, stimulation of the cells with CpG ODN did not activate NF-κB activity (figure 12C). Consistent with this, degradation of IκBα was not observed in CpG ODN-stimulated CD34$^+$ cells, as determined by immunoblot analysis. However, the addition of an ERK inhibitor (U0126) or a p38 inhibitor (SB203580) showed approximately 60% inhibition of IL-8 production in CD34+ cells stimulated with CpG DNA [37]. The partial suppression may be due to other pathways which can activate AP-1 signals. Further study is necessary to clearly AP-1 activation pathways in CpG DNA-stimulated CD34$^+$ cells.

EFFECT OF SIGNALING INHIBITORS ON CPG ODN-INDUCED IL-8 EXPRESSION IN CD34$^+$ CELLS

CpG ODN has been shown to stimulate several signaling pathways, including ERK1/2 and NF-κB in macrophages and other immune cells [53-55]. As shown in figure 13A, treatment of CD34$^+$ cells with CpG ODN induced activation of phosphorylated ERK1/2 and p38. Next, we determined the pharmacological sensitivities of these pathways that might have contributed to the expression of IL-8 in CD34$^+$ cells after CpG ODN exposure. Figure 13B shows that MEK1/2 inhibitor U0126 and p38 inhibitor SB203580 significantly inhibited the CpG ODN-induced increase of IL-8 production. The ERK inhibitor (U0126) or p38 inhibitor

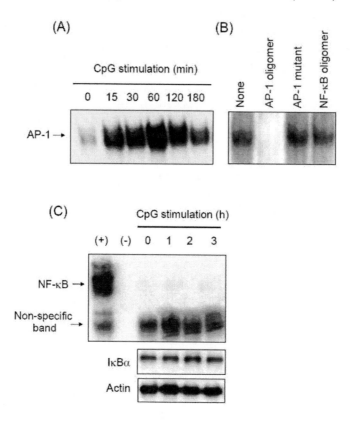

Figure 12. CpG ODN activates AP-1 signals in CD34$^+$ cells. CD34$^+$ cells were stimulated with CpG ODN (10 μM) for the indicated periods of time. (A) AP-1 activity was assessed by electrophoretic mobility shift assay (EMSA). (B) Competition assay for AP-1 was performed using each oligomer to the nuclear extracts of CD34$^+$ cells. (C) NF-κB DNA binding activity was also assessed by EMSA at the indicated times. Immunoblots for concurrent IκBα and actin under the same condition are provided beneath each EMSA time point. (+) represents a positive control, where CD34$^+$ cells were treated with TNF-α (20 ng/ml) for 3 h. (-) represents negative control. These results are representatives of three independent experiments. [37]

(SB203580) prevented CpG DNA-mediated phosphorylation of ERK1/2 or p38 in CD34$^+$ cells (figure 13C). However, NF-κB inhibitor PDTC had no effect on the CpG ODN-stimulated IL-8 expression. To confirm that the inhibition of NF-κB activity had no effect on the CpG ODN-stimulated IL-8 expression, transfection with retrovirus-IκBα-AA was performed. Our recent study showed that activation of NF-κB signals was completely inhibited when the CD34$^+$ cells were transfected with retrovirus-IκBα-AA. In this condition, IL-8 production in response to CpG ODN was not attenuated in NF-κB-suppressed CD34$^+$ cells (control, 0.6 ± 0.3 ng/ml; CpG, 10.1 ± 1.5 ng/ml; CpG + retrovirus-IκBα-AA, 10.2 ± 0.8 ng/ml; mean ± SEM, n=3) [37]. These results suggest that CpG ODN up-regulates IL-8 in CD34$^+$ cells through the activation of MAPK signaling pathways. It is of interest to note that the stimulation with CpG ODN did not activate NF-κB signals in CD34$^+$ cells. In the previous study, infection of CD34$^+$ cells with live *E. coli* activated NF-κB signals [13]. This difference might have been due to the fact that CpG DNA constitutes only a small part of *E. coli*, suggesting that live *E. coli* may involve a variety of signaling pathways. Although CD34+ cells are homogeneous in CD34 expression, there is a possibility that CD34+ cells may be still heterogeneous. Therefore, target cells for CpG DNA may be minor population. This might be one of the causes why CpG DNA-induced NF-κB activation was undetectable.

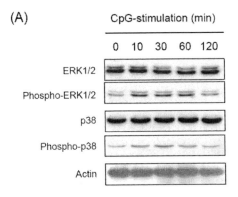

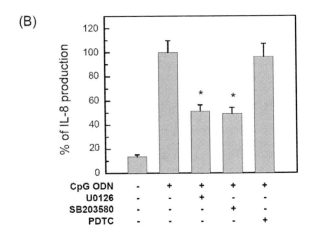

Figure 13. CpG ODN activates MAPK in CD34+ cells. (A) After CD34+ cells were stimulated with CpG ODN (10 μM) for the indicated times, cell lysates were prepared and subjected to immunoblot analysis for ERK1/2 and p38. (B) CD34+ cells were treated with U0126 (50 μM), SB203580 (10 μM) or PDTC (100 μM) for 30 min, followed by CpG ODN treatment (10 μg/ml). ELISA analysis of IL-8 production 24 h, following CpG ODN treatment (mean ± SEM, n = 5; *$P < 0.05$ compared with group treated CpG ODN only). [37]

COSTIMULATION WITH LPS AND CPG SYNERGISTICALLY UP-REGULATES IL-8 IN CD34+ CELLS

Simultaneous exposure to different antigenic components of bacteria, such as LPS and lipoprotein or CpG DNA plus LPS, has been shown to synergistically act to induce cytokine production in cultured immune cells and in intact animals [56,57]. Recently, a study demonstrated that costimulation of TLR4 and TLR2 or TLR9 induced synergistic release of the Th1 cytokines, IFN-γ and TNF-α [58]. We also showed that costimulation of CD34+ cells with CpG DNA and LPS led to a synergistic increase of IL-8 expression [37]. Although different TLRs are known to induce distinct cellular and systemic responses to infection, TLR4 and TLR9 induce similar proinflammatory responses [56]. Considering LPS-mediated TLR4 activation in many cells [59], it is quite possible that the increase of IL-8 expression was mediated by TLR4 in LPS-stimulated CD34+ cells, indicating cooperation between TLR9 and TLR4 in stimulation of immune response in the cells.

Results obtained from our studies may have important implications in host defense and gene therapy strategies. In particular, a new role of CpG DNA and $CD34^+$ cells in systemic bacterial infection is possible. To date, LPS has been the major focus in studying the Gram-negative sepsis. The fact that CpG DNA was also active in inducing proinflammatory response in $CD34^+$ cells may suggest its involvement in the development and/or progression of sepsis. This is particularly highlighted by the fact that LPS and CpG have a synergistic effect in inducing IL-8 response in $CD34^+$ cells [37]. The results also have important implications in $CD34^+$ gene transfer. The fact that expression plasmid had a direct CpG-mediated biological effect on $CD34^+$ cells raises not only a safety concern, but also suggests caution in interpreting experimental data. Furthermore, attention should be paid to distinguish the therapeutic gene-mediated biological effect from the CpG-mediated nonspecific effect. Strategies are currently being developed to modify the plasmid expression vectors to decrease CpG immunostimulatory activity.

LOW MOLECULAR WEIGHT POLYETHYLENIMINE IS EFFICIENT FOR TRANSFECTION OF HUMAN UMBILICAL CORD BLOOD-DERIVED CD34$^+$ CELLS

Hematopoietic stem cells have recently emerged as potential gene and cell therapy vehicles. Viral systems such as lentivirus and parvovirus B19 have been used for gene delivery into hematopoietic cells. However, due to the inherent safety issues of viral vectors [60], researchers are currently seeking safe and efficient nonviral gene delivery systems. Cationic liposomes [61] and electroporation [62] have been studied as promising nonviral gene delivery systems for hematopoietic progenitors or stem cells, but the use of cationic liposomes is limited by toxicity and low transfection efficiency [63]. Moreover, electroporation is often followed by apoptotic and necrotic cell death [64]. Polyethylenimine (PEI), a nonviral cationic polymer, has been studied as a gene delivery vector. PEI molecules with higher molecular weights (>20,000) have been commonly used for delivery of genes in various adherent cell lines including NIH 3T3, HeLa, and HepG2 cells [65]. PEI 22K (MW 22,000) was shown to be more effective than cationic liposomes or electroporation for transgene expression in human embryonic stem cells [66]. PEI 25K yielded high transfection activity and prolonged organ expression in mice [67]. However, few studies have examined the transfection efficiency of PEI in hematopoietic and progenitor cells. We tested whether PEI (0.8–750 K) could enhance cellular gene delivery and transfection activity in hematopoietic and human cord blood-derived $CD34^+$ cells, and found that PEI 2K (MW

2,000) significantly increased the efficiency of gene delivery to various human hematopoietic cell lines and cord blood CD34$^+$ cells with little cytotoxicity [68]. In particular, the lower molecular weight PEI 2K can potentially be applied at the optimal N/P ratio for the effective, safe gene modification of hematopoietic and cord blood CD34$^+$ cells [68].

CONCLUSION

Umbilical cord blood has emerged as an alternative source of hematopoietic CD34$^+$ cells for allogeneic stem cell transplantation. Since bacteremia induced by *E. coli* is considered one of the complications of transplantation, we have discussed immunological responses of CD34$^+$ stem cells to bacterial infection in this chapter. CD34$^+$ cells and their cultured cells infected with *E. coli* induced the expression of several proinflammatory cytokines via NF-κB pathway. Expression of the proinflammatory cytokines was mainly generated from granulocytes-macrophage lineages. In addition, we showed first evidence that TLR9 molecules are constitutively expressed in CD34$^+$ cells. Exposure of CD34$^+$ cells to CpG ODN resulted in a time- and dose-dependent increase of IL-8 expression, and activation of phosphorylated ERK1/2 and p38 MAPK. In addition, CpG ODN stimulated AP-1, but not NF-κB signals. Moreover, costimulation with LPS and CpG synergistically up-regulates IL-8 in CD34$^+$ cells. These results suggest that CpG DNA, acting on TLR9, activates CD34$^+$ cells to express IL-8 through MAPK-dependent and NF-κB-independent pathways. In addition, these results may have important implications in host defense and gene therapy strategies. In particular, a new role of CpG DNA and CD34$^+$ cells in systemic bacterial infection is possible. Furthermore, attention should be paid to distinguish the therapeutic gene-mediated biological effect from the CpG-mediated nonspecific effect. Strategies are currently being developed to modify the plasmid expression vectors to decrease CpG immunostimulatory activity.

ACKNOWLEDGMENTS

This work has been collaborated with Yu-Kyoung Oh (School of Life Sciences and Biotechnology, Korea University) and Myung-Ju Ahn (Division of Hematology-Oncology, Department of Medicine, Samsung Medical Center, Sungkyunkwan University School of Medicine), South Korea.

REFERENCES

[1] Ogawa M. Differentiation and proliferation of hematopoietic stem cells. *Blood.* 1993;81:2844-2853.

[2] Broxmeyer HE, Gluckman E, Auerbach A, Douglas GW, Friedman H, Cooper S, Hangoc G, Kurtzberg J, Bard J, Boyse EA. Human umbilical cord blood: a clinically

useful source of transplantable hematopoietic stem/progenitor cells. *Int. J. Cell Cloning.* 1990;8:76-89.

[3] Emerson SG., Sieff CA, Wang EA, Wong G.G., Clark SC, Nathan DG. Purification of fetal hemopoietic progenitors and demonstration of recombinant multipotential colony-stimulating activity. *J. Clin. Invest.* 1985;76:1286-1290.

[4] Saavedra S, Sanz GF, Jarque I, Moscardó F, Jiménez C, Lorenzo I, Martín G, Martínez J, De La Rubia J, Andreu R, Mollá S, Llopis I, Fernández MJ, Salavert M, Acosta B, Gobernado M, Sanz MA. Early infections in adult patients undergoing unrelated donor cord blood transplantation. *Bone Marrow Transplant.* 2002;30:937-943.

[5] Kolb-Mäurer A, Goebel W. Susceptibility of hematopoietic stem cells to pathogens: role in virus/bacteria tropism and pathogenesis. *FEMS Microbiol. Lett.* 2003;26:203-207.

[6] Kolb-Mäurer A, Wilhlem M, Weissinger F, Bröcker, EB, Goebel W. Interaction of human hematopoietic stem cells with bacterial pathogens. *Blood.* 2002;100:3703-3709.

[7] Mullen CA, Nair J, Sandesh S, Chan KW. Fever and neutropenia in pediatric hematopoietic stem cell transplant patients. *Bone Marrow Transplant.* 2000;25:59-65.

[8] Azuma I. Inducer of cytokines in vivo: overview of field and romurtide experience. *Int. J. Immunopharmacol.* 1992;14:487-496.

[9] Salazar-Mather TP, Hokeness KL. Calling in the troops: regulation of inflammatory cell trafficking through innate cytokine/chemokine networks. *Viral Immunol.* 2003;16:291-306.

[10] Suzuki K, Nakaji S, Yamada M, Totsuka M, Sato K, Sugawara K. Systemic inflammatory response to exhaustive exercise. Cytokine kinetics. *Exerc. Immunol. Rev.* 2002;8:6-48.

[11] Janeway CA Jr., Travers P, Walport M, Shlomchik MJ. Innate immunity: In Immunobiology, 8th Edn. Edinburgh: Churchill Livingstone 2001;35-91.

[12] Van Amersfoort ES, Van Berkel TJ, Kuiper J. Receptors, mediators, and mechanisms involved in bacterial sepsis and septic shock. *Clin. Microbiol. Rev.* 2003;6:379-414.

[13] Kim JM, Oh YK, Kim YJ, Yoon J, Ahn MJ. *Escherichia coli* up-regulates proinflammatory cytokine expression in granulocyte/macrophage lineages of CD34+ stem cells via p50 homodimeric NF-κB. *Clin. Exp. Immunol.* 2004;137:341-350.

[14] Waage A, Steinshamn S. Cytokine mediators of septic infections in the normal and granulocytopenic host. *Eur. J. Haematol.* 1993;50:243-249.

[15] Rollins BJ. Chemokines. *Blood.* 1997;90:909-928.

[16] Lee HS, Jang MY, Choi JH, Lee YY, Park HB, Lee YS, Kim SW, Ahn MJ. Proliferation, apoptosis and telomerase activity in human cord blood CD34+ cells cultured with various cytokine combinations. *J. Microbiol. Biotechnol.* 2003;13:422-428.

[17] Arnalich F, Garcia-Palomero E, López J, Jiménez M, Madero R, Renart J, Vázquez JJ, Montiel C. Predictive value of nuclear factor-κB activity and plasma cytokine levels in patients with sepsis. *Infect. Immun.* 2000;68:1942-1945.

[18] Elewaut D, DiDonato JA, Kim JM, Truong F, Eckmann L, Kagnoff MF. NF-kappa B is a central regulator of the intestinal epithelial cell innate immune response induced by infection with enteroinvasive bacteria. *J. Immunol.* 1999; 163:1457-1466.

[19] Hawiger J. Innate immunity and inflammation: a transcriptional paradigm. *Immunol. Res.* 2001;23:99-109.

[20] Kim JM, Kim JS, Lee LY, Kim YJ, Youn HJ, Kim IY, Chee YJ, Oh YK, Kim N, Jung HC, Song IS. Vacuolating cytotoxin in *Helicobacter pylori* water-soluble proteins

upregulates chemokine expression in human eosinophils via Ca2+ influx, mitochondrial reactive oxygen intermediates, and NF-κB activation. *Infect. Immun.* 2007;75:3373-3381.

[21] Tato CM, Hunter CA. Host-pathogen interactions: subversion and utilization of the NF-κB pathway during infection. *Infect. Immun.* 2002;70:3311-3317.

[22] Baeuerle PA, Henkel T. Function and activation of NF-κB in the immune system. *Annu. Rev. Immunol.* 1994;12:141-179.

[23] Baldwin AS. The NF-κB and IκB proteins: new discoveries and insights. *Annu. Rev. Immunol.* 1996;14:649-683.

[24] Thanos D, Maniatis T. NF-κB: a lesson in family values. *Cell.* 1995;80:529-532.

[25] Carter RS, Pennington KN, Ungurait BJ, Ballard DW. In vivo identification of inducible phosphoacceptors in the IKKgamma/NEMO subunit of human IkappaB kinase. *J. Biol. Chem.* 2003;278:19642-19648.

[26] Tang ED, Wang CY, Xiong Y, Guan KL. A role for NF-kappaB essential modifier/IkappaB kinase-gamma (NEMO/IKKgamma) ubiquitination in the activation of the IkappaB kinase complex by tumor necrosis factor-alpha. *J. Biol. Chem.* 2003;278:37297-37305.

[27] Karin M, Ben-Neriah Y. Phosphorylation meets ubiquitination: the control of NF-κB activity. *Annu. Rev. Immunol.* 2000;18:621-663.

[28] Liou HC, Hsia CY. Distinctions between c-Rel and other NF-kappaB proteins in immunity and disease. *Bioessays.* 2003;25:767-780.

[29] Ouaaz F, Arron J, Zheng Y, Choi Y, Beg AA. Dendritic cell development and survival require distinct NF-kappaB subunits. *Immunity.* 2002;16:257-270.

[30] Grumont R, Hochrein H, O'Keeffe M, Gugasyan R, White C, Caminschi I, Cook W, Gerondakis S. c-Rel regulates interleukin 12 p70 expression in CD8(+) dendritic cells by specifically inducing p35 gene transcription. *J. Exp. Med.* 2001;194:1021-1032.

[31] May MJ, D'Acquisto F, Madge LA, Glöckner J, Pober JS, Ghosh S. Selective inhibition of NF-kappaB activation by a peptide that blocks the interaction of NEMO with the IkappaB kinase complex. *Science.* 2000;289:1550-1554.

[32] Fitzgerald KA, Rowe DC, Barnes BJ, Caffrey DR, Visintin A, Latz E, Monks B, Pitha PM, Golenbock DT. LPS-TLR4 signaling to IRF-3/7 and NF-kappaB involves the toll adapters TRAM and TRIF. *J. Exp. Med.* 2003;198:1043-1055.

[33] Lonsdorf AS, Kuekrek H, Stern BV, Boehm BO, Lehmann PV, Tary-Lehmann M. Intratumor CpG-oligodeoxynucleotide injection induces protective antitumor T cell immunity. *J. Immunol.* 2003;171:3941-3946.

[34] Means TK, Hayashi F, Smith KD, Aderem A, Luster AD. The Toll-like receptor 5 stimulus bacterial flagellin induces maturation and chemokine production in human dendritic cells. *J. Immunol.* 2003;170:5165-5175.

[35] Krieg AM, Yi AK, Matson S, Waldschmidt TJ, Bishop GA, Teasdale R, Koretzky GA, Klinman DM. CpG motifs in bacterial DNA trigger direct B-cell activation. *Nature.* 1995;374:546-549.

[36] Moseman EA, Liang X, Dawson AJ, Panoskaltsis-Mortari A, Krieg AM, Liu YJ, Blazar BR, Chen W. Human plasmacytoid dendritic cells activated by CpG oligodeoxynucleotides induce the generation of CD4+CD25+ regulatory T cells. *J. Immunol.* 2004;173:4433-4442.

[37] Kim JM, Kim NI, Oh YK, Kim YJ, Youn J, Ahn MJ. CpG oligodeoxynucleotides induce interleukin-8 expression in CD34+ cells via mitogen-activated protein kinase-dependent and NF-κB-independent pathways. *Int. Immunol.* 2005;17:1525-1531.

[38] Akira S, Hemmi H. Recognition of pathogen-associated molecular patterns by TLR family. *Immunol. Lett.* 2003;85:85-95.

[39] Hemmi H, Takeuchi O, Kawai T, Kawai T, Kaisho T, Sato S, Sanjo H, Matsumoto M, Hoshino K, Wagner H, Takeda K, Akira S. A Toll-like receptor recognizes bacterial DNA. *Nature*. 2000;408:740-745.

[40] Takeshita F, Leifer CA, Gursel I, Ishii KJ, Takeshita S, Gursel M, Klinman DM Cutting edge: role of Toll-like receptor 9 in CpG DNA-induced activation of human cells. *J. Immunol.* 2001;167:3555-3558.

[41] Lee S, Hong J, Choi SY, Oh SB, Park K, Kim JS, Karin M, Lee SJ. CpG oligodeoxynucleotides induce expression of proinflammatory cytokines and chemokines in astrocytes: the role of c-Jun N-terminal kinase in CpG ODN-mediated NF-kappaB activation. *J. Neuroimmunol.* 2004;153:50-63.

[42] Takeda K, Kaisho T, Akira S. Toll-like receptors. *Annu. Rev. Immunol.* 2003;21:335-376.

[43] Ballas ZK, Rasmussen WL, Krieg AM. Induction of NK activity in murine and human cells by CpG motifs in oligodeoxynucleotides and bacterial DNA. *J. Immunol.* 1996;157:1840-1845.

[44] Hartmann G., Weeratna RD, Ballas ZK, Payette P, Blackwell S, Suparto I, Rasmussen WL, Waldschmidt M, Sajuthi D, Purcell RH, Davis HL, Krieg AM. Delineation of a CpG phosphorothioate oligodeoxynucleotide for activating primate immune responses in vitro and in vivo. *J. Immunol.* 2000;164:1617-1624.

[45] Kato A, Ogasawara T, Homma T, Batchelor J, Imai S, Wakiquchi H, Saito H, Matsumoto K. CpG oligodeoxynucleotides directly induce CXCR3 chemokines in human B cells. *Biochem. Biophys. Res. Commun.* 2004;320:1139-1147.

[46] Sivori S, Falco M, Della Chiesa M, Carlomagno S, Vitale M, Moretta L, Moretta A. CpG and double-stranded RNA trigger human NK cells by Toll-like receptors: induction of cytokine release and cytotoxicity against tumors and dendritic cells. *Proc. Natl. Acad. Sci. U. S. A.* 2004;101:10116-10121.

[47] Ahmad-Nejad P, Hacker H, Rutz M., Bauer S, Vabulas RM, Wagner H. Bacterial CpG-DNA and lipopolysaccharides activate Toll-like receptors at distinct cellular compartments. *Eur. J. Immunol.* 2002;32:1958-1968.

[48] Krieg AM. Direct immunologic activities of CpG DNA and implications for gene therapy. *J. Gene Med.* 1999;1:56-63.

[49] Kim JM, Jung HY, Lee JY, Youn J, Lee CH, Kim KH. Mitogen-activated protein kinase and activator protein-1 dependent signals are essential for *Bacteroides fragilis* enterotoxin-induced enteritis. *Eur. J. Immunol.* 2005;35:2648-2657.

[50] Hipskind RA, Rao VN, Mueller CG., Reddy ES, Nordheim A. Ets-related protein Elk-1 is homologous to the c-fos regulatory factor p62TCF. *Nature*. 1991;354:531-534.

[51] Lamph WW, Wamsley P, Sassone-Corsi P, Verma IM. Induction of proto-oncogene JUN/AP-1 by serum and TPA. *Nature*. 1988;334:629-631.

[52] Lee JY, Park HR, Oh YK, Kim YJ, Youn J, Han HS, Kim JM. Effects of transcription factor activator protein-1 on interleukin-8 expression and enteritis in response to *Clostridium difficile* toxin A. *J. Mol. Med.* 2007;85:1393-1404.

[53] Ashkar AA, Rosenthal KL. Toll-like receptor 9, CpG DNA and innate immunity. *Curr. Mol. Med.* 2002;2:545-556.

[54] Stovall SH, Yi AK, Meals EA, Talati AJ, Godambe SA, English BK. Role of vav1- and src-related tyrosine kinases in macrophage activation by CpG DNA. *J. Biol. Chem.* 2004;279:13809-13816.

[55] Takeshita F, Gursel I, Ishii KJ, Suzuki K, Gursel M, Klinman DM. Signal transduction pathways mediated by the interaction of CpG DNA with Toll-like receptor 9. *Semin. Immunol.* 2004;16:17-22.

[56] Li J, Ma Z, Tang ZL, Stevens T, Pitt B, Li S. CpG DNA-mediated immune response in pulmonary endothelial cells. *Am. J. Physiol. Lung Cell Mol. Physiol.* 2004;287:552-558.

[57] Yi AK, Yoon JG., Hong SC, Redford T W, Krieg AM. Lipopolysaccharide and CpG DNA synergize for tumor necrosis factor-alpha production through activation of NF-kappaB. *Int. Immunol.* 2001;13:1391-1404.

[58] Equils O, Schito ML, Karahashi H, Madak Z, Yarali A, Michelsen KS, Sher A, Arditi M. Toll-like receptor 2 (TLR2) and TLR9 signaling results in HIV-long terminal repeat trans-activation and HIV replication in HIV-1 transgenic mouse spleen cells: implications of simultaneous activation of TLRs on HIV replication. *J. Immunol.* 2003;170:5159-5164.

[59] Miller SI, Ernst RK, Bader MW. LPS, TLR4 and infectious disease diversity. *Nat. Rev. Microbiol.* 2005;3:36-46.

[60] Maguire-Zeiss KA, Federoff HJ. Safety of viral vectors for neurological gene therapies. *Curr. Opin. Mol. Ther.* 2004;6:473-481.

[61] Keller H, Yunxu C, Marit G, Pla M, Reiffers J, Thèze J, Froussard P. Transgene expression, but not gene delivery, is improved by adhesion-assisted lipofection of hematopoietic cells. *Gene Ther.* 1999; 93-938.

[62] Van Tendeloo VF, Ponsaerts P, Lardon F, Nijs G, Lenjou M, Van Broeckhoven C, Van Bockstaele DR, Berneman ZN. Highly efficient gene delivery by mRNA electroporation in human hematopoietic cells: superiority to lipofection and passive pulsing of mRNA and to electroporation of plasmid cDNA for tumor antigen loading of dendritic cells. *Blood.* 2001;98:49-56.

[63] Hirko A, Tang F, Hughes JA. Cationic lipid vectors for plasmid DNA delivery. *Curr. Med. Chem.* 2003 1185-1193.

[64] Pinero J., M. Lopez-Baena, T. Ortiz, F. Cortes. Apoptotic and necrotic cell death are both induced by electroporation in HL60 human promyeloid leukaemia cells. *Apoptosis.* 1997;2:330-336.

[65] Oh YK, Suh D, Kim JM, Choi HG., Shin K, Ko JJ. Polyethylenimine-mediated cellular uptake, nucleus trafficking and expression of cytokine plasmid DNA. *Gene Ther.* 2002;9:1627-1632.

[66] Eiges R, Schuldiner M, Drukker M, Yanuka O, Itskovitz-Eldor J, Benvenisty N. Establishment of human embryonic stem cell-transfected clones carrying a marker for undifferentiated cells. *Curr. Biol.* 2001;11:514-518.

[67] Oh YK, Kim JP, Yoon H, Kim JM, Yang JS, Kim CK. Prolonged organ retention and safety of plasmid DNA administered in polyethylenimine complexes. *Gene Ther.* 2001;8:1587-1592.

[68] Shin JY, Suh D, Kim JM, Choi HG, Kim JA, Ko JJ, Lee YB, Kim JS, Oh YK. Low molecular weight polyethylenimine for efficient transfection of human hematopoietic and umbilical cord blood-derived CD34+ cells. *Biochimica et Biophyica Acta.* 2005;1725:377-384.

In: Encyclopedia of Stem Cell Research (2 Volume Set)
Editor: Alexander L. Greene

ISBN: 978-1-61761-835-2
© 2012 Nova Science Publishers, Inc.

Chapter XVIII

ENDOTHELIAL PROGENITOR CELLS: FROM BENCH TO BEDSIDE

Jeremy Ben-Shoshan and Jacob George
The Department of Cardiology and the Cardiovascular Research Center,
Tel Aviv Medical Center, Sackler Faculty of Medicine, Tel Aviv, Israel

ABSTRACT

Cell-based restoration of tissue blood supply for the treatment of ischemic cardiovascular diseases has been profoundly examined during the last decade. The recent discovery of a bone marrow-derived scarce population of endothelial progenitor cells (EPCs), capable of participating in postnatal formation of new blood vessels, has thus gained considerable attention. Substantial efforts are still being made in order to identify the phenotype of these putative cells. Meanwhile, growing evidence obtained from both animal and primary human studies point to the tremendous potential of bone marrow-derived progenitor cells as diagnostic and therapeutic tools. Nevertheless, the long term clinical benefits of progenitor cell mobilization or delivery still remain to be further elucidated. In the present chapter, we describe the phenotypical and functional characterization of EPCs known so far, as well as their value as diagnostic markers of vascular dysfunction. Additionally, we review the data accumulated from animal studies and pilot clinical trials regarding cell-based angiogenic therapy. Eventually, we discuss the potential hurdles to be taken into account as well as potential strategies for the amelioration of the angiogenic properties of EPCs.

Keywords- endothelial progenitor cells, bone marrow, peripheral blood, mobilization, cell-based therapy, cardiovascular diseases

1. Introduction

Until the previous decade, the formation of new blood vessels, a process designated as vasculogenesis, was thought to take place merely in the embryo, during cardiovascular development. Neovascularization of adult tissues was attributed to a different mechanism, termed angiogenesis, consisting of sprouting and elongation of existing vessels due to reorganization and proliferation of local mature endothelial cells[1]. This notion has changed after the characterization of a population of circulating endothelial progenitor cells (EPCs) in adult peripheral blood (PB)[2]. EPCs were then described as bone marrow (BM) derived cells, capable of migrating towards areas of neovascularization, proliferating and differentiating into mature endothelial cells. Numerous subsequent works have indeed reinforced this dogma and demonstrated the involvement of EPCs in postnatal vessel formation in various ischemic conditions.

The recognition of the huge potential hidden in adult progenitor cells as a regenerative tool, has led to multiple animal studies which addressed the efficacy and safety of cell-based therapy for ischemic cardiovascular diseases. One major strategy that was widely tested is based on increasing mobilization of progenitor cells from the BM compartment to the circulation, in order to eventually promote their homing into injured tissues. An additional approach consists of transplantation of progenitor cells, either locally or systemically to contribute to ischemic organ blood restoration. Along with tissue regeneration one objective of those studies was to promote blood flow renewal and tissue reperfusion by increasing local accumulation of EPCs. The promising results achieved in these studies paved the way to pilot clinical trials which assessed growth factor-induced mobilization or transfer of BM-progenitor cells in different ischemic diseases. The central issues tested during these trials included the most suitable cell population as well as mode and time of delivery to be employed in order to obtain optimal outcome. Simultaneously, various molecular and structural approaches, such as genetic modulation as well as combination of cellular and structural elements, have been recently considered to improve the regenerative potential of progenitor cells.

2. EPC Phenotype

In the embryo, the vascular network originates from two cellular sources: the angioblast and the hematopoietic stem cell. These two cell types mutually share several antigenic determinants including CD34, CD117 (c-Kit), vascular endothelial growth factor receptor-2 (VEGFR2) and angiopoietin-1 receptor (Tie2), and are suggested to arise from a common precursor, termed hemangioblast[3]. The hemangioblast, endowed with long term proliferative capacity and bilineage differentiation potential, persists into adulthood and contributes to the homeostasis and repair of the hematopoietic and endothelial lineages[4,5]. During differentiation the hemangioblast gives rise to angioblasts and subsequently to EPCs. However, the precise points of diversion as well as the surface markers that specifically characterize EPCs still remain controversial. In general, $CD34^+/VEGFR2^+/CD45^-$ circulating cells, which account for about 0.01% of peripheral blood mononuclear cells (PBMCs), appear to appropriately mirror a subpopulation of progenitor cells capable of differentiating to endothelial but not to hematopoietic lineage[6,7]. According to several studies these cells might be termed 'early' EPCs, and differ from 'late' EPCs, which apparently lose stem cell markers such as CD133[3] and express endothelial lineage cell markers including platelet-endothelial cell adhesion molecule-1 (PECAM-1/CD31), von-Willebrand factor (vWF), vascular endothelial (VE) cadherin and endothelial nitric oxide synthase (eNOS)[2].

3. FUNCTIONAL PROPERTIES OF EPCs

3.1. Mobilization

The local cellular response in ischemic areas, results in an increase of plasma levels of various growth factors and cytokines. The main regulator of this process is hypoxia-inducible factor (HIF), a transcription factor stabilized and active under low oxygen levels that consequently drives the expression of multiple factors, mediating cellular survival and adaptation to hypoxic conditions[8]. The transcriptome of HIF includes various factors that play central roles in the release of EPCs from the BM and mobilization to the ischemic site. For instance, vascular endothelial growth factor (VEGF) and plancental growth factor (PlGF), which are abundantly expressed in ischemic tissues, trigger activation of matrix metaloproteinases (MMPs) in the BM[9,10]. Activation of MMP-9 results in cleavage of membrane bound Kit ligand (mKit-L) on BM stromal cells surface into soluble Kit ligand (sKit-L). sKit-L then bind to c-Kit receptor on progenitor cells, enhancing their proliferation and mobilization to the bloodstream[11]. Another well established key player in progenitor cells mobilization is granulocyte colony-stimulating factor (G-CSF)[12], which stimulates progenitor cell proliferation and the release of elastase and cathepsin-G from neutrophils[13]. These proteinases disintgegrate adhesive interactions between progenitor and stromal cells, as vascular cell adhesion molecules-1 (VCAM-1)/very late antigen-4 (VLA-4)[14] and stromal cell-derived factor-1 (SDF-1)/CXCR-4[15], which function as retention signals within the BM, allowing EPC migration to the circulation.

In the bloodstream, EPCs circulate toward chemotactic stimuli which emanate from ischemic tissues. SDF-1, a C-X-C chemokine ligand regulated by HIF, is the principal mediator of progenitor cell recruitment, including EPCs. High plasma levels of SDF-1 appear to reverse the SDF-1 gradient across the BM barrier, forcing CXCR-4$^+$ cells to exit the BM compartment[16,17]. In fact, SDF-1 expression in the bone marrow appears to be down-regulated time-dependently with the increase in peripheral blood circulating progenitor cells[18]. Following SDF-1 binding to the CXCR-4 receptor, EPCs circulate through SDF-1 gradient to areas of rapid vascular expansion[17]. VEGF plays also a pivotal role in chemo-attraction of EPCs towards target organs[19,9]. Recently, VEGF-induced migration of EPCs was demonstrated to be mediated by both VEGFR1 (flt-1) and VEGFR2 (flk-1), whereas mature endothelial cells primarily migrate via VEGFR2[10]. Other endogenous migration pathways, such as EPO/EPO-receptor[20], have also been shown to play important roles in migration and accumulation of EPCs.

3.2. Homing

Recruitment and integration of EPCs at the target site occurs through a multistep process, comprising adhesion, transmigration and incorporation into functional vascular networks. The ischemic local environment induces an increased expression of multiple adhesion molecules on endothelial cells that take part in attachment of circulating EPCs. One of the major elements responsible for rolling and initial cell arrest of EPCs are selectins, expressed on stimulated endothelial cells[21, 22, 23]. Likewise, β2-integrins, which are abundantly expressed on the surface of EPCs, play a crucial role in adhesion of EPCs to endothelial cells and trans-endothelial invasion, by binding to intercellular adhesion molecule-1 (ICAM-1)[24,14]. In addition to the interaction between CXCR-4 and CXCL-12 mentioned previously, the binding between CXC chemokine receptor-2 (CXCR-2), expressed on the surface of EPCs, and its ligand CXCL1, expressed by various cell types in vascularized sites, were recently found to be of importance in the local adhesion and homing of EPCs to injured vessels[25].

Incorporation into growing vessels necessitates penetration of EPCs through the extracellular matrix. EPCs secrete various proteolytic enzymes that are essential determinants of this migratory process. MMP-2 and MMP-9 are both produced by EPCs and assist in their tissue invasion via extracellular component degradation[26]. Interestingly, VEGF, which is abundantly secreted by activated EPCs, was shown to increase MMPs production by resident endothelial and smooth muscle cells, potentially contributing indirectly to the integration of EPCs within tissues [27, 28]. The protease cathepsin L (CathL) is also highly expressed in EPCs, in contrast with mature endothelial cells, and plays a central role in matrix degradation, invasion and homing of EPCs[29].

3.3. Differentiation

Following homing in ischemic tissues, EPCs incorporate into capillaries and small arteries and differentiate into mature endothelial cells. Various cell transplantation experiments employing methods of genetic labeling have demonstrated integration of delivered EPCs into host vessels [2, 30], pointing at the ability of these cells to contribute to the process of tissues vascularization. In these studies, the endothelial phenotype of the transferred EPCs was confirmed, ruling out the possibility of random, non-functional, engraftment of the cells into the growing vessels. The phenotypic characterization of the cells was based mainly on in-situ co-localization of the transferred cells and endothelial typical markers such as VEGFR-2, PECAM-1 and vWF. In some cases, the stability and maturation of EPCs containing-vessel were validated by the recognition of adjacent mural smooth muscle cells or pericytes [31, 32]. Eventually, the exact course of the endogenous conversion of EPCs into mature endothelial cells probably varies from that observed *in vitro* and thus still remains to be further elucidated.

4. Ex-vivo Expansion of EPCs

Cell-based therapy mainly consists of ex-vivo expansion of adult progenitor cells and subsequent systemic or local transplantation of the enriched population. The PB and the BM comprise the major sources for isolation of EPCs. The mononuclear cells (MNCs) fraction can be separated from the general cell population, based on density gradient. EPCs can be then enriched by direct cell sorting (i.e. flow cytometry or magnetic beads), using either a single or combination of antibodies directed against specific surface proteins. Distinct marker-based methods of characterization are currently employed in order to assess and isolate EPCs [2, 33, 3, 6]. However, the quantity and quality of EPCs achieved by sorting methods is frequently limited. Therefore, whole MNCs culture is commonly employed as a starting population for efficient *in-vitro* selective expansion of EPCs. MNCs are plated on fibronectin/collagen coated dishes for 2-3 days and the hematopoietic non-adherent cell fraction is removed. Adherent cells are then maintained in endothelial selective medium supplemented by pro-angiogenic cytokines (ex. VEGF, bFGF, GM-CSF). After 3-5 additional days, early clusters of elongated, spindle shaped attached cells originates and will generally persist for 2 weeks in culture. At days 12-21, a distinct 'late' cell outgrowth appears, characterized by a cobblestone endothelial-like appearance, which rapidly proliferate from colonies to a confluent monolayer [34]. These cells abundantly express markers such as VEGFR2, vWF and CD31 but not hematopoietic or monocyte/macrophage specific cell surface antigen such as CD45 and CD14 [35]. Additionally, these late outgrowth EPCs demonstrate endothelial properties like endocytosis of acetylated low-density lipoprotein and binding of Ulex europaeus agglutinin-1. Based on their paracrine activity, EPCs can be further distinguished by their tendency to secrete soluble angiogenic factors as VEGF, IGF-1 and interleukin 8 [36] and to produce nitric oxide in response to acetylcholine (Ach) or VEGF [2]. Eventually, the function of EPCs is typically confirmed *in vitro* by the ability of the cells to form capillary-like tubes when seeded on matrix components.

5. Induced Mobilization of EPCs

As mentioned above, the hypoxic environment within ischemic tissues endorses cytokine-mediated trafficking and recruitment of EPCs. Consistent with this observation, multiple studies have evaluated the use of various cytokines and growth factors in order to improve the accumulation of EPCs in injured tissues. The factors used for this purpose are angiogenic cytokines, endogenously elevated during ischemia, which exhibit beneficial effects *in vitro* on the proliferation, migration and adhesive capacity of EPCs. One of the major factors employed as a promoter of progenitor cell mobilization for angiogenic therapy is VEGF, the plasma levels of which were found to directly correlate with circulating EPCs number[37,38]. In fact, VEGF administration has been found to efficiently increase EPC levels and consequent neovascularization, both in animal models[39] and pilot clinical trials[19]. Local delivery of SDF-1, an additional key regulator of EPC trafficking, was also shown to improve vessel formation and tissue perfusion by augmenting regional accumulation of EPC[40,18].

Treatment with Erythropoietin (Epo) in various disorders has also been associated with increased levels and improved functional properties of circulating EPCs [20,41].

BM-derived progenitor cell recruitment is also influenced by cytokines that promote granulocyte proliferation and mobilization. Both granulocyte-colony stimulating factor (G-CSF) [42,43] and granulocyte macrophage-colony stimulating factor (GM-CSF)[44] have been shown to induce EPC mobilization from the bone marrow compartment. Additionally, genetic cell-labeling techniques have demonstrated integration of G-CSF and GM-CSF-mobilized progenitors into the growing vasculature of ischemic tissues. These growth factors promote angiogenesis also by stimulating angiogenic factor release from resident cells in ischemic tissue, that further enhance homing of EPCs[45]. Interestingly, combined therapy of G-CSF with bFGF led to an additive increase of capillary networks in mice ischemic limbs, compared to either strategy alone[46]. Likewise, combined treatment with G-CSF/GM-CSF[47] and GM-CSF/SDF-1[31] were found to increase systemic levels of pro-angiogenic factors, subsequently contributing to developing vessels.

Several studies have shown that estrogen modulates the levels of circulating EPCs as well as their mitogenic activity, resulting in enhanced reendothelization and improved vasculoprotective properties of reconstituted endothelium[48,49]. These effects of estrogen were found to be eNOS-dependent (a key regulator of EPC release from the BM[50]), and to occur predominantly through the estrogen alpha and beta receptors[51]. The anti-apoptotic effects of estrogen on EPCs were associated to an increased telomerase activity and enhanced VEGF secretion.

Interestingly, mobilization of EPCs was found to be affected also by some pharmacological agents. The cholesterol-lowering drugs HMG-CoA reductase inhibitors (statins) affect coronary blood flow and myocardial ischemia through unclear mechanisms. Recently, statins were found to stimulate BM-EPC mobilization and EPC-mediated vascularization, comparably to VEGF, leading to improved left ventricular (LV) function after myocardial infarction in mice[52,53]. In a study conducted on type-2 diabetic patients, the PPARgamma-agonist rosiglitazone was shown to increase EPC numbers and enhance their migratory capacity[54]. Similarly, in response to ischemic stress, mice treated with angiotensin-converting enzyme (ACE) inhibitor displayed increased SDF-1 gradient-mediated EPC mobilization with increased angiogenic capacity[55]. These findings could potentially contribute to the understanding of the improved endothelial function evident in these studies.

Finally, several reports have documented the beneficial effects of physical training on EPC numbers. Different terms of endurance training in healthy subjects, as well as in patients with various degrees of coronary artery disease, led to a considerable increase in circulating EPCs[56]. The increase in circulating EPCs was correlated with serum VEGF levels, nitric oxide synthesis or vascular function[57].

6. EPCs AS DIAGNOSTIC MARKERS OF VASCULAR DYSFUNCTION

The pathogenesis underlying a large majority of cardiovascular diseases is associated with endothelial dysfunction[58]. In the presence of hyperlipidemia, hypertension, diabetes or inflammation the blood vessel is predisposed to a permanent disruption of its endothelial integrity. Consequently, the vascular wall is exposed to increased vascular shear stress, leukocyte and platelet adhesion, thrombosis, oxidative stress, smooth muscle proliferation and, eventually, atherosclerotic lesion formation.

6.1. Ischemic Vascular Disorders

It has been hypothesized that risk-factor–induced endothelial dysfunction may eventually lead to the exhaustion of a restricted storage of BM-derived progenitors, which participate in vascular maintenance. This conception is supported by studies which correlate age-associated cardiac morbidity with a reduction and dysfunction of BM-EPCs[59]. The contribution of EPCs to the maintenance of the endothelium was indirectly demonstrated by the evaluation of EPC number and function in patients with cardiovascular disorders, or ones that are prone by having several risk factors. A negative correlation was demonstrated between EPC levels and the occurrence of cardiac events[59,60]. Indeed, circulating EPC number was found to predict vascular reactivity impairment more efficiently than conventional risks factors. Likewise, EPCs isolated from patients with coronary artery disease or multiple cardiovascular risk factors exhibited impaired pro-angiogenic properties with increased senescence, compared to controls[61,62].

Under ischemic conditions, EPC levels in the circulation often rise, apparently as a compensatory mechanism to promote revascularization. Acute myocardial infarction induces EPC mobilization to the blood stream, peaking on day 7, in parallel to the elevation in VEGF plasma levels[37]. Interestingly, the functional improvement and infarct dimension in these patients correlated with the capacity of EPCs to differentiate, as defined by CD31 and VEGFR-2 expression[63]. In chronic heart failure (CHF) patients, the number of EPCs correlate with TNFα plasma levels[64]. Additionally, EPC levels among patients with CHF appear to be independent predictors of all-cause mortality[65]. Elevated EPC number was noted also in patients with unstable angina pectoris, compared to stable angina patients and in association with systemic inflammation[66]. Similarly, in patients with cardiac syndrome X, defined as angina-like chest pains with normal coronary arteries, elevated numbers of EPCs were measured, but with impaired capillary formation capacity, consistent with the impaired endothelial function that is found those patients[67].

Another setting in which the protective effects of EPCs was demonstrated is invasive interventions, such as heart transplantation and percutaneous coronary intervention (PCI). EPCs contributed to endothelial regeneration in murine autologous vein graft model[68] and human cardiac allografts[69]. Complications such as allograft vasculopathy were associated with lower levels of circulating EPCs[68]. Patients undergoing implantation of intracoronary stents also rely on a competent endothelial regeneration, in order to prevent neo-intimal formation followed by in-stent restenosis[70]. In this context, a negative correlation was found between the incidence and severity of diffuse in-stent restenosis and circulating EPC number and adhesiveness. Collectively, these findings point to the potential importance of EPCs in vascular homeostasis and restoration.

6.2. Peripheral Vascular Diseases (PVD)

EPCs are involved also in the pathophysiology of various peripheral vascular diseases (PVD). For example, impaired arterial perfusion, hemoglobin A1C levels and fasting glucose values in diabetes patients negatively correlate with the number and proliferative capacity of EPCs [71, 72, 73]. Additionally, the migratory and adhesive properties of diabetic EPCs are considerably compromised. The underlying mechanisms include overexpression of thrombospondin-1[74] and down-regulated expression of NOS in EPCs as well as inability of diabetic EPCs to respond to VEGF and SDF-1 chemo-attractant signals[75]. Patients with chronic renal failure and essential hypertension were also characterized by a low number and function of EPCs[76]. These observations may partially account for the increased CV disease risk in the patients.

7. Cell-Based Approaches for Therapeutic Angiogenesis

The main rational of BM-based is that increasing numbers of EPCs within ischemic areas could potentially enhance their integration in the growing vasculature and thus improve revascularization. Consequently, the options of transplantation or endogenous mobilization of EPCs have been widely investigated during the last decade.

7.1. Animal Studies

Experimental myocardial infarction studies have shown that transendocardial administration of autologous PB-MNCs[76], PB-CD31$^+$ cells[78] or BM-MNCs[79] accelerate the formation of new vessels in the infarct area and enhance left ventricular ejection fraction (LVEF) 3-6 weeks after implantation. Similar results were achieved in murine myocardial infarction models using injection of autologous BM-MNCs[80] or Lin-/c-Kit+ cells[81]. Additionaly, intramyocardial[82] or systemic[43,77] injection of human CD34$^+$ cells to nude rats was also associated with increased capillary density and cardiac performance.

Transplantation of EPCs was evaluated in animal hind-limb ischemia models. In those studies, both intramuscular injection of autologous BM-MNCs[83] or systemic injection of human PB-MNCs [30, 39, 84] were associated with increased capillary formation and limb rescue. After cerebral ischemia EPCs contributed to the infarct border and choroide plexus neovascularization, despite the complex structure and rare turnover of the cerebral endothelium[85]. Importantly, the ability of progenitor cells to incorporate into sites of neovascularization has been successfully confirmed during those experiments.

EPC-based therapeutic neovascularization has protective effects also in different non-ischemic cardiovascular diseases. Transfer of EPCs to rats with dilated cardiomyopathy (DCM)[86] results in an improved cardiac performance as well as reduced scar tissue and thickened ventricular walls. Beneficial effects were documented also in doxorubicin-induced cardiomyopathy in rats following EPC administration[87]. Interestingly, diabetic neuropathy was also found to be reversed in diabetic nude rats treated with human EPCs[88].

7.2. Clinical Trials

Following the results from animal studies, several groups have conducted clinical trials aiming to evaluate the safety and efficacy of strategies based on progenitor cell transfer or mobilization. The large majority of these trials enrolled either patients with myocardial infarction or no-option cardiac patients and these trials lack of appropriate large, controlled and randomized cohorts. Herein are present the results of several recent, studies some of which included a randomized, double blind designs.

7.2.1. Acute Myocardial Infarction (AMI)

An improvement in cardiac function attained by means of cell-therapy has come from studies using autologous BM-derived cells after AMI. The TOPCARE-AMI (transplantation of progenitor cells and regeneration enhancement in acute myocardial infarction) trial[89] evaluated the efficacy and safety of intra-coronary catheter-based administration of PB-MNCs (n=30) versus BM-MNCs (n=29), in post-MI patients after percutaneous revascularization. In this study, ex-vivo expansion of three days directed more than 90% of the implanted cells towards the endothelial lineage. At 4 months of follow-up, LV angiography showed an increase in ejection fraction and a decrease in end-systolic volumes in both groups. After 12 months, magnetic resonance imaging (MRI) confirmed the evident improvement and showed reduced infarct size, as well as absence of reactive hypertrophy, suggesting a well established functional LV regeneration.

The randomized and controlled BOOST (bone marrow transfer to enhance ST-elevation infarct regeneration) trial [90] tested injection of autologous BM-MNCs in the infract-related artery in 30 post-MI patients, 5 days after coronary stenting. At 6 months follow-up, cardiac MRI revealed enhanced global LV ejection fraction, compared to 30 control patients treated with optimal medical therapy. Likewise, at this time point, cell transfer was associated with an improved LV systolic function predominantly nearby the necrotic myocardium. However, at 18 months follow-up, no long-term benefit on LV systolic function was documented compared with the control group[91]. In another study, this same group[92] demonstrated incorporation of up to 39% of the implanted cells in the myocardium employing fluoro-deoxy-glucose and 3D photon emission tomography imaging.

The REPAIR-AMI (reinfusion of enriched progenitor cells and infarct remodeling in AMI) trial was a multi-center, double-blind, placebo-controlled, randomized study that included 204 patients at 17 different medical centers in Germany and Switzerland[93]. Post-

MI patients (n=58) were randomized to receive an intracoronary infusion of autologous BM-MNCs or placebo, 3 to 6 days after AMI and primary PCI. At 4 months, the cell-treated patient group which started with a baseline ejection fraction of less than 49% or alternately were treated by cell injection 5 days after MI, showed a significant improvement in functional peformance, compared to placebo. Intracoronary Doppler analysis revealed a restoration of microvascular function of the infarct-related artery associated with an improvement in vascular conductance capacity[94]. The study failed to detect a statistically significant difference in clinical end points. However, treated patients exhibited a tendency toward a reduction of the composite of death, MI, or repeat revascularization (21% vs 30%).

Several studies have reported no beneficial effects of BMC transplantation for AMI. For example, one of the main randomized, controlled trial[95] enrolled 47 patients with AMI treated with PCI for intracoronary injection of autologous BM-MNCs and 50 control subjects, in which no injection was performed. After 6 months of follow up, the groups did not differ significantly in LV ejection fraction, LV end-diastolic volume or infarct size and had similar rates of adverse events.

Finally, a recent meta-analysis that evaluated the controlled trials reporting on intracoronary cell therapy in patients with AMI, did report of a marginal although statistically signficant benefit of cell transfer on cardiac function and remodeling[96]. The authors emphasized the need for further multicenter randomized trials to fully evaluate the contribution of intracoronary cell therapy on overall and event-free long-term survival.

7.2.2. Chronic Ischemic Heart Failure

Progenitor cells transfer was utilized also for the treatment of heart failure patients. The examined cohorts in these studies consisted of 5-19 patients and trans-myocardial and intracoronary delivery of BM-derived progenitors was employed[97, 98, 99, 100, 101]. At follow-up periods of 3-12 months, the investigators reported improved myocardial perfusion and oxygen consumption as well as increased left ventricular ejection fraction and wall motion. From the clinical standpoint, several studies reported higher life quality of the patients according to the New York Heart Association (NYHA) classification, namely, less chest discomfort on physical activity. Notably, no significant complications neither ventricular arrhythmias were reported during these trials. Evidently these small studies and their results can, at this stage only regarded anecdotal.

7.2.3. Progenitor Cell Mobilization

As mentioned previously, different cytokines and growth factors induce EPC mobilization and have been shown to have beneficial effects on the progression of ischemic diseases in animal experiments[102]. Subsequently, cytokine-based treatment, mainly G-CSF administration, have been investigated in attempt to circumvent the invasive interventions required for cell transplantation. Two of the different controlled randomized (non-double-blinded) trials[103,104] including 20 and 50 AMI patients tested the effects of subcutaneously injected G-CSF (5-10 µg/kg/day for 4-6 days) compared to placebo. G-CSF promoted mobilization of PB-EPCs. A partial follow-up of 4-6 months revealed an improved left ventricular dimension and function in G-CSF-treated patients.

However, two large cohort studies[105,106] have undermined the former results regarding G-CSF effects. In the STEM-MI (stem cell mobilization induced by subcutaneous G-CSF to improve cardiac regeneration after acute ST-elevation MI) and REVIVAL-2 (regenerate vital myocardium by vigorous activation of BM stem cells) studies, 72 and 114 patients after MI and successful reperfusion by primary percutaneous revascularization entered a randomized, double-blind, placebo-controlled trial, respectively. Patients were randomly assigned to receive either a daily dose of G-CSF treatment (10 µg/kg/day s.c. for 5-6 days) or placebo. At 6 months, both studies concluded that G-CSF did not lead to an improved recovery of ventricular function or infarct size, compared to placebo.

In the MAGIC trial[107], 60 patients with MI who underwent coronary stenting were prospectively randomised into three groups; G-CSF followed by infusion of the collected progenitor cells-enriched PB-MNCs, G-CSF alone, and control group. At 6 months, exercise capacity, myocardial perfusion, and systolic function were improved in patients treated with G-CSF and cell infusion, compared to the other groups. Finally, at 2 years follow-up, the combined therapy was more efficient for cardiac functional rehabilitation and remodeling than G-CSF alone but both groups failed to show significant overall improvement compared to control.

8. POTENTIAL OBSTACLES IN BM-BASED THERAPY

Relying on the accumulating data obtained from the preclinical and clinical studies to this end, clinical implementation of EPC-based therapy will require different hurdles to be addressed. Initially, the phenotype of EPCs will have to undergo standardization in order to properly interpret the results achieved in different studies. Furthermore, as mentioned above, cardiovascular diseases are closely related to impaired function and number of EPCs. Thus, in order to conduct efficient autologous cell-therapy in those patients, improved techniques for ex-vivo expansion will be required.

Different experimental studies were conducted to test the influence of EPCs on the development of the atherosclerosis yielding equivocal results. Most of the data achieved so far originate from experiments with ApoE knockout mice that develop accelerated spontaneous atherosclerosis[108]. Delivery of EPCs isolated from young $ApoE^{-/-}$ mice efficiently prevented plaque progression in adult atherosclerotic $ApoE^{-/-}$ recipients[61]. Conversely, intravenous EPC injection in age-matched $ApoE^{-/-}$ mice model was shown to contribute to atherosclerotic lesion size and decrease plaque stability[109]. Both studies reported EPC engraftment in recipient arteries and an increase in systemic inflammation markers, following cell transfer. Potential explanation may come from studies showing that BM cells may differentiate into smooth muscle cells and contribute vessel wall remodeling[110]. An additional potentially disturbing side effect of cell therapy is of calcifications observed following trans-myocardial implantation of unselected BM cells in a rat MI model[111]. Interestingly, this observation was not noticed using clonally expanded BMCs. There are also conflicting results on the impact of EPCs on allograft vasculopathy[112,113]. Thus, considerable attention should be payed to the phenotype and route of delivery of the transferred cells.

The follow-up periods of the cell therapy clinical trials did not reveal any consistent untoward adverse events, such as pro-arrhythmic effects or myocardial calcification. However, an unexpected, increase of in-stent restenosis and a greater loss of luminal diameter were observed in patients who received G-CSF during the MAGIC trial[107]. The authors hypothesized that BMC differentiation into smooth muscle cells within the stented artery might have contribute to the restenosis. Nevertheless, the following trials addressed this issue and conclude that G-CSF treated patients, following coronary stent implantation, are not likely to develop increased restenosis. An additional concern regarding pro-angiogenic therapies, such as cell transfer or cytokine administration, is related to the occurrence of malignant angiogenic neoplasia or, the vascularization of occult tumors. This point deserves special attention considering the growing evidence supporting the involvement of EPCs in tumor neovascularization[114].

A large part of the clinical trials conducted so far lacked appropriate controls, randomization and blinding and were performed on small cohorts, followed-up for short periods of time. Moreover, discrete cell phenotypes and delivery modes were employed, complicating the evaluation of progenitor cell benefits between studies. Eventually, since the minority of the trials actually followed progenitor's fate within the treated tissues, it is difficult to interpret the true contribution of the cells to the existing cardiac recovery process.

9. Future Prospectives

Various strategies have been proposed in order to enhance the potential contribution of EPCs to the formation of new vessels. Genetic manipulations were recently suggested to modify the expression of angiogenic/anti-angiogenic genes in EPCs. In fact, overexpression of factors, such as VEGF[39], was shown to markedly improve the activity of EPCs. In addition, the use of various biodegradable scaffolds for proper organization and mobilization of EPCs as well as EPC-seeded arterial stents have also gained attention during recent years [115,116]. Eventually, the clinical implementation of standard treatment strategies based on EPC-mediated increase in angiogenesis still demands a more profound understanding of the molecular mechanisms and cellular interactions involved in EPC function. Such an understanding will allow more efficient isolation, *in vitro* manipulations as well as delivery methods of EPCs.

Conclusion

Postnatal bone-marrow contains progenitor cells capable of mobilizing towards peripheral blood and homing to ischemic areas. Subsequently, the cells incorporate into growing vessels and differentiate into mature endothelial cells. The extent of the migration of progenitor cells depends on cytokine gradients and might be controlled by different factors and pharmacological agents. The number and function of EPCs are altered in various cardiovascular pathologies in which vascular dysfunction plays a prominent role. The therapeutic benefit of EPC transfer was demonstrated in numerous animal studies and pioneering clinical trials. Yet, larger, randomized and controlled trials will be required to fully assess the potential safety and efficacy of these progenitor cells for the future treatment of cardiovascular diseases.

REFERENCES

[1] Risau W. Mechanisms of angiogenesis. 1997;386(6626):671-674.
[2] Asahara T, Murohara T, Sullivan A, et al. Isolation of Putative Progenitor Endothelial Cells for Angiogenesis. *Science.* 1997;275(5302):964-966.
[3] Peichev M, Naiyer AJ, Pereira D, et al. Expression of VEGFR-2 and AC133 by circulating human CD34+ cells identifies a population of functional endothelial precursors. *Blood.* 2000;95(3):952-958.
[4] Harraz M, Jiao C, Hanlon HD, et al. CD34- Blood-Derived Human Endothelial Cell Progenitors. *Stem Cells.* 2001;19(4):304-312.
[5] Pelosi E, Valtieri M, Coppola S, et al. Identification of the hemangioblast in postnatal life. *Blood.* 2002;100(9):3203-3208.
[6] George J, Shmilovich H, Deutsch V, et al. Comparative Analysis of Methods for Assessment of Circulating Endothelial Progenitor Cells. *Tissue Engineering.* 2006;12(2):331-335.
[7] Timmermans F, Van Hauwermeiren F, De Smedt M, et al. Endothelial Outgrowth Cells Are Not Derived From CD133+ Cells or CD45+ Hematopoietic Precursors. *Arterioscler Thromb Vasc Biol.* 2007;27(7):1572-1579.
[8] Wang G, Semenza G. Characterization of hypoxia-inducible factor 1 and regulation of DNA binding activity by hypoxia. *J. Biol. Chem.* 1993;268(29):21513-21518.
[9] Eriksson U, Alitalo K. VEGF receptor 1 stimulates stem-cell recruitment and new hope for angiogenesis therapies. *Nat. Med.* 2002;8(8):775-777.
[10] Li B, Sharpe EE, Maupin AB, et al. VEGF and PlGF promote adult vasculogenesis by enhancing EPC recruitment and vessel formation at the site of tumor neovascularization. *FASEB J.* 2006;20(9):1495-1497.
[11] Heissig B, Hattori K, Dias S, et al. Recruitment of Stem and Progenitor Cells from the Bone Marrow Niche Requires MMP-9 Mediated Release of Kit-Ligand. *Cell.* 2002;109(5):625-637.
[12] Kang H-J, Kim H-S, Zhang S-Y, et al. Effects of intracoronary infusion of peripheral blood stem-cells mobilised with granulocyte-colony stimulating factor on left ventricular systolic function and restenosis after coronary stenting in myocardial infarction: the MAGIC cell randomised clinical trial. *The Lancet.* 2004;363(9411):751-756.
[13] Lapidot T. Current understanding of stem cell mobilization: The roles of chemokines, proteolytic enzymes, adhesion molecules, cytokines, and stromal cells. *Experimental Hematology.* 2002;30(9):973-981.
[14] Yoon C-H, Hur J, Oh I-Y, et al. Intercellular Adhesion Molecule-1 Is Upregulated in Ischemic Muscle, Which Mediates Trafficking of Endothelial Progenitor Cells. *Arterioscler. Thromb. Vasc. Biol.* 2006;26(5):1066-1072.
[15] Levesque J-P, Hendy J, Takamatsu Y, et al. Disruption of the CXCR4/CXCL12 chemotactic interaction during hematopoietic stem cell mobilization induced by GCSF or cyclophosphamide. *J. Clin. Invest.* 2003;111(2):187-196.

[16] Hattori K, Heissig B, Tashiro K, et al. Plasma elevation of stromal cell-derived factor-1 induces mobilization of mature and immature hematopoietic progenitor and stem cells. *Blood.* 2001;97(11):3354-3360.

[17] Ceradini DJ, Kulkarni AR, Callaghan MJ, et al. Progenitor cell trafficking is regulated by hypoxic gradients through HIF-1 induction of SDF-1. *Nat. Med.* 10(8):858-864.

[18] De Falco E, Porcelli D, Torella AR, et al. SDF-1 involvement in endothelial phenotype and ischemia-induced recruitment of bone marrow progenitor cells. *Blood.* 2004;104(12):3472-3482.

[19] Kalka C, Masuda H, Takahashi T, et al. Vascular Endothelial Growth Factor165 Gene Transfer Augments Circulating Endothelial Progenitor Cells in Human Subjects. *Circ. Res.* 2000;86(12):1198-1202.

[20] Bahlmann FH, De Groot K, Spandau JM, et al. Erythropoietin regulates endothelial progenitor cells. *Blood.* 2004;103(3):921-926.

[21] Vajkoczy P, Blum S, Lamparter M, et al. Multistep Nature of Microvascular Recruitment of Ex Vivo-expanded Embryonic Endothelial Progenitor Cells during Tumor Angiogenesis. *J. Exp. Med.* %R 10.1084/jem.20021659. 2003;197(12):1755-1765.

[22] Biancone L, Cantaluppi V, Duo D, et al. Role of L-Selectin in the Vascular Homing of Peripheral Blood-Derived Endothelial Progenitor Cells. *J. Immunol.* 2004;173(8):5268-5274.

[23] Nishiwaki Y, Yoshida M, Iwaguro H, et al. Endothelial E-Selectin Potentiates Neovascularization via Endothelial Progenitor Cell-Dependent and -Independent Mechanisms. *Arterioscler Thromb Vasc Biol* 2007;27(3):512-518.

[24] Chavakis E, Aicher A, Heeschen C, et al. Role of {beta}2-integrins for homing and neovascularization capacity of endothelial progenitor cells. *J. Exp. Med.* %R 10.1084/jem.20041402. 2005;201(1):63-72.

[25] Hristov M, Zernecke A, Bidzhekov K, et al. Importance of CXC Chemokine Receptor 2 in the Homing of Human Peripheral Blood Endothelial Progenitor Cells to Sites of Arterial Injury. *Circ. Res.* 2007;100(4):590-597.

[26] Yoon C-H, Hur J, Park K-W, et al. Synergistic Neovascularization by Mixed Transplantation of Early Endothelial Progenitor Cells and Late Outgrowth Endothelial Cells: The Role of Angiogenic Cytokines and Matrix Metalloproteinases. *Circulation* 2005;112(11):1618-1627.

[27] Zucker S, Mirza, H., Conner, C.E., Lorenz, A.F., Drews, M.H., Bahou, W.F., Jesty, J. Vascular endothelial groth factor induces tissue factor and matrix metalloproteinase production in endothelial cells: Conversion of prothrombin to thrombin results in progelatininase a activation and cell proliferation. *International Journal of Cancer.* 1998;75(5):780-786.

[28] Wang H, Keiser JA. Vascular Endothelial Growth Factor Upregulates the Expression of Matrix Metalloproteinases in Vascular Smooth Muscle Cells : Role of flt-1. *Circ. Res.* 1998;83(8):832-840.

[29] Urbich C, Heeschen C, Aicher A, et al. Cathepsin L is required for endothelial progenitor cell-induced neovascularization. *Nat. Med.* 2005;11(2):206-213.

[30] Kalka C, Masuda H, Takahashi T, et al. Transplantation of ex vivo expanded endothelial progenitor cells for therapeutic neovascularization. *Proceedings of the National Academy of Sciences.* 2000;97(7):3422-3427.

[31] Atluri P, Liao GP, Panlilio CM, et al. Neovasculogenic Therapy to Augment Perfusion and Preserve Viability in Ischemic Cardiomyopathy. *Ann. Thorac. Surg.* 2006;81(5):1728-1736.

[32] Shepherd BR, Enis DR, Wang F, et al. Vascularization and engraftment of a human skin substitute using circulating progenitor cell-derived endothelial cells. *FASEB J.* 2006;20(10):1739-1741.

[33] Shi Q, Rafii S, Wu MH-D, et al. Evidence for Circulating Bone Marrow-Derived Endothelial Cells. *Blood.* 1998;92(2):362-367.

[34] Hur J, Yoon C-H, Kim H-S, et al. Characterization of Two Types of Endothelial Progenitor Cells and Their Different Contributions to Neovasculogenesis. *Arterioscler Thromb Vasc Biol* 2004;24(2):288-293.

[35] Yoder MC, Mead LE, Prater D, et al. Redefining endothelial progenitor cells via clonal analysis and hematopoietic stem/progenitor cell principals. *Blood.* 2007;109(5):1801-1809.

[36] Urbich C, Aicher A, Heeschen C, et al. Soluble factors released by endothelial progenitor cells promote migration of endothelial cells and cardiac resident progenitor cells. *Journal of Molecular and Cellular Cardiology.* 2005;39(5):733-742.

[37] Shintani S, Murohara T, Ikeda H, et al. Augmentation of Postnatal Neovascularization With Autologous Bone Marrow Transplantation. *Circulation.* 2001;103(6):897-903.

[38] Gill M, Dias S, Hattori K, et al. Vascular Trauma Induces Rapid but Transient Mobilization of VEGFR2+AC133+ Endothelial Precursor Cells. *Circ. Res.* 2001;88(2):167-174.

[39] Iwaguro H, Yamaguchi J-i, Kalka C, et al. Endothelial Progenitor Cell Vascular Endothelial Growth Factor Gene Transfer for Vascular Regeneration 10.1161/hc0602.103673. *Circulation.* 2002;105(6):732-738.

[40] Yamaguchi J-i, Kusano KF, Masuo O, et al. Stromal Cell-Derived Factor-1 Effects on Ex Vivo Expanded Endothelial Progenitor Cell Recruitment for Ischemic Neovascularization. *Circulation.* 2003;107(9):1322-1328.

[41] George J, Goldstein, E., Abashidze, A., Wexler, D., Hamed, S., Shmilovich, H., Deutsch, V., Miller, H., Keren, G., Roth, A. Erythropoietin promotes endothelial progenitor cell proliferative and adhesive properties in a PI 3-kinase-dependent manner. *Cardiovascular Res.* 2005;68(2):299-306.

[42] Takahashi T, Kalka, C., Masuda, H., Chen, D., Silver, M., Kearney, M., Magner, M., Isner, J.M., Asahara, T. Ischemia- and cytokine-induced mobilization of bone marrow-derived endothelial progenitor cells for neovascularization. *Nat. Med.* 1999;5(4):434-438.

[43] Kocher AA, Schuster MD, Szabolcs MJ, et al. Neovascularization of ischemic myocardium by human bone-marrow-derived angioblasts prevents cardiomyocyte apoptosis, reduces remodeling and improves cardiac function. *Nat. Med.* 2001;7(4):430-436.

[44] Natori T, Sata M, Washida M, et al. G-CSF stimulates angiogenesis and promotes tumor growth: potential contribution of bone marrow-derived endothelial progenitor cells. *Biochemical and Biophysical Research Communications.* 2002;297(4):1058-1061.

[45] Ohki Y, Heissig B, Sato Y, et al. Granulocyte colony-stimulating factor promotes neovascularization by releasing vascular endothelial growth factor from neutrophils. *FASEB J.* 2005:04-3496fje.

[46] Jeon, O., Hwang, K.C., Yoo, K.J. & Kim, B.S. (2006) Combined sustained delivery of basic fibroblast growth factor and administration of granulocyte colony-stimulating factor: synergistic effect on angiogenesis in mouse ischemic limbs. *J Endovasc Ther* 13(2), 175-181.

[47] Bruno S, Bussolati B, Scacciatella P, et al. Combined administration of G-CSF and GM-CSF stimulates monocyte-derived pro-angiogenic cells in patients with acute myocardial infarction. *Cytokine.* 2006;34(1-2):56-65.

[48] Strehlow K, Werner N, Berweiler J, et al. Estrogen Increases Bone Marrow-Derived Endothelial Progenitor Cell Production and Diminishes Neointima Formation. *Circulation.* 2003;107(24):3059-3065.

[49] Iwakura A, Luedemann C, Shastry S, et al. Estrogen-Mediated, Endothelial Nitric Oxide Synthase-Dependent Mobilization of Bone Marrow-Derived Endothelial Progenitor Cells Contributes to Reendothelialization After Arterial Injury. *Circulation.* 2003.

[50] Aicher A, Heeschen C, Mildner-Rihm C, et al. Essential role of endothelial nitric oxide synthase for mobilization of stem and progenitor cells. *Nat Med.* 2003;9(11):1370-1376.

[51] Hamada H, Kim MK, Iwakura A, et al. Estrogen Receptors {alpha} and {beta} Mediate Contribution of Bone Marrow-Derived Endothelial Progenitor Cells to Functional Recovery After Myocardial Infarction. *Circulation.* 2006;114(21):2261-2270.

[52] Llevadot J, Murasawa S, Kureishi Y, et al. HMG-CoA reductase inhibitor mobilizes bone marrow-derived endothelial progenitor cells. *J. Clin. Invest.* 2001;108(3):399-405.

[53] Vasa M, Fichtlscherer S, Adler K, et al. Increase in Circulating Endothelial Progenitor Cells by Statin Therapy in Patients With Stable Coronary Artery Disease. *Circulation.* 2001;103(24):2885-2890.

[54] Pistrosch F, Herbrig K, Oelschlaegel U, et al. PPAR[gamma]-agonist rosiglitazone increases number and migratory activity of cultured endothelial progenitor cells. *Atherosclerosis.* 2005;183(1):163-167.

[55] Wang C-H, Verma S, Hsieh IC, et al. Enalapril increases ischemia-induced endothelial progenitor cell mobilization through manipulation of the CD26 system. *Journal of Molecular and Cellular Cardiology.* 2006;41(1):34-43.

[56] Laufs U, Werner N, Link A, et al. Physical Training Increases Endothelial Progenitor Cells, Inhibits Neointima Formation, and Enhances Angiogenesis. *Circulation.* 2004;109(2):220-226.

[57] Steiner S, Niessner A, Ziegler S, et al. Endurance training increases the number of endothelial progenitor cells in patients with cardiovascular risk and coronary artery disease. *Atherosclerosis.* 2005;181(2):305-310.

[58] Lusis AJ. Atherosclerosis. *Nature.* 2000;407(6801):233-241.

[59] Hill JM, Zalos G, Halcox JPJ, et al. Circulating Endothelial Progenitor Cells, Vascular Function, and Cardiovascular Risk. *N Engl J Med.* 2003;348(7):593-600.

[60] Werner N, Kosiol S, Schiegl T, et al. Circulating Endothelial Progenitor Cells and Cardiovascular Outcomes. *N. Engl. J. Med.* 2005;353(10):999-1007.

[61] Rivard A, Fabre J-E, Silver M, et al. Age-Dependent Impairment of Angiogenesis. *Circulation.* 1999;99(1):111-120.

[62] Rauscher FM, Goldschmidt-Clermont PJ, Davis BH, et al. Aging, Progenitor Cell Exhaustion, and Atherosclerosis. *Circulation.* 2003;108(4):457-463.

[63] Numaguchi Y, Sone T, Okumura K, et al. The Impact of the Capability of Circulating Progenitor Cell to Differentiate on Myocardial Salvage in Patients With Primary Acute Myocardial Infarction. *Circulation.* 2006;114(1_suppl):I-114-119.

[64] Valgimigli M, Rigolin GM, Fucili A, et al. CD34+ and Endothelial Progenitor Cells in Patients With Various Degrees of Congestive Heart Failure. *Circulation.* 2004;110(10):1209-1212.

[65] Michowitz Y, Goldstein E, Wexler D, et al. Circulating endothelial progenitor cells and clinical outcome in patients with congestive heart failure. *Heart.* 2007;93(9):1046-1050.

[66] George J, Goldstein E, Abashidze S, et al. Circulating endothelial progenitor cells in patients with unstable angina: association with systemic inflammation. *Eur. Heart J.* 2004;25(12):1003-1008.

[67] Shmilovich H, Deutsch V, Roth A, et al. Circulating endothelial progenitor cells in patients with cardiac syndrome X. *Heart* 2007;93(9):1071-1076.

[68] Xu Q, Zhang Z, Davison F, et al. Circulating Progenitor Cells Regenerate Endothelium of Vein Graft Atherosclerosis, Which Is Diminished in ApoE-Deficient Mice. *Circ. Res.* 2003;93(8):e76-86.

[69] Simper D, Wang S, Deb A, et al. Endothelial Progenitor Cells Are Decreased in Blood of Cardiac Allograft Patients With Vasculopathy and Endothelial Cells of Noncardiac Origin Are Enriched in Transplant Atherosclerosis. *Circulation.* 2003;108(2):143-149.

[70] George J, Herz I, Goldstein E, et al. Number and Adhesive Properties of Circulating Endothelial Progenitor Cells in Patients With In-Stent Restenosis. *Arterioscler. Thromb. Vasc. Biol.* 2003;23(12):e57-60.

[71] Tepper OM, Galiano RD, Capla JM, et al. Human Endothelial Progenitor Cells From Type II Diabetics Exhibit Impaired Proliferation, Adhesion, and Incorporation Into Vascular Structures. *Circulation.* 2002;106(22):2781-2786.

[72] Loomans CJM, de Koning EJP, Staal FJT, et al. Endothelial Progenitor Cell Dysfunction: A Novel Concept in the Pathogenesis of Vascular Complications of Type 1 Diabetes. *Diabetes.* 2004;53(1):195-199.

[73] Fadini GP, Miorin M, Facco M, et al. Circulating Endothelial Progenitor Cells Are Reduced in Peripheral Vascular Complications of Type 2 Diabetes Mellitus. *J. Am. Coll. Cardiol.* 2005;45(9):1449-1457.

[74] Ii M, Takenaka H, Asai J, et al. Endothelial Progenitor Thrombospondin-1 Mediates Diabetes-Induced Delay in Reendothelialization Following Arterial Injury. *Circ. Res.* 2006;98(5):697-704.

[75] Segal MS, Shah R, Afzal A, et al. Nitric Oxide Cytoskeletal-Induced Alterations Reverse the Endothelial Progenitor Cell Migratory Defect Associated With Diabetes. *Diabetes.* 2006;55(1):102-109.

[76] Choi J-H, Kim KL, Huh W, et al. Decreased Number and Impaired Angiogenic Function of Endothelial Progenitor Cells in Patients With Chronic Renal Failure. *Arterioscler. Thromb. Vasc. Biol.* 2004;24(7):1246-1252.

[77] Kawamoto A, Tkebuchava T, Yamaguchi J-I, et al. Intramyocardial Transplantation of Autologous Endothelial Progenitor Cells for Therapeutic Neovascularization of Myocardial Ischemia. *Circulation.* 2003;107(3):461-468.

[78] Kamihata H, Matsubara H, Nishiue T, et al. Improvement of Collateral Perfusion and Regional Function by Implantation of Peripheral Blood Mononuclear Cells Into Ischemic Hibernating Myocardium. *Arterioscler. Thromb. Vasc. Biol.* 2002;22(11):1804-1810.

[79] Fuchs S, Baffour R, Zhou YF, et al. Transendocardial delivery of autologous bone marrow enhances collateral perfusion and regional function in pigs with chronic experimental myocardial ischemia. *Journal of the American College of Cardiology.* 2001;37(6):1726-1732.

[80] Kobayashi T, Hamano K, Li T-S, et al. Enhancement of Angiogenesis by the Implantation of Self Bone Marrow Cells in a Rat Ischemic Heart Model. *Journal of Surgical Research.* 2000;89(2):189-195.

[81] Orlic D, Kajstura J, Chimenti S, et al. Bone marrow cells regenerate infarcted myocardium. *Nature.* 2001;410(6829):701-705.

[82] Kawamoto A, Gwon H-C, Iwaguro H, et al. Therapeutic Potential of Ex Vivo Expanded Endothelial Progenitor Cells for Myocardial Ischemia. *Circulation.* 2001;103(5):634-637.

[83] Ikenaga S, Hamano K, Nishida M, et al. Autologous Bone Marrow Implantation Induced Angiogenesis and Improved Deteriorated Exercise Capacity in a Rat Ischemic Hindlimb Model. *Journal of Surgical Research.* 2001;96(2):277-283.

[84] Iba O, Matsubara H, Nozawa Y, et al. Angiogenesis by Implantation of Peripheral Blood Mononuclear Cells and Platelets Into Ischemic Limbs. *Circulation.* 2002;106(15):2019-2025.

[85] Zhang ZG, Zhang L, Jiang Q, et al. Bone Marrow-Derived Endothelial Progenitor Cells Participate in Cerebral Neovascularization After Focal Cerebral Ischemia in the Adult Mouse. *Circ. Res.* 2002;90(3):284-288.

[86] Werner L, Deutsch V, Barshack I, et al. Transfer of endothelial progenitor cells improves myocardial performance in rats with dilated cardiomyopathy induced following experimental myocarditis. *Journal of Molecular and Cellular Cardiology.* 2005;39(4):691-697.

[87] Hamed S, Barshack I, Luboshits G, et al. Erythropoietin improves myocardial performance in doxorubicin-induced cardiomyopathy. *Eur. Heart J.* 2006;27(15):1876-1883.

[88] Naruse K, Hamada Y, Nakashima E, et al. Therapeutic Neovascularization Using Cord Blood-Derived Endothelial Progenitor Cells for Diabetic Neuropathy. *Diabetes.* 2005;54(6):1823-1828.

[89] Schachinger V, Assmus B, Britten MB, et al. Transplantation of progenitor cells and regeneration enhancement in acute myocardial infarction: Final one-year results of the TOPCARE-AMI Trial. *Journal of the American College of Cardiology.* 2004;44(8):1690-1699.

[90] Wollert KC, Meyer GP, Lotz J, et al. Intracoronary autologous bone-marrow cell transfer after myocardial infarction: the BOOST randomised controlled clinical trial. *The Lancet.* 2004;364(9429):141-148.

[91] Meyer GP, Wollert KC, Lotz J, et al. Intracoronary Bone Marrow Cell Transfer After Myocardial Infarction: Eighteen Months' Follow-Up Data From the Randomized, Controlled BOOST (BOne marrOw transfer to enhance ST-elevation infarct regeneration) Trial. *Circulation.* 2006;113(10):1287-1294.

[92] Hofmann M, Wollert KC, Meyer GP, et al. Monitoring of Bone Marrow Cell Homing Into the Infarcted Human Myocardium. *Circulation.* 2005;111(17):2198-2202.

[93] Schachinger V, Erbs S, Elsasser A, et al. Intracoronary Bone Marrow-Derived Progenitor Cells in Acute Myocardial Infarction. *N. Engl. J. Med.* 2006;355(12):1210-1221.

[94] Erbs S, Linke A, Schachinger V, et al. Restoration of Microvascular Function in the Infarct-Related Artery by Intracoronary Transplantation of Bone Marrow Progenitor Cells in Patients With Acute Myocardial Infarction: The Doppler Substudy of the Reinfusion of Enriched Progenitor Cells and Infarct Remodeling in Acute Myocardial Infarction (REPAIR-AMI) Trial. *Circulation.* 2007;116(4):366-374.

[95] Lunde K, Solheim S, Aakhus S, et al. Intracoronary Injection of Mononuclear Bone Marrow Cells in Acute Myocardial Infarction. *N. Engl. J. Med.* 2006;355(12):1199-1209.

[96] Lipinski MJ, Biondi-Zoccai GGL, Abbate A, et al. Impact of Intracoronary Cell Therapy on Left Ventricular Function in the Setting of Acute Myocardial Infarction: A Collaborative Systematic Review and Meta-Analysis of Controlled Clinical Trials. *J. Am. Coll. Cardiol.* 2007;50(18):1761-1767.

[97] Fuchs S, Satler LF, Kornowski R, et al. Catheter-based autologous bone marrow myocardial injection in no-option patients with advanced coronary artery disease: A feasibility study. *Journal of the American College of Cardiology.* 2003;41(10):1721-1724.

[98] Tse H-F, Kwong Y-L, Chan JKF, et al. Angiogenesis in ischaemic myocardium by intramyocardial autologous bone marrow mononuclear cell implantation. *The Lancet.* 2003;361(9351):47-49.

[99] Stamm C, Westphal B, Kleine H-D, et al. Autologous bone-marrow stem-cell transplantation for myocardial regeneration. *The Lancet.* 2003;361(9351):45-46.

[100] Perin EC, Dohmann HFR, Borojevic R, et al. Transendocardial, Autologous Bone Marrow Cell Transplantation for Severe, Chronic Ischemic Heart Failure. *Circulation.* 2003;107(18):2294-2302.

[101] Perin E. Transendocardial injection of autologous mononuclear bone marrow cells in end-stage ischemic heart failure patients: one-year follow-up. *International Journal of Cardiology.* 2004;95(Supplement 1):S45-S46.

[102] Minatoguchi S, Takemura G, Chen X-H, et al. Acceleration of the Healing Process and Myocardial Regeneration May Be Important as a Mechanism of Improvement of Cardiac Function and Remodeling by Postinfarction Granulocyte Colony-Stimulating Factor Treatment. *Circulation.* 2004;109(21):2572-2580.

[103] Ince H, Petzsch M, Kleine HD, et al. Prevention of Left Ventricular Remodeling With Granulocyte Colony-Stimulating Factor After Acute Myocardial Infarction: Final 1-year Results of the Front-Integrated Revascularization and Stem Cell Liberation in Evolving Acute Myocardial Infarction by Granulocyte Colony-Stimulating Factor (FIRSTLINE-AMI) Trial. *Circulation.* 2005;112(9_suppl):I-73-80.

[104] Valgimigli M, Rigolin GM, Fucili A, et al. CD34+ and Endothelial Progenitor Cells in Patients With Various Degrees of Congestive Heart Failure. *Circulation.* 2004;110(10):1209-1212.

[105] Ripa RS, Jorgensen E, Wang Y, et al. Stem Cell Mobilization Induced by Subcutaneous Granulocyte-Colony Stimulating Factor to Improve Cardiac Regeneration After Acute ST-Elevation Myocardial Infarction: Result of the Double-Blind, Randomized, Placebo-Controlled Stem Cells in Myocardial Infarction (STEMMI) Trial. *Circulation.* 2006;113(16):1983-1992.

[106] Zohlnhofer D, Ott I, Mehilli J, et al. Stem Cell Mobilization by Granulocyte Colony-Stimulating Factor in Patients With Acute Myocardial Infarction: A Randomized Controlled Trial. *JAMA.* 2006;295(9):1003-1010.

[107] Kang H-J, Kim H-S, Koo B-K, et al. Intracoronary infusion of the mobilized peripheral blood stem cell by G-CSF is better than mobilization alone by G-CSF for improvement of cardiac function and remodeling: 2-Year follow-up results of the Myocardial Regeneration and Angiogenesis in Myocardial Infarction with G-CSF and Intra-Coronary Stem Cell Infusion (MAGIC Cell) 1 trial. *American Heart Journal.* 2007;153(2):237.e231-237.e238.

[108] Zhang SH, Reddick RL, Piedrahita JA, et al. Spontaneous hypercholesterolemia and arterial lesions in mice lacking apolipoprotein E. *Science.* 1992;258(5081):468-471.

[109] George J, Afek A, Abashidze A, et al. Transfer of Endothelial Progenitor and Bone Marrow Cells Influences Atherosclerotic Plaque Size and Composition in Apolipoprotein E Knockout Mice. *Arterioscler Thromb Vasc Biol* 2005;25(12):2636-2641.

[110] Caplice NM, Bunch TJ, Stalboerger PG, et al. Smooth muscle cells in human coronary atherosclerosis can originate from cells administered at marrow transplantation. *Proceedings of the National Academy of Sciences.* 2003;100(8):4754-4759.

[111] Yoon Y-S, Park J-S, Tkebuchava T, et al. Unexpected Severe Calcification After Transplantation of Bone Marrow Cells in Acute Myocardial Infarction. *Circulation.* 2004;109(25):3154-3157.

[112] Hu Y, Davison F, Zhang Z, et al. Endothelial Replacement and Angiogenesis in Arteriosclerotic Lesions of Allografts Are Contributed by Circulating Progenitor Cells. *Circulation.* 2003;108(25):3122-3127.

[113] Hillebrands J-L, Klatter FA, van Dijk WD, et al. Bone marrow does not contribute substantially to endothelial-cell replacement in transplant arteriosclerosis. *Nat. Med.* 2002;8(3):194-195.

[114] Davidoff AM, Ng CYC, Brown P, et al. Bone Marrow-derived Cells Contribute to Tumor Neovasculature and, When Modified to Express an Angiogenesis Inhibitor, Can Restrict Tumor Growth in Mice. *Clin. Cancer Res.* 2001;7(9):2870-2879.

[115] Matsumura G, Miyagawa-Tomita S, Shin'oka T, et al. First Evidence That Bone Marrow Cells Contribute to the Construction of Tissue-Engineered Vascular Autografts In Vivo. *Circulation.* 2003;108(14):1729-1734.

[116] Shirota T, Yasui H, Shimokawa H, et al. Fabrication of endothelial progenitor cell (EPC)-seeded intravascular stent devices and in vitro endothelialization on hybrid vascular tissue. *Biomaterials.* 2003;24(13):2295-2302.

In: Encyclopedia of Stem Cell Research (2 Volume Set) ISBN: 978-1-61761-835-2
Editor: Alexander L. Greene © 2012 Nova Science Publishers, Inc.

Chapter XIX

MESENCHYMAL STEM CELLS IN VASCULAR THERAPY

Gael Y. Rochefort[*]
LAB.P.ART., EA3852, IFR 135, UFR Medecine, Universite François Rabelais, France

ABSTRACT

Mesenchymal stem cells (MSCs) constitute a heterogeneous population of undifferentiated and committed multipotential cells. They serve *in vitro* and *in vivo* as precursors for bone marrow stroma, bone, fat, cartilage, muscle (smooth, cardiac and skeletal) and neural cells. They are able to home upon engraftment to a number of microenvironments, capable of extensive proliferation and of producing large number of differentiated progenitors to repair functionally tissue after injury. MSCs are usually isolated from adult bone marrow but can also be isolated from several other tissues, such as fetal liver, adult circulating blood, umbilical cord blood, placenta or adipose tissue. Furthermore, MSCs present several immuno-regulatory characteristics with immuno-suppressive effects that induce a tolerance and could be therapeutic for reduction of graft-versus-host disease, rejection and modulation of inflammation. Since MSCs follow a vascular smooth muscle differentiation pathway, their therapeutic potential has been widely investigated in the treatment of vascular diseases. Indeed, MSCs can participate in the development of new vessels from pre-existing vascular walls (angiogenesis), in the induction of new vascular networks (vasculogenesis), in the collateral artery growth (arteriogenesis) or in plastic and reconstructive surgery applications. These cells can promote vascular growth by incorporating into vessels' wall, but they also may function as supporting factors by producing paracrine vascular promoting factors. In this chapter, the mesenchymal stem cells isolation, culture and characterization, but also their potential use in vascular therapy, in both human and animal models, are reported and discussed, whereas perspectives in angiogenesis, vasculogenesis, arteriogenesis or vascular engineering are explored.

---

[*] Tel. (+33) 247 366 091; gael.rochefort@gmail.com

I. INTRODUCTION

The biology of stem cells and progenitors is currently one of the most promising fields of investigation, with a very broad potential of application in the field of regenerative medicine. Most of the stem cell and progenitor studies were initially focused on the contribution of a mixed cell population, composed of poorly characterized stem cells among a larger population of support cells, on the tissue regeneration after injection. Next, the specific role of characterized and defined stem cell populations like mesenchymal stem cells (MSCs) was assessed *in-situ* or after local injections, with in particular the role of MSCs during cardiopulmonary remodeling. At last, many recent studies were focused on the stem cell angiogenic potential and on their paracrine action during the initial development of pathologies. This is particularly true in the vascular biology field, where many studies were interested in the participation of various stem cell types, such as MSCs, in angiogenesis and the revascularization of specific organs, like lungs, heart or peripheral vessels.

Arterial remodeling, characterized either by an expansive remodeling (by widening) or by a constrictive remodeling (by a diameter reduction), is an important factor that can be observed under various pathological conditions involving a lot of different cells, such as smooth muscle cells. The origin of the smooth muscle cells in several vascular remodeling is not clearly established. These cells can indeed come from a local proliferation of the smooth muscle cells that are present in the vessel media at the lesion level, but these cells can also come from the differentiation of stem cells or progenitors that are also present in the vessel media or from circulating progenitors. The therapeutic use of stem cells to repair an organ or tissue degenerative lesion becomes thus a very attractive possibility.

Adult stem cells are constitutively present in most tissues and organs, including the skin, lungs, the liver, the heart and the bone marrow, thus authorizing local tissue regeneration during physiological or pathological processes. The bone marrow is composed of hematopoietic stem cells (HSCs) closely associated to a bone marrow stroma responsible for their survival, their proliferation, their self-renewal and their differentiation into mature blood cells. This stromal tissue is mainly made up of stromal cells, which follow a vascular smooth muscle differentiation, osteoblasts, adipocytes and endothelial cells, all deriving from the differentiation of MSCs. These multipotent stem cells have also the capacity to give rise to chondrocytes and to differentiate into other cell types, such as hepatocytes or nervous-related cells. These stem cells represent a heterogeneous population of cells having very variable characteristics according to studies, culture conditions and species. Moreover, MSCs have a strong proliferation potential as well as immuno-modulating capacity allowing these cells to become powerful tools in the treatment of pathologies by cell therapy.

II. WHAT IS A STEM CELL?

A. Definitions and Ontogenesis

Definition: The classic definition of a stem cell is an entity that meets the basic characteristics of self-renewal, clonality, multi-potentiality, generation of differentiated cells, and *in vivo* functional reconstitution of a given tissue [1]. Admittedly, this definition may be satisfactory for embryonic stem cells (ES) or the primordial stem cells, the zygote, but this definition is not applicable in all occurrences and is best used as a guide to help describe cellular attributes.

Indeed, stem cells have varying degrees of potential, ranging from the totipotency (ability to form the whole embryo and its annexes, i.e. the trophoblast of the placenta or the amnios) of the fertilized oocyte (the zygote), to the pluripotency (ability to form all tissues from the three germ layers) of ES cells, to the multipotency (capacity to differentiate into a limited range of cell lineages appropriate to their location) of most tissues derived stem cells, and at last to the unipotency (only able to generate one cell type) of progenitor cells such as intestinal epithelial precursors, gastric epithelial precursors or spermatogonial cells of the testis [2]. Thus, a more complete description of a stem cell includes a consideration of replication capacity, clonality, and potency.

Self-renewal: Stem cells are often described with expressions such as "immortal", "unlimited", "continuous", and "capable of extensive proliferation". All these terms, used to describe the stem cell's replicative or proliferative capacity, must be probably best used sparingly if at all.

Clonality: This important characteristic is the idea that stem cells are clonogenic entities, where a single stem cell has the capacity to create more stem cells with the same capacities. Indeed, the best cellular preparation would be a high purified clonal population of stem cells, but it must be recognized that most cellular stem cell preparations, that do not derive from a single cell, may be a mixed population containing stem cells and a separate population of "supportive" cells required for the propagation of the purported stem cells.

Potency: This basic and widely accepted characteristic is supported by the idea of a lineage hierarchy of each cell type. Thus, the primordial totipotent stem cell generates among other things multipotent stem cells, which then generate multiple types of differentiated cells with distinct morphologies and gene expression patterns.

Plasticity: This idea is based on the fact that restrictions in cell fates are not permanent but are flexible and reversible. In that way, a terminally differentiated somatic cell can be reverse to another committed cell fate by dedifferentiation. A related concept is that of trans-differentiation, where a functional cells from a tissue, organ, or lineage can be generated from another cell type that is distinct from that of the founding stem cell. Important issues are to known whether the cells supposed to dedifferentiate and trans-differentiate are clonal or not, and whether the mechanism by which they form the functional cell requires fusion.

Tissue reconstitution: The best assessment of this characteristic is to purify a population of cells, transplant a single cell into an acceptable host without any intervening *in vitro* culture, and observe self-renewal and tissue, organ, or lineage reconstitution. Admittedly, this type of *in vivo* reconstitution assay is not well defined for many types of adult stem cells, but this developmental potential remains to be accurately defined for *in vitro* assays. Nevertheless, this clonal assay should be the standard by which fetal and adult stem cells should be evaluated because it removes doubts about contamination with other cell types.

Ontogenesis: The concept of stem cells came from the hematopoietic system where the short blood cells lifetime and the high need of renewal require a quick, high and continuous generation of blood cells to avoid aplasia. This blood cells production is provided by the bone marrow hematopoietic stem cells (HSC) that are able to self-renew and to engender the whole blood lineage.

B. Totipotent Stem Cells

The first cell of life, the zygote (the fertilized egg) is also the first totipotent stem cell and has the exclusive ability to generate an entire organism from the three germ layers to the embryonic annexes. This totipotency is retained by early progeny of the zygote up to the eight-cell stage of the morula. Subsequently, cell differentiation results in the formation of a blastocyst composed of two cell types. The first one, the outer trophoblast cells, is composed of multipotent cells and generates the embryonic annexes. Indeed, trophectoderm stem cells have been isolated, and these only generate cells of the trophectoderm lineage. The second cell type, the undifferentiated inner cells commonly referred to as the "inner cell mass", generates ES cells and embryonic germinal stem cells (EG) that are no longer totipotent but pluripotent and retain the ability to develop into all cell types of the embryo proper [3]. ES and EG cells generate all somatic lineages as well as germ cells but rarely if ever contribute to the trophectoderm, extra-embryonic endoderm, or extra-embryonic mesoderm. Importantly, no totipotent stem cell has been isolated from early embryo.

C. Pluripotent Stem Cells

Researches on pluripotent stem cells, which are able to form all tissues from the three germ layers, dates back to the early 1970s with mouse ES cells, and is now widely extended to other species. Pluripotent stem cell lines have been generated from human livestock (review in [4]) but also from model organisms, such as chicken [5, 6], hamster [7], rabbit [8, 9] and rat [10-13]; however, only mouse and chicken ES cells have proven capable of colonizing the germ line. The establishment of ES cell lines from nonhuman primates, including rhesus monkey [14, 15], common marmoset (*Callithrix jacchus* [16]), and cynomolgus monkey (*Macaca fascicularis* [3, 17]) is also of major importance for human stem cell research.

To date, three pluripotent stem cell types have been fully establish, including embryonic carcinoma cells (EC), embryonic stem (ES) cells and primordial germ (PG) cells.

EC: Embryonic carcinoma cells were firstly generated from a mouse germ-line tumor, called teratocarcinomas [18], and were then established as cell lines [19-21] in the early 1970s. This "funny little tumor" produced benign teratomas or malignant teratocarcinomas [22, 23] after transplantation to extra-uterine sites of appropriate mouse strains. When clonally isolated, EC cells retained the differentiation capacity and could produce derivatives of all three primary germ layers, including ectoderm, mesoderm, and endoderm. Furthermore, when introduced into the inner cell mass of early embryos, EC cells were able to participate in embryonic development and to generate chimeric mice [24].

However, EC cells demonstrated chromosomal aberrations [25], lost their ability to differentiate [26], or differentiated *in vitro* only under specific conditions [27] and with chemical inducers such as dimethyl sulphoxide or retinoic acid [28]. The undifferentiated state maintenance was also relied only on cultivation with feeder cells [29]. Furthermore, EC cells only sporadically colonized the germ line after transfer into early blastocysts [30]. All these data suggested that the EC cells had undergone cellular changes during the transient tumorigenic state *in vivo*, and thus partially retain the pluripotent capacities of early embryonic cells (see [31] for review).

ES: Embryonic stem cell lines are originated from the inner cell mass and can be maintained *in vitro* without any apparent or significant loss of differentiation potential, even after several hundred divisions. The demonstration of their pluripotency was made *in vivo* by their introduction into a mouse blastocyst in the early 1980s. The resulting mouse chimera demonstrated that the introduced ES cells could contribute to all cell lineages including the germ line [32]. *In vitro*, mouse ES cells also showed the capacity to generate various somatic cell types from the three germ layers [33-35]. ES cells were finally found to generate germ cell lines *in vitro* only in the early 2000s [36-38]. ES cells are characterized by the high proliferation ability, by *in vitro* differentiation capacities [39], by the presence of stem cell markers typical of other stem cell lines, and by the capacity to erase gene imprints.

PG: The third embryonic cell type with pluripotent capabilities is the primordial germ cells, which form normally within the developing genital ridges. Isolation and cultivation of mouse PG cells on feeder cells led to the establishment of mouse embryonic germ cell lines [40-42]. Once transferred into blastocysts, these cells can contribute to somatic and germ cell lineages in chimeric animals [40-43]. Finally, PG cells retain the capacity to erase gene imprints.

D. Multipotent Stem Cells

Multipotent stem cells have the fundamental capacity to differentiate into a limited range of cell lineages appropriate to their location. Most tissues derived stem cells self-renew and generate single stem cell-derived daughter cells that are able to differentiate *in vitro* and *in vivo* into more than one cell type. Several examples are now known, include hematopoietic stem cells (HSC), neural stem cells (NSC), endothelial progenitor cells (EPC), or mesenchymal stem cells (MSC). Multipotent stem cells also contribute to the generation of differentiated progeny *in vivo* even in the absence of tissue damage [44].

HSC: Hematopoietic stem cells, the first tissue-specific stem cells to be prospectively isolated [45], are one of the most stem cells used in routine clinical, with extensive use of grafts and transplantations in the treatment of a variety of blood cell diseases such as leukemias or autoimmune disorders [46]. In fact, HSCs were extensively reported to repopulate the tissue of origin when transplanted in a damaged recipient. In the hematopoietic system, HSCs reside at the top of the hematopoietic hierarchy and give rise to several functional cells. All these distinct types are produced from HSCs in successive differentiation processes, producing intermediary increasingly committed progenitor cells. Because of the very short life span of most cells, mature blood cell production is an ongoing process and the estimated production reaches 1.5×10^6 blood cells every second in an adult human. In that case, this high turnover rate necessitates profound homeostatic control mechanisms where the primary level is the HSC itself.

EPC: As epithelial tissue comprises 60% of the differentiated tissue types in mammals, epithelial stem cells and EPCs need to reach a high proliferative potential when a broad array of diseases, injuries and wounds are surrounded [47]. EPCs were first identified in the late 1990s as a population of postnatal mononuclear blood cells that adopted an adherent, endothelial morphology when cultured for 7 days in endothelial growth medium [48]. Like endothelial cells, these isolated cells incorporated acetylated DiI-LDL, expressed several markers in common with endothelial cells such as CD34, CD31, vascular endothelial growth factor receptor 2 and Tie2. To date, the circulating EPC contributions to angiogenesis in tumors, ischaemic injury or other diseases, and their usefulness in the repair of wounded hearts and limbs remain under intense investigation.

NSC: Neural stem cells can generate neural tissue or are derived from the nervous system, have the ability to self-renew, and can generate other cells than themselves through asymmetric cell division [49]. Neural stem cells are more frequent in the developing mammalian nervous system but are retained in the adult nervous system of all mammalian organisms, including humans. A variety of neural dysfunctions are now candidates for NSC-based cell therapy, including many neurodegenerative diseases such as Parkinson's disease, Alzheimer's diseases, and genetic disorders such as Batten's, Gaucher's, and Tay Sach's diseases. The potential for tissue repair is not restricted to the replacement of neurons, and a promising approach is the generation of oligodendrocytes from stem cells to promote repair in diseases such as multiple sclerosis [50].

MSC: mesenchymal stem cells are multipotent stem cells that can be differentiated into several cells types, including fibroblasts, osteoblasts, chondroblasts, and adipocytes. More information regarding this multipotent cell type is given below.

E. Unipotent Stem Cells

Unipotent stem cells are probably best described as progenitors. Indeed, progenitors are typically the descendants of stem cells; they are more constrain in their differentiation potential or capacity for self-renewal and can only produce one type of differentiated descendant that is no more a stem cell. Intestinal epithelial precursors, gastric epithelial precursors or satellites cells, which conduct to the formation of muscle fibers, are some example of progenitors.

F. Between Differentiation and Self-Renewing: The Stem Cell Niche

The first stem cell niche, the bone marrow HSC niche, was first formally laid by Schofield in 1978 after an analysis of findings on the spleen colony-forming cell (CFU-S) [51]. Schofield proposed that stem cells are fixed tissue cells that are prevented from differentiation and continue to proliferate as stem cells within a functionally and spatially characterized "niche", where the micro-anatomic environment, composed of neighboring stromal cells, supports and instructs stem cells. However, the stem cell niche concept was largely neglected until its recent resurgence with Drosophila studies [52].

A stem cell niche is an interactive structural unit, composed of tissue cells, extracellular substrates and micro-environmental cells that nurture stem cells and enable them to maintain their undifferentiated state capacities and tissue homeostasis [53]. An appropriate spatio-temporal dialog occurs between stem cells and niche cells in order to fulfill lifelong demands for differentiated cells and to facilitate cell-fate decisions in a proper spatiotemporal manner. Niche cells provide a sheltering environment that sequesters stem cells from differentiation, apoptotic, or other stimuli that would challenge stem cell reserves. The niche also safeguards against excessive stem cell production that could lead to cancer. Stem cells must be periodically activated to produce progenitors or transit amplifying cells that are committed to produce mature cell lineages. Thus, the hallmark of a functional niche is to maintain a balance between stem cell quiescence and activity, with key signaling and molecular cross-talk events that occurred in the right place at the right time [54, 55]. Interactions with other cell types and the components of the extracellular matrix are believed to control the stem cell survival and self-renewal, the progeny production and the generation of the committed cells.

G. Stemness

The core stem cell properties of self-renewal and common molecular processes underlying the generation of differentiated progeny are referred in the literature by "stemness". Although stems cells in different cellular microenvironments or niches will by necessity have different physiological demands and therefore distinct molecular programs, there are likely certain genetic characteristics specific to and shared by all stem cells.

Stem cells appear to have the capacity to sense a broad range of growth factors and signaling molecules and to express many of the downstream signaling components involved in the transduction of these signals, including TGFβ, Notch, Wnt, and Jak/Stat family members. Stem cells also express many molecules according to the establishment of their specialized cell cycles. Thus, most quiescent adult stem cells express compounds related to maintaining cell cycle arrest, whereas stem cells rapid cycling, as is the case for example for ES cells, depends on molecules connected to progression through cell cycle checkpoints. There is considerable evidence that stem cells express high levels of telomerase enzyme and with higher activity, and present significantly remodeled chromatin involving DNA methylases or transcriptional repressors of histone deacetylase. Finally, most stem cells have the molecular and functional characteristic to be resistant to stress mediated by the expression of multi-drug resistance transporters, protein-folding machinery, ubiquitin, and detoxifier systems [3].

Identification of cell surface and molecular markers has proven critical to define the molecular basis of stem cell balance between self-renewal and determination/commitment toward lineages. In the future, it may be possible to define stem cells as a whole and individually entity by their molecular identities, and thus to precisely describe the stemness concept [3].

III. MESENCHYMAL STEM CELLS

A. Origin

1. Historical Identification

Mesenchymal stem cells (MSC) were first identified by Alexander Friedenstein who described undifferentiated progenitors cells in adult bone marrow [56-58]. When seeding at low density in liquid medium containing serum, bone marrow cells from rabbits or rodents, formed after few days discrete colonies containing plastic-adherent, non phagocytic, elongated cells that resemble to fibroblasts. Such colony being generated from a single cell was called colony-forming unit-fibroblasts (CFU-F). When seeded individually under the renal capsule of semi-syngeneic animals, each colony generated after a few weeks fibrous tissue, bone and bone-containing bone marrow. Friedenstein also observed by using chimerical animals that fibrous tissue and bone cells were of donor origin, while marrow hematopoietic cells within the bony spaces were provided by the host. He hypothesized that the bone marrow contains a population of progenitors capable to generate *in vivo* fibrous tissue and bone, and that the CFU-F-generated bone-containing tissue express cellular and/or molecular components proving the adequate microenvironment for HSC homing and growth. Friedenstein was thus the first to conjecture the existence of stem cell niches within the bone marrow.

Then in the early 1990s, Arnold Caplan defined MSCs as cells that would give rise not only to bone and marrow stroma, but also to cartilage, tendon, and muscle [59]. During the course of the years, these cells received several designations and abbreviations. Maureen Owen used in 1988 the term of "Stromal Stem Cells" to underline the fact that MSCs are generated from the stromal layer of long-term bone marrow cultures [60, 61]. In 1997, Darwin Prockop proposed that the abbreviation of MSC could stands for either "Mesenchymal Stem Cell" or "Marrow Stromal Cell", because of their capacity to serve also as niche for other types of stem cells such as HSCs [62]. James Dennis used in 1999 the term of "Mesenchymal Progenitor Cell" to indicate that this cell type may not represent an authentic category of stem cells but be closer to progenitor/transit amplifying cells situated downstream of the stem cell compartment [63]. Pamela Gehron Robey and Paolo Bianco used in the early 2000s the term of "Skeletal Stem Cell" to emphasize the specificity for MSCs to give rise to the different cellular components of skeletal tissues [64-67]. Finally, Catherine Verfaillie's team described a cell population that may represent a more primitive cell type with differentiation potential larger than that of MSCs, and they designated it as "Mesodermal Progenitor Cells" [68] and "Multipotent Adult Progenitor Cells" (MAPCs) [69].

2. Source

a) Various Species

MSC, or progenitor cells with similar features, can be isolated from many different species.

The best characterized are those of human [67, 70-75], murine [76-78] and rat [79-81] origin but MSCs from guinea pigs, cats [82], baboons [83], sheep [84], dogs [85], pigs [86,

87], cows [88] and horses [89, 90] provide a better opportunity to test their therapeutic potential in large mammal systems.

b) Tissue Localization

MSCs are widely distributed with a variable proportion in several fetal and adult tissues. However, MSCs are often a rare population in these tissues.

Adult bone marrow: The most well studied and accessible source of MSCs is the adult bone marrow [70, 76, 78, 91]. MSCs are a rare population of the bone marrow microenvironment, present in a low frequency that may represent 0.01-0.0001% of the adult human bone marrow nucleated cells [74, 75].

Other adult tissues: To date, cells with mesenchymal stem cell characteristics were isolated from several tissues such as spleen [92], liver [92, 93], kidney [92], pancreas [92, 94], lung [92], smooth muscle [92], skeletal muscle [91, 95, 96], aorta [92], vena cava [92], brain [92], thymus [92], dental pulp [97], deciduous teeth [96], scalp tissue and hair follicle [98, 99], periosteum [95, 96], trabecular bone [96], adipose tissue [95, 96, 100] and synovium [95, 96].

Fetal tissues: MSCs have also been isolated from several fetal tissues including fetal liver [101-103], fetal bone marrow [102, 103], fetal thymus [104], fetal lung [102], fetal spleen [102] and fetal pancreas [105]. MSCs can also be isolated with a variable proportion from several parts of the placenta including chorionic villi of the placenta [73-75, 106], amniotic fluid [107], umbilical cord blood collections [108] and umbilical cord vein [72, 109].

Blood sample: Blood samples are of particular importance because of the facility to be obtained. Thus, MSCs were described in the peripheral blood of normal adults [71, 110] and healthy women during or following pregnancy [111], where they may be of fetal origin and may persist for more than 60 years [56, 112]. MSCs can also been isolated from fetal blood [71, 103] and from fresh umbilical cord blood [108, 113, 114] and cryopreserved cord blood [115].

c) Mobilization

The term of mobilization indicates the recruitment into the bloodstream after treatment (chemotherapy, cytokine injection) or physiopathological events, and the enhancement of the physiological release of stem cells and progenitors from reservoirs, such as the bone marrow, in response to stress signals during injury and inflammation. Currently, mobilized cells are the preferable and major source of stem and progenitor cells because of the higher yield of these cells and decreased procedural risks compared with harvested BM cells [116]. Less known than the HSC mobilization, the MSC specific mobilization process might be initiated by repeated stimulation with cytokines such as granulocyte colony-stimulating factor (G-CSF) or granulocyte-macrophage colony-stimulating factor (GM-CSF) [110, 117, 118], or recently by several physiopathological circumstances, such as chronic hypoxia [79], myocardial infarction or encephalopathy [119].

Thus, after injection of G-CSF during the development of hypoxic encephalopathy in mice, MSCs were found mobilized in the blood system, homed into damaged zones and committed into specialized elements [119]. After myocardial infarction and G-CSF treatment in lethally irradiated mice, MSCs were found mobilized and expressed cardiomyogenic markers [120]. Finally, chronic hypoxia has been shown to increase the circulating concentration of MSCs without increasing the circulating hematopoietic progenitor cells concentration [79].

B. Culture

1. Isolation

There are as many different isolation procedures as there are tissue sources, species and publications, but we have summarized the MSC procedure outlines.

The bone marrow-derived MSCs are obtained from bone shafts. Typically, cells are aspirated into a syringe containing anticoagulant, wash with medium or with phosphate-buffered saline and cultured at a density of 10^4 to 10^5 cells/cm^2. The first change of medium is performed between 2 and 3 days after initial plating and adherent cells are cultured during 2 to 3 weeks until they reach 80%–90% confluence. Tissue-derived MSCs are usually obtained after enzymatic digestion. The tissue is washed several times, mechanically minced and then enzymatically digested (with trypsin and/or collagenase). Digested tissue is filtered through cell strainer to eliminate undigested fragments, washed and then cultured at a density of 10^5 to 10^6 cells/cm^2. At last, blood-derived MSCs (from umbilical cord blood or from peripheral blood) are obtained after a low-density fraction separation (e.g. Ficoll). The mononuclear cell fraction is washed and then cultured at a density of 10^6 to 10^7 cells/cm^2.

Some authors also optimize their isolation procedures with a subpopulation fraction enrichment (depletion or enrichment), with red cells disruption, with dish coating (e.g. fibronectin, gelatin or collagen), or with growth factor and cytokine supplementation.

2. CFU-F

Contributions to our understanding of stromal precursor cells were provided by Friedenstein, Owen, and colleagues. Indeed, they demonstrated the growth of colonies of cells morphologically resembling to fibroblasts when single cell suspensions of bone marrow were explanted at low densities (10^4 to 10^5 cells/cm^2). In liquid cultures generated from single-cell suspensions, colonies were formed, each derived from a single precursor cell termed the colony-forming-unit fibroblast (CFU-F) and described as rapidly adherent, non-phagocytic clonogenic cells capable of extended proliferation in vitro [58, 121]. When these cells were plated at higher densities, the colonies merged early and grew as monolayer.

To visualize and enumerate CFU-F, cells are usually stained with Giemsa solution, washed and then air-dried. CFU-F colonies are typically between 1 and 8mm in diameter and are scored macroscopically.

3. A Heterogeneous Population

When grown *in vitro* in fetal calf serum, culture-expanded MSCs form characteristic adherent, fibroblast-like colonies that may be expanded further in the presence of various growth factors [122, 123] and thus appear to be homogeneous according to a number of criteria. The morphology is usually that of elongated cells with, in particular in murine cultures, thin filopodial extensions. However, the homogeneity of the cultured cell population depends on culture conditions.

Initial cell growing populating is consisted of cells with two different morphologies: one population with a fibroblastic, spindle-shaped morphology and another with an epithelioid, polygonal morphology. After passaging, the epithelioid population disappears rapidly from culture and it is no longer found thereafter. The fibroblastic population of cells continues to proliferate, even after numerous passages [75]. These single-cell derived colonies are morphologically heterogeneous and contain a mixture of small and larger cells [68, 124]. The proliferative activity of MSC appears to be directly proportional to their differentiation potential but both cell types are similarly efficient in supporting cultures of hematopoietic stem cells [56]. Small cells, about 7μm in diameter and spindle-shaped with large nuclear-to-cytoplasmic ratio, are in the G0-G1 phase of the cell cycle and, after a lag phase, these cells rapidly renew; whereas large cells, about 15μm in diameter and widespread, slowly renew [124, 125]. The selection of adherent cells by day 2-4 [70] and the passages, required to get rid of contaminating hematopoietic cells (usually 1-2 passages for human, but 4-6 for murine cultures), may lead to a more homogeneous population.

The population heterogeneity is better assessed on freshly isolated cells or, at least, on cells cultured for short spans of time. The proliferative capacity and differentiation potential heterogeneity were greatly revealed by clonal studies of human bone marrow cells. Thus, Pittenger and co-workers [70] but also Muraglia and collaborators [126] both proved that only one third of the human MSC clones studied were tripotential and were able to differentiate into osteoblasts, chondrocytes and adipocytes, whereas the clones generated by the team of Phinney differed widely in their expression of alkaline phosphatase, an osteoblast marker [76]. In 2002 and using immortalized human MSCs, Okamoto *et al.* found that only a minority of the generated clones were multipotential [127]. At last, the generation of bone-like tissue *in vitro* did not appear to reflect the capacity of forming bones *in vivo* [128] and only 50% of these clones had the ability to form bone *in vivo* [123]. However, this apparent heterogeneity is not translated into a distinctive and specific phenotype (see below) and only few phenotypical studies report heterogeneity. Thus, Gronthos and collaborators used the membrane expression of alkaline phosphatase within a human Stro-1$^+$ MSC subset to discriminate a population of cells with a restricted differentiation potential into osteoblastic cells [129]. Finally, the human STRO-1$^+$ MSC subpopulation was also reported to have a higher engraftment potential in spleen, bone marrow and kidneys, a lower engraftment potential in lungs, and a lesser hematopoiesis-supportive capacity than the Stro-1$^-$ MSC subset [130].

Taken together, all these data indicate that MSCs constitute a heterogeneous cell population that may reflects a hierarchy of stem and transit amplifying cells as described for HSCs. In 2000, Muraglia *et al.* proposed a hierarchy model based on clonogenic studies, where early tripotent mesenchymal progenitors display a sequential loss of lineage potentials and generate osteo-chondrogenic progenitors, which, in turn, give rise to osteogenic precursors [126].

4. Phenotype

To date, no specific immuno-phenotypic markers have been identified to allow the phenotypic isolation of MSCs, but in contrast, MSCs express a wide variety of antigens presented by many other cell types. Therefore, the MSC identification is based on an extensive panel of markers, including differentiation and lineage specific markers, adhesion molecules, extracellular matrix, and growth factor receptors [122, 131, 132]. MSCs are most homogeneously accepted positive for CD13, CD29, CD44, CD49a, CD49e, CD73 (SH3 and SH4), CD90, CD105 (SH2), CD106, CD166 and HLA ABC but are negative for the hematopoietic and/or endothelial markers CD31, CD34, CD45 and HLA DR [70, 74, 133, 134]. Nevertheless, few antigens appear to be present on cell subsets only [135, 136], and to add confusion to the issue of MSC specific markers, there are evidences that some molecules are variably expressed depending on time in culture and the extent of MSC multipotency [56, 137].

C. Properties

1. Growth and Self-Renewing

The proliferation potential: In vitro, human CFU-Fs show extensive proliferation capacity, giving rise to colonies that can reach several millimeters in diameter, but the MSC proliferation is restricted by the Hayflick's limit of 50 cell doublings [70, 138], with shortened telomeres and lacking telomerases [139]. Although, when transfected with the catalytic unit of the telomerase, MSCs then obtained are displaying improved proliferation, hematopoiesis-supportive capacity and differentiation potential *in vitro* [131, 140]. *In vivo*, extensive proliferation can be observed only in models with intense mesenchymal turnover such as osteogenesis imperfecta [141].

Tritiated thymidine continuous labeling of fresh bone marrow harvested cell reveals that CFU-Fs are not cycling *in vivo* [57], and their subsequent development into colonies and their entry into the cell cycle depend on serum growth factors *in vitro* [142]. In fact, higher cell doublings might be achieved when adding specific growth factors (e.g., fibroblast growth factor-2) to the basal culture medium [143]. Cell seeding density also plays a critical role in the MSC expansion capacity, because a higher expansion profile (2,000-fold expansion) is obtained when MSCs are plated at very low density (1.5-3 cells/cm^2) whereas a lower expansion profile (60-fold expansion) is observed when cells are plated at higher density (12 cells/cm^2) [124].

The self-renewal capacity: This ability to generate identical copies of themselves through mitotic division over extended periods is one of the defining characteristics of a stem cell and the MSC absolute self-renewal potential remains unclear, due in large part to the different methods employed to derive MSC populations. *In vitro*, some CFU-Fs can be expanded many times, and *in vivo*, ossicle formation capacity is transferable for up to five passages [144]. However, the demonstration of the self-renewal capacity of multipotential cells can be made only in models with sufficient and systemic cell renewal such as osteogenesis imperfecta. To date, there are no experiments in such models where cells from reconstituted tissues (e.g. cartilage, bone, or other tissues) from a primary recipient were injected into a secondary recipient to show that the multipotential reconstituting activity had been maintained in the primary recipient and transferable to the second.

2. The Bone Marrow Microenvironment and Hematopoiesis Support

The bone marrow hematopoiesis niche can be subdivided into a hematopoietic cell compartment and a stroma compartment, which is mainly composed of fibroblasts, adipocytes, nerves, and the bone marrow's vascular system [54, 56]. However, mesenchymal cells are always found in fetal liver and in fetal bone marrow as early as 9 weeks of gestation before the onset of definitive hematopoiesis [145-148]. MSCs are also reported to circulate in fetal blood in high numbers from at least 7 weeks gestation. The circulating fetal MSC rate is at its highest level early in the first trimester and declines to around 0.0001% during the second trimester [103]. Thus, MSCs might contribute to the establishment of hematopoiesis [56].

The supporting role of marrow stromal cells in hematopoiesis was firstly evidenced by Friedenstein, who reported the formation of bone-like structures ("ossicles") when marrow stromal cells were transplanted under the capsule kidney, and where the donor stroma was colonized by hematopoietic cells deriving from the host [149]. Furthermore, donor HSCs engrafted in the host stromal microenvironment during clinical bone marrow transplantation *in vivo*, whereas MSCs supported hematopoiesis *in vitro* for periods longer than 6 months in Dexter cultures [150] and thus allowed the generation of all lineage, including myeloid, lymphoid, and megakaryocytic cells [56].

The hematopoietic bone marrow microenvironment is composed of osteoblasts and their extra-cellular products, adipocytic cells and several ad-luminal mural stromal cells with smooth muscle characteristics, including endothelial cells, capillary pericytes, parasinusal myoid cells, adventitial reticular cells, barrier cells [54, 151-155]. All these cells might derive from MSCs since they are able to differentiate into osteoblasts, adipocytes, vascular smooth muscle-like stroma, and more controversially into endothelial cells [156, 157].

3. Lineage Differentiation

During the embryonic development, the neuron-ectodermal lineage gives rise to the peripheral and central nervous systems, but also to the epithelial lineage which will become epidermal tissue, and partially to muscles (muscles of the iris, the arrector pili muscles attached to hairs, and the myoepithelial cells of the lacrimal, salivary, sweat and mammary glands) [158, 159]. Mesoderm gives rise to muscles (skeletal, cardiac, visceral and vascular smooth muscles), bone, cartilage, blood and connective tissue [160]. Pancreas and liver cells derive from the endoderm layer [3, 161, 162].

a) Mechanism

Adult stem cells are able to differentiate into cells of the tissue in which they reside; however, this committed fate dogma has been extended during the last few years with several evidences for the multi-lineage differentiation potential of many stem cell types including MSCs [163]. In fact, MSCs are not only able to differentiate into limb-bud mesodermal tissues, including osteoblasts, chondroblasts, adipocytes, fibroblasts and skeletal myoblasts [62, 70, 133, 164, 165], but they are also able to acquire characteristics of cell lineages outside the limb-bud, such as endothelial cells [69, 166], neural cells [167-169], and cells of the endoderm [1, 69, 170, 171], *in vitro* and *in vivo* [172-174].

In the early 2000s, Markus Loeffler and his team proposed a single cell-based stochastic model to describe the stem cell organization and to explain the cell kinetic and functional stem cell heterogeneity, flexibility and reversibility of cellular properties, self-organized regeneration after damage, fluctuating activity and competition of stem cell clones, and microenvironment dependency of stem cell quality [175-177]. To illustrate the flexibility and reversibility concept, they postulated that stem cells might change their proliferative status, change their lineage specification, lose and subsequently re-acquire their self-renewal potential. In fact, the MSC differentiation potential does not appear to be an irreversible process because cells apparently terminally differentiated may shift their differentiation pathway when placed in specific *in vitro* conditions [178]. Thus, for examples adipocytes may turn into osteoblasts, osteoblasts into chondrocytes, chondrocytes into adipocytes, and so on [179].

This lineage reversibility does not result from the selection of a subset because it has been reported at the single cell (clonal) level; and furthermore several lineage characteristics are reported to be expressed at the same time indicating an intermediate state between several lineages. Indeed, MSCs express simultaneously, at the mRNA or protein level, adipocytic and chondrocytic and/or osteoblastic or vascular smooth muscle markers [178], but also present structures specific for vascular smooth muscle cells and adipocytes [180]. This property of plasticity, implying de-differentiation and reprogramming, might be explained by the stimulation of several distinct lineage-specific transcription factors already activated in primitive stem cells and thus by making cells receptive to extrinsic factors (hormones, cytokines, cell contacts…).

Recently, the bone marrow stem cells trans-differentiation was discussed after the observation of spontaneous fusion of stem cells to adopt the phenotype of the recipient cells. Moreover, cell fusion is reported to be a frequent rather than rare event and up to 1% of human MSCs were recovered as bi-nucleated cells [181, 182]. However, other studies demonstrated that stem-cell plasticity is a true characteristic of stem cells and can be achieved without cell fusion [173, 183].

Whatever the degree of differentiation of the cell undergoing the differentiation shift, plasticity has major functional consequences: it removes the theoretical requirement of hierarchy and self-renewal since it makes possible for a daughter cell to recover the full differentiation potential of the mother MSC at the origin of the clone.

b). Ectodermal Tissues

The ectoderm is the start of a tissue that covers the body surface. It emerges first and forms the outermost of the germ layers. The ectoderm forms several tissues, including the central nervous system, retina and lens, cranial bones, ganglia and nerves, pigment cells, head connective tissue, epidermis, hair, mammary glands.

Skin-related tissue: The skin, perhaps the largest organ in the body, is composed by three layers, the dermis, the epidermis and the hypodermis, and has several physiological functions. Indeed, skin keeps organs in place, stops pathogens entering, helps in the prevention of getting burnt, prevents unregulated water loss, is almost waterproof, is sensitive to touch and pain, regulates body temperature through homeostasis, makes vitamin D and melanin, and finally has an excretory role in removing urea.

When co-cultured directly or indirectly with heat-shocked human sweat gland cells, human MSCs differentiate into gland cells. Indeed, carcinoembryonic antigen, a specific marker of the sweat gland which is not expressed elsewhere in the normal skin [184, 185], and cytokeratin 19, a structural protein of intermediate filaments which is expressed in both ductal and secretory cells of normal human sweat glands [184], are both expressed by MSCs after both the direct and indirect co-culture differentiation conditions [186]. When implanted subcutaneously into nude mice, human MSCs produce E-cadherin and contribute to the development of hair follicles by forming epithelial-like cells *in vitro* and *in vivo*, by following a mesenchymal to epithelial transition [187, 188]. Furthermore, the hair follicle may represent a suitable, accessible source for MSCs [99, 187].

Like other stem cells, MSCs are also widely and successfully used in the treatment of extensive wounds and deep burn injury [189, 190]. Indeed, the transplantation of bone marrow MSCs allows the regeneration of the dermis in wound healing and the reduction of scar formation [191-193]. In addition, MSCs are able to migrate *in vivo*, proliferate and differentiate into either matrix epithelial cells (which form the hair shaft) or cornified keratinocytes (which form skin) in response to epidermal damage [187]. At last, here are several protocols that allow stem cells to differentiate into the keratinocyte lineage *in vitro* [194].

Central nervous system-related tissue: During the brain development, neurons migrate from the neural tubes and differentiate into various neural cells and satellite cells. It has long been established that mature neurons lack their proliferation potential, but in 1992, Reynolds and Weiss [195] isolated for the first time the multipotential stem cells from the striatum of adult human brain and induced them into neural cells *in vitro*. Although further researchers showed that only a very few sites, such as the sub-ventricular zone, may contain neural stem cells (NSC), this discovery necessitated revision of classical assumptions of neuronal theory and problems associated with regeneration. Indeed, NSCs are present in the brain during the entire life span of mammals and humans; they can be isolated and differentiated into all three types of neural cells. NSCs might offer some wonderful perspectives for cell therapy of neurodegenerative diseases and injuries of the central nervous system, but on the other hand, the problems of immunological compatibility of allogeneic NSCs remain unsolved, as are the ethical problems. Recently, MSCs were reported to possess the potential of *in vitro* differentiation into NeuN-expressing neurons and astrocytes expressing glial fibrillary acidic protein (GFAP) when cultured under appropriate conditions [168], but also *in vivo*, after implantation into the brain tissue [167, 169].

As a matter of fact, MSCs were reported to express neural markers at baseline [196-198], and their neural differentiation into glial and neuron-like cells can be easily obtained after co-culturing with NSCs or with stimulating culture media and factors [196-203], whereas some groups failed to show glial and neural markers [204, 205]. Several methods of induction were developed to differentiate human or rodent MSCs into neuron-like cells [168, 196, 204, 206], including combinations of different growth factors and retinoic acid [207]. MSCs thus acquired new morphological characteristics, neural markers, and electrophysiological properties compatible with a neuronal differentiation [208].

After infusion into a rat brain, MSCs can engraft, migrate and survive without any evidence of an inflammatory response or rejection [202]. Injected MSCs react to brain microenvironment signals, differentiate into glia and neurons [202, 203], and promote restoration and regeneration of the nervous tissue after brain or spinal cord injuries [203, 209-211].

Eye-related tissue: The retinal pigment epithelium (RPE) is the pigmented cell layer just outside the retina that contains retinal visual cells, and is firmly attached to the underlying choroid and overlying retinal visual cells. The RPE is composed of a single layer of hexagonal cells that are densely packed with pigment granules. When viewed from the outer surface, these cells are smooth and hexagonal in shape. When seen in section, each cell consists of an outer non-pigmented part containing a large oval nucleus and an inner-pigmented portion, which extends as a series of straight thread-like processes between the rods, this being especially the case when the eye is exposed to light.

When co-cultured *in vitro* with retina or sub-retinal cells, or when cultured with epidermal growth factor and activin A, MSCs were able to generate cells expressing markers for photoreceptors like opsin [212], rhodopsin and recoverin [213]. Recently, MSCs were also reported to have the ability to adopt a RPE-like morphology *in* vivo after sub-retinal grafting into normal adult rats and into RPE degenerative rat model. MSCs thus adopted the hexagonal morphology of RPE cells, and expressed the epithelial marker cytokeratin after transplantation [214]. Finally, MSCs made contacts with adjacent recipient cells, expressed the tight junction protein ZO-1 [215], and retinal cell-specific markers including calbindin and rhodopsin [216].

c) Mesodermal Tissues

The mesoderm germ layer is forming in triploblastic animals during gastrulation, where some of the cells migrating inward to contribute an additional layer between the endoderm and the ectoderm. The formation of a mesoderm led to the formation of a coelom where organs formed inside can freely move, grow, and develop independently of the body wall while fluid cushions protects them from shocks. The mesoderm forms several tissues, including skeletal muscles, skeleton, dermis of skin, connective tissue, urogenital system, heart, blood (lymph cells), and spleen.

Adipocytic lineage: The primary role of adipocytes is to store energy and to break down this stored lipid into free fatty acids when energy is required. Adipocytes also play a major role in the control of metabolism through secretion of paracrine and endocrine hormones that have effects on feeding behavior, metabolism, insulin sensitivity and secretion, and reproductive and immune functions [217]. Finally, adipose tissue has a major impact on energy flux, plasma lipid levels, and rates of glucose uptake.

During the embryonary development, the adipose lineage arises from a multipotent stem cell population of mesodermal origin residing in the vascular stroma of adipose tissue, and undergoes a multi-step differentiation process, comprising an initial commitment step and then a subsequent activation program resulting in the adipocyte phenotype. Factors that initiate this process are now identified and secreted by the vascular stromal population and/or adipocytes. These factors are now used *ex vivo* to induce the commitment of MSCs to the adipose lineage [218, 219].

MSCs express small amounts of the crucial transcription factors that promote adipogenesis, such as CCAAT-enhancer-binding protein α (C/EBPα) and peroxisome proliferator-activated receptor γ (PPARγ) [220-224], but also osteogenic factors such as RUNX2, MSX2, DLX5, and osterix [225-227]. As factors of one lineage repress factors of the other lineages, thereby maintaining the undifferentiated state, the balance may be tipped under appropriate conditions leading to a cascade that promotes one cell fate while repressing other possible fates. Indeed, RUNX2 represses adipogenesis, and furthermore cells with suppressed Runx2 show enhanced adipocyte development [228], whereas mice lacking PPARγ have increased bone mass while PPARγ agonists decrease bone density in normal mice [229-231].

C/EBPα and PPARγ proteins, already present in uncommitted MSCs [232, 233], may be induced after the treatment with a differentiation cocktail and promote the adipocytic differentiation [234]. Insulin is classically viewed as a promoter of adipogenesis when using low concentrations, whereas high concentrations of insulin activate the IGF-I receptor, have a mitogenic effect and slightly inhibit adipogenesis [235]. Serums, insulin, dexamethasone, indomethacin and 3-isobutyl-1-methylxanthine (IBMX) are thus classically used to induce the differentiation of MSCs into the adipose lineage. Then, the adipogenic differentiation is usually shown by cellular accumulation of large lipid vacuoles, visualized after Oil Red O staining that has an excitation wavelength of 485 and an emission wavelength of 595 nm. The gene and protein expression of all factors that are involved in regulation of the differentiation process during adipogenic conversion may also be assessed by reverse-transcription and Western blotting [79, 236-238].

Osteogenic lineage: Bones are rigid organs that form part of the skeleton of vertebrates. One of the first functions of the skeleton is to hold up the body and supports muscles and soft organs. Bones enclose and protect the brain, spinal cord, lungs, heart, pelvic viscera and bone marrow. Bones provide the rigid attachment and leverage that allow skeletal muscle movements. Red bone marrow is the major producer of blood cells, including most cells of the immune system. The skeleton is also the body's main mineral reservoir; it stores calcium and phosphate and releases them according to the body's physiological needs. Finally, bones buffer the blood against excessive pH changes by absorbing or releasing alkaline mineral salts.

During early development, neural crest cells give rise to the cranio-facial skeleton whereas the axial skeleton (spine, sternum, rib cage) is derived from sclerotome cells that came from somites, and finally, the lateral-plate mesoderm give rise to the appendicular skeletal components (limbs) [239]. In the postnatal state, cells with osteogenic potential like MSCs persist in the bone marrow and play an integral part in bone growth and remodeling, as well as bone repair. After migration of cells with osteogenic potential (mesenchymal cells) to the site of future skeletogenesis, the process of bone development is followed by mesenchymal-epithelial interactions that lead to condensation or aggregation of MSCs and subsequent differentiation into either the chondrogenic or osteogenic lineage.

Thus, several strategies were extensively used to direct the *in vitro* differentiation of MSCs into the osteogenic and chondrocytic lineages for tissue repair [134, 240, 241]. The first of them was to develop a defined culture medium for directing osteogenic differentiation of MSCs *in vitro*. Thus, several exogenous cytokines and growth factors were used, including various isoforms of bone morphogenic protein (BMP) which are all members of the transforming growth factor-β (TGF-β) superfamily [242-245], interleukin-6 (IL-6) [246], growth hormone [247], leptin [248], sortilin [249], and transglutaminase [250]. In addition to cytokines and growth factors, several non-proteinaceous chemical compounds have also been used to promote stem cell differentiation into the osteogenic lineage *in vitro*, including prostaglandin E_2 (a natural eicosanoid) [251, 252], 1,25-dihydroxyvitamin D3 (the active form of vitamin D3 also known as calcitriol) [253], L-ascorbic acid (vitamin C) [254], dexamethasone (a synthetic steroid) [254-257], β-glycerol phosphate [257], the synthetic potent inducer TAK-778 [258, 259], and statins [260-262]. Another strategy to direct osteogenic differentiation of MSCs *in vitro* was to co-culture the stem cells with a different stem cell population. Indeed, co-culture with chondrocytes is reported to have a positive effect on the osteogenic differentiation of MSCs [250, 263, 264], but also co-culture with myeloma cells [265], vascular endothelial cells [266, 267], calvarial dura mater cells [268, 269], non-adherent bone marrow cells [270] and differentiated osteoblasts [254, 262], bone sialoprotein [271], osteopontin [272], osteocalcin [273], osteonectin [254] and osteocrin [274].

To promote osteogenic differentiation *in vivo*, MSCs were firstly seeded *in vitro* on extracellular matrices such as hydroxyapatite and then subcutaneously implanted *in vivo* into NOD/SCID mice, subsequently observing bone formation [275]. Next, MSCs were used to repair segmental bone defects of critical size in various animal models, including rabbit, sheep, rat, mice, goat, pig and dog [276-285]. Then, MSCs infused *in situ* into irradiated mice with osteogenesis imperfecta were able to promote the formation of functional bone and cartilage [141]. Similarly, with children suffering of osteogenesis imperfecta, infused MSCs were not only able to engrafted without any side effect, but they also increased the osteoblast number three months after, the formation of new lamellar bone and the total body mineral content [286]. After that and especially for orthopedic applications, natural or synthetic biomaterials were used as carriers for MSC delivery [287], with the use of nonporous, biologically inert materials (ceramics or titanium), and porous, resorbable and osteoconductive biomaterials (hydroxyapatite and tricalcium phosphate) [288, 289]. The next step was to use cell-matrix compounds, composed of MSCs seeded on hydroxyapatite/ tricalcium phosphate ceramics [290] or poly-L-lactide-co-glycolide [291], which were successfully used *in vivo* to repair critical segmental bone defects in animals but also in humans with large bone defects [292], to reconstruct a phalanx [293], or to repair a mandible [294].

Chondrogenic lineage: Cartilage is a type of dense connective tissue composed of collagenous fibers and/or elastic fibers, and chondrocytes, all embedded in a matrix of gel-like ground substance. Cartilage is avascular and serves several functions, including providing a framework for bone deposition, and supplying smooth surfaces for the movement of articulating bones. Cartilage is found in many places in the body including joints, rib cage, ear, nose, bronchial tubes and between inter-vertebral discs. During embryonic development, cartilage is enclosed in a dense connective tissue called the perichondrium, which also contains the cartilage cell precursors (chondroblasts), and is afterward replaced by bone (ossification) or remains unossified during the whole of life (joint cartilage).

To promote the chondrogenic differentiation of MSCs *in vitro*, two different strategies were adapted from the original method of the "pellet" culture system [295, 296]. This system is based on the aggregation of MSCs into a conical tube and the culture of pelleted cells with a defined serum-free medium. Indeed, "alginate bead" culture system, that maintained the differentiated phenotype of encapsulated cells over times, allows freshly isolated articular chondrocytes but also MSCs to synthesize *in vitro* a matrix similar to that of native articular cartilage and to maintain their chondrogenic phenotype for as long as eight months [297-299]. The second strategy to induce chondrogenesis *in vitro* is to allow MSCs to form a compact cell pellet in conical tubes (by gently centrifugation) and to incubate them with a chemically defined serum-free medium, consisting of high-glucose Dulbecco modified Eagle medium supplemented with insulin, transferrin, selenious acid, linoleic acid, ascorbate 2-phosphate, dexamethasone and TGF-β [295, 296]. The chondrogenic differentiation is finally checked by the Safranin O or toluidine blue specific staining of cartilage glycosaminoglycans on formalin-fixed paraffin or resin embedded aggregates, whereas up-regulation of both type II and X collagens is also usually confirmed.

In vivo, undifferentiated MSCs have been used to repair full-thickness, joint cartilage defects in animal models using various carrier matrices [300-304] since local injections of chondrocyte suspension inducing clinical benefits were described [305], allowing the development of MSC-based strategies to induce *in situ* differentiation of mesenchymal progenitors into cartilage [306, 307]. Thus, evidence of regeneration of the injured knee meniscus after medial menisciectomy and resection of the anterior crucial ligament was observed when allogeneic MSCs were injected into goats in combination with hyaluronan carrier [308]. Furthermore, goats treated in that way showed a significant decrease of bone resorption with subchondral bone remodeling, osteophyte formation and cartilage destruction, and a better preservation of the joint lining, without any signs of inflammation or immune rejection [308]. This kind of cartilage regeneration is also reported in rabbit with the full reparation of joint cartilage defect after injection of autologous MSCs dispersed in a type I collagen gel [302], or with the reparation of osteochondral defects after injection of MSC-loaded phosphate and hyaluronan deriving from sponges [309]. Like with the osteogenic lineage differentiation, the chondrogenic differentiation is promoted when using poly-L-lactic acid and poly-L-lactide-co-glycolide synthetic polymers [310, 311]. In a rat model, MSCs have been successfully used to repair intervertebral discs after local injection with a reported 100% cell viability [312]. Autologous MSC injection was also successfully realized to treat patients with osteoarthritis [303], showing the feasibility of MSC therapy for cartilage repair in human.

Finally, the mostly effective strategy to treat joint cartilage defects might be to use the combination of bioactive tridimensional matrices and scaffolds, osteoinductive growth factors and cytokines (such as the bone morphogenetic protein-2), and injection of MSCs [313-317].

Tendon: A tendon is a tough band of fibrous connective tissue that connects muscle to bone, or muscle to muscle and that is designed to withstand tension. Tendons are similar to ligaments except that ligaments join one bone to another. Tendons and muscles work together and can only exert a pulling force. Tendons are composed mainly of water, type-I collagen and tenocytes or tendinocytes, which are inactive fibrocytes. Minor fibrillar collagens, fibril-associated collagens and proteoglycans are present in small quantities and are critical for tendon structure. Most of the strength of tendon is due to the vertical, hierarchical arrangement of densely packed collagen fibrils. Tenocytes are specialized fibroblasts responsible for the maintenance of collagen structure; they produce collagen molecules that aggregate end-to-end and side-to-side to produce collagen fibrils. Blood vessels may be visualized within the endotendon running parallel to collagen fibers, with occasional branching transverse anastomoses. After tendon injury, rehabilitation and repair are long processes that could easily last eight to twelve weeks. During this time, immobilization and protected motion are required because the inability to return to full function early puts the healing tendon at risk of complications.

Recently, several animal and human studies have evaluated the efficiency of MSC local injections in tendon repair [318, 319]. Indeed, local injection of autologous MSCs in a type I collagen gel significantly improved tendon repair [320]. Unexpectedly almost 30% of the MSC grafted tendons demonstrated evidences of ectopic tendon formation in the regenerating repair site [320], but unfortunately, the maximum force and maximum stress for the MSCs grafted repairs were only around 30% of normal control [320]. When implanted into long gap defects in the rabbit Achilles tendon, biochemical and histological analysis revealed that MSCs collagen composites improved biomechanical properties, tissue architecture and functionality of the tendon after injury [321]. Furthermore, 12 weeks after surgery, the repaired tissue presented a modulus and maximum stress around one third of normal values [321].

Tendon and ligament tissue regeneration may be enhanced by using exogenous growth or differentiation factors (GDF), members of the TGF-beta factor super-family implicated in tendon formation, including GDF-5, GDF-6 and GDF-7 [322]. Scaffold alone, but also scaffolds seeded with poly-lactide-co-glycolide have also the potential to regenerate and repair gap defect of Achilles tendon and to restore structure and function [323, 324]. MSC viability in culture, but also biomechanics and histological appearance 12 weeks after surgery, may as well be improved by have an adequate cell-to-collagen ratio (around 40.10^3 cells/mg collagen) [325]. Finally, 12 weeks after surgery, biomechanics and cellular organization of patellar tendon repairs may be significantly improved by the introduction of MSCs into a gel-sponge composite, and by the mechanical stimulation with a matched strain signal [325].

Skeletal muscle lineage: Skeletal muscle is the contractile and voluntary tissue of the body deriving from the mesodermal layer. Its function is to produce force and cause motion, either locomotion or movement within internal organs. The skeletal muscle cell or fiber, which is the main compound of the muscle, contains myofibrils and sarcomeres, composed of actin and myosin. Muscle fibers, surrounded by endomysium, are bound together by perimysium into bundles called fascicles, whereas bundles are enclosed in a sheath of epimysium and grouped together to form muscle. The body musculature, composed of approximately 650 muscles in the human body, is thus arranged in discrete muscles and attached to skeletal tissue by tendons.

Skeletal mature muscles also contain mononuclear progenitor cells, referred as satellite cells, which are localized between the basal lamina and sarcolemma. Satellite cells are able to re-enter the cell cycle, to differentiate and fuse to augment existing muscle fibers and to form new fibers. These cells are involved in the normal growth of muscle, as well as regeneration following injury or disease [326, 327]. In addition to satellite cells, others progenitor cells, known to be involved in muscle regeneration, are present in skeletal muscle [328, 329]. Indeed, side population progenitors, MSCs and HSCs may play a role during the muscle regeneration process [330-332]. Furthermore, several studies have reported that MSCs have the potential to differentiate into muscle fibers but also to contribute to the replenishment of the satellite cell compartment [333-337].

In vitro, differentiation of MSCs into skeletal muscle cells may be obtained after incubation with various chemical compounds, including 5-azacytidine, basic fibroblast growth factor, forskolin, platelet-derived growth factor or neuregulin [81, 211, 338-340], but also vascular endothelial growth factor, insulin-like growth factor [338] or amphotericin B [76, 341]. During the skeletal differentiation process, adjacent MSCs fused, formed multinucleated myotubes [64, 76, 341-343] and express several markers, including Pax3, Pax7, Myo-D, myogenin, Myf5 and the myogenic regulatory factor 4 [64, 338, 339, 344, 345]. Finally, after differentiation *in vitro*, MSCs were able to differentiate into contractile myotubes [333, 346]. Although the conversion of MSCs into skeletal muscle cells *in vitro* is a rare event [338], this allows the establishment of the differentiation mechanism and thus allows a better understanding of the regeneration muscle process performed by satellite cells, particularly in the awareness of the local signals released by damaged muscles [81].

Differentiation of MSCs into skeletal muscle was also widely reported after infusion *in vivo*. Ferrari et al. thus have demonstrated for the first time in 1998 that, after infusion, BM-derived stem cells (i.e. a majority of HSC) migrate into muscle degeneration areas, differentiate into myogenic cells contribute to the skeletal muscle regeneration [334]. After that, Gussoni *et al.* reported that infused adult BM stem cells in the mdx mouse, an animal model of Duchenne's muscular dystrophy, were able to migrate into skeletal muscles, incorporate and partial restore the dystrophin expression in the affected muscle [328]. This benefit from HSC transplantation to restore muscle structure and function has opened several perspectives in the treatment of congenital skeletal muscle defects, such as muscular dystrophy and other myopathies, and numerous authors have intended to explore the specific muscle restoration potential of MSCs *in vivo* [172, 347]. Adult MSCs contributed to myofibers, restored sarcolemmal expression of dystrophin, acted as long-term persisting functional satellite cells when administrated into mdx mouse muscle and thus providing evidences for their potential clinical use in human Duchenne muscular dystrophy [337, 348], but also during muscle regeneration after injury [347]. Although, like *in vitro*, the *in vivo* conversation of MSCs into satellite cells or skeletal muscle only occurs in a limited amount of fibers, varying between less than 1 and to a maximum of 10% [349-352], all data clearly indicated a significant muscle regeneration providing hopes for the treatment of muscle degenerative disorders using MSCs transplantation therapy.

Cardiac muscle lineage: Cardiac muscle is a type of involuntary mononucleated and striated muscle found exclusively within the heart. Its function is to pump blood through the circulatory system by contracting. Whereas skeletal muscle contracts in response to nerve stimulation, cardiac muscle is myogenic and is able of self-excitable stimulating contraction without a requisite electrical impulse coming from the central nervous system. Indeed, an isolated cardiac muscle cell will contract rhythmically at a steady rate, and if two or more cardiac muscle cells are in contact, whichever one contracts first will stimulate the other to contract, and so on. This transmission of impulses is allowed by specialized intercellular connections, called intercalated discs, which conduct electrochemical potentials directly between the cytoplasms of adjacent cells via gap junctions. Since cardiac muscle is myogenic, specialized pacemaker cells in the sinoatrial node normally determine the overall rate of contractions, with an average resting pulse of 72 beats per minute, and serve only to modulate and coordinate contractions. This inherent contractile activity is heavily regulated by the autonomic nervous system. Thus, the central nervous system does not directly create the impulses that contract the heart, but only sends modulatory signals to speed up (sympathetic nervous system) or slow down (parasympathetic nervous system) the heart rate. If synchronization of cardiac muscle contraction is disrupted for some reason (e.g. during a heart attack), uncoordinated contraction can result, leading to fibrillation.

The cardiovascular system begins to develop during the third week in human embryonic development, in the extra-embryonic mesoderm of the yolk sac. Thus, blood islands in the splanchnopleuric mesoderm of the yolk sac wall begin to anastamose and form the initial vascular network. After that, embryonic vasculature, forming a primitive vascular network, extends towards and anastamoses to establish a primitive circulatory system. The heart is thus materialized initially in the embryonic disc as a simple paired tube inside the forming pericardial cavity. When the embryonic disc folds, the embryonic heart is carried into the correct anatomical position in the chest cavity, whereas small regions differentiate into "blood islands" throughout the mesoderm, which supply both blood vessels (walls) and fetal red blood cells. A key aspect of heart development is the septation of the heart into separate chambers. Indeed, the initial primitive heart tube develops a series of constrictions and expansions, and then loops and folds into a characteristic "S" shape, whereas it is internally divided by septae into four separate chambers.

After birth, the adult mammalian heart is not able to regenerate extensively the large number of cardiomyocytes lost after diseases (e.g. infarction). After adaptative mechanisms, such as hypertrophy that is initially beneficial but becomes detrimental at the end, the only curative option is the heart transplantation that is limited by donor availability and transplant rejection. Thus, stem cell-based strategies, including differentiation of stem cells or reactivation of resident myocardial cells, are currently investigated for their potential to reconstitute the myocardium and regenerate the heart.

Several studies have shown that MSCs, once exposed to a variety of physiologic or non-physiologic stimuli, differentiate into cells displaying several features of cardiomyocytes-like cells [333, 342, 353-359]. Thus, after culturing with chemicals, including 5-azacytidine, amphotericin B or oxytocin, or after co-culturing with cardiomyocytes, *in vitro* differentiated MSCs exhibit a myotubes-like structure spontaneously beating. The cardiomyocytes-like phenotype was demonstrated by the exhibition of a characteristic ultrastructure with typical sarcomeres, atrial granules and a centrally positioned nucleus, and by the production of peptides and the expression of multiple structural and contractile proteins, including myosin heavy chain, beta-actin, desmin, phospholamban, adrenergic and muscarinic receptors, connexin 43, titin, and troponins C, I and T [342, 354-361]. Thus, co-culture experiments demonstrated that a cell-to-cell contact with cardiomyocytes *in vitro* might relay a "cardiac environmental signals" that promote extensively the MSC differentiation into a cardiomyogenic lineage [358, 359, 362, 363]. At last, differentiated MSCs into cardiomyogenic lineage cells display gap junction with a cell-to-cell coupling, but also sinus node–like and ventricular cell–like action potentials [333, 364, 365].

In vivo, injected MSCs can be tracked with the help an iron fluorophore-particle labeling and the use of magnetic resonance fluoroscopy, or using after transfection with a tag gene (e.g. luciferase or GFP). Indeed, after cardiac damage, injected MSCs into the myocardium of experimental models (e.g. myocardial cryoinjury, infarction) were able to engraft, to differentiate into cardiomyocytes and induce angiogenesis [342, 366-370]. Furthermore, some groups have reported improved cardiac function and myocardial perfusion after injection of autologous MSCs in a myocardial infarction pig model [355, 366, 367]. Following animal studies, the first randomized clinical trial assessing the effect of intra-coronary infusion of autologous BM-derived progenitor cells was carried out in 2004. Sixty patients with myocardial infarction were thus enrolled and 30 of them received autologous BM cells. After 6 month, the left ventricular systolic function was enhanced, with increased left ventricular ejection fraction and reduced end-systolic volume, only in the BM cell group, without adverse clinical events (e.g. pro-arrhythmic effects or in-stent restenosis) [371]. Also in 2004, another randomized clinical trial was carried out in 69 patients with acute myocardial infarction. Thirty-four of them received an intra-coronary injection of autologous BM-derived MSCs during the percutaneous coronary intervention procedure. Three months after, the left ventricular function was improved in the BM-derived MSC injection group, with an improved left ventricle perfusion and decreased perfusion defects, suggesting that MSCs may improve the ventricle remodeling by supplying viable cardiomyocytes or paracrine factors [372]. Finally, Miyahara and colleagues have reported in 2006 that purified and fully characterized MSCs were able to form a thick striatum containing newly formed vessels, undifferentiated cells and few cardiomyocytes, after transplantation onto the coronary ligated scarred myocardium, and improved cardiac function [373].

Hematopoietic supporting stroma and vascular-smooth muscle-like lineage: In the bone marrow, the structural and physiological support for hematopoietic cells is provided by the bone marrow stroma, which consists of a heterogeneous population of cells following a vascular smooth muscle cell differentiation pathway [374]. Within the bone marrow stromal niche, MSCs provide cell contacts and release growth factors, chemokines and extracellular matrix molecules that regulate the survival, self-renewal, migration and differentiation of HSCs into all hematopoietic lineages [56].

In fact, MSC-derived long-term cultures but also immortalized stromal lines express cytoskeletal and extracellular matrix proteins specific for vascular smooth muscle cells [375-380]. The earliest reported and constitutively expressed markers in culture are the α-smooth muscle actin (ASMA) and the fibronectin isoforms, both strongly express in smooth muscle cells [381-383]. Then, other cytoskeletal vascular smooth muscle cell-specific markers appear later, including vinculin, metavinculin, h-caldesmon, l-caldesmon, h1-calponin, SM22α and smooth muscle actinin [380-382, 384]. Finally, when fully differentiated into a vascular smooth muscle cell phenotype, MSCs express contractile protein, including desmin and smooth muscle myosin heavy chain 1 and 2 [384]. MSCs also express extracellular matrix proteins observed on vascular smooth muscle cells, including thrombospondin and laminin [380, 384]. Indeed, MSC differentiation in culture appears to recapitulate the developmental program of vascular smooth muscle cells differentiation.

Kidney and urogenital-related tissues: Part of the urinary system, the kidneys are bean-shaped excretory organs in and filter wastes (such as urea and uric acid) from the blood and excrete them, along with water, as urine. The kidneys also regulate the pH, by eliminating H ions concentration, the water composition of the blood, and the plasma volume. They regulate the blood pressure by a homeostatic process involving the rennin-angiotensin system and aldosterone. At last, the kidneys secrete a variety of hormones, including erythropoietin, urodilatin and vitamin D.

In humans, the two kidneys are located in the posterior part of the abdomen on each side of the spine, with the right just below the liver and the left below the diaphragm and adjacent to the spleen. An adrenal gland (also called the suprarenal gland) is found above each kidney. Kidney development, also called nephrogenesis, proceeds from the intermediate mesoderm through a series of three successive phases, each marked by the development of a more advanced pair of kidneys. The first of them, the pronephros, appears approximately on day 22 of human gestation and is considered nonfunctional in mammals because it cannot excrete waste from the embryo. The second, the mesonephros, is similar to the kidneys of aquatic amphibians and fishes. At last, the third, the metanephros, develops during the fifth week of gestation to form the ureteric bud, the metanephric duct and the ureter, and undergoes a series of branching to form the collecting duct system of the kidney [385].

The kidneys may be affected by several congenital diseases and disorders, including congenital hydronephrosis, congenital obstruction of urinary tract, duplicated ureter, horseshoe kidney, polycystic kidney disease, renal dysplasia or unilateral small kidney, and acquired diseases and disorders, including diabetic nephropathy, glomerulonephritis, hydronephrosis, interstitial nephritis, kidney stones, kidney tumors, lupus nephritis, nephrotic syndrome, pyelonephritis or renal failure. In the early 2000s, some experiments have reported that BM-derived cells were able to give rise to renal cells *in vitro* and *in vivo* [386]. Indeed, after transplantation of GFP-labeled BM-derived cells (i.e. a majority of HSCs), Imasawa *et al.* but also Ito *et al.* were able to trace and localized the GFP-positive cells in glomeruli, in the periglomerular space, and in the kidney interstitium, and to demonstrate that BM-derived cells differentiate into mesangial cells [387, 388]. After detection of Y chromosome in female kidney after sex-mismatched transplantation, Poulsom *et al.* and Krause *et al.* reported that BM cells exhibited a tubular epithelial phenotype, expressed the epithelial markers CAM5.2 and may thus partially contribute to the renal cell turnover [389, 390]. Then, the MSC contribution in kidney remodeling was first suggested by Iwano *et al.* and El Kossi *et al.* [391, 392]. Then, the presence of cytokeratin expressing and Y chromosome containing tubular epithelial cells in female kidneys of male recipients was confirmed *in vivo* supporting the hypothesis that extra-renal stem cells participate in the injured kidney regeneration [393]. After intravenous infusion, MSCs were monitored *in vivo* [394, 395], engrafted into the damaged kidney and differentiated into tubular epithelial cells, thereby restoring renal structure and function after acute renal failure [174, 396, 397].

d) Endodermal Tissues

Endoderm is one of the germ layers forming the inner layer of the gastrula during animal embryogenesis. Endoderm forms several tissues, including whole digestive tube epithelial lining (excepting part of the mouth, pharynx and the terminal part of the rectum, which are lined by involutions of the ectoderm), all digestive tube glands lining cells (liver and pancreas), auditory tube epithelium, tympanic cavity, trachea, bronchi, and lungs air cells, urinary bladder, thyroid gland follicles and thymus.

Gastrointestinal tract related tissues: The gastrointestinal tract is the system of organs that takes in food, digests it to extract energy and nutrients, and expels the remaining waste. The major functions of the gastrointestinal tract are digestion and excretion. The gastrointestinal tract is connected with other endoderm-derived digestion-related organs, including the liver, which secretes bile into the small intestine via the biliary system and employs the gall-bladder as a reservoir, and the pancreas, which secretes bicarbonate and several enzymes, including trypsin, chymotrypsin, lipase, and pancreatic amylase, as well as nucleolytic enzymes (deoxyribonuclease and ribonuclease), into the small intestine.

In a normal human adult male, the gastrointestinal tract is approximately 6.5 meters long (20 feet) and consists of the upper and lower gastrointestinal tracts, but it may also be divided into foregut, midgut, and hindgut, reflecting the endoderm-derived embryological origin of each segment of the tract. The upper gastrointestinal tract, consisting of the mouth, pharynx, esophagus, and stomach, roughly corresponds to the derivatives of the foregut, with the exception of the first part of the duodenum. The lower gastrointestinal tract, comprising the intestines and anus, derives from the midgut for the lower duodenum and the first half of the transverse colon, and from the hindgut for the second half of the transverse colon and the upper part of the anal canal.

Since the epithelial cell lineage turnover within the gastrointestinal tract is a constant process, occurring every 2–7 days, it must be highly regulated by multipotent stem cells, which give rise to all gastrointestinal epithelial cell lineages and can regenerate the entire intestinal crypts and gastric glands under normal homeostasis but also after damage [398]. Next to the gastrointestinal side population cells [395, 398-400], recent reports illustrated that BM-derived cells were also able to incorporate into the small intestine pericryptal fibroblast region and to contribute to the intestinal regeneration after sex-mismatched BM transplants in human [399-401] and in animals [395, 402, 403] by forming myofibroblasts, fibroblasts, epithelial cells, smooth muscle cells and endothelial cell lineages. At last, BM-derived stem cells were also reported to express cytokeratin vimentin in the damage area and to be involved in the stomach regeneration in rats after ethanol-induced mucosal injury [404].

Liver lineage: The liver plays a major role in metabolism and has a number of functions in the body, including glycogen storage, plasma protein synthesis, and drug detoxification. Coming from an endoderm-derived part of the foregut called hepatic diverticulum, the liver produces bile and performs several functions, including the carbohydrate metabolism regulation (gluconeogenesis, glycogenolysis and glycogenesis), lipid and cholesterol metabolism, the detoxification and the production of insulin and coagulation factors. The liver, composed of hepatocytes that act as unipotential stem cells, and of bipotential stem cells, called oval cells that can differentiate into either hepatocytes or cholangiocytes, is among the few internal human organs capable of natural regeneration of lost tissue, and only 25% of remaining liver is enough to regenerate a whole liver.

Aside the different types of fetal and adult liver (stem) cells already identified, several types of BM-derived stem cells were reported to have the capacity to differentiate towards hepatocytic cells under appropriate *in vitro* conditions. A liver specific gene expression (cytokeratins 8 and 18, alpha-feto-protein, albumin, tryptophan-2,3-dioxygenase, tyrosine amino-transferase and the c-Met receptor for hepatocyte growth factor) was thus observed after induction by the hepatocyte growth factor HGF or the epidermal growth factor EGF, in culture with MSCs [405-412], for HSCs [413, 414], and for MAPCs from rat, mouse or human [170]. After co-cultures with hepatocytes, BM-derived stem cells were shown to express hepatic specific markers as well, and to adopt a metabolic activity [114, 408, 410, 415, 416].

In vivo, BM and liver transplantation were used to trace the origin of the liver repopulating cells during liver regeneration, and thus to observe that BM-derived HSCs may under certain conditions act as the progenitors of several types of liver cells, including oval cells, hepatocytes and cholangiocytes [93, 417]. At last, the *in vivo* differentiation of MSCs was also confirmed recently [406, 416].

Pancreas lineage: Deriving from two separate ventral and dorsal buds of the duodenum, the pancreas is an organ in the digestive and endocrine system which is both exocrine (secreting pancreatic juice containing digestive enzymes) and endocrine (islets of Langerhans that product several important hormones, including insulin, glucagon, and somatostatin). Due to the importance of its enzyme contents, injuring the pancreas is a very dangerous situation and several diseases or disorders may affect the pancreas, including tumors and cancer, insulinoma, cystic fibrosis, diabetes, exocrine pancreatic insufficiency, hemosuccus pancreaticus, pancreatitis and pancreatic pseudocyst. Among them, diabetes is one of the leading causes of morbidity and mortality in many countries caused by absolute insulin deficiency due to an autoimmune destruction of insulin secreting pancreatic β cells (type 1) or by a relative insulin deficiency due to decreased insulin sensitivity (type 2). Replacement of pancreatic β-cells, with the transplantation of islets of Langerhans, is already representing an ideal treatment [418, 419] but is restricted to a limited number of patients due the lack human islet donor tissues. Generation of insulin-producing cells from stem cells may thus represent an attractive alternative.

Within pancreatic islets and in non-endocrine compartments of the pancreas, some multipotent stem cells have been described [105, 420-422] and have the capacity to differentiate into pancreatic islet-like structures [423, 424]. Furthermore, cells that do not reside within the pancreas have been differentiated into pancreatic endocrine hormone-producing cells *in vitro* and *in vivo*, including embryonic stem cells [161, 423, 425], hepatic oval cells [426, 427], spleen-derived cells [428] or the central nervous system [429]. BM-derived stem cells could also play a supportive role in pancreas regeneration *in vivo* rather than participate in the differentiation of endocrine cells themselves [430]. However, human or rodent MSCs were reported to have the potential to differentiate *in vitro* into insulin, glucagon and somatostatin-secreting cells but also *in vivo* to reverse hyperglycemia in animal models of diabetes [431, 432], and to express the islet pancreatic transcription factors Nkx-2.2, Nkx-6.1, Pax-4, Pax-6, Isl-1 and Ipf-1 [412, 421, 432].

Lung-related tissue: In mammalians, the lung has the largest surface area, which reaches a final gas diffusion area of 70 m^2 in human lung, compared to the next largest epithelial organ, the skin, which has a surface area of about 40 times less. This essential respiration organ in air-breathing vertebrates is able to transport oxygen from the atmosphere into the bloodstream, to excrete carbon dioxide from the bloodstream into the atmosphere, and thus to support a systemic oxygen consumption ranging between 250 mL/min at rest to 5,500 mL/min during exercise. This gaze exchange is accomplished in the mosaic of specialized cells that form millions of tiny, exceptionally thin-walled air sacs called alveoli. A matching capillary network is also developed in close apposition to the alveolar surface, which can accommodate a blood flow rising from 4 to 40 L/min during the transition from rest to maximal exercise.

Coming from a ventral appendage of the endodermal epithelium lining the floor of the primitive embryonic anterior pharynx, the lung divides laterally into two buds and begins dichotomous branching into the surrounding splanchnic mesenchyme. The lung development is divided into four chronological stages, with the pseudoglandular stage (bronchial and respiratory tree development, undifferentiated primordial system formation), the canalicular stage (terminal sacs and vascularization development), the terminal sac stage (terminal sac number and vascularization increase, type I and II cells differentiation), and the alveolar stage (terminal sacs development into mature alveolar ducts and alveoli) [433, 434]. The mature lung comprises at least 40 morphologically differentiated cell lineages [435]. Thus, the larynx is lined with squamous epithelium and the upper airways are lined with ciliated columnar cells and mucus-secreting cells. Clara cells line the lower airways and alveolar type 1 and 2 epithelial cells line the alveoli and surround some pulmonary neuroendocrine cells situated in small foci. The pulmonary interstitium contains several specialized lineages of mesenchymal origin, including fibroblasts, myofibroblasts, and smooth muscle cells. At last, the lung also contains vascular, lymphatic and neuronal components [436]. Therefore, the development of the conducting airway and alveolar regions are suggested to be derived from different populations of stem cells, an airway stem cell population and a lung parenchyma stem cell population [92, 437-440].

Resident stem/progenitor cells have been described in specific regions in the proximal airway of the lung, including proximal airway epithelial progenitor cells [441, 442], bronchiolar epithelial progenitor cells [439] and alveolar epithelial stem cells [438, 443]. However, several groups have recently described the capacity of non-resident stem cells to differentiate into alveolar epithelial cells *in vitro*. For example, Rippon *et al.*, reported the differentiation of murine ES cells into distal airway epithelium after a three-step differentiation protocol incorporating an activin A treatment, a serum-free medium incubation and a commercially available lung-specific medium [444]. The MSC ability to differentiation into airway epithelium *in vitro* was described by Wang *et al.* when co-cultured with airway epithelial cells [445]. Moreover, when transduced with a virus construct expressing the cystic fibrosis trans-membrane regulator (CFTR), the gene corrected autologous MSCs were demonstrated to contribute to apical chloride secretion in response to cAMP agonist stimulation, suggesting the possibility of developing cell-based therapy for human cystic fibrosis [445]. At last, after intravenous injection into bleomycin-induced pulmonary fibrosis sex-mismatched animals, BM-derived bleomycin-resistant MSCs were reported to engraft the lung, to exhibit an epithelium-like morphology, to express type 1 alveolar epithelial cell specific markers (*Lycopersicon esculentum* lectin, aquaporin-5 and T1α) and to reduce inflammation and collagen deposition in lung tissue [446, 447].

4. Immunosuppressive Properties

In recent years, several observations reported that MSCs could exert immuno-regulatory activity, such as immuno-suppression by inhibiting T-cell responses to both polyclonal stimuli and their cognate peptide [448-450]. On study state, MSCs constitutively express low surface densities of MHC class I molecules and are negative for MHC class II and for co-stimulatory molecules (e.g. CD40, CD80 and CD86), both up-regulated by inflammatory stimuli [451, 452]. Indeed, because MSCs are generally considered as poorly immunogenic cells, they are of great importance in the view of potential utilization for therapeutic purposes (e.g. hematopoietic stem/progenitor cell engraftment or graft-versus-host disease).

MSCs and T-lymphocytes: In 1984, the group of Ildstad was the first to postulate that the transplantation of incompatible BM-derived stem cells into a mismatched recipient could induce tolerance to allogeneic or xenogeneic grafts [453]. However, the clear demonstration of T cells proliferation inhibition induced by MSCs was only reported in 2002 [448, 454]. After that, other reports showed that the MSC anti-proliferative activity does not appear to be antigen specific and targets both primary and secondary T-cell responses, but may still exert some selectivity because it appears to discriminate between cellular responses to allo-antigens and recall antigens [449, 454, 455]. Both suppression of T cell proliferation and their accumulation in the G0 phase of the cell cycle did not require MHC restriction, but could also be mediated by allogeneic MSCs [450]. Suppression of T cells proliferation induced by MSCs depends on a cross talk between the two cell populations, on the production of inflammatory cytokines, such as IFN-γ and IL-1β [448, 455, 456], and on the decreased production of Th1 cytokines [457]. Several MSC-derived molecules have been proposed to exert immuno-modulatory activity on T cell responses, including TGF-β1, HGF, IL-10, indoleamine 2,3-dioxygenase and prostaglandin E2 [448, 456, 458-461].

MSCs and B-lymphocytes: Only few studies addressed the effects of MSCs on B cell function. However, in 2005, Glennie *et al.* but also Augello *et al.* both reported that MSCs inhibit B cell proliferation, instigated in part by a physical contact between the 2 cell types and in part by a soluble factors released by MSCs in the culture supernatant [450, 457]. Deng *et al.* also reported that allogeneic MSC inhibited B cell activation, proliferation and IgG secretion, with enhanced CD40 and CD40 ligand expression, on BXSB-derived B cells, which is an experimental model for human systemic lupus erythematosus [462]. Finally, Corcione *et al.* described a study in which proliferation of B cells, stimulated and activated with anti-Ig antibodies, soluble CD40 ligand and cytokines (IL-2 and IL-4), was inhibited by MSCs in a manner depending on MSC-derived soluble factors released upon their cross talk with B cells [463].

MSCs and NK cells: As for T and B cells, interactions between MSCs and NK cells, which are major effectors in the elimination of virus-infected and malignant cells, induced an inhibition of the IL-2- or IL-15-driven NK proliferation, but also a reduced production of IL-15-induced cytokines (IFN-c, IL-10 and TNF-α) [456, 464, 465]. Similarly, soluble factors, including TGF-β1 and prostaglandin E2 have been suggested to play a role in the MSC-mediated suppression of NK cell proliferation [466].

MSCs and dendritic cells: The main function of dendritic cells is to process antigen material and present it on their surface to other cells of the immune system. The antigen presenting capacity might thus be altered by MSCs to promote their immuno-modulatory effects. Indeed, MSCs have been reported to inhibit the maturation of monocyte-derived myeloid dendritic cells, by down-regulating the surface expression of CD11c, CD83, MHC class II and co-stimulatory molecules, and by reducing the production of IL-12 [461, 465, 467, 468]. Ones again, the MSC-induced inhibition of dendritic cells differentiation and function is mediated by soluble factors (prostaglandin E2) and cell-to-cell contacts [459, 468, 469]. Thus, the MSC-induced inhibition of T lymphocyte proliferation may not only be the result of a direct suppressive effect on T cells, but may also be caused by an inhibitory effect on dendritic cell maturation, activation and antigen presentation.

MSC immunological effects in vivo: Several *in vivo* studies have reported the immuno-modulatory effects of MSCs. Indeed, infusion of MSCs delayed the rejection of skins allografts in a non-human model of organ transplantation [454], attenuates experimental autoimmune encephalomyelitis (a model of human multiple sclerosis) [470], and has beneficial effects in different human diseases including graft-versus-host disease, breast cancer, osteogenesis imperfecta, metachromatic leukodystrophy, Hurler syndrome, hematological malignancies and stroke [471-475]. However, some doubts rose from recent *in vivo* experiments about the reported MSC immuno-privilege, indicating that in some cases, administration of allogeneic MSCs into an MHC-mismatched host may result in their rejection or failed to prevent graft-versus-host disease [452, 475-477].

D. Capacities

1. Homing and Domiciliation

After systemic administration, MSCs are detected in bone, bone marrow, spleen, and cartilage, which localization is in agreement with the *in vitro* differentiation potential, but also in liver, lungs, kidneys [80, 478-480]. When intravenously injected, the donor MSC contribution in recipient bone and BM was estimated in mice and represent 5% of the total cell content after 5 months [141]. Labeled MSCs were also collected and recovered from BM and spleen 6 weeks after transplantation of galactosidase labeled human MSCs into pre-immune fetal sheep [172]. After transplantation into sub-lethally irradiated mice, more than half injected GFP-labeled MSCs were recovered from BM after 24 hours [480], and around 10-20% in BM within 3-10 weeks after infusion [481]. After infusion, MSCs were still detected after 12 weeks in NOD/SCID mice in lungs, kidneys, liver, intestine and brain, in addition to bone, bone marrow and spleen [130] but also after 1 year in baboons [83]. At last, differentiated human MSCs were detected after birth in a number of tissues, with tissue-specific differentiation into myocytes, cardiomyocytes and thymic stroma, in addition to bone marrow stroma, chondrocytes and adipocytes, after intraperitoneal injected in pre-immune sheep fetus [172].

All these studies allowed several issues to be raised. Firstly, after intravenous injection, MSCs are immediately trapped in the lungs [80, 478], suggesting that the number of cells arriving to the target organ, in particular bone marrow and bone, might be extremely limited, while the intra-BM route was not reported to be more effective [482]. Secondly, the steady state MSC turnover in the mesenchymal system is small (years are for example needed to the complete bone renewal), but it may dramatically increase in normal period of growth or after injury [59, 138]. Therefore, the recipient condition is a critical parameter in the MSC homing capacity, such as irradiation, which allows a significant MSC homing increase [341, 357, 480]. Thirdly, the MSC detection in a given tissue after infusion does not necessarily mean engraftment, but at least indicate cell survival in tissue [66, 483]. Finally, some of the detected cells after transplantation might be the result of cell fusion with *in situ* cells, such as striated myocytes, cardiomyocytes, Purkinje cells and hepatocytes [182, 343, 347, 348, 484], whereas specific differentiation of MSC without fusion are reported for hepatocytes [173].

2. Tissue Regeneration

Tissue regeneration is a cardinal stem cell property that has been partially confirmed for MSCs, especially for bone repair. Transgenic mice, with mutated collagen 1 gene leading to a phenotype of fragile bones resembling osteogenesis imperfecta, were reported to have a significant increase in bone collagen and mineral content 1 month after transplantation with BM-derived MSC from normal mice [485]. Similarly in human, local administration of autologous MSCs allows the healing of large bone defects [292] and increase the growth velocity of body length of young patients with osteogenesis imperfecta 4-6 weeks after transplantation [286, 486]. MSCs may also be used in several other diseases because of their assumed large differentiation potential as described above, including for example vascular diseases or skeletal and cardiac muscle disorders.

3. Oxygen Sensing

Oxygen concentration, and particularly hypoxia, is associated with critical role in the placenta development [487], during the early human embryogenesis [488], at birth (ductus arteriosus and foramen ovale closures) [489], in adult to optimize the matching of regional blood flow and ventilation in the lung with a physiological mechanism called hypoxic pulmonary vasoconstriction, and during virtually all known diseases. Within the BM, adult stem cells are also exposed to low oxygen and the mean oxygen concentration of the BM has been reported to be around 7% at steady state [490]. Mathematical models have indicated the existence of a gradient across the marrow from the rather well oxygenated sinuses to the relatively hypoxic areas near the bone endosteum [491], and HSCs are reported to be in an undifferentiated state in BM hypoxic niches and to expanse and differentiate along an oxygen gradient [492]. Furthermore, hypoxia has been shown to improve HSC survival, enhance self-renewal [493] and stimulate the formation of granulocytic-monocytic progenitors [494]. The BM is also the residence place of MSCs and oxygen has been shown to modulate some MSC characteristics as well. In particular, culturing MSCs at reduced oxygen tension (5-8%) increased *in vitro* their bone-forming potential [495], their adipogenesis potential [496, 497], their chondrogenesis potential [498, 499], and promote their mobilization into peripheral blood [79]. On the other hand, a hypoxic condition (2% of oxygen or less) compared to the physiological condition (7% of oxygen), is reported to inhibit strongly MSC chondrogenesis and osteogenesis *in vitro* [500] and to induce apoptosis [501].

Finally, since oxygen might have a regulatory role in growth kinetic and some differentiation pathways, several precautions should be taken when reading nearly all MSC-related reports, especially when *in vitro* experiments are set up at an oxygen concentration corresponding to that of the ambient air, because such oxygen level conditions probably several-fold surpass those found under physiological conditions [502, 503].

IV. VASCULAR THERAPIES

There are a number of clinical situations where the recipient site may not be amenable to a direct MSC transplantation, such as vascular diseases. Moreover, several factors limit the vascular tissue engineering, such as the availability of a suitable and abundant source of tissue. Since MSCs are multipotent and their number can be expanded in culture, there has been much interest in their clinical potential for tissue repair, especially as a potential source for generating mesenchyme cells in the vascular wall such as smooth muscle cells (SMC) or for the construction of vascular grafts. When transplanted into the heart, MSCs can differentiate into SMCs and contribute to vascular remodeling *in vivo* [504, 505], suggesting that some micro-environmental signals may be important in promoting differentiation to a SMC phenotype. However, the effects of vascular micro-environmental factors on MSCs or the *in vitro* factors needed to undergo SMC differentiation are not yet fully understood.

Several physiological or pathological processes may contribute to modify the normal vessel. Arteriogenesis refers to an increase in the diameter of existing arterial vessels. Angiogenesis is a physiological and normal process, involving the growth of new blood vessels from pre-existing vessels, which can be observed in a normal process such as in growth and development, as well as in wound healing, but also during the tumors transition from a dormant state to a malignant state. At last, vasculogenesis is the process of blood vessel formation occurring by a *de novo* production of endothelial cells, when endothelial precursor cells (angioblasts) migrate and differentiate in response to local signals to form new blood vessels. Vasculogenesis is thus observed during the embryologic development but also in adult during the neo-vascularization of a tumor or during the revascularization process of an avascularized area following trauma (e.g. cardiac ischemia).

A. The Normal Vessel

The normal arterial wall, consisting of concentric layers that surround the arterial lumen, is divided into three well-defined layers having each distinctive composition of cells and extracellular matrix, including the layer immediately adjacent to the lumen called the intima, the middle layer known as the media, and the outermost layer referred as the arterial adventitia. Two concentric layers of elastin demarcate these three layers, known as the internal elastic lamina that separates the intima from the media, and the external elastic lamina that separates the media from the adventitia. Lining the luminal surface of arteries, a single contiguous layer of endothelial cells sits on a basement membrane of extracellular matrix and proteoglycans that is bordered by the internal elastic lamina. Although some SMCs are occasionally found in the intima, the principal cellular component, forming a functional barrier between flowing blood and the arterial wall stroma, is constituted by endothelial cells of this anatomic layer. The media layer is composed principally by SMCs arranged in layers, where the number of layers is depending on the arterial size. SMCs are held together by an extracellular matrix, composed of elastic fibers, collagen and proteoglycans, which may be supplied by an increasing content of elastin typically observed within larger arteries. At last, the outermost layer of the artery, the adventitia, is typically composed of a loose matrix of elastin, SMCs, fibroblasts, and collagen, where most of the neural input into blood vessels also traverses through the adventitia. Previously considered inactive with respect to vascular homeostasis, the adventitia is now playing an important role in controlling vascular remodeling and nitric oxide bioactivity, through the production of reactive oxygen species.

Like all the other organs, cells of the vessels must receive nutrients and oxygen and reject wastes. Most of the time, vascular cells directly carry out their exchanges with circulating blood, but for vessels of larger diameter, the nutrition of cells constituting the vascular wall can be assured at the same time by blood circulating in the vessel but also starting from a capillary system: the vasa vasorum. This capillary network, bringing nutrients to cells furthest away from the vessel lumen, is present in all arteries comprising more than 29 lamellate units. The vasa vasorum can moreover bring a certain number of mediators and hormones in more or less direct contact with SMCs of largest arteries.

B. Mesenchymal Stem Cells Implication in Vascular Remodeling

Within the framework of a vascular therapy, MSCs could be integrated into the muscular layer of the vascular wall and they may be differentiated into in smooth muscular cells. They may also transdifferentiate into endothelial cells and thus contribute to the vessel intima. At last, these cells could incorporate the arterial adventitia like pericytes and secrete cytokines and growth factors to act in an indirect way on a more extended portion of the vessel by paracrine stimulation.

1. MSCs and the Smooth Muscle Differentiation

a) Bone Marrow Stroma and Vascular Smooth Muscle Phenotype

Within the bone marrow, the structural and physiological support of hematopoietic cells is provided by the bone marrow stroma, which is composed of a heterogeneous population of cells that follow a vascular smooth muscle differentiation pathway [374]. In the bone marrow stroma niche *in vivo*, MSCs provide cellular contacts and produce growth factors, chemokines and extracellular matrix molecules that control survival, self-renewal, transfer and differentiation of HSCs into all hematopoietic cells [56]. *In vitro*, after long-term culture, MSCs but also MSCs derived cell-lines express cytoskeleton-associated and extracellular matrix specific proteins that are found on smooth muscle cells [375-380]. In MSC culture, the first and most constitutively expressed markers are the alpha-smooth muscle actin and fibronectin isoforms, which are both strongly expressed in smooth muscle cells [382, 383]. Then, other cellular markers found in smooth muscle cells appear belatedly in MSCs under culture, including the vinculin, the metavinculin, the h-caldesmon, the l-caldesmon, the h1-calponin, SM22α and the smooth muscle actinin [380, 381, 384]. At last and more lately, MSCs express smooth muscle specific contractile proteins, such as desmin or smooth muscle heavy chains 1 and 2 [384]. Moreover, MSCs produce a smooth muscle-like extracellular matrix, made up of thrombospondin 1 and laminin [384]. Thus, after long-term culture, MSCs seem to acquire a smooth muscle phenotype with the sequential expression of developmental markers.

This differentiation pathway might seem to be astonishing for the hematopoietic stroma and not related to a known function of the smooth muscle cells. However, some analyzes revealed a functional significance. Indeed, hematopoietic supporting stroma cells synthesize a great number of cytokines and adhesion molecules that are essential to hematopoiesis, but these cells also play a critical role in the hematopoietic cell migration by modifying the endothelial cell junction organization [266, 506] and by producing a SDF-1 gradient [507]. This dual role, the mediator synthesis and the progenitor traffic control, is a reminiscence of the two functions described for smooth muscle cells, passing from a synthetic to a contractile phenotype [384]. Thus, the synthetic phenotype would be characteristic of an immature cell (MSCs under the differentiation course), while the contractile phenotype would be characteristic of a mature and completely differentiated cell, such as smooth muscle cells from the vascular media layer.

b) The Smooth Muscle Differentiation

In vivo, mediators expressed and/or secreted by endothelial cells seem to play a role in the smooth muscle cell recruitment and differentiation [384, 508-510]. The cell recruitment might be induced by several released factors, such as PDGF, tissue factor and endoglin [511], and by the expression of transcription factors, such as MEF-2C (myocyte-specific enhancer-binding Factor-2C) [512]. The future smooth muscle differentiation cell would be controlled by a balance between activators (TGF-β, IGF, endothelin I, angiotensin II, heparan sulfate, laminin, type IV collagen, retinoic acid) and inhibitors (PDGF, interferon γ, fibronectin) [374]. Moreover, the cellular aspect seems to be important in the differentiation process since the alpha-smooth muscle actin and other cytoskeletal proteins are expressed in response to an extracellular matrix and to stretching [513].

Smooth muscle markers (alpha-smooth muscle actin, vimentin, desmin, myosins, calponin, metavinculin) are classically induced *in vitro* when culturing MSCs in a Dexter-type medium (basic medium supplemented with in particular fetal calf serum, horse serum and cortisol) [377]. However, other studies reported a smooth muscle phenotype induction after incubating stromal cells in another differentiation medium (basic medium supplemented with fetal calf serum and β-mercaptoethanol) [514], with the induction of various markers (alpha-smooth muscle actin, SM22α, h-caldesmon, h1-calponin). Moreover, these authors also showed that the ascorbic acid was a potential smooth muscle differentiation inductor [514]. On the other hand, the dimethyl sulfoxide was reported to inhibit the MSC to smooth muscle differentiation [515].

Studies about the MSC *in vitro* culture conditions had allow to point out the importance of many cytokines (TGF-β, EGF, IL-1, IL-6, TNF-α, bFGF, PDGF) in these stromal cells long-term maintenance and differentiation [122, 123, 516]. Moreover, these cytokines induce a variety of effects according to culture conditions (presence or not of serum, presence or not of adhesion molecules covering the dish, liquid or semi-solid culture medium, sorted-cells or not). Although few specific studies were specifically interested in the MSC to smooth muscle differentiation, it is probable that autocrine secreted TGF-β [517] and PDGF both play a modulating role in coordination with extracellular matrix molecules [346]. Thus, TGF-β and a

TGF-β activator, the thrombospondin 1, would stimulate of the production of alpha-smooth muscle actin in fibroblasts and myofibroblasts [375, 380, 518], while PDGF-β would reduce the alpha-smooth muscle actin expression [346].

c) Markers of the Smooth Muscle Differentiation

The MSC *in vitro* acquisition of a smooth muscle phenotype, with the acquisition of specific markers, is currently well established. However, the presence of various markers is only one stage towards the acquisition of a complete smooth muscle phenotype and it is necessary to determine if MSC differentiated in smooth muscle cells have the fundamental capacity of the smooth muscle: the contraction.

One of the methods allowing the evaluation the contraction capacity is to place cells into a collagen or glycosaminoglycan matrix and to measure its shortening. Thus, Young and colleagues reported the rabbit MSC contraction capacity in a collagen matrix [321]; however, the contraction degree was not evaluated. Then, a quantitative analysis of the MSC contraction within a collagen and glycosaminoglycan composite matrix was reported where authors showed without ambiguity the contraction capacity of rabbit and dog bone marrow-derived MSC after culture into a Dexter-type medium (smooth muscle differentiation medium) [519]. At last, Kinner and collaborators showed in 2002 that human MSCs (characterized by their differentiation capacity along the three reference lineages) had a contraction capacity correlated to their alpha-smooth muscle actin content [346]. These authors also reported that the MSC contraction within a collagen matrix after culture into a Dexter-type medium was completely inhibited by cytochalasin-D (a cytoskeletal actin depolymerizing agent), partially inhibited by PDGF-β and potentiated by TGF-β [346].

Many studies remain to be carried out to determine whether all MSCs have this contraction capacity or if a particular cell fraction is selected during *in vitro* cultures. Moreover, since contractile proteins associated to the smooth muscle phenotype, such as the alpha-smooth muscle actin or myosins, are not sufficient to obtain contractile smooth muscle cells from MSCs, it would be important to study the presence of other markers associated with the smooth muscle cell functionality, such as the calcium homeostasis or the electrophysiological profile.

Some teams were thus interested in the calcium-signaling pathway in MSCs [140, 520-522]. In undifferentiated MSCs, the cytosolic calcium is thus reported to be released mainly from endoplasmic reticulum stocks. Moreover, this calcium is preferentially released through inositol-1,4,5-triphosphate sensitive endoplasmic receptors and not or little through ryanodine sensitive endoplasmic receptors. At last, a little part of the intracellular calcium might come inside cells mainly through plasma membrane calcium channels (store-operated calcium channels) [521]. Undifferentiated MSCs were also reported to show calcium oscillations mainly from sodium-calcium exchangers (NCX1, 2 and 3) and plasma membrane calcium pumps [140, 521], but not from plasma membrane voltage-operated calcium channels [522]. However, no specific study regarding the calcium-signaling pathway was made concerning the particular context of the MSC to smooth muscle differentiation.

The study of the MSC electrophysiological profile characterizing the membrane potential at rest and their capacity to be depolarized authorizing the contraction, could allow to determine which smooth muscle cell type might be obtained after differentiation. Thus, ionic channels usually reported on smooth muscle cells, such as the large-conductance calcium-activated potassium channel (BKca), and Kv2.1 or Kv1.5 sub-units, ionic exchanges (e.g. NCX-1, 2 or 3), are also found within the MSC membrane [521, 523, 524]. However, since these ionic channels are largely expressed in the majority of smooth muscle cell types (vascular, mesenteric, bronco-tracheal or uterine), they do not allow any discrimination.

2. MSCs and Endothelial Trans-Differentiation

Beside their integration in the vessel media layer and their smooth muscle differentiation, MSCs could also participate to the vessel intima layer and (trans)-differentiate into endothelial cells. Likewise, studies showed that endothelial cells and progenitors could differentiate into smooth muscle cells under TGF-β induction [525-527]; it was brought back a MSC "trans-differentiation" into endothelial cells *in vitro* coming from human bone marrow [528] or from human umbilical cord blood [529]. Even if the conversion of a cellular type towards another seems to be a rare event, with a conversion frequency estimated between 0,01 and 0,03% [530], it was also reported cells presenting at the same time an endothelial phenotype (von Willebrand factor expression), and a smooth muscle phenotype (alpha-smooth muscle actin expression) [526, 530].

This *in vitro* trans-differentiation was associated with a epithelial to mesenchymal transition, characterized by a cell-to-cell contact disruption [530], an endothelial markers differential expression (VE-cadherin, von Willebrand factor, Tie-1 and 2, VCAM-1) and by the capacity to form a tubular network structure [528, 529]. At last, various growth factors were also associated to this endothelial trans-differentiation, such as VEGF, TGF-β, EGF, PDGF or hydrocortisone [528, 529, 531]. Thus, this capacity adds a clinical advantage to the MSC use with an aim of vascular therapy.

3. Growth Factor Release and Paracrine Effects of MSCs

Practically all information regarding the cytokine production by stromal cells and MSCs come from *in vitro* studies on cultured cells. Indeed, it is currently difficult to correlate these *in vitro* results with a potential *in vivo* role of each cytokine. Moreover, it is currently not clearly established if MSCs, coming from various tissue sources, are presenting a specific cytokine production profile, and if there is a cytokine regionalization within the same tissue [56].

One of the first observations was to show the MSC capacity to produce cytokines maintaining HSCs in quiescence or inducing their self-renewal rather than their differentiation. Indeed, MSCs are reported to excrete the following molecules: SCF, LIF, SDF-1, BMP-4, Flt-3 ligand, TGF-β [74, 532-534]. MSCs produce a broad variety of interleukins (IL-1, IL-6, IL-7, IL-8, IL-11, IL-12, IL-14, and IL-15) and, when they are cultivated in the presence of IL-1a, MSCs also produce cytokines acting on more mature hematopoietic progenitors, such as the GM-CSF and G-CSF [534]. Studies also brought back the existence of a "dialog" between HSCs and MSCs, osteoblasts and stromal cells, allowing the regulation the hematopoietic cells production [535-537].

MSC paracrine secretions thus play a fundamental role in the bone marrow microenvironment; however, these cytokine secretions can also play an important role during angiogenesis and arteriogenesis. In 2004, Kinnaird and colleagues showed that MSCs could secrete angiogenic factors *in vitro*, such as VEGF, bFGF, PGF and MCP-1 [538, 539]. These authors also reported a beneficial effect of the MSC local injection on the vascular perfusion in a model of lower limb ischemia by MSC paracrine secretions *in situ* of VEGF and bFGF. Furthermore, this ischemia protection mechanism, characterized by an apoptosis reduction and an angiogenesis increase after injection of MSC, was also reported with a bFGF and TGF-α secretion in a model of acute renal ischemia [174] or in a model of myocardial infarction [373, 540, 541]. Thus, even if a low number of MSCs integrates the new vessels architecture [174, 373, 538-541], MSCs are capable of long-term survival after injection, to exhibit immunosuppressive activities, to reduce fibrosis (scar formation), to inhibit apoptosis, to induce angiogenesis and to stimulate mitosis and differentiation of cells leading to tissue repair by their of bioactive molecule secretion [542].

C. Stem Cell Implication during Angiogenesis, Vasculogenesis and Arteriogenesis

Vascular remodeling and in particular arterial remodeling can be observed under various pathological conditions whatever the touched organ, causing the widening (expansive remodeling) or the reduction (constrictive remodeling) of the vessel diameter. All vascular remodeling are important physiological and pathological mechanisms in the tissue perfusion adaptation that lead to structural and functional modifications of the vascular wall. These processes are characterized by a smooth muscle cell hypertrophy or hyperplasia within the media layer of preexistent vessels, but also by a complete remodeling of the vasculature with disappearance of some vessels by apoptose and with appearance of new vessels by angiogenesis or vasculogenesis.

Smooth muscle cells that play a critical role during these vascular remodeling may have a variable origin. Indeed, these cells can come from the local proliferation of smooth muscle cells that are already present in the vessel media layer at the lesion level, but these cells may also come from the differentiation of endogenous stem cells and progenitors that are present in the vessel media layer or from circulating progenitors.

1. Stem Cell Implication during Pulmonary Remodeling

a) Mechanisms of the Pulmonary Vascular Development

The pulmonary vascularization is formed according to two distinct mechanisms: angiogenesis and vasculogenesis. During vasculogenesis, local endogenous progenitors proliferate to form a loose complex of cells being used as starting point to the development of new vessels. After the cellular network formation, proliferative cells are assembled to form tubular structures, while the later development by angiogenesis leads to the formation of the final vascular tree. Angiogenesis is the process by which new vessels emergent starting from preexistent vessels. It is a complex process directed by growth factors that stimulate the endothelial cell proliferation, which control the vascular lumen formation, and which direct the recruitment of perivascular components (pericytes and smooth muscle cells) towards the vascular wall [543, 544]. Angiogenesis thus allows the extension of preexistent vessels but also the establishment of links between close structures.

Although there is a debate regarding the exact chronology of the pulmonary vascular network formation mechanisms, both angiogenesis and vasculogenesis play essential roles. Many studies actually showed that proximal vessels were initially formed by budding starting from a preexistent vessel (angiogenesis), while the distal vessels were formed *de novo* starting from splanchnopleuric-derived mesenchymal progenitors (vasculogenesis) [545, 546].

The stem cell and progenitor participation during the vascular vessel formation starts to be supported since Summer and his team has successfully isolated a stem cell population from embryonic lungs [440]. After characterization, this heterogeneous population was composed of hematopoietic cells and non-hematopoietic cells, and allowed endothelial and smooth muscle cells to be obtained. HSC- and MSC-like stem cells were also brought back as being present within the pulmonary tissue where they could participate to the constitutive replacement of the pulmonary parenchyma, the epithelium and pulmonary vessels, but also during several pathologies like pulmonary hypertension, pulmonary fibrosis or emphysema.

b) Stem Cells and Pulmonary Vascular Pathologies

The purpose of several studies was to show the stem cell contribution to the pathogenesis of many adult pulmonary diseases by contributing to a hyper-proliferative response with phenotypical and functional differentiations into alveolar, endothelial or smooth muscle cells. On the other hand, the stem cell contribution to the pulmonary tissue remodeling can also be defective, thus contributing to decrease the tissue repair.

Pulmonary arterial hypertension: Pulmonary hypertension is characterized by an abnormal function of endothelial cells, causing a sustained vasoconstriction and a pulmonary vessel remodeling [547], but it is also characterized by a high pulmonary blood pressure with a pulmonary vascular resistance increase, leading to a right cardiac insufficiency. In addition to an abnormal endothelial cell functionality, the pulmonary vascular remodeling is characterized by an intima thickening, a media hypertrophy, a smooth muscle cell hyperplasia and by plexiform lesions blocking pulmonary capillaries [548]. The pulmonary vessel sustained vasoconstriction was a long time considered as the principal cause of the pulmonary pressure rise; however, during the 10 last years, many data gave evidences that an exuberant angiogenesis also contributed to the development of the pathology. Thus, Tuder and collaborators were among the first to bring back the expression of angiogenic molecules within plexiform lesions from patients suffering of severe pulmonary arterial hypertension, with a VEGF over-expression leading to an excessive proliferation of local or circulating endothelial cells [549-551].

Then, as the pulmonary mesenchyme is a vascular precursor source [552] and as various types of progenitors capable of vascular differentiation are circulating constitutively in the bloodstream, the contribution of these stem cells during the plexiform lesion development was suspected but not yet clearly established [553]. Thus, Hashimoto and collaborators showed in 2004 that some pulmonary fibroblasts came from bone marrow derived progenitors [554], while Davie reported the presence of $c-kit^+$ progenitors (probably HSCs) around remodeled pulmonary arteries in a bovine model of hypoxia-induced pulmonary hypertension [555]. At last, even if $Sca-1^+$ $c-kit^+$ vascular progenitors not coming from bone marrow were detected in the mouse vessel adventitia [556], Hayashida concluded that bone marrow stem cells (i.e. HSCs) were mobilized into the peripheral blood and could contribute to pulmonary vascular remodeling in a model of hypoxia-induced pulmonary hypertension in the bone marrow transplanted transgenic GFP mouse [557].

The intravenous injection of MSCs or endothelial progenitors genetically modified to express the endothelial nitric oxide synthase attenuated the monocrotaline-induced pulmonary hypertension, with improvement of the animal survival and restoration of the pulmonary microvasculature structure and function [558, 559].

Asthma: Contrary to the pulmonary hypertension, the pulmonary angiogenesis contribution was brought back since more than one ten years in the airway remodeling of the patients suffering from bronchial asthma [560]. Indeed, bronchial biopsies coming from children and adult patients suffering from moderate to severe asthma showed a vessel number increase that was correlated to the expression of several angiogenic factors and their receptors [561, 562]. In the same way, asthmatic patients presented an airways chronic inflammation whose severity is correlated to the disease severity [563]. Thus, great concentrations of angiogenesis and inflammation related growth factors, such as VEGF or angiopoietin 1 [564], were found in pulmonary tissue and were reported to cause a vascular patency variation but also modifications of the vessels fenestration [565].

MSCs, but also HSCs, that both have the capacity to differentiate into endothelial cells [166, 528], could intervene in the asthmatic angiogenesis. Moreover, bone marrow hematopoiesis sites can be stimulated by circulating factors produced during the airways inflammation [566], leading to the mobilization of inflammatory cells and various progenitors. Such cells could play an important role in the airway chronic inflammatory response by attenuating immunological responses [476], or by initiating the epithelium [567], collagen [554], blood vessels [568] and muscular cells smooth [569] remodeling.

Idiopathic pulmonary fibrosis and emphysema: The idiopathic pulmonary fibrosis and the emphysema are two pulmonary pathology examples where the stem cells contribution is defective in the local cellular regeneration with in particular an abnormal localization and differentiation of these stem cells within the pulmonary tissue.

The idiopathic pulmonary fibrosis could be the result of an initial lesion, inducing an inflammatory response or an activation of alveolar epithelial cells leading to a rise in the cytokine rate, an inappropriate signalization of the epithelial and mesenchymal cells and a disorganization of tissue repair [570, 571]. Although this disease is usually characterized by a small artery muscularization, Cosgrove and collaborators reported a strong reduction in the vessel density associated with an aberrant angiogenesis after pulmonary tissue histological observation [572]. In the same way, Ebina and collaborators reported an absence of vessels in pulmonary fibrosis zone with fibroblastic proliferation [573]. These myofibroblasts could also derive from preexistent intra-pulmonary mesenchymal precursors, but also from circulating progenitors such as MSCs or HSCs [574].

Emphysema and chronic obstructive pulmonary disease are also characterized they by a pulmonary blood vessel rarefaction, with a parenchyma destruction, an apoptose increase and an airway widening and fibrosis [575-577]. The origin of the cells contributing to the final fibrosis is discussed, with a pulmonary origin [578] or a bone marrow origin [554, 579]. The treatment would consist in the stimulation of an intact epithelium formation and in the fibroblastic proliferation suppression with in particular a correction of the local or bone marrow derived stem cell deficiency.

2. Stem Cell Implication during Cardiac Remodeling

The cardiomyocyte loss after a myocardial infarction causes a contractile function loss, since the necrotic area is replaced by fibroblasts forming an uncontractile scar tissue. Furthermore, the surrounding myocardium remodeling is itself critical and raise the cardiac insufficiency [580]. The fetal cardiomyocyte or skeletal myoblasts transplantation was proposed as a future method to treat myocardial infarctions [581-584].

a) Cellular Therapy of Myocardial Infarction

Several authors showed that the direct injection, within the coronary arteries, of a bone marrow derived heterogeneous stem cell population or MSCs could represent a simple but effective approach in the heart attack treatment. Thus, Strauer reported in 2002 a clinical study with 20 patients in the treatment of myocardial infarction [585]. After right and left catheterization, coronary angiography and left ventriculography, patients underwent a balloon angioplasty. Five to 9 days after the acute infarction, bone marrow cells were aspired and the mononuclear fraction, able to generate MSCs *in vitro*, was transplanted within the infarcted zone using a small balloon angioplasty. Tree months after, the comparison of both groups, treated by standard therapy or by cell transplantation, showed a significant positive effect of the cellular treatment on the cardiac function and on the infarcted zone regression. At last, the perfusion defect within the myocardium, detected by thallium scintigraphy, was considerably decreased in the cell treated group [585].

Another study on the use of the cellular therapy for the treatment of the myocardium acute infarction was carried out by the team of Chen in 2004 [372]. Sixty-nine patients, presenting a beginning of infarction since less than 12 hours and undergoing emergency angiography and angioplasty, were recruited in a randomized clinical study to receive or not autologous MSCs after bone marrow aspiration realized during the urgency examination. Ten days after the cardiac event, the adherent mononuclear fraction, cultivated *in vitro* to obtain MSCs, was injected through the coronary artery near the infarcted zone, while the other group of patients received a physiological solution. After a regular echocardiogram, echocardiography and positron emission tomography, the percentage of hypokinetic, akinetic, and dyskinetic segments significantly decreased in the cell-treated group after 3 months in comparison with the control group and with the beginning of the study. At last, the left ventricular ejection fraction was higher in the cell treated group compared to patients who received a physiological solution [372].

A randomized clinical study reported by the group of Wollert allowed to evaluate by echocardiography the effectiveness of the local injection of autologous adherent bone marrow cells (mainly MSCs) for the acute myocardial infarction treatment [371]. After angioplasty, patients were randomly separated in two groups to receive the traditional post-infarction treatment or an *in situ* injection of autologous cells cultivated *in vitro* during 4 to 8 days. Although authors could not highlight significant differences between the two groups regarding the left ventricular volumes in systole and diastole, they reported after 6 months a significant beneficial effect of the cellular therapy on the right ventricular ejection fraction and on the mobility of the ventricular wall surrounding the infarcted zone. Authors thus suggested that autologous adherent bone marrow cells could be injected *in situ* to improve the restoration of the ventricular function among patients presenting a myocardial infarction [371].

However, while experimental and clinical studies tend to support an improvement of cardiac repair by the cellular therapy, many points remain to be clear up; including 1/the optimal cellular type corresponding to the patient clinical profile, 2/the mechanism inducing the cardiac function improvement, 3/the cell survival optimization, 4/the development of less traumatic administration techniques, and 5/the potential benefits of cell transplantation in non-ischemic heart failure. Moreover, recent studies showed that adult stem cells (cardiomyocytes or bone marrow stem cells) fail to integrate electromechanically within the recipient heart, while cardiac stem cells and cardiac-precommitted ES cells could allow a true regeneration of the necrotic myocardium [586].

b) Mechanisms of Cardiac Repair

All these results, as well as others presenting similar studies [587, 588], show that the bone marrow stem cell therapy is feasible and sure, and could contribute to the tissue regeneration after myocardial infarction. Nevertheless, several aspects remain controversial: what kind of stem cells is appropriate to the patients? When these cells should be transplanted to patients? How the transplanted cell viability may be supervised? What is the action mechanism of the transplanted stem cells: secretion of growth factors or cell-to-cell interactions?

Some studies were thus interested in the cell type allowing the post-infarction cardiac function improvement after transplantation. Based on the cell therapeutic effectiveness and on the fact that an unpurified mononuclear cell population avoided cell expansion problems but was inevitably composed of a small percentage of pluripotent cells diluted among an enormous quantity of committed cells, some authors supposed that the preliminary culture of a bone marrow cell population composed of MSCs and endothelial progenitors could support at the same time the cardiomyogenesis (by MSCs) and the angiogenesis (by endothelial progenitors) on the level of the infarcted zone [589]. These authors thus enrolled patients presenting a recent or old myocardial infarction treated by angioplasty. Autologous MSCs and endothelial progenitors, selected *in vitro* during 7 days, were injected into the left coronary artery during catheterization and allowed a heart contractility improvement in one or more myocardial segments previously nonviable, while this improvement was not found in the group controls. Results indicated that the two cell type used (MSCs and endothelial progenitors) had a positive effect on the myocardial contractility mainly with patients presenting a recent myocardial infarction [589].

Perin *et al.* have evaluated the potential effect of a bone marrow-derived mononuclear cell transplantation on neo-vascularization and on the cardiac functionality loss prevention leading to the myocardial infarction in patients with cardiac ischemia [590]. They thus treated chronic coronary patients, who had a left ventricular ejection fraction lower than 40% and who were ineligible for a percutaneous or surgical revascularization, by cell therapy. Patients received local injections of bone marrow-derived mononuclear autologous cells during the cardiac catheterization intervention with electromechanical cartography of the ventricle right allowing the viable ventricular zone identification. Two and 4 months after, patients treated by cell therapy presented a cardiac function improvement [590] and an increased myocardial perfusion and exercise capacity [591].

At last, to determine if the myocardial regeneration observed after a stem cell injection was due to a cardiomyocyte differentiation or to the formation of new vessels, two animal studies reported the MSC effects on cardiac cytoprotection. The first study, based on a myocardial infarction experimental model after ligation of the left anterior descending coronary artery in rats, showed that the injection of MSCs in the infarcted myocardial zone increased the release of angiogenic factors, such as SDF-1, bFGF or VEGF [540]. Moreover, these authors reported a capillary density rise in animals treated with MSCs. Thus, this team supposed that the cardiac cytoprotection effects caused by the MSC injection were mainly due to a paracrine-induced angiogenesis [540]. The second study was interested in the angiogenic roles of MSCs in the myocardium regeneration after experimental infarction in rats [373]. A MSC monolayer, cultured *in vitro* on a detachable support and transplanted onto the scarred myocardium, allowed the formation of a thick stratum that included newly formed vessels, undifferentiated cells and few cardiomyocytes. Moreover, the stem cell layer secreted paracrine factors inducing angiogenesis. Thus, authors evidenced that MSCs could regenerate the myocardium by acting on angiogenesis and cardiac cytoprotection induced by paracrine factors. Furthermore, MSCs were also reported to be integrated into tissue and to be differentiated in cardiomyocytes and vascular cells [373].

3. Stem Cell Implication during Systemic Vascular Remodeling

Beside cardiopulmonary pathologies with an abnormal vascularization, ischemic effects can touch other organs or tissues inducing a reduction of the blood circulation by obstruction (atherosclerosis and obliterating arteriopathy of the lower limbs, renal ischemia). The treatment consists in tracking techniques, in angioplasty, in arterial bypass surgery or at last in the member amputation. Since many years, studies patients touched by vascular ischemia showed the spontaneous development of a collateral vascularization replacing the normal circulation [592-596]. Several approaches emerged to stimulate these spontaneous reparation mechanisms, in particular by activating the growth of compensatory blood vessels attenuating a too weak blood flow. Thus, most studies had concentrated on the stem and progenitor cell participation in two distinct types to reduce ischemia, such as the formation of new collateral vessels starting from preexistent vascular structures (angiogenesis) [597] or the growth and the enlargement of thin capillaries already present and functional (arteriogenesis) [598].

a) Atherosclerosis

Atherosclerosis is a phenomenon physiological of blood vessel ageing with loss of elasticity that begins with the embryonic life and that is considerably accelerated by cardiovascular risk factors (smoking, cholesterol, arterial hypertension, diabetes, sedentary, alcohol, heredity, age and gender). Thin arterial lesions can be observed as early as 20 years of age, while several various development stages were identified involving an intimal remodeling of the large and medium blood vessels (aorta and its branches, coronary, cerebral or lower limbs arteries) and an accumulation of lipids, complex carbohydrates, blood and blood products, fat tissues and mineral deposits.

The traditional hypothesis [599], which assumes that the smooth muscle cells forming atherosclerotic lesions would come from the vessel media layer after migration towards a neointimal space, is currently questioned since there are many evidence showing that these smooth muscle cells could also come from circulating progenitors [600]. The HSC participation in the atherosclerosis development was reported in 2002 by Sata [601] who gave the bases for the development of new strategies in the vascular pathology treatment by directing the mobilization, the domiciliation, the differentiation and the proliferation of bone marrow derived progenitors. Then other authors explored the immunophenotypical profile of cells found in atherosclerotic lesions of Apo-E mice [556]. They thus reported that a great number of these cells exhibited stem cell markers (Sca-1, C-kit, CD34, Flk1), indicating that many stem cell types, including endothelial progenitors, MSCs and HSCs, may participate in the formation of atherosclerotic vascular remodeling. Moreover, when Sca-1^+ cells were injected onto the adventitia surrounding remodeled zones, these cells were found within atherosclerotic intimal lesions, thus showing their migration and their participation in the development of atherosclerotic lesions [556].

Recent studies reported the migration of stem cells coming from the vascular wall towards atherosclerotic lesion sites [602, 603], such as MSCs [604]. Since MSCs have the capacities to modulate the proliferation and the migration of smooth muscle cells and to differentiate into endothelial cells [605], MSCs could thus contribute to the atherosclerotic smooth muscle layer and could contribute to form a fibromuscular cap stabilizing the vulnerable atherosclerotic plaque. After bone marrow transplantation [606] or in an atherosclerosis mouse model [607], donor cells were found in vascular zones with atherosclerotic plaques but not in normal zones, indicating that this cell domiciliation could require inflammatory signals. Thus, since stem cells participate in the renewal and the generation of vascular tissues, a deregulation of these stem cells could play a part in the atherosclerosis development.

b) Vascular Stenosis

Arterial (re)stenosis is a physiopathological phenomenon that may occur after an angioplasty, an arteriotomy, or a bypass in human and in experimental animal models of vascular lesions, that induces a partial or complete occlusion of the arterial lumen and thus often requires a new revascularization procedure. The vascular damage, with intimal and medial cell loss, the internal elastic lamina fragmentation and the architectural tissue lesions, leads to an excessive repair and to the proliferation and the migration of smooth muscle cells, inducing a neointimal hyperplasia [608, 609]. Recent studies evidenced that the vascular function depended not only on the cells within the vessels, but also that stenosis and restenosis were also significantly modulated by bone marrow-derived stem cells [610]. Thus, some authors supposed that restenosis could be prevented by an early vessel repair under the influence of stem cells, such as endothelial progenitors or MSCs.

An interesting study was carried out by using endogenous endothelial progenitors where authors surgically implanted anti-CD34 coated stents and reported that circulating endothelial progenitors were captured on the stent surface leading to a prevention of a thrombus formation and restenosis [611]. A similar study in clinical situation was initiated in 2006 to determine the effects of the endothelial progenitor capture on stents, coupled with a statine-induced mobilization [612].

Many studies were also interested in the potential role of MSCs in the restenosis vascular process. Indeed, MSCs injected into the blood circulation 15 minutes before the induction of a vascular lesion were reported to have the capacity to domiciliate at the site lesion and in particular in vasa vasorum containing adventitial zones, in a rat coronary arteriotomy model [608]. Moreover, Han reported in 2001 the contribution of MSCs to a neointimal formation in a mouse model of iliac artery scratch lesion [613]. These authors also showed that 56% of the alpha-smooth muscle actin positive cells from the neointima were bone marrow stem cells. At last, these results, regarding the MSC acquisition of a smooth muscle profile during vascular lesions, were also confirmed by Tanaka *et al.* [610].

4. Stem Cell Implication during Tumor Vasculature Development

At the opposite of beneficial effects of such mechanisms reducing ischemia, the formation of the tumor vasculature is harmful since it allows the tumor to grow and leads to metastasis.

In 1971, Folkman was the first to postulate that the tumor growth and the development of metastases were angiogenesis dependant processes [614]. After what, various stages of the tumor development were reported [615] and showed that several genetic and epigenetic changes occurred in tumor cells, and revealed the microenvironment role in the malignity development. Indeed, tumors are made up of neoplastic cells and a stroma composed of fibroblasts, myofibroblasts, endothelial cells, pericytes and infiltrated hematopoietic cells. These tumor associated cells are supposed to control critical processes in the tumor progression, such as the tumor cell evolution, the anti-tumor immunity, the extracellular matrix remodeling, the angiogenesis and the metastasis invasion [616-619]. Thus, hematopoietic cells exhibit several functions in the tumor development, by decreasing the tumor immunogenicity and by stimulating the neoplastic progression [620].

In addition to stimulate the tumor cell growth and migration, the hematopoietic cells were reported to secrete factors inducing the tumor angiogenesis, allowing the generation of blood vessels with the tumor and providing nutrients and oxygen needed to the tumor growth. Angiogenesis was for a long time considered as a critical stage in the tumor growth, thus representing a key target in anti-tumor strategies [621, 622]. Many studies brought back the bone marrow-derived stem cell participation in the tumor angiogenesis, including MSCs, HSCs and endothelial progenitors. However, the specific stem cell type accused and the exact function of these cells in the tumor vessel formation remain irresolute and discussed.

The endothelial progenitor contribution to the tumor angiogenesis was reported in 2001 by Lyden, when he used a tumor xenograft murine model [623]. Other authors also proposed that this endothelial progenitor mobilization, from the bone marrow towards tumor sites, required the activation of the matrix metalloproteinase-9 [624]. However, De Palma reported that only a few number of endothelial progenitors integrated within new vessels was really detected and that a majority of bone marrow-derived cells found in tumor vessels was found localized in perivascular zones, attesting of a preferentially paracrine role rather than structural [625]. At last, another study reported that 4.9% of the total endothelial cells in tumor vessels came from the bone marrow [626].

Recently, some studies also studied the MSC potential role in the tumor angiogenesis. One pioneer study thus evidenced that MSCs could be integrated in tumor vessels [627]. MSCs were also reported to support the tumor growth *in vivo* [628]. Then, MSCs were suggested to have a positive role on the development of preexistent tumors, but also to have a tumor-initiating role. According to this concept, MSCs would fuse with muted cells leading to a tumor formation. In this case, bone marrow stem cells would be at the same time tools and targets for an anti-tumor therapy.

5. MSCs and Vascular Engineering

The increasing request for vascular grafts, in particular for vessels with a diameter lower than 5 mm, generated a growing interest for the artificial vascular prosthesis engineering. During 30 years, several synthetic materials, such as expanded polytetrafluoroethylene (ePTFE) and polyurethane, have been used to engineer small diameter vessels, but unfortunately, they did not lead to satisfactory patency, mainly because of a strong thrombosis [629]. This approach was then improved by seeding the prosthesis internal face with endothelial cells, thus reducing thrombosis [630-632]. Furthermore, vascular prosthesis seeded with smooth muscle and endothelial cells revealed a higher patency than unseeded covered prosthesis [633, 634], but thrombosis and restenosis of these prosthesis however remained notable [635]. The reasons could be a loss of the smooth muscle or endothelial cell functions during their *ex vivo* expansion, or a loss of cells *in vivo* by prosthesis partial washing caused by vascular flow.

Endothelial progenitors were first used to seed prosthesis, with an excellent patency after 130 days in a ovine carotid graft model [636]. However, these endothelial progenitors were not able to generate smooth muscle cells, indicating that this lonely cell type was not sufficient to regenerate a complete vascular structure. An alternative approach was then initiated by using MSCs to replace smooth muscle or endothelial cells. In 2005, Cho reported the use of bone marrow-derived adherent stem cells, differentiated in culture into smooth muscle or endothelial cells, to seed a vascular prosthesis [637, 638], while Kanki-Horimoto used β-galactosidase transduced MSCs to seed the internal face of a small diameter vascular prosthesis [639]. Taken together, these results evidenced that both MSC derived smooth muscle and endothelial cells contributed to the regeneration of the three vascular layers (intima, media and adventitia) and improved the small diameter vessel patency. However, we do not know yet if undifferentiated MSCs seeding on vascular prosthesis can differentiate *in vivo* into smooth muscle and endothelial cells.

a) Various Materials

Most of materials used currently to develop small diameter vascular grafts consist of synthetic or natural polymers with variable thickness, porosity, elasticity and density degrees. One of the first studies interested in the impact of these several parameters on the vascular patency showed that a low pore diameter promoted the cell growth and the vascular graft patency [629]. Thus, several studies were conducted with microporous vascular substitutes, such as the expanded polytetrafluoroethylene, allowing small diameter vessels (a few millimeters) to be successfully seeded with bone marrow derived stem cells [637]. A polypropylene carbonate matrix seeded with MSCs was also used to form small diameter vessels (2 mm) [640] because of its excellent compatibility its biological resorption [641].

Other materials, such as poly-glycolic acid polymers, were also reported to have a good MSC adhesion capacity and a gradual degradation allowing its physiological replacement by tissue [642]. Various resorbable materials were thus successfully seeded by MSCs, such as poly-L-lactic acid polymers [643], poly-lactic-Co-glycolic acid polymers [644, 645] or sodium arginate matrix [645]. Other new bioabsorbable matrices were used as cell culture support before being implanted *in vivo*. These synthetic polymer vascular substitutes, composed of 4-hydroxy-butyric acid, supported cell culture *in vitro* and after may be colonized by vascular cells after *in vivo* implantation [646]. Moreover, this substitute allowed the concentric cell growth of several overlaid layers. At last, authors reported a complete resorption of the synthetic material after 169 days, allowing the establishment of vascular structures without the long-term foreign material presence [646].

Other authors also reported the use of biological matrices where endogenous cells were eliminated by detergents (Triton) [638]. The resulting biological matrix, composed of collagen fibers, elastin and extracellular matrix molecules, was seeded with bone marrow-derived stem cells *in vitro* differentiated into smooth muscle and endothelial cells. After *in vivo* implantation, this vascular substitute conducted to a complete and functional vascular wall [638]. The major advantage of this substitute is its biological source (sometimes autologous), but above all this decellularized material limits the inflammation risk [647].

b) The Mechanical Stress Impact

Many studies showed that a mechanical environment controlled the smooth muscle cell characteristics. *In vivo*, smooth muscle cells within vascular walls reside typically in a dynamic environment with a vascular flow where they are guided in a particular direction and where they exhibit a contractile phenotype, which is crucial for the vascular tissue properties [648]. However, vascular smooth muscular tissues, produced *in vitro* with conventional culture techniques, could not be functional since cells are not lined up [649, 650] and exhibit a synthetic phenotype instead of a contractile phenotype [651, 652].

Several mechanical constraints can be found into vascular walls according to their localization. For example, the blood vessel rectilinear part is mainly subjected to a cyclic mechanical force following a circumferential direction, while junction or diameter change zones (e.g. aneurism) are subjected to isotropic constraints. To determine the relative contribution of each mechanical force on smooth muscle cell effects and regulation mechanisms, several equipments were developed. Thus, cells were cultured on two dimension deformable substrates (e.g. silicone membranes) where mechanical forces can be applied to stretch the substrate according to only one or several axes in the same plan. Three dimension systems were then used to mimic the pulsatile nature of the blood flow into a vascular substitute tube whose internal face was seeded with cells. These studies evidenced the importance of mechanical signals in the smooth muscle cell phenotype regulation in two dimensions systems [653-655] and in the smooth muscle cell proliferation and migration in three dimensions systems [648, 656, 657]. Thus, the design of vascular substitutes under mechanical constraints led to the improvement of the vascular patency, with an enhancement of the collagen production and with an increased protection against mechanical strains [633, 658].

At last, the induction the expression of smooth muscle-related properties were reported for MSC when cultured under mechanical stresses produced in these culture systems [659, 660]. Thus, the contractile protein expression (actin and myosin) was preferentially induced by the pressure constraints whereas shear-stress forces induced by the pulsatile component of flow did not induce this protein expression [659].

c) Towards the Realization of a Functional and Complete Vessel

Researches for a perfect complete and functional biocompatible vessel model started in 1986 when Weinberg and Bell designed for the first time an artery with multiple concentric layers around a Dacron mesh and where the vascular lumen was limited by endothelial cells [661]. Then in 1999, Niklason was among the first to report the *in vitro* constitution of a complete vessel starting from a poly-glycolic acid biodegradable matrix seeded with smooth muscle cells cultivated under pulsatile conditions [633]. After incubation during 8 weeks in a bioreactor under a radial pulsatile stress, this synthetic vessel presented concentric smooth muscle layers that could be recovered by an endothelial cell monolayer. At last, these authors also reported the absence of stenosis or dilation and an excellent patency up to 24 days after the substitution of a miniature swine femoral artery portion [633]. This *in vitro* engineered new concept of artificially vessels was also used by Hoerstrup who sequentially seeded fibroblasts and endothelial cells. Then, the resulting graft was placed under natural mechanical conditions of pulsatile flow, pressure and forces of shearing [662].

Taken together and considering our current knowledge regarding the MSC differentiation capacities into smooth muscle cells but also the technical possibilities to engineer arteries with several concentric layers, why a complete and functional vessel is not yet engineered and used in human? One of the problems could be the need to maintain a controlled growth of the new vessel allowing its growth and its remodeling capacities, but also preserving a biocompatibility [643, 663]. This difficulty could be overcome by using autologous stem cells, ensuring the biocompatibility and maintaining a proliferative potential. Another obstacle may be the requirement to cultivate these cells *in vitro* under an adequate flow in a growing medium containing animal-derived proteins and growth factors while these vascular substitutes will have to be implanted into men. However, this could be over-passed by the future arrival of serum-free culture medium.

Thus, the use of MSCs to engineer synthetic vessels is right at its beginning. Models currently used showed the utility to recreate conditions mimicking the morphological and the biological environment.

CONCLUSION

A better knowledge of the factors intervening in the MSC mobilization, domiciliation and differentiation is of obvious potential interest to use these cells in therapy. In the same way, the intrinsic roles of these cells in the vascular remodeling processes in response to chemotactic signals released by injured tissues remain to be determined. Lastly, MSCs improve significantly the biocompatibility of vascular prosthesis, and furthermore allow a complete and functional arterial wall to be recreated. Thus, the use of MSCs as a product for cell therapies remains a future prospect, since these cells exhibit a great plasticity and biocompatibility authorizing them to colonize many tissues, to survive and release many cytoprotective and angiogenic factors.

MSCs also exhibit a great capacity to domiciliate into several tissues. At last, their differentiation potential into vascular smooth muscle cells and their ability to response to mechanical stress authorize them to be used extensively for regenerative vascular therapies, like cardiac vascular endoprosthesis or valvular and vessel biocompatible prosthesis.

REFERENCES

[1] Verfaillie, C.M., Adult stem cells: assessing the case for pluripotency. *Trends Cell Biol*, 2002. 12(11): p. 502-8.
[2] Preston, S.L., et al., The new stem cell biology: something for everyone. *Mol. Pathol.*, 2003. 56(2): p. 86-96.
[3] Wobus, A.M. and K.R. Boheler, Embryonic stem cells: prospects for developmental biology and cell therapy. *Physiol. Rev.*, 2005. 85(2): p. 635-78.
[4] Prelle, K., et al., Establishment of pluripotent cell lines from vertebrate species--present status and future prospects. *Cells Tissues Organs*, 1999. 165(3-4): p. 220-36.
[5] Pain, B., et al., Long-term in vitro culture and characterisation of avian embryonic stem cells with multiple morphogenetic potentialities. *Development*, 1996. 122(8): p. 2339-48.
[6] Chang, I.K., et al., Production of germline chimeric chickens by transfer of cultured primordial germ cells. *Cell Biol. Int.*, 1997. 21(8): p. 495-9.
[7] Doetschman, T., P. Williams, and N. Maeda, Establishment of hamster blastocyst-derived embryonic stem (ES) cells. *Dev. Biol.*, 1988. 127(1): p. 224-7.
[8] Graves, K.H. and R.W. Moreadith, Derivation and characterization of putative pluripotential embryonic stem cells from preimplantation rabbit embryos. *Mol. Reprod. Dev.*, 1993. 36(4): p. 424-33.
[9] Schoonjans, L., et al., Pluripotential rabbit embryonic stem (ES) cells are capable of forming overt coat color chimeras following injection into blastocysts. *Mol. Reprod. Dev.*, 1996. 45(4): p. 439-43.
[10] Iannaccone, P.M., et al., Pluripotent embryonic stem cells from the rat are capable of producing chimeras. *Dev. Biol.*, 1994. 163(1): p. 288-92.
[11] Brenin, D., et al., Rat embryonic stem cells: a progress report. *Transplant Proc.*, 1997. 29(3): p. 1761-5.
[12] Vassilieva, S., et al., Establishment of SSEA-1- and Oct-4-expressing rat embryonic stem-like cell lines and effects of cytokines of the IL-6 family on clonal growth. *Exp. Cell Res.*, 2000. 258(2): p. 361-73.
[13] Buehr, M., et al., Rapid loss of Oct-4 and pluripotency in cultured rodent blastocysts and derivative cell lines. *Biol. Reprod.*, 2003. 68(1): p. 222-9.

[14] Thomson, J.A., et al., Isolation of a primate embryonic stem cell line. *Proc. Natl. Acad. Sci. USA,* 1995. 92(17): p. 7844-8.

[15] Pau, K.Y. and D.P. Wolf, Derivation and characterization of monkey embryonic stem cells. *Reprod. Biol. Endocrinol.*, 2004. 2: p. 41.

[16] Thomson, J.A., et al., Pluripotent cell lines derived from common marmoset (Callithrix jacchus) blastocysts. *Biol. Reprod.*, 1996. 55(2): p. 254-9.

[17] Suemori, H., et al., Establishment of embryonic stem cell lines from cynomolgus monkey blastocysts produced by IVF or ICSI. *Dev. Dyn,* 2001. 222(2): p. 273-9.

[18] Stevens, L.C., Origin of testicular teratomas from primordial germ cells in mice. *J. Natl. Cancer Inst*, 1967. 38(4): p. 549-52.

[19] Kahan, B.W. and B. Ephrussi, Developmental potentialities of clonal in vitro cultures of mouse testicular teratoma. *J. Natl. Cancer Inst.*, 1970. 44(5): p. 1015-36.

[20] Jacob, S.W. and R. Herschler, Pharmacology of DMSO. *Cryobiology*, 1986. 23(1): p. 14-27.

[21] Gearhart, J.D. and B. Mintz, Contact-mediated myogenesis and increased acetylcholinesterase activity in primary cultures of mouse teratocarcinoma cells. *Proc. Natl. Acad. Sci. USA*, 1974. 71(5): p. 1734-8.

[22] Stevens, L.C., The development of transplantable teratocarcinomas from intratesticular grafts of pre- and postimplantation mouse embryos. *Dev. Biol.*, 1970. 21(3): p. 364-82.

[23] Evans, M.J., The isolation and properties of a clonal tissue culture strain of pluripotent mouse teratoma cells. *J. Embryol. Exp. Morphol.*, 1972. 28(1): p. 163-76.

[24] Skarnes, W.C., et al., Capturing genes encoding membrane and secreted proteins important for mouse development. *Proc. Natl. Acad. Sci. USA*, 1995. 92(14): p. 6592-6.

[25] Papaioannou, V.E., et al., Fate of teratocarcinoma cells injected into early mouse embryos. *Nature,* 1975. 258(5530): p. 70-73.

[26] Berstine, E.G., et al., Alkaline phosphatase activity in mouse teratoma. *Proc. Natl. Acad. Sci. USA*, 1973. 70(12): p. 3899-903.

[27] Nicolas, J.F., et al., [Mouse teratocarcinoma: differentiation in cultures of a multipotential primitive cell line (author's transl)]. *Ann. Microbiol.* (Paris), 1975. 126(1): p. 3-22.

[28] McBurney, M.W., et al., Control of muscle and neuronal differentiation in a cultured embryonal carcinoma cell line. *Nature*, 1982. 299(5879): p. 165-7.

[29] Martin, G.R. and M.J. Evans, The morphology and growth of a pluripotent teratocarcinoma cell line and its derivatives in tissue culture. *Cell*, 1974. 2(3): p. 163-72.

[30] Mintz, B. and K. Illmensee, Normal genetically mosaic mice produced from malignant teratocarcinoma cells. *Proc. Natl. Acad. Sci. USA*, 1975. 72(9): p. 3585-9.

[31] Andrews, P.W., From teratocarcinomas to embryonic stem cells. *Philos. Trans R Soc. Lond B Biol. Sci.*, 2002. 357(1420): p. 405-17.

[32] Bradley, A., et al., Formation of germ-line chimaeras from embryo-derived teratocarcinoma cell lines. *Nature*, 1984. 309(5965): p. 255-6.

[33] Evans, M.J. and M.H. Kaufman, Establishment in culture of pluripotential cells from mouse embryos. *Nature,* 1981. 292(5819): p. 154-6.

[34] Wobus, A.M., et al., Characterization of a pluripotent stem cell line derived from a mouse embryo. *Exp. Cell Res.*, 1984. 152(1): p. 212-9.

[35] Doetschman, T.C., et al., The in vitro development of blastocyst-derived embryonic stem cell lines: formation of visceral yolk sac, blood islands and myocardium. *J. Embryol. Exp. Morphol.*, 1985. 87: p. 27-45.

[36] Hubner, K., et al., Derivation of oocytes from mouse embryonic stem cells. *Science*, 2003. 300(5623): p. 1251-6.

[37] Toyooka, Y., et al., Embryonic stem cells can form germ cells in vitro. *Proc. Natl. Acad. Sci. USA*, 2003. 100(20): p. 11457-62.

[38] Geijsen, N., et al., Derivation of embryonic germ cells and male gametes from embryonic stem cells. *Nature*, 2004. 427(6970): p. 148-54.

[39] Rohwedel, J., et al., Primordial germ cell-derived mouse embryonic germ (EG) cells in vitro resemble undifferentiated stem cells with respect to differentiation capacity and cell cycle distribution. *Cell Biol. Int.*, 1996. 20(8): p. 579-87.

[40] Labosky, P.A., D.P. Barlow, and B.L. Hogan, Embryonic germ cell lines and their derivation from mouse primordial germ cells. *Ciba Found Symp.*, 1994. 182: p. 157-68; discussion 168-78.

[41] Labosky, P.A., D.P. Barlow, and B.L. Hogan, Mouse embryonic germ (EG) cell lines: transmission through the germline and differences in the methylation imprint of insulin-like growth factor 2 receptor (Igf2r) gene compared with embryonic stem (ES) cell lines. *Development*, 1994. 120(11): p. 3197-204.

[42] Stewart, C.L., I. Gadi, and H. Bhatt, Stem cells from primordial germ cells can reenter the germ line. *Dev. Biol.*, 1994. 161(2): p. 626-8.

[43] Matsui, Y., K. Zsebo, and B.L. Hogan, Derivation of pluripotential embryonic stem cells from murine primordial germ cells in culture. *Cell*, 1992. 70(5): p. 841-7.

[44] Verfaillie, C.M., M.F. Pera, and P.M. Lansdorp, Stem cells: hype and reality. *Hematology* (Am Soc Hematol Educ Program), 2002: p. 369-91.

[45] Spangrude, G.J., S. Heimfeld, and I.L. Weissman, Purification and characterization of mouse hematopoietic stem cells. *Science*, 1988. 241(4861): p. 58-62.

[46] Weissman, I.L., Translating stem and progenitor cell biology to the clinic: barriers and opportunities. *Science*, 2000. 287(5457): p. 1442-6.

[47] Rheinwald, J.G. and H. Green, Serial cultivation of strains of human epidermal keratinocytes: the formation of keratinizing colonies from single cells. *Cell*, 1975. 6(3): p. 331-43.

[48] Asahara, T., et al., Isolation of putative progenitor endothelial cells for angiogenesis. *Science*, 1997. 275(5302): p. 964-7.

[49] Gage, F.H., Mammalian neural stem cells. *Science*, 2000. 287(5457): p. 1433-8.

[50] Gage, F.H., Structural plasticity: cause, result, or correlate of depression. *Biol. Psychiatry*, 2000. 48(8): p. 713-4.

[51] Schofield, R., The relationship between the spleen colony-forming cell and the haemopoietic stem cell. *Blood Cells*, 1978. 4(1-2): p. 7-25.

[52] Lin, H., The stem-cell niche theory: lessons from flies. *Nat. Rev. Genet*, 2002. 3(12): p. 931-40.

[53] Spradling, A., D. Drummond-Barbosa, and T. Kai, Stem cells find their niche. *Nature*, 2001. 414(6859): p. 98-104.

[54] Kopp, H.G., et al., The bone marrow vascular niche: home of HSC differentiation and mobilization. *Physiology* (Bethesda), 2005. 20: p. 349-56.

[55] Moore, K.A. and I.R. Lemischka, Stem cells and their niches. *Science*, 2006. 311(5769): p. 1880-5.

[56] Dazzi, F., et al., The role of mesenchymal stem cells in haemopoiesis. *Blood Rev.*, 2006. 20(3): p. 161-71.

[57] Friedenstein, A.J., et al., Precursors for fibroblasts in different populations of hematopoietic cells as detected by the in vitro colony assay method. *Exp. Hematol.*, 1974. 2(2): p. 83-92.

[58] Friedenstein, A.J., et al., Origin of bone marrow stromal mechanocytes in radiochimeras and heterotopic transplants. *Exp. Hematol.*, 1978. 6(5): p. 440-4.

[59] Caplan, A.I., Mesenchymal stem cells. *J. Orthop Res.*, 1991. 9(5): p. 641-50.

[60] Owen, M., Marrow stromal stem cells. *J. Cell Sci. Suppl.*, 1988. 10: p. 63-76.

[61] Owen, M. and A.J. Friedenstein, Stromal stem cells: marrow-derived osteogenic precursors. Ciba Found Symp, 1988. 136: p. 42-60.

[62] Prockop, D.J., Marrow stromal cells as stem cells for nonhematopoietic tissues. *Science,* 1997. 276(5309): p. 71-4.

[63] Dennis, J.E., et al., A quadripotential mesenchymal progenitor cell isolated from the marrow of an adult mouse. *J. Bone Miner Res.*, 1999. 14(5): p. 700-9.

[64] Bhagavati, S. and W. Xu, Isolation and enrichment of skeletal muscle progenitor cells from mouse bone marrow. *Biochem. Biophys. Res. Commun.*, 2004. 318(1): p. 119-24.

[65] Bianco, P. and P. Gehron Robey, Marrow stromal stem cells. *J. Clin. Invest,* 2000. 105(12): p. 1663-8.

[66] Bianco, P., et al., Bone marrow stromal stem cells: nature, biology, and potential applications. *Stem Cells,* 2001. 19(3): p. 180-92.

[67] Kuznetsov, S.A., et al., Circulating skeletal stem cells. *J. Cell Biol.*, 2001. 153(5): p. 1133-40.

[68] Reyes, M., et al., Purification and ex vivo expansion of postnatal human marrow mesodermal progenitor cells. *Blood,* 2001. 98(9): p. 2615-25.

[69] Jiang, Y., et al., Pluripotency of mesenchymal stem cells derived from adult marrow. *Nature*, 2002. 418(6893): p. 41-9.

[70] Pittenger, M.F., et al., Multilineage potential of adult human mesenchymal stem cells. *Science,* 1999. 284(5411): p. 143-7.

[71] Zvaifler, N.J., et al., Mesenchymal precursor cells in the blood of normal individuals. *Arthritis Res.*, 2000. 2(6): p. 477-88.

[72] Covas, D.T., et al., Isolation and culture of umbilical vein mesenchymal stem cells. *Braz. J. Med. Biol. Res.,* 2003. 36(9): p. 1179-83.

[73] In 't Anker, P.S., et al., Isolation of mesenchymal stem cells of fetal or maternal origin from human placenta. *Stem Cells*, 2004. 22(7): p. 1338-45.

[74] Zhang, Y., et al., Comparison of mesenchymal stem cells from human placenta and bone marrow. *Chin. Med. J.* (Engl), 2004. 117(6): p. 882-7.

[75] Miao, Z., et al., Isolation of mesenchymal stem cells from human placenta: Comparison with human bone marrow mesenchymal stem cells. *Cell Biol. Int.*, 2006. 30(9): p. 681-7.

[76] Phinney, D.G., et al., Plastic adherent stromal cells from the bone marrow of commonly used strains of inbred mice: variations in yield, growth, and differentiation. *J. Cell Biochem.*, 1999. 72(4): p. 570-85.

[77] Baddoo, M., et al., Characterization of mesenchymal stem cells isolated from murine bone marrow by negative selection. *J. Cell Biochem.*, 2003. 89(6): p. 1235-49.

[78] Tropel, P., et al., Isolation and characterisation of mesenchymal stem cells from adult mouse bone marrow. *Exp. Cell Res.*, 2004. 295(2): p. 395-406.

[79] Rochefort, G.Y., et al., Multipotential mesenchymal stem cells are mobilized into peripheral blood by hypoxia. *Stem Cells*, 2006. 24(10): p. 2202-8.

[80] Rochefort, G.Y., et al., Influence of hypoxia on the domiciliation of mesenchymal stem cells after infusion into rats: possibilities of targeting pulmonary artery remodeling via cells therapies? *Respir Res.*, 2005. 6: p. 125.

[81] Santa Maria, L., C.V. Rojas, and J.J. Minguell, Signals from damaged but not undamaged skeletal muscle induce myogenic differentiation of rat bone-marrow-derived mesenchymal stem cells. *Exp. Cell Res.*, 2004. 300(2): p. 418-26.

[82] Martin, D.R., et al., Isolation and characterization of multipotential mesenchymal stem cells from feline bone marrow. *Exp. Hematol.*, 2002. 30(8): p. 879-86.

[83] Devine, S.M., et al., Mesenchymal stem cells are capable of homing to the bone marrow of non-human primates following systemic infusion. *Exp. Hematol.*, 2001. 29(2): p. 244-55.

[84] Airey, J.A., et al., Human mesenchymal stem cells form Purkinje fibers in fetal sheep heart. *Circulation*, 2004. 109(11): p. 1401-7.

[85] Silva, G.V., et al., Mesenchymal stem cells differentiate into an endothelial phenotype, enhance vascular density, and improve heart function in a canine chronic ischemia model. *Circulation,* 2005. 111(2): p. 150-6.

[86] Moscoso, I., et al., Differentiation "in vitro" of primary and immortalized porcine mesenchymal stem cells into cardiomyocytes for cell transplantation. *Transplant Proc.*, 2005. 37(1): p. 481-2.

[87] Bosch, P., S.L. Pratt, and S.L. Stice, Isolation, characterization, gene modification, and nuclear reprogramming of porcine mesenchymal stem cells. *Biol. Reprod.*, 2006. 74(1): p. 46-57.

[88] Bosnakovski, D., et al., Isolation and multilineage differentiation of bovine bone marrow mesenchymal stem cells. *Cell Tissue Res.*, 2005. 319(2): p. 243-53.

[89] Worster, A.A., et al., Effect of transforming growth factor beta1 on chondrogenic differentiation of cultured equine mesenchymal stem cells. *Am. J. Vet. Res.*, 2000. 61(9): p. 1003-10.

[90] Ringe, J., T. Haupl, and M. Sittinger, [Mesenchymal stem cells for tissue engineering of bone and cartilage]. *Med. Klin.* (Munich), 2003. 98 Suppl 2: p. 35-40.

[91] Howell, J.C., et al., Pluripotent stem cells identified in multiple murine tissues. *Ann. NY Acad. Sci.,* 2003. 996: p. 158-73.

[92] da Silva Meirelles, L., P.C. Chagastelles, and N.B. Nardi, Mesenchymal stem cells reside in virtually all post-natal organs and tissues. *J. Cell Sci.*, 2006. 119(Pt 11): p. 2204-13.

[93] Herrera, M.B., et al., Isolation and Characterization of a Stem Cell Population from Adult Human Liver. *Stem Cells*, 2006.

[94] Seeberger, K.L., et al., Expansion of mesenchymal stem cells from human pancreatic ductal epithelium. *Lab. Invest,* 2006. 86(2): p. 141-53.

[95] Yoshimura, H., et al., Comparison of rat mesenchymal stem cells derived from bone marrow, synovium, periosteum, adipose tissue, and muscle. *Cell Tissue Res.*, 2006.

[96] Barry, F.P. and J.M. Murphy, Mesenchymal stem cells: clinical applications and biological characterization. *Int. J. Biochem. Cell Biol.*, 2004. 36(4): p. 568-84.

[97] Pierdomenico, L., et al., Multipotent mesenchymal stem cells with immunosuppressive activity can be easily isolated from dental pulp. *Transplantation,* 2005. 80(6): p. 836-42.

[98] Shih, D.T., et al., Isolation and characterization of neurogenic mesenchymal stem cells in human scalp tissue. *Stem Cells,* 2005. 23(7): p. 1012-20.

[99] Hoogduijn, M.J., E. Gorjup, and P.G. Genever, Comparative characterization of hair follicle dermal stem cells and bone marrow mesenchymal stem cells. *Stem Cells Dev.*, 2006. 15(1): p. 49-60.

[100] Moon, M.H., et al., Human adipose tissue-derived mesenchymal stem cells improve postnatal neovascularization in a mouse model of hindlimb ischemia. *Cell Physiol. Biochem.*, 2006. 17(5-6): p. 279-90.

[101] Dan, Y.Y., et al., Isolation of multipotent progenitor cells from human fetal liver capable of differentiating into liver and mesenchymal lineages. *Proc. Natl. Acad. Sci. USA,* 2006. 103(26): p. 9912-7.

[102] In 't Anker, P.S., et al., Mesenchymal stem cells in human second-trimester bone marrow, liver, lung, and spleen exhibit a similar immunophenotype but a heterogeneous multilineage differentiation potential. *Haematologica,* 2003. 88(8): p. 845-52.

[103] Campagnoli, C., et al., Identification of mesenchymal stem/progenitor cells in human first-trimester fetal blood, liver, and bone marrow. *Blood,* 2001. 98(8): p. 2396-402.

[104] Rzhaninova, A.A., S.N. Gornostaeva, and D.V. Goldshtein, Isolation and phenotypical characterization of mesenchymal stem cells from human fetal thymus. *Bull. Exp. Biol. Med.*, 2005. 139(1): p. 134-40.

[105] Hu, Y., et al., Isolation and identification of mesenchymal stem cells from human fetal pancreas. *J. Lab. Clin. Med.*, 2003. 141(5): p. 342-9.

[106] Igura, K., et al., Isolation and characterization of mesenchymal progenitor cells from chorionic villi of human placenta. *Cytotherapy,* 2004. 6(6): p. 543-53.

[107] Tsai, M.S., et al., Isolation of human multipotent mesenchymal stem cells from second-trimester amniotic fluid using a novel two-stage culture protocol. *Hum. Reprod.*, 2004. 19(6): p. 1450-6.

[108] Erices, A., P. Conget, and J.J. Minguell, Mesenchymal progenitor cells in human umbilical cord blood. *Br. J. Haematol.*, 2000. 109(1): p. 235-42.

[109] Kim, J.W., et al., Mesenchymal progenitor cells in the human umbilical cord. *Ann. Hematol.*, 2004. 83(12): p. 733-8.

[110] Villaron, E.M., et al., Mesenchymal stem cells are present in peripheral blood and can engraft after allogeneic hematopoietic stem cell transplantation. *Haematologica,* 2004. 89(12): p. 1421-7.

[111] O'Donoghue, K., et al., Identification of fetal mesenchymal stem cells in maternal blood: implications for non-invasive prenatal diagnosis. *Mol. Hum. Reprod.,* 2003. 9(8): p. 497-502.

[112] O'Donoghue, K., et al., Microchimerism in female bone marrow and bone decades after fetal mesenchymal stem-cell trafficking in pregnancy. *Lancet,* 2004. 364(9429): p. 179-82.

[113] Romanov, Y.A., V.A. Svintsitskaya, and V.N. Smirnov, Searching for alternative sources of postnatal human mesenchymal stem cells: candidate MSC-like cells from umbilical cord. *Stem Cells,* 2003. 21(1): p. 105-10.

[114] Lee, O.K., et al., Isolation of multipotent mesenchymal stem cells from umbilical cord blood. *Blood,* 2004. 103(5): p. 1669-75.

[115] Lee, M.W., et al., Mesenchymal stem cells from cryopreserved human umbilical cord blood. *Biochem. Biophys. Res. Commun.,* 2004. 320(1): p. 273-8.

[116] Kassis, I., et al., Isolation of mesenchymal stem cells from G-CSF-mobilized human peripheral blood using fibrin microbeads. *Bone Marrow Transplant,* 2006. 37(10): p. 967-76.

[117] Kucia, M., et al., Tissue-specific muscle, neural and liver stem/progenitor cells reside in the bone marrow, respond to an SDF-1 gradient and are mobilized into peripheral blood during stress and tissue injury. *Blood Cells Mol. Dis.,* 2004. 32(1): p. 52-7.

[118] Fernandez, M., et al., Detection of stromal cells in peripheral blood progenitor cell collections from breast cancer patients. *Bone Marrow Transplant,* 1997. 20(4): p. 265-71.

[119] Zyuz'kov, G.N., et al., Role of stem cells in adaptation to hypoxia and mechanisms of neuroprotective effect of granulocytic colony-stimulating factor. *Bull. Exp. Biol. Med.,* 2005. 140(5): p. 606-11.

[120] Kawada, H., et al., Nonhematopoietic mesenchymal stem cells can be mobilized and differentiate into cardiomyocytes after myocardial infarction. *Blood,* 2004. 104(12): p. 3581-7.

[121] Latsinik, N.V., et al., [The stromal colony-forming cell (CFUf) count in the bone marrow of mice and the clonal nature of the fibroblast colonies they form]. *Ontogenez,* 1986. 17(1): p. 27-36.

[122] Gronthos, S. and P.J. Simmons, The growth factor requirements of STRO-1-positive human bone marrow stromal precursors under serum-deprived conditions in vitro. *Blood,* 1995. 85(4): p. 929-40.

[123] Kuznetsov, S.A., A.J. Friedenstein, and P.G. Robey, Factors required for bone marrow stromal fibroblast colony formation in vitro. *Br. J. Haematol.,* 1997. 97(3): p. 561-70.

[124] Colter, D.C., et al., Rapid expansion of recycling stem cells in cultures of plastic-adherent cells from human bone marrow. *Proc. Natl. Acad. Sci. USA,* 2000. 97(7): p. 3213-8.

[125] Colter, D.C., I. Sekiya, and D.J. Prockop, Identification of a subpopulation of rapidly self-renewing and multipotential adult stem cells in colonies of human marrow stromal cells. *Proc. Natl. Acad. Sci. USA*, 2001. 98(14): p. 7841-5.

[126] Muraglia, A., R. Cancedda, and R. Quarto, Clonal mesenchymal progenitors from human bone marrow differentiate in vitro according to a hierarchical model. *J. Cell Sci.*, 2000. 113 (Pt 7): p. 1161-6.

[127] Okamoto, T., et al., Clonal heterogeneity in differentiation potential of immortalized human mesenchymal stem cells. *Biochem. Biophys. Res. Commun.*, 2002. 295(2): p. 354-61.

[128] Satomura, K., et al., Osteogenic imprinting upstream of marrow stromal cell differentiation. *J. Cell Biochem.*, 2000. 78(3): p. 391-403.

[129] Gronthos, S., et al., Differential cell surface expression of the STRO-1 and alkaline phosphatase antigens on discrete developmental stages in primary cultures of human bone cells. *J. Bone Miner Res.*, 1999. 14(1): p. 47-56.

[130] Bensidhoum, M., et al., Homing of in vitro expanded Stro-1- or Stro-1+ human mesenchymal stem cells into the NOD/SCID mouse and their role in supporting human CD34 cell engraftment. *Blood,* 2004. 103(9): p. 3313-9.

[131] Simmons, P.J., et al., Vascular cell adhesion molecule-1 expressed by bone marrow stromal cells mediates the binding of hematopoietic progenitor cells. *Blood,* 1992. 80(2): p. 388-95.

[132] Simmons, P.J. and B. Torok-Storb, Identification of stromal cell precursors in human bone marrow by a novel monoclonal antibody, STRO-1. *Blood,* 1991. 78(1): p. 55-62.

[133] Haynesworth, S.E., M.A. Baber, and A.I. Caplan, Cell surface antigens on human marrow-derived mesenchymal cells are detected by monoclonal antibodies. *Bone,* 1992. 13(1): p. 69-80.

[134] Barry, F., et al., The SH-3 and SH-4 antibodies recognize distinct epitopes on CD73 from human mesenchymal stem cells. *Biochem. Biophys. Res. Commun.*, 2001. 289(2): p. 519-24.

[135] De Ugarte, D.A., et al., Differential expression of stem cell mobilization-associated molecules on multi-lineage cells from adipose tissue and bone marrow. *Immunol. Lett.*, 2003. 89(2-3): p. 267-70.

[136] Vogel, G., Biotechnology. Stem cells lose market luster. *Science*, 2003. 299(5614): p. 1830-1.

[137] Vogel, W., et al., Heterogeneity among human bone marrow-derived mesenchymal stem cells and neural progenitor cells. *Haematologica,* 2003. 88(2): p. 126-33.

[138] Bruder, S.P., N. Jaiswal, and S.E. Haynesworth, Growth kinetics, self-renewal, and the osteogenic potential of purified human mesenchymal stem cells during extensive subcultivation and following cryopreservation. *J. Cell Biochem.*, 1997. 64(2): p. 278-94.

[139] Banfi, A., et al., Replicative aging and gene expression in long-term cultures of human bone marrow stromal cells. *Tissue Eng.*, 2002. 8(6): p. 901-10.

[140] Kawano, S., et al., Ca(2+) oscillations regulated by Na(+)-Ca(2+) exchanger and plasma membrane Ca(2+) pump induce fluctuations of membrane currents and potentials in human mesenchymal stem cells. *Cell Calcium.*, 2003. 34(2): p. 145-56.

[141] Pereira, R.F., et al., Cultured adherent cells from marrow can serve as long-lasting precursor cells for bone, cartilage, and lung in irradiated mice. *Proc. Natl. Acad. Sci. USA,* 1995. 92(11): p. 4857-61.

[142] Castro-Malaspina, H., et al., Characterization of human bone marrow fibroblast colony-forming cells (CFU-F) and their progeny. *Blood,* 1980. 56(2): p. 289-301.

[143] Bianchi, G., et al., Ex vivo enrichment of mesenchymal cell progenitors by fibroblast growth factor 2. *Exp. Cell Res.,* 2003. 287(1): p. 98-105.

[144] Bonyadi, M., et al., Mesenchymal progenitor self-renewal deficiency leads to age-dependent osteoporosis in Sca-1/Ly-6A null mice. *Proc. Natl. Acad. Sci. USA,* 2003. 100(10): p. 5840-5.

[145] Klein, A.K., et al., Characterization of canine fetal lymphohematopoiesis: studies of CFUGM, CFUL, and CFUF. *Exp. Hematol.,* 1983. 11(4): p. 263-74.

[146] Van den Heuvel, R.L., et al., Stromal stem cells (CFU-f) in yolk sac, liver, spleen and bone marrow of pre- and postnatal mice. *Br. J. Haematol.,* 1987. 66(1): p. 15-20.

[147] Charbord, P., et al., Early ontogeny of the human marrow from long bones: an immunohistochemical study of hematopoiesis and its microenvironment. *Blood,* 1996. 87(10): p. 4109-19.

[148] Mendes, S.C., C. Robin, and E. Dzierzak, Mesenchymal progenitor cells localize within hematopoietic sites throughout ontogeny. *Development,* 2005. 132(5): p. 1127-36.

[149] Friedenstein, A.J., S. Piatetzky, II, and K.V. Petrakova, Osteogenesis in transplants of bone marrow cells. *J. Embryol. Exp. Morphol.,* 1966. 16(3): p. 381-90.

[150] Dexter, T.M., T.D. Allen, and L.G. Lajtha, Conditions controlling the proliferation of haemopoietic stem cells in vitro. *J. Cell Physiol.,* 1977. 91(3): p. 335-44.

[151] Gupta, P., et al., Structurally specific heparan sulfates support primitive human hematopoiesis by formation of a multimolecular stem cell niche. *Blood,* 1998. 92(12): p. 4641-51.

[152] Calvi, L.M., et al., Osteoblastic cells regulate the haematopoietic stem cell niche. *Nature,* 2003. 425(6960): p. 841-6.

[153] Shi, S. and S. Gronthos, Perivascular niche of postnatal mesenchymal stem cells in human bone marrow and dental pulp. *J. Bone Miner Res.,* 2003. 18(4): p. 696-704.

[154] Moore, K.A., Recent advances in defining the hematopoietic stem cell niche. *Curr. Opin. Hematol.,* 2004. 11(2): p. 107-11.

[155] Arai, F., A. Hirao, and T. Suda, Regulation of hematopoietic stem cells by the niche. *Trends Cardiovasc. Med.,* 2005. 15(2): p. 75-9.

[156] Charbord, P., [The hematopoietic stem cell and the stromal microenvironment]. *Therapie,* 2001. 56(4): p. 383-4.

[157] Chagraoui, J., et al., Fetal liver stroma consists of cells in epithelial-to-mesenchymal transition. *Blood,* 2003. 101(8): p. 2973-82.

[158] Fuchs, E. and C. Byrne, The epidermis: rising to the surface. *Curr. Opin. Genet Dev.,* 1994. 4(5): p. 725-36.

[159] Lo, L., L. Sommer, and D.J. Anderson, MASH1 maintains competence for BMP2-induced neuronal differentiation in post-migratory neural crest cells. *Curr. Biol.,* 1997. 7(6): p. 440-50.

[160] Baron, M., Induction of embryonic hematopoietic and endothelial stem/progenitor cells by hedgehog-mediated signals. *Differentiation*, 2001. 68(4-5): p. 175-85.

[161] Soria, B., In-vitro differentiation of pancreatic beta-cells. *Differentiation*, 2001. 68(4-5): p. 205-19.

[162] Gupta, S., Hepatocyte transplantation. *J. Gastroenterol. Hepatol.*, 2002. 17 Suppl 3: p. S287-S293.

[163] Herzog, E.L., L. Chai, and D.S. Krause, Plasticity of marrow-derived stem cells. *Blood*, 2003. 102(10): p. 3483-93.

[164] Fridenshtein, A., [Stromal bone marrow cells and the hematopoietic microenvironment]. *Arkh Patol*, 1982. 44(10): p. 3-11.

[165] Gronthos, S. and P.J. Simmons, The biology and application of human bone marrow stromal cell precursors. *J. Hematother.*, 1996. 5(1): p. 15-23.

[166] Reyes, M., et al., Origin of endothelial progenitors in human postnatal bone marrow. *J. Clin. Invest.*, 2002. 109(3): p. 337-46.

[167] Brazelton, T.R., et al., From marrow to brain: expression of neuronal phenotypes in adult mice. Science, 2000. 290(5497): p. 1775-9.

[168] Sanchez-Ramos, J., et al., Adult bone marrow stromal cells differentiate into neural cells in vitro. *Exp. Neurol.*, 2000. 164(2): p. 247-56.

[169] Zhao, L.X., et al., Modification of the brain-derived neurotrophic factor gene: a portal to transform mesenchymal stem cells into advantageous engineering cells for neuroregeneration and neuroprotection. *Exp. Neurol.*, 2004. 190(2): p. 396-406.

[170] Schwartz, R.E., et al., Multipotent adult progenitor cells from bone marrow differentiate into functional hepatocyte-like cells. *J. Clin. Invest.*, 2002. 109(10): p. 1291-302.

[171] Sata, M., et al., The role of circulating precursors in vascular repair and lesion formation. *J. Cell Mol. Med.*, 2005. 9(3): p. 557-68.

[172] Liechty, K.W., et al., Human mesenchymal stem cells engraft and demonstrate site-specific differentiation after in utero transplantation in sheep. *Nat. Med.* 2000. 6(11): p. 1282-6.

[173] Sato, Y., et al., Human mesenchymal stem cells xenografted directly to rat liver are differentiated into human hepatocytes without fusion. *Blood*, 2005. 106(2): p. 756-63.

[174] Togel, F., et al., Administered mesenchymal stem cells protect against ischemic acute renal failure through differentiation-independent mechanisms. *Am. J. Physiol. Renal. Physiol*, 2005. 289(1): p. F31-42.

[175] Loeffler, M. and I. Roeder, Tissue stem cells: definition, plasticity, heterogeneity, self-organization and models--a conceptual approach. *Cells Tissues Organs*, 2002. 171(1): p. 8-26.

[176] Loeffler, M. and I. Roeder, Conceptual models to understand tissue stem cell organization. *Curr. Opin. Hematol.*, 2004. 11(2): p. 81-7.

[177] Roeder, I. and M. Loeffler, A novel dynamic model of hematopoietic stem cell organization based on the concept of within-tissue plasticity. *Exp. Hematol.*, 2002. 30(8): p. 853-61.

[178] Song, L. and R.S. Tuan, Transdifferentiation potential of human mesenchymal stem cells derived from bone marrow. *Faseb J.*, 2004. 18(9): p. 980-2.

[179] Park, S.R., R.O. Oreffo, and J.T. Triffitt, Interconversion potential of cloned human marrow adipocytes in vitro. *Bone*, 1999. 24(6): p. 549-54.

[180] Dennis, J.E., et al., The STRO-1+ marrow cell population is multipotential. *Cells Tissues Organs*, 2002. 170(2-3): p. 73-82.

[181] Terada, N., et al., Bone marrow cells adopt the phenotype of other cells by spontaneous cell fusion. *Nature*, 2002. 416(6880): p. 542-5.

[182] Spees, J.L., et al., Differentiation, cell fusion, and nuclear fusion during ex vivo repair of epithelium by human adult stem cells from bone marrow stroma. *Proc. Natl. Acad. Sci. USA*, 2003. 100(5): p. 2397-402.

[183] Wurmser, A.E., et al., Cell fusion-independent differentiation of neural stem cells to the endothelial lineage. *Nature*, 2004. 430(6997): p. 350-6.

[184] Saga, K., Structure and function of human sweat glands studied with histochemistry and cytochemistry. *Prog. Histochem. Cytochem.*, 2002. 37(4): p. 323-86.

[185] Shikiji, T., et al., Keratinocytes can differentiate into eccrine sweat ducts in vitro: involvement of epidermal growth factor and fetal bovine serum. *J. Dermatol. Sci.*, 2003. 33(3): p. 141-50.

[186] Li, H., et al., Adult bone-marrow-derived mesenchymal stem cells contribute to wound healing of skin appendages. *Cell Tissue Res.*, 2006. 326(3): p. 725-736.

[187] Borue, X., et al., Bone marrow-derived cells contribute to epithelial engraftment during wound healing. *Am. J. Pathol.*, 2004. 165(5): p. 1767-72.

[188] Wu, M., et al., Differentiation potential of human embryonic mesenchymal stem cells for skin-related tissue. *Br. J. Dermatol.*, 2006. 155(2): p. 282-91.

[189] Ronfard, V., et al., Long-term regeneration of human epidermis on third degree burns transplanted with autologous cultured epithelium grown on a fibrin matrix. *Transplantation*, 2000. 70(11): p. 1588-98.

[190] Shi, C., et al., Stem cells and their applications in skin-cell therapy. *Trends Biotechnol*, 2006. 24(1): p. 48-52.

[191] Gharzi, A., A.J. Reynolds, and C.A. Jahoda, Plasticity of hair follicle dermal cells in wound healing and induction. *Exp. Dermatol.*, 2003. 12(2): p. 126-36.

[192] Chunmeng, S. and C. Tianmin, Effects of plastic-adherent dermal multipotent cells on peripheral blood leukocytes and CFU-GM in rats. *Transplant Proc.*, 2004. 36(5): p. 1578-81.

[193] Deng, W., et al., Allogeneic bone marrow-derived flk-1+Sca-1- mesenchymal stem cells leads to stable mixed chimerism and donor-specific tolerance. *Exp. Hematol.*, 2004. 32(9): p. 861-7.

[194] Heng, B.C., et al., Directing stem cells into the keratinocyte lineage in vitro. *Exp. Dermatol.*, 2005. 14(1): p. 1-16.

[195] Reynolds, B.A. and S. Weiss, Generation of neurons and astrocytes from isolated cells of the adult mammalian central nervous system. *Science*, 1992. 255(5052): p. 1707-10.

[196] Woodbury, D., et al., Adult rat and human bone marrow stromal cells differentiate into neurons. *J. Neurosci. Res.*, 2000. 61(4): p. 364-70.

[197] Tondreau, T., et al., Bone marrow-derived mesenchymal stem cells already express specific neural proteins before any differentiation. *Differentiation*, 2004. 72(7): p. 319-26.

[198] Minguell, J.J., et al., Nonstimulated human uncommitted mesenchymal stem cells express cell markers of mesenchymal and neural lineages. *Stem Cells Dev.*, 2005. 14(4): p. 408-14.

[199] Long, X., et al., Neural cell differentiation in vitro from adult human bone marrow mesenchymal stem cells. *Stem Cells Dev.,* 2005. 14(1): p. 65-9.

[200] Magaki, T., K. Kurisu, and T. Okazaki, Generation of bone marrow-derived neural cells in serum-free monolayer culture. *Neurosci. Lett.*, 2005. 384(3): p. 282-7.

[201] Tao, H., R. Rao, and D.D. Ma, Cytokine-induced stable neuronal differentiation of human bone marrow mesenchymal stem cells in a serum/feeder cell-free condition. *Dev. Growth Differ*, 2005. 47(6): p. 423-33.

[202] Azizi, S.A., et al., Engraftment and migration of human bone marrow stromal cells implanted in the brains of albino rats--similarities to astrocyte grafts. *Proc. Natl. Acad. Sci. USA,* 1998. 95(7): p. 3908-13.

[203] Munoz-Elias, G., et al., Adult bone marrow stromal cells in the embryonic brain: engraftment, migration, differentiation, and long-term survival. *J. Neurosci.*, 2004. 24(19): p. 4585-95.

[204] Deng, W., et al., In vitro differentiation of human marrow stromal cells into early progenitors of neural cells by conditions that increase intracellular cyclic AMP. *Biochem. Biophys. Res. Commun.*, 2001. 282(1): p. 148-52.

[205] Wehner, T., et al., Bone marrow-derived cells expressing green fluorescent protein under the control of the glial fibrillary acidic protein promoter do not differentiate into astrocytes in vitro and in vivo. *J. Neurosci.*, 2003. 23(12): p. 5004-11.

[206] Kim, B.J., et al., Differentiation of adult bone marrow stem cells into neuroprogenitor cells in vitro. *Neuroreport,* 2002. 13(9): p. 1185-8.

[207] Abouelfetouh, A., et al., Morphological differentiation of bone marrow stromal cells into neuron-like cells after co-culture with hippocampal slice. *Brain Res.*, 2004. 1029(1): p. 114-9.

[208] Mareschi, K., et al., Neural differentiation of human mesenchymal stem cells: Evidence for expression of neural markers and eag K+ channel types. *Exp. Hematol.*, 2006. 34(11): p. 1563-72.

[209] Mori, K., et al., Functional recovery of neuronal activity in rat whisker-barrel cortex sensory pathway from freezing injury after transplantation of adult bone marrow stromal cells. *J. Cereb. Blood Flow Metab.*, 2005. 25(7): p. 887-98.

[210] Zhao, L.R., et al., Human bone marrow stem cells exhibit neural phenotypes and ameliorate neurological deficits after grafting into the ischemic brain of rats. *Exp. Neurol.*, 2002. 174(1): p. 11-20.

[211] Dezawa, M., et al., Specific induction of neuronal cells from bone marrow stromal cells and application for autologous transplantation. *J. Clin. Invest*, 2004. 113(12): p. 1701-10.

[212] Chiou, S.H., et al., A novel in vitro retinal differentiation model by co-culturing adult human bone marrow stem cells with retinal pigmented epithelium cells. *Biochem. Biophys. Res. Commun.*, 2005. 326(3): p. 578-85.

[213] Kicic, A., et al., Differentiation of marrow stromal cells into photoreceptors in the rat eye. *J. Neurosci.*, 2003. 23(21): p. 7742-9.

[214] Arnhold, S., et al., Transplantation of bone marrow-derived mesenchymal stem cells rescue photoreceptor cells in the dystrophic retina of the rhodopsin knockout mouse. *Graefes Arch. Clin. Exp. Ophthalmol.*, 2006.

[215] Arnhold, S., et al., Adenovirally transduced bone marrow stromal cells differentiate into pigment epithelial cells and induce rescue effects in RCS rats. *Invest. Ophthalmol. Vis. Sci.*, 2006. 47(9): p. 4121-9.

[216] Tomita, M., et al., Bone marrow-derived stem cells can differentiate into retinal cells in injured rat retina. *Stem Cells*, 2002. 20(4): p. 279-83.

[217] Kershaw, E.E. and J.S. Flier, Adipose tissue as an endocrine organ. *J. Clin. Endocrinol. Metab.*, 2004. 89(6): p. 2548-56.

[218] Otto, T.C. and M.D. Lane, Adipose development: from stem cell to adipocyte. *Crit. Rev. Biochem. Mol. Biol.*, 2005. 40(4): p. 229-42.

[219] Rosen, E.D. and O.A. MacDougald, Adipocyte differentiation from the inside out. *Nat. Rev. Mol. Cell Biol.*, 2006. 7(12): p. 885-96.

[220] Neubauer, M., et al., Basic fibroblast growth factor enhances PPARgamma ligand-induced adipogenesis of mesenchymal stem cells. *FEBS Lett.*, 2004. 577(1-2): p. 277-83.

[221] Ogawa, R., et al., Adipogenic differentiation by adipose-derived stem cells harvested from GFP transgenic mice-including relationship of sex differences. *Biochem. Biophys. Res. Commun.*, 2004. 319(2): p. 511-7.

[222] Pakala, R., et al., Peroxisome proliferator-activated receptor gamma: its role in metabolic syndrome. *Cardiovasc. Radiat. Med.*, 2004. 5(2): p. 97-103.

[223] She, H., et al., Adipogenic transcriptional regulation of hepatic stellate cells. *J. Biol. Chem.*, 2005. 280(6): p. 4959-67.

[224] Tominaga, S., et al., Negative regulation of adipogenesis from human mesenchymal stem cells by Jun N-terminal kinase. *Biochem. Biophys. Res. Commun.*, 2005. 326(2): p. 499-504.

[225] Spinella-Jaegle, S., et al., Sonic hedgehog increases the commitment of pluripotent mesenchymal cells into the osteoblastic lineage and abolishes adipocytic differentiation. *J. Cell Sci.*, 2001. 114(Pt 11): p. 2085-94.

[226] Bennett, C.N., et al., Regulation of osteoblastogenesis and bone mass by Wnt10b. *Proc. Natl. Acad. Sci. USA,* 2005. 102(9): p. 3324-9.

[227] Suh, J.M., et al., Hedgehog signaling plays a conserved role in inhibiting fat formation. *Cell Metab.*, 2006. 3(1): p. 25-34.

[228] Jeon, M.J., et al., Activation of peroxisome proliferator-activated receptor-gamma inhibits the Runx2-mediated transcription of osteocalcin in osteoblasts. *J. Biol. Chem.*, 2003. 278(26): p. 23270-7.

[229] Akune, T., et al., PPARgamma insufficiency enhances osteogenesis through osteoblast formation from bone marrow progenitors. *J. Clin. Invest.*, 2004. 113(6): p. 846-55.

[230] Ali, A.A., et al., Rosiglitazone causes bone loss in mice by suppressing osteoblast differentiation and bone formation. *Endocrinology,* 2005. 146(3): p. 1226-35.

[231] Kawaguchi, H., et al., Distinct effects of PPARgamma insufficiency on bone marrow cells, osteoblasts, and osteoclastic cells. *J. Bone Miner Metab.*, 2005. 23(4): p. 275-9.

[232] Gimble, J.M., et al., Peroxisome proliferator-activated receptor-gamma activation by thiazolidinediones induces adipogenesis in bone marrow stromal cells. *Mol. Pharmacol.*, 1996. 50(5): p. 1087-94.

[233] Ahdjoudj, S., et al., Reciprocal control of osteoblast/chondroblast and osteoblast/adipocyte differentiation of multipotential clonal human marrow stromal F/STRO-1(+) cells. *J. Cell Biochem.*, 2001. 81(1): p. 23-38.

[234] Rosen, E.D. and B.M. Spiegelman, Molecular regulation of adipogenesis. *Annu. Rev. Cell Dev. Biol.*, 2000. 16: p. 145-71.

[235] Janderova, L., et al., Human mesenchymal stem cells as an in vitro model for human adipogenesis. *Obes. Res.*, 2003. 11(1): p. 65-74.

[236] Scavo, L.M., et al., Insulin-like growth factor-I stimulates both cell growth and lipogenesis during differentiation of human mesenchymal stem cells into adipocytes. *J. Clin. Endocrinol. Metab.*, 2004. 89(7): p. 3543-53.

[237] Kim, S.J., et al., Human adipose stromal cells expanded in human serum promote engraftment of human peripheral blood hematopoietic stem cells in NOD/SCID mice. *Biochem. Biophys. Res. Commun.*, 2005. 329(1): p. 25-31.

[238] Lin, T.M., et al., Accelerated growth and prolonged lifespan of adipose tissue-derived human mesenchymal stem cells in a medium using reduced calcium and antioxidants. *Stem Cells Dev.*, 2005. 14(1): p. 92-102.

[239] Olsen, B.R., A.M. Reginato, and W. Wang, Bone development. *Annu. Rev. Cell Dev. Biol.*, 2000. 16: p. 191-220.

[240] Long, M.W., Osteogenesis and bone-marrow-derived cells. *Blood Cells Mol. Dis.*, 2001. 27(3): p. 677-90.

[241] Fibbe, W.E., Mesenchymal stem cells. A potential source for skeletal repair. *Ann. Rheum. Dis.*, 2002. 61 Suppl 2: p. ii29-31.

[242] Ramoshebi, L.N., et al., Tissue engineering: TGF-beta superfamily members and delivery systems in bone regeneration. *Expert. Rev. Mol. Med.*, 2002. 2002: p. 1-11.

[243] Canalis, E., A.N. Economides, and E. Gazzerro, Bone morphogenetic proteins, their antagonists, and the skeleton. *Endocr. Rev.*, 2003. 24(2): p. 218-35.

[244] Rawadi, G., et al., BMP-2 controls alkaline phosphatase expression and osteoblast mineralization by a Wnt autocrine loop. *J. Bone Miner Res.*, 2003. 18(10): p. 1842-53.

[245] Sykaras, N. and L.A. Opperman, Bone morphogenetic proteins (BMPs): how do they function and what can they offer the clinician? *J. Oral Sci.*, 2003. 45(2): p. 57-73.

[246] Taguchi, Y., et al., Interleukin-6-type cytokines stimulate mesenchymal progenitor differentiation toward the osteoblastic lineage. *Proc. Assoc. Am. Physicians*, 1998. 110(6): p. 559-74.

[247] Kroger, H., E. Soppi, and N. Loveridge, Growth hormone, osteoblasts, and marrow adipocytes: a case report. *Calcif. Tissue Int.*, 1997. 61(1): p. 33-5.

[248] Thomas, T., et al., Leptin acts on human marrow stromal cells to enhance differentiation to osteoblasts and to inhibit differentiation to adipocytes. *Endocrinology*, 1999. 140(4): p. 1630-8.

[249] Maeda, S., et al., Sortilin is upregulated during osteoblastic differentiation of mesenchymal stem cells and promotes extracellular matrix mineralization. *J. Cell Physiol.*, 2002. 193(1): p. 73-9.

[250] Nurminskaya, M., et al., Chondrocyte-derived transglutaminase promotes maturation of preosteoblasts in periosteal bone. *Dev. Biol.*, 2003. 263(1): p. 139-52.

[251] Raisz, L.G., C.C. Pilbeam, and P.M. Fall, Prostaglandins: mechanisms of action and regulation of production in bone. *Osteoporos Int,* 1993. 3 Suppl 1: p. 136-40.

[252] Weinreb, M., A. Grosskopf, and N. Shir, The anabolic effect of PGE2 in rat bone marrow cultures is mediated via the EP4 receptor subtype. *Am. J. Physiol.*, 1999. 276(2 Pt 1): p. E376-83.

[253] van Leeuwen, J.P., et al., Vitamin D control of osteoblast function and bone extracellular matrix mineralization. *Crit. Rev. Eukaryot. Gene Expr.*, 2001. 11(1-3): p. 199-226.

[254] zur Nieden, N.I., G. Kempka, and H.J. Ahr, In vitro differentiation of embryonic stem cells into mineralized osteoblasts. *Differentiation*, 2003. 71(1): p. 18-27.

[255] Rogers, J.J., et al., Differentiation factors induce expression of muscle, fat, cartilage, and bone in a clone of mouse pluripotent mesenchymal stem cells. *Am. Surg.*, 1995. 61(3): p. 231-6.

[256] Buttery, L.D., et al., Differentiation of osteoblasts and in vitro bone formation from murine embryonic stem cells. *Tissue Eng,* 2001. 7(1): p. 89-99.

[257] Sottile, V., A. Thomson, and J. McWhir, In vitro osteogenic differentiation of human ES cells. *Cloning Stem Cells*, 2003. 5(2): p. 149-55.

[258] Notoya, K., et al., Enhancement of osteogenesis in vitro and in vivo by a novel osteoblast differentiation promoting compound, TAK-778. *J. Pharmacol. Exp. Ther.*, 1999. 290(3): p. 1054-64.

[259] Rosa, A.L. and M.M. Beloti, TAK-778 enhances osteoblast differentiation of human bone marrow cells. *J. Cell Biochem.*, 2003. 89(6): p. 1148-53.

[260] Sugiyama, M., et al., Compactin and simvastatin, but not pravastatin, induce bone morphogenetic protein-2 in human osteosarcoma cells. *Biochem. Biophys. Res. Commun.*, 2000. 271(3): p. 688-92.

[261] Ohnaka, K., et al., Pitavastatin enhanced BMP-2 and osteocalcin expression by inhibition of Rho-associated kinase in human osteoblasts. *Biochem. Biophys. Res. Commun.*, 2001. 287(2): p. 337-42.

[262] Phillips, B.W., et al., Compactin enhances osteogenesis in murine embryonic stem cells. *Biochem. Biophys. Res. Commun.*, 2001. 284(2): p. 478-84.

[263] Gerstenfeld, L.C., et al., Osteogenic differentiation is selectively promoted by morphogenetic signals from chondrocytes and synergized by a nutrient rich growth environment. *Connect. Tissue Res.*, 2003. 44 Suppl 1: p. 85-91.

[264] Gerstenfeld, L.C., et al., Chondrocytes provide morphogenic signals that selectively induce osteogenic differentiation of mesenchymal stem cells. *J. Bone Miner Res.*, 2002. 17(2): p. 221-30.

[265] Karadag, A., A.M. Scutt, and P.I. Croucher, Human myeloma cells promote the recruitment of osteoblast precursors: mediation by interleukin-6 and soluble interleukin-6 receptor. *J. Bone Miner Res.*, 2000. 15(10): p. 1935-43.

[266] Villars, F., et al., Effect of HUVEC on human osteoprogenitor cell differentiation needs heterotypic gap junction communication. *Am. J. Physiol. Cell Physiol.*, 2002. 282(4): p. C775-85.

[267] Zhou, J., et al., [Research in use of vascular endothelial cells to promote osteogenesis of marrow stromal cells]. *Sheng Wu Yi Xue Gong Cheng Xue Za Zhi*, 2003. 20(3): p. 447-50.

[268] Greenwald, J.A., et al., Biomolecular mechanisms of calvarial bone induction: immature versus mature dura mater. *Plast. Reconstr. Surg.*, 2000. 105(4): p. 1382-92.

[269] Spector, J.A., et al., Co-culture of osteoblasts with immature dural cells causes an increased rate and degree of osteoblast differentiation. *Plast. Reconstr. Surg.*, 2002. 109(2): p. 631-42; discussion 643-4.

[270] Aubin, J.E., Osteoprogenitor cell frequency in rat bone marrow stromal populations: role for heterotypic cell-cell interactions in osteoblast differentiation. *J. Cell Biochem.*, 1999. 72(3): p. 396-410.

[271] Bianco, P., et al., Expression of bone sialoprotein (BSP) in developing human tissues. *Calcif Tissue Int,* 1991. 49(6): p. 421-6.

[272] Helder, M.N., A.L. Bronckers, and J.H. Woltgens, Dissimilar expression patterns for the extracellular matrix proteins osteopontin (OPN) and collagen type I in dental tissues and alveolar bone of the neonatal rat. *Matrix,* 1993. 13(5): p. 415-25.

[273] Bronckers, A.L., et al., Developmental appearance of Gla proteins (osteocalcin) and alkaline phosphatase in tooth germs and bones of the rat. *Bone Miner*, 1987. 2(5): p. 361-73.

[274] Thomas, G., et al., Osteocrin, a novel bone-specific secreted protein that modulates the osteoblast phenotype. *J. Biol. Chem.*, 2003. 278(50): p. 50563-71.

[275] Krebsbach, P.H., et al., Bone formation in vivo: comparison of osteogenesis by transplanted mouse and human marrow stromal fibroblasts. *Transplantation*, 1997. 63(8): p. 1059-69.

[276] Kon, E., et al., Autologous bone marrow stromal cells loaded onto porous hydroxyapatite ceramic accelerate bone repair in critical-size defects of sheep long bones. *J. Biomed. Mater. Res.*, 2000. 49(3): p. 328-37.

[277] Petite, H., et al., Tissue-engineered bone regeneration. *Nat. Biotechnol.*, 2000. 18(9): p. 959-63.

[278] Chen, F., et al., Injectable bone. *Br. J. Oral. Maxillofac. Surg.*, 2003. 41(4): p. 240-3.

[279] Chang, S.C., et al., Cranial repair using BMP-2 gene engineered bone marrow stromal cells. *J. Surg. Res.*, 2004. 119(1): p. 85-91.

[280] Schantz, J.T., et al., Repair of calvarial defects with customised tissue-engineered bone grafts II. Evaluation of cellular efficiency and efficacy in vivo. *Tissue Eng*, 2003. 9 Suppl 1: p. S127-39.

[281] Dai, K.R., et al., Repairing of goat tibial bone defects with BMP-2 gene-modified tissue-engineered bone. *Calcif Tissue Int*, 2005. 77(1): p. 55-61.

[282] Li, Z., et al., Repair of sheep metatarsus defects by using tissue-engineering technique. *J. Huazhong Univ. Sci. Technolog. Med. Sci.,* 2005. 25(1): p. 62-7.

[283] Meinel, L., et al., Silk implants for the healing of critical size bone defects. *Bone*, 2005. 37(5): p. 688-98.

[284] Brodke, D., et al., Bone grafts prepared with selective cell retention technology heal canine segmental defects as effectively as autograft. *J. Orthop. Res.*, 2006. 24(5): p. 857-66.

[285] Yoon, E., et al., In Vivo Osteogenic Potential of Human Adipose-Derived Stem Cells/Poly Lactide-Co-Glycolic Acid Constructs for Bone Regeneration in a Rat Critical-Sized Calvarial Defect Model. *Tissue Eng*, 2006.

[286] Horwitz, E.M., et al., Transplantability and therapeutic effects of bone marrow-derived mesenchymal cells in children with osteogenesis imperfecta. *Nat. Med.*, 1999. 5(3): p. 309-13.

[287] Cancedda, R., et al., Tissue engineering and cell therapy of cartilage and bone. *Matrix Biol.*, 2003. 22(1): p. 81-91.

[288] Rose, F.R. and R.O. Oreffo, Bone tissue engineering: hope vs hype. *Biochem. Biophys. Res. Commun.*, 2002. 292(1): p. 1-7.

[289] Vats, A., et al., Scaffolds and biomaterials for tissue engineering: a review of clinical applications. *Clin. Otolaryngol. Allied Sci.*, 2003. 28(3): p. 165-72.

[290] Bruder, S.P., et al., Bone regeneration by implantation of purified, culture-expanded human mesenchymal stem cells. *J. Orthop. Res.*, 1998. 16(2): p. 155-62.

[291] El-Amin, S.F., et al., Integrin expression by human osteoblasts cultured on degradable polymeric materials applicable for tissue engineered bone. *J. Orthop. Res.*, 2002. 20(1): p. 20-8.

[292] Quarto, R., et al., Repair of large bone defects with the use of autologous bone marrow stromal cells. *N. Engl. J. Med.*, 2001. 344(5): p. 385-6.

[293] Vacanti, C.A., et al., Replacement of an avulsed phalanx with tissue-engineered bone. *N. Engl. J. Med.*, 2001. 344(20): p. 1511-4.

[294] Warnke, P.H., et al., Growth and transplantation of a custom vascularised bone graft in a man. *Lancet*, 2004. 364(9436): p. 766-70.

[295] Johnstone, B., et al., In vitro chondrogenesis of bone marrow-derived mesenchymal progenitor cells. *Exp. Cell Res.*, 1998. 238(1): p. 265-72.

[296] Yoo, J.U., et al., The chondrogenic potential of human bone-marrow-derived mesenchymal progenitor cells. *J. Bone Joint Surg. Am.*, 1998. 80(12): p. 1745-57.

[297] Kavalkovich, K.W., et al., Chondrogenic differentiation of human mesenchymal stem cells within an alginate layer culture system. *In Vitro Cell Dev. Biol. Anim.*, 2002. 38(8): p. 457-66.

[298] Lee, J.W., et al., Chondrogenic differentiation of mesenchymal stem cells and its clinical applications. *Yonsei Med. J.*, 2004. 45 Suppl: p. 41-7.

[299] Yang, I.H., et al., Comparison of phenotypic characterization between "alginate bead" and "pellet" culture systems as chondrogenic differentiation models for human mesenchymal stem cells. *Yonsei Med. J.*, 2004. 45(5): p. 891-900.

[300] Caplan, A.I., et al., Principles of cartilage repair and regeneration. *Clin. Orthop. Relat. Res.*, 1997(342): p. 254-69.

[301] Murphy, J.M., et al., Stem cell therapy in a caprine model of osteoarthritis. *Arthritis Rheum.*, 2003. 48(12): p. 3464-74.

[302] Wakitani, S., et al., Mesenchymal cell-based repair of large, full-thickness defects of articular cartilage. *J. Bone Joint Surg. Am.*, 1994. 76(4): p. 579-92.

[303] Wakitani, S., et al., Human autologous culture expanded bone marrow mesenchymal cell transplantation for repair of cartilage defects in osteoarthritic knees. *Osteoarthritis Cartilage*, 2002. 10(3): p. 199-206.

[304] Wakitani, S. and T. Yamamoto, Response of the donor and recipient cells in mesenchymal cell transplantation to cartilage defect. *Microsc. Res.Tech.*, 2002. 58(1): p. 14-8.
[305] Brittberg, M., et al., Treatment of deep cartilage defects in the knee with autologous chondrocyte transplantation. N Engl J Med, 1994. 331(14): p. 889-95.
[306] Jorgensen, C., et al., Stem cells for repair of cartilage and bone: the next challenge in osteoarthritis and rheumatoid arthritis. *Ann. Rheum. Dis.*, 2001. 60(4): p. 305-9.
[307] Schultz, O., et al., Emerging strategies of bone and joint repair. *Arthritis Res.*, 2000. 2(6): p. 433-6.
[308] Yamasaki, T., et al., Meniscal regeneration using tissue engineering with a scaffold derived from a rat meniscus and mesenchymal stromal cells derived from rat bone marrow. *J. Biomed. Mater. Res. A*, 2005. 75(1): p. 23-30.
[309] Gao, J., et al., Repair of osteochondral defect with tissue-engineered two-phase composite material of injectable calcium phosphate and hyaluronan sponge. *Tissue Eng.*, 2002. 8(5): p. 827-37.
[310] Caterson, E.J., et al., Three-dimensional cartilage formation by bone marrow-derived cells seeded in polylactide/alginate amalgam. *J. Biomed. Mater. Res.*, 2001. 57(3): p. 394-403.
[311] Tuan, R.S., G. Boland, and R. Tuli, Adult mesenchymal stem cells and cell-based tissue engineering. *Arthritis Res. Ther.*, 2003. 5(1): p. 32-45.
[312] Crevensten, G., et al., Intervertebral disc cell therapy for regeneration: mesenchymal stem cell implantation in rat intervertebral discs. *Ann. Biomed. Eng.*, 2004. 32(3): p. 430-4.
[313] Reddi, A.H., Role of morphogenetic proteins in skeletal tissue engineering and regeneration. *Nat. Biotechnol.*, 1998. 16(3): p. 247-52.
[314] van Beuningen, H.M., et al., Differential effects of local application of BMP-2 or TGF-beta 1 on both articular cartilage composition and osteophyte formation. *Osteoarthritis Cartilage*, 1998. 6(5): p. 306-17.
[315] Aung, T., et al., Chondroinduction of mouse mesenchymal stem cells in three-dimensional highly porous matrix scaffolds. *J. Biomed. Mater. Res.*, 2002. 61(1): p. 75-82.
[316] Ikeuchi, M., et al., Recombinant human bone morphogenetic protein-2 promotes osteogenesis within atelopeptide type I collagen solution by combination with rat cultured marrow cells. *J. Biomed. Mater. Res.*, 2002. 60(1): p. 61-9.
[317] Girotto, D., et al., Tissue-specific gene expression in chondrocytes grown on three-dimensional hyaluronic acid scaffolds. *Biomaterials*, 2003. 24(19): p. 3265-75.
[318] Awad, H.A., et al., Autologous mesenchymal stem cell-mediated repair of tendon. *Tissue Eng.*, 1999. 5(3): p. 267-77.
[319] Ringe, J., et al., Stem cells for regenerative medicine: advances in the engineering of tissues and organs. *Naturwissenschaften*, 2002. 89(8): p. 338-51.
[320] Awad, H.A., et al., Repair of patellar tendon injuries using a cell-collagen composite. *J. Orthop. Res.*, 2003. 21(3): p. 420-31.
[321] Young, R.G., et al., Use of mesenchymal stem cells in a collagen matrix for Achilles tendon repair. *J. Orthop. Res.*, 1998. 16(4): p. 406-13.

[322] Wolfman, N.M., et al., Ectopic induction of tendon and ligament in rats by growth and differentiation factors 5, 6, and 7, members of the TGF-beta gene family. *J. Clin. Invest.*, 1997. 100(2): p. 321-30.

[323] Ouyang, H.W., et al., The efficacy of bone marrow stromal cell-seeded knitted PLGA fiber scaffold for Achilles tendon repair. *Ann. NY Acad. Sci.*, 2002. 961: p. 126-9.

[324] Ouyang, H.W., et al., Knitted poly-lactide-co-glycolide scaffold loaded with bone marrow stromal cells in repair and regeneration of rabbit Achilles tendon. *Tissue Eng*, 2003. 9(3): p. 431-9.

[325] Juncosa-Melvin, N., et al., Effects of cell-to-collagen ratio in mesenchymal stem cell-seeded implants on tendon repair biomechanics and histology. *Tissue Eng*, 2005. 11(3-4): p. 448-57.

[326] Zammit, P. and J. Beauchamp, The skeletal muscle satellite cell: stem cell or son of stem cell? *Differentiation*, 2001. 68(4-5): p. 193-204.

[327] Charge, S.B. and M.A. Rudnicki, Cellular and molecular regulation of muscle regeneration. *Physiol. Rev.*, 2004. 84(1): p. 209-38.

[328] Gussoni, E., et al., Dystrophin expression in the mdx mouse restored by stem cell transplantation. *Nature*, 1999. 401(6751): p. 390-4.

[329] Polesskaya, A., P. Seale, and M.A. Rudnicki, Wnt signaling induces the myogenic specification of resident CD45+ adult stem cells during muscle regeneration. *Cell*, 2003. 113(7): p. 841-52.

[330] Majka, S.M., et al., Distinct progenitor populations in skeletal muscle are bone marrow derived and exhibit different cell fates during vascular regeneration. *J. Clin. Invest*, 2003. 111(1): p. 71-9.

[331] Williams, J.T., et al., Cells isolated from adult human skeletal muscle capable of differentiating into multiple mesodermal phenotypes. *Am. Surg.*, 1999. 65(1): p. 22-6.

[332] Young, H.E., et al., Human reserve pluripotent mesenchymal stem cells are present in the connective tissues of skeletal muscle and dermis derived from fetal, adult, and geriatric donors. *Anat Rec.*, 2001. 264(1): p. 51-62.

[333] Wakitani, S., T. Saito, and A.I. Caplan, Myogenic cells derived from rat bone marrow mesenchymal stem cells exposed to 5-azacytidine. *Muscle Nerve*, 1995. 18(12): p. 1417-26.

[334] Ferrari, G., et al., Muscle regeneration by bone marrow-derived myogenic progenitors. *Science*, 1998. 279(5356): p. 1528-30.

[335] Bittner, R.E., et al., Recruitment of bone-marrow-derived cells by skeletal and cardiac muscle in adult dystrophic mdx mice. *Anat. Embryol.* (Berl), 1999. 199(5): p. 391-6.

[336] LaBarge, M.A. and H.M. Blau, Biological progression from adult bone marrow to mononucleate muscle stem cell to multinucleate muscle fiber in response to injury. *Cell*, 2002. 111(4): p. 589-601.

[337] De Bari, C., et al., Skeletal muscle repair by adult human mesenchymal stem cells from synovial membrane. *J. Cell Biol.*, 2003. 160(6): p. 909-18.

[338] Muguruma, Y., et al., In vivo and in vitro differentiation of myocytes from human bone marrow-derived multipotent progenitor cells. *Exp. Hematol.*, 2003. 31(12): p. 1323-30.

[339] Dezawa, M., Insights into autotransplantation: the unexpected discovery of specific induction systems in bone marrow stromal cells. *Cell Mol. Life Sci.*, 2006. 63(23): p. 2764-72.

[340] Dezawa, M., et al., Bone marrow stromal cells generate muscle cells and repair muscle degeneration. *Science*, 2005. 309(5732): p. 314-7.

[341] Wu, G.D., et al., Migration of mesenchymal stem cells to heart allografts during chronic rejection. *Transplantation*, 2003. 75(5): p. 679-85.

[342] Toma, C., et al., Human mesenchymal stem cells differentiate to a cardiomyocyte phenotype in the adult murine heart. *Circulation*, 2002. 105(1): p. 93-8.

[343] Schulze, M., et al., Mesenchymal stem cells are recruited to striated muscle by NFAT/IL-4-mediated cell fusion. *Genes Dev.*, 2005. 19(15): p. 1787-98.

[344] Mizuno, H., et al., Myogenic differentiation by human processed lipoaspirate cells. *Plast Reconstr. Surg.*, 2002. 109(1): p. 199-209; discussion 210-1.

[345] Gang, E.J., et al., In vitro mesengenic potential of human umbilical cord blood-derived mesenchymal stem cells. *Biochem. Biophys. Res. Commun.*, 2004. 321(1): p. 102-8.

[346] Kinner, B., J.M. Zaleskas, and M. Spector, Regulation of smooth muscle actin expression and contraction in adult human mesenchymal stem cells. *Exp. Cell Res.*, 2002. 278(1): p. 72-83.

[347] Shi, D., et al., Myogenic fusion of human bone marrow stromal cells, but not hematopoietic cells. *Blood*, 2004. 104(1): p. 290-4.

[348] Goncalves, M.A., et al., Human mesenchymal stem cells ectopically expressing full-length dystrophin can complement Duchenne muscular dystrophy myotubes by cell fusion. *Hum. Mol. Genet.*, 2006. 15(2): p. 213-21.

[349] Mendell, J.R., et al., Myoblast transfer in the treatment of Duchenne's muscular dystrophy. *N. Engl. J. Med.*, 1995. 333(13): p. 832-8.

[350] Miller, R.G., et al., Myoblast implantation in Duchenne muscular dystrophy: the San Francisco study. *Muscle Nerve*, 1997. 20(4): p. 469-78.

[351] Neumeyer, A.M., et al., Pilot study of myoblast transfer in the treatment of Becker muscular dystrophy. *Neurology*, 1998. 51(2): p. 589-92.

[352] Sorrentino, V., Stem cells and muscle diseases. *J. Muscle. Res. Cell Motil.*, 2004. 25(3): p. 225-30.

[353] Makino, S., et al., Cardiomyocytes can be generated from marrow stromal cells in vitro. *J. Clin. Invest.*, 1999. 103(5): p. 697-705.

[354] Bittira, B., et al., In vitro preprogramming of marrow stromal cells for myocardial regeneration. *Ann. Thorac. Surg.*, 2002. 74(4): p. 1154-9; discussion 1159-60.

[355] Min, J.Y., et al., Transplantation of embryonic stem cells improves cardiac function in postinfarcted rats. *J. Appl. Physiol.*, 2002. 92(1): p. 288-96.

[356] Cheng, F., et al., Induced differentiation of human cord blood mesenchymal stem/progenitor cells into cardiomyocyte-like cells in vitro. *J. Huazhong Univ. Sci. Technolog Med. Sci.*, 2003. 23(2): p. 154-7.

[357] Erices, A.A., et al., Human cord blood-derived mesenchymal stem cells home and survive in the marrow of immunodeficient mice after systemic infusion. *Cell Transplant*, 2003. 12(6): p. 555-61.

[358] Fukuda, K., Application of mesenchymal stem cells for the regeneration of cardiomyocyte and its use for cell transplantation therapy. *Hum. Cell*, 2003. 16(3): p. 83-94.

[359] Rangappa, S., et al., Cardiomyocyte-mediated contact programs human mesenchymal stem cells to express cardiogenic phenotype. *J. Thorac. Cardiovasc. Surg.*, 2003. 126(1): p. 124-32.

[360] Vanelli, P., et al., Cardiac precursors in human bone marrow and cord blood: in vitro cell cardiogenesis. *Ital. Heart J.*, 2004. 5(5): p. 384-8.

[361] Xu, W., et al., Mesenchymal stem cells from adult human bone marrow differentiate into a cardiomyocyte phenotype in vitro. *Exp. Biol. Med.* (Maywood), 2004. 229(7): p. 623-31.

[362] Yoon, J., et al., Transdifferentiation of mesenchymal stem cells into cardiomyocytes by direct cell-to-cell contact with neonatal cardiomyocyte but not adult cardiomyocytes. *Ann. Hematol.*, 2005. 84(11): p. 715-21.

[363] Wang, T., et al., Cell-to-cell contact induces mesenchymal stem cell to differentiate into cardiomyocyte and smooth muscle cell. Int J Cardiol, 2005.

[364] Potapova, I., et al., Human mesenchymal stem cells as a gene delivery system to create cardiac pacemakers. *Circ. Res.,* 2004. 94(7): p. 952-9.

[365] Valiunas, V., et al., Human mesenchymal stem cells make cardiac connexins and form functional gap junctions. *J. Physiol.*, 2004. 555(Pt 3): p. 617-26.

[366] Min, J.J., et al., In vivo bioluminescence imaging of cord blood derived mesenchymal stem cell transplantation into rat myocardium. Ann Nucl Med, 2006. 20(3): p. 165-70.

[367] Min, J.Y., et al., Significant improvement of heart function by cotransplantation of human mesenchymal stem cells and fetal cardiomyocytes in postinfarcted pigs. *Ann. Thorac. Surg.*, 2002. 74(5): p. 1568-75.

[368] Shake, J.G., et al., Mesenchymal stem cell implantation in a swine myocardial infarct model: engraftment and functional effects. *Ann. Thorac. Surg.*, 2002. 73(6): p. 1919-25; discussion 1926.

[369] Dick, A.J., et al., Magnetic resonance fluoroscopy allows targeted delivery of mesenchymal stem cells to infarct borders in Swine. *Circulation*, 2003. 108(23): p. 2899-904.

[370] Kraitchman, D.L., et al., In vivo magnetic resonance imaging of mesenchymal stem cells in myocardial infarction. *Circulation,* 2003. 107(18): p. 2290-3.

[371] Wollert, K.C., et al., Intracoronary autologous bone-marrow cell transfer after myocardial infarction: the BOOST randomised controlled clinical trial. *Lancet,* 2004. 364(9429): p. 141-8.

[372] Chen, S.L., et al., Effect on left ventricular function of intracoronary transplantation of autologous bone marrow mesenchymal stem cell in patients with acute myocardial infarction. *Am. J. Cardiol.*, 2004. 94(1): p. 92-5.

[373] Miyahara, Y., et al., Monolayered mesenchymal stem cells repair scarred myocardium after myocardial infarction. *Nat. Med.*, 2006. 12(4): p. 459-65.

[374] Dennis, J.E. and P. Charbord, Origin and differentiation of human and murine stroma. *Stem Cells*, 2002. 20(3): p. 205-14.

[375] Charbord, P., et al., Analysis of the microenvironment necessary for engraftment: role of the vascular smooth muscle-like stromal cells. *J. Hematother. Stem Cell Res.*, 2000. 9(6): p. 935-43.

[376] Charbord, P., et al., The Hematopoietic Microenvironment: Phenotypic and Functional Characterization of Human Marrow Vascular Stromal Cells. *Hematol.*, 1999. 4(3): p. 257-282.

[377] Galmiche, M.C., et al., Stromal cells from human long-term marrow cultures are mesenchymal cells that differentiate following a vascular smooth muscle differentiation pathway. *Blood,* 1993. 82(1): p. 66-76.

[378] Lerat, H., et al., Role of stromal cells and macrophages in fibronectin biosynthesis and matrix assembly in human long-term marrow cultures. *Blood*, 1993. 82(5): p. 1480-92.

[379] Li, J., et al., Nontransformed colony-derived stromal cell lines from normal human marrows. II. Phenotypic characterization and differentiation pathway. *Exp. Hematol.*, 1995. 23(2): p. 133-41.

[380] Remy-Martin, J.P., et al., Vascular smooth muscle differentiation of murine stroma: a sequential model. *Exp. Hematol.*, 1999. 27(12): p. 1782-95.

[381] Glukhova, M.A., M.G. Frid, and V.E. Koteliansky, Developmental changes in expression of contractile and cytoskeletal proteins in human aortic smooth muscle. *J. Biol. Chem.*, 1990. 265(22): p. 13042-6.

[382] Glukhova, M.A., et al., Expression of fibronectin variants in vascular and visceral smooth muscle cells in development. *Dev. Biol.*, 1990. 141(1): p. 193-202.

[383] Slomp, J., et al., Differentiation, dedifferentiation, and apoptosis of smooth muscle cells during the development of the human ductus arteriosus. *Arterioscler. Thromb. Vasc. Biol.*, 1997. 17(5): p. 1003-9.

[384] Owens, G.K., Regulation of differentiation of vascular smooth muscle cells. *Physiol. Rev.*, 1995. 75(3): p. 487-517.

[385] Davies, J.A., The Kidney Development Database. *Dev. Genet.*, 1999. 24(3-4): p. 194-8.

[386] Imai, E. and T. Ito, Can bone marrow differentiate into renal cells? *Pediatr. Nephrol.*, 2002. 17(10): p. 790-4.

[387] Imasawa, T., et al., The potential of bone marrow-derived cells to differentiate to glomerular mesangial cells. *J. Am. Soc. Nephrol.,*. 2001. 12(7): p. 1401-9.

[388] Ito, T., et al., Bone marrow is a reservoir of repopulating mesangial cells during glomerular remodeling. *J. Am. Soc. Nephrol.*, 2001. 12(12): p. 2625-35.

[389] Poulsom, R., et al., Bone marrow contributes to renal parenchymal turnover and regeneration. *J. Pathol.*, 2001. 195(2): p. 229-35.

[390] Krause, D.S., et al., Multi-organ, multi-lineage engraftment by a single bone marrow-derived stem cell. *Cell*, 2001. 105(3): p. 369-77.

[391] Iwano, M., et al., Evidence that fibroblasts derive from epithelium during tissue fibrosis. *J. Clin. Invest.*, 2002. 110(3): p. 341-50.

[392] El Kossi, M.M. and A.M. El Nahas, Stem cell factor and crescentic glomerulonephritis. *Am. J. Kidney Dis.*, 2003. 41(4): p. 785-95.

[393] Gupta, S., et al., A role for extrarenal cells in the regeneration following acute renal failure. *Kidney Int,* 2002. 62(4): p. 1285-90.

[394] Bos, C., et al., In vivo MR imaging of intravascularly injected magnetically labeled mesenchymal stem cells in rat kidney and liver. *Radiology*, 2004. 233(3): p. 781-9.

[395] Semont, A., et al., Mesenchymal stem cells increase self-renewal of small intestinal epithelium and accelerate structural recovery after radiation injury. *Adv. Exp. Med. Biol.*, 2006. 585: p. 19-30.

[396] Morigi, M., et al., Mesenchymal stem cells are renotropic, helping to repair the kidney and improve function in acute renal failure. *J. Am. Soc. Nephrol.*, 2004. 15(7): p. 1794-804.

[397] Szczypka, M.S., et al., Rare incorporation of bone marrow-derived cells into kidney after folic acid-induced injury. *Stem Cells*, 2005. 23(1): p. 44-54.

[398] Brittan, M. and N.A. Wright, Gastrointestinal stem cells. *J. Pathol.*, 2002. 197(4): p. 492-509.

[399] Brittan, M., et al., Bone marrow derivation of pericryptal myofibroblasts in the mouse and human small intestine and colon. *Gut*, 2002. 50(6): p. 752-7.

[400] Matsumoto, T., et al., Increase of bone marrow-derived secretory lineage epithelial cells during regeneration in the human intestine. *Gastroenterology*, 2005. 128(7): p. 1851-67.

[401] Okamoto, R., et al., Damaged epithelia regenerated by bone marrow-derived cells in the human gastrointestinal tract. *Nat. Med.*, 2002. 8(9): p. 1011-7.

[402] Brittan, M., et al., A regenerative role for bone marrow following experimental colitis: contribution to neovasculogenesis and myofibroblasts. *Gastroenterology*, 2005. 128(7): p. 1984-95.

[403] Rizvi, A.Z., et al., Bone marrow-derived cells fuse with normal and transformed intestinal stem cells. *Proc. Natl. Acad. Sci. USA*, 2006. 103(16): p. 6321-5.

[404] Komori, M., et al., Efficiency of bone marrow-derived cells in regeneration of the stomach after induction of ethanol-induced ulcers in rats. *J. Gastroenterol.*, 2005. 40(6): p. 591-9.

[405] Oh, S.H., et al., Hepatocyte growth factor induces differentiation of adult rat bone marrow cells into a hepatocyte lineage in vitro. *Biochem. Biophys. Res. Commun.*, 2000. 279(2): p. 500-4.

[406] Avital, I., et al., Isolation, characterization, and transplantation of bone marrow-derived hepatocyte stem cells. *Biochem. Biophys. Res. Commun.*, 2001. 288(1): p. 156-64.

[407] Miyazaki, M., et al., Improved conditions to induce hepatocytes from rat bone marrow cells in culture. *Biochem. Biophys. Res. Commun.*, 2002. 298(1): p. 24-30.

[408] Okumoto, K., et al., Differentiation of bone marrow cells into cells that express liver-specific genes in vitro: implication of the Notch signals in differentiation. *Biochem. Biophys. Res. Commun.*, 2003. 304(4): p. 691-5.

[409] Lee, K.D., et al., In vitro hepatic differentiation of human mesenchymal stem cells. *Hepatology*, 2004. 40(6): p. 1275-84.

[410] Kang, X.Q., et al., Rat bone marrow mesenchymal stem cells differentiate into hepatocytes in vitro. *World J. Gastroenterol.*, 2005. 11(22): p. 3479-84.

[411] Lange, C., et al., Hepatocytic gene expression in cultured rat mesenchymal stem cells. *Transplant Proc.*, 2005. 37(1): p. 276-9.

[412] Moriscot, C., et al., Human bone marrow mesenchymal stem cells can express insulin and key transcription factors of the endocrine pancreas developmental pathway upon genetic and/or microenvironmental manipulation in vitro. *Stem Cells*, 2005. 23(4): p. 594-603.

[413] Theise, N.D., et al., Liver from bone marrow in humans. *Hepatology*, 2000. 32(1): p. 11-6.

[414] Fiegel, H.C., et al., Liver-specific gene expression in cultured human hematopoietic stem cells. *Stem Cells*, 2003. 21(1): p. 98-104.

[415] Lange, C., et al., Liver-specific gene expression in mesenchymal stem cells is induced by liver cells. *World J. Gastroenterol*, 2005. 11(29): p. 4497-504.

[416] Seo, M.J., et al., Differentiation of human adipose stromal cells into hepatic lineage in vitro and in vivo. *Biochem. Biophys. Res. Commun.*, 2005. 328(1): p. 258-64.

[417] Petersen, B.E., et al., Bone marrow as a potential source of hepatic oval cells. *Science*, 1999. 284(5417): p. 1168-70.

[418] Shapiro, A.M., et al., Islet transplantation in seven patients with type 1 diabetes mellitus using a glucocorticoid-free immunosuppressive regimen. *N. Engl. J. Med.*, 2000. 343(4): p. 230-8.

[419] Shapiro, A.M., C. Ricordi, and B. Hering, Edmonton's islet success has indeed been replicated elsewhere. *Lancet*, 2003. 362(9391): p. 1242.

[420] Schwitzgebel, V.M., et al., Expression of neurogenin3 reveals an islet cell precursor population in the pancreas. *Development*, 2000. 127(16): p. 3533-42.

[421] Eberhardt, M., et al., Multipotential nestin and Isl-1 positive mesenchymal stem cells isolated from human pancreatic islets. *Biochem. Biophys. Res. Commun.*, 2006. 345(3): p. 1167-76.

[422] Zulewski, H., et al., Multipotential nestin-positive stem cells isolated from adult pancreatic islets differentiate ex vivo into pancreatic endocrine, exocrine, and hepatic phenotypes. *Diabetes*, 2001. 50(3): p. 521-33.

[423] Zulewski, H., Stem cells with potential to generate insulin producing cells in man. *Swiss Med Wkly*, 2006. 136(41-42): p. 647-54.

[424] Bonner-Weir, S. and A. Sharma, Pancreatic stem cells. *J. Pathol.*, 2002. 197(4): p. 519-26.

[425] D'Amour, K.A., et al., Efficient differentiation of human embryonic stem cells to definitive endoderm. *Nat. Biotechnol.*, 2005. 23(12): p. 1534-41.

[426] Zalzman, M., et al., Reversal of hyperglycemia in mice by using human expandable insulin-producing cells differentiated from fetal liver progenitor cells. *Proc. Natl. Acad. Sci. USA*, 2003. 100(12): p. 7253-8.

[427] Sapir, T., et al., Cell-replacement therapy for diabetes: Generating functional insulin-producing tissue from adult human liver cells. *Proc. Natl. Acad. Sci. USA*, 2005. 102(22): p. 7964-9.

[428] Kodama, S., et al., Islet regeneration during the reversal of autoimmune diabetes in NOD mice. *Science*, 2003. 302(5648): p. 1223-7.

[429] Hori, Y., et al., Differentiation of insulin-producing cells from human neural progenitor cells. *PLoS Med.*, 2005. 2(4): p. e103.

[430] Hess, D., et al., Bone marrow-derived stem cells initiate pancreatic regeneration. *Nat. Biotechnol.*, 2003. 21(7): p. 763-70.

[431] Oh, S.H., et al., Adult bone marrow-derived cells trans-differentiating into insulin-producing cells for the treatment of type I diabetes. *Lab. Invest.*, 2004. 84(5): p. 607-17.

[432] Timper, K., et al., Human adipose tissue-derived mesenchymal stem cells differentiate into insulin, somatostatin, and glucagon expressing cells. *Biochem. Biophys. Res. Commun.*, 2006. 341(4): p. 1135-40.

[433] Gomi, T., et al., Stages in the development of the rat lung: morphometric, light and electron microscopic studies. *Kaibogaku Zasshi,* 1994. 69(4): p. 392-405.

[434] Yamada, Y., et al., Bone regeneration following injection of mesenchymal stem cells and fibrin glue with a biodegradable scaffold. *J. Craniomaxillofac. Surg.*, 2003. 31(1): p. 27-33.

[435] Engelhardt, J.F., Stem cell niches in the mouse airway. *Am. J. Respir. Cell Mol. Biol.*, 2001. 24(6): p. 649-52.

[436] Cardoso, W.V., Molecular regulation of lung development. *Annu. Rev. Physiol.*, 2001. 63: p. 471-94.

[437] in 't Anker, P.S., et al., Nonexpanded primary lung and bone marrow-derived mesenchymal cells promote the engraftment of umbilical cord blood-derived CD34(+) cells in NOD/SCID mice. *Exp. Hematol.*, 2003. 31(10): p. 881-9.

[438] Reddy, R., et al., Isolation of a putative progenitor subpopulation of alveolar epithelial type 2 cells. *Am. J. Physiol. Lung Cell Mol. Physiol.*, 2004. 286(4): p. L658-67.

[439] Kim, C.F., et al., Identification of bronchioalveolar stem cells in normal lung and lung cancer. *Cell*, 2005. 121(6): p. 823-35.

[440] Summer, R., et al., Embryonic lung side population cells are hematopoietic and vascular precursors. *Am. J. Respir. Cell Mol. Biol.*, 2005. 33(1): p. 32-40.

[441] Boers, J.E., A.W. Ambergen, and F.B. Thunnissen, Number and proliferation of basal and parabasal cells in normal human airway epithelium. *Am. J. Respir. Crit. Care Med.*, 1998. 157(6 Pt 1): p. 2000-6.

[442] Duan, D., et al., Lef1 transcription factor expression defines airway progenitor cell targets for in utero gene therapy of submucosal gland in cystic fibrosis. *Am. J. Respir. Cell Mol. Biol.*, 1998. 18(6): p. 750-8.

[443] Danto, S.I., et al., Reversible transdifferentiation of alveolar epithelial cells. *Am. J. Respir. Cell Mol. Biol.*, 1995. 12(5): p. 497-502.

[444] Rippon, H.J., et al., Derivation of distal lung epithelial progenitors from murine embryonic stem cells using a novel three-step differentiation protocol. *Stem Cells,* 2006. 24(5): p. 1389-98.

[445] Wang, G., et al., Adult stem cells from bone marrow stroma differentiate into airway epithelial cells: potential therapy for cystic fibrosis. *Proc. Natl. Acad. Sci. USA*, 2005. 102(1): p. 186-91.

[446] Kotton, D.N., et al., Bone marrow-derived cells as progenitors of lung alveolar epithelium. *Development,* 2001. 128(24): p. 5181-8.

[447] Ortiz, L.A., et al., Mesenchymal stem cell engraftment in lung is enhanced in response to bleomycin exposure and ameliorates its fibrotic effects. *Proc. Natl. Acad. Sci. USA*, 2003. 100(14): p. 8407-11.

[448] Di Nicola, M., et al., Human bone marrow stromal cells suppress T-lymphocyte proliferation induced by cellular or nonspecific mitogenic stimuli. *Blood*, 2002. 99(10): p. 3838-43.

[449] Krampera, M., et al., Bone marrow mesenchymal stem cells inhibit the response of naive and memory antigen-specific T cells to their cognate peptide. *Blood*, 2003. 101(9): p. 3722-9.

[450] Glennie, S., et al., Bone marrow mesenchymal stem cells induce division arrest anergy of activated T cells. Blood, 2005. 105(7): p. 2821-7.

[451] Tintut, Y., et al., Multilineage potential of cells from the artery wall. *Circulation*, 2003. 108(20): p. 2505-10.

[452] Eliopoulos, N., et al., Allogeneic marrow stromal cells are immune rejected by MHC class I- and class II-mismatched recipient mice. *Blood*, 2005. 106(13): p. 4057-65.

[453] Ildstad, S.T. and D.H. Sachs, Reconstitution with syngeneic plus allogeneic or xenogeneic bone marrow leads to specific acceptance of allografts or xenografts. *Nature*, 1984. 307(5947): p. 168-70.

[454] Bartholomew, A., et al., Mesenchymal stem cells suppress lymphocyte proliferation in vitro and prolong skin graft survival in vivo. *Exp. Hematol.* 2002. 30(1): p. 42-8.

[455] Potian, J.A., et al., Veto-like activity of mesenchymal stem cells: functional discrimination between cellular responses to alloantigens and recall antigens. *J. Immunol.*, 2003. 171(7): p. 3426-34.

[456] Aggarwal, S. and M.F. Pittenger, Human mesenchymal stem cells modulate allogeneic immune cell responses. *Blood*, 2005. 105(4): p. 1815-22.

[457] Augello, A., et al., Bone marrow mesenchymal progenitor cells inhibit lymphocyte proliferation by activation of the programmed death 1 pathway. *Eur. J. Immunol.*, 2005. 35(5): p. 1482-90.

[458] Meisel, R., et al., Human bone marrow stromal cells inhibit allogeneic T-cell responses by indoleamine 2,3-dioxygenase-mediated tryptophan degradation. *Blood*, 2004. 103(12): p. 4619-21.

[459] Barry, F.P., et al., Immunogenicity of adult mesenchymal stem cells: lessons from the fetal allograft. Stem Cells Dev., 2005. 14(3): p. 252-65.

[460] Plumas, J., et al., Mesenchymal stem cells induce apoptosis of activated T cells. *Leukemia*, 2005. 19(9): p. 1597-604.

[461] Ryan, J.M., et al., Mesenchymal stem cells avoid allogeneic rejection. *J. Inflamm.* (Lond), 2005. 2: p. 8.

[462] Deng, W., et al., Effects of allogeneic bone marrow-derived mesenchymal stem cells on T and B lymphocytes from BXSB mice. *DNA Cell Biol.*, 2005. 24(7): p. 458-63.

[463] Corcione, A., et al., Human mesenchymal stem cells modulate B-cell functions. *Blood*, 2006. 107(1): p. 367-72.

[464] Krampera, M., et al., Role for interferon-gamma in the immunomodulatory activity of human bone marrow mesenchymal stem cells. *Stem Cells,* 2006. 24(2): p. 386-98.

[465] Spaggiari, G.M., et al., Mesenchymal stem cell-natural killer cell interactions: evidence that activated NK cells are capable of killing MSCs, whereas MSCs can inhibit IL-2-induced NK-cell proliferation. *Blood*, 2006. 107(4): p. 1484-90.

[466] Sotiropoulou, P.A., et al., Interactions between human mesenchymal stem cells and natural killer cells. *Stem Cells,* 2006. 24(1): p. 74-85.

[467] Zhang, W., et al., Effects of mesenchymal stem cells on differentiation, maturation, and function of human monocyte-derived dendritic cells. *Stem Cells Dev.,* 2004. 13(3): p. 263-71.

[468] Jiang, X.X., et al., Human mesenchymal stem cells inhibit differentiation and function of monocyte-derived dendritic cells. *Blood,* 2005. 105(10): p. 4120-6.

[469] Beyth, S., et al., Human mesenchymal stem cells alter antigen-presenting cell maturation and induce T-cell unresponsiveness. *Blood,* 2005. 105(5): p. 2214-9.

[470] Zappia, E., et al., Mesenchymal stem cells ameliorate experimental autoimmune encephalomyelitis inducing T-cell anergy. *Blood,* 2005. 106(5): p. 1755-61.

[471] Horwitz, E.M., et al., Isolated allogeneic bone marrow-derived mesenchymal cells engraft and stimulate growth in children with osteogenesis imperfecta: Implications for cell therapy of bone. *Proc. Natl. Acad. Sci. USA*, 2002. 99(13): p. 8932-7.

[472] Koc, O.N., et al., Allogeneic mesenchymal stem cell infusion for treatment of metachromatic leukodystrophy (MLD) and Hurler syndrome (MPS-IH). *Bone Marrow Transplant,* 2002. 30(4): p. 215-22.

[473] Koc, O.N., et al., Rapid hematopoietic recovery after coinfusion of autologous-blood stem cells and culture-expanded marrow mesenchymal stem cells in advanced breast cancer patients receiving high-dose chemotherapy. *J. Clin. Oncol.,* 2000. 18(2): p. 307-16.

[474] Lazarus, H.M., et al., Cotransplantation of HLA-identical sibling culture-expanded mesenchymal stem cells and hematopoietic stem cells in hematologic malignancy patients. *Biol. Blood Marrow Transplant,* 2005. 11(5): p. 389-98.

[475] Nauta, A.J., et al., Donor-derived mesenchymal stem cells are immunogenic in an allogeneic host and stimulate donor graft rejection in a nonmyeloablative setting. *Blood,* 2006. 108(6): p. 2114-20.

[476] Le Blanc, K., et al., Treatment of severe acute graft-versus-host disease with third party haploidentical mesenchymal stem cells. *Lancet,* 2004. 363(9419): p. 1439-41.

[477] Sudres, M., et al., Bone marrow mesenchymal stem cells suppress lymphocyte proliferation in vitro but fail to prevent graft-versus-host disease in mice. *J. Immunol.,* 2006. 176(12): p. 7761-7.

[478] Gao, J., et al., The dynamic in vivo distribution of bone marrow-derived mesenchymal stem cells after infusion. *Cells Tissues Organs,* 2001. 169(1): p. 12-20.

[479] Barbash, I.M., et al., Systemic delivery of bone marrow-derived mesenchymal stem cells to the infarcted myocardium: feasibility, cell migration, and body distribution. *Circulation,* 2003. 108(7): p. 863-8.

[480] Francois, S., et al., Local irradiation not only induces homing of human mesenchymal stem cells at exposed sites but promotes their widespread engraftment to multiple organs: a study of their quantitative distribution after irradiation damage. *Stem Cells,* 2006. 24(4): p. 1020-9.

[481] Dahir, G.A., et al., Pluripotential mesenchymal cells repopulate bone marrow and retain osteogenic properties. *Clin. Orthop. Relat. Res.,* 2000(379 Suppl): p. S134-45.

[482] Mahmud, N., et al., Studies of the route of administration and role of conditioning with radiation on unrelated allogeneic mismatched mesenchymal stem cell engraftment in a nonhuman primate model. *Exp. Hematol.*, 2004. 32(5): p. 494-501.

[483] Javazon, E.H., K.J. Beggs, and A.W. Flake, Mesenchymal stem cells: paradoxes of passaging. *Exp. Hematol.*, 2004. 32(5): p. 414-25.

[484] Alvarez-Dolado, M., et al., Fusion of bone-marrow-derived cells with Purkinje neurons, cardiomyocytes and hepatocytes. *Nature*, 2003. 425(6961): p. 968-73.

[485] Pereira, R.F., et al., Marrow stromal cells as a source of progenitor cells for nonhematopoietic tissues in transgenic mice with a phenotype of osteogenesis imperfecta. *Proc. Natl. Acad. Sci. USA*, 1998. 95(3): p. 1142-7.

[486] Horwitz, E.M., et al., Clinical responses to bone marrow transplantation in children with severe osteogenesis imperfecta. *Blood,* 2001. 97(5): p. 1227-31.

[487] Genbacev, O. and R.K. Miller, Post-implantation differentiation and proliferation of cytotrophoblast cells: in vitro models--a review. Placenta, 2000. 21 Suppl A: p. S45-9.

[488] Jauniaux, E., et al., In-vivo measurement of intrauterine gases and acid-base values early in human pregnancy. *Hum. Reprod.*, 1999. 14(11): p. 2901-4.

[489] Kiserud, T., Physiology of the fetal circulation. *Semin. Fetal. Neonatal. Med.*, 2005. 10(6): p. 493-503.

[490] Ishikawa, Y. and T. Ito, Kinetics of hemopoietic stem cells in a hypoxic culture. *Eur. J. Haematol.*, 1988. 40(2): p. 126-9.

[491] Chow, D.C., et al., Modeling pO(2) distributions in the bone marrow hematopoietic compartment. I. Krogh's model. *Biophys. J.,* 2001. 81(2): p. 675-84.

[492] Cipolleschi, M.G., P. Dello Sbarba, and M. Olivotto, The role of hypoxia in the maintenance of hematopoietic stem cells. *Blood*, 1993. 82(7): p. 2031-7.

[493] Danet, G.H., et al., Expansion of human SCID-repopulating cells under hypoxic conditions. *J. Clin. Invest.*, 2003. 112(1): p. 126-35.

[494] Taneja, R., et al., Effects of hypoxia on granulocytic-monocytic progenitors in rats. Role of bone marrow stroma. *Am. J. Hematol.*, 2000. 64(1): p. 20-5.

[495] Lennon, D.P., J.M. Edmison, and A.I. Caplan, Cultivation of rat marrow-derived mesenchymal stem cells in reduced oxygen tension: effects on in vitro and in vivo osteochondrogenesis. *J. Cell Physiol.*, 2001. 187(3): p. 345-55.

[496] Fink, T., et al., Induction of adipocyte-like phenotype in human mesenchymal stem cells by hypoxia. *Stem Cells*, 2004. 22(7): p. 1346-55.

[497] Honczarenko, M., et al., Human bone marrow stromal cells express a distinct set of biologically functional chemokine receptors. *Stem Cells*, 2006. 24(4): p. 1030-41.

[498] Moussavi-Harami, F., et al., Oxygen effects on senescence in chondrocytes and mesenchymal stem cells: consequences for tissue engineering. *Iowa Orthop J.*, 2004. 24: p. 15-20.

[499] Robins, J.C., et al., Hypoxia induces chondrocyte-specific gene expression in mesenchymal cells in association with transcriptional activation of Sox9. *Bone*, 2005. 37(3): p. 313-22.

[500] Malladi, P., et al., Effect of reduced oxygen tension on chondrogenesis and osteogenesis in adipose-derived mesenchymal cells. *Am. J. Physiol. Cell Ph*ysiol., 2006. 290(4): p. C1139-46.

[501] Zhu, W., et al., Hypoxia and serum deprivation-induced apoptosis in mesenchymal stem cells. *Stem Cells,* 2006. 24(2): p. 416-25.

[502] Grayson, W.L., et al., Effects of hypoxia on human mesenchymal stem cell expansion and plasticity in 3D constructs. *J. Cell Physiol.,* 2006. 207(2): p. 331-9.

[503] Martin-Rendon, E., et al., Transcriptional profiling of human cord blood CD133+ and cultured bone marrow mesenchymal stem cells in response to hypoxia. *Stem Cells,* 2006.

[504] Gojo, S., et al., In vivo cardiovasculogenesis by direct injection of isolated adult mesenchymal stem cells. *Exp. Cell Res.,* 2003. 288(1): p. 51-9.

[505] Mangi, A.A., et al., Mesenchymal stem cells modified with Akt prevent remodeling and restore performance of infarcted hearts. *Nat. Med.,.* 2003. 9(9): p. 1195-201.

[506] Massas, R. and D. Benayahu, Parathyroid hormone effect on cell-to-cell communication in stromal and osteoblastic cells. *J. Cell Biochem.,* 1998. 69(1): p. 81-6.

[507] Bleul, C.C., et al., A highly efficacious lymphocyte chemoattractant, stromal cell-derived factor 1 (SDF-1). *J. Exp. Med.,* 1996. 184(3): p. 1101-9.

[508] Thayer, J.M., et al., Formation of the arterial media during vascular development. *Cell Mol. Biol. Res.,* 1995. 41(4): p. 251-62.

[509] Owens, G.K., S.M. Vernon, and C.S. Madsen, Molecular regulation of smooth muscle cell differentiation. *J. Hypertens. Suppl.,* 1996. 14(5): p. S55-64.

[510] Hungerford, J.E. and C.D. Little, Developmental biology of the vascular smooth muscle cell: building a multilayered vessel wall. *J. Vasc. Res.,* 1999. 36(1): p. 2-27.

[511] Li, D.Y., et al., Defective angiogenesis in mice lacking endoglin. *Science,* 1999. 284(5419): p. 1534-7.

[512] Lin, Q., et al., Requirement of the MADS-box transcription factor MEF2C for vascular development. *Development,* 1998. 125(22): p. 4565-74.

[513] Yang, Y., et al., Embryonic mesenchymal cells share the potential for smooth muscle differentiation: myogenesis is controlled by the cell's shape. *Development,* 1999. 126(13): p. 3027-33.

[514] Arakawa, E., et al., A mouse bone marrow stromal cell line, TBR-B, shows inducible expression of smooth muscle-specific genes. *FEBS Lett,* 2000. 481(2): p. 193-6.

[515] Hegner, B., et al., Differential regulation of smooth muscle markers in human bone marrow-derived mesenchymal stem cells. *J. Hypertens,* 2005. 23(6): p. 1191-202.

[516] Andrades, J.A., et al., A recombinant human TGF-beta1 fusion protein with collagen-binding domain promotes migration, growth, and differentiation of bone marrow mesenchymal cells. *Exp. Cell Res.,* 1999. 250(2): p. 485-98.

[517] Sensebe, L., et al., Cytokines active on granulomonopoiesis: release and consumption by human marrow myoid [corrected] stromal cells. *Br. J. Haematol.,* 1997. 98(2): p. 274-82.

[518] Jeon, E.S., et al., Sphingosylphosphorylcholine induces differentiation of human mesenchymal stem cells into smooth-muscle-like cells through a TGF-beta-dependent mechanism. *J. Cell Sci.,* 2006. 119(Pt 23): p. 4994-5005.

[519] Cai, D., et al., Lapine and canine bone marrow stromal cells contain smooth muscle actin and contract a collagen-glycosaminoglycan matrix. *Tissue Eng,* 2001. 7(6): p. 829-41.

[520] Kawano, S., et al., ATP autocrine/paracrine signaling induces calcium oscillations and NFAT activation in human mesenchymal stem cells. *Cell Calcium*, 2006.

[521] Kawano, S., et al., Characterization of Ca(2+) signaling pathways in human mesenchymal stem cells. *Cell Calcium*, 2002. 32(4): p. 165-74.

[522] Zahanich, I., et al., Molecular and functional expression of voltage-operated calcium channels during osteogenic differentiation of human mesenchymal stem cells. *J. Bone Miner Res.*, 2005. 20(9): p. 1637-46.

[523] Heubach, J.F., et al., Electrophysiological properties of human mesenchymal stem cells. *J. Physiol.*, 2004. 554(Pt 3): p. 659-72.

[524] Li, G.R., et al., Characterization of ionic currents in human mesenchymal stem cells from bone marrow. *Stem Cells*, 2005. 23(3): p. 371-82.

[525] Amberger, A., et al., Reversible expression of sm alpha-actin protein and sm alpha-actin mRNA in cloned cerebral endothelial cells. *FEBS Lett*, 1991. 287(1-2): p. 223-5.

[526] Arciniegas, E., et al., Transforming growth factor beta 1 promotes the differentiation of endothelial cells into smooth muscle-like cells in vitro. *J. Cell Sci.*, 1992. 103 (Pt 2): p. 521-9.

[527] DeRuiter, M.C., et al., Embryonic endothelial cells transdifferentiate into mesenchymal cells expressing smooth muscle actins in vivo and in vitro. *Circ. Res.*, 1997. 80(4): p. 444-51.

[528] Oswald, J., et al., Mesenchymal stem cells can be differentiated into endothelial cells in vitro. *Stem Cells*, 2004. 22(3): p. 377-84.

[529] Gang, E.J., et al., In vitro endothelial potential of human UC blood-derived mesenchymal stem cells. *Cytotherapy*, 2006. 8(3): p. 215-27.

[530] Frid, M.G., V.A. Kale, and K.R. Stenmark, Mature vascular endothelium can give rise to smooth muscle cells via endothelial-mesenchymal transdifferentiation: in vitro analysis. *Circ. Res.*, 2002. 90(11): p. 1189-96.

[531] Yamashita, J., et al., Flk1-positive cells derived from embryonic stem cells serve as vascular progenitors. *Nature*, 2000. 408(6808): p. 92-6.

[532] Haynesworth, S.E., M.A. Baber, and A.I. Caplan, Cytokine expression by human marrow-derived mesenchymal progenitor cells in vitro: effects of dexamethasone and IL-1 alpha. *J. Cell Physiol.*, 1996. 166(3): p. 585-92.

[533] Majumdar, M.K., et al., Human marrow-derived mesenchymal stem cells (MSCs) express hematopoietic cytokines and support long-term hematopoiesis when differentiated toward stromal and osteogenic lineages. *J. Hematother. Stem. Cell Res.*, 2000. 9(6): p. 841-8.

[534] Majumdar, M.K., et al., Phenotypic and functional comparison of cultures of marrow-derived mesenchymal stem cells (MSCs) and stromal cells. *J. Cell Physiol.*, 1998. 176(1): p. 57-66.

[535] Ahmed, N., et al., Effect of bone morphogenetic protein-6 on haemopoietic stem cells and cytokine production in normal human bone marrow stroma. *Cell Biol. Int.*, 2001. 25(5): p. 429-35.

[536] Petit, I., et al., G-CSF induces stem cell mobilization by decreasing bone marrow SDF-1 and up-regulating CXCR4. *Nat. Immunol.*, 2002. 3(7): p. 687-94.

[537] Taichman, R.S., et al., Augmented production of interleukin-6 by normal human osteoblasts in response to CD34+ hematopoietic bone marrow cells in vitro. *Blood*, 1997. 89(4): p. 1165-72.

[538] Kinnaird, T., et al., Marrow-derived stromal cells express genes encoding a broad spectrum of arteriogenic cytokines and promote in vitro and in vivo arteriogenesis through paracrine mechanisms. *Circ. Res.*, 2004. 94(5): p. 678-85.

[539] Kinnaird, T., et al., Local delivery of marrow-derived stromal cells augments collateral perfusion through paracrine mechanisms. *Circulation*, 2004. 109(12): p. 1543-9.

[540] Tang, Y.L., et al., Paracrine action enhances the effects of autologous mesenchymal stem cell transplantation on vascular regeneration in rat model of myocardial infarction. *Ann. Thorac. Surg.*, 2005. 80(1): p. 229-36; discussion 236-7.

[541] Tang, Y.L., et al., Autologous mesenchymal stem cell transplantation induce VEGF and neovascularization in ischemic myocardium. *Regul. Pept.*, 2004. 117(1): p. 3-10.

[542] Caplan, A.I. and J.E. Dennis, Mesenchymal stem cells as trophic mediators. *J. Cell Biochem.*, 2006. 98(5): p. 1076-84.

[543] Wakelee, H.A. and J.H. Schiller, Targeting angiogenesis with vascular endothelial growth factor receptor small-molecule inhibitors: novel agents with potential in lung cancer. *Clin. Lung Cancer*, 2005. 7 Suppl 1: p. S31-8.

[544] Thebaud, B., et al., Vascular endothelial growth factor gene therapy increases survival, promotes lung angiogenesis, and prevents alveolar damage in hyperoxia-induced lung injury: evidence that angiogenesis participates in alveolarization. *Circulation*, 2005. 112(16): p. 2477-86.

[545] deMello, D.E., et al., Early fetal development of lung vasculature. *Am. J. Respir. Cell Mol. Biol.*, 1997. 16(5): p. 568-81.

[546] Anderson-Berry, A., et al., Vasculogenesis drives pulmonary vascular growth in the developing chick embryo. *Dev. Dyn.*, 2005. 233(1): p. 145-53.

[547] Mitani, Y., et al., Vascular smooth muscle cell phenotypes in primary pulmonary hypertension. *Eur. Respir. J.*, 2001. 17(2): p. 316-20.

[548] Ghamra, Z.W. and R.A. Dweik, Primary pulmonary hypertension: an overview of epidemiology and pathogenesis. *Cleve Clin. J. Med.*, 2003. 70 Suppl 1: p. S2-8.

[549] Tuder, R.M., et al., Exuberant endothelial cell growth and elements of inflammation are present in plexiform lesions of pulmonary hypertension. *Am. J. Pathol*, 1994. 144(2): p. 275-85.

[550] Tuder, R.M., et al., Expression of angiogenesis-related molecules in plexiform lesions in severe pulmonary hypertension: evidence for a process of disordered angiogenesis. *J. Pathol.*, 2001. 195(3): p. 367-74.

[551] Hyvelin, J.M., et al., Inhibition of Rho-kinase attenuates hypoxia-induced angiogenesis in the pulmonary circulation. *Circ. Res.*, 2005. 97(2): p. 185-91.

[552] Akeson, A.L., et al., Embryonic vasculogenesis by endothelial precursor cells derived from lung mesenchyme. *Dev. Dyn.*, 2000. 217(1): p. 11-23.

[553] Sata, M., Role of circulating vascular progenitors in angiogenesis, vascular healing, and pulmonary hypertension: lessons from animal models. *Arterioscler. Thromb. Vasc. Biol.*, 2006. 26(5): p. 1008-14.

[554] Hashimoto, N., et al., Bone marrow-derived progenitor cells in pulmonary fibrosis. *J. Clin. Invest.*, 2004. 113(2): p. 243-52.

[555] Davie, N.J., et al., Hypoxia-induced pulmonary artery adventitial remodeling and neovascularization: contribution of progenitor cells. *Am. J. Physiol. Lung Cell Mol. Physiol.*, 2004. 286(4): p. L668-78.

[556] Hu, Y., et al., Abundant progenitor cells in the adventitia contribute to atherosclerosis of vein grafts in ApoE-deficient mice. *J. Clin. Invest.*, 2004. 113(9): p. 1258-65.

[557] Hayashida, K., et al., Bone marrow-derived cells contribute to pulmonary vascular remodeling in hypoxia-induced pulmonary hypertension. *Chest,* 2005. 127(5): p. 1793-8.

[558] Kanki-Horimoto, S., et al., Implantation of mesenchymal stem cells overexpressing endothelial nitric oxide synthase improves right ventricular impairments caused by pulmonary hypertension. *Circulation*, 2006. 114(1 Suppl): p. I181-5.

[559] Zhao, Y.D., et al., Rescue of monocrotaline-induced pulmonary arterial hypertension using bone marrow-derived endothelial-like progenitor cells: efficacy of combined cell and eNOS gene therapy in established disease. *Circ. Res.,* 2005. 96(4): p. 442-50.

[560] Li, X. and J.W. Wilson, Increased vascularity of the bronchial mucosa in mild asthma. *Am. J. Respir. Crit. Care Med.*, 1997. 156(1): p. 229-33.

[561] Hoshino, M., Y. Nakamura, and Q.A. Hamid, Gene expression of vascular endothelial growth factor and its receptors and angiogenesis in bronchial asthma. *J. Allergy Clin. Immunol.*, 2001. 107(6): p. 1034-8.

[562] Favre, C.J., et al., Expression of genes involved in vascular development and angiogenesis in endothelial cells of adult lung. *Am. J. Physiol. Heart Circ Physiol.*, 2003. 285(5): p. H1917-38.

[563] Salvato, G., Quantitative and morphological analysis of the vascular bed in bronchial biopsy specimens from asthmatic and non-asthmatic subjects. *Thorax*, 2001. 56(12): p. 902-6.

[564] McDonald, D.M., Angiogenesis and remodeling of airway vasculature in chronic inflammation. *Am. J. Respir. Crit. Care Med.*, 2001. 164(10 Pt 2): p. S39-45.

[565] Roberts, W.G. and G.E. Palade, Neovasculature induced by vascular endothelial growth factor is fenestrated. *Cancer Res.*, 1997. 57(4): p. 765-72.

[566] Denburg, J.A., et al., Systemic aspects of allergic disease: bone marrow responses. *J. Allergy Clin. Immunol.*, 2000. 106(5 Suppl): p. S242-6.

[567] Delplanque, A., et al., Epithelial stem cell-mediated development of the human respiratory mucosa in SCID mice. *J. Cell Sci.*, 2000. 113 (Pt 5): p. 767-78.

[568] Kamihata, H., et al., Improvement of collateral perfusion and regional function by implantation of peripheral blood mononuclear cells into ischemic hibernating myocardium. *Arterioscler. Thromb. Vasc. Biol.*, 2002. 22(11): p. 1804-10.

[569] Yeh, E.T., et al., Transdifferentiation of human peripheral blood CD34+-enriched cell population into cardiomyocytes, endothelial cells, and smooth muscle cells in vivo. *Circulation*, 2003. 108(17): p. 2070-3.

[570] Crystal, R.G., et al., Future research directions in idiopathic pulmonary fibrosis: summary of a National Heart, Lung, and Blood Institute working group. *Am. J. Respir. Crit. Care Med.*, 2002. 166(2): p. 236-46.

[571] Selman, M., et al., Idiopathic pulmonary fibrosis: pathogenesis and therapeutic approaches. *Drugs*, 2004. 64(4): p. 405-30.

[572] Cosgrove, G.P., et al., Pigment epithelium-derived factor in idiopathic pulmonary fibrosis: a role in aberrant angiogenesis. *Am. J. Respir. Crit. Care Med.*, 2004. 170(3): p. 242-51.

[573] Ebina, M., et al., Heterogeneous increase in CD34-positive alveolar capillaries in idiopathic pulmonary fibrosis. *Am. J. Respir. Crit Care Med.*, 2004. 169(11): p. 1203-8.

[574] Epperly, M.W., et al., Bone marrow origin of myofibroblasts in irradiation pulmonary fibrosis. *Am. J. Respir. Cell Mol. Biol.*, 2003. 29(2): p. 213-24.

[575] Voelkel, N.F. and R.M. Tuder, Hypoxia-induced pulmonary vascular remodeling: a model for what human disease? *J. Clin. Invest.*, 2000. 106(6): p. 733-8.

[576] Wiebe, B.M. and H. Laursen, Lung morphometry by unbiased methods in emphysema: bronchial and blood vessel volume, alveolar surface area and capillary length. *Apmis*, 1998. 106(6): p. 651-6.

[577] Taraseviciene-Stewart, L., et al., Is alveolar destruction and emphysema in chronic obstructive pulmonary disease an immune disease? *Proc. Am. Thorac. Soc.*, 2006. 3(8): p. 687-90.

[578] Abe, S., et al., Lung cells transplanted to irradiated recipients generate lymphohematopoietic progeny. *Am. J. Respir. Cell Mol. Biol.*, 2004. 30(4): p. 491-9.

[579] Dunsmore, S.E. and S.D. Shapiro, The bone marrow leaves its scar: new concepts in pulmonary fibrosis. *J. Clin. Invest.*, 2004. 113(2): p. 180-2.

[580] Ambrose, J.A., Myocardial ischemia and infarction. *J. Am. Coll Cardiol.*, 2006. 47(11 Suppl): p. D13-7.

[581] Soonpaa, M.H., et al., Formation of nascent intercalated disks between grafted fetal cardiomyocytes and host myocardium. *Science*, 1994. 264(5155): p. 98-101.

[582] Murry, C.E., et al., Skeletal myoblast transplantation for repair of myocardial necrosis. *J. Clin. Invest.*, 1996. 98(11): p. 2512-23.

[583] Taylor, D.A., et al., Regenerating functional myocardium: improved performance after skeletal myoblast transplantation. *Nat. Med.*, 1998. 4(8): p. 929-33.

[584] Tomita, S., et al., Autologous transplantation of bone marrow cells improves damaged heart function. *Circulation*, 1999. 100(19 Suppl): p. II247-56.

[585] Strauer, B.E., et al., Repair of infarcted myocardium by autologous intracoronary mononuclear bone marrow cell transplantation in humans. *Circulation*, 2002. 106(15): p. 1913-8.

[586] Menasche, P., Stem cells for clinical use in cardiovascular medicine: current limitations and future perspectives. *Thromb. Haemost*, 2005. 94(4): p. 697-701.

[587] Assmus, B., et al., Transplantation of Progenitor Cells and Regeneration Enhancement in Acute Myocardial Infarction (TOPCARE-AMI). *Circulation*, 2002. 106(24): p. 3009-17.

[588] Stamm, C., et al., Autologous bone-marrow stem-cell transplantation for myocardial regeneration. *Lancet*, 2003. 361(9351): p. 45-6.

[589] Katritsis, D.G., et al., Transcoronary transplantation of autologous mesenchymal stem cells and endothelial progenitors into infarcted human myocardium. *Catheter Cardiovasc. Interv.*, 2005. 65(3): p. 321-9.

[590] Perin, E.C., et al., Transendocardial, autologous bone marrow cell transplantation for severe, chronic ischemic heart failure. *Circulation*, 2003. 107(18): p. 2294-302.

[591] Perin, E.C., et al., Improved exercise capacity and ischemia 6 and 12 months after transendocardial injection of autologous bone marrow mononuclear cells for ischemic cardiomyopathy. *Circulation,* 2004. 110(11 Suppl 1): p. II213-8.

[592] Mc, D.D. and J.M. Potter, A method for the study of arterial anastomoses. *J. Anat,.* 1950. 84(4): p. 327-8.

[593] Urschel, H.C., Jr. and E.J. Roth, Small arterial anastomoses: I. Nonsuture. *Ann. Surg.*, 1961. 153: p. 599-610.

[594] Urschel, H.C., Jr. and E.J. Roth, Small arterial anastomoses: II. Suture. *Ann. Surg.*, 1961. 153: p. 611-6.

[595] Fulton, W.F., The Dynamic Factor in Enlargement of Coronary Arterial Anastomoses, and Paradoxical Changes in the Subendocardial Plexus. *Br. Heart J.*, 1964. 26: p. 39-50.

[596] Fulton, W.F., The Time Factor in the Enlargement of Anastomoses in Coronary Artery Disease. *Scott .Med. J.*, 1964. 9: p. 18-23.

[597] Risau, W., Mechanisms of angiogenesis. *Nature,* 1997. 386(6626): p. 671-4.

[598] Heil, M. and W. Schaper, Influence of mechanical, cellular, and molecular factors on collateral artery growth (arteriogenesis). *Circ. Res.*, 2004. 95(5): p. 449-58.

[599] Ross, R., The pathogenesis of atherosclerosis: a perspective for the 1990s. *Nature,* 1993. 362(6423): p. 801-9.

[600] Simper, D., et al., Smooth muscle progenitor cells in human blood. *Circulation,* 2002. 106(10): p. 1199-204.

[601] Sata, M., et al., Hematopoietic stem cells differentiate into vascular cells that participate in the pathogenesis of atherosclerosis. *Nat. Med.*, 2002. 8(4): p. 403-9.

[602] Campbell, J.H., J.L. Efendy, and G.R. Campbell, Novel vascular graft grown within recipient's own peritoneal cavity. *Circ. Res.*, 1999. 85(12): p. 1173-8.

[603] Montfort, M.J., et al., Adult blood vessels restore host hematopoiesis following lethal irradiation. *Exp. Hematol.*, 2002. 30(8): p. 950-6.

[604] Covas, D.T., et al., Mesenchymal stem cells can be obtained from the human saphena vein. *Exp. Cell Res.*, 2005. 309(2): p. 340-4.

[605] Wu, X., et al., Mesenchymal stem cells participating in ex vivo endothelium repair and its effect on vascular smooth muscle cells growth. *Int. J. Cardiol.*, 2005. 105(3): p. 274-82.

[606] Caplice, N.M., et al., Smooth muscle cells in human coronary atherosclerosis can originate from cells administered at marrow transplantation. *Proc. Natl. Acad. Sci. USA*, 2003. 100(8): p. 4754-9.

[607] Shimizu, K., et al., Host bone-marrow cells are a source of donor intimal smooth-muscle-like cells in murine aortic transplant arteriopathy. *Nat. Med.*, 2001. 7(6): p. 738-41.

[608] Forte, A., et al., Molecular analysis of arterial stenosis in rat carotids. *J. Cell Physiol.*, 2001. 186(2): p. 307-13.

[609] Xu, Y., et al., Role of bone marrow-derived progenitor cells in cuff-induced vascular injury in mice. *Arterioscler. Thromb. Vasc. Biol.*, 2004. 24(3): p. 477-82.

[610] Tanaka, K., et al., Diverse contribution of bone marrow cells to neointimal hyperplasia after mechanical vascular injuries. *Circ. Res.*, 2003. 93(8): p. 783-90.

[611] Aoki, J., et al., Endothelial progenitor cell capture by stents coated with antibody against CD34: the HEALING-FIM (Healthy Endothelial Accelerated Lining Inhibits Neointimal Growth-First In Man) Registry. *J. Am. Coll Cardiol.*, 2005. 45(10): p. 1574-9.

[612] Silber, S., Capturing circulating endothelial progenitor cells: a new concept tested in the HEALING studies. *Minerva Cardioangiol.*, 2006. 54(1): p. 1-3.

[613] Han, C.I., G.R. Campbell, and J.H. Campbell, Circulating bone marrow cells can contribute to neointimal formation. *J. Vasc. Res.*, 2001. 38(2): p. 113-9.

[614] Folkman, J., et al., Isolation of a tumor factor responsible for angiogenesis. *J. Exp. Med.*, 1971. 133(2): p. 275-88.

[615] Hanahan, D. and R.A. Weinberg, The hallmarks of cancer. *Cell*, 2000. 100(1): p. 57-70.

[616] Vakkila, J. and M.T. Lotze, Inflammation and necrosis promote tumour growth. *Nat. Rev. Immunol.*, 2004. 4(8): p. 641-8.

[617] Mueller, M.M. and N.E. Fusenig, Friends or foes - bipolar effects of the tumour stroma in cancer. *Nat. Rev. Cancer*, 2004. 4(11): p. 839-49.

[618] Bergers, G. and L.E. Benjamin, Tumorigenesis and the angiogenic switch. *Nat. Rev. Cancer*, 2003. 3(6): p. 401-10.

[619] Condeelis, J. and J.W. Pollard, Macrophages: obligate partners for tumor cell migration, invasion, and metastasis. *Cell*, 2006. 124(2): p. 263-6.

[620] de Visser, K.E., A. Eichten, and L.M. Coussens, Paradoxical roles of the immune system during cancer development. *Nat. Rev. Cancer*, 2006. 6(1): p. 24-37.

[621] Carmeliet, P., Angiogenesis in life, disease and medicine. *Nature*, 2005. 438(7070): p. 932-6.

[622] Ferrara, N. and R.S. Kerbel, Angiogenesis as a therapeutic target. *Nature*, 2005. 438(7070): p. 967-74.

[623] Lyden, D., et al., Impaired recruitment of bone-marrow-derived endothelial and hematopoietic precursor cells blocks tumor angiogenesis and growth. *Nat. Med.*, 2001. 7(11): p. 1194-201.

[624] Heissig, B., et al., Recruitment of stem and progenitor cells from the bone marrow niche requires MMP-9 mediated release of kit-ligand. *Cell*, 2002. 109(5): p. 625-37.

[625] De Palma, M., et al., Targeting exogenous genes to tumor angiogenesis by transplantation of genetically modified hematopoietic stem cells. *Nat. Med.*, 2003. 9(6): p. 789-95.

[626] Peters, B.A., et al., Contribution of bone marrow-derived endothelial cells to human tumor vasculature. *Nat. Med.*, 2005. 11(3): p. 261-2.

[627] Sun, B., et al., Correlation between melanoma angiogenesis and the mesenchymal stem cells and endothelial progenitor cells derived from bone marrow. *Stem. Cells Dev.*, 2005. 14(3): p. 292-8.

[628] Zhu, W., et al., Mesenchymal stem cells derived from bone marrow favor tumor cell growth in vivo. *Exp. Mol. Pathol.*, 2006. 80(3): p. 267-74.

[629] Campbell, C.D., D. Goldfarb, and R. Roe, A small arterial substitute: expanded microporous polytetrafluoroethylene: patency versus porosity. *Ann. Surg.*, 1975. 182(2): p. 138-43.
[630] Lepidi, S., et al., In vivo regeneration of small-diameter (2 mm) arteries using a polymer scaffold. *Faseb J.*, 2006. 20(1): p. 103-5.
[631] Jarrell, B.E., et al., Use of an endothelial monolayer on a vascular graft prior to implantation. Temporal dynamics and compatibility with the operating room. *Ann. Surg.*, 1986. 203(6): p. 671-8.
[632] Herring, M.B., et al., Seeding arterial prostheses with vascular endothelium. The nature of the lining. *Ann. Surg.*, 1979. 190(1): p. 84-90.
[633] Niklason, L.E., et al., Functional arteries grown in vitro. *Science,* 1999. 284(5413): p. 489-93.
[634] Yu, H., et al., Smooth muscle cells improve endothelial cell retention on polytetrafluoroethylene grafts in vivo. *J. Vasc. Surg.*, 2003. 38(3): p. 557-63.
[635] L'Heureux, N., et al., A completely biological tissue-engineered human blood vessel. *Faseb J.,* 1998. 12(1): p. 47-56.
[636] Kaushal, S., et al., Functional small-diameter neovessels created using endothelial progenitor cells expanded ex vivo. *Nat. Med,.* 2001. 7(9): p. 1035-40.
[637] Cho, S.W., et al., Small-diameter blood vessels engineered with bone marrow-derived cells. *Ann. Surg.*, 2005. 241(3): p. 506-15.
[638] Cho, S.W., et al., Vascular patches tissue-engineered with autologous bone marrow-derived cells and decellularized tissue matrices. *Biomaterials,* 2005. 26(14): p. 1915-24.
[639] Kanki-Horimoto, S., et al., Synthetic vascular prosthesis impregnated with genetically modified bone marrow cells produced recombinant proteins. *Artif. Organs*, 2005. 29(10): p. 815-9.
[640] Zhang, J., et al., Engineering of vascular grafts with genetically modified bone marrow mesenchymal stem cells on poly (propylene carbonate) graft. *Artif. Organs*, 2006. 30(12): p. 898-905.
[641] Chisholm, M.H., D. Navarro-Llobet, and Z. Zhou, Poly(propylene carbonate). 1. More about Poly(propylene carbonate) Formed from the Copolymerization of Propylene Oxide and Carbon Dioxide Employing a Zinc Glutarate Catalyst. *Macromolecules,* 2002. 35(17): p. 6494-6504.
[642] Kadner, A., et al., A new source for cardiovascular tissue engineering: human bone marrow stromal cells. *Eur. J. Cardiothorac. Surg.*, 2002. 21(6): p. 1055-60.
[643] Matsumura, G., et al., First evidence that bone marrow cells contribute to the construction of tissue-engineered vascular autografts in vivo. *Circulation,* 2003. 108(14): p. 1729-34.
[644] Cho, S.W., et al., Smooth muscle-like tissues engineered with bone marrow stromal cells. *Biomaterials,* 2004. 25(15): p. 2979-86.
[645] Cassell, O.C., et al., The influence of extracellular matrix on the generation of vascularized, engineered, transplantable tissue. *Ann. NY Acad. Sci*, 2001. 944: p. 429-42.

[646] Stock, U.A., et al., Patch augmentation of the pulmonary artery with bioabsorbable polymers and autologous cell seeding. *J. Thorac. Cardiovasc. Surg.*, 2000. 120(6): p. 1158-67; discussion 1168.

[647] Wilson, G.J., et al., Acellular matrix: a biomaterials approach for coronary artery bypass and heart valve replacement. *Ann. Thorac. Surg.*, 1995. 60(2 Suppl): p. S353-8.

[648] Kim, B.S. and D.J. Mooney, Scaffolds for engineering smooth muscle under cyclic mechanical strain conditions. *J. Biomech. Eng.*, 2000. 122(3): p. 210-5.

[649] Dartsch, P.C. and H. Hammerle, Orientation response of arterial smooth muscle cells to mechanical stimulation. *Eur. J. Cell Biol.*, 1986. 41(2): p. 339-46.

[650] Dartsch, P.C., H. Hammerle, and E. Betz, Orientation of cultured arterial smooth muscle cells growing on cyclically stretched substrates. *Acta Anat* (Basel), 1986. 125(2): p. 108-13.

[651] Thyberg, J., Differentiated properties and proliferation of arterial smooth muscle cells in culture. *Int. Rev. Cytol.*, 1996. 169: p. 183-265.

[652] Osol, G., Mechanotransduction by vascular smooth muscle. *J. Vasc. Res.*, 1995. 32(5): p. 275-92.

[653] Baskin, L., P.S. Howard, and E. Macarak, Effect of physical forces on bladder smooth muscle and urothelium. *J. Urol.*, 1993. 150(2 Pt 2): p. 601-7.

[654] Birukov, K.G., et al., Stretch affects phenotype and proliferation of vascular smooth muscle cells. *Mol. Cell Biochem.*, 1995. 144(2): p. 131-9.

[655] Reusch, P., et al., Mechanical strain increases smooth muscle and decreases nonmuscle myosin expression in rat vascular smooth muscle cells. *Circ. Res.*, 1996. 79(5): p. 1046-53.

[656] Niklason, L.E., et al., Morphologic and mechanical characteristics of engineered bovine arteries. *J. Vasc. Surg.*, 2001. 33(3): p. 628-38.

[657] Niklason, L.E. and R.S. Langer, Advances in tissue engineering of blood vessels and other tissues. *Transpl. Immunol.*, 1997. 5(4): p. 303-6.

[658] Kim, B.S., et al., Cyclic mechanical strain regulates the development of engineered smooth muscle tissue. *Nat. Biotechnol.*, 1999. 17(10): p. 979-83.

[659] Kobayashi, N., et al., Mechanical stress promotes the expression of smooth muscle-like properties in marrow stromal cells. *Exp. Hematol.*, 2004. 32(12): p. 1238-45.

[660] Kurpinski, K., et al., Regulation of vascular smooth muscle cells and mesenchymal stem cells by mechanical strain. *Mol. Cell Biomech.*, 2006. 3(1): p. 21-34.

[661] Weinberg, C.B. and E. Bell, A blood vessel model constructed from collagen and cultured vascular cells. *Science*, 1986. 231(4736): p. 397-400.

[662] Hoerstrup, S.P., et al., Tissue engineering of small caliber vascular grafts. *Eur. J. Cardiothorac. Surg.*, 2001. 20(1): p. 164-9.

[663] Hoerstrup, S.P., et al., Living, autologous pulmonary artery conduits tissue engineered from human umbilical cord cells. *Ann. Thorac. Surg.*, 2002. 74(1): p. 46-52; discussion 52.

In: Encyclopedia of Stem Cell Research (2 Volume Set) ISBN: 978-1-61761-835-2
Editor: Alexander L. Greene © 2012 Nova Science Publishers, Inc.

Chapter XX

HUMAN EMBRYONIC STEM CELLS: KEY CHARACTERISTICS AND MAIN APPLICATIONS IN DISEASE RESEARCH

Kathryn Cherise Davidson[*,1,2,3,4], *Mirella Dottori*[1,2] *and Alice Pébay*[1,2]

[1]Centre for Neuroscience, University of Melbourne,
Parkville, Australia
[2]Department of Pharmacology, the University of Melbourne,
Parkville, Australia
[3]Monash Institute for Medical Research, Monash University, and the
Australian Stem Cell Centre, Clayton, Australia
[4]Department of Pharmacology, University of Washington, Seattle, WA, US

ABSTRACT

Embryonic stem cells (ESC), derived from the inner cell mass of pre-implantation mammalian embryos, are primordial, pluripotent cells capable of both self-renewal and further differentiation into the three primary germ lineages, ectoderm, endoderm, and mesoderm, which give rise to all cells types found within an adult organism. Once established in culture, ESC lines can be propagated indefinitely without undergoing a restriction in developmental potential and thereby can provide an unlimited source of cells for exploitation. Since ESC were first isolated from mouse blastocysts in 1981 [1], they have become a vital tool for the study of development and diseases. The derivation of human ESC (hESC) nearly twenty years later generated considerable interest and excitement as researchers predicted their broad utility for human studies and cellular therapies [2, 3]. Understanding the mechanisms that govern stem cell self-renewal and differentiation is of fundamental significance to cellular and developmental biology. The knowledge gained from such research is anticipated to lead to major biomedical

---

[*] Author for correspondence. Tel: +61 3 83443988; Fax: +61 3 93494432; E-mail: davidsok@u.washington.edu

outcomes. This review aims to summarize the current knowledge on hESC characterization, and will discuss the potential applications of hESC in disease research.

INTRODUCTION

Human embryonic stem cells (hESC) are pluripotent cells derived from the human blastocyst prior to their commitment to form differentiated cells [2, 4]. *In vitro* cultured hESC are round in appearance, have a high nucleus to cytoplasm ratio, and form relatively flat, compact colonies with distinct cell borders and well-defined colony edges. They also pile up in within the interior of the colony if allowed to expand for several days. Individual cells often exhibit large nucleoli, suggestive of active transcription and protein synthesis during active cell proliferation. Representative images of hESC illustrate the typical morphology of a colony and individual cells in Figure 1.

The techniques originally used for hESC derivation and maintenance are very similar to the conditions used to isolate and propagate mouse ESC. However, these methods have progressed from culture in the presence of serum to serum-free, and more recently xeno-free conditions, with advances towards eliminating the feeder component completely. Indeed serum-free culture on feeders using enzymatic means of passage has become the preferred culture method for routine propagation of hESC. Serum-free, feeder-free culture conditions using Matrigel and Knockout Serum Replacement (KSR)-based medium dominate the literature and have become accepted practice in most hESC laboratories. Ultimately, researchers would like to achieve fully defined conditions for hESC derivation and propagation in order to work towards clinically acceptable sources of cells. Given the rate of improvement in culture methods to date, this will likely be achieved in the near future, though modification of traditional culture methods will require substantial evidence of maintenance of pluripotency and stable karyotype through extended passage in several hESC lines.

Due to their ability to differentiate into most cell types of the body, hESC show great promises for human therapies. In particular, hESC and their derivatives are predicted to have the greatest impact in two principle applications: 1) as a renewable source of material for use in regenerative medicine, and 2) as *in vitro* models for the study of development and disease. As we approach a decade of hESC research following the first derivation, we have gained extensive insights into the basic biology of these cells and developed techniques to generate cell types of clinical significance. However, hESC technology still faces many hurdles that will need to be overcome before any potential clinical application could be generated involving transplant of ESC-derivatives. In this review, we will summarize the key characteristics of hESC; we will consider the main applications of hESC in disease research and discuss the advantages and limitations of current hESC technology. We will also discuss the role somatic cell nuclear transfer and disease-specific hESC lines will play in the next generation of hESC research.

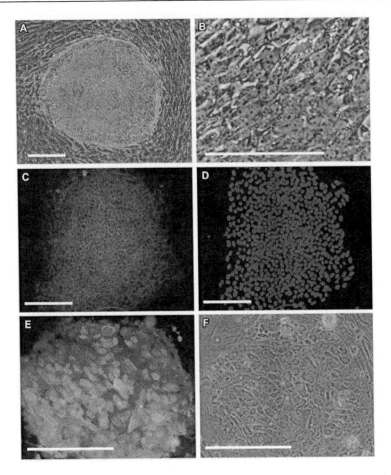

Figure 1. Typical hESC morphology and marker staining. Brightfield image of a hESC colony growing on MEF feeders (day 5) is compact with well defined colony boundary and piled-up cells within the colony interior (A). High magnification brightfield image showing individual cell morphology of live hESC: cells are round with dark nucleoli, high nuclear to cytoplasm ratio, distinct borders and bright glowing areas between cells indicative of secreted extracellular matrix (B). In green, CD9 immunostaining of a hESC colony cultured on Matrigel (day 6) (C) and corresponding DAPI stain (D). HESC colony (day 3) immunolabeled with Oct4 (red) and GCTM2 (green) (E) and corresponding brightfield image (F). Scalebar = 500 µm in (A) and 200 µm in (B-F).

1. CHARACTERIZATION OF HUMAN EMBRYONIC STEM CELLS

Our concept of qualities that define pluripotent hESC has evolved over the years as more hESC lines have been isolated and cultured under a variety of conditions. With mouse ESC lines, pluripotency can be evaluated by the ability of ESC to contribute to somatic tissues of the three primary lineages, as well as the germline, when injected into pre-implantation embryos [5]. This is considered the "gold standard" assay for pluripotency. Ethical considerations prevent such embryo assays in the human and likewise prohibit injection of hESC into embryos of other species for the purpose of generating a chimeric organism.

Instead, a number of key features have been identified that collectively demonstrate pluripotency in cultured hESC. Characteristics of hESC include: (1) evidence of pluripotency *in vitro* and/or *in vivo* as determined by the ability to give rise to cell types representative of the three primary germ lineages; (2) prolonged propagation and expansion *in vitro* without loss of pluripotency; (3) stable, diploid karyotype over extended periods of culture (which will be discussed in a later part of this chapter); (4) high level of telomerase activity as measured by expression of hTERT, the catalytic component of telomerase; (5) expression of known transcripts and protein markers of pluripotent stem cells [2, 4, 6-8].

1.1. Expression of Human Embryonic Stem Cell Markers

A number of stem cell markers have been identified; however, most of these markers can also be detected on other tissue types. Thus, accurate determination of hESC marker expression must be confirmed by using a panel of markers (Table 1).

Cell Surface Markers

The most well-documented markers used to characterize hESC (in bold in Table 1) consists largely of markers previously used to characterize human embryonic carcinoma (hEC) cells and mouse ESC [3]. A number of cell surface markers recognize glycolipids or glycoproteins expressed on the surface of hESC. To date, all hESC lines characterized share similar expression of these particular markers, which include the glycolipid antigens Stage Specific Embryonic Antigen (SSEA)-3 and SSEA-4 and the high molecular weight keratin sulphate proteoglycans TRA-1-60 and TRA-1-81 (named after the Battle of Trafalgar, not "Tumor Rejection Antigen") [2, 3, 6, 8, 31, 32]. TRA-1-60 and TRA-1-81 react with carbohydrate residues of the keratin sulphate/chondroiton sulphate cell surface/pericellular matrix proteoglycan, while Germ Cell Tumor Monoclonal-2 (GCTM-2) and TG343 antibodies detect epitopes on the protein core of the same antigen [9, 10, 33, 34]. The functional significance of these antigens is unknown; however expression of all these markers decreases significantly following spontaneous or induced differentiation *in vitro* [11] (Davidson, unpublished data). In addition, the tetraspanin transmembrane protein CD9, which is involved in cell adhesion, embryo implantation, and integrin signaling, is highly expressed in mouse and human ESC [35, 36]. Its expression also decreases upon differentiation, making it a reliable marker for pluripotent hESC [12, 37, 38].

Enzymatic Markers

Alkaline phosphatases are ubiquitous in many species ranging from prokaryotes to mammals, indicating that these enzymes perform important biological functions. Several alkaline phosphatase (AP) isozymes are expressed in a tissue-specific manner (placental, embryonic, and intestinal), while one AP is tissue-nonspecific and especially abundant in liver, kidney, and bone [39-41]. HESC express high levels of the liver/bone/kidney isozyme of alkaline phosphatase, as do other pluripotent cells such as primordial germ cells and embryonic carcinoma (EC) cells [2, 3, 11, 13, 42, 43]. For quantitative assessment of cell surface AP, TRA-2-49 and TRA-2-54 antibodies are often used; other AP assays are acceptable although these may only yield positive or negative results rather than quantitative data [11, 13].

Table 1. Characteristic markers of hESC

Marker	human ESC
Cell Surface Markers	
SSEA-1	−
SSEA-3	+
SSEA-4	+
TRA-1-60 [1,2]	+
TRA-1-81 [1,2]	+
GCTM-2 [1,3]	+
TG343 [1,3]	+
CD9 (TG30) [4]	+
Podocalyxin	+
CD133 (Prominin, AC133)	+
E-cadherin	+
Thy-1 (CD-90)	+
gp130	+/−
Transcription Factors	
Oct4	+
Nanog	+
Sox2	+
FoxD3 (Genesis)	+/−
Rex1 (Zfp42)	+/−
UTF-1	+
STAT3	+/−
Enzyme Activity	
Alkaline phosphatase [5]	+
Telomerase	+
Other Molecular Markers	
Cripto (TDGF1) [6]	+
FGF4	+/−
GDF3	+
Cx43 [7]	+
Cx45 [7]	+
Nodal	+
Lefty	+

Key: (+) expressed, (−) not expressed, (+/−) inconsistent reports of expression according to the literature, NR = non-reactive species. Markers in bold are the best known and most documented hESC markers which have also been shown to down-regulate upon differentiation.
References: [2-4, 6, 8-30].
[1] Target antigen is a 200kDa cell surface/pericellular matrix keratin sulphate/chondroiton sulphate proteoglycan containing extensive O-linked carbohydrates. [2] Antibody reacts with the carbohydrate epitopes. [3] Antibody reacts with the core protein of the proteoglycan. [4] CD9 is the antigen detected by TG30 antibody [5] Alkaline phosphatase often detected with TRA-2-54 or TRA-2-49 antibodies in human cells. [6] Cripto is a cell-surface associated protein that can also act as a secreted ligand. [7] Connexin 43 and 45 are transmembrane proteins involved in gap junction intercellular communication.

The capacity of hESC to proliferate indefinitely is accompanied by a high level of telomerase activity, which effectively maintains chromosomal length and prevents cellular senescence [44-46]. Most diploid somatic cells do not express telomerase and enter replicative senescence after a finite period of proliferation *in vitro* [47]. Some adult stem cell populations, such as hematopoietic stem cells, express telomerase *in vivo*, but do not maintain this expression when cultured *in vitro* [48, 49]. In hESC, as in cells of the early embryo, hTERT, the catalytic subunit of the telomerase, is expressed at high levels and down-regulated upon differentiation [2, 50, 51]. Chromosome telomeres have been reported to fluctuate in various hESC lines, ranging from 7 to 12 Kb in one study [8], but remain well above the senescence length. Because hESC exhibit high telomerase activity, maintain telomere length, and proliferate indefinitely in culture, they are considered immortal.

Molecular Markers

The POU domain transcription factor, Oct4, is expressed in pluripotent cell populations such as early embryo cells, blastomeres, and germ cells as well as in EC cells, embryonic germ (EG) cells, and ESC *in vitro* [52-56]. In particular, its expression in the ICM of blastocysts and cultured ESC has been demonstrated for mouse, primate, and human [57-61]. In addition to Oct4, the transcription factors Sox2 and Nanog are also highly expressed in ESC and other pluripotent cells [62-64]. These three transcription factors are essential for maintaining cells of the ICM *in vivo* and ESC *in vitro* in both human and mouse; all are down-regulated during differentiation [65-68]. Because of the functional significance of Oct4, Nanog, and Sox2 in regulating self-renewal, they are used as intracellular markers of hESC.

1.2. Assays for Pluripotency

In addition to their ability to being cultured for long periods of time in the undifferentiated state, hESC can also differentiate into cells of the three primary germ layers *in vivo* and *in vitro* [2, 4, 69]. HESC undergo rigorous tests to demonstrate their pluripotency in this regard. In contrast to mouse ESC, hESC can also reportedly differentiate into extraembryonic cell types such as trophectoderm and extraembryonic endoderm [2, 4], although in terms of pluripotency, differentiation into extraembryonic tissues is not a requirement. When injected into muscle, testis, or under the renal capsule of severe combined immunodeficiency (SCID) mice, hESC form teratomas containing tissues representative of all three germ lineages [2, 4]. This is the standard *in vivo* test of pluripotency (see Figure 2).

In vitro methods of differentiation may involve (1) spontaneous differentiation from high-density hESC colonies expanded without passage for several weeks, (2) spontaneous differentiation as embryoid bodies (EB) grown in suspension culture, or (3) directed differentiation in conditions devised specifically, and often empirically, for enriched or selective differentiation towards a particular lineage (Figure 2). Mixed populations of differentiated cells that arise from these conditions are often identified by their protein marker expression and/or characteristic morphology (such as beating cardiac muscle). Alternatively, a simple approach is to isolate RNA from an entire mixture of differentiated cells and look for expression of transcripts indicative of each lineage. Methods of *in vitro* differentiation not only provide valuable tools to interrogate the pluripotency of hESC lines, but are an important element of efforts to develop cell replacement therapies.

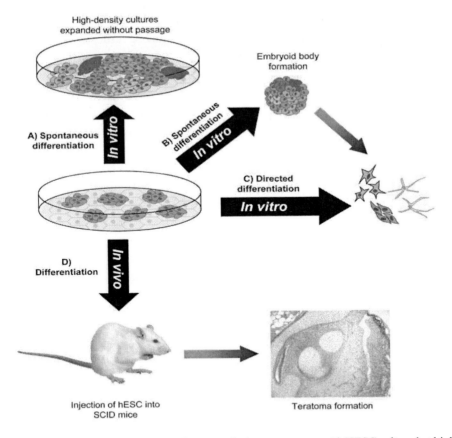

Figure 2. Schematic diagram of *in vitro* and *in vivo* pluripotency assays. A) HESC cultured at high density without passage for several weeks undergo spontaneous differentiation into cell types of all three germ lineages. Undifferentiated cells also continue to expand under these conditions, resulting in a heterogeneous mixture of undifferentiated and differentiated progeny. B) If grown in suspension culture as embryoid bodies (EB), hESC also differentiate spontaneously *in vitro* into cells indicative of the three primary lineages. EB may also contain some residual undifferentiated cells. C) HESC may also be differentiated *in vitro* towards a particular lineage using directed differentiation techniques. Pluripotency is confirmed if differentiation can be directed towards cells of all three germ lineages. D) The *in vivo* assay for pluripotency involves injection of hESC into immuno-compromised (SCID) mice to induce teratoma formation. Pluripotent hESC give rise to teratomas consisting of a variety of differentiated tissues which contain cell types from all three primary lineages. *In vitro* assays of pluripotency (A-C) may utilize RNA and/or protein expression to identify transcripts/markers indicative of the three germ lineages. Teratoma assays (D) rely primarily on histological determination of cell types found within the benign tumors.

2. EMBRYONIC STEM CELLS, PREREQUISITES FOR CLINICAL APPLICATION

2.1. Chromosomal Stability

A key feature that has traditionally distinguished hESC from hEC cells is their retention of a stable, diploid karyotype over prolonged periods of time, provided they are cultured under optimal conditions (and were isolated from a karyotypically normal embryo). In the past, this was true for hESC cultured for several years on mouse feeder layers in the presence of serum [70, 71]. Recently though, a number of reports indicate that hESC cultured under more defined conditions (often feeder-free and/or serum-free and with enzymatic passage) present abnormal karyotypes with much greater frequency [70-73]. In terms of hESC characteristics however, a normal karyotype has always been, and continues to be, an important requirement for lines to be considered "normal", "of good quality" and suitable for potential clinical applications.

2.2. Animal-Free Culture

Traditionally hESC have been derived and cultured in the presence of fetal calf serum (FCS). Although complex and poorly defined, serum culture conditions form the basis for some of the most characterized and reliable hESC information currently available. Conventional hESC serum culture medium incorporates 20% FCS and may also include fibroblast growth factor (FGF)-2 [2, 4, 14, 36]. Attempts to substitute human serum in place of FCS have been met with limited success [74] and still present clear disadvantages in terms of expense, need for pathogen testing, variability between batches, and lack of defined content. Efforts have focused on finding suitable alternatives for the serum component altogether rather than using human serum in hESC culture medium.

In recent years the requirement for serum has been successfully overcome by substituting the serum component in hESC media with a proprietary serum-free supplement called Knockout Serum Replacement (KSR), which consists in an undefined mixture of animal proteins [75], in combination with FGF-2. Since its first description in 2000 by Amit *et al.*, the serum-free method of hESC culture using KSR+FGF-2 has been incorporated into most hESC laboratories worldwide and allows for propagation of hESC on a larger scale than was previously possible using serum conditions [50, 76-78]. Existing hESC have been successfully sub-cultured in serum-free conditions and new cell lines have been isolated using serum-free media (SR-containing or similar, all contain FGF-2) [79-82]. KSR-containing medium (KSR medium) has proved effective in maintaining hESC growth and pluripotency over long-term culture on feeders. Table 2 lists in detail the progressive refinements in derivation and culture of hESC published since their initial isolation in 1998. In general, the conditions for hESC culture have evolved over time from poorly defined serum-containing medium to serum-free and, more recently, chemically defined medium.

With this shift to serum-free culture has also followed a movement away from labor-intensive mechanical transfer of hESC colonies towards more straightforward enzymatic/low-calcium buffer methods of passage (Table 2). Concerns have been raised about the genetic stability of hESC cultured for prolonged periods of time under serum-free conditions using these passage techniques [70, 71, 73, 83]. Aneuploidies, in particular those involving chromosome 12 or 17, have been detected independently by several labs using similar serum-free culture methods for different hESC lines (summarized in Table 3). Interestingly, these two chromosomes are also often duplicated in germ cell tumors [84-86]. The mechanism behind the apparent increased predisposition to aneuploidy is unknown, and opinions vary as to whether the serum-free medium or dissociation method (or combination thereof) is to blame. The nonrandom nature of the most frequently observed karyotypic abnormalities suggests a selective advantage of these aneuploid hESC in culture; however, whether there are contributing factors that promote an increased rate of mutation or genetic instability under particular conditions has yet to be determined. Certainly a number of publications also describe prolonged propagation of karyotypically normal hESC in serum-free medium on various types of feeder layers (comprehensive list in Table 2) [15, 76, 87, 88]. One trend is clear though, hESC cultured under standard serum conditions and passaged with mechanical transfer rarely exhibit the karyotypic aberrations that have been observed repeatedly in serum-free conditions.

Although the majority of publications detailing serum-free propagation of hESC utilize KSR+FGF medium, KSR still contains undefined complex animal components, albeit less variable than serum. Chemically defined media (devoid of KSR) for hESC culture have been described, though few have demonstrated long-term maintenance of genetically stable hESC lines. Pébay and colleagues used a HEPES-buffered DMEM basal medium supplemented with sphingosine-1-phosphate (S1P) and platelet-derived growth factor (PDGF) to maintain undifferentiated growth of hESC on MEFs for >80 passages [88]. HESC propagated under these conditions presented normal karyotypes after approximately 12 months (58 passages) in culture. Vallier *et al.* reported maintenance for 10 passages only in chemically defined medium using tissue culture surfaces pre-coated with FCS [109]. Ludwig *et al.* successfully propagated hESC on various matrices in a novel chemically defined medium, TeSR1, (KSR-free) supplemented with FGF-2, TGF-β1 and other factors; however two hESC lines derived in this condition became aneuploid within less than 30 passages [114]. Yao *et al.* described maintenance of hESC for >20 passages in a DMEM/F12 basal medium containing FGF-2 and nutrient supplements N2 and B27, with a normal karyotype obtained at passage 22 [117]. Lu *et al.* also reported maintenance of hESC for >20 passages using a different chemically defined media containing FGF-2, Wnt-3a, and April/BAFF, with normal karyotypes obtained at passage 23 [116].

Efficient isolation and establishment of hESC lines has remained largely dependent on the use of a fetal-derived feeder cell layer, most commonly MEFs, although human fetal and placental tissues and post-natal foreskin fibroblasts have also been utilized as feeder layers in an effort to move towards xeno-free conditions [87, 91, 93, 94, 96]. There are also reports of hESC-derived fibroblasts that support undifferentiated growth of autogenic and allogenic hESC [98, 100, 103, 118]. Some adult tissues have demonstrated the capacity to maintain hESC when used as feeders, such as marrow stromal cells, fallopian tube epithelial cells, uterine endometrial cells, and to some degree adult skin (depending on cell line); however, in general, tissues of fetal origin are considered superior sources of feeder cells [74, 91, 92, 97]. Table 2 includes details of known feeder layers used for hESC culture and derivation. Feeder density varies from 2-7 x 10^4 cells/cm^2 for serum-cultured hESC according to the majority of methods published (WiCell Protocols 2003 http://www.wicell.org ; ES Cell International Methodology Manual 2005 http://www.escellinternational.com/stemcellprod/training.htm; http://www.mcb.harvard.edu/melton/hues/HUES_manual.pdf [accessed] 2006). Some

Table 2. Summary of conditions for hESC culture

Cell line(s)	Substrate	Der	Key medium components	Passage method	Characterization SCM	Characterization Plurip	Characterization Karyo	Reference
H1,H7,H9,H13,H14	MEF	Y	20% FCS	dispase, MT, collagenase	Y	T	Y	[2]
HES1,HES2	MEF	Y	20% FCS	dispase, MT	Y	T,IV	Y	[4]
BG01,02,03,04	MEF	Y	20% FCS +1000U/ml hLIF +4ng/ml FGF	MT	Y	EB[1]	Y	[14]
H9.1,H9.2	MEF	N	20% KSR +4ng/ml FGF2	collagenase	Y	T	Y	[76]
hES-NCL1	MEF, Matrigel [2]	Y	*Derivation*: 10% FCS *Culture*: 10-20% KSR +4ng/ml FGF2	collagenase	Y	IV,T	Y	[77]
Miz-hES4-8, 10-13	MEF	Y	20% KSR +4ng/ml FGF2	MT	Y	EB,T	Y/N[3]	[82]
SA002,FC018,AS034 AS038,SA121,SA181 AS034.1 (subclone)	MEF	Y	VitroHES (serum-free) +4ng/ml FGF2	MT	Y	EB,IV,T[4]	Y/N[4]	[81]
HUES1-17	MEF	Y	8-10% KSR, 8-10% plasmanate +5ng/ml FGF2 +12ng/ml hLIF	trypsin	Y	EB,T	Y/N[5]	[80]
HES2,HES3,HES4	MEF	N	DMEM/HEPES +10uM S1P +20ng/ml PDGF-AB	MT	Y	T,IV	Y	[88]

Key: Der = condition used for derivation (Yes or No); Characterization: SCM = stem cell marker expression (Yes or No); Plurip = assay for pluripotency (EB = Embryoid body, T = teratoma formation, IV = *in vitro* monolayer differentiation); Karyo = normal karyotype (Yes or No), Ref = Reference

Abbreviations: AFT (adult fallopian tube), CDM (chemically defined medium), CM (conditioned medium), CN (collagen), ECM (extracellular matrix preparation), FCS (fetal calf serum), FN (fibronectin), HEF (hESC-derived feeders), hLIF (human LIF), KGF (keratinocyte growth factor), KSR (knockout serum replacement), LN (Laminin), MT (mechanical transfer), N/D (not described), NIC (nicotinamide), VN (vitronectin)

[1] No endoderm lineage. [2] hESC derived on MEF, then transferred to matrigel/MEF CM culture conditions as described by Xu *et al.* (2001). [3] Of the 9 lines derived, 1 had an abnormal karyotype. [4] All hESC lines gave rise to cells positive for markers indicative of the three germ lineages *in vitro*; in teratoma assay FC018 & AS038 resulted in fluid-filled cysts while the other lines yielded normal teratomas containing cells of all the lineages. SA002 & FC018 were aneuploid, while the other lines were karyotypically normal. [5] Initial karyotype normal for all 17 lines tested after long-term culture (range P7-P20), but 3 of 4 lines tested after long-term culture (>P29) acquired significant karyotypic abnormalities.

Cell line(s)	Substrate	Der	Key medium components	Passage method	SCM	Plurip	Karyo	Reference
Miz-hES1,2,3	STO	Y	Derivation: 20% FCS +2000U/ml hLIF +4ng/ml FGF2 Culture: 20% KSR +4ng/ml FGF2	MT	Y	EB,T	Y	[89]
MB01-09	STO	Y	Derivation: 20% FCS +2000U/ml hLIF +4ng/ml FGF2 Culture: 20% KSR +4ng/ml FGF2	MT, collagenase	Y	EB	Y	[90]
HES3, HES4	AFT epithelial cells, fetal muscle, fetal skin	N	20% FCS	MT		T	Y	[91]
Novel	fetal muscle	Y	20% human serum [6]	MT	Y	T	Y	[91]
HES3,HES4	fetal muscle, fetal skin D551, adult skin	N	20% FCS or 20% KSR +4-8ng/ml FGF2	dispase, MT	Y	T	Y	[74]
H1	human marrow stromal cells	N	20% KSR +4ng/ml FGF2	collagenase, trypsin	Y	EB,IV [7]	Y	[92]
I-6, I-3, H9	foreskin fibroblasts	N	15% KSR +4ng/ml FGF2	collagenase	Y	EB,T	Y	[87]
HS181	foreskin fibroblasts	Y	20% FCS +1ug/ml hLIF	dispase, MT	Y	T	Y	[93]
HS293,HS306	foreskin fibroblasts	Y	20% KSR +8ng/mlFGF2	MT	Y	EB,T	Y	[94]
SA611	foreskin fibroblasts	Y	20% human serum +10ng/ml FGF2	MT, TrypLE Select	Y	IV,T	Y	[95]
H1,H9,HSF1,HSF6	placental fibroblasts	N	20% KSR +4ng/ml FGF2	collagenase	Y	N/D	N/D	[96]
UCSF1,UCSF2	placental fibroblasts	Y	20% KSR +12ng/ml FGF2	MT, collagenase	Y	EB,T	Y	[96]

[6] Maintained hESC poorly beyond 10 passages. [7] Pluripotency was assessed by EB formation and visual observation of differentiated cell morphology induced by retinoic acid (RA) treatment. Examination of EBs and RA-differentiated cells for markers/transcripts indicative of the three primary germ layers was presumably not carried out.

Table 2. (Continued)

Cell line(s)	Substrate	Der	Key medium components	Passage method	Characterization SCM	Characterization Plurip	Characterization Karyo	Reference
Miz-hES9,14,15	human uterine endometrial cells	Y	20% KSR +4ng/ml FGF	N/D	Y	EB,T	Y	[97]
Miz-hES1,2,3	STO	Y	*Derivation:* 20% FCS +2000U/ml hLIF Culture: 20% KSR +4ng/ml FGF2	MT	Y	EB,T	Y	[89]
H1	hESC-DF	N	20% KSR +4ng/ml FGF2	collagenase	Y	EB,T	Y	[98]
SH7	hESC-DF	Y	20% KSR +4-8ng/ml FGF2	collagenase	Y	N/D	N/D	[98]
HES2,3,4	ΔE-MEF, Matrigel [8]	N	15% KSR +4-8ng/ml FGF2	collagenase	Y	T	Y	[99]
H1,hES-NCL1	hESC-DF	N	20% KSR +4ng/ml FGF2	collagenase	Y	IV,T	Y	[100]
H1,hES-NCL1	Matrigel	N	hESC-DF CM (20% KSR +4ng/ml FGF2)	collagenase	Y	N/D	N/D	[100]
H1	Matrigel, LN	N	MEF CM (20% KSR +4ng/ml FGF2)	collagenase	Y	EB,T	Y	[15]
H1,H7,H9	Matrigel	N	MEF CM (20% KSR +8ng/ml FGF2)	collagenase	Y	EB,T	Y/N	[37]
BG01,02,03	Matrigel, FN	N	MEF CM (20% KSR +4ng/ml FGF2)	EDTA-free trypsin	Y	N/D	Y	[101]
H1	Matrigel	N	NIH/3T3-Nog CM (20%KSR +4ng/ml FGF2)	collagenase	Y	N/D	N/D	[102]
H1,H7,H9	Matrigel	N	HEF-TERT CM (20%KSR +8ng/mlFGF2)	collagenase	Y	EB	Y	[103]
H1,hES-NCL1	human serum	N	hESC-DF CM (20% KSR +8ng/ml FGF)	collagenase	Y	IV,T	Y	[104]
H1,H7,H9	MEF ECM	N	8% KSR, 8% plasmanate +16ng/ml FGF2 +20ng/ml hLIF	MT, trypsin	Y	EB	Y	[105]

[8] ΔE-MEF are MEFs immortalized via infection with E6 and E7 genes from human papillomavirus (HPV16). hESC were cultured on ΔE-MEF and also transferred to matrigel with ΔE-MEFCM. [9] When cultured in this media, hESC morphology changed to irregular monolayer appearance rather than regular tightly clustered colonies, however cells stained positive for stem cell markers and formed teratomas when injected under the renal capsule of nude mice.

Cell line(s)	Substrate	Der	Key medium components	Passage method	Characterization SCM	Characterization Plurip	Characterization Karyo	Reference
ACT-14	MEF ECM	Y	(same as above)	MT, trypsin	Y	EB	Y	[105]
HSF6	LN	N	KSR +50ng/ml Activin +50ng/ml KGF +10mM NIC [9]	collagenase	Y	EB,T	Y	[106]
H1,BGN1,BGN2	Matrigel	N	20% KSR +4ng/ml FGF2 +2uM BIO[10]	None[10]	Y	EB	N/D	[107]
I-6,I-3,H9	human FN	N	20% KSR +0.12ng/ml TGFβ1 +4ng/ml FGF2 +/- 1000U/ml hLIF	collagenase	Y	EB,T	Y	[79]
H1,BGN1,BGN2	Matrigel	N	20% KSR +4ng/ml FGF +25ng/ml Activin	collagenase	Y	EB	N/D	[108]
H9	FCS	N	CDM +12ng/ml FGF2 +10ng/ml Activin [11]	collagenase	Y	EB	Y/N	[109]
UCSF1	human placental LN	N	X-VIVO 10 +80ng/ml FGF2[12]	collagenase	Y	EB	Y	[96]
H1	Matrigel, LN	N	X-VIVO 10 +80ng/ml FGF2	collagenase	Y	EB,T	Y	[110]
H7,H9	Matrigel	N	20% KSR +40ng/ml FGF2	collagenase	Y	EB,T	Y	[111]
H1,H7,H9,H14	Matrigel	N	20% KSR +100ng/ml FGF2	dispase	Y	T	Y	[112]
H1,H9,H14	Matrigel	N	20% KSR +40ng/ml FGF2 +500ng/ml Noggin	dispase	Y	EB,T	Y	[113]

[10]Cultured for 7 days only without passage. [11]CDM: 50% IMDM, 50% F12 NUT-MIX, 7ug/ml insulin, 15ug/ml transferrin, 450uM momothioglycerol, 5mg/ml BSA [115]; supportive capacity of this medium was demonstrated for 10 passages only. [12]X-VIVO 10 is a proprietary defined medium. [13]Key components include FGF2, LiCl, GABA, pipecolic acid, and TGFβ1. [14]WA15 initially showed a normal karyotype, but acquired trisomy 12 by 7 months; WA16 was aneuploid at the time of first karyotype analysis.

Table 2. (Continued)

Cell line(s)	Substrate	Der	Key medium components	Passage method	SCM	Plurip	Karyo	Reference
H1	Matrigel	N	20% KSR +40ng/ml FGF2 +500ng/ml Noggin	collagenase	Y	IV	Y	[102]
H1,H7,H9,H14	Matrigel	N	TeSR1 defined medium[13]	dispase	Y	T	Y	[114]
WA15,WA16	CN,FN,VN,LN	Y	TeSR1 defined medium[13]	MT, dispase	Y	N/D	N[14]	[114]
H9,BG01	FN	N	HESCO[15] +4ng/ml FGF2 +100ng/ml Wnt3a +100ng/ml April/BAFF	collagenase, trypsin-EDTA	Y	EB,T	Y	[116]
H1,HSF6	Matrigel	N	N2/B27-CDM[16] +20ng/ml FGF2	dispase	Y	T,IV	Y	[117]

[15]HESCO is a defined DMEM/F12 based medium supplemented with insulin, transferrin, albumin, cholesterol lipid, and growth factors; hESC were maintained for 8 passages only in this medium. [16]N2/B27-CDM is comprised of basal DMEM/F12 (1:1) plus 1X N2 and 1X B27 supplements (both Gibco).

laboratories adjust feeder densities depending on the serum content of the medium [36]. Regardless of the precise density, the feeder component is an important aspect of hESC culture.

Once hESC lines are established in culture, feeder-free propagation is possible using various matrices (such as Matrigel, fibronectin, or laminin), growth factors, and feeder-conditioned medium (although whether feeder-conditioned medium qualifies as "feeder-free" is debatable) [15, 37, 77, 100-104, 119]. Specific factors that feeder cells contribute to the culture system have yet to be fully characterized, however the fact that feeder-conditioned medium supports hESC growth is evidence that the key factors are secreted. Genuine feeder-free methods of hESC propagation have also been described using similar matrices and unconditioned KSR-medium supplemented with a range of growth factor combinations. These conditions tend to incorporate high concentrations (40-100 ng/ml) of FGF-2 in the medium [96, 110, 111] and may also include the BMP-antagonist, Noggin [102, 113]. Several other groups have also described successful maintenance of hESC in KSR-medium including Activin in combination with FGF-2 or other growth factors [106, 108, 109]. Clearly, FGF and Activin/Nodal/TGFβ1 emerge as strong candidates for feeder-secreted maintenance factors from the existing literature [79]. Feeder-free conditions are also summarized in Table 2.

Table 3. Chromosomal abnormalities reported in cultured hESC lines

hESC line(s)	Mutation(s)	Reference
HUES1	+2q	[80]
HUES3, HUES4	+12	[80]
HUES5, HUES9	inv9 [1]	[80]
H14, H1.1A (subclone)	+12	[73]
H7.S9, H14.S9	+17	[73]
H1.1B (subclone), H7.S6	other [2]	[73]
H1, H7, H9	+20 [3]	[37]
SA002	+13	[81]
FC018	Triploid (XXY)	[81]
Miz-hES13	+3	[82]
HS237	Isodicentric (X)(q21)	[121]
BG01	+12,+17/ +12, +17, +X	[71]
BG02	+17	[71]
BG02	+12, +14, +17, +X	[71]
BG02	+12, +14, +17, +20, +X	[71]
BG01	+17q	[120]
H1, H7, H9, SA002/2.5	other [2]	[120]
HES2	other [2]	[70]
HES3	+12	[70]
HS181	+i(12) isochromosome	[122]
WA15	+12	[114]
WA	16+X [4]	[114]
FES22	+17	[123]
FES30	+X	[123]
H13	+17	[124]
H9	+X	[124]

Table 3. (Continued)

hESC line(s)	Mutation(s)	Reference
H1	+12, +17/ +12, +17 +X	[72]
H1	+12/ +17/ +12, +17	[72]
H14	+12/ +i(12)	[72]
H7	+X, +20, other [2]	[72]
HUES5	+XX, +12, +14, +17/+12,+14,+17	[72]
HUES6, HUES14	other [2]	[72]
HUES7	+12,+17/+X,+12,+17/+7,+12,+17	[72]
HUES10	+X, +9, +12, +17	[72]
HUES13	+7, +12	[72]
HUES17	+12, +17	[72]
Shef1	+3	[72]
Shef1	+i(12)	[72]
Shef4	+17	[72]
Shef5	+20	[72]

Note: The two most common chromosomal anueploidies reported in hESC involve chromosome 12 (in green) and 17 (in blue). All lines except SA002, SA002/2.5, FC018, Miz-hES13, WA16 have previously yielded normal karyotypes, thus the chromosomal abnormality occurred during *in vitro* expansion of the lines and may be linked to culture techniques that deviate from the established methods which historically have supported genetically stable hESC.

[1]inv9 (p11q13) is a frequently observed chromosomal variant of no clinical significance. [2]"other" refers to various unique and/or complex chromosomal amplifications, deletions, and rearrangements. [3]authors state this was the most common karyotypic abnormality but imply that other mutations were also detected. [4]This particular cell line was abnormal at the time of the first karyotypes analysis, therefore it is not known whether the karyotypic insult occurred early during *in vitro* culture or whether it originated from the blastocyst from which the hESC line was derived.

It is interesting to note that several laboratories have independently experienced recurrent karyotypic abnormalities in previously stable hESC lines upon long-term culture in serum-free and feeder-free conditions [71, 73, 101, 120], while others have reported lower levels (approximately 20%) of aneuploidy under the same conditions [37] (Table 3). This suggests that serum-free and/or feeder-free culture environment may present a selective advantage for abnormal or adapted hESC within the population, in contrast to serum/MEF conditions in which hESC line have proven remarkably genetically stable over long-term culture (several years). Whether these karyotypic changes are a result of passage method (and subsequent likelihood of separation into single cells), medium composition, substrate, or some other unknown cellular stress remains speculation, although there seems to be an association between long-term serum-free, feeder-free conditions and genetic instability.

During the early stages of inner cell mass outgrowth, hESC are extremely vulnerable to the microenvironment and must be provided with optimal culture conditions. The feeder component at this stage has traditionally been necessary for efficient success rates of derivation, however Klimanskaya *et al.* reported successful isolation of one hESC line using an extracellular matrix preparation from MEFs with a similar efficiency to reports using feeders [105]. Although the preparation does not contain live MEFs, it may still contain hormones, lipids, and other stable molecules, and arguably still contains uncharacterized MEF-components. The only case of genuinely defined feeder-free conditions for hESC derivation was reported in 2006 and utilized a combination of human collagen IV, fibronectin, laminin, and vitronectin matrices with TeSR1 medium containing human growth factors [114]. This study described derivation efficiencies similar to those published using traditional feeder conditions, but after 4 and 7 months respectively the two new hESC lines presented aneuploid karyotypes. Therefore, despite significant advances in feeder-free culture methods, the lack of examples in the literature of feeder-free hESC derivation illustrates the importance of the feeder substrate for ICM outgrowth and early establishment of genetically stable hESC lines.

2.3. Tumorigenicity and Immune Response

An essential prerequisite to the use of hESC in human therapy is that the cells do not present a risk of tumorigenicity once transplanted into humans. Indeed, while the ordinary proof of concept of hESC pluripotency is the formation of teratomas containing tissues representative of the three germ layers, this outcome must be avoided for therapy. Another essential prerequisite to the use of hESC for therapy is that hESC must not induce an immune response after transplantation. Data suggest that due to the current culture systems (which rely on animal products), hESC and hESC-derived progenitors incorporate the nonhuman sialic acid Neu5Gc (Neu5Gc), against which most humans carry circulating antibodies [125]. These data thus suggest the potential of hESC to induce an immune response following transplantation [125], even if unlikely [126].

2.4. Functional

Lastly, a fundamental requirement for cell-replacement therapy is that hESC-derived cells will need to be functional. This aspect has not yet been thoroughly studied in hESC; however as we will see later in the chapter (part 3.1), mouse ESC give us a positive insight into hESC ability to be functional after transplantation.

3. SIGNIFICANCE OF STEM CELL RESEARCH

In some aspects hESC resemble other pluripotent cell populations, such as hEC cells, derived from germ cell tumors called teratocarcinomas, and human embryonic germ (hEG) cells, isolated from the gonadal ridge of 5-9 week old fetal tissue, as well as ESC from other species [3]. These pluripotent cells share similar patterns of marker expression; however, several factors distinguish hESC from hEC and hEG cells. HEC cells frequently carry gross chromosomal abnormalities and aneuploidies, in contrast to hESC which exhibit a stable and normal karyotype. HEG cells differ from hESC with respect to several key markers, such as SSEA-1 and SSEA-3, and are more difficult to propagate in their undifferentiated state for extended periods of time (greater than 2-3 months). Although hEG cells can form EBs containing ectodermal, endodermal, and mesodermal lineages, they do not yield teratomas *in vivo* and fail to give rise *in vitro* to certain cell types readily found in spontaneously differentiated hESC cultures, such as contracting cardiomyocytes [127]. These important features of hESC (pluripotency and genetic stability) offer a clear advantage over other pluripotent cell populations for development of therapeutic applications.

Stem cells are predicted to have the greatest impact in two principle applications: 1) as an unlimited source of material for use in regenerative medicine, and 2) as *in vitro* models for the study of development and diseases.

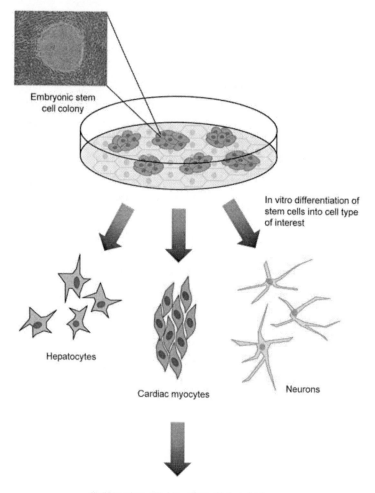

Figure 3. Therapeutic applications of human embryonic stem cells for regenerative medicine.

3.1. Potential Stem Cell Therapies

Regenerative Medicine –Cell Replacement

Because of their ability to differentiate into any cell type, hESC have generated much interest as a possible renewable source of cells for therapeutic transplantation (Figure 3). Potential use in regenerative medicine has lead many researchers to focus on expanding undifferentiated embryonic stem cells under xeno-free conditions and developing techniques to direct differentiation efficiently towards lineages of particular significance, such as pancreatic islet cells [128-130], neurons [131-133], cardiomyocytes [134], and hepatocytes [135, 136].

In fact, cell therapy has been carried out in animal models of disease using several ESC-derived cell types, with notable success in treating central nervous system (CNS) disease [137], stroke [138], damaged liver [139], diabetes [140-142], and cardiovascular disease [143]. Derivatives of hESC may also have clinical applications as tools with which to identify gene targets for novel drugs, to screen new compounds for toxicity and teratogenicity, and to deliver gene therapy.

There are several key issues that need to be examined for hESC derivatives to be successfully used in cell replacement. These issues include integration of donor cells into host tissue, their differentiation to functional mature cell types and their ongoing survival. The function of the donor cells needs to also be appropriately regulated in the host tissue. For example, transplantation of insulin producing cells requires appropriate release of insulin levels into the blood stream in response to blood glucose. Likewise, donor neuronal cells in an injury site require their correct innervation and targeting of host cells, as well as receiving input signals from the endogenous neural circuitry. Thus, transplantation studies aimed to replace or replenish endogenous cells, require careful and thorough analyses to address all the necessary requirements to achieve complete repair of the diseased or injured host tissue.

Vehicles to Provide Factors to Rescue a Diseased State

Transplantation of hESC and their derivatives may also be therapeutically used as vehicles to secrete factors involved in repair of endogenous host environment. A study by Lee and colleagues [144], showed that transplantation of hESC-derived neural stem cells in a rodent model of the neurodegenerative Sandhoff disease resulted in significantly reduced neuropathology. Sandhoff disease is a genetic disorder whereby a deficiency in the brain enzyme beta-hexosaminidase results in the accumulation of lipids causing severe neurotoxicity. Lee and colleagues (2007) found that the substantial recovery observed in the transplanted rodents was not directly due to neuronal replacement of the donor cells but rather their production of beta-hexosaminidase [144]. It is known that hESC-derived neural progenitors secrete factors, such as Wnt proteins [145], that may also provide support to the endogenous cellular microenvironment. In addition, several donor stem cell types, as well as other cell types, can be genetically modified to release specific factors [146-149]. As the technology for genetically modifying hESC and their derivatives has been developed and optimized [150], researchers may now be able to genetically engineer hESC to secrete specific factors required for repair.

Somatic Cell Nuclear Transfer

Once successful cell therapies have been developed, hESC could theoretically offer a solution to the use of immunosuppressive therapy in transplantation by using somatic cell nuclear transfer (SCNT, also known as "therapeutic cloning") to produce patient-matched hESC lines. SCNT involves removing the nucleus from a donated oocyte and replacing it with the nucleus from a somatic cell of a patient. The SCNT "embryo" can be stimulated to divide *in vitro* to give rise to a blastocyst, from which ESC can be isolated for regenerative medicine applications. ESC produced using SCNT embryos should be genetically identical to the person who donated the nuclear genetic material. SCNT differs from traditional "cloning" in that the *intent* is not to produce a living cloned organism (termed "reproductive cloning"), which would require transfer of the embryo to a womb, but rather to produce a patient-specific ESC line which can be used for the purpose of cell transplant therapy (Figure 4). SCNT-derived ESC and their cell derivatives could also be used for other research purposes, such as drug screening to best predict the most effective treatments for a patient with a particular genetic disease.

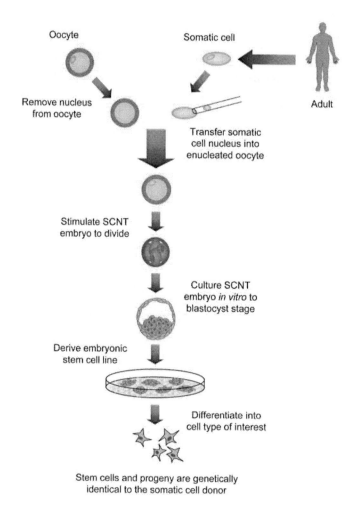

Figure 4. In the future, somatic cell nuclear transfer (SCNT) could circumvent the need for immunosuppressive therapy in recipients of hESC-based cell transplants. SCNT involves removing the nucleus from a donated oocyte and replacing it with the nucleus from a somatic cell. The SCNT embryo can be stimulated to divide *in vitro* to give rise to a blastocyst, from which ESC can be isolated. ESC, as well as their differentiated progeny, produced using SCNT embryos should be genetically identical to the person who donated the somatic cell nucleus.

Proof of principle studies carried out in the mouse by Munsie *et al.* (2000) demonstrated that mouse ESC lines isolated from SCNT embryos were in fact pluripotent, evidenced by their ability to contribute to all three germ layers in teratomas and chimeric mice [151]. This work was confirmed by Wakayama and colleagues, who also generated nuclear transfer-derived (nt) mouse ESC from SCNT embryos using another somatic donor cell type [152]. Rideout and colleagues took the work a step further and were able to create ntESC from immuno-deficient Rag2 knockout mice, correct the genetic defect *in vitro* via homologous recombination, then use the corrected mouse ESC for cell therapy [153]. The genetically repaired ESC were differentiated into functional hematopoietic precursors for cellular transplant using two methods: 1) *in vivo* by using tetraploid embryo complementation to generate mice as bone marrow donors and 2) *in vitro* by differentiating the ESC to hematopoietic stem cells [153]. Both methods resulted in successful engraftment and some degree of functional immune improvement, although additional host manipulation was necessary to enhance engraftment of the *in vitro* ESC-derived hematopoietic population. The study proved in principle that combined therapeutic cloning and gene therapy is possible. Using a different disease model, Barberi and colleagues successfully transplanted ntESC-derived dopaminergic neurons into parkinsonian mice and found improvements in the behavioral phenotype following treatment, demonstrating the functionality of ntESC-derivatives and efficacy of therapeutic cloning in an animal model of CNS disease [154]. These animal studies have set the stage for SCNT-based therapies to be investigated along with hESC-derived cell therapy as potential treatments for human diseases. Indeed, human SCNT blastocysts have been produced with surprisingly high efficiency using adult fibroblast donor cells [155].

3.2. Human Embryonic Stem Cells as Models for Research

Models for Development

Because of their embryonic origin, hESC exhibit properties similar to cells of the inner cell mass and not surprisingly share characteristics related to pluripotency. hESC provide an *in vitro* model system to study early developmental processes, such as lineage specification, differentiation, and tissue patterning, especially in cases where these is a significant difference between mouse and human embryology. Given the physical limitations of studying human post-implantation embryonic development *in vivo*, hESC provide a suitable cellular model for research into fertility, embryo metabolism, developmental diseases, and birth defects. hESC offer an advantage over multipotent fetal-derived stem cells for such studies in that they can be propagated indefinitely *in vitro*, whereas fetal stem cells (FSC) require periodic isolation from a regular source of fetal tissue, which can be difficult to obtain due to ethical constraints.

However, hESC cultured *in vitro* also differ from the early developing embryo from which they were derived. In the embryo, ICM cells occupy a transient stage of development and progressively become restricted to more committed cell fates as development proceeds. Embryonic stem cells are maintained somewhat artificially *in vitro* in this primitive state. Although the expression profile (transcriptional and protein) of hESC resembles that of the inner cell mass cells [6, 156], they are clearly not the same. Re-establishing a three-dimensional structure in the mouse by culturing mouse ESC as embryoid bodies cannot recapitulate embryonic development, but does result in sequential expression of gene cohorts associated with gastrulation, primitive streak formation, and lineage specification [157]. However embryoid bodies established spontaneously from hESC are often disorganized and variable in their morphology, interior cellular structures, and transcriptional profiles [158, 159]. Given the right inductive conditions, hESC differentiate towards many critical developmental stages found in the early embryo, however this too occurs in a variable fashion [69]. Thus, even though hESC exhibit pluripotent characteristics and are receptive to early inductive signaling events similar to cells of the early embryo, they lack the ability to fully regulate and reorganize developmental processes once removed from the embryonic environment. However, the *in vitro* culture environment provides a unique setting to enable control of extrinsic cytokines and/or growth factors in order to study effects on cellular differentiation. This allows for a systematic approach to dissecting signaling pathways involved in early development that might otherwise prove too complex and difficult to examine in whole embryo studies.

Models for Cancer

In vitro cultured stem cells, like other cultured cells, are susceptible to epigenetic modifications, karyotypic insult, and adaptations that may lead to a selective advantage and thus genetic changes within cell populations over time. In this way, hESC may acquire characteristics of their cancerous counterparts, embryonic carcinoma (EC) cells, as reported by several groups working with aneuploid hESC [70, 73]. Even normal hESC can give rise to tumors *in vivo* when exposed to a certain microenvironment. Furthermore, there is evidence that cancer initiation *in vivo* may result from oncogenic mutations in long-lived stem cells residing within adult tissues [160]. Some cancers, such as leukemia, brain, and breast cancer, appear to consist of a small subset of self-renewing cancer stem cells that are responsible for long-term tumor growth [161]. By studying ESC and EC cells in culture, we may also discover important intrinsic and extrinsic pathways that control cancer initiation. This work may lead to the development of novel drugs to target cancer stem cells in order to reduce the rate of recurrence commonly associated with particular cancers.

Models for Disease Progression

With greater access to preimplantation genetic diagnosis (PGD) prior to embryo transfer, many couples seeking embryo biopsy may chose to donate embryos carrying a known genetic defect for use in derivation of hESC lines. Alternatively, it may be discovered after the fact that embryos from which hESC were derived contained a genetic abnormality with a known disease association. Already hESC lines have been established with the following genetic disorders: adrenoleukodystrophy, cystic fibrosis, Duchenne and Becker muscular dystrophy, Fanconi anemia, fragile-X syndrome, Huntington disease, Marfan syndrome, myotonic dystrophy, neurofibromatosis type I, and thalassemia [162-164]. Disease-specific stem cell lines may also be derived from a person afflicted with a disease using SCNT in the absence of a genetic test. Regardless of the derivation method, hESC lines with genetic disorders provide *in vitro* models to study the molecular and cellular disturbances and complicated etiology associated with human diseases. These hESC lines could also be used in functional drug-screening, especially for conditions which lack a suitable animal model in which to test compounds for efficacy prior to clinical trials.

CONCLUSION

Despite the fact that most hESC lines have been characterized by immunological, molecular and biological analyses to determine stem cell phenotype and differentiation capacity, only a few lines have been examined thoroughly by more than one laboratory, and little systematic comparison of cell lines has been carried out. Various transcriptome analyses of hESC highlight both similarities and differences among/between lines, although most studies have examined only two or three cell lines [16, 101, 165, 166]. Clearly there is a need for more comparative characterization of hESC lines in order to address these many variations. Furthermore, different hESC lines vary in the ease with which they can be propagated under equivalent culture conditions. A recent comparison of nine hESC lines identified some considerable differences in growth, adaptation to bulk culture conditions (KSR medium, enzymatic passage), cloning efficiency, karyotypic stability, and transfection efficiency [124]. Differences between hESC lines are not surprising given that hESC do not originate from an inbred population (as do mouse ESC) and that hESC have been isolated from embryos of various stages of preimplantation development (from early to late blastocyst, and in some cases even late morula). However, if variations are identified in growth and/or differentiation properties of certain hESC lines, some lines may prove more suitable for particular applications than others. In an effort to establish a comprehensive set of standards for characterization of hESC, the International Stem Cell Initiative (ISCI) undertook a comparative analysis of 75 hESC lines through a collaborative study involving 17 laboratories across eleven countries [167, 168]. Such comparative information will be a valuable addition to existing studies of hESC lines. In addition, comparative hESC studies should endeavor to utilize quantitative analyses when possible, since much characterization to date has been qualitative. Lastly, before therapy could use hESC, one will need to find a way to cultivate hESC in a larger scale than currently available.

HESC undoubtedly provide an invaluable tool to study human embryology and to develop cell replacement therapies. However, almost 10 years after the first report of hESC maintenance *in vitro*, very little of hESC biology is truly understood. For instance, the current knowledge on the signaling pathways involved in hESC maintenance is slowly improving and a few intracellular signaling pathways are now emerging as essential to hESC maintenance of pluripotency, self-renewal and survival (see [169] for review). We regard this particular field of research as extremely valuable, as the characterization of the signals involved in pluripotency, self-renewal, survival and differentiation of hESC is a fundamental requirement to a proper design of an optimal system for hESC maintenance as well as to hESC manipulation for future cell therapies.

ACKNOWLEDGMENTS

This work was supported by the University of Melbourne and the Australian Stem Cell Centre.

REFERENCES

[1] Evans, M.J. and M.H. Kaufman, *Establishment in culture of pluripotential cells from mouse embryos.* Nature, 1981. 292(5819): p. 154-6.
[2] Thomson, J.A., et al., *Embryonic stem cell lines derived from human blastocysts.* Science, 1998. 282(5391): p. 1145-7.
[3] Pera, M.F., B. Reubinoff, and A. Trounson, *Human embryonic stem cells.* J Cell Sci, 2000. 113 (Pt 1): p. 5-10.
[4] Reubinoff, B.E., et al., Embryonic stem cell lines from human blastocysts: somatic differentiation in vitro. Nat Biotechnol, 2000. 18(4): p. 399-404.
[5] Bradley, A., et al., *Formation of germ-line chimaeras from embryo-derived teratocarcinoma cell lines.* Nature, 1984. 309(5965): p. 255-6.
[6] Henderson, J.K., et al., Preimplantation human embryos and embryonic stem cells show comparable expression of stage-specific embryonic antigens. Stem Cells, 2002. 20(4): p. 329-37.
[7] Laslett, A.L., A.A. Filipczyk, and M.F. Pera, *Characterization and culture of human embryonic stem cells.* Trends Cardiovasc Med, 2003. 13(7): p. 295-301.
[8] Carpenter, M.K., E. Rosler, and M.S. Rao, *Characterization and differentiation of human embryonic stem cells.* Cloning Stem Cells, 2003. 5(1): p. 79-88.
[9] Badcock, G., et al., *The human embryonal carcinoma marker antigen TRA-1-60 is a sialylated keratan sulfate proteoglycan.* Cancer Res, 1999. 59(18): p. 4715-9.
[10] Cooper, S., et al., Biochemical properties of a keratan sulphate/chondroitin sulphate proteoglycan expressed in primate pluripotent stem cells. J Anat, 2002. 200(Pt 3): p. 259-65.
[11] Draper, J.S., et al., Surface antigens of human embryonic stem cells: changes upon differentiation in culture. J Anat, 2002. 200(Pt 3): p. 249-58.
[12] Cai, J., et al., Assessing self-renewal and differentiation in human embryonic stem cell lines. Stem Cells, 2006. 24(3): p. 516-30.
[13] Andrews, P.W., et al., Comparative analysis of cell surface antigens expressed by cell lines derived from human germ cell tumours. Int J Cancer, 1996. 66(6): p. 806-16.
[14] Mitalipova, M., et al., *Human embryonic stem cell lines derived from discarded embryos.* Stem Cells, 2003. 21(5): p. 521-6.
[15] Xu, C., et al., *Feeder-free growth of undifferentiated human embryonic stem cells.* Nat Biotechnol, 2001. 19(10): p. 971-4.
[16] Abeyta, M.J., et al., Unique gene expression signatures of independently-derived human embryonic stem cell lines. Hum Mol Genet, 2004. 13(6): p. 601-8.
[17] Pera, M.F., et al., *Isolation and characterization of human ES cells*, in *Embryonic Stem Cells: A Practical Approach*, E. Notarianni and M.J. Evans, Editors. 2006, Oxford University Press: Oxford. p. 238-259.

[18] Schopperle, W.M. and W.C. Dewolf, The Tra-1-60 and Tra-1-81 Human Pluripotent Stem Cell Markers Are Expressed on Podocalyxin in Embryonal Carcinoma. Stem Cells, 2006.
[19] Brivanlou, A.H., et al., *Stem cells. Setting standards for human embryonic stem cells.* Science, 2003. 300(5621): p. 913-6.
[20] Cai, J., et al., Development of antibodies to human embryonic stem cell antigens. BMC Dev Biol, 2005. 5: p. 26.
[21] Rho, J.Y., et al., Transcriptional profiling of the developmentally important signalling pathways in human embryonic stem cells. Hum Reprod, 2006. 21(2): p. 405-12.
[22] Noaksson, K., et al., *Monitoring differentiation of human embryonic stem cells using real-time PCR.* Stem Cells, 2005. 23(10): p. 1460-7.
[23] Brandenberger, R., et al., *MPSS profiling of human embryonic stem cells.* BMC Dev Biol, 2004. 4: p. 10.
[24] Sato, N., et al., *Molecular signature of human embryonic stem cells and its comparison with the mouse.* Dev Biol, 2003. 260(2): p. 404-13.
[25] Zeng, X., et al., *Properties of pluripotent human embryonic stem cells BG01 and BG02.* Stem Cells, 2004. 22(3): p. 292-312.
[26] Ginis, I., et al., *Differences between human and mouse embryonic stem cells.* Dev Biol, 2004. 269(2): p. 360-80.
[27] Clark, A.T., et al., Human STELLAR, NANOG, and GDF3 genes are expressed in pluripotent cells and map to chromosome 12p13, a hotspot for teratocarcinoma. Stem Cells, 2004. 22(2): p. 169-79.
[28] Richards, M., et al., *The transcriptome profile of human embryonic stem cells as defined by SAGE.* Stem Cells, 2004. 22(1): p. 51-64.
[29] Clark, A.T., et al., Spontaneous differentiation of germ cells from human embryonic stem cells in vitro. Hum Mol Genet, 2004. 13(7): p. 727-39.
[30] Wei, C.L., et al., Transcriptome profiling of human and murine ESCs identifies divergent paths required to maintain the stem cell state. Stem Cells, 2005. 23(2): p. 166-85.
[31] Andrews, P.W., et al., Three monoclonal antibodies defining distinct differentiation antigens associated with different high molecular weight polypeptides on the surface of human embryonal carcinoma cells. Hybridoma, 1984. 3(4): p. 347-61.
[32] Kannagi, R., et al., Stage-specific embryonic antigens (SSEA-3 and -4) are epitopes of a unique globo-series ganglioside isolated from human teratocarcoma cells. Embo J, 1983. 2(12): p. 2355-61.
[33] Cooper, S., et al., A novel keratan sulphate proteoglycan from a human embryonal carcinoma cell line. Biochem J, 1992. 286 (Pt 3): p. 959-66.
[34] Pera, M.F., et al., Analysis of cell-differentiation lineage in human teratomas using new monoclonal antibodies to cytostructural antigens of embryonal carcinoma cells. Differentiation, 1988. 39(2): p. 139-49.
[35] Oka, M., et al., CD9 is associated with leukemia inhibitory factor-mediated maintenance of embryonic stem cells. Mol Biol Cell, 2002. 13(4): p. 1274-81.
[36] Pera, M.F., et al., *Isolation, characterization, and differentiation of human embryonic stem cells.* Methods Enzymol, 2003. 365: p. 429-46.
[37] Rosler, E.S., et al., *Long-term culture of human embryonic stem cells in feeder-free conditions.* Dev Dyn, 2004. 229(2): p. 259-74.
[38] Skottman, H., et al., Gene expression signatures of seven individual human embryonic stem cell lines. Stem Cells, 2005. 23(9): p. 1343-56.

[39] Whyte, M.P., et al., Alkaline phosphatase: placental and tissue-nonspecific isoenzymes hydrolyze phosphoethanolamine, inorganic pyrophosphate, and pyridoxal 5'-phosphate. Substrate accumulation in carriers of hypophosphatasia corrects during pregnancy. J Clin Invest, 1995. 95(4): p. 1440-5.

[40] Manes, T., et al., Genomic structure and comparison of mouse tissue-specific alkaline phosphatase genes. Genomics, 1990. 8(3): p. 541-54.

[41] Terao, M. and B. Mintz, *Cloning and characterization of a cDNA coding for mouse placental alkaline phosphatase.* Proc Natl Acad Sci U S A, 1987. 84(20): p. 7051-5.

[42] Andrews, P.W., et al., Two monoclonal antibodies recognizing determinants on human embryonal carcinoma cells react specifically with the liver isozyme of human alkaline phosphatase. Hybridoma, 1984. 3(1): p. 33-9.

[43] MacGregor, G.R., B.P. Zambrowicz, and P. Soriano, Tissue non-specific alkaline phosphatase is expressed in both embryonic and extraembryonic lineages during mouse embryogenesis but is not required for migration of primordial germ cells. Development, 1995. 121(5): p. 1487-96.

[44] Allsopp, R.C., et al., *Telomere length predicts replicative capacity of human fibroblasts.* Proc Natl Acad Sci U S A, 1992. 89(21): p. 10114-8.

[45] Blackburn, E.H., et al., *Recognition and elongation of telomeres by telomerase.* Genome, 1989. 31(2): p. 553-60.

[46] Harley, C.B., et al., *The telomere hypothesis of cellular aging.* Exp Gerontol, 1992. 27(4): p. 375-82.

[47] Hayflick, L. and P.S. Moorhead, *The serial cultivation of human diploid cell strains.* Exp Cell Res, 1961. 25: p. 585-621.

[48] Yui, J., C.P. Chiu, and P.M. Lansdorp, Telomerase activity in candidate stem cells from fetal liver and adult bone marrow. Blood, 1998. 91(9): p. 3255-62.

[49] Chiu, C.P., et al., Differential expression of telomerase activity in hematopoietic progenitors from adult human bone marrow. Stem Cells, 1996. 14(2): p. 239-48.

[50] Lebkowski, J.S., et al., Human embryonic stem cells: culture, differentiation, and genetic modification for regenerative medicine applications. Cancer J, 2001. 7 Suppl 2: p. S83-93.

[51] Wright, W.E., et al., Telomerase activity in human germline and embryonic tissues and cells. Dev Genet, 1996. 18(2): p. 173-9.

[52] Ezeh, U.I., et al., Human embryonic stem cell genes OCT4, NANOG, STELLAR, and GDF3 are expressed in both seminoma and breast carcinoma. Cancer, 2005. 104(10): p. 2255-65.

[53] Okamoto, K., et al., A novel octamer binding transcription factor is differentially expressed in mouse embryonic cells. Cell, 1990. 60(3): p. 461-72.

[54] Palmieri, S.L., et al., Oct-4 transcription factor is differentially expressed in the mouse embryo during establishment of the first two extraembryonic cell lineages involved in implantation. Dev Biol, 1994. 166(1): p. 259-67.

[55] Scholer, H.R., et al., Oct-4: a germline-specific transcription factor mapping to the mouse t-complex. Embo J, 1990. 9(7): p. 2185-95.

[56] Scholer, H.R., et al., *New type of POU domain in germ line-specific protein Oct-4.* Nature, 1990. 344(6265): p. 435-9.

[57] Abdel-Rahman, B., et al., *Expression of transcription regulating genes in human preimplantation embryos.* Hum Reprod, 1995. 10(10): p. 2787-92.

[58] Hansis, C., J.A. Grifo, and L.C. Krey, *Oct-4 expression in inner cell mass and trophectoderm of human blastocysts.* Mol Hum Reprod, 2000. 6(11): p. 999-1004.

[59] Mitalipov, S.M., et al., *Oct-4 expression in pluripotent cells of the rhesus monkey.* Biol Reprod, 2003. 69(6): p. 1785-92.

[60] Rosner, M.H., et al., A POU-domain transcription factor in early stem cells and germ cells of the mammalian embryo. Nature, 1990. 345(6277): p. 686-92.

[61] Verlinsky, Y., et al., *Isolation of cDNA libraries from individual human preimplantation embryos.* Mol Hum Reprod, 1998. 4(6): p. 571-5.

[62] Chambers, I., et al., Functional expression cloning of Nanog, a pluripotency sustaining factor in embryonic stem cells. Cell, 2003. 113(5): p. 643-55.

[63] Collignon, J., et al., A comparison of the properties of Sox-3 with Sry and two related genes, Sox-1 and Sox-2. Development, 1996. 122(2): p. 509-20.

[64] Niwa, H., Molecular mechanism to maintain stem cell renewal of ES cells. Cell Struct Funct, 2001. 26(3): p. 137-48.

[65] Avilion, A.A., et al., Multipotent cell lineages in early mouse development depend on SOX2 function. Genes Dev, 2003. 17(1): p. 126-40.

[66] Hyslop, L., et al., Downregulation of NANOG induces differentiation of human embryonic stem cells to extraembryonic lineages. Stem Cells, 2005. 23(8): p. 1035-43.

[67] Mitsui, K., et al., The homeoprotein Nanog is required for maintenance of pluripotency in mouse epiblast and ES cells. Cell, 2003. 113(5): p. 631-42.

[68] Nichols, J., et al., Formation of pluripotent stem cells in the mammalian embryo depends on the POU transcription factor Oct4. Cell, 1998. 95(3): p. 379-91.

[69] Schuldiner, M., et al., From the cover: effects of eight growth factors on the differentiation of cells derived from human embryonic stem cells. Proc Natl Acad Sci U S A, 2000. 97(21): p. 11307-12.

[70] Herszfeld, D., et al., CD30 is a survival factor and a biomarker for transformed human pluripotent stem cells. Nat Biotechnol, 2006. 24(3): p. 351-7.

[71] Mitalipova, M.M., et al., *Preserving the genetic integrity of human embryonic stem cells.* Nat Biotechnol, 2005. 23(1): p. 19-20.

[72] Baker, D.E., et al., *Adaptation to culture of human embryonic stem cells and oncogenesis in vivo.* Nat Biotechnol, 2007. 25(2): p. 207-15.

[73] Draper, J.S., et al., *Recurrent gain of chromosomes 17q and 12 in cultured human embryonic stem cells.* Nat Biotechnol, 2004. 22(1): p. 53-4.

[74] Richards, M., et al., Comparative evaluation of various human feeders for prolonged undifferentiated growth of human embryonic stem cells. Stem Cells, 2003. 21(5): p. 546-56.

[75] Price, P.J. and M.D. Goldsborough, Embryonic stem cell serum replacement., in International Patent Application. 1998.

[76] Amit, M., et al., Clonally derived human embryonic stem cell lines maintain pluripotency and proliferative potential for prolonged periods of culture. Dev Biol, 2000. 227(2): p. 271-8.

[77] Stojkovic, M., et al., Derivation of human embryonic stem cells from day-8 blastocysts recovered after three-step in vitro culture. Stem Cells, 2004. 22(5): p. 790-7.

[78] Strelchenko, N., et al., *Morula-derived human embryonic stem cells.* Reprod Biomed Online, 2004. 9(6): p. 623-9.

[79] Amit, M., et al., *Feeder layer- and serum-free culture of human embryonic stem cells.* Biol Reprod, 2004. 70(3): p. 837-45.

[80] Cowan, C.A., et al., *Derivation of embryonic stem-cell lines from human blastocysts.* N Engl J Med, 2004. 350(13): p. 1353-6.

[81] Heins, N., et al., *Derivation, characterization, and differentiation of human embryonic stem cells.* Stem Cells, 2004. 22(3): p. 367-76.

[82] Kim, S.J., et al., *Efficient derivation of new human embryonic stem cell lines.* Mol Cells, 2005. 19(1): p. 46-53.

[83] Buzzard, J.J., et al., *Karyotype of human ES cells during extended culture.* Nat Biotechnol, 2004. 22(4): p. 381-2; author reply 382.

[84] Atkin, N.B. and M.C. Baker, *Specific chromosome change, i(12p), in testicular tumours?* Lancet, 1982. 2(8311): p. 1349.

[85] Rodriguez, E., et al., *Molecular cytogenetic analysis of i(12p)-negative human male germ cell tumors.* Genes Chromosomes Cancer, 1993. 8(4): p. 230-6.

[86] Skotheim, R.I., et al., New insights into testicular germ cell tumorigenesis from gene expression profiling. Cancer Res, 2002. 62(8): p. 2359-64.

[87] Amit, M., et al., *Human feeder layers for human embryonic stem cells.* Biol Reprod, 2003. 68(6): p. 2150-6.

[88] Pebay, A., et al., Essential roles of sphingosine-1-phosphate and platelet-derived growth factor in the maintenance of human embryonic stem cells. Stem Cells, 2005. 23(10): p. 1541-8.

[89] Park, J.H., et al., Establishment and maintenance of human embryonic stem cells on STO, a permanently growing cell line. Biol Reprod, 2003. 69(6): p. 2007-14.

[90] Park, S.P., et al., Establishment of human embryonic stem cell lines from frozen-thawed blastocysts using STO cell feeder layers. Hum Reprod, 2004. 19(3): p. 676-84.

[91] Richards, M., et al., Human feeders support prolonged undifferentiated growth of human inner cell masses and embryonic stem cells. Nat Biotechnol, 2002. 20(9): p. 933-6.

[92] Cheng, L., et al., Human adult marrow cells support prolonged expansion of human embryonic stem cells in culture. Stem Cells, 2003. 21(2): p. 131-42.

[93] Hovatta, O., et al., A culture system using human foreskin fibroblasts as feeder cells allows production of human embryonic stem cells. Hum Reprod, 2003. 18(7): p. 1404-9.

[94] Inzunza, J., et al., Derivation of human embryonic stem cell lines in serum replacement medium using postnatal human fibroblasts as feeder cells. Stem Cells, 2005. 23(4): p. 544-9.

[95] Ellerstrom, C., et al., *Derivation of a xeno-free human embryonic stem cell line.* Stem Cells, 2006. 24(10): p. 2170-6.

[96] Genbacev, O., et al., Serum-free derivation of human embryonic stem cell lines on human placental fibroblast feeders. Fertil Steril, 2005. 83(5): p. 1517-29.

[97] Lee, J.B., et al., Establishment and maintenance of human embryonic stem cell lines on human feeder cells derived from uterine endometrium under serum-free condition. Biol Reprod, 2005. 72(1): p. 42-9.

[98] Wang, Q., et al., *Derivation and growing human embryonic stem cells on feeders derived from themselves.* Stem Cells, 2005. 23(9): p. 1221-7.

[99] Choo, A., et al., Immortalized feeders for the scale-up of human embryonic stem cells in feeder and feeder-free conditions. J Biotechnol, 2006. 122(1): p. 130-41.

[100] Stojkovic, P., et al., An autogeneic feeder cell system that efficiently supports growth of undifferentiated human embryonic stem cells. Stem Cells, 2005. 23(3): p. 306-14.

[101] Brimble, S.N., et al., Karyotypic stability, genotyping, differentiation, feeder-free maintenance, and gene expression sampling in three human embryonic stem cell lines derived prior to August 9, 2001. Stem Cells Dev, 2004. 13(6): p. 585-97.

[102] Wang, G., et al., Noggin and bFGF cooperate to maintain the pluripotency of human embryonic stem cells in the absence of feeder layers. Biochem Biophys Res Commun, 2005. 330(3): p. 934-42.

[103] Xu, C., et al., Immortalized fibroblast-like cells derived from human embryonic stem cells support undifferentiated cell growth. Stem Cells, 2004. 22(6): p. 972-80.

[104] Stojkovic, P., et al., Human-serum matrix supports undifferentiated growth of human embryonic stem cells. Stem Cells, 2005. 23(7): p. 895-902.

[105] Klimanskaya, I., et al., *Human embryonic stem cells derived without feeder cells.* Lancet, 2005. 365(9471): p. 1636-41.

[106] Beattie, G.M., et al., *Activin A maintains pluripotency of human embryonic stem cells in the absence of feeder layers.* Stem Cells, 2005. 23(4): p. 489-95.

[107] Sato, N., et al., Maintenance of pluripotency in human and mouse embryonic stem cells through activation of Wnt signaling by a pharmacological GSK-3-specific inhibitor. Nat Med, 2004. 10(1): p. 55-63.

[108] James, D., et al., TGF{beta}/activin/nodal signaling is necessary for the maintenance of pluripotency in human embryonic stem cells. Development, 2005. 132(6): p. 1273-82.

[109] Vallier, L., M. Alexander, and R.A. Pedersen, Activin/Nodal and FGF pathways cooperate to maintain pluripotency of human embryonic stem cells. J Cell Sci, 2005. 118(Pt 19): p. 4495-509.

[110] Li, Y., et al., Expansion of human embryonic stem cells in defined serum-free medium devoid of animal-derived products. Biotechnol Bioeng, 2005. 91(6): p. 688-98.

[111] Xu, C., et al., Basic fibroblast growth factor supports undifferentiated human embryonic stem cell growth without conditioned medium. Stem Cells, 2005. 23(3): p. 315-23.

[112] Levenstein, M.E., et al., Basic fibroblast growth factor support of human embryonic stem cell self-renewal. Stem Cells, 2006. 24(3): p. 568-74.

[113] Xu, R.H., et al., Basic FGF and suppression of BMP signaling sustain undifferentiated proliferation of human ES cells. Nat Methods, 2005. 2(3): p. 185-90.

[114] Ludwig, T.E., et al., *Derivation of human embryonic stem cells in defined conditions.* Nat Biotechnol, 2006. 24(2): p. 185-7.

[115] Johansson, B.M. and M.V. Wiles, Evidence for involvement of activin A and bone morphogenetic protein 4 in mammalian mesoderm and hematopoietic development. Mol Cell Biol, 1995. 15(1): p. 141-51.

[116] Lu, J., et al., *Defined culture conditions of human embryonic stem cells.* Proc Natl Acad Sci U S A, 2006. 103(15): p. 5688-93.

[117] Yao, S., et al., Long-term self-renewal and directed differentiation of human embryonic stem cells in chemically defined conditions. Proc Natl Acad Sci U S A, 2006. 103(18): p. 6907-12.

[118] Yoo, S.J., et al., Efficient culture system for human embryonic stem cells using autologous human embryonic stem cell-derived feeder cells. Exp Mol Med, 2005. 37(5): p. 399-407.

[119] Carpenter, M.K., et al., Properties of four human embryonic stem cell lines maintained in a feeder-free culture system. Dev Dyn, 2004. 229(2): p. 243-58.

[120] Maitra, A., et al., *Genomic alterations in cultured human embryonic stem cells.* Nat Genet, 2005. 37(10): p. 1099-103.

[121] Inzunza, J., et al., Comparative genomic hybridization and karyotyping of human embryonic stem cells reveals the occurrence of an isodicentric X chromosome after long-term cultivation. Mol Hum Reprod, 2004. 10(6): p. 461-6.

[122] Imreh, M.P., et al., In vitro culture conditions favoring selection of chromosomal abnormalities in human ES cells. J Cell Biochem, 2006.
[123] Mikkola, M., et al., Distinct differentiation characteristics of individual human embryonic stem cell lines. BMC Dev Biol, 2006. 6: p. 40.
[124] Ware, C.B., A.M. Nelson, and C.A. Blau, *A Comparison of NIH-Approved Human ESC Lines.* Stem Cells, 2006. 24(12): p. 2677-84.
[125] Martin, M.J., et al., *Human embryonic stem cells express an immunogenic nonhuman sialic acid.* Nat Med, 2005. 11(2): p. 228-32.
[126] Cerdan, C., et al., Complement targeting of nonhuman sialic acid does not mediate cell death of human embryonic stem cells. Nat Med, 2006. 12(10): p. 1113-4; author reply 1115.
[127] Turnpenny, L., et al., Evaluating human embryonic germ cells: concord and conflict as pluripotent stem cells. Stem Cells, 2006. 24(2): p. 212-20.
[128] Assady, S., et al., *Insulin production by human embryonic stem cells.* Diabetes, 2001. 50(8): p. 1691-7.
[129] Baharvand, H., et al., *Generation of insulin-secreting cells from human embryonic stem cells.* Dev Growth Differ, 2006. 48(5): p. 323-32.
[130] Xu, X., et al., *Endoderm and pancreatic islet lineage differentiation from human embryonic stem cells.* Cloning Stem Cells, 2006. 8(2): p. 96-107.
[131] Schulz, T.C., et al., Differentiation of human embryonic stem cells to dopaminergic neurons in serum-free suspension culture. Stem Cells, 2004. 22(7): p. 1218-38.
[132] Schulz, T.C., et al., *Directed neuronal differentiation of human embryonic stem cells.* BMC Neurosci, 2003. 4: p. 27.
[133] Yan, Y., et al., Directed differentiation of dopaminergic neuronal subtypes from human embryonic stem cells. Stem Cells, 2005. 23(6): p. 781-90.
[134] Mummery, C., et al., *Cardiomyocyte differentiation of mouse and human embryonic stem cells.* J Anat, 2002. 200(Pt 3): p. 233-42.
[135] Lavon, N., O. Yanuka, and N. Benvenisty, *Differentiation and isolation of hepatic-like cells from human embryonic stem cells.* Differentiation, 2004. 72(5): p. 230-8.
[136] Shirahashi, H., et al., *Differentiation of human and mouse embryonic stem cells along a hepatocyte lineage.* Cell Transplant, 2004. 13(3): p. 197-211.
[137] Ben-Hur, T., et al., Transplantation of human embryonic stem cell-derived neural progenitors improves behavioral deficit in Parkinsonian rats. Stem Cells, 2004. 22(7): p. 1246-55.
[138] Buhnemann, C., et al., Neuronal differentiation of transplanted embryonic stem cell-derived precursors in stroke lesions of adult rats. Brain, 2006. 129(Pt 12): p. 3238-48.
[139] Heo, J., et al., Hepatic precursors derived from murine embryonic stem cells contribute to regeneration of injured liver. Hepatology, 2006. 44(6): p. 1478-86.
[140] Blyszczuk, P., et al., Expression of Pax4 in embryonic stem cells promotes differentiation of nestin-positive progenitor and insulin-producing cells. Proc Natl Acad Sci U S A, 2003. 100(3): p. 998-1003.
[141] Hori, Y., et al., Growth inhibitors promote differentiation of insulin-producing tissue from embryonic stem cells. Proc Natl Acad Sci U S A, 2002. 99(25): p. 16105-10.
[142] Soria, B., A. Skoudy, and F. Martin, From stem cells to beta cells: new strategies in cell therapy of diabetes mellitus. Diabetologia, 2001. 44(4): p. 407-15.
[143] Yang, Y., et al., VEGF enhances functional improvement of postinfarcted hearts by transplantation of ESC-differentiated cells. J Appl Physiol, 2002. 93(3): p. 1140-51.

[144] Lee, J.P., et al., Stem cells act through multiple mechanisms to benefit mice with neurodegenerative metabolic disease. Nat Med, 2007. 13(4): p. 439-47.
[145] Davidson, K.C., et al., Wnt3a regulates survival, expansion, and maintenance of neural progenitors derived from human embryonic stem cells. Mol Cell Neurosci, 2007.
[146] Suzuki, M., et al., GDNF secreting human neural progenitor cells protect dying motor neurons, but not their projection to muscle, in a rat model of familial ALS. PLoS ONE, 2007. 2(1): p. e689.
[147] Li, W., et al., Bcl-2 engineered MSCs inhibited apoptosis and improved heart function. Stem Cells, 2007. 25(8): p. 2118-27.
[148] Lee, H.J., et al., Human neural stem cells over-expressing VEGF provide neuroprotection, angiogenesis and functional recovery in mouse stroke model. PLoS ONE, 2007. 2(1): p. e156.
[149] Babaie, Y., et al., Analysis of OCT4 dependent transcriptional networks regulating self renewal and pluripotency in human embryonic stem cells. Stem Cells, 2006.
[150] Costa, M., et al., *A method for genetic modification of human embryonic stem cells using electroporation.* Nat Protoc, 2007. 2(4): p. 792-6.
[151] Munsie, M.J., et al., Isolation of pluripotent embryonic stem cells from reprogrammed adult mouse somatic cell nuclei. Curr Biol, 2000. 10(16): p. 989-92.
[152] Wakayama, T., et al., Differentiation of embryonic stem cell lines generated from adult somatic cells by nuclear transfer. Science, 2001. 292(5517): p. 740-3.
[153] Rideout, W.M., 3rd, et al., Correction of a genetic defect by nuclear transplantation and combined cell and gene therapy. Cell, 2002. 109(1): p. 17-27.
[154] Barberi, T., et al., Neural subtype specification of fertilization and nuclear transfer embryonic stem cells and application in parkinsonian mice. Nat Biotechnol, 2003. 21(10): p. 1200-7.
[155] French, A.J., et al., Development of Human cloned Blastocysts Following Somatic Cell Nuclear Transfer (SCNT) with Adult Fibroblasts. Stem Cells, 2008.
[156] Itskovitz-Eldor, J., et al., Differentiation of human embryonic stem cells into embryoid bodies compromising the three embryonic germ layers. Mol Med, 2000. 6(2): p. 88-95.
[157] Hirst, C.E., et al., Transcriptional profiling of mouse and human ES cells identifies SLAIN1, a novel stem cell gene. Dev Biol, 2006. 293(1): p. 90-103.
[158] Bhattacharya, B., et al., Comparison of the gene expression profile of undifferentiated human embryonic stem cell lines and differentiating embryoid bodies. BMC Dev Biol, 2005. 5: p. 22.
[159] Odorico, J.S., D.S. Kaufman, and J.A. Thomson, *Multilineage differentiation from human embryonic stem cell lines.* Stem Cells, 2001. 19(3): p. 193-204.
[160] Reya, T., et al., *Stem cells, cancer, and cancer stem cells.* Nature, 2001. 414(6859): p. 105-11.
[161] Gudjonsson, T. and M.K. Magnusson, *Stem cell biology and the cellular pathways of carcinogenesis.* Apmis, 2005. 113(11-12): p. 922-9.
[162] Mateizel, I., et al., Derivation of human embryonic stem cell lines from embryos obtained after IVF and after PGD for monogenic disorders. Hum Reprod, 2006. 21(2): p. 503-11.
[163] Pickering, S.J., et al., Generation of a human embryonic stem cell line encoding the cystic fibrosis mutation deltaF508, using preimplantation genetic diagnosis. Reprod Biomed Online, 2005. 10(3): p. 390-7.
[164] Verlinsky, Y., et al., *Human embryonic stem cell lines with genetic disorders.* Reprod Biomed Online, 2005. 10(1): p. 105-10.

[165] Rao, R.R., et al., *Comparative transcriptional profiling of two human embryonic stem cell lines.* Biotechnol Bioeng, 2004. 88(3): p. 273-86.

[166] Sperger, J.M., et al., Gene expression patterns in human embryonic stem cells and human pluripotent germ cell tumors. Proc Natl Acad Sci U S A, 2003. 100(23): p. 13350-5.

[167] Andrews, P.W., et al., The International Stem Cell Initiative: toward benchmarks for human embryonic stem cell research. Nat Biotechnol, 2005. 23(7): p. 795-7.

[168] Adewumi, O., et al., Characterization of human embryonic stem cell lines by the International Stem Cell Initiative. Nat Biotechnol, 2007. 25(7): p. 803-16.

[169] Wong, R.C. and A. Pebay, *Signaling pathways invovled in the maintenance of human embryonic stem cells.* Journal of Stem Cells, 2006. 1(4): p. 271-282.

Chapter XXI

ESTABLISHMENT OF INDIVIDUAL-SPECIFIC ES CELLS FROM ADULT SOMATIC CELLS BY NUCLEAR TRANSFER

Sayaka Wakayama and Teruhiko Wakayama[*]
RIKEN Center for Developmental Biology
Minatojima-minamimachi, Kobe, Japan

ABSTRACT

Cloning methods are now well described and becoming routine. Yet the frequency at which cloned offspring are produced still remains below 10%, irrespective of the nucleus donor species or cell type. Especially in the mouse, only a few laboratories have obtained clones from adult somatic cells, and most mouse strains never succeed in producing cloned mice. On the other hand, nuclear transfer can be used to generate embryonic stem (ntES) cell lines from a subject's own somatic cells. We have shown that ntES cells can be generated relatively easily from a variety of mouse genotypes and cell types of both sexes, even though it may be more difficult to generate clones directly. Several reports have already demonstrated that ntES cells can be used in regenerative medicine in order to rescue immunodeficient or infertile phenotypes. This technique can also be applied for preservation of genetic resource of mouse strains instead of embryos, oocytes or spermatozoa. However, if ntES cells have abnormalities, such as those associated with the offspring produced by reproductive cloning, then their scientific and medical utilities could prove to be limited. Fortunately, turned out to be a groundless fear, for these ntES cells were able to differentiate into all functional embryonic tissues *in vivo*. Moreover, they were identical to fertilized-derived ES cells in terms of their expression of pluripotency markers, pattern of tissue-dependent differentially DNA methylated regions and global gene expression. These similarities of ntES cells and ES cells indicate that murine therapeutic cloning by somatic cell nuclear transfer can provide a reliable model for preclinical stem cell research. Nuclear transfer requires a large number of fresh

---

[*] Tel: 81-78-306-3049; Fax:81-78-306-3095; E-mail: teru@cdb.riken.jp

oocytes, which gives rise to fundamental ethical concerns surrounding its potential applications in human cells, as fresh oocytes must be obtained from a healthy female donor. This review seeks to describe the phenotype, application, possible abnormalities and resolution of ethical problem of cloned mice and ntES cell lines.

1. INTRODUCTION

Since it was first reported in 1997 [1], somatic cell cloning has been demonstrated in several mammalian species. While cloning efficiencies can range from 0 to 20%, rates of just 1–2% are typical in mice (i.e. one or two live offspring are produced per one hundred initial embryos). Moreover, many abnormalities in mice cloned from somatic cells have been reported, such as abnormal gene expression in embryos [2-4], abnormal placenta [5], obesity [6, 7] and early death [8]. Such abnormalities notwithstanding, success in generating cloned offspring has opened new avenues of investigation. It also provides a valuable tool that basic research scientists have employed to study complex processes, such as genomic reprogramming, imprinting and embryonic development. A number of potential agricultural and clinical applications are also being explored, including therapeutic cloning for human cells, tissues and organ replacement, as well as the reproductive cloning of farm animals.

There is also a great deal of interest in the possible application of human embryonic stem (ES) cells in regenerative medicine, as ES cells are envisioned to be a potential source for cell replacement therapies. However, as with any allogeneic material, ES cells derived from fertilized blastocysts and the progeny of such cells inevitably face the risk of immunorejection on transplantation. It has been proposed that ES cells derived from embryos cloned from the host patient's own cell nuclei represent a potential solution to the problem of rejection, as any replacement cells would be genetically identical to the host's own somatic cell nuclei [9-11]. We have previously shown that those nuclear transfer derived ES-like cell lines are capable of differentiating into all three germ layers *in vitro* or into spermatozoa and oocytes in chimeric mice [12]. This was the first demonstration that those ES-like cells have the same potential as ES cells from fertilized blastocysts. To distinguish nuclear transfer-derived ES cell lines from those derived from fertilized embryos, the former are referred to as nuclear transfer ES cell (ntES cell) lines [12]. These techniques have now been applied not only to preliminary medical research [13], but also to basic biological research, such as the preservation of genetic resources of infertile mouse strains instead of preserving such resources in the embryo, oocyte or spermatozoa [14].

However, ntES cell have given rise to ethical objections in humans, such as concerns that fresh oocytes must be donated by healthy women, and that the cloned embryos are deprived of their potential to develop into a complete human being. To avoid such objections, several approaches have been tried and some parts of the problem successfully solved. This review describes features of cloning and ntES cell technology for both basic and applied investigation.

2. SOMATIC CELL NUCLEAR CLONING

2.1. History of Somatic Cell Cloning

The first report of cloned mammals was in mice [15]. This report described the production of three mice (one male and two females) by coordinated microinjection of inner cell mass (ICM) cell nuclei into zygotes and immediate removal of the pre-existing pronuclei. However, this report was controversial. All subsequent investigators failed to reproduce the experiment [16]. Until the end of the 1980s, only the nuclei of 1- or 2-cell embryos had been shown to be capable of programming full mouse development following the transfer into an enucleated zygote or 2-cell embryo blastomere [17, 18].

The first demonstrably reproducible cloning of a mammal (sheep) was achieved by transferring the 8-cell stage embryonic nuclei into the recipient unfertilized eggs (oocytes), instead of transferring 1- or 2-cell embryos [19]. It is probable that in mammalian cloning the oocyte represents a more viable recipient than the zygote [20]. Thereafter, the techniques of mammalian cloning were developed and more mature cells began to be used as donors. Ten years later, Campbell *et al.* reported cloned sheep derived from an established embryonic cell line [21]. Using these techniques, the same group later reported the first somatic-cell cloned animal [1].

Cumulina, the first cloned mouse derived from adult somatic-cell nuclei, was achieved using a piezo-actuated injection system in 1997 [22]. Works on Cumulina and contemporaneously cloned mice demonstrated, for the first time, that mammalian clones were fertile and could produce normal offspring [22].

At the outset this technique proved difficult to reproduce in other laboratories. Now, however, several laboratories continuously reproduce cloned mice and currently, cumulus cells [22], tail tip cells (probably fibroblasts) [5, 23], Sertoli cells [24], fetal cells [25, 26], and ES cells [27] are routinely used to produce cloned mice. NKT cells [28], post-mitotic cells such as granulocytes [29], primordial germ cells [30], hematopoietic stem cells [31], mesenchymal stem cells [32], and fetal neuronal cells [33] as well as new born neuronal stem cell [32, 34] have also been used. Interestingly, the genetic background of the mouse strain is very important [26, 35]. Thus far, only hybrid mice and 129 strain have been used successfully as sources of donor nuclei (either somatic or ES cell) or recipient oocytes.

Since the first success of mammalian cloning [1], the success rate did not improve, even thought a great number of researchers took up the challenge. Meanwhile, recent molecular analyses of cloned embryos have revealed abnormal epigenetic modification, such as DNA methylation and histone modification [36-38]. Therefore, the prevention of such epigenetic errors has been expected to lead to an improvement in the success rate of animal cloning. There are a number of reports concerning 5-azacytidine, an inhibitor of DNA methylation, and Trichostatin A (TSA), an inhibitor of histone deacetylase, treatments [39]. Although the *in vitro* developmental potential was increased significantly by these drugs, they did not achieve full term development. Moreover, because those drugs are very toxic, each drug must be examined for the appropriate exposure timing, concentration and duration. Recently, we identified the optimal conditions for TSA in a study in which a 5-50 nM TSA-treatment for 10 h following oocyte activation led to more than a 5-fold increase in the success rate of mouse cloning from cumulus cells without obvious abnormalities [40] (Figure 1). We have found that TSA can also be used to produce cloned mice even from outbred strain [41]. Thus, our findings provide a new approach for a practical improvement of mouse cloning techniques and insight into the reprogramming of somatic nuclei.

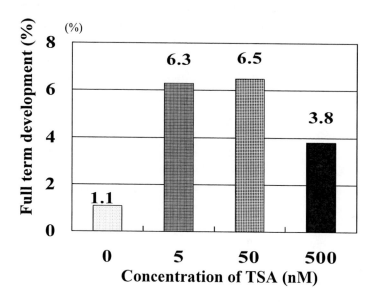

Figure 1. Effect of trichostatin A (TSA) treatment on cloned embryo development to full term. The success rates of obtaining full term cloned mice were significantly improved when cloned embryos were cultured with 5-50 nM TSA for 10 h.

2.2. The Abnormality of Cloned Mice

One striking and possibly diagnostic effect of mouse cloning is that it generates offspring with placentas that are enlarged 2- to 3-fold relative to those of their non-cloned counterparts [5, 42] (Figure 2). The effect is, to our knowledge, universal and occurs irrespective of the nucleus donor source and method of nuclear transfer. This placental enlargement is predominantly due to the exaggerated development of the basal layer: spongiotrophoblasts, giant trophoblasts and especially glycogen cells [42]. Moreover, placental zonation seems to be disrupted by the apparent invasion of spongiotrophoblasts and glycogen cells into the labyrinthine layer. These abnormalities presumably reflect a dysregulation of gene function in cells of the trophectodermal lineage, which may be accounted for by aberrant reprogramming – the failure to completely reset the differentiated state of the host cell [42, 43].

Abnormalities in cloned offspring have also been reported: when an inbred mouse strain was used for the donor, most of the cloned mice died soon after birth by respiratory catastrophe [5, 27], while those from a hybrid mouse strain did not [8]. However, with significant variance across strains, the postpubertal body mass of clones becomes significantly greater than that of the non-cloned controls from approximately 8–10 weeks of age [7], and these clones have elevated plasma leptin and insulin [6]. The increase in body mass is not a consequence of low activity or increased dietary intake, as behavioral assays do not show any significant difference between the cloned and the control animals. Hence, the difference in body mass may be due to lower basal energy expenditure in the clones [6].

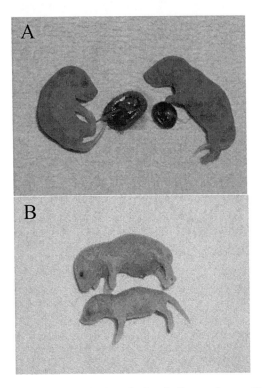

Figure 2. Abnormality of cloned mice. A. all cloned mice (left) were born with an extremely large size placenta compare to control (right). B. Eyes were open in some of the cloned mice at birth.

Although the imprinted gene expression patterns appeared normal in the apparently "normal" cloned mice [44], they still exhibited epigenetic defects [38, 45, 46 43], often including premature death [8]. DNA microarray analysis revealed that 4%–12% of the expressed genes in the cloned placentas differed in expression level from the controls [43, 47]. Another evidence of a cloning difference is X chromosome inactivation (XCI), which may also be perturbed during nuclear reprogramming. In cloned animals that are generated from female donor nuclei, XCI appears to be normal, i.e. random. This means that the inactive X chromosome from the donor nucleus must have been reactivated, after which the embryo must have re-established random activation of maternal and paternal chromosomes. Placental XCI is usually skewed in clones with the inactive X chromosome [48], but we found that even the bodies of cloned mice exhibited skewed X-inactivation [46]. However, those abnormalities seem to indicate epigenetic reprogramming errors, not DNA damage, because they were not transmitted to the next generation [6, 49, 50].

The fact that cloned embryos exhibit such abnormal methylation and yet are able to develop into pups indicates that the success of mammalian cloning is not critically sensitive to a perfect maintenance of the methylation state. Interestingly, those epigenetic abnormalities were corrected with increased age and became close to those of normal mice [51]. In conclusion, for cloned mice abnormalies, the cloned mouse is not a perfect copy of the original mouse in terms of placental development, body weight or the methylation status of genomic DNA [38].

3. ntES Cells

The first successes in generating these ES-like cell lines from somatic cells via nuclear transfer reported have been performed in the cow [52], and then the mouse [53, 54]. These ES-like cell lines are believed to possess the same capacities for unlimited differentiation and self-renewal as conventional ES cell lines derived from normal embryos produced by fertilization. We have previously shown that those nuclear transfer derived ES-like cell lines are capable of differentiating into all three germ layers *in vitro* or into spermatozoa and oocytes in chimeric mice [12]. This was the first demonstration that those ES-like cells have the same potential as ES cells from fertilized blastocysts. To distinguish nuclear transfer-derived ES cell lines from those derived from fertilized embryos, the former are referred to as nuclear transfer ES cell (ntES cell) lines [12]. Interestingly, ntES cell lines can be established with success rates 10 times higher than reproductive cloning [12, 55-57]. Therapeutic cloning is thus at least an order of magnitude more successful than reproductive cloning [11].

3.1. Establishment of ntES Cell Lines from Individuals

It has been proposed that ntES cells derived from the host patient's own cells represent a potential solution to the problem of immunorejection, as any replacement cells would be genetically identical to the host's own [9-11, 13, 58]. Therefore , it is important to know the possible effects of the genotype of the particular animal strain or sex of the donor nucleus. Such factors often affect the successful full-term development of cloned animals [26, 35]. For example, the success rate of cloned mice depends on the mouse genotype: hybrid genotypes are more tolerant of cloning than inbred genotypes, such as C57BL/6 and C3H/He, which are in common use in mouse genetic studies, but which have never been cloned successfully [26, 35]. In contrast to cloning mice, ntES cell lines can be established irrespective of mouse genotypes, cell type or sex as sources of donor nuclei with a higher success rate (Figures 3 and 4). When inbred and F1 genotypes were compared, the rate of development to the blastocyst stage and the frequency of ntES cell derivation were significantly better when F1 cumulus cells were used as the donor nucleus. However, this difference was only seen when the data were compared from reconstructed oocytes, which probably suggests that the overall success rate appears to depend primarily on preimplantation development; once embryos have reached the blastocyst stage, the genotype differences are no longer significant [57]. Surprisingly, it has been shown that even differentiated neuron and lymphocyte cells can be used to establish an ntES cell line (0.1–2%), although in previous studies these cells failed to produce any cloned offspring [12, 59-61].

Recently, we have found that TSA can improve the success rate of reproductive cloning (see previous section). When TSA was used for ntES cell experiments, it also significantly improved the ntES cells establishment [40], but we must further examine the effect of TSA before use in human being due to the potential toxicity of this drug.

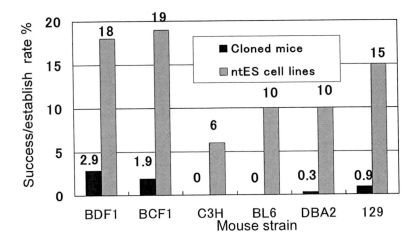

Figure 3. Comparison of the success rate of cloned mice and establishment rate of ntES cell lines. The rate of ntES cell establishment is nearly 10 times higher than the rate of producing cloned mice. Interestingly, ntES cell lines can be established even from unclonable mouse strains, such as C3H or C57BL/6 (BL6).

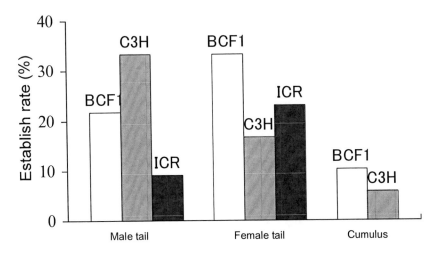

Figure 4. Comparison of the ntES cell establishment rate between males and females, and between tail and cumulus cells. The establishment rate between males and females exhibited no difference, but when it was compared between the tail cells and cumulus cells, usually tail cells displayed the better rate.

3.2. Normality of ntES Cells

It remains unclear whether these somatically derived ntES cells are identical to the ES cells derived from early, normally fertilized embryos. Most ntES cell lines differentiate into germ cells in chimeric mice [12, 55, 57], the strongest evidence to date that these cells have the same potential as ES cells. By contrast, most, if not all, cloned animals show serious fetal and postnatal abnormalities, perhaps resulting from defects or incomplete genomic reprogramming [2-4], as mentioned above. As ntES cell lines are established using the same procedures, it is possible that they will also exhibit epigenetic defects. Thus, either most ntES cell lines have been established from cloned embryos with negligible reproductive potential, or most cloned embryos die during or after implantation because of abnormal placental development, which does not involve ES cells. If these somatic ntES cell lines have inherent abnormalities, such as epigenetic defects, there may be potential risks in their clinical use and the scientific discoveries based on these ntES cells might be of limited utility. For example, we have found that the potential of ntES cell nuclei for creating full-term cloned offspring by second nuclear transfer differed among the ntES cell lines, even when the cell lines were derived from the same individual at the same time [56] (Figure 5). Thus, ntES cell lines show different potential not only according to their genetic background, but also epigenetic differences between each line, even among those from the same individual.

To evaluate the characteristics of ntES cells, we established more than 150 ntES cell lines from adult somatic cells of several mouse strains [57] and examined the pluripotency and karyotype, physical damage of DNA by nuclear transfer, similarity of ntES cells by tissue-dependent and differentially methylated region assay, similarity of ntES cells by grovel gene expression analysis, and differentiation potential into functional embryonic tissues by tetraploid chimera formation assay(Table 1) [55]. As a result, we have demonstrated that these ntES cells were identical to fertilized ES cells in their expression of pluripotency markers and tissue-dependent differentially DNA methylated regions of all 26 examined loci. In the karyotype experiments, we found that a few cell lines had a low percentage of the normal karyotype, but most of the examined ntES cell lines were within the normal range. It is impossible to judge whether these ntES cell lines were heterogeneous from the beginning or whether the abnormalities arose because of the culture conditions.

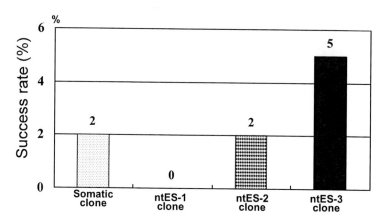

Figure 5. Comparison of the cloned mice success rate between somatic cell and 3 ntES cell lines derived from the same individual. In this experiment, all donor cells (somatic and 3 ntES cell lines) were derived from the same individual. However, the success rate of the cloned mice was significantly different between cell lines. This suggests that each ntES cell line has different potential or differently reprogrammable nuclei for the production of cloned mice after nuclear transfer.

Establishment of Individual-Specific ES Cells...

Table 1. Comparison of cell marker, gene expression, genetic and epigenetic normality and differentiation potential between ES and ntES cell

Cell type	Nuclear normality		Gene expression normality (compare between ES and ntES)			Epigenetic normality	Differentiation potential	
	Chromosome damage	DNA damage	ES cell marker	Microarray	HiCEP	DNA methylation	In vitro	4n chimera
ES	None	None	All positive	No difference	No difference	Normal	Good	Live offspring
ntES	None	None	All positive			Normal	Good	Live offspring

Thus, karyotype analysis is a prerequisite for ensuring the normalcy of ntES cell lines, as with fertilized ES cells. However, similar abnormalities are often found in mouse or human ES cells [62, 63], so these abnormalities do not seem to be specific for ntES cell lines. In addition, the sequential ntES cell establishment data indicates that the process of nuclear transfer or the physical treatment in itself did not cause the abnormalities in the ntES cell lines, even when nuclear transfer was repeated 10 times. Moreover, interestingly, the establishment rate of the re-ntES cell increased with the increase in the number of the repeated times (Figure 6).

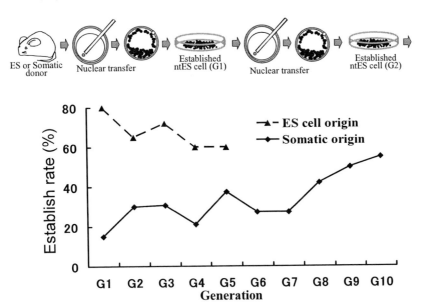

Figure 6. Establishment of re-ntES cell lines from ntES cell nuclei. To test the physical damage by nuclear transfer, it was repeated up to ten times. However, even when the nuclear transfer was repeated 10 times, the karyotype and pulipotency of those re-ntES cell lines did not show any abnormalities. As a control, fertilized derived ES cell were used and nuclear transfer repeated 5 times.

This data may suggest that early generation ntES cell lines still have some epigenetic abnormalities, and these difference were corrected by serial nuclear transfer and/or re-reprogramming. The DNA microarray profiles and high-coverage gene expression profiling

(HiCEP) [64] experiments demonstrate that all ES cells (ntES cell or control fertilized ES cell) derived in the same laboratory are similar to each other, but are different from the other commercially available ES cell lines, such as E14 and ESVJ. Only insignificant differences in gene expression between the ntES cell and other ES cell lines were found here, with the minor differences probably resulting from subtle variations in sample-to-sample preparations. Smith *et al.* and Brambrink *et al.* also demonstrated that bovine and mouse cloned embryonic cells closely resemble naturally fertilized embryos, respectively, using global gene expression profiles [65, 66]. Even if ntES cells may inherit some undetectable epigenetic abnormalities, the similarities of ntES cells and ES cells in terms of molecular and other characteristics indicate that murine therapeutic cloning can provide a reliable model for preclinical stem cell research.

Finally, we examined the differentiation potential of ntES cells by tetraploid complementation analysis. If ntES cells are able to differentiate normally to all embryonic cell types, the resulting 4n chimeric mice should have healthy phenotypes: which would be the strongest evidence for the normality of ntES cells. We found the rates of generating healthy offspring derived from ntES cell or ES cell lines to be similar [55], and all of these mice display germline transmission at adulthood (Table 1). Thus, our experiment clearly demonstrates that, like fertilized ES cells, ntES cells can differentiate into all normal embryonic tissues *in vivo*.

3.3. Why Are ntES Cells Normal?

To establish an ntES cell line, a cloned blastocyst must be cultured for more than one month *in vitro*. During this period, survival of the cloned embryo and early stage derivative is independent of most developmentally related gene expression and placental development; it might be able to proceed reprogramming gradually to obtain the normal pattern of gene expression. Another possibility is that some of the cloned embryos possess only a few normally reprogrammed cells [2, 4] and these few cells are insufficient to sustain a viable term fetus. However, viable ntES cells can be established even from these few normal cells during a period of one month of culture. Alternatively, in reproductive cloning, the cloned embryos must express all the appropriate genes and exhibit relatively normal placental development immediately after implantation. This more stringent set of criteria may account for the higher developmental failure rates of presumably incompletely reprogrammed cloned embryos following implantation. At the very least the data suggest that this therapeutic cloning approach appears to be a powerful and reliable method for establishing ES cells, which cells importantly display nearly identical biological characteristics to normally fertilized ES cells.

3.4. Applications of ntES Cell Techniques

Embryonic stem cells derived by nuclear transfer are genetically identical to the donor and are potentially useful for therapeutic application. Therefore, therapeutic cloning may improve the treatment of neurodegenerative diseases, blood disorders or diabetes, since therapy for these diseases is currently limited by the availability and immunocompatibility of tissue transplants [9-11, 13]. We have demonstrated that dopaminergic and serotonergic neurons can be generated from ntES cells derived from tail tip cells [12]. Rideout *et al.* reported that therapeutic cloning combined with gene therapy was able to treat a form of combined immune deficiency in mice [13]. They made one ntES cell line from an immune deficient mutant mouse. First, the ntES cell with mutated alleles was repaired by homologous recombination, thereby restoring normal gene structure. They then transplanted those ntES cells to the immunodeficient mouse. In addition, Barberi *et al.* reported an interesting study that showed that mouse-tail or cumulus-cell derived ntES cells could be differentiated into neural cells at even higher efficiencies than fertilization derived ES cells [58].

Additionally, ntES techniques can be applied to biological science as a new tool of investigation. We have demonstrated that cloned mice can be generated from the nucleus of ntES cells by a second nuclear transfer [12, 14, 56]. Unfortunately, the success rate was no improvement over that for somatic cell cloning. To overcome this low efficiency in the production of cloned animals, complementation with tetraploid embryos was employed, in which ntES cells were injected into the tetraploid blastocyst. As a result, almost all parts of the chimeric offspring, including germ cells, originated from the ntES cells. The offspring were referred to as the ES mouse [67, 68] or the clonal mouse [69]. Using this technique, monoclonal mice have been generated from ntES cells derived from B and T lymphocyte nuclei [60]. The ntES cell techniques can also be used for the characterization of very rare cells in the body. If ntES cells from these rare cell nuclei are established once, the cells can proliferate infinitely. It is hypothesized that an odorant receptor gene chosen from thousands is controlled by DNA rearrangements in olfactory sensory neurons, such as lymphocyte nuclei. However, this could not demonstrated due to the very low number of specific differentiated cells. Li *et al.* and Eggan *et al.* generated ntES cells from the nucleus of a single olfactory sensory neuron and demonstrated that odorant receptor gene choice is reset by nuclear transfer and is not accompanied by genomic alterations [59, 61]. On the other hand, ntES cell techniques can be used to assess tumorigenic and developmental potential. The ntES cell lines have also been established from embryonal carcinoma (EC) cells or melanoma cell nuclei, but chimeric mice from ntES cells developed cancer with higher frequency. It has been demonstrated that non-reprogrammable genetic modifications define the tumorigenic potential [70, 71].

The genetically modified mouse is a powerful tool for research in the fields of medicine and biology. However, infertility was listed as a phenotypic trait in more than half of the mutants described in one large-scale ethyl-nitrosourea (ENU) mutagenesis study [72]. This is a challenge worth the undertaking, as the ability to maintain such types of mutant mice as genetic resources would afford numerous crucial advantages to research in human infertility and the biology of reproduction. Unfortunately, the success rate of somatic cell cloning is very low. Even in cases in which the cloning of a sterile mouse is successful, due to the non-reproductive nature of the phenotype, it will still be necessary to clone all subsequent generations. This represents another significant potential barrier, as the success rate of cloning from cloned mice decreases for each successive generation after the first nuclear transfer [73]. Although the ntES cell establishment rate is nearly 10 times higher than the success rate of cloned mice, unfortunately, the conversion from somatic cells to ntES cells does not increase the overall success rate of cloning [12, 57]. However, we were ultimately able to obtain cloned mice from six out of seven individuals by using either somatic cells or ntES cells (Figure 7). Therefore, although the use of ntES cells as donor nuclei does not assure a superior success rate for mouse cloning over that for somatic cells, we recommend the establishment of ntES cell lines at the same time to preserve and clone a valuable individual. These can be used as an unlimited source of donor nuclei for nuclear transfer and therefore complement conventional somatic cell nuclear transfer cloning approaches [56].

Another example is that we have found a mutant, hermaphrodite, sterile mouse in our ICR mouse breeding colony. ICR is one of the most difficult strains to use in cloning [41, 74]. As a result, cloned mice have not been established. Fortunately, ntES cell lines from a tail tip fibroblast of the infertile mouse have been successfully established. However, the mutant mouse died accidentally before the ntES cell lines were analyzed and the Y chromosome abnormality was revealed. Since then we have tried to make cloned mice from ntES cell nuclei, but again, we could not obtain full-term offspring. As the offspring from the ntES cell lines were not obtained by conventional nuclear transfer, we have tried to make chimeric mice by either using diploid embryos or tetraploid embryos. Using the tetraploid complementation method, we obtained two ES mice which consisted mostly of diploid ntES cells with abnormal Y chromosomes. Furthermore, they were phenotypically male and were proven infertile, but they were not hermaphrodites. They also lacked spermatogenetic cells, although the seminiferous tubules contained Sertoli cells.

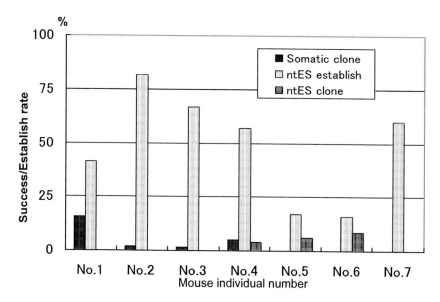

Figure 7. Production of cloned mice from 7 individual mice by somatic or ntES cell nuclear transfer. In the first nuclear transfer, cloned mice were obtained from 4 out of 7 donor mice (No. 1 to 4), and ntES cell lines were established from all of the mice at the same time. By second nuclear transfer using ntES cells as the donor nuclei, cloned mice were obtained from 2 out of 3 remaining donor mice (No. 5 and 6). Only one donor mouse (No. 7) failed to produce a cloned mouse either by somatic or ntES cell cloning.

In the diploid chimera, the animal with the highest contribution of ntES cells in terms of the coat color was infertile. Interestingly, one diploid chimeric male transmitted most of its genes to the next generation via the ntES cells. Thus, ntES cells can maintain the mutant gene, but neither cloning nor tetraploid complementation chimera construction could rescue the lineage of the original infertile hermaphrodite male [14].

4. AVOIDING ETHICAL PROBLEMS WITH NTES CELL

Among the fundamental ethical objections to human ntES cell research are the following. (1) fresh oocytes must be harvested from healthy women, and (2) the embryos are denied their potential to develop offspring. Several different approaches have been proposed to overcome these ethical objections, which can be categorized into three different type of methods. 1. Use lethally vulnerable embryos or use embryos without destroying them. For example, parthenogenetically activated embryos can be used to establish ES cell lines without the destruction of "normal" embryos, because they lack a paternal genome and invariably die [75, 76]. However, this method can only be used for healthy women and the differentiation potential of such ES cells is poor. To generate patient-specific ES cells, genetically altered donor nuclei have been used for nuclear transfer in a mouse model [77], in which the cloned embryos lack a gene essential for trophoblast development. This can prevent implantation without interfering with ES cell potency. Recently, Egli et al., successfully established ntES cell lines using enucleated polyspermic mouse zygotes, which also can not develop due to the triploid phenotype [78]. Alternatively, ES cell lines could be established non-destructively by removing single blastomeres from fertilized embryos, but this can only be applied to subsequent generations, not to treatment of the patient [79, 80].

Category 2; reprogram somatic cell without use oocytes. One of these approaches is the cell fusion between pluripotent stem cells (e.g. ES cells) and somatic cell [81, 82]. Although such fused cell become tetraploid, somatic cell nuclei are significantly reprogrammed and exhibit pluripotency. The other approach uses ES-like pluripotent stem cell lines, which have been established directly from somatic cells by retroviral infection rather than by NT [83, 84]. In these two situations, there is no need for embryo production or destruction, although it does require genetic modification of the cell lines. However, Verlinsky and colleagues have developed a new method they call "stembrid technology" [85-87]. This is based on the hybridization of adult somatic cells with enucleated cell of hES cells, which leads to a pluripotent state without contamination with hES cell nucleus. Using this technique, they have established a hES cell line repository that includes over 100 normal genotype cell lines [86].

Category 3; create oocytes from ES cells or use the oocytes of other species, which has shown great promise toward addressing the chronic scarcity of human oocytes for use in nuclear transfer studies. These studies can be accomplished either through the artificial creation of oocytes by *in vitro* differentiation [88] or through non-human oocytes, such as those of the cow or rabbit [89, 90], which have the potential to be reprogrammed using human somatic cell nuclei to establish human ntES cell lines. However fundamental questions remain as to whether artificial oocytes have the same developmental potential as natural oocytes, and whether ntES cells and their rabbit mitochondria-containing derivatives would be tolerated by a human host's immune system on transplantation.

Thus, so far several approaches have been reported, all of which have merits and demerits for establishing cell lines. We have also tried the following 3 approaches to avoid or at least minimize the ethical problems associated with ES cell establishment.

4.1. Improvement of Parthenogenetic ES Cells by Nuclear Transfer

Parthenogenesis is the process by which an oocyte develops into an embryo without being fertilized by a spermatozoon. Although such embryos lack the potential to develop to full term, they can be used to establish parthenogenetic embryonic stem (pES) cells for autologous cell therapy in females without needing to destroy normally competent embryos. Such pES cells may be more acceptable ethically for the treatment of human patients. For primates, it has already been demonstrated that pES cells can be differentiated into all three embryonic germ cell lines *in vitro* [75]. However, there are several negative reports of the application of pES cells. When chimeric mouse offspring were generated from parthenogenetic and fertilized embryos, they showed postnatal growth retardation; moreover, the cell lineages of the parthenogenetic cells were restricted, particularly in the formation of mesoderm and endoderm [91-94]. To resolve and improve the differentiation potential, we tried to re-establish pES cells using nuclear transfer and ntES techniques. As a result, the *in vivo* differentiation potentials of nt-pES cells were significantly (two to five times) better than the original pES cells, judged by the production of chimeric mice (Figure 8). Although we could not detect alteration in the differentially methylated sequences of the examined imprinted genes, it may be that some epigenetic modifications in the nt-pES cell nuclei occurred after nuclear transfer. Interestingly, in the heart and liver, the nt-pES cells only contributed a percentage of approximately 4%, which is consistent with previous work [91, 92, 95].

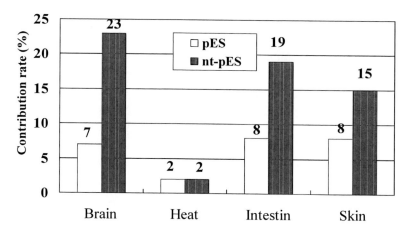

Figure 8. Comparison of the contribution rate between pES and nt-pES cells in chimeric mice. When pES cell were re-established as nt-pES cells by nuclear transfer, the contribution rate in chimeric mice was significantly increased in certain organs (brain, intestine and skin).

It is possible that the effects of NT differ between internal organs or that paternal gene expression is required in particular organs, and this could not be reversed by the NT procedure. So far, NT techniques have required additional oocytes; however, in this study, only eight oocytes per line were required for establishment (a mean of 12.4% from oocytes), because of the high success rate of the growing of the nt-pES cell lines. Although these nuclei maintained parthenogenetic phenotypes, those cloned embryos are still destined to perish, so ES cell derivation may be performed without any need of destroying potential individuals. This would help to overcome the ethical objections to the sacrifice of normal embryos. We have also established a useful tool for investigating the effect of epigenetic modifications, because these nt-pES cells permit the possibility of investigating the roles of imprinted genes.

4.2 Efficient Establishment of ES Cell Lines from Single Blastomeres and Polar Bodies

With improvements in micromanipulation techniques, biopsies of human embryos are now carried out routinely in assisted reproductive technology clinics for the purpose of preimplantation genetic diagnosis [96-98]. If ES cells could be established from these biopsied blastomeres, then the babies' own ES cells would be available to them at birth. There have been several reports of attempts to establish ES cell lines from single blastomeres [99, 100] or preblastocysts [101].

In 1996, Delhaise et al. first reported that ES-like cell lines could be established from single blastomeres [99]. However, they could establish only one cell line from the blastomeres of uncompacted eight-cell embryos separated by disaggregation. Although this cell line had a normal karyotype, it did not lead to germline transmission in chimeric mice. This suggested that the establishment of ES cell lines from single blastomeres is neither simple nor easy. However, recently, Chung et al. [79] reported that five ES cell lines and seven trophoblast stem cell lines were established from single blastomeres from eight-cell mouse embryos. The same group succeeded in establishing human ES cell lines from the blastomeres of 8–10-cell embryos [80]. The isolated blastomeres were each aggregated with a small clump of previously established GFP-expressing ES cells, plated onto MEFs, and cultured in ES cell growth medium. After the cells had proliferated, the GFP-negative cells were separated from the GFP-positive ES cells. However, the overall success rates in both mice and humans were only 4% and 2%, respectively (five ES cell lines from 125 attempts in mice and two ES cell lines from 91 attempts in humans). The authors suggested that such ES cell co-culture was critical to the success of this system, but it was unclear whether this was attributable to substances secreted by the ES cells or a requirement for cell–cell contact, the latter of which may increase the risk of contamination. Nevertheless, this research points to the potential for banking autologous ES cell lines, although the technique clearly needs improvement if it is to be applied to human regenerative medicine.

We also reported a simple and highly efficient method of establishing mouse ES cell lines from single blastomeres at the same time, in which single blastomeres are simply plated onto a feeder layer of mouse embryonic fibroblasts with modified ES cell medium.[102] A total of 112 ES cell lines were established from two-cell (establishment rate, 50%–69%), early four-cell (28%–40%), late four-cell (22%), and eight-cell (14%–16%) stage embryos (Figure 9). Most of the cell lines examined maintained normal karyotypes and expressed markers of pluripotency, including germline transmission in chimeric mice. The best outcomes were achieved with early four-cell embryos: 40% produced ES cell lines and 67% of biopsied embryos went on to full-term development, which are similar to the survival rates achieved with intact blastocysts.

In contrast to previous work, our method did not require aggregation with other ES cells, so this success rate is probably attributable to the new ES cell medium [103], which contains KSR and ACTH instead of FCS. It has been considered that FCS contains potential differentiation factors, whereas KSR lacks such factors and thus provides a differentiation-factor-free growing environment for ES cells [103]. It seems that this medium can support single blastomere development, even 2- to 8-cell stage embryos, to allow the establishment of blastocysts and ES cells more efficiently than the method which is based on aggregation with other ES cells.

In addition, we successfully established ES cells from first and second polar bodies (Figure 10) [102]. The first and second polar bodies, which can be obtained from the oocyte or zygote without its destruction, are degenerate and make no known contribution to life in nature. We have previously demonstrated that these polar bodies have normal developmental potential as female gametes [104, 105]. If the first and second polar bodies can be used to establish ES cell lines, the destruction of the donor oocyte, like that of the biopsied embryo, can be avoided. We also successfully established 18 parthenogenetic ES cell lines from first (36%–40%) and second polar bodies (33%), the nuclei of which were reconstructed into embryos by nuclear transfer.

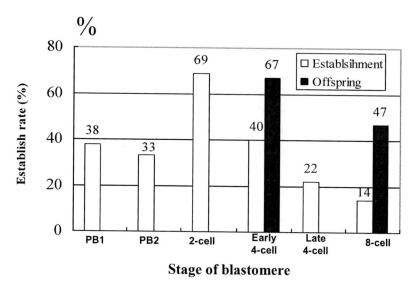

Figure 9. ES cell establishment from polar body (PB) or single blastomeres, and production of offspring from biopsied embryos. Newly developed ES cell culture media can support ES cell derivation from single blastomeres of 2-cell to 8-cell stage embryos, with quite a higher establishment rate. Moreover, if one uses nuclear transfer techniques, then even polar bodies can be used to establish ES cell lines.

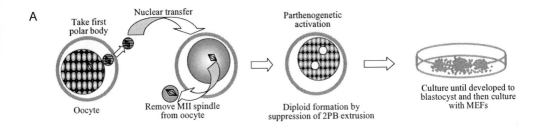

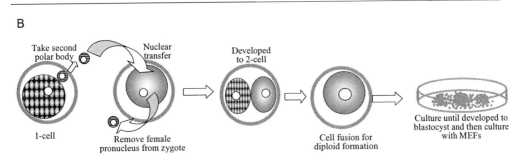

Figure 10. Method for establishment of pES cell lines from first or second polar bodies. A. First polar bodies were transferred into enucleated oocytes, and reconstructed oocytes were parthenogenetically activated. To make diploid cells, second polar body extrusion suppressed by cytochalasin B. B. Second polar bodies were transferred into enucleated zygotes. The next day, when the reconstructed embryo develops to the 2-cell stage, blastomeres were electrically fused with each other to make diploid cells.

In conclusion, our results suggest that the single cells of all early stage embryos or polar bodies can potentially be converted into ES cells without any special treatment. For humans, this suggests that embryo biopsy for preimplantation genetic diagnosis may offer the additional benefit of allowing autologous ES cell lines to be established.

4.3. Establishment of ntES Cell Lines from Aged, Fertilization-Failure Mouse Oocytes

Human *in vitro* fertilization (IVF) is now routinely performed in infertility clinics with high success (60-70% in human, over 70% in mice) [106-108], but some oocytes often fail to fertilize, for unknown reasons. This might be because the oocytes have innate defects rather than because of sperm dysfunction [109]. These unfertilized oocytes continue to age *in vitro* and often show abnormalities such as metaphase spindle disassembly [110-112]. Although intracytoplasmic sperm injection (ICSI) can be used to inseminate these unfertilized oocytes—so-called "rescue ICSI"—[113, 114], the oocytes lose developmental potential rapidly over time [115, 116]. However, if such aged fertilization failure (AFF) oocytes could be used to generate ntES cell lines, then this could reduce or even eliminate ethical concerns over oocyte donation and embryo destruction. Here we tested whether mouse AFF oocytes could be used instead of fresh oocytes as recipients of somatic cell nuclei [117].

The success rate of the nuclear transfer procedure (pseudo-pronuclear formation) and development to the morula or blastocyst stage was significantly lower in the AFF oocytes than in fresh oocytes. However, the rate of establishment of ntES cell lines from cloned morulae or blastocyst stage embryo was similar or even higher than those of fresh oocytes (6% vs 7%, Figure 11) [117]. All of the established cell lines stained positive for the ES cell-specific markers alkaline phosphatase, Oct3/4 and Nanog. When karyotypes of randomly selected cell lines were examined, all the examined cell lines were within the normal ranges. Importantly, tetraploid chimeric mice derived from these ntES cell demonstrated that these ntES cell lines had normal differentiation potential into functional organs.

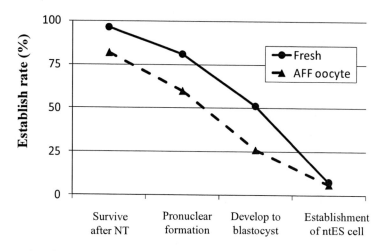

Figure 11. Comparison between fresh and AFF oocytes in embryo development and ntES cell establishment. When AFF oocytes were used as recipients, each of the outcome measures showed lower success rates than when fresh oocytes were used. However, the final rate of establishment of ntES cell lines was almost the same between fresh and AFF oocytes.

Table 2. Establishment of ntES cell lines, production of cloned and ICSI offspring using AFF oocytes

Type of Exp.	Type of oocyte	No. used oocytes	No. embryos developed to blastocyst (%)	No. established cell lines (%)	No. embryos developed to 2-cell (%)	No. of offspring (%)
ntES	AFF	430	112 (26)	27 (6)	-	-
	24h stored	73	24 (33)	4 (5)	-	-
	Fresh	162	83 (51)	12 (7)	-	-
Clone	AFF	797	-	-	357 (45)	0
	Fresh	162	-	-	119 (73)	3 (1.9)

AFF: Aged, fertilization failure oocytes.

For practical use in humans, as NT is inefficient, it might be necessary to transport AFF oocytes from other clinics to increase the number of oocytes available. Mouse oocytes can survive functionally when stored at room temperature, but not at 37°C or 4°C [111]. Surprisingly, even when oocytes are stored at room temperature for one day, they retain their capacity for genomic reprogramming and can be used to establish ntES cell lines from several different mouse strains (Table 2). Thus, in theory, AFF human oocytes could be pooled among nearby clinics by simple storage at room temperature.

On the other hand, if these cloned embryos have the potential to develop to full term, a second ethical problem, i.e. "the embryos are denied their potential to develop to establish ntES cell lines" might arguably still remain. Therefore, we also examined the full term developmental potential of cloned embryos produced from AFF oocytes. However, none of the cloned embryos developed to full term when AFF oocytes were used (Table 2). It appears the genomic reprogramming potential of AFF oocytes is sufficient to generate ntES cells, but not for full term development. Thus they might serve as a basic science tool, for example to detect the reprogramming factors by comparing between fresh and AFF oocytes [117].

CONCLUSION

Recently, several new methods were proposed to create patient-specific ES cells that would not elicit ethical objections. However, thus far, ntES cells are the most similar type of pluripotent stem cells to fertilized derived ES cells without genetic modification of the original donor nucleus. It is still too early to judge which of these approaches is the most promising, but it seems clear that a deeper understanding of nuclear reprogramming will be needed if therapeutic cloning is to become a clinical reality.

REFERENCES

[1] Wilmut I, Schnieke AE, McWhir J, et al. Viable offspring derived from fetal and adult mammalian cells. *Nature.* 1997;385:810-813.

[2] Boiani M, Eckardt S, Scholer HR, et al. Oct4 distribution and level in mouse clones: consequences for pluripotency. *Genes Dev.* 2002;16:1209-1219.

[3] Bortvin A, Eggan K, Skaletsky H, et al. Incomplete reactivation of Oct4-related genes in mouse embryos cloned from somatic nuclei. *Development.* 2003;130:1673-1680.

[4] Kishigami S, Hikichi T, Van Thuan N, et al. Normal specification of the extraembryonic lineage after somatic nuclear transfer. *FEBS Lett.* 2006;580:1801-1806.

[5] Wakayama T, Yanagimachi R. Cloning of male mice from adult tail-tip cells. *Nat. Genet.* 1999;22:127-128.

[6] Tamashiro KL, Wakayama T, Akutsu H, et al. Cloned mice have an obese phenotype not transmitted to their offspring. *Nat. Med.* 2002;8:262-267.

[7] Tamashiro KL, Wakayama T, Blanchard RJ, et al. Postnatal growth and behavioral development of mice cloned from adult cumulus cells. *Biol. Reprod.* 2000;63:328-334.

[8] Ogonuki N, Inoue K, Yamamoto Y, et al. Early death of mice cloned from somatic cells. *Nat. Genet.* 2002;30:253-254.

[9] Gurdon JB, Colman A. The future of cloning. *Nature.* 1999;402:743-746.

[10] Mombaerts P. Therapeutic cloning in the mouse. *Proc. Natl. Acad. Sci. USA.* 2003;100 Suppl 1:11924-11925.

[11] Wakayama T. On the road to therapeutic cloning. *Nat. Biotechnol.* 2004;22:399-400.

[12] Wakayama T, Tabar V, Rodriguez I, et al. Differentiation of embryonic stem cell lines generated from adult somatic cells by nuclear transfer. *Science.* 2001;292:740-743.

[13] Rideout WM, 3rd, Hochedlinger K, Kyba M, et al. Correction of a genetic defect by nuclear transplantation and combined cell and gene therapy. *Cell.* 2002;109:17-27.

[14] Wakayama S, Kishigami S, Van Thuan N, et al. Propagation of an infertile hermaphrodite mouse lacking germ cells by using nuclear transfer and embryonic stem cell technology. *Proc. Natl. Acad. Sci. USA.* 2005;102:29-33.

[15] Illmensee K, Hoppe PC. Nuclear transplantation in Mus musculus: developmental potential of nuclei from preimplantation embryos. *Cell.* 1981;23:9-18.

[16] McGrath J, Solter D. Nuclear transplantation in the mouse embryo by microsurgery and cell fusion. *Science.* 1983;220:1300-1302.

[17] Robl JM, Gilligan B, Critser ES, et al. Nuclear transplantation in mouse embryos: assessment of recipient cell stage. *Biol. Reprod.* 1986;34:733-739.

[18] Tsunoda Y, Yasui T, Shioda Y, et al. Full-term development of mouse blastomere nuclei transplanted into enucleated two-cell embryos. *J. Exp. Zool.* 1987;242:147-151.

[19] Willadsen SM. Nuclear transplantation in sheep embryos. *Nature.* 1986;320:63-65.

[20] Wakayama T, Tateno H, Mombaerts P, et al. Nuclear transfer into mouse zygotes. *Nat. Genet.* 2000;24:108-109.

[21] Campbell KH, McWhir J, Ritchie WA, et al. Sheep cloned by nuclear transfer from a cultured cell line. *Nature.* 1996;380:64-66.

[22] Wakayama T, Perry AC, Zuccotti M, et al. Full-term development of mice from enucleated oocytes injected with cumulus cell nuclei. *Nature.* 1998;394:369-374.

[23] Ogura A, Inoue K, Takano K, et al. Birth of mice after nuclear transfer by electrofusion using tail tip cells. *Mol. Reprod. Dev.* 2000;57:55-59.

[24] Ogura A, Inoue K, Ogonuki N, et al. Production of male cloned mice from fresh, cultured, and cryopreserved immature Sertoli cells. *Biol. Reprod.* 2000;62:1579-1584.

[25] Ono Y, Shimozawa N, Ito M, et al. Cloned mice from fetal fibroblast cells arrested at metaphase by a serial nuclear transfer. *Biol. Reprod.* 2001;64:44-50.

[26] Wakayama T, Yanagimachi R. Mouse cloning with nucleus donor cells of different age and type. *Mol. Reprod. Dev.* 2001;58:376-383.

[27] Wakayama T, Rodriguez I, Perry AC, et al. Mice cloned from embryonic stem cells. *Proc. Natl. Acad. Sci. USA.* 1999;96:14984-14989.

[28] Inoue K, Wakao H, Ogonuki N, et al. Generation of cloned mice by direct nuclear transfer from natural killer T cells. *Curr. Biol.* 2005;15:1114-1118.

[29] Sung LY, Gao S, Shen H, et al. Differentiated cells are more efficient than adult stem cells for cloning by somatic cell nuclear transfer. *Nat. Genet.* 2006.

[30] Miki H, Inoue K, Kohda T, et al. Birth of mice produced by germ cell nuclear transfer. *Genesis.* 2005;41:81-86.

[31] Inoue K, Ogonuki N, Miki H, et al. Inefficient reprogramming of the hematopoietic stem cell genome following nuclear transfer. *J. Cell Sci.* 2006;119:1985-1991.

[32] Inoue K, Noda S, Ogonuki N, et al. Differential developmental ability of embryos cloned from tissue-specific stem cells. *Stem Cells.* 2007;25:1279-1285.

[33] Yamazaki Y, Makino H, Hamaguchi-Hamada K, et al. Assessment of the developmental totipotency of neural cells in the cerebral cortex of mouse embryo by nuclear transfer. *Proc. Natl. Acad. Sci USA.* 2001;98:14022-14026.

[34] Mizutani E, Ohta H, Kishigami S, et al. Developmental ability of cloned embryos from neural stem cells. *Reproduction.* 2006;132:849-857.

[35] Inoue K, Ogonuki N, Mochida K, et al. Effects of donor cell type and genotype on the efficiency of mouse somatic cell cloning. *Biol. Reprod.* 2003;69:1394-1400.

[36] Dean W, Santos F, Stojkovic M, et al. Conservation of methylation reprogramming in mammalian development: aberrant reprogramming in cloned embryos. *Proc. Natl. Acad. Sci. USA.* 2001;98:13734-13738.

[37] Kang YK, Koo DB, Park JS, et al. Aberrant methylation of donor genome in cloned bovine embryos. *Nat. Genet.* 2001;28:173-177.

[38] Ohgane J, Wakayama T, Kogo Y, et al. DNA methylation variation in cloned mice. *Genesis.* 2001;30:45-50.

[39] Enright BP, Kubota C, Yang X, et al. Epigenetic characteristics and development of embryos cloned from donor cells treated by trichostatin A or 5-aza-2'-deoxycytidine. *Biol. Reprod.* 2003;69:896-901.

[40] Kishigami S, Mizutani E, Ohta H, et al. Significant improvement of mouse cloning technique by treatment with trichostatin A after somatic nuclear transfer. *Biochem. Biophys. Res. Commun.* 2006;340:183-189.

[41] Kishigami S, Bui HT, Wakayama S, et al. Successful mouse cloning of an outbred strain by trichostatin A treatment after somatic nuclear transfer. *J. Reprod. Dev.* 2007;53:165-170.

[42] Tanaka S, Oda M, Toyoshima Y, et al. Placentomegaly in cloned mouse concepti caused by expansion of the spongiotrophoblast layer. *Biol. Reprod.* 2001;65:1813-1821.

[43] Kohda T, Inoue K, Ogonuki N, et al. Variation in gene expression and aberrantly regulated chromosome regions in cloned mice. *Biol. Reprod.* 2005;73:1302-1311.

[44] Inoue K, Kohda T, Lee J, et al. Faithful expression of imprinted genes in cloned mice. *Science.* 2002;295:297.

[45] Humpherys D, Eggan K, Akutsu H, et al. Epigenetic instability in ES cells and cloned mice. *Science.* 2001;293:95-97.

[46] Senda S, Wakayama T, Yamazaki Y, et al. Skewed X-inactivation in cloned mice. *Biochem. Biophys. Res. Commun.* 2004;321:38-44.

[47] Humpherys D, Eggan K, Akutsu H, et al. Abnormal gene expression in cloned mice derived from embryonic stem cell and cumulus cell nuclei. *Proc. Natl. Acad. Sci. USA.* 2002;99:12889-12894.

[48] Eggan K, Akutsu H, Hochedlinger K, et al. X-Chromosome inactivation in cloned mouse embryos. *Science.* 2000;290:1578-1581.

[49] Ohta H, Wakayama T. Generation of normal progeny by intracytoplasmic sperm injection following grafting of testicular tissue from cloned mice that died postnatally. *Biol. Reprod.* 2005;73:390-395.

[50] Shimozawa N, Ono Y, Kimoto S, et al. Abnormalities in cloned mice are not transmitted to the progeny. *Genesis.* 2002;34:203-207.

[51] Senda S, Wakayama T, Arai Y, et al. DNA methylation errors in cloned mice disappear with advancement of aging. *Cloning Stem Cells.* 2007;9:293-302.

[52] Cibelli JB, Stice SL, Golueke PJ, et al. Transgenic bovine chimeric offspring produced from somatic cell-derived stem-like cells. *Nat. Biotechnol.* 1998;16:642-646.

[53] Kawase E, Yamazaki Y, Yagi T, et al. Mouse embryonic stem (ES) cell lines established from neuronal cell-derived cloned blastocysts. *Genesis.* 2000;28:156-163.

[54] Munsie MJ, Michalska AE, O'Brien CM, et al. Isolation of pluripotent embryonic stem cells from reprogrammed adult mouse somatic cell nuclei. *Curr. Biol.* 2000;10:989-992.

[55] Wakayama S, Jakt ML, Suzuki M, et al. Equivalency of nuclear transfer-derived embryonic stem cells to those derived from fertilized mouse blastocysts. *Stem Cells.* 2006;24:2023-2033.

[56] Wakayama S, Mizutani E, Kishigami S, et al. Mice cloned by nuclear transfer from somatic and ntES cells derived from the same individuals. *J. Reprod. Dev.* 2005;51:765-772.

[57] Wakayama S, Ohta H, Kishigami S, et al. Establishment of male and female nuclear transfer embryonic stem cell lines from different mouse strains and tissues. *Biol. Reprod.* 2005;72:932-936.

[58] Barberi T, Klivenyi P, Calingasan NY, et al. Neural subtype specification of fertilization and nuclear transfer embryonic stem cells and application in parkinsonian mice. *Nat. Biotechnol.* 2003;21:1200-1207.

[59] Eggan K, Baldwin K, Tackett M, et al. Mice cloned from olfactory sensory neurons. *Nature.* 2004;428:44-49.

[60] Hochedlinger K, Jaenisch R. Monoclonal mice generated by nuclear transfer from mature B and T donor cells. *Nature.* 2002;415:1035-1038.

[61] Li J, Ishii T, Feinstein P, et al. Odorant receptor gene choice is reset by nuclear transfer from mouse olfactory sensory neurons. *Nature.* 2004;428:393-399.

[62] Mitalipova MM, Rao RR, Hoyer DM, et al. Preserving the genetic integrity of human embryonic stem cells. *Nat. Biotechnol.* 2005;23:19-20.

[63] Suzuki H, Kamada N, Ueda O, et al. Germ-line contribution of embryonic stem cells in chimeric mice: influence of karyotype and in vitro differentiation ability. *Exp. Anim.* 1997;46:17-23.

[64] Fukumura R, Takahashi H, Saito T, et al. A sensitive transcriptome analysis method that can detect unknown transcripts. *Nucleic Acids Res.* 2003;31:e94.

[65] Brambrink T, Hochedlinger K, Bell G, et al. ES cells derived from cloned and fertilized blastocysts are transcriptionally and functionally indistinguishable. *Proc. Natl. Acad. Sci. USA.* 2006;103:933-938.

[66] Smith SL, Everts RE, Tian XC, et al. Global gene expression profiles reveal significant nuclear reprogramming by the blastocyst stage after cloning. *Proc. Natl. Acad. Sci. USA.* 2005;102:17582-17587.

[67] Nagy A, Gocza E, Diaz EM, et al. Embryonic stem cells alone are able to support fetal development in the mouse. *Development.* 1990;110:815-821.

[68] Wang Z, Jaenisch R. At most three ES cells contribute to the somatic lineages of chimeric mice and of mice produced by ES-tetraploid complementation. *Dev. Biol.* 2004;275:192-201.

[69] Li J, Ishii T, Wen D, et al. Non-equivalence of cloned and clonal mice. *Curr. Biol.* 2005;15:R756-757.

[70] Blelloch RH, Hochedlinger K, Yamada Y, et al. Nuclear cloning of embryonal carcinoma cells. *Proc. Natl. Acad. Sci. USA.* 2004;101:13985-13990.

[71] Hochedlinger K, Blelloch R, Brennan C, et al. Reprogramming of a melanoma genome by nuclear transplantation. *Genes Dev.* 2004;18:1875-1885.

[72] Hrabe de Angelis MH, Flaswinkel H, Fuchs H, et al. Genome-wide, large-scale production of mutant mice by ENU mutagenesis. *Nat. Genet.* 2000;25:444-447.

[73] Wakayama T, Shinkai Y, Tamashiro KL, et al. Cloning of mice to six generations. *Nature.* 2000;407:318-319.

[74] Saito M, Saga A, Matsuoka H. Production of a cloned mouse by nuclear transfer from a fetal fibroblast cell of a mouse closed colony strain. *Exp. Anim.* 2004;53:467-469.

[75] Cibelli JB, Grant KA, Chapman KB, et al. Parthenogenetic stem cells in nonhuman primates. *Science.* 2002;295:819.

[76] Hikichi T, Wakayama S, Mizutani E, et al. Differentiation potential of parthenogenetic embryonic stem cells is improved by nuclear transfer. *Stem Cells.* 2007;25:46-53.

[77] Meissner A, Jaenisch R. Generation of nuclear transfer-derived pluripotent ES cells from cloned Cdx2-deficient blastocysts. *Nature.* 2006;439:212-215.

[78] Egli D, Rosains J, Birkhoff G, et al. Developmental reprogramming after chromosome transfer into mitotic mouse zygotes. *Nature.* 2007;447:679-685.

[79] Chung Y, Klimanskaya I, Becker S, et al. Embryonic and extraembryonic stem cell lines derived from single mouse blastomeres. *Nature.* 2006;439:216-219.

[80] Klimanskaya I, Chung Y, Becker S, et al. Human embryonic stem cell lines derived from single blastomeres. *Nature.* 2006;444:481-485.

[81] Cowan CA, Atienza J, Melton DA, et al. Nuclear reprogramming of somatic cells after fusion with human embryonic stem cells. *Science.* 2005;309:1369-1373.

[82] Matsumura H, Tada M, Otsuji T, et al. Targeted chromosome elimination from ES-somatic hybrid cells. *Nat. Methods.* 2007;4:23-25.

[83] Okita K, Ichisaka T, Yamanaka S. Generation of germline-competent induced pluripotent stem cells. *Nature.* 2007;448:313-317.

[84] Takahashi K, Yamanaka S. Induction of pluripotent stem cells from mouse embryonic and adult fibroblast cultures by defined factors. *Cell.* 2006;126:663-676.

[85] Strelchenko N, Kukharenko V, Shkumatov A, et al. Reprogramming of human somatic cells by embryonic stem cell cytoplast. *Reprod. Biomed. Online.* 2006;12:107-111.

[86] Verlinsky Y, Strelchenko N, Kukharenko V, et al. Repository of human embryonic stem cell lines and development of individual specific lines using stembrid technology. *Reprod. Biomed. Online.* 2006;13:547-550.

[87] Verlinsky Y, Strelchenko N, Shkumatov A, et al. Cytoplasmic cell fusion: Stembrid technology for reprogramming pluripotentiality. *Stem cell reviews.* 2006;2:297-299.

[88] Hubner K, Fuhrmann G, Christenson LK, et al. Derivation of oocytes from mouse embryonic stem cells. *Science.* 2003;300:1251-1256.

[89] Chen Y, He ZX, Liu A, et al. Embryonic stem cells generated by nuclear transfer of human somatic nuclei into rabbit oocytes. *Cell Res.* 2003;13:251-263.

[90] Dominko T, Mitalipova M, Haley B, et al. Bovine oocyte cytoplasm supports development of embryos produced by nuclear transfer of somatic cell nuclei from various mammalian species. *Biol. Reprod.* 1999;60:1496-1502.

[91] Fundele R, Norris ML, Barton SC, et al. Systematic elimination of parthenogenetic cells in mouse chimeras. *Development.* 1989;106:29-35.

[92] Fundele RH, Norris ML, Barton SC, et al. Temporal and spatial selection against parthenogenetic cells during development of fetal chimeras. *Development.* 1990;108:203-211.

[93] Nagy A, Paldi A, Dezso L, et al. Prenatal fate of parthenogenetic cells in mouse aggregation chimaeras. *Development.* 1987;101:67-71.

[94] Paldi A, Nagy A, Markkula M, et al. Postnatal development of parthenogenetic in equilibrium with fertilized mouse aggregation chimeras. *Development.* 1989;105:115-118.

[95] Allen ND, Barton SC, Hilton K, et al. A functional analysis of imprinting in parthenogenetic embryonic stem cells. *Development.* 1994;120:1473-1482.

[96] Geber S, Winston RM, Handyside AH. Proliferation of blastomeres from biopsied cleavage stage human embryos in vitro: an alternative to blastocyst biopsy for preimplantation diagnosis. *Hum. Reprod.* 1995;10:1492-1496.

[97] Handyside AH, Kontogianni EH, Hardy K, et al. Pregnancies from biopsied human preimplantation embryos sexed by Y-specific DNA amplification. *Nature.* 1990;344:768-770.

[98] Staessen C, Platteau P, Van Assche E, et al. Comparison of blastocyst transfer with or without preimplantation genetic diagnosis for aneuploidy screening in couples with advanced maternal age: a prospective randomized controlled trial. *Hum. Reprod.* 2004;19:2849-2858.

[99] Delhaise F, Bralion V, Schuurbiers N, et al. Establishment of an embryonic stem cell line from 8-cell stage mouse embryos. *Eur. J. Morphol.* 1996;34:237-243.

[100] Wilton LJ, Trounson AO. Biopsy of preimplantation mouse embryos: development of micromanipulated embryos and proliferation of single blastomeres in vitro. *Biol. Reprod.* 1989;40:145-152.

[101] Tesar PJ. Derivation of germ-line-competent embryonic stem cell lines from preblastocyst mouse embryos. *Proc. Natl. Acad. Sci. USA.* 2005;102:8239-8244.

[102] Wakayama S, Hikichi T, Suetsugu R, et al. Efficient establishment of mouse embryonic stem cell lines from single blastomeres and polar bodies. *Stem Cells.* 2007;25:986-993.

[103] Ogawa K, Matsui H, Ohtsuka S, et al. A novel mechanism for regulating clonal propagation of mouse ES cells. *Genes Cells.* 2004;9:471-477.

[104] Wakayama T, Hayashi Y, Ogura A. Participation of the female pronucleus derived from the second polar body in full embryonic development of mice. *J. Reprod. Fertil.* 1997;110:263-266.

[105] Wakayama T, Yanagimachi R. The first polar body can be used for the production of normal offspring in mice. *Biol. Reprod.* 1998;59:100-104.

[106] Chen HL, Copperman AB, Grunfeld L, et al. Failed fertilization in vitro: second day micromanipulation of oocytes versus reinsemination. *Fertil Steril.* 1995;63:1337-1340.

[107] Nagy ZP, Joris H, Liu J, et al. Intracytoplasmic single sperm injection of 1-day-old unfertilized human oocytes. *Hum. Reprod.* 1993;8:2180-2184.

[108] Toyoda Y, Yokoyama M, Hoshi T. Studies on the fertilization of mouse eggs in vitro. *Japanese journal of Animal Reproduction.* 1971;16:152-157.

[109] Bedford JM, Kim HH. Sperm/egg binding patterns and oocyte cytology in retrospective analysis of fertilization failure in vitro. *Hum. Reprod.* 1993;8:453-463.

[110] Kunathikom S, Makemaharn O, Suksompong S, et al. Chromosomal analysis of "failed-fertilized" human oocytes resulting from in-vitro fertilization and intracytoplasmic sperm injection. *J. Med. Assoc. Thai.* 2001;84:532-538.

[111] Wakayama S, Thuan NV, Kishigami S, et al. Production of offspring from one-day-old oocytes stored at room temperature. *J. Reprod. Dev.* 2004;50:627-637.

[112] Wang WH, Meng L, Hackett RJ, et al. The spindle observation and its relationship with fertilization after intracytoplasmic sperm injection in living human oocytes. *Fertil Steril.* 2001;75:348-353.

[113] Sjogren A, Lundin K, Hamberger L. Intracytoplasmic sperm injection of 1 day old oocytes after fertilization failure. *Hum. Reprod.* 1995;10:974-975.

[114] Tsirigotis M, Nicholson N, Taranissi M, et al. Late intracytoplasmic sperm injection in unexpected failed fertilization in vitro: diagnostic or therapeutic? *Fertil Steril.* 1995;63:816-819.

[115] Chen C, Kattera S. Rescue ICSI of oocytes that failed to extrude the second polar body 6 h post-insemination in conventional IVF. *Hum. Reprod.* 2003;18:2118-2121.

[116] Kuczynski W, Dhont M, Grygoruk C, et al. Rescue ICSI of unfertilized oocytes after IVF. *Hum. Reprod.* 2002;17:2423-2427.

[117] Wakayama S, Suetsugu R, Thuan NV, et al. Establishment of mouse embryonic stem cell lines from somatic cell nuclei by nuclear transfer into aged, fertilization-failure mouse oocytes. *Curr. Biol.* 2007;17:R120-121.

Chapter XXII

OCULAR LIMBAL STEM CELL BIOLOGY AND TRANSPLANTATION

Ali R. Djalilian[1], Nariman Nassiri[1], Chi-Chao Chan[2]
[1]Department of Ophthalmology, University of Illinois at Chicago, Chicago, IL, US
[2]Laboratory of Immunology, NEI/NIH, Bethesda, MD, US

INTRODUCTION

The cornea is covered by a continuous renewing stratified squamous epithelium. Like stem cells of other epithelial surfaces that reside in a special region (niche) throughout adulthood, the corneal epithelial stem cells are localized in the basal layer of the corneoscleral junction, known as the limbus [1-3]. These stem cells are important prerequisite for corneal epithelial homeostasis. Meanwhile, the ocular surface is an ideal site to conduct epithelial stem cell research due to the unique compartmentalization of the corneal stem cells in the limbus allowing the study of the proliferative and nonproliferative population of cells, regulatory factors (growth or inhibitor), and mechanism of the differentiation and migration of epithelial cells. Elucidation of the biology of stem cells of corneal epithelia has led to better therapeutic strategies in treatment of patients with a group of ocular surface diseases caused by limbal stem cell deficiency, manifesting with abnormal conjunctival epithelial ingrowths (conjunctivalization) over the cornea, vascularization, and ultimately visual loss. The objective of this chapter is to review the basic biology of corneal epithelial stem cells and their clinical application in limbal stem cell transplantation.

OCULAR SURFACE

The surface of the eye comprises of a transparent cornea in the center and a thin conjunctiva in the periphery, the border between the two, known as corneoscleral junction, or limbus. The conjunctiva extends from the corneal limbus up to the mucocutaneous junction at the lid margin. It is divided anatomically into bulbar, forniceal and palpebral regions (Figure

1). The cornea, conjunctiva and limbus are covered by a stratified, squamous, nonkeratinizing epithelium on the surface of the eye. The precorneal tear film, neural innervations, and protective blink reflex help to sustain environment favorable for the ocular surface epithelium. The cornea consists of epithelial, stromal and endothelial layers (Figure 2).

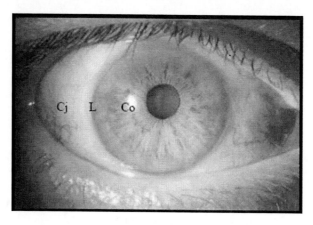

Figure 1. The conjunctiva (Cj), cornea (Co) and the limbus (L).

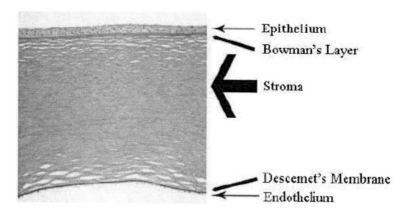

Figure 2. The corneal epithelium is the outermost layer of the cornea. The stroma, the middle and thickest layer, is composed of organized layers of collagen and stromal keratocyte cells. The inner most layer is the endothelium.

The cornea is the gateway of external images into the eye. A healthy cornea is responsible for more than two thirds of the total refractive power of the eye to focus light on the cornea. So, the clarity of the cornea is important for its physiological requirements. It also serves as a protective barrier to prevent the entrance of pathogens. The corneal epithelium includes from its superficial aspects, about 1-3 layers of flattened squamous cells. The superficial cells contain extensive microvilli, called microplicae that increase the cell surface area and facilitate their close association with the precorneal tear film. The lateral tight junction between the superficial cells avoids the entrance of harmful substances. Beneath the superficial layer are 2-3 layers of suprabasal or wing cells with lateral wing-like extensions; these cells are not capable of further cell division. The innermost layer of the corneal epithelium is a single layer of columnar cells, called basal cells. They can undergo cell division to produce the wing and squamous cells. They also secrete several matrix molecules that are incorporated into the underlying basement membrane and stroma, organize the hemidesmosomes that maintain stable attachment to the underlying basement membrane and finally, organize the more transient cell-matrix attachments called focal complexes that are important in mediating cell migration in response to an injury. Between the corneal epithelia and the stroma, there is a basement membrane and an additional collagenous layer known as Bowman's layer. Beneath the Bowman's layer, the stroma is located. It constitutes of more than 90% of the entire cornea. It consists of corneal fibroblasts (keratocytes), which are responsible for producing and organizing the stromal extracellular matrix (ECM). The stroma acts as a structural support for the cornea as well as maintaining the corneal transparency.

The stroma overlies another basement membrane known as Descemet's membrane. Beneath this membrane is a single layer of flattened cells, called corneal endothelium. These are connected with tight junctions. The endothelium plays an important role in the corneal transparency. It pumps the fluids and nutrients into the stroma. Furthermore, the nutrients diffuse passively through the stroma nourishing the keratocytes and corneal epithelium.

Both corneal and conjunctival epithelia are in a state of constant renewal and regeneration. Conjunctival and corneal epithelial cells have been shown to belong to two distinct lineages [4]. Unlike corneal epithelial, conjunctival epithelium consists of both nongoblet epithelial cells as well as mucin-secreting goblet cells. Both populations of cells originate from mutual bipotent progenitor cells [5, 6]. It has been shown that conjunctival forniceal region is the site of conjunctival stem cells. However, conjunctival stem cells are also likely to be present in other regions of the conjunctiva [5, 6].

Limbus is a 1.5-2 cm wide area between the cornea and conjunctiva. It has been proposed that basal layer of the limbus is the residing site of corneal epithelial stem cells which are responsible for the continuous renewal of the corneal epithelium [3, 7-10].

BASAL LIMBUS AS THE RESIDING REGION FOR CORNEAL EPITHELIAL STEM CELLS (CESCs)

As one of the earliest documentation of corneal epithelial wound healing in living eye, Mann [11] described that cells migrate from the limbal area towards the injured area. They noted a sliding of pigment from the limbal region towards the epithelial defect of rabbit corneal epithelium that had been wounded by simple trauma or chemical injury.

The concept of the limbus location of the corneal epithelial stem cells was first proposed by Davanger and Evensen [1]. Goldberg et al. demonstrated that limbal papillary structure (*palisades of Vogt*) is the likely location for the proliferative reservoir of corneal epithelial cells [12]. Since then, numerous surveys have supported the limbal location of stem cells.

Experimental Evidence for the Limbal Location of CESCs

(1) Keratins as a group of intracellular cytoskeletal proteins are synthesized by almost all epithelial surfaces. The analysis of these water-soluble proteins gives valuable

information about the level of differentiation and lineage of epithelial cells. Keratin 3 (K3) and Keratin 12 (K12) have been proposed as tissue-specific keratins of corneal epithelia [2, 3, 13]. They are not expressed in the conjunctival epithelium. It has been shown that K3 and K12 are expressed by more differentiated corneal epithelial cells. They are synthesized throughout the entire cornea epithelium and suprabasal limbal epithelium, whereas limbal basal epithelium lack these keratins and instead express the more primitive keratin 14 (K14) indicating their less differentiated state. This evidence coupled with the finding of circumferential migration and a centripetal movement of cells from the limbus towards the central cornea during re-epitheliazation of injured human eyes suggests that corneal epithelial stem cells are positioned in limbal basal epithelium [14]. Since then, further studies have confirmed these findings [15-18].

(2) *In vitro* studies have demonstrated that limbal basal epithelial cells have a higher proliferation potential in culture than those epithelial cells in the periphery and center of the cornea [19, 20]. Additionally, it has been shown that limbal basal epithelial cells respond to central corneal wounds and to differentiation-inducing agents with much higher proliferative rates compared to the central corneal epithelial cells [2, 21]. Furthermore, limbal and central corneal epithelial cells have different responses to growth factors, retinoic acid, and calcium [10, 22, 23]. DNA Labeling studies have demonstrated that the peripheral cornea undergoes more active DNA synthesis [24]. Furthermore, Barrandon and Green classified epidermal keratinocytes into three distinct colonies in terms of size and proliferation capacity [25]. 'Holoclone' colonies are the largest and with the highest proliferative capacity. They consist less than 5% of cells in each colony differentiating; these are considered to be stem cells. 'Paraclone' colonies have poorest proliferative capacity. They consist the highest percentage of differentiating cells and considered to be abortive colonies of terminally differentiated cells (TDCs). 'Meroclone' clonies with intermediate characteristics are considered to be a reservoir of transient amplifying cells (TACs). Pellegrini et al. have demonstrated that only limbal basal cells are able to become holoclone colonies, whereas central corneal epithelia can only give rise to paraclone and meroclone clonies [26].

(3) One of the intrinsic characteristics of the corneal stem cells is label-retaining or slow-cycling. Both tritiated thymidine and bromodeoxyuridine have been applied in studies to identify this property [3, 28-29]. In these experiments, the DNA of cells in S-phase is labeled over several days by continuous treatment of mice with label. Then, the treatment is stopped and the mice are allowed to grow and mature. After two months, when the epithelial cells have gone through multiple cell division, the label begins to dissipate within cells. However, the cells that do not divide and thus retain the label for long periods of time are known as label retaining or slow-cycling cells. It has been shown that these cells are located at the limbal region in the basal cell population [3].

(4) Surgical removal of rabbit limbal epithelia results in defective corneal epithelial regeneration with abnormal conjunctival epithelial ingrowths over the cornea

[30].This is suggestive of limited capacity of corneal epithelial wound healing in the absence of limbal epithelium.

(5) Yuspa et al. demonstrated that there can be two sorts of proliferative basal cells in terms of their response to phorbol ester tumor promoters [31]. Tumor promoter-sensitive subpopulation is those that stop proliferating and initiate terminal differentiation in the presence of phorbol ester tumor promoters. These are considered of more differentiated TACs. On the other hand, tumor promoter-resistant continues proliferation in the exposure to phorbol ester tumor promoters and may be the target of carcinogenic substances; these can be considered stem cells. Kruse and Tseng revealed that a considerable population of tumor promter-resistent cell is positioned in the limbal epithelium compared with central corneal epithelium [21]. Additionally, phorbol esters induce proliferation in corneal epithelial cells, subsequently exhausting the proliferative capacity of TACs and causing terminal differentiation. Conversely, limbal stem cells retain their proliferative capacity after removal of phorbol ester [21].

Clinical Evidence for the Limbal Location of CESCs

(1) The clinical evidence for the limbal location of corneal epithelial stem cells comes from a group of ocular surface diseases with partial or complete limbal stem cell deficiency due to injuries to their limbus. This results in corneal epithelial regeneration with non-corneal epithelium from conjunctiva (conjunctivalization), vascularization and ultimately visual loss. On the other hand, Kenyon and Tseng have shown that the normal corneal epithelia can be reconstituted by autograft limbal tissue transplantation [32]. Later studies have demonstrated that transplantation of cultured limbal cells to also be sufficient for restoring a normal corneal epithelium in patients or animals with conjunctivalization of the cornea [33, 34, 35].

(2) Further clinical evidence comes from the idea that almost all corneal neoplasm originate from the limbus and virtually never from the central corneal epithelium [36]. Any error in DNA replication at the level of stem cells will be passed on unlimitedly to the daughter cells. This coupled with the fact that most tumors arise from stem cells [37] are suggestive of the idea that stem cells reside at the limbus.

The above experimental and clinical evidence indicate that corneal epithelial stem cells are exclusively located at the limbal basal epithelium.

CHARACTERISTICS OF LIMBAL STEM CELLS

The following properties which have been applied to other stem cells, can also be applied to CESCs:

Undifferentiated phenotype: The concept of stemness indicates poor differentiation. Limbal basal stem cells have long been recognized as primitive in terms of differentiation markers [3]. Entering the differentiation pathway means removal of cell from the stem cell population.

Unlimited (compared with life-time of the host) proliferative and self-renewal capacity: To maintain both the corneal epithelial cell mass under normal as well as wound healing states, limbal stem cells must have unlimited proliferative capacity, giving rise to progenitor cells that enter the differentiation pathway. Tissue-specific stem cells are also defined by their ability to self-renew. Differentiated cells are generally short-lived; they are produced from a small pool of long-lived stem cells that last throughout life [38, 39]. However, there is universal acceptance that stem cells are capable of unlimited self-renewal. Cell division within the stem cells are naturally asymmetric leading to production of daughter cells, one remains as its parent and serves to replenish the stem cell pool, whereas the other daughter cell is destined for differentiation pathway to become rapidly-dividing transit TACs [3,40]. These TACs constitute the majority of the proliferative cell population in corneal /limbal epithelium [41]. Before leaving the proliferative section, TACs undergo a limited number of cell divisions to become more terminally differentiated, known as TDCs or post-mitotic cells (PMCs).

Infrequent proliferation in the steady state: Although stem cells have high proliferative capacity, under steady state conditions they exhibit extremely low rates of proliferation [7] indicative of low mitotic activity. Label-retaining or slow cycling is one of the intrinsic properties of stem cells [27, 28, 42].

Pluripotency (Transdifferentiation)

Transdifferentiation or plasticity means the differentiation of an adult tissue-specific stem cell into another type of cell or tissue. It has been shown that basal epithelial cells form the adult cornea under an appropriate microenvironment can give rise to hair follicles [43, 44]. Under the right environmental cues, K3/K12 positive corneal epithelial cells can stop making corneal keratins and begin expressing keratin 5 and K14 as expressed in the basal cells of the limbus and epidermis. These cells can further give rise to hair follicles. These experiments are suggestive of pluripotent nature of corneal epithelial cells [43, 44].

Discrete microenvironment or niche: The concept of niche was first introduced by Schofield in 1978 [47]. Niche, as a Germen word meaning nest, is a specific microenvironment in which adult stem cells reside in their tissue of origin. It consists of a healthy organized microenvironment in which various factors, such as secreted cytokines, extracellular matrix and intercellular adhesion. Within a niche, stem cells are able to maintain their unique properties. Specific niche cells may provide an environment to protect stem cells from differentiation stimuli, apoptotic stimuli, and any other external insult. Additionally, it preserves stem cells against excessive proliferation leading to malignancies. The mentioned characteristics of niche necessitate that the limbal environment be different from the one in the cornea to provide an appropriate environment for residency of stem cells. Compared with cornea, which is avascular, the limbus has blood supply providing needed nutrients and growth factors [48,49]. The basement membrane beneath the CESCs has a distinct ECM composition in terms of laminin isoforms [50], collagen type 4 alfa chain [50], and the AE27 bone marrow antigen [51].

Due to the importance of stem cell within niche, they are protected in different ways. The undulated basement membrane at the limbus not only increase the surface area for contact with the basement membrane but also provide noticeable protection from possible shearing forces [52]. A rich deposit of pigments on the Limbal basal cell offer photoprotection against possible DNA damage via ultraviolet radiation and subsequent generation of oxygen radicals. Additionally, indirect immunohistochemical findings are suggestive of the prominent accumulation of stem cells in the superior and inferior zones where they are naturally protected by eyelids. In addition, Bell's phenomenon as defense mechanism also helps for further protection.

IDENTIFICATION OF STEM CELLS

Although a number of markers have been suggested to be as potential markers for limbal stem cells, a definite marker has not been established to date. Therefore, the identification of limbal stem cells is largely based on indirect evidence. Having specific markers leads to better purification and analysis of these cells while allowing the establishment of diagnostic criteria for disease stages caused by limbal stem cell deficiency. Currently, the proposed molecular markers for CESCs can be classified as (1) Positive markers: those associated to stem cells, such as p63 (2) Negative markers (differentiated markers): those that are absent or poorly expressed in limbal basal cells, such as K3 [2, 13, 44]. While the markers do not have to be present exclusively on cells of the ocular surface, their presence, absence or relative expression allows the enrichment and/or isolation of corneal stem cells.

CLINICAL APPLICATION OF LIMBAL STEM CELLS

The basal limbal stem cells are necessary for corneal epithelial regeneration. The clinical application of limbal stem cells has been most pertinent to a group of ocular surface diseases caused by limbal stem cell deficiency (LSCD) [54]. LSCD can be both partial and complete. The clinical symptoms include conjunctivalization, recurrent corneal epithelial defects, corneal neovascularization, secondary stromal scarring, and ultimately corneal blindness.

Based on the pathogenic nature of limbal involvement, corneal surface diseases can be divided in two categories (Table 3).

Table 1. Stem cell-associated markers in limbal and corneal epithelia immunohistochemical and/or immunofluorescence (adapted from Chen et al. 2004 [53])

Markers	Limbal epithelium (stem cell)		Corneal epithelium	
	Basal	Suprabasal	Basal	Suprabasal
P63	+++	±	±	-
Integrin alpha9	+++	±	-	-
ABCG2	+++	±	-	-
NGF receptor (TrkA)	+++	++	+++	++
Alpha-Enolase	+++	+	++	+
Na/K ATPase	+++	+	++	+
Carbonic anhydrase	+++	+	++	+
Cytochrome oxidase	+++	+	++	+
Vimentin	+++	+	+++	+++
Keratin 19	+++	+	+++	+++

NGF: nerve growth factor; -: no expression; ±: very weak expression; +: weak expression; ++: moderate expression; +++: strong expression.

Table 2. Differentiation markers in limbal and corneal epithelia, immunohistochemical and/or immunofluorescence (adapted from Chen et al. 2004 [53])

Markers	Limbal epithelium		Corneal epithelium	
	Basal	Suprabasal	Basal	Suprabasal
K3/K12	-	+++	+++	+++
Connexin 43	-	+++	+	+++
Connexin 50	-	+++	-	+++
Involucrin	-	+++	+	+++
Nestin	-	+++	+	+++
NGF receptor (p75^{NTR})	-	+++	+++	+++

NGF: nerve growth factor; -: no expression; ±: very weak expression; +: weak expression; ++: moderate expression; +++: strong expression.

Table 3. Ocular Surface Diseases Caused by Limbal Stem Cell Deficiency

Category 1. Destruction of limbal epithelial stem cell population

    a. Chemical or thermal injuries.
    b. Multiple surgeries or cryotherapies of the limbus.
    c. Stevens-Johnson syndrome.
    d. Contact-lens-induced keratopathy.
    e. Severe microbial infection.

Category 2. Dysfunction of stromal microenvironment of limbal epithelial stem cells

a. Aniridia (hereditary)
b. Keratitis associated with multiple endocrine deficiencies (hereditary)
c. Neurotrophic keratopathy (neuronal or ischemic)
d. Chronic limbitis or peripheral corneal inflammation and ulceration.
e. Ptergium and Pseudopterygium.
f. Idiopahtic keratopathy

Adapted from Puangsricharern V., and Tseng SC. Cytologic evidence of corneal diseases with limbal stem cell deficiency. Ophthalmology 1995; 20: 192.

Category 1 includes those with a definite pathogenic etiology for destruction of limbal epithelial stem cells, which can be detected by the history. On the other hand, *Category 2* represents limbal stem cells dysfunction due to gradual loss of the limbal stem cell function. The pathogenesis might be due to genetic, microenvironmental and/or regulatory factors affecting limbal stem cells. Currently, limbal stem cell transplantation is the treatment of choice for LSCD (Figure 3A and B: clinical successful LSC transplantation- before and after surgery).

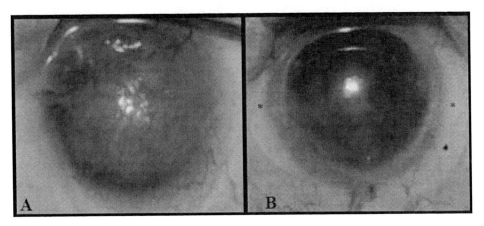

Figure 3. A patient with limbal stem cell deficiency due to Stevens-Johnson syndrome before (A) and after (B) limbal stem cell transplantation. The limbal grafts are visible in the peripheral cornea (*). (Photos courtesy of Dr Edward J. Holland).

It has been shown to be effective in 50-90% of cases depending on the underlying cause and the severity of involvement [55-57]. In localized or unilateral cases where enough healthy limbal tissue can be provided by the patient, a limbal autograft is indicated. On the other hand, in cases with bilateral LSCD, allogenic limbal grafts should be applied. As the use of allogenic grafts is associated with the risk of graft rejection, the long-term success with this procedure is highly dependent on the prevention of immunologic rejection as well as maintenance of healthy ocular tear film. Thus, HLA-matching and long-term systemic and/or immunosuppression should be considered and applied. Studies, with less than optimal immunosuppression have shown that about 50% of allogenic grafts fail within 3 to 5 year [58, 59]. On the other hand, other studies with more complete immunsuppressive regimens have indicated greater long-term success rate for allogenic grafts [57, 60].

Limbal Stem-Cell Transplantation

Although the long-term application of immunosuppression may accompany significant complications [61, 62], there is still debate on the necessity of long-term immunosuppression. Recently, Djalilian et al demonstrated the presence of donor epithelial cells up to 3.5 years after limbal allograft transplantation [63]. Previously, long-term donor survival has been reported in patients receiving immunosuppression [64]. These findings indicated that the long-term success of limbal allograft transplantation is dependant on the survival of the donor stem cells which in turn requires adequate immunosuppression to prevent rejection. This is in contrast to other previous studies which had suggested that transplanted limbal stem cells do not survive in the long run [65-69].

The use of *ex vivo* expanded autologous or allogeneic limbal stem cells grown on amniotic membrane or similar carriers have provided a new strategy for the treatment of limbal stem cell deficiency [26, 70-73]. It has been shown that the cultivated limbal stem cells retain their in vivo properties following expansion in cell culture [74]. Thus, only small amount of tissue is required for *ex vivo* expansion, which reduces the risk of iatrogenic limbal stem cell deficiency secondary to surgical removal of tissue in donor eye.

CONCLUSION

The corneal epithelium is a continuously renewing epithelium that is integral for the clarity of the cornea and thus clear vision. The corneal epithelial stem cells reside in the basal layer of the limbus and can be subjected to various insults leading to diseases known as limbal stem cell deficiency. Understanding the basic biology of limbal stem cells has led to significant advancement in the treatment of patients with limbal stem cell deficiency. Currently, limbal stem cell transplantation is the treatment of choice for these disorders. Future studies will likely uncover the precise pathways controlling limbal stem cells growth and differentiation, thus leading to novel therapeutic strategies for ocular surface regeneration.

REFERENCES

[1] Davanger M., Evensen A., Role of pericorneal papillary structure in renewal of corneal epithelium. *Nature* 1971; 229: 560-561.
[2] Schermer A, Galvin S, Sun TT. Differetiation-related expression of a major 64k corneal keratin in vivo and in culture suggests limbal location of corneal epithelial stem cells. *J. Cell Biol.* 1986; 103: 49-62.
[3] Cotsarelis G, Cheng SZ, Dong G, Sun TT, Lavker RM (1989). Existence of slow cycling limbal basal epithelial cells that can be preferentially stimulated to proliferate: implications on epithelial stem cells. *Cell* 57:201-9.
[4] Wei ZG, Sun TT, Lavker RM. Rabbit conjunctival and corneal epithelial cells belong to two separate lineages. *Invest. Ophthalmol. Vis. Sci.* 1996; 37: 523-33

[5] Wei ZG, Wu RL, Lavker RM, Sun TT. In vitro growth and differentiation of rabbit bulbar, fornix and palpebral conjunctival epithelia. Implications on conjunctival epithelial transdifferentiation and stem cells. *Invest. Ophthalmol. Vis. Sci.* 1993; 34: 1814-28.

[6] Wei ZG, Lin T, Sun TT, Lavker RM. Clonal analysis of the in vivo differentiation potential of keratinocyre. *Invest. Ophthalmol. Vis. Sci.* 1997, 38: 753-61.

[7] Dua HS, Azuara-Blanco A. Limbal stem cells of the cornea epithelium. *Sur. Ophthalmol.* 2000; 44: 415-25.

[8] Thoft RA, Wiley LA, Sundarraj N. The multipotential cells of the limbus. *Eye*, 1989; 3: 109-13.

[9] Dua HS. Stem cells of the ocular surface: scientific principles and clinical applications. *Br. J. Ophthalmolo.* 1995; 79: 968-9.

[10] Tseng SC. Regulation and clinical implications of corneal epithelial stem cells. *Mol. Biol. Rep.* 1996; 23: 47-58.

[11] Mann I. A study of epithelial regeneration in the living eye. *Br. J. Ophthalmol.* 1944; 28: 26-40.

[12] Goldberg M.F., Bron A.J. Limbal palisades of Vogt. Trans. AM. *Ophthalmol. Soc.* 1982; 80: 155-171.

[13] Kurpakus MA, Stock EL, Jones JC. Expression of 55-kD/64-kD corneal keratins in ocular surface epithelium. *Invest. Ophthalmol. Vis. Sci.* 1990; 31: 448-56.

[14] Lemp M.A. and Mathers W.D. Corneal epithelial cell movement in humans. *Eye* 1989; 3: 438-445.

[15] Kiritoshi A., SundarRaj N, Thoft R.A. Differentiation in cultured Limbal epithelium as defined by keratin expression. *Invest. Ophthalmol. Vis. Sci.* 1991; 32: 3073-3077.

[16] Kurpakus M.A, Maniaci M.T, Esco M. Expression of keratins K12, K4 and K14 during development of ocular surface epithelium. *Curr. Eye Res.* 1994; 13: 805-814.

[17] Liu C.Y., Zhu G., Westerhausen-Larson, A., Converse, R., Kao, C.W., Sun T.T., Kao, W.W., 1993. Cornea-specific expression of K12 keratin during mouse development. *Curr. Eye Res.* 12, 963-974.

[18] Matic M., Petrov I.N., Chen S., Wang C., Dimitrijevich S.D., Wolosin J.M., Stem cells of the corneal epithelium lack connexins and metabolite transfer capacity. *Differentiation* 1997; 61: 251-260.

[19] Ebato B., Friend J., and Thoft R. A. Comparison of limbal and peripheral human corneal epithelium in tissue culture. *Invest. Ophthalmol. Vis. Sci.* 1988; 29: 1533-1537.

[20] Lindberg K. et al. In vitro propagation of human ocular surface epithelial cells for transplantation. *Invest. Ophthalmol. Vis. Sci.* 1993; 34: 2672-2679.

[21] Kruse FE. and Tseng SC. A tumor promoter-resistant subpopulation of progenitor cells is larger in limbal epithelium than in corneal epithelium. *Invest. Ophthalmol. Vis. Sci.* 1993; 34: 2501-2511.

[22] Kruse FE. and Tseng SC. Retinoic acid regulates clonal growth and differentiation of cultured limbal and peripheral corneal epithelium. *Invest. Ophthalmol. Vis. Sci.* 1994; 35:2405-2420.

[23] Kruse FE and Tseng S.C. Growth factors modulate clonal growth and differentiation of cultured rabbit limbal and corneal epithelium. *Invest. Ophthalmol. Vis. Sci.* 1993; 34:1963-1976.

[24] Hanna C. and O'Brien J. E. Cell production and migration in the epithelial layer of the cornea. *Arch. Ophthalmol.* 1960; 64: 536-539.

[25] BarrandonY. and Green H. Three clonal type of keratinocyte with different capacities for multicaption. *Proc. Natl. Acad. Sci. USA.* 1987; 84: 2302-2306.

[26] Pellegrini G., Golisano O., Paterna P., Lambiase A., Bonini S., Rama P. and De Luca M. Location and clonal analysis of stem cells and their differentiated progeny in the human ocular surface. *J. Cell Biol.* 1999; 145: 769-782.

[27] Cotsarelis G., Cheng SZ., Dong G., Sun TT., and Lavker RM. Existance of slow-cycling limbal epithelia basal cells that can be preferentiallt stimulate to proliferate: implications on epithelia stem cells. *Cell* (Cambridge, Mass.) 1989; 57: 201-209.

[28] Lavker Rm. and Sun TT. Epithelial stem cells: the eye provides a vision. *Eye* 2003; 17: 937-942.

[29] Lavker RM., Tseng SC. and Sun TT. Corneal epithelial stem cells at the limbus: looking at some old problems from a new angle. *Exp. Eye Res.* 2004; 78: 433-436.

[30] Huang A.J. and Tseng S.C. Corneal epithelial wound healing in the absence Limbal epithelium. *Invest. Ophthalmol. Vis.Sci.* 1991; 32: 96-105.

[31] Yuspa SH, Ben T, Hennings H, Lichti U. Divergent responses in epidermal basal cells exposed to the tumor promoter 12-O-tetradecanoylphorbol-13-acetate. *Cancer Res.* 1982; 42: 2344-9.

[32] Kenyon K.R and Tseng S.C. Limbal autograft transplantation for ocular surface diordes. *Ophthalmol.* 1989; 96: 709-722.

[33] Pires RT., Chokshi A. and Tseng SC. Amniotic membrane transplantation or conjunctival limbal autograft fro limbal stem cell deficiency induced by 5-fluorouracil in glaucoma surgeries. *Cornea* 2000; 19: 284-287.

[34] Stenevi U., Hanson C., Claesson M., Corneliusson E. and EK S. Survival of transplanted human corneal stem cells. *Acta Ophthalmol. Scand.* 2002; 80: 105-109.

[35] Tsai R.J., Sun T., and Tseng S.C. Comparison of limbal and conjunctival autograft transplantation in corneal surface reconstruction in rabbits. *Ophthalmology* 1990; 97: 446-455.

[36] Waring GO 3rd, Roth AM, EKins MB. Clinical and pathologic description of 17 cases of corneal intraepithelial neoplasia. *Am. J. Ophthalmol.* 1984; 97: 547-59.

[37] Reya T, Morrison SJ, Clarke MF, Weissman IL, Stem cells, cancer, and cancer stem cells. *Nature* 2001; 414: 105-11.

[38] Dexter TM, Spooncer E. Growth and differentiation in the hematopoitic system. *Annu. Rev. Cell Biol.* 1989; 3: 423-441.

[39] Jones PH. Epithelial stem cells. *Bioessays* 1997; 19: 683-690.

[40] Morrison SJ, Shah NM, Anderson DJ. Regulatory mechanisms in stem cell biology. *Cell* 1997; 88: 287-98.

[41] Lehrer M.S., Sunn T.T., Lavker R.M., Strategies of epithelial repair: modulation of stem cell and transit amplifying cell proliferation. *J. Cell Sci.* 1998; 111: 2867-2875.

[42] Lavker R.M., Wei Z.G. and Sun T.T. Phorbol ester preferentially stimulates mouse fornical conjunctival and limbal epithelial cells to proliferate in vivo. *Invest. Ophthalmol. Vis. Sci.* 1998; 39: 301-307.

[43] Ferraris C., Chevalier G., Favier B., Jahoda CA. and Dhouailly D. Adult corneal epithelium basal cells possess the capacity to activate epidermal, pilosebaceous and sweat gland genetic program in response to embryonic dermal stimuli. *Development.* 2000; 127: 5487-5495.

[44] Pearton DJ., Ferraris C. and Dhouailly D. Transdifferentiation of corneal epithelium: evidence for lineage between the segregation of epiderma stem cells and induction of hair follicles during embryogenesis. *Int. J. Dev. Boil.* 2004; 48: 197-202.

[45] Orkin SH. Diversification of haematopoietic stem cells to specific lineages. *Nat. Rev. Genet.* 2000; 1: 57-64.

[46] Watt FM. Epidermal stem cells: markers patterning and the control of stem cell fate. *Philos. Trans. R. Soc/ Lond. B Biol. Sci.* 1998; 353: 831-837.

[47] R. Schofield, *Blood cells* 1978; 4: 7.

[48] Gipson IK. The epithelial basement membrane zone of the limbus. *Eye* 1989; 3:132-40.

[49] Zieske JD. Perpetuation of stem cells in the eye. *Eye* 1994; 8:163-9.

[50] Ljubimov AV, Burgeson RE, Bokowski RJ, Michael AF, Sun TT, Kenney MC. Human corneal basement memberane heterogeneity: topographical differences in expression of type 4 collagen and laminin isoforms. *Lab. Invest* 1995; 72: 461-73.

[51] Kolega J, Manabe M, Sun TT. Basement membrane etrogeneity and variation in corneal epithelial differentiation. *Differentiation* 1989; 42: 54-63.

[52] Gipson IL. The epithelial basement membrane zone of the limbus. *Eye* 1989; 3: 132-40.

[53] Chen Z, de Pavia CS, Luo L, Kretzer FL, Pflugfelder SC, Li DQ. Characteristics of putative stem cell phenotype in human limbal epithelia. *Stem cells* 2004; 22: 355-66.

[54] Tseng SC. and Sun TT. Corneal Surgery: Theory, Technique, and Tissue (F.S. Brightbill, ed.), *Mosby-Year Book*, Inc., St. louis, Missouri, pp. 0-18.

[55] Holland EJ. Epithelial transplantation for the management of severe ocular surface disease. *Trans Am Ophthalmol Soc.* 1996; 94: 677-743.

[56] Holland EJ, Schwartz GS. The evolution of epithelial transplantation for severe ocular surface disease and a proposed classification system. *Cornea* 1996; 15: 549-556.

[57] Holland EJ, Djalilian AR, Schwartz GS. Management of aniridic keratopathy with keratolimbal allograft-a limbal stem cell transplantation technique. *Ophthalmology.* 2003; 110: 125-130.

[58] Ilari L, Daya SM. Long-term outcomes of keratolimbal allograft for the treatment of sever ocular surface disorders. *Ophthalmology* 2002; 109: 1278-84.

[59] Solomon A, Ellies P, Anderson DF, Touhami A, Gruererich M, Espana EM, et al. Long-term outcomes of keratolimbal allograft with or without penetrating keratoplasty for total limbal stem cell deficiency. *Ophthalmology* 2002; 109: 1159-66.

[60] Reinhard T, Spelsberg H, Henke L, et al. Long-term results of allogeneic penetrating limbo-keratoplast in total limbal stem cell deficiency. *Ophthalmology.* 2004; 11: 775-782.

[61] Frangie JP, Leibowitz HM. *Steroids. Int. Ophthalmol.* 1993; 33: 9-29.

[62] Barraquer J. Immunosuppression agents in penetrating keratoplasty. *Am. J. Ophthalmol.* 1985; 100: 61-64.

[63] Djalilian AR, Mahesh SP, Koch CA, et. Al. Survival of donor epithelial cells after limbal stem cell transplantation. *Inest. Ophthalmol. Vis. Sci.* 2005; 46: 803-807.

[64] Shimazaki J, Kaido M, Shinozaki N, et. al. Evidence of long-term survival of donor-derived cells after Limbal allograft transplantation. *Invest Ophthalmol Vis. Sci.* 1999; 40: 1664-1668.

[65] Henderson TR, Coster DJ, Williams KA. The lomg-term outcomes of Limbal allografts: the search for surviving cells. *Br. J. Ophthalmol.* 2001; 8:604-609.

[66] Williams KA, Brereton HM, Aggarwal R, et al. Use of DNA polymorphisms and polymerase chain reaction to examine the survival of human Limbal stem cell allograft. *Am. J. Ophthalmol.* 1995; 120: 342-350.

[67] Henderson TR, Mc Cal SH, Taylor GR, Noble BA. Do transplanted corneal Limbal stem cells survive in vivo long-term?-possible techniques to detect donor cell survival by polymerase chain reaction with the amelogenin gene and Y-specific probes. *Eye.* 1997; 11: 779-785.

[68] Henderson TR, Findlay I, Matthews PL, Noble BA. Identifying the origin of single corneal cells by DNA fingerprinting. Part 1: implications for corneal Limbal allografting. *Cornea.* 2001; 20: 400-403.

[69] Henderson TR, Findlay I, Matthews PL, Noble BA. Identifying the origin of single corneal cells by DNA fingerprinting. Part 2: implications for corneal Limbal allografting. *Cornea.* 2001; 20: 404-407.

[70] Kiozumi N. Inatomi T, Suzuki T, Sotozono C, Kinoshita S. Cultivated corneal epithelial stem cell transplantation in ocular surface disorders. *Ophthalmology* 2001; 108: 1569-74.

[71] Pellegrini G, Traverso CE, Franzi AT, Zingrian M, Cancedda R, DeLuca M. Long-term restoration of amaged corneal surfaces with autologous cultivated corneal epithelium. *Lancet* 1997; 349: 990-3.

[72] Schwab IR, Reyes M, Isseroff RR. Successful transplantation of bioengineered tissue replacement in patients with ocular surface disease. *Cornea* 2000; 19: 421-6.

[73] Tsai RJ, Li LM, Chen JK. Reconstruction of damaged corneas by transplantation of autologous limbal epithelial cells. *N. Eng. J. Med.* 2000; 343: 86-93.

[74] 74. Meller D, Pires RT, Tseng SC. Ex vivo preservation and expansion of human limbal epithelial stem cells on aminiotic membrane cultures. *Br. J. Ophthalmol.* 2002; 86: 463-71.

[75] Coster DJ, Aggawal RK, Williams KA. Surgical management of ocular surface disorders using conjunctival and stem cell allografts. *Br. J. Ophthalmol.* 1995; 79: 977-82.

In: Encyclopedia of Stem Cell Research (2 Volume Set) ISBN: 978-1-61761-835-2
Editor: Alexander L. Greene © 2012 Nova Science Publishers, Inc.

Chapter XXIII

PARACRINE, AUTOCRINE AND INTRACRINE PATTERNING FOR CARDIOVASCULAR REPAIR WITH HUMAN MESENCHYMAL STEM CELLS: ROLE OF NEW CHEMISTRY FOR REGENERATIVE MEDICINE

Carlo Ventura[*], *Silvia Cantoni, Francesca Bianchi and Claudia Cavallini*

Laboratory of Molecular Biology and Stem Cell Engineering,
Institute of Cardiology – National Institute of Biostructures and Biosystems,
University of Bologna, Italy, and Bioscience Institute,
Falciano, Repubblica di San Marino

ABSTRACT

Acute myocardial infarction and extensive loss of cardiomyocytes may progress toward heart failure despite revascularization procedures and pharmacological treatments. Initial studies supported the concept that bone marrow cells may hold the promise of rebuilding the injured heart from its component elements, offering a valid alternative to the ultimate resort of heart transplantation. However, stem cell biology turned out to be considerably more complex that initially expected. Different stem cell populations, including mesenchymal stem cells, adipose- and amniotic fluid-derived stem cells, and cardiac-resident stem cells have been progressively characterized. It is increasingly becoming evident that secretion of specific growth factors from transplanted stem cells may activate angiogenic, antiapoptotic and antifibrotic paracrine patterning, playing a

---

[*] Address correspondence to: Carlo Ventura, Laboratory of Molecular Biology and Stem Cell Engineering - National Institute of Biostructures and Biosystems, University of Bologna, Italy. S. Orsola - Malpighi Hospital, Institute of Cardiology, Pavilion 21, Via Massarenti N. 9, Bologna 40138, Italy. Tel. +39-051-340339; Fax: +39-051-344859; E-mail: cvent@libero.it or carlo.ventura@unibo.it

major role in cardiac repair. Released growth factors may also act in an autocrine fashion on cell surface receptors to prime differentiating decisions and orchestrate a complex interplay with the recipient tissue. The stem cell nucleus itself harbors the potential for intrinsic signal transduction pathways. The term "intracrine" has been proposed for growth regulatory peptides acting within their cell of synthesis on the nuclear envelope, or subnuclear components to drive targeted lineage commitment.

Multiple randomized clinical trials of autologous bone marrow cells are on the way in acute myocardial infarction. However, based on the complexity of stem cell biology, it is not surprising that the results of these trials showed modest, transient, or no improvement in cardiac performance. These hurdles raise the larger question as to whether our efforts to provide mechanistic basis for cardiovascular cell therapy should be more closely related to the biology of wound healing than regenerative medicine. Cardiovascular commitment and secretion of trophic mediators are extremely low-yield processes in both adult and embryonic stem cells. Cell-based phenotypic- and pathway-specific screens of natural and synthetic compounds will provide a number of molecules achieving selective control of stem cell growth and differentiation. Novel hyaluronan mixed esters of butyric and retinoic acids have been recently synthesized, emerging as new tools for manipulation of cardio/vasculogenic gene expression through the modulation of targeted signaling pathways and chromatin-remodeling enzymes. These molecules have coaxed both murine embryonic and human mesenchymal stem cells towards cardiovascular decision and paracrine secretion of bioactive factors, remarkably enhancing the rescuing potential of human stem cells in in vivo animal models of myocardial infarction. This new chemistry may ultimately pave the way to promising approaches in tissue engineering and cardiovascular repair.

Keywords: stem cells, cardiovascular repair, new molecules, regenerative medicine

INTRODUCTION

Myocardial infarction and inherited cardiomyopathies kill myocardial cells. In the adult mammalian heart, the damaged area forms a scar tissue, which impairs cardiac performance. For millions of patients every year the progression of heart damage towards heart failure is a grim reminder that current treatments are not a substitute for the irreversible loss of cardiomyocytes. Despite the development of therapeutic strategies and electrophysiological and surgical treatments, heart failure remains one of the major causes of mortality in the Western world. So far, the ultimate resort for heart failure is heart transplantation.

In the last decade, major advances in molecular and cellular biology had a significant impact on our understanding of stem cell growth and differentiation ensuing in substantial hope for the emerging new field of "regenerative medicine". As one of the least self-renewing organs in the human body, the heart would greatly take advantage of the ability of stem or progenitor cells to behave as pluripotent, self-renewable elements that can be committed to multiple cell lineages.

Nevertheless, cardiogenesis is one of the earliest and most complex morphogenetic events in the embryo, and is still poorly understood at the molecular level. An effective cell therapy for cardiac failure should therefore rely on the identification of the molecular mechanisms underlying a cardiogenic/angiogenic decision within suitable pluripotent cells committable both to myocardial and endothelial lineages, the two major cell types needed to repair a damaged heart. A growing body of evidence suggest that the potential improvement elicited by different types of stem cells in *in vivo* animal models of tissue damage (i.e. heart, and vessels) may also be largely affected by the release of a broad spectrum of "trophic factors" acting in a paracrine fashion as angiogenetic, antiapoptotic and antifibrotic molecules [1-7]. These findings suggest the potential therapeutic effect of specific "paracrine pathways" in improving the overall function in injured tissues. It is now clear that released growth factors may also act in an "autocrine" fashion on cell surface receptors of their secreting cells to afford further regulation of stem cell growth and fate specification [8]. Intriguingly, a number of growth regulatory peptides may also act in an "intracrine fashion" within their cell of synthesis coupling to nuclear receptors and chromatin binding sites to trigger nuclear signaling and transcriptional activation of tissue-restricted genes [8-10].

Based on the above, it is conceivable that affording a significant repair of a damaged myocardium is not simply an issue of stem cell transdifferentiation. Indeed, the attainment of a myocardial fate is an extremely low-yield process, even in longstanding *in vitro* models of cardiogenesis, including the well-characterized mouse embryonic stem (ES) cells. The use of virus-mediated gene transfer technologies to obtain cells transduced with cardiogenetic genes is still a cumbersome approach that may perturb normal homeostasis in both engineered cells and recipient tissues, and is not readily envisionable in humans. Therefore, future strategies in sight of a cell therapy of damaged hearts will require the development of new molecules with "differentiating logics", turning cardiogenesis into a high-throughput differentiating response.

These considerations raise the larger question as to whether strategies providing realistic underpinning for cardiovascular cell therapy (the rescue of failing hearts) should be more closely related to the biology of wound healing than regenerative medicine. This would imply a substantial shift in the paradigm of uniquely relying in stem cell transdifferentiation, and prompt further efforts in taking a glimpse on the overall paracrine patterning of secreted growth factors (secretome) that may be released from stem cells to enhance endogenous angiogenesis and remarkably counteract apoptosis and scar tissue formation in a recipient myocardium.

The present review will cover recent developments using the most extensive studies for cardiac repair. We will also focus on the emerging role of chemistry in the identification of natural products and the synthesis of multicomponent-multitarget molecules harboring both differentiating and paracrine logics for stem cell therapy of heart failure.

FINDING THE PROPER PROGENITOR

A major commitment in *in vitro* and *in vivo* studies on cardiogenesis and cardiac repair is assessing the potential for both cardiac and endothelial differentiation in putative pluripotent cells.

Embryonic Stem Cells

Besides the ethical debate, the use of human ES cells in stem cell therapy is hampered by significant technical challenges, including the isolation of fully competent ventricular cardiomyocytes and the consequences of their implantation in the infarcted myocardium. When mouse ES cells are grown in suspension in the absence of leukemia inhibitory factor (LIF), they aggregate into "embryoid bodies" which spontaneously differentiate into multiple cell types, including cardiomyocytes and endothelial cells [11, 12]. However, spontaneous differentiation is generally inefficient (less than 0.1%), ensuing into heterogeneous populations of undifferentiated and differentiated cells. This heterogeneity is a substantial bias in both biological studies of cardiogenetic programs and potential cell-based therapy *in vivo*. A major caveat is the tumorigenicity of ES cells. This is an unacceptable outcome, which deserves considerable efforts to obtain highly purified preparations of ES-derived cardiomyocytes that are free of undifferentiated, potentially tumorigenic stem cells. Another hurdle is that ES cells may be rejected by immune system or undergo potential epigenetic modifications and phenotypic drifts within the hostile environment of an infarcted myocardium.

Hematopoietic Stem Cells

Adult stem cells display a considerably wider spectrum of plasticity than previously expected, and it is now evident that they can give raise to multiple cell lineages suitable for regenerative medicine. A longstanding and well-established source of adult stem cells is the bone marrow.

Bone marrow-derived hematopoietic stem cells isolated from mice constitutively expressing enhanced green fluorescent protein (EGFP+) have been injected into the border zone of wild type mice subjected to acute myocardial infarction. These studies provided evidence for a remarkable regeneration of the infarct with EGFP+ cells [13]. In particular, colocalization of EGFP fluorescence with immunostaining for cardiac and vascular markers was associated with improvement in echocardiographic and hemodynamic indices of left ventricular performance. These findings led to further studies aiming at identifying readily accessible populations of autologous cells that might regenerate the heart. As a result, the initial findings were severely challenged in subsequent investigations, demonstrating that mouse hematopoietic bone marrow cells failed to differentiate into cardiac myocytes and repair infarcted hearts [14-16]. These controversies energized the field prompting further efforts in identifying suitable cardiogenic progenitors with potential applications in human cell therapy of heart failure. To this end, recent evidence suggests that age and disease states in humans affect the collection of sufficient healthy autologous bone marrow-derived hematopoietic stem cells for transplantation [17], which will decrease the ability of autologous cells to improve ventricular function after a myocardial infarction. Moreover, bone marrow mononuclear cells from patients with ischemic heart disease exhibit a significantly lower rescuing potential than cells from healthy subjects [18]. These findings suggest that further efforts in cardiac cell therapy will involve the identification of alternative sources of pluripotent cells, which can be committed both to myocardial and vascular fates, and then implanted in infarcted hearts even in an allogenic setting.

Human Mesenchymal Stem Cells

Human mesenchymal stem cells (hMSCs) have been first isolated from adult bone marrow (BMhMSCs) and have shown a great potential for cell therapy. These cells possess pluripotent capabilities, proliferate rapidly, induce angiogenesis, and differentiate into myogenic cells [19]. BMhMSCs have also been shown to differentiate into cardiomyocytes when injected into healthy murine hearts or cocultured with adult rat ventricular cardiomyocytes [20.21], suggesting that BMhMSCs may afford highly effective cell therapy of heart failure. So far, a major limitation in eterologous stem cell therapy of failing hearts is immunorejection. Interestingly, transplanted allogeneic hMSCs can be detected in recipients at extended time points, indicating a lack of immune recognition and clearance [22]. A role for hMSCs in reducing the incidence and severity of graft-versus-host disease (GVHD) during allogeneic transplantation has recently been reported, although the mechanisms remain to be elucidated. Coculture of hMSCs with purified subpopulations of immune cells revealed that hMSCs altered the cytokine secretion profile of dendritic cells (DCs), naive and effector T cells (T helper 1 [T(H)1] and T(H)2), and natural killer (NK) cells to induce a more anti-inflammatory or tolerant phenotype [22]. In actual fact, hMSCs coaxed mature type 1 DCs (DC1) to decrease tumor necrosis factor alpha (TNF-alpha) secretion and mature DC2 to increase interleukin-10 (IL-10) secretion; hMSCs decreased interferon gamma (IFN-gamma) secretion from T(H)1 cells, and led the T(H)2 cells to increase secretion of IL-4. hMSCs also caused an increase in the proportion of regulatory T cells (T(Regs)) and decreased secretion of IFN-gamma from the NK cells. Recent evidence suggests that enhanced production of prostaglandin E2 (PGE(2)) may have a major impact in the tolerogenic properties of hMSCs, since these cells expressed high PGE(2) in co-cultures and inhibitors of PGE(2) production mitigated hMSC-mediated immune modulation [22].

Results of a randomized study of swine BMMSCs, administered to infarcted pigs, indicated that cellular transplantation resulted in long-term engraftment, profound reduction in scar formation, and near-normalization of cardiac function [23]. Although transplanted cells were prepared from an allogeneic donor they were not rejected, suggesting a major practical advance for widespread application of hMSCs in the cell therapy of failing hearts. Recently, human "Unrestricted Somatic Stem Cells (USSCs)" isolated from umbilical cord blood have been proposed as an earlier cell type than multipotent hMSCs, possibly representing their precursor cells, displaying a great potential to differentiate into myogenic cells and induce angiogenesis [24]. Accordingly, a preclinical study using USSCs indicated substantial cardiac repair and functional recovery in a porcine model of myocardial infarction [25].

Despite these encouraging findings, the use of bone marrow-derived cells is potentially hampered by high degree of viral infection and significant decline in cell viability and differentiation with age. Besides bone marrow, the human dental pulp includes a clonogenic, rapidly proliferating population of mesenchymal stem cells (DPhMSCs) sharing an immunophenotype similar to BMhMSCs [26]. Fetal membranes may also represent tissues of particular interest for their role in preventing fetus rejection and their early embryologic origin, which may entail progenitor potential. Phenotypic and gene expression studies revealed mesenchymal stem cell-like profiles in both amnion and chorion cells of fetal membranes (FMhMSCs) [27]. These observations suggest that alternative hMSCs may prove rewarding in the rescue of injured hearts. Within this context, we have recently provided evidence that both DPhMSCs and FMhMSCs spontaneously exhibited a low-yield commitment to cardiac marker-expressing cells *in vitro* [28]. Moreover, transplantation of FMhMSCs into the hearts of rats subjected to acute myocardial infarction led to near-normalization of myocardial performance and significant reduction in scar tissue formation [28]. The cardiovascular differentiation of FMhMSCs and their rescuing potential in infarcted rat hearts were remarkably enhanced by cell pretreatment *ex vivo* in the presence of a hyaluronan mixed ester of butyric and retinoic acids (HBR) [28], a novel agent encompassing both differentiating and paracrine patterning developed in our laboratory (see below in this review).

Resident Myocardial Progenitors

Cardiomyocytes in the adult mammalian heart have long been considered as terminally differentiated cells within a tissue devoid of regenerative potential. This view has been recently overthrown. Beltrami *et al.* detected c-kit positive cells in the adult rat heart and succeeded in their ex vivo expansion [29]. When injected into infarcted myocardium, these cells differentiated into cardiomyocytes, smooth muscle and endothelial cells, rescuing the majority of the infarcted tissue [29]. Myocardial repair occurred in spite of the fact that these cells were smaller than typical cardiomyocytes without evident sarcomeric-like features [29]. Another study isolated Sca-1 positive cells in the adult mouse heart [30]. In vitro culture of these cells in the presence of the demethylating agent 5-azacytidine induced their differentiation into cardiac marker-expressing cells. Subsequent injection into acutely ischemic mouse hearts led to significant cardiac repair that appeared to be partially dependent on cell fusion [30]. Laugwitz *et al.* demonstrated that cells expressing islet-1 (isl1), a transcription factor contributing to a second wave of cardiomyocyte formation during development, could be detected in the newborn hearts of mice, rats and humans [31]. Purified isl1+ cells cocultured with cardiomyocytes exhibited both cardiogenic gene expression and cardiomyocyte features [31]. Whether isl+1 cells may hold promises for cardiac repair applications will mainly depend on whether the much rarer isl1+ cells in the adult rat could be isolated, expanded and differentiated to cardiomyocytes.

Recently, Beltrami *et al.* grew and cloned finite cell lines obtained from adult human liver, heart and bone marrow and named them human Multipotent Adult Stem Cells (hMASCs) [32]. Cloned hMASCs, obtained from the three different tissues, expressed the pluripotent state-specific transcription factors *Oct-4*, *NANOG* and *REX1*, displayed telomerase activity, and exhibited a wide range of differentiation potential, as shown both at a morphological and functional level [32]. In neurogenic medium, hMASCs acquired electrophysiological properties indicative of functional differentiation toward neuronal phenotypes [32]. In conditioned media, hMASCs showed organized filaments of α-actinin and α-sarcomeric actin. Gap-junctions were demonstrated by the presence of connexin-43 in proximity to cell-to-cell contact sites. Ryanodine receptors were organized in tubular structures interdigitating α-actinin filaments, suggesting their localization in the developing sarcoplasmic reticulum [32]. L-Type calcium channels were also identified in differentiated cells. In separate experiments hMASCs could also be committed to endodermic differentiation, acquiring some hepatocytic functions such as the abilities to store glycogen, to produce albumin, and to exhibit an inducible cytochrome P450 activity. hMASCs maintained a human diploid DNA content, and shared a common gene expression signature, as compared to several somatic cell lines and irrespectively of the tissue of isolation. In particular, the pathways regulating stem cell self-renewal/maintenance, such as Wnt, Hedgehog and Notch, were transcriptionally active [32]. On the whole, these results indicate the adult heart, like other adult organs encompasses pluripotent cells that can be expanded *in vitro* and induced to acquire morphological and functional features of mature cells even embryologically not related to the tissue of origin.

Lessons from Clinical Trials

Most of clinical trials involving bone marrow for myocardial repair have been uncontrolled or used non-randomized controls for comparison and have been focused on bone marrow mononuclear cells, a heterogeneous population of hematopoietic and hMSCs containing less than 0.1% stem cells. As reviewed in detail elsewhere [33], cells have both been delivered intracoronary to patients with recent myocardial infarction or subjected to catheter-based intramyocardial injection into patients with chronic ischemic disease and old infarcts. Interestingly these trials indicated that cell delivery was feasible and devoid of significant complications. However, while several studies reported improved ventricular function and perfusion, recent double-blind, randomized, placebo-controlled trials in patients receiving intracoronary unfractionated bone marrow cells within 24 hours of acute infarction reported modest [34] or no improvement in ejection fraction [35,36]. Nevertheless, enhanced infarct shrinkage was detected with magnetic resonance imaging, suggesting that several degree of cardiac repair might have occurred [35]. An important cautionary note was raised by a recent randomized clinical trial showing that an increase in cardiac performance following bone marrow cell transfer in patients in patients with acute myocardial infarction was short-lived, and that the difference with the control group receiving optimal post-infarction therapy was significant after six months but not after 18 months [37].

On the whole, the results from these clinical studies indicate that additional randomized, controlled clinical trials should be warranted to explore the efficacy of stem cell transplantation as a novel therapy for myocardial infarction and failure.

Clearly, more efficient and selective strategies are needed to direct the proliferation and the differentiation of stem cells to produce homogeneous populations of particular cell types (i.e. cardiomyocytes, endothelial and smooth muscle cells). Strategies to enhance the release of throphic mediators with paracrine angiogenic antiapoptotic and antifibrotic properties should also be envisioned. These requirements highlight the crucial role of basic science studies unraveling the molecular plight impacting the process of cardiogenesis, the generation of high yields of cardiovascular elements, and secretome regulation from suitable precursor cells.

MOLECULAR DISSECTION OF CARDIOGENESIS: A MAJOR REQUIREMENT FOR FURTHER STEPS IN CARDIAC CELL THERAPY

Stem cell fate is fashioned at multiple interconnected levels and is controlled by a complex interplay between cell signaling, nucleosomal assembly, the establishment of multifaceted transcriptional motifs and the temporal and spatial organization of chromatin in loops and domains. It's now clear that a selected number of lineage-restricted transcription factors, including the "zinc finger-containing" GATA-4 and the homeodomain Nkx-2.5 are essential for cardiogenesis in different animal species, including humans [38-40]. However, the identification of genes and signaling patterning recruited for the expression of cardiogenic transcription factors is only partially exploited. The analysis of cardiac lineage commitment in mouse ES cells and *in vivo* models of cardiac differentiation revealed that a number of crucial growth factors are released from precursor cells, acting in an autocrine fashion on specific plasma membrane receptors to prime a cardiogenic decision. In this regard, we have found that the prodynorphin gene, encoding for the dynorphin family of endorphin peptides, was expressed in pluripotent mouse embryonal carcinoma cells, acting as a major conductor for their differentiation into cardiomyocytes [41]. In our subsequent studies using mouse ES cells, we found that dynorphin B, a natural agonist of κ opioid receptors, was synthesized and secreted by undifferentiated ES cells [42]. The secreted peptide acted in an autocrine loop on plasma membrane endorphin receptors to trigger the activation and subcellular redistribution of targeted protein kinase C (PKC) isozymes, a signaling response that emerged as a major molecular trait in cardiogenesis [42]. Intriguingly, immunoreactive dynorphin B was consistently detectable within undifferentiated cells and was remarkably enhanced in ES-derived cardiomyocytes, spreading throughout the cytoplasm and gatering around the nucleus [43], suggesting that endorphins may also act intracellularly. We found that nuclei isolated from undifferentiated ES cells express k endorphin receptors and that their stimulation activated nuclear-resident PKC isozymes leading to the transcription of genes encoding cardiogenic transcription factors [43]. The term "intracrine" has been proposed for the action of a peptide hormone either within its cell of synthesis or after internalization. An intracrine must retain the potential of being found in the extracellular space producing a response after binding to a membrane receptor like a traditional endocrine, paracrine or autocrine. Besides this, a putative intracrine factor must be found in association with one or more intracellular organelles not associated with secretory or degratory structures (these may arguably be viewed as extensions of the extracellular space). Our finding that a cardiogenic program may be recapitulated by a nuclear endorphinergic system, suggests that cardiogenesis may also be orchestrated by self-sustaining intracrine loops behaving as long-lived signals that impart features characteristic of differentiation, growth regulation and cell memory.

Besides endorphins and their related signals, other crucial growth factors and signaling patterning have been found to act in an autocrine/intracrine fashion to orchestrate cell growth and differentiation. These include the Wnt pathway, the renin-angiotensin system, VEGF, BDNF, and FGF-2. Most of these systems have been found to have an important role in cardiac and/or vascular differentiation. The interested reader is referred to our recent review on this field [8].

MULTICOMPONENT-MULTITARGET MOLECULES, A NEW CHEMISTRY FOR STEM CELL THERAPY

Stem cell fate is orchestrated both by intrinsic modulators (i.e. the expression of genes and tissue-restricted transcription factors, signaling pathway) and the extracellular environment (niche).

Design and Synthesis of Novel Differentiating Agents

Recent developments in the area of stem cell research have been boosted by an increasing understanding of transcriptional regulation and epigenetic modifications, including histone acetylation, DNA methylation and chromatin remodeling. This is a crucial issue, since the rescuing potential of cardiac stem cell therapy is severely limited by the fact that stem cell-derived cardiomyocytes withdraw early from the cell cycle and by the low yield of cardiogenic commitment. The development of molecules affording high-throughput of cardiogenesis from pluripotent cells would have obvious therapeutic potential and is an emerging new field in regenerative medicine.

We have recently developed hyaluronan mixed esters with retinoic and butyric acid, and provided evidence that these compounds (HBR) act as novel differentiating agents eliciting a remarkable increase in the yield of cardiomyocytes derived from mouse ES cells [44]. The rationale for the synthesis of these novel glycoconjugates is discussed in detail elsewhere [44]. Briefly, the CD44 HA receptor is highly expressed by cardiogenic cells [45] and cardiogenesis is abrogated by disruption of hyaluronan synthase-2 [46]. HA promotes CD44-dependent angiogenesis [47]. HA-binding proteins translocate to the nucleus, priming cell growth and differentiation [48-51]. Hence, HA may regulate cardiovascular commitment, acting as a carrier for HA-grafting synthetic compounds, such as butyrate (BU) and retinoic acid (RA). BU, inhibits histone deacetylases, increasing transcription factor accessibility to target *cis*-acting regulatory sites [52], and drives both endothelial and cardiac fates [53]. Grafting of RA into HBR is supported by the occurrence of abnormal heart development following RXRalpha gene inactivation [54,55] and by RA-mediated increase in ES cardiogenesis [56] and mammalian vascular development [57]. Notably, histone deacetylase inhibitors enhance RXR/RAR heterodimer action, and major developmental patterns in stem cells [58]. In our study, HBR remarkably increased the expression of the cardiac lineage-promoting genes GATA-4, Nkx-2.5, and prodynorphin [44], enhancing the synthesis and secretion of dynorphin B. Nuclear run-off transcription analyses indicated that these effects occurred at the transcriptional level. The activation of such a cardiogenic program of gene transcription was associated with an increase in the expression of the cardiac specific genes MHC and MLC-2V, giving raise to high yields of spontaneously beating ES-derived cardiomyocytes. HBR failed to affect the transcription rate of MyoD and neurogenin1 [44], two genes involved in skeletal myogenesis and neuronal determination, respectively, indicating that a novel generation of mixed esters of hyaluronan may be proposed to selectively organize lineage patterning in ES cells.

These results demonstrate the potential for chemically modifying the gene program of cardiac differentiation in ES cells without the aid of gene transfer technologies and may pave the way for novel approaches in tissue engineering and myocardial regeneration.

Recently, we have used HBR to successfully enhance the commitment of BMhMSCs, as well as DPhMSCs and FMhMSCs, towards a cardiovascular decision *in vitro* [28]. As reported above in this review, a limited percentage (about 1%) of these populations of hMSCs spontaneously differentiated in culture into cardiac marker expressing cells [28]. In each cell population, HBR remarkably increased both GATA-4 and Nkx-2.5 mRNA expression, leading to high yields of cells expressing cardiac specific markers, including sarcomeric myosin heavy chain, α-sarcomeric actinin, and connexin 43. Flow cytometry analysis revealed that about 36% of HBR-exposed FMhMSCs differentiated in α-sarcomeric actinin positive cells, as compared to about 15% of BMhMSCs exposed to the hyaluronan mixed ester [28]. HBR treatment also enhanced the gene expression of Vascular Endothelial Growth Factor (VEGF), KDR, encoding for a major VEGF receptor, and Hepatocyte Growth Factor (HGF) [28]. Consonant with the pivotal role of these genes in both endothelial tissue formation (vasculogenesis) and sprouting of new blood vessels from pre-existing vessels (angiogenesis), stem cell exposure to the glycoconjugate gave raise to von Willebrand factor (vWF)-expressing endothelial cells [28]. Also in the attainment of an endothelial fate, FMhMSCs proved to be more responsive to HBR (more than 40% of vWF+ cells), compared to HBR-pretread BMhMSCs (about 18%). Interestingly, HBR primed a remarkable and sustained (more than 14 days) increase in the secretion of both VEGF and HGF [28]. To this end, BMhMSCs overexpressing Akt have been shown to inhibit ventricular remodeling and restore cardiac function mainly through paracrine mechanisms involving an increase in the expression of VEGF, FGF-2, and HGF genes and enhanced secretion of their related products [59,60]. Accordingly, monolayered adipose tissue-derived mesenchymal stem cells repaired scarred myocardium in infarcted rat hearts acting as trophic mediators for paracrine angiogenic pathways [61]. Under our experimental conditions, the differentiating and paracrine effects primed by HBR *in vitro* were remarkably more pronounced in FMhMSCs than in BMhMSCs or DPhMSCs. Transplantation of FMhMSCs preconditioned *ex vivo* with HBR into the hearts of rats subjected to acute myocardial infarction by coronary ligation led to complete normalization of myocardial performance and dramatic reduction in scar formation [28]. The injection of HBR-treated cells was followed by a significant increase in density of capillaries negative for anti-human vWF, compared to the capillary density observed in the tissue transplanted with untreated cells. Both VEGF, and HGF not only possess angiogenic but also cardioprotective effects, including antiapoptotic, mitogenic and antifibrotic activities [62,63]. HGF gene transfer into the myocardium improved myocardial function and geometry [64], in particular owing to antifibrotic effects through inhibition of transforming growth factor-β expression. Thus, enhanced *in vivo* release of VEGF and HGF by HBR-pretreated FMhMSCs may have contributed both to the observed angiogenic response and the reduction of infarct size and scar formation through antiapoptic and antifibrotic paracrine actions. Besides this, in the hearts injected with HBR-exposed FMhMSCs, the yield of cells positively stained with a human-specific anti-vWF antibody remarkably exceeded the number of vWF-positive cells detected in samples from the untreated group [28]. A consistent organization of human vWF positive cells into erythrocyte containing capillary vessels was only observed in hearts transplanted with HBR-treated FMhMSCs. Hence, the endothelial lineage commitment primed by HBR *in vitro* was retained within the transplanted cells in the infarcted myocardium, suggesting that HBR-treated cells may also contribute to neovascularization and heart rescue through their ability to generate capillary-like structures. A consistent amount of the transplanted cells that had been pretreated with HBR also exhibited a colocalization of connexin 43 and cardiac troponin I with a human mitochondrial protein [28].

Noteworthy, xenogeneic FMhMSC transplantation was devoid of immune rejection and did not require immunosuppressant procedures. This observation and the finding that FMhMSCs exhibited larger differentiating and paracrine repsonses to HBR compared to DPhMSCs or BMhMSCs may be relevant for future development of new chemistry designed for targeting stem cell fate and therapy. In fact, the use of FMhMSCs may circumvent the hurdles of collecting healthy autologous bone marrow cells from aged and/or diseased patients [17]. FMhMSCs do not induce allogeneic or xenogeneic lymphocyte proliferation and actively suppress lymphocyte responsiveness [65]. Moreover, FMhMSC transplantation in neonatal swine and rats resulted in human microchimerism in various organs and tissues [65]. Therefore, the combined use of novel chemical agents and tolerogenic human msenchymal stem cells isolated from alternative sources to the bone marrow may offer promise for unprecedented "of the shelf" strategies of cardiovascular cell therapy. Within this context, cell-based phenotypic assays and the screening of wide ranging signaling pathways elicited by synthetic small molecules and natural products have recently provided useful tools for both orienting cell lineage and gaining insights into the molecular patterning underlying targeted fate specification. In particular, the screening of large combinatorial chemical libraries of synthetic small molecules indicated that diaminopyrimidine compounds, named cardiogenols, could selectively induce mouse embryonal carcinoma and ES cells to adopt a cardiogenic fate [66].

THE CONCEPT OF "NICHE" AND THE DEVELOPMENT OF NANOFABRICATED SCAFFOLDS

Stem cell commitment may be regulated not only by chemical but physical stimuli and by the cell shape itself. Both external and internal forces regulate cell shape creating a complex and still poorly defined habitat, the "niche". During *in vivo* embryonic development, not only biochemical soluble signals, but also macromolecular components of the extracellular matrix (ECM) ma play an important role in defining and guiding multiple differentiation processes. Besides providing a physical support, the ECM also displays an array of macromolecular cues that orchestrate cell proliferation and differentiation. Culturing mouse ES cells in various semi-interpenetrating polymer networks made of collagen, fibronectin and laminin is providing evidence that both composition and strength of the supporting matrix is essential in stem cell differentiation [67]. In recent years remarkable progress has been done in the engineering of biomaterials with the aim of creating multiscale 3D architectures to promote tissue repair and regeneration. The urgent needs for nanosized and nanostructured polymeric biomaterials to mimic natural cellular environment affording better control of cellular patterning for targeted biomedical applications, has driven researchers towards the design of more advanced biomaterial nanofabrication technologies. Through the application of nanotechnology in medicine, it has become possible to design smart, multi-functional implants composed of polymeric structures with suitable architectures, bioactive signaling factors and cells, which can interact with the surrounding micro-environment and facilitate tissue regeneration. When stem cells are combined with bioactive materials, a major breakthrough is expected, since such a combination would remarkably increase both the differentiation potential and the secretion of "trophic" factors involved in tissue repair and survival.

Tissue engineering using 3D polymeric scaffolds will conceivably offer an alternative approach to the direct cell injection for tissue repair. The 3D artificial structures (functionalized with bioactive molecules and growth factors) could replace the damaged tissue and provide a temporary support for resident or implanted cells, thus recreating a niche properly influencing stem cell homing, self-renewal and differentiation. There is now increasing hope that within these scaffolds transplanted stem cells may be able to mimic their ability to replicate and migrate out of the niche towards the sites of cell replacement where they differentiate. The design of synthetic materials that mimic natural stem cell microenvironments may be a potentially powerful tool both to understand and control stem cell function. Research in this field is still very limited, and artificial niches for stem cells have been developed mainly using artificial proteins with applications limited to neural stem cells [68-71]. It is now evident that novel scaffolds can be fabricated with the aim of creating an "integrated niche" encompassing both the stem cells and differentiating molecules suitable for attaining a high-throughput of cell differentiation and paracrine release of trophic mediators [61,72,73]. Stem cell culture on micro-nanopatterned substrates has provided evidence that stem cells can "sense" substrate features or topography at micro-nanoscale level adjusting the degree of cell spreading against the substrate and their fates in relation to the physical patterning of the substrate itself [74]. It is well recognized that 3D nanofibrous structures mimicking the extracellular environment play a role in modulating cellular response. Nanofiber fabrication at present is dominated by electrospinning technology [72,73]. Novel electrospun nanofibrous polymeric scaffolds with adjustable fiber size and orientation are expected to offer a structurally bio-mimetic environment to stem cells, therefore improving both their culturing conditions and the output of clinically transplantable cells.

Stem Cell Differentiation by Physical Stimuli

Stem cell commitment, and the resulting development of lineage-specific characteristics, have been shown to be affected by cell shape [74-78]. Internal and external forces regulate cell shape and studies have shown that cell shape can control apoptosis, gene expression, and protein synthesis, in addition to stem cell fate [77-79]. Studies in which physical and/or chemical changes of the stem cell are tracked throughout differentiation in an attempt to deduce the inherent forces would be a logical extension of these discoveries. Another logical consequence of this perception should be the development of studies aiming at assessing whether specific physical stimuli can be "delivered" to cultured stem cells in the attempt to change their fate and terminal differentiation. A variety of studies using internal and external forces in the nN to pN range have been exploited by the aid of atomic force microscopy (AFM), optical tweezers, magnetic tweezers, and magnetic twisting cytometry, posing the basis to measure the structural and nanomechanical properties of growth and differentiation at the single cell level [80,81]. Within this context we have shown that exposure of mouse ES cells to sinusoidal extremely low-frequency magnetic fields (50 Hz, 0.8 mTrms) remarkably increased the expression of the cardiogenic genes GATA-4 and Nkx-2.5 ensuing in a high yield of spontaleously beating cardiomyocytes [82]. Magnetic fields also enhanced prodynorphin mRNA expression and the levels of dynorphin B, in both embryoid bodies (EBs) and ES-derived cardiomyocytes, and in their incubation media [82]. Interestingly, nuclear run-off analyses performed in isolated ES nuclei indicated that the MF action occurred at the transcriptional level [82]. This finding is particularly rewarding, due to the autocrine/intracrine roles of the prodynorphin gene and its related product dynorphin B in ES cells cardiogenesis. The observation that cell fate may be orchestrated by magnetic fields opens the new perspective of using magnetic energy to direct the differentiation processes of stem cells into a specific cellular phenotype without the aid of gene transfer or chemical-based technologies. These findings also prompt future investigations to shed additional light on the molecular events underlying the differentiating response primed by MF in ES cells and to assess whether such a response may be dependent on the field characteristics including MF intensity, frequency and wave shape.

CONCLUSION

For many years the idea of regenerating the heart has been skeptically regarded. The recent findings in stem cell research open an optimistic scenario for cardiac cell therapy. However, we believe that this hope is for the future. A note of caution is currently worth sounding and a number of interrelated general challenges remain to be addressed, including:

High-Throughput Bioprocess Development and Improved Downstream Processing

Bioprocess development involves the design and practical demonstration of scaleable, reproducible and regulatory-compliant processes. This implies significant modification, improvement and re-testing of current strategies of stem cell culturing and cardiovascular commitment complying with all standards of Good Manufacturing Practice (GMP). In particular, the current state-of-the-art is hampered by low-yield processing in stem cell expansion and differentiation that may lead to unacceptable performance on scale-up. These general problems are particularly relevant in extremely low-yield processes, such as cardiogenesis, causing a severe delay in reaching a stable and acceptable manufacturing process, prolonging time to both clinic and market.

Development of Novel Multicomponents-Multitargets Molecules Harboring Both Differentiating and Paracrine Logics

The current logics in chemical manipulation of stem cell fate for tissue repair are to apply single powerful natural or synthetic factors to trigger and/or enhance the onset of phenotypic processes. Future efforts will be based on the design, synthesis and development of single-multitarget or multicomponent-multitarget molecules capable to enter the stem cells and act through a timely release of the assembled moieties to affect both cardio/vasulogenic signaling and secretome patterning. the secretion of trophic mediators of tissue repair. These developments will provide a major breakthrough towards the integration of transcriptional therapies and stem cell therapy for the rescue of damaged heart. Another major technological and commercial impact is that these molecules, like the stem cells, must be produced under GMP conditions and that all chemical synthesis will start from GMP-grade reagents. These features will support the definition and control of parameters critical to biomanufacturing, particularly in downstream recovery and purification and in formulation, and help ensure that safe, stable, economically produced biopharmaceuticals for stem cell manipulation are successfully brought to market. This understanding may also contribute to the development of biopharmaceuticals in which manufacturability is built into the molecules during early discovery.

Integration of Nanofabrications and Stem Cell Therapy

Stem cells are defined by their function in complex microenvironments that are just beginning to be defined. The architecture of these anatomic sites in molecular, cellular and developmental terms has provided insight into how tissues are formed and maintained throughout life. They now provide an opportunity for examining settings of disease and offering a distinct group of possible therapeutic interventions. The development of novel nanofabricated scaffolds will deeply impact on our understanding of stem cell niches to explore unifying principles and identify opportunities for application in both stem cell culturing and tissue regeneration. This will result in an additional high-technology output from GMP cell factories.

Analytical Methodologies for Control of Bioprocessing and Differentiation Efficiencies

The development of high-throughput screening techniques, and array biochips will have a significant impact in the establishment of improved analytical methods and tools for the design, analysis and control of bioprocessing through measurement of critical parameters. Another impact of the establishment of analytical methodologies is that they will form "predictive tools" to give a forecast output of a change to a bioprocess. Such predictive and risk-based tools are important in bioprocess development to assist in achieving a stable process (i.e. cardiovascular commitment and paracrine release of growth factors suitable for cardiovascular repair). To this end, high-throughput analytical methods will help development of cardiovascular cell therapy at a number of scales including: (i) Molecular – predicting the impact of molecular characteristics on processing decisions, performance and product properties; (ii) Cellular – the impact of cellular characteristics on processing efficiency; (iii) Unit operation – predicting the behaviour of unit operations and sequences of operations at scale.

The field of regenerative medicine is moving extremely quickly, involving both clinical expectations and economical interests. In order to gain real perspectives for cardiac repair, we need to bring together cell biologists, clinicians, chemists, physics, and engineers to expand our knowledge on the fundamental biology of stem cells and strategies of bioprocessing and scale up within a GMP environment. If these efforts are successful, stem cells may become a tool for improving the health of millions of people suffering for heart failure.

ACKNOWLEDGMENTS

This work was supported by Ministero della Sanità (attività di Ricerca Finalizzata – 2006, "Il buon uso dell'organo"). Activity was performed in cooperation with and supported by "Centro Nazionale Trapianti", Rome, Italy, within the context of the "Italian Transplant Research Network".

REFERENCES

[1] Kim, DH; Yoo, KH; Choi, KS; Choi, J; Choi, SY; Yang, SE; Yang, YS; Im, HJ; Kim, KH; Jung, HL; Sung, KW; Koo, HH. Gene expression profile of cytokine and growth factor during differentiation of bone marrow-derived mesenchymal stem cell. *Cytokine,* 2005, *31,* 119-126.

[2] Mayer, H; Bertram, H; Lindenmaier, W; Korff, T; Weber, H; Weich, H. Vascular endothelial growth factor (VEGF-A) expression in human mesenchymal stem cells:

autocrine and paracrine role on osteoblastic and endothelial differentiation. *J. Cell. Biochem.,* 2005, *95,* 827-839.

[3] Kinnaird, T; Stabile, E; Burnett, MS; Lee, CW; Barr, S; Fuchs, S; Epstein SE. Marrow-derived stromal cells express genes encoding a broad spectrum of arteriogenic cytokines and promote in vitro and in vivo arteriogenesis through paracrine mechanisms. *Circ. Res.,* 2004, *94,* 678-685.

[4] Caplan, AI; Dennis, JE. Mesenchymal stem cells as trophic mediators. *J. Cell. Biochem.,* 2006, *98,* 1076-1084.

[5] Mangi, AA; Noiseux, N; Kong, D; He, H; Rezvani, M; Ingwall, JS; Dzau, VJ. Mesenchymal stem cells modified with Akt prevent remodeling and restore performance of infarcted hearts. *Nat. Med.,* 2003, *9,* 1195-1201.

[6] Tang, YL; Zhao, Q; Zhang, YC; Cheng, L; Liu, M; Shi, J; Yang, YZ; Pan, C; Ge, J; Phillips, MI. Autologous mesenchymal stem cell transplantation induce VEGF and neovascularization in ischemic myocardium. *Regul. Pept.,* 2004, *117,* 3-10.

[7] Nagaya, N; Kangawa, K; Itoh, T; Iwase, T; Murakami, S; Miyahara, Y; Fujii, T; Uematsu, M; Ohgushi, H; Yamagishi, M; Tokudome, T; Mori, H; Miyatake, K; Kitamura, S. Transplantation of mesenchymal stem cells improves cardiac function in a rat model of dilated cardiomyopathy. *Circulation,* 2005, *112,* 1128-1135.

[8] Ventura, C; Branzi, A. Autocrine and intracrine signaling for cardiogenesis in embryonic stem cells: a clue for the development of novel differentiating agents. *Handb. Exp. Pharmacol.,* 2006, *174,* 123-146.

[9] Re, RN; Cook, JL. An intracrine view of angiogenesis. *Bioessays,* 2006, *28,* 943-953.

[10] Re, RN. Intracellular renin and the nature of intracrine enzymes. *Hypertension,* 2003, *42,* 117-122.

[11] Doetschman, TC; Eistetter, H; Katz, M; Schmidt, W; Kemier, R. The in vitro development of blastocyst-derived embryonic stem cell lines: formation of visceral yolk sac, blood islands and myocardium. *J. Embryol. Exp. Morphol.,* 1985, *87,* 27-45.

[12] Maltsev, VA; Rohwedel, J; Hescheler, J; Wobus AM. Embryonic stem cells differentiate in vitro into cardiomyocytes representing sinusoidal, atrial and ventricular cell types. *Mech. Dev.,* 1993, *44,* 41-50.

[13] Orlic, D; Kajstura, J; Chimenti, S; Jakoniuk, I; Anderson, SM; Li, B; Pickel, J; McKay, R; Nadal-Ginard, B; Bodine, DM; Anversa, P. Bone marrow cells regenerate infarcted myocardium. *Nature,* 2001, *410,* 701-705.

[14] Balsam, LB; Wagers, AJ; Christensen, JL; Kofidis, T; Weissman, IL; Robbins RC. Haematopoietic stem cells adopt mature haematopoietic fates in ischaemic myocardium. *Nature,* 2004, *428,* 668-673.

[15] Murry, CE; Soonpaa, MH; Reinecke, H; Nakajima, H; Nakajima, HO; Rubart, M; Pasumarthi, KBS; Virag, JI; Bartelmez, SH; Poppa, V; Bradford, G; Dowell, JD; Williams, DA; Field, LJ. Haematopoietic stem cells do not transdifferentiate into cardiac myocytes in myocardial infarcts. *Nature,* 2004, *428,* 664-668.

[16] Nygren, JM; Jovinge, S; Breitbach, M; Sawen, P; Roll, W; Hescheler, J; Taneera, J; Fleischmann, BK; Jacobsen, SE. Bone marrow-derived hematopoietic cells generate cardiomyocytes at a low frequency through cell fusion, but not transdifferentiation. *Nat. Med.,* 2004, *10,* 494-501.

[17] Scheubel, RJ; Zorn. H; Silber, RE; Kuss, O; Morawietz, H; Holtz, J; Simm, A. Age-dependent depression in circulating endothelial progenitor cells in patients undergoing coronary artery bypass grafting. *J. Am. Coll. Cardiol.*, 2003, *42*, 2073–2080.

[18] Heeschen, C; Lehmann, R; Honold, J; Assmus, B; Aicher, A; Walter, DH; Martin, H; Zeiher, AM; Dimmeler, S. Profoundly reduced neovascularization capacity of bone marrow mononuclear cells derived from patients with chronic ischemic heart disease. *Circulation*, 2004, *109*, 1615–1622.

[19] Pittenger, MF; Martin, BJ. Mesenchymal stem cells and their potential as cardiac therapeutics. *Circ. Res.*, 2004, *95*, 9-20.

[20] Toma, C; Pittenger, MF; Cahill, KS; Byrne, BJ; Kessler, PD. Human mesenchymal stem cells differentiate to a cardiomyocyte phenotype in the adult murine heart. *Circulation*, 2002, *105*, 93-98.

[21] Rangappa, S; Entwistle, JW; Wechsler, AS; Kresh, JY. Cardiomyocyte-mediated contact programs human mesenchymal stem cells to express cardiogenic phenotype. *J. Thorac. Cardiovasc. Surg.*, 2003, 126, 124-132.

[22] Aggarwal, S; Pittenger, MF. Human mesenchymal stem cells modulate allogeneic immune cell responses. *Blood*, 2005, *105*, 1815-1822.

[23] Amado, LC; Saliaris, AP; Schuleri, KH; St John, M; Xie, JS; Cattaneo, S; Durand, DJ; Fitton, T; Kuang, JQ; Stewart, G; Lehrke, S; Baumgartner, WW; Martin, BJ; Heldman, AW; Hare, JM. Cardiac repair with intramyocardial injection of allogeneic mesenchymal stem cells after myocardial infarction. *Proc. Natl. Acad. Sci. USA*, 2005, *102*, 11474-11479.

[24] Kogler, G; Sensken, S; Airey, JA; Trapp, T; Muschen, M; Feldhahn, N; Liedtke, S; Sorg, RV; Fischer, J; Rosenbaum, C; Greschat, S; Knipper, A; Bender, J; Degistirici, O; Gao, J; Caplan, AI; Colletti, EJ; Almeida-Porada, G; Muller, HW; Zanjani, E; Wernet, P. A new human somatic stem cell from placental cord blood with intrinsic pluripotent differentiation potential. *J. Exp. Med.*, 2004, *200*, 123-135.

[25] Kim, BO; Tian, H; Prasongsukarn, K; Wu, J; Angoulvant, D; Wnendt, S; Muhs, A; Spitkovsky, D; Li, RK. Cell transplantation improves ventricular function after a myocardial infarction: a preclinical study of human unrestricted somatic stem cells in a porcine model. *Circulation*, 2005, *112(9 Suppl)*, I96-104.

[26] Gronthos, S; Mankani, M; Brahim, J; Gehron Robey, P; Shi, S. Postnatal human dental pulp stem cells (DPSCs) in vitro and in vivo. *Proc. Natl. Acad. Sci. USA*, 2000, *97*, 13625-13630.

[27] In 't Anker, PS; Scherjon, SA; Kleijburg-van der Keur, C; de Groot-Swings, GM; Claas, FH; Fibbe, WE; Kanhai, HH. Isolation of mesenchymal stem cells of fetal or maternal origin from human placenta. *Stem Cells*, 2004, *22*, 1338-1345.

[28] Ventura, C; Cantoni, S; Bianchi, F; Lionetti, V; Cavallini, C; Scarlata, I; Foroni, L; Maioli, M; Bonsi, L; Alviano, F; Fossati, V; Bagnara, GP; Pasquinelli, G; Recchia, FA; Perbellini, A. Hyaluronan mixed esters of butyric and retinoic Acid drive cardiac and endothelial fate in term placenta human mesenchymal stem cells and enhance cardiac repair in infarcted rat hearts. *J. Biol. Chem.*, 2007, *282*, 14243-14252.

[29] Beltrami, AP; Barlucchi, L; Torella, D; Baker, M; Limana, F; Chimenti, S; Kasahara, H; Rota, M; Musso, E; Urbanek, K; Leri, A; Kajstura, J; Nadal-Ginard, B; Anversa, P.

Adult cardiac stem cells are multipotent and support myocardial regeneration. *Cell,* 2003, *114*, 763-776.

[30] Oh, H; Bradfute, SB; Gallardo, TD; Nakamura, T; Gaussin, V; Mishina, Y; Pocius, J; Michael, LH; Behringer, RR; Garry, DJ; Entman, ML; Schneider, MD. Cardiac progenitor cells from adult myocardium: homing, differentiation, and fusion after infarction. *Proc. Natl. Acad. Sci. USA,* 2003, *100*, 12313-12318.

[31] Laugwitz, KL; Moretti, A; Lam, J; Gruber, P; Chen, Y; Woodard, S; Lin, LZ; Cai, CL; Lu, MM.; Reth, M; Platoshyn, O; Yuan, JX; Evans, S; Chien, KR. Postnatal isl1+ cardioblasts enter fully differentiated cardiomyocyte lineages. *Nature,* 2005, *433*, 647-653.

[32] Beltrami, A; Cesselli, D; Bergamin, N; Marcon, P; Rigo, S; Puppato, E; D'Aurizio, F; Verardo, R; Piazza, S; Pignatelli, A; Poz, A; Baccarani, U; Damiani, D; Fanin, R; Mariuzzi, L; Finato, N; Masolini, P; Burelli, S; Belluzzi, O; Schneider, C; Beltrami, CA. Multipotent cells can be generated in vitro from several adult human organs (heart, liver and bone marrow). *Blood,* 2007 prepublished online May 24, 2007; DOI 10.1182/blood-2006-11-055566

[33] Dimmeler, S; Zeiher, AM; Schneider, MD. Unchain my heart: the scientific foundations of cardiac repair. *J. Clin. Invest.,* 2005, *115*, 572-583.

[34] Cleland, JG; Freemantle, N; Coletta, AP; Clark, AL. Clinical trials update from the American Heart Association: REPAIR-AMI, ASTAMI, JELIS, MEGA, REVIVE-II, SURVIVE, and PROACTIVE. *Eur. J. Heart. Fail.,* 2006, *8*, 105-110.

[35] Janssens, S; Dubois, C; Bogaert, J; Theunissen, K; Deroose, C; Desmet, W; Kalantzi, M; Herbots, L; Sinnaeve, P; Dens, J; Maertens, J; Rademakers, F; Dymarkowski, S; Gheysens, O; Van Cleemput, J; Bormans, G; Nuyts, J; Belmans, A; Mortelmans, L; Boogaerts, M; Van de Werf, F. Autologous bone marrow-derived stem-cell transfer in patients with ST-segment elevation myocardial infarction: double-blind, randomised controlled trial. *Lancet,* 2006, *367*, 113-121.

[36] Lunde, K; Solheim, S; Aakhus, S; Arnesen, H; Abdelnoor, M; Forfang, K. ASTAMI investigators. Autologous stem cell transplantation in acute myocardial infarction: The ASTAMI randomized controlled trial. Intracoronary transplantation of autologous mononuclear bone marrow cells, study design and safety aspects. *Scand. Cardiovasc. J.,* 2005, *39*, 150-158.

[37] Meyer, GP; Wollert, KC; Lotz, J; Steffens, J; Lippolt, P; Fichtner, S; Hecker, H; Schaefer, A; Arseniev, L; Hertenstein, B; Ganser, A; Drexler, H. Intracoronary bone marrow cell transfer after myocardial infarction: eighteen months' follow-up data from the randomized, controlled BOOST (BOne marrOw transfer to enhance ST-elevation infarct regeneration) trial. *Circulation,* 2006, *113*, 1287-1294.

[38] Grepin, C; Robitaille, L; Antakly, T; Nemer, M. Inhibition of transcription factor GATA-4 expression blocks in vitro cardiac muscle differentiation. *Mol. Cell. Biol.,* 1995, *15*, 4095-4102.

[39] Biben, C; Harvey, RP. Homeodomain factor Nkx-2.5 controls left/right asimmetric expression of bHLH gene eHand during heart development. *Genes Dev.,* 1997, *11*, 1357-1369.

[40] Schott, JJ; Benson, DW; Basson, CT; Pease, W; Silberbach, GM; Moak, JP; Maron, BJ; Seidman, CE; Seidman, JG. Congenital heart disease caused by mutations in the transcription factor Nkx-2.5. *Science,* 1998, *281*, 108-111.

[41] Ventura, C; Maioli, M. Opioid peptide gene expression primes cardiogenesis in embryonal pluripotent stem cells. *Circ. Res.,* 2000, *87*, 189-194.

[42] Ventura, C; Zinellu, E; Maninchedda, E; Fadda, M; Maioli, M. Protein kinase C signaling transduces endorphin-primed cardiogenesis in GTR1 embryonic stem cells. *Circ. Res.,* 2003, *92*, 617-622.

[43] Ventura, C; Zinellu, E; Maninchedda, E; Maioli, M. Dynorphin B is an agonist of nuclear opioid receptors coupling nuclear protein kinase C activation to the transcription of cardiogenic genes in GTR1 embryonic stem cells. *Circ. Res.,* 2003, *92*, 623-629.

[44] Ventura, C; Maioli, M; Asara, Y; Santoni, D; Scarlata, I; Cantoni, S; Perbellini, A. Butyric and retinoic mixed ester of hyaluronan. A novel differentiating glycoconjugate affording a high throughput of cardiogenesis in embryonic stem cells. *J. Biol. Chem.,* 2004, *279*, 23574-23579.

[45] Wheatley, SC; Isacke, CM; Crossley, PH. Restricted expression of the hyaluronan receptor, CD44, during postimplantation mouse embryogenesis suggests key roles in tissue formation and patterning. *Development,* 1993, *119*, 295–306.

[46] Camenisch, TD; Spicer, AP; Brehm-Gibson, T; Biesterfeldt, J; Augustine, ML; Calabro, A Jr; Kubalak, S; Klewer, SE; McDonald, JA. Disruption of hyaluronan synthase-2 abrogates normal cardiac morphogenesis and hyaluronan-mediated transformation of epithelium to mesenchyme. *J. Clin. Invest.,* 2000, *106*, 349-360.

[47] Takahashi, Y; Li, L; Kamiryo, M; Asteriou, T; Moustakas, A; Yamashita, H; Heldin P. Hyaluronan fragments induce endothelial cell differentiation in a CD44- and CXCL1/GRO1-dependent manner. *J. Biol. Chem.,* 2005, *280*, 24195–24204.

[48] Savani, RC; Cao, G; Pooler, PM; Zaman, A; Zhou, Z; DeLisser, HM. Differential involvement of the hyaluronan (HA) receptors CD44 and receptor for HA-mediated motility in endothelial cell function and angiogenesis. *J. Biol. Chem.,* 2001, *276*, 36770-36778.

[49] Tammi, R; Rilla, K; Pienimaki, JP; MacCallum, DK; Hogg, M; Luukkonen, M; Hascall, VC; Tammi, M. Hyaluronan enters keratinocytes by a novel endocytic route for catabolism. *J. Biol. Chem.,* 2001, *276*, 35111–35122.

[50] Majumdar, M; Meenakshi, J; Goswami, SK; Datta, K. Hyaluronan binding protein 1 (HABP1)/C1QBP/p32 is an endogenous substrate for MAP kinase and is translocated to the nucleus upon mitogenic stimulation. *Biochem. Biophys. Res. Commun.,* 2002, *291*, 829-837.

[51] Grammatikakis, N; Grammatikakis, A; Yoneda, M; Yu, Q; Banerjee, SD; Toole, BP. A novel glycosaminoglycan-binding protein is the vertebrate homologue of the cell cycle control protein, Cdc37. *J. Biol. Chem.,* 1995, *270*, 16198-16205.

[52] Wolffe, AP; Pruss, D. Targeting chromatin disruption: Transcription regulators that acetylate histones. *Cell,* 1996, *84*, 817-819.

[53] Illi, B; Scopece, A; Nanni, S; Farsetti, A; Morgante, L; Biglioli, P; Capogrossi, MC; Gaetano, C. Epigenetic histone modification and cardiovascular lineage programming

in mouse embryonic stem cells exposed to laminar shear stress. *Circ. Res.,* 2005, *96,* 501-508.

[54] Kastner, P; Grondona, JM; Mark, M; Gansmuller, A; LeMeur, M; Decimo, D; Vonesch, JL; Dolle, P; Chambon, P. Genetic analysis of RXR alpha developmental function: convergence of RXR and RAR signaling pathways in heart and eye morphogenesis. *Cell,* 1994, *78,* 987-1003.

[55] Sucov, HM; Dyson, E; Gumeringer, CL; Price, J; Chien, KR; Evans, RM. RXR alpha mutant mice establish a genetic basis for vitamin A signaling in heart morphogenesis. *Genes Dev.,* 1994, *8,* 1007-1018.

[56] Wobus, AM; Kaomei, G; Shan, J; Wellner, MC; Rohwedel, J; Ji, G; Fleischmann, B; Katus, HA; Hescheler, J; Franz, WM. Retinoic acid accelerates embryonic stem cell-derived cardiac differentiation and enhances development of ventricular cardiomyocytes. *J. Mol. Cell. Cardiol.,* 1997, *29,* 1525–1539.

[57] Lai, L; Bohnsack, BL; Niederreither, K; Hirschi, KK. Retinoic acid regulates endothelial cell proliferation during vasculogenesis. *Development,* 2003, *130,* 6465-6474.

[58] Dilworth, FJ; Fromental-Ramain, C; Yamamoto, K; Chambon, P. ATP-driven chromatin remodeling activity and histone acetyltransferases act sequentially during transactivation by RAR/RXR In vitro. *Mol. Cell,* 2000, *6,* 1049-1058.

[59] Gnecchi, M; He, H; Noiseux, N; Liang, OD; Zhang, L; Morello, F; Mu, H; Melo, LG; Pratt, RE; Ingwall, JS; Dzau, VJ. Evidence supporting paracrine hypothesis for Akt-modified mesenchymal stem cell-mediated cardiac protection and functional improvement. *FASEB J.,* 2006, *20,* 661-669.

[60] Noiseux, N; Gnecchi, M; Lopez-Ilasaca, M; Zhang, L; Solomon, SD; Deb, A; Dzau, VJ; Pratt, RE. Mesenchymal stem cells overexpressing Akt dramatically repair infarcted myocardium and improve cardiac function despite infrequent cellular fusion or differentiation. *Mol. Ther.,* 2006, *14,* 840-850.

[61] Miyahara, Y; Nagaya, N; Kataoka, M; Yanagawa, B; Tanaka, K; Hao, H; Ishino, K; Ishida, H; Shimizu, T; Kangawa, K; Sano, S; Okano, T; Kitamura, S; Mori, H. Monolayered mesenchymal stem cells repair scarred myocardium after myocardial infarction. *Nat. Med.,* 2006, *12,* 459-465.

[62] Nakamura, T; Nishizawa, T; Hagiya, M; Seki, T; Shimonishi, M; Sugimura, A; Tashiro, K; Shimizu, S. Molecular cloning and expression of human hepatocyte growth factor. *Nature,* 1989, *342,* 440-443.

[63] Nakamura, T; Mizuno, S; Matsumoto, K; Sawa, Y; Matsuda, H; Nakamura, T. Myocardial protection from ischemia/reperfusion injury by endogenous and exogenous HGF. *J. Clin. Invest.,* 2000, *106,* 1511-1519.

[64] Li, Y; Takemura, G; Kosai, K; Yuge, K; Nagano, S; Esaki, M; Goto, K; Takahashi, T; Hayakawa, K; Koda, M; Kawase, Y; Maruyama, R; Okada, H; Minatoguchi, S; Mizuguchi, H; Fujiwara, T; Fujiwara, H. Postinfarction treatment with an adenoviral vector expressing hepatocyte growth factor relieves chronic left ventricular remodeling and dysfunction in mice. *Circulation,* 2003, *107,* 2499-2506.

[65] Bailo, M; Soncini, M; Vertua, E; Signoroni, PB; Sanzone, S; Lombardi, G; Arienti, D; Calamani, F; Zatti, D; Paul, P; Albertini, A; Zorzi, F; Cavagnini, A; Candotti, F;

Wengler, GS; Parolini, O. Engraftment potential of human amnion and chorion cells derived from term placenta. *Transplantation,* 2004, *78,* 1439-1448.

[66] Wu X, Ding S, Ding Q, Gray NS, Schultz PG. Small molecules that induce cardiomyogenesis in embryonic stem cells. *J. Am. Chem. Soc.,* 2004, *126,* 1590-1591.

[67] Battista, S; Guarnieri, D; Borselli, C; Zeppetelli, S; Borzacchiello, A; Mayol, L; Gerbasio, D; Keene, DR; Ambrosio, L; Netti, PA. The effect of matrix composition of 3D constructs on embryonic stem cell differentiation. *Biomaterials,* 2005, *26,* 6194-6207.

[68] Bhang, SH; Lim, JS; Choi, CY; Kwon, YK; Kim, BS. The behavior of neural stem cells on biodegradable synthetic polymers. *J. Biomater. Sci. Polym. Ed.,* 2007, *18,* 223-239.

[69] Gelain, F; Bottai, D; Vescovi, A; Zhang S. Designer self-assembling Peptide nanofiber scaffolds for adult mouse neural stem cell 3-dimensional cultures. *PLoS ONE,* 2006, 1:e119.

[70] Willerth, SM; Arendas, KJ; Gottlieb, DI; Sakiyama-Elbert, SE. Optimization of fibrin scaffolds for differentiation of murine embryonic stem cells into neural lineage cells. *Biomaterials,* 2006, *27,* 5990-6003.

[71] Yim, EK; Leong, KW. Proliferation and differentiation of human embryonic germ cell derivatives in bioactive polymeric fibrous scaffold. *J. Biomater. Sci. Polym. Ed.,* 2005, *16,* 1193-1217.

[72] Boudriot, U; Goetz, B; Dersch, R; Greiner, A; Wendorff, JH. Role of electrospun nanofibers in stem cell technologies and tissue engineering. *Macromol. Symp.,* 2005, *225,* 9-16.

[73] Zhang, YZ; Venugopal, J; Huang, ZM; Lim, CT; Ramakrishna, S. Characterization of the surface biocompatibility of the electrospun PCL-collagen nanofibers using fibroblasts. *Biomacromolecules,* 2005, *6,* 2583-2589.

[74] McBeath, R; Pirone, DM; Nelson, CM; Bhadriraju, K; Chen, CS. Cell shape, cytoskeletal tension, and RhoA regulate stem cell lineage commitment. *Dev. Cell,* 2004, *6,* 483-495.

[75] Roskelley, C; Desprez, P; Bissell, M. Extracellular Matrix-Dependent Tissue-Specific Gene Expression in Mammary Epithelial Cells Requires both Physical and Biochemical Signal Transduction. *Proc. Nat. Acad. Sci. USA,* 1994, *91,* 12378-12382.

[76] Watt, FM; Jordan, PW; O'Neill, CH. Cell Shape Controls Terminal Differentiation of Human Epidermal Keratinocytes. *Proc. Nat. Acad. Sci. USA,* 1988, *85,* 5576-5580.

[77] Spiegelman, BM; Ginty, CA. Fibronectin modulation of cell shape and lipogenic gene expression in 3T3-adipocytes. *Cell,* 1983, *35,* 657-666.

[78] Chen, CS; Mrksich, M; Huang, S; Whitesides, GM; Ingber, DE. Geometric control of cell life and death. *Science,* 1997, *276,* 1425-1428.

[79] Thomas, CH; Collier, JH; Sfeir, CS; Healy, KE. Engineering gene expression and protein synthesis by modulation of nuclear shape. *Proc. Natl. Acad. Sci. USA,* 2002, *99,* 1972-1977.

[80] Tan, JL; Tien, J; Pirone, DM; Gray, DS; Bhadriraju, K; Chen, CS. Cells lying on a bed of microneedles: an approach to isolate mechanical force. *Proc. Natl. Acad. Sci. USA,* 2003, *100,* 1484-1489.

[81] Coughlin, MF; Stamenovic, D. A prestressed cable network model of the adherent cell cytoskeleton. *Biophys. J.,* 2003, *84*, 1328-1336.
[82] Ventura, C; Maioli, M; Asara, Y; Santoni, D; Mesirca, P; Remondini, D; Bersani, F. Turning on stem cell cardiogenesis with extremely low frequency magnetic fields. *FASEB J.,* 2005, *19*, 155-157.

Chapter XXIV

YIN AND YANG OF ADULT STEM CELLS: CURE-ALL FOR THERAPY OR ROOTS FOR CANCER?

Christian Dani, Cédric Darini and Annie Ladoux[*]
Institute of Signaling Biology Development and Cancer,
University of Nice Sophia-Antipolis, CNRS UMR
NICE Cedex, France

ABSTRACT

Stem cells have raised hope for patients and doctors to cure diseases devoid of any appropriate treatment. Adult stem cells have been identified in several organs including bone marrow, brain, skin, muscle, intestine, liver and adipose tissue where they interact with their micro environment to maintain specific properties such as the capacity to seemingly indefinitely self-renew, i.e., divide and create additional stem cells. They also retain the ability to differentiate along, at least, one or multiple lineages to generate and to properly control the turnover of cells bearing an assigned function.

Thus, they play a critical role to maintain and repair organ systems, but when their ability to divide and/or differentiate is disrupted, certain diseases such as cancers may result.

Considerable efforts have been put in the identification of markers that specifically define stem cells within an organ and cancer stem cells within a population of tumor cells, allowing prospective isolation and evaluation of their potential either to regenerate a functional organ or to drive a terrible disease.

This review will focus on the characterization and the isolation of mesenchymal stem cells. They represent invaluable tools to regenerate an accurate biological function within an organ and thus display a great therapeutic potential if carefully monitored.

---

[*] Corresponding author: email: ladoux@unice.fr, tel: 33 4 92 07 64 37, Fax: 33 4 92 07 64 04

We will then consider the concept of cancer stem cells, evaluate their implication in the progression of solid tumors and will propose tools designed specifically to target and kill this population.

INTRODUCTION

Stem cells differ from other kinds of cells in the body. All stem cells, regardless of their source, have three general properties: they are capable of dividing and renewing themselves for long periods, they are unspecialised as they don't have any assigned function and they can choose to become one of the many different types of cells present in the body, depending on signals they receive from their environment.

Adult stem cells have been found in many adult tissues, such as the bone marrow, brain, gut... [1, 2]. All adult stem cells are multipotent progenitors able to self–renew, that reside within a given organ. They are also able to generate very specialized cells involved in the proper function of their host organ, thus contributing to its maintenance and regeneration. Indeed, normal stem cells are tissue-specific and represent unrelated entities that display distinctive molecular signatures and undergo separate differentiation pathways. Among the different stem cells that have been identified in adults, mesenchymal stem cells (MSCs) represent a very unique population as they could be isolated from different organs [3]. The bone marrow is the most widely used stem cell source but multipotent stem cells have been identified in many adult tissues including adipose tissue, placenta, blood chord, pancreas ... [4, 5].

Our purpose is to provide information on the differentiation ability of MSCs to evaluate their attractive potential for therapy, but also to illustrate how deregulation in the fundamental properties of stem cells, including MSCs, can lead to severe malignant disorders.

MESENCHYMAL STEM CELLS

Molecular Characterization and Differentiation Properties of Mesenchymal Stem Cells

Minimal identification criteria for MSCs issued from different origins were defined upon three properties: (i) their ability to remain plastic-adherent when maintained in standard culture conditions, (ii) their cell-surface marker expression and (iii) their differentiation potential [6].

Phenotypically, MSCs express a number of markers such as CD105, CD73, CD44, CD90 and CD106 but lack expression of CD45, CD34 and C14. However, none of them are specific to MSCs and there is variable expression for some of them. For example MSCs isolated from human adipose tissue express CD49d but not CD106 whereas MSCs isolated from bone-marrow express CD106 but not CD49d. Two alternatives can explain this observation: a variation in tissue source or more likely the method used for isolation and culture of these cells [7]. Indeed, cell surface markers expressed by adipose tissue-derived MSCs resemble those of bone marrow-derived MSCs. Direct comparisons between both immunophenotypes revealed at least more than 90% homology, strongly indicating that the two cell populations are related. Due to the lack of a specific and universal molecular marker to identify adult stem cells, functional assays are required and remain to be designed to ascertain their presence within a tissue.

Several papers report on the *in vitro* differentiation potential of adipose-derived MSCs towards various functional lineages including adipocytes, osteoblasts, chondrocytes and endothelial cells (for recent reviews see Casteilla and Dani [8] and Schaffer *et al.* [9]). More remarkably, functional cardiomyocyte-like cells were obtained from culture of adipose tissue stromal cells [10]. As MSCs derived from human adipose tissue isolated in our lab express myogenic markers, determination of a skeletal myogenic potential was undertaken. These cells were not able to form myotubes *in vitro* and direct contact with primary muscle cells was necessary for myotube formation ([11] and C. Dechesne and C. Dani, unpublished data).

Under specific culture conditions, adipose-derived MSCs seem to be able to undergo neurogenic, pancreatic and hepatic differentiation. However, information available is still scant and further evidence from functional studies is necessary to establish if MSCs derived from human adipose tissues present a putative "non-mesenchymal differentiation potential", valuable for future clinical applications. Indeed, this vast differentiation potential may reflect the importance of MSCs in the maintenance of the many organs from which they have been isolated.

The Adipose Tissue as a Source of MSCs for Regenerative Medicine

Considering the diversity of pathologies devoid of effective pharmacological treatments and the wide differentiation spectra of these cells, identification and purification of MSCs for medical purposes have raised up huge enthusiasm with a view to putative benefits for patients. However, stem cells are rare in adult tissues and thus, difficult to isolate and to maintain *ex vivo*. As adipose tissue allows the extraction of a large volume of tissue with limited invasive surgery, this tissue appeared as an attractive stem-cell source alternative and adipose tissue derived-stem cells offer tremendous potential for regenerative medicine. First, Zuk and colleagues reported the existence of a cell population able to undergo *in vitro* differentiation into different mesenchymal cell types, in human adipose tissue harvested by liposuction [12]. Then, by analogy with mesenchymal stem cell isolated from bone marrow, cells arising from the cultures of stroma vascular fraction of adipose tissue were termed stem cells, although self-renewal and multipotentiality at a clonal level were not established until recently [13-15]. Then, MSCs derived from adipose tissue were also named ADSC (adipose tissue-derived stromal cells), or hMADS (human Multipotent Adipose Derived Stem) cells after confirmation of the stem cell features i.e., self-renewal and multipotency at the clonal level.

Indeed, these cells display an *in vivo* regeneration potential that has recently been reported. ADSC and hMADS cells have the capacity to participate in muscle regeneration [13, 16], to form bone after transplantation in mice [17] and to promote neovascularization after transplantation of into animal models [18]. These findings highlight the concept that adipose tissue represents a new source of stem cells presenting a therapeutic potential that is worth considering.

Beneficial Properties of Mesenchymal Stem Cells for a Therapeutic Use

Several groups have reported that MSCs, including those derived from human adipose tissue, are non immunogenic and effective in inducing tolerance [13, 19]. The mechanisms by which adipose-derived MSCs escape immune surveillance remain unclear but there are likely to be several. For example, the analysis of the major histocompatibility complex proteins revealed low expression levels for HLA class-I molecules, while HLA class-II molecules could not be detected. This observation strongly supports an absence of immune recognition.

Beside the deficiency in immune recognition, immunosuppressive properties were described for MSCs derived from human and mouse bone marrow [20]. This immunosuppression mechanism is likely to occur via the production of cytokines, such as IL-4, IL-10 and TGF-β involved in the inhibition of alloreactive lymphocyte proliferation. These two mechanisms can act alternately or concomitantly.

The non immunogenic properties of MSCs make them a suitable tool for heterologous transplantation and their immunosuppressive activity has been successfully tested in animal models of autoimmunity [21].

Detrimental Properties of Mesenchymal Stem Cells for a Therapeutic Use

However, systemic immunosuppression might exhibit adverse effects favoring tumor growth. This possibility has been clearly demonstrated by Djouad and collaborators showing that co implantation of MSCs and tumor cells promoted the development of a tumor in a mouse model [22]. More recently, involvement of MSCs has been demonstrated to promote breast cancer metastasis [23]. These findings underscore the roles of the micro environment and of the chemokine networks in tumor progression. Therefore, caution applies for the therapeutic use of MSCs in the context of the putative malignant behavior of these cells.

hMADS cells do not display any malignant potential as transplantation of up to fifty million cells did not induce any tumor formation in Nude mice (A. Ladoux and C. Dani, unpublished data). However, extensive expansion, that is a prerequisite for evaluating the therapeutic potential in ongoing clinical trials, could expose MSCs to mutations. It has been reported that *in vitro* expanded human bone marrow-derived MSCs can spontaneously create clones (around 15% of the cases) presenting characteristics of transformed cells, including abnormal karyotype and anchorage independence. These clones did not present a strong tumorigenic potential when injected in Nude mice. After numerous passages, mouse MSCs proceed to a transformed state and form tumors *in vivo* [24]. Therefore, it is critical to carefully and systematically assess that MSCs display a non-transformed phenotype before any transplantation. By means of which criteria remains a crucial open question?

The ability to assign at MSCs the origin of some tumors remains limited. Liposarcomas are the most common diagnoses of soft tumors. These tumors occur in adipose depots, and it has been recently reported that adipocyte precursors exhibit chromosomal features close to those of liposarcomas [25]. However, there is no direct evidence so far, that adipose derived MSCs are at the origin of liposarcomas. Ewing tumor (ET), a tumor of bone and soft tissues, is characterized by the fusion of EWS gene with FLI1 gene creating a chimeric oncoprotein that behaves as an aberrant transcription regulator [26]. Recently Tirode et al. provided evidence supporting the possibility that MSCs could be one of the origins of Ewing's sarcoma family tumors, although expression of neural markers by these tumors was shown [27]. These authors showed that inhibition of EWS/FLI1 in Ewing tumor cell lines induced their adipocyte and osteogenic differentiation whereas the ectopic expression of EWS/FLI1 in MSCs blocked these differentiations. Indeed, the authors didn't show that transfection of the chimeric oncoprotein in MSCs could transform them into putative cancer stem cells whereas this process was inefficient in other adult stem cells.

Altogether these data indicate that MSCs that can be easily obtained from adult donors, are extraordinary tools presenting a strong interest for therapeutic purposes. A better characterization of this cell population and of its immune privilege is requested as it is mandatory for host tolerance but can drive malignant disorders. This reveals a weakness that has to be circumvented before the medical use of these cells and indicates that any *in vivo* treatment will have to be conducted under strict control. So far, no indisputable evidence implicating directly MSCs in the generation of cancer stem cells has been reported. This is not the case for other adult stem cells.

CANCER STEM CELLS

Tumors consist of a heterogeneous population of cells: a small proportion of proliferating cells and a majority representing differentiated daughter cells. The coexistence of different cell types harboring different properties within a tumor cell population has raised the hypothesis that a hierarchy was governing the tumorigenic potential.

The concept of cancer stem cells i.e., the existence, within a given tumor, of a minor population of crucial cells laying within an appropriate micro environment to fuel tumors and possessing an indefinite proliferative potential resembling self-renewal of stem cells, arise in the 19th century and is receiving increasing support [28]. The existence of cancer stem cells was first described for leukemia and more recently these cells were found in solid tumors [29]. They are also frequently referred to as "tumor-initiating cells" or TICs.

Despite considerable efforts displayed to characterize them, they still remain largely unknown and misunderstood.

Origin of Cancer Stem Cells

The origin of cancer stem cells is still under debate. Neoplasic processes develop as a consequence of alterations affecting three families of genes: oncogenes, tumor-suppressor genes and stability genes [30]. Cancer stem cells have been proposed to derive from normal cells presenting stem cells properties that accumulated genetic and epigenetic aberrations, as suggested for Ewing tumors [27]. Others presented evidences for an alteration of progenitor cells already committed within a specific lineage. Although these two possibilities are not mutually exclusive, the difficulty in settling for one or the other resides in the current poor knowledge of normal adult stem cells and/or progenitors identities, including MSCs. They have been described in different organs but their molecular characterization is difficult to achieve and the co-existence of different types of stem cells within an organ has to be taken in account, as for example the bone marrow contains both hematopoietic stem cells (HSCs) and MSCs.

Tissue-specific stem cells or progenitors of stem cells consist in long-lived cells normally undergoing a limited number of cell divisions. They reside in a micro environment, designed as "niche", which is suited to maintain both the stem cell pool and stem cell properties [1]. They can be affected by genetic mutations, transformation and/or deregulation of self-renewal pathways which represent the main source for disorders [31]. As a direct consequence, these cells present, at least, a selective growth and/or survival advantage. In addition, changes in the differentiation potential of stem cells or progenitors cells can also be considered as a fundamental alternative mechanism contributing to tumor development and can occur concomitantly with proliferation deregulation. These alterations may also result in different homing properties and the modifications or the absence of interactions between cancer stem cells and their niches further support the development and dissemination of the cancer stem cell phenotype.

Physiological Definition of Cancer Stem Cells

It has been well documented that leukemia development was sustained by a small fraction of cells likely to proliferate extensively. In the sixties, several teams showed that myeloma cells were displaying a clonogenic potential either *in vitro* in semi solid growth conditions [32] or *in vivo* after transplantation [33]. When few cells were implanted in immunodeficient mice, regeneration potential confirmed that these cells were able to generate a tumor bearing characteristics similar to the parental tumor. For long, the detection of cancer stem cells within tumors has been based upon these functional assays which contributed to reveal a tremendous vast diversity in cancer stem cell populations. This reflected the differences in clonogenecity among normal HSCs, and pointed out the pathway or the progenitor that were affected by malignancy [29]. They are still currently used as they are absolutely essential to ascertain the clonal and the tumorigenic potential of putative cancer stem cells.

Isolation of Cancer Stem Cells Further Confirmed Their Diversity and Their Heterogeneous Origin

The first isolation of cancer stem cells was reported by Dick and colleagues who showed that, in acute myelogenic leukaemia (AML), the clonogenic and malignant potentials were the feature of a precise population comprising a minute number of cells that were purified as CD34+ CD38- [34].

Then considerable efforts were put to identify specific membrane markers providing clues for easier isolation and therefore characterization of cancer stem cells. Another strategy consisted in defining specific functions assigned to cancer stem cells with interest for identification and further isolation of living cell populations.

In solid tumors, the first evidence for the presence of cancer stem cells based on cell-surface marker expression came from studies performed in human breast carcinoma. Using Fluorescence Activated Cell Sorter (FACS), carcinoma cells were fractionated upon CD44 and CD24 expression. Cells defined by the phenotype CD44+ CD24- were able to form tumors when implanted in the mammary fat pad of NOD/SCID mice that exhibited similar morphologic and immunophenotypic heterogeneity than the parental tumor [35]. Furthermore engrafted tumors could be serially transplanted providing the clearest possible evidence for a self-renewal capacity.

CD44 is a cell adhesion protein that undergoes dramatic structural and functional changes during neoplasic processes. The expression of CD44 multiple isoforms and the resulting haluronic acid binding pattern can dramatically influence tumor growth and development. For example CD44 influences proper homing of AML leukemia stem cells to their environmental niche and is essential to maintain them in a "primitive state" [36]. In solid tumors, CD44 positive cells were detected in colorectal cancer [37], in prostate [38] in head and neck carcinomas [39] and in pancreas [40] where they are considered as putative cancer stem cells. Interestingly, the population of pancreatic cancer cells displaying CD44 and CD24 positive labeling was the most tumorigenic while this potential was assigned to the CD44 positive, CD24 negative cells in breast cancer.

The analysis of CD44 expression gave useful information to understand the origin of cancer stem cells.

- On one hand, expression of CD44 larger isoform seemed to be a hallmark of epithelial stem cells [41] and in breast, all luminal and basal epithelial cancer cells were shown positive for CD44 [42]. Thus the association of CD44 expression with epithelial TICs supported the hypothesis that these cells derived from normal stem cells or progenitors that accumulated enough mutations to prevent them from properly controlling their growth.
- On the other hand, CD44 positive cells were identified as putative TICs in pancreatic adenocarcinoma [40] but no CD44 isoform has been detected in pancreatic aciniar cells [41]. This simple observation pointed out that, under certain circumstances, cancer stem cells might not just derive from a normal counterpart subjected to genetic alterations but that other mechanisms accounted for the malignant potential of TICs. Taken together these observations revealed multiple origins for cancer stem cells. Their development resulted from several independent alterations that target normal adult stem cells as well as other cell types.

CD44 doesn't represent a unique molecular signature for cancer stem cells. TICs displaying a strong CD133 labeling, could be isolated first from brain tumors and represented cells bearing the capacity of self-renewal and proliferation, while the CD133 negative cells counterpart did not [43]. CD133 expression was not restricted to brain TICs and was found in

TICs from colon, prostate or liver [44]. CD133 is believed to be the human orthologue of mouse prominin. It is a transmembrane glycoprotein that is expressed in microvillis. CD133 expression was detected in normal human neural stem cells [45] and in normal primitive cells of the hematopoietic, epithelial and endothelial lineages [46] and its expression declined with differentiation [45, 47, 48]. Thus CD133 expression in glioma cancer stem cells may reflect a direct lineage with normal neural stem cells. Although the expression of CD44 or CD133 in tumor cells is sufficient to define TICs population, these two markers can be co-expressed in cells displaying cancer stem cell properties [38, 49].

Additional identification strategies based on the existence of a "functional signature" for cancer stem cells were designed to provide quick and efficient alternatives for direct isolation of the cancer stem cell population.

It has been reported that cancer stem cells represent a population able to escape to chemotherapy treatments because they express high levels of multi drug resistance proteins including the ATP-binding cassette (ABCG2) transporter [50, 51]. This feature was used to select a cell-population called "Side Population" (SP), able to actively pump-out the fluorescent dye Hoechst 33342, when analyzed by FACS. The SP population has been described in normal adult stem cells although the biological significance of this property is not understood in this case. In cancer stem cells, SP cells are likely responsible for resistance to cytotoxic drugs and tumor escape.

Another promising purification strategy to identify and isolate TICs exploits the expression of cytosolic aldehyde dehydrogenase (ALDH), an enzyme implicated in the metabolism of a wide variety of aliphatic aldehydes that confers resistance to alkylating agents. Fluorescent substrates that allowed purification of cells expressing high levels of ALDH have been developed. This strategy was first successfully applied to isolate normal human and murine hematopoietic progenitors. An associated expression of ALDH with CD133 further defined long term reconstituting hematopoietic stem cells [52]. The presence of ALDH expressing cells was assigned to the cancer stem cell pool in some solid tumors. The phenotypic characterization of colorectal cancer revealed that CD133 positive population contained a small subset of cells displaying high ALDH activity as well as CD44 and epithelial-specific antigen labeling [37]. In retinoblastoma, ALDH was detected in cells expressing ABCG2 transporter and was shown to represent the SP fraction of cancer cells [53].

Thus identification of a molecular or a functional signature for TICs allowed their isolation and purification. It provided crucial information supporting the existence of different origins for these populations. It also revealed that there was not a unique cancer stem cell and contributed to testify of the vast diversity of cancer stem cells.

Heterogeneity of Cancer Stem Cells within a Tumor

Recent studies indicate that purification of cells upon expression of cell surface markers, as previously described, much more consists in an enriched population of tumorigenic cells but doesn't necessary represent a pure population of cancer stem cells. We already noticed that stem cell populations could be defined according to different molecular and/or functional criteria.

Evidence for the existence of distinct populations of cancer stem cells were presented in an elegant study performed in pancreatic cancers [49]. The cancer stem cell population was restricted to CD133 positive cells that could reproduce the original tumor in permissive recipients with a very high efficiency. Within this cell population, the authors analyzed the role played by CXCR4, a membrane receptor for a peptide involved in cell migration: stromal cell-derived factor 1. They could associate an invasive phenotype responsible for tumor metastasis to the CD133+ CXCR4+ population while the CD133+ CXCR4- population represented cells that have few propensities to disseminate. Hermann and collaborators did not include the marker combination CD44+ CD24+ ESA+ used by Li *et al.* [40], but they mentioned an overlap between the two populations which sustained the diversity of stem cells within pancreatic tumors.

Another example of heterogeneity within a cancer stem cell population came out from analysis of the molecular signature of breast cancer stem cells. CD44+ CD24- cells presented a gene expression profile that resembled that of stem cells [42]. However, the authors hypothesized that these CD44+ cells might be subject to evolution and able to change their phenotype as the main population of cells present in distant metastasis consisted in CD24+ cells.

Taken together, these observations point out two essential notions: (i) different populations of TICs exist within a tumor and (ii) cells presenting the highest metastatic potential do not exactly match the primary stem cell population of the original tumor and/or require evolution.

Pathways Contributing to Self-Renewal Deregulation in Cancer Stem Cells

Several signaling pathways described to play a crucial role in embryonic stem cells for maintenance of pluripotency or to control proper organ developments were also reported being activated in different tumor types. They include JAK/STAT, Notch, MAPK/ERK, PI3K/AKT, NF-κB, Wnt, TGF-β and Hedgehog pathways [30, 54, 55]. Beside them, tumor suppressor genes such as *PTEN* (phosphatase and tensin homolog on chromosome 10) and *TP53* (tumor protein p53) have also been implicated in the regulation of cancer stem cell self-renewal [56]. Different types of alterations leading to dysfunction within these pathways have been reported and were shown to cooperate to increase the tumor incidence. Examples from the literature depict a wide range of effects in the transformation processes that may lead to the acquisition of cancer stem cell properties. We will focus to determine precisely their direct involvement in conferring tumoral potential to cancer stem cells because activation of these pathways has often been studied within a whole tumor.

In this regard, convincing results indicated that a pathway can be activated without conferring stem cell properties to normal progenitors. This was illustrated by JAK2 V617F mutations within the JAK/STAT pathway. This mutation was found in most of the patients with polycythemia vera and myeloproliferative disorders and led to constitutive activation of the kinase [57]. Expression of this mutation in hematopoietic cell lines induced autonomous cell growth [58]. When hematopoietic stem cells bearing this mutation were injected into SCID mice, this disease was not transplantable, indicating that this mutation did not confer self-renewal capacity to HSCs [59]. This example illustrates that the JAK2 V617F mutation probably consists in a major step towards the acquisition of malignant properties, but that it is not sufficient to produce TICs.

The CD44+ CD24- population of breast cancer cell displayed up-regulation of both Wnt and TGF-β signaling pathways [42]. Although no specific mutation could be associated to activation of TGF-β pathway, it was shown that TGF-β treatment activated this pathway in CD44 positive cells giving them at least a more mesenchymal appearance and a more invasive phenotype. Again, no clear evidence that activation of this pathway was involved in self-renewal of breast cancer stem cell could be established so far.

p53 gene mutations are encountered in a wide variety of cancers displaying different origins. The resulting p53 protein doesn't function properly and fails in reducing the progression through the cell cycle of cells harboring DNA damage, presenting oncogenic mutations or submitted to various stresses [60]. p53 controls a large number of genes involved in cell division, apoptosis and genetic stability, and their improper expression has severe consequences for the homeostasis of a tissue and its role in self-renewal was assessed in neural stem cells [61]. p53 was expressed in the neural stem cell niche in the brain. Invalidation of the mouse *p53* gene resulted both in a larger cell number and an increased proliferation in the neural stem cells of the subventricular zone. No effect was measured on the differentiation potential of these cells. Similar results were reported for HSCs [62]. Disruption in the negative control exerted by p53 on stem cell self-renewal probably consists in an important step in tumor initiation.

Activation of Wnt signaling pathway represents one of the most documented examples linking major genetic or epigenetic defect to up-regulation of a specific signaling pathway and self-renewal. This pathway is essential for the maintenance of self-renewal of hematopoietic stem cells and progenitors and for the maintenance of normal intestinal epithelial cells [31]. Several genes have been targeted for mutations, mainly the adenomatosis polyposis coli (APC) or the β-catenin genes. As a direct consequence of aberrant β-catenin accumulation in the nucleus, controlled growth is abrogated and cell differentiation is impaired. This process leads to development of aggressive tumors that, in the case of $Apc^{min}/+$ mutant mice, resulted from proliferation of the stem cell progeny [63]. Absence of functional APC protein was associated with 90% of colon cancer and 76% of gastric carcinomas while β-catenin aberrant expression was found in 64% of gastric polyps and 48% of small intestinal carcinomas [54]. Activation of this pathway is also detected in melanomas, brain tumors and chronic myeloid leukaemia.

Wnt canonical pathway activation has been shown to induce CD133 expression through binding of β-catenin to TCF/LEF sites present in CD133 promoter [64]. CD44 was also reported to be a target of this pathway [65, 66]. Thus, it is not surprising to find a strong tumorigenic potential associated with cells expressing CD133 or CD44. However, in colon cancer two recent studies identified TICs as cells expressing CD133, no association with deregulation in the Wnt pathway, which is associated with a vast majority of gastro-intestinal malignancies, was documented [46, 67].

Up-regulation of the Hedgehog signaling pathway was first described in a human glioma cell line [68] and was further documented in sporadic and familial basal-cell carcinoma where it resulted from a loss of functional PTCH1, the Hedgehog receptor that behaves as a tumor suppressor gene involved in a fine tune regulation of the Hedgehog pathway [69]. In human glioma, CD133 high expression was show to define the TICs population [70]. Maintenance of self-renewal and tumorigeneicity within this population was assigned to a strong activation of the Hedgehog signaling pathway. Furthermore grade III glioma presented a stemness signature associated with an increased expression of a sub-group of stemness genes such as *Nanog, Oct-4, Sox2* and *Bmi* that are inherent to embryonic stem cell features. This stemness signature is lost in higher grade gliomas probably because of dilution of cancer stem cells in the tumor pool as suggested by the authors. Alternatively, one could consider that any evolution of this stemness signature might also represent a pool of cancer stem cells that were subjected to evolution. Such a stemness signature was detected in teratocarcinomas where its activation largely contributed to self-renewal of germ cancer cells [71]. These tumors represent classic stem cell tumors and are serially transplantable in immunodeficient mice. Maintenance of the malignant stem cell pool was depending on Oct-4 expression levels, a transcription factor required to maintain pluripotency of embryonic stem cells [72] and whose ectopic expression was shown sufficient to induce dysplasia in epithelial tissues [73].

This overview shows the diversity of pathways that are involved in the evolution towards carcinogenesis. Although activation of these pathways is well established for the bulk tumor, considerable efforts are needed to identify the signaling pathways involved in the development of cells responsible for malignancies. Mutations and up-regulations were identified in several pathways but they were not always directly responsible for the acquisition of cancer stem cell properties. In other cases, these properties could result from concomitant activation of several signaling pathways. A focus on their precise involvement will pin point the defects that create a specific cancer stem cell and represent an interesting approach to propose adapted treatments targeting directly this population.

Further Requirements to Characterize Cancer Stem Cells and Kill Them

The ability of stem cells to change their phenotype and the possibility that different stem cell populations can co-exist within the same tumor depict the cell fraction essential to eradicate to cure cancer even more difficult to target and to hit.

The first anti tumoral strategies were directed against the whole tumor. Radiation therapies and/or chemotherapies were efficient to shrink it by killing the majority of the proliferating cancer cells. Anti angiogenic therapies were efficient to block nutrient supply therefore reducing tumor growth, but they provided the tumor cells with a more hypoxic environment that was shown to strongly favor stem cell maintenance [74]. Differentiation therapies were first initiated to process leukemia and induced the maturation of cancer cells. Unfortunately, none of these therapies was efficient to eradicate this small portion of cells that could reinitiate tumor growth as soon as they are discontinued [30, 75].

- Thus the challenge for physicians might consist in defining proper medical strategies adapted to kill the different stem cell populations involved both in primary tumor growth and in development of metastasis. As, depending on their origin and on their tumorigenic potential, a vast diversity of cancer stem cells exists, tailor-made treatments must be considered.
- The first step is to identify the origin of the molecular insult responsible for cancer in each patient and to determine the resulting molecular signature associated with one proper tumor. This strategy is promising as it has been shown that reintroduction of a functional wild type p53 protein expression was leading efficiently to tumor regression *in vivo* in *p53* null mice [76, 77]. Targeting AML leukemic stem cells using an antibody directed against CD44 resulted in modifications of interactions with their micro environment that were efficient to eradicate them [36]. Although this approach has not been reported efficient for solid tumors so far, it represents another example of a strategy presenting an interesting potential for therapy. Its limit relies on the ability to discriminate between the different CD44 isoforms expressed in normal and malignant stem cells as CD44 is ubiquitously expressed.
- The second step consists in choosing the best strategy to target a de-regulated signaling pathway or specific sub-populations of cells. Several molecular inhibitors were identified to block efficiently a specific signaling pathway *in vitro* [75, 78]. Before any possible prescription to patients, their toxicity *in vivo* and their specificity to target cancer stem cells but not normal stem cells have to be carefully evaluated. The delivery of interfering RNAs remains another very attractive alternative. The limit of this strategy remains the development of efficient and non toxic delivery systems to cancer stem cells.

Cancer stem cells identity and behavior still stand as an enigma. The development of animal models contributed already to a better understanding of neoplasic processes development. Indeed, new models are requested to assess stemness properties and propensity to change the phenotype of TICs. They will represent a great advantage to select this (these) population(s) specifically and to follow its (their) evolution. They will also provide crucial information to adapt the best strategies to target and eradicate TICs, as well as models to validate the best therapeutic approaches.

CONCLUSION

These last 10 years, considerable information arose in the stem cell field. Stem cells, especially adult MSCs, appeared very promising as potent pharmaceutical tools to treat diseases lacking any effective therapy. They display advantage of ruling out ethical concerns raised by embryonic stem cells and they can be isolated in large amounts from adipose tissue that represents an accessible source. A better knowledge and characterization of these cells may lead to an effective modulation of their immune properties to facilitate an *in vivo* utilization and to avoid the development of unwanted neoplasic processes. The origin of cancer stem cells and their characterization is still under debate. Regarding their diversity and their unusual phenotypic change behavior, they represent a challenge for physicians. A better knowledge of this population is of primary importance to propose efficient therapeutic alternatives able to eradicate them and to efficiently cure cancer.

ACKNOWLEDGMENTS

Our lab receives financial support from Association pour la Recherche contre le Cancer (ARC) (Grant number: 3721) and a special grant from ARC and Institut National du Cancer (INCA) (Grant number: 07/1616/23-11/NGNC).

We thank Pascal Peraldi and Eric Lingueglia for critical reading of the manuscript, Mansour Djedaini for expert technical assistance and our colleagues for helpful suggestions and discussions.

REFERENCES

[1] Fuchs E, Tumbar T, Guasch G. Socializing with the neighbors: stem cells and their niche. *Cell*. 2004;116(6):769-78.

[2] Barry FP, Murphy JM. Mesenchymal stem cells: clinical applications and biological characterization. *Int. J. Biochem. Cell Biol.* 2004;36(4):568-84.

[3] Dennis JE, Charbord P. Origin and differentiation of human and murine stroma. *Stem Cells*. 2002;20(3):205-14.

[4] Verfaillie CM. Adult stem cells: assessing the case for pluripotency. *Trends Cell Biol.* 2002;12(11):502-8.

[5] da Silva Meirelles L, Chagastelles PC, Nardi NB. Mesenchymal stem cells reside in virtually all post-natal organs and tissues. *J. Cell Sci.* 2006;119(Pt 11):2204-13.

[6] Dominici M, Le Blanc K, Mueller I, et al. Minimal criteria for defining multipotent mesenchymal stromal cells. The International Society for Cellular Therapy position statement. *Cytotherapy*. 2006;8(4):315-7.

[7] Mitchell JB, McIntosh K, Zvonic S, et al. Immunophenotype of human adipose-derived cells: temporal changes in stromal-associated and stem cell-associated markers. *Stem Cells*. 2006;24(2):376-85.

[8] Casteilla L, Dani C. Adipose tissue-derived cells: from physiology to regenerative medicine. *Diabetes Metab*. 2006;32(5 Pt 1):393-401.

[9] Schaffler A, Buchler C. Concise review: adipose tissue-derived stromal cells--basic and clinical implications for novel cell-based therapies. *Stem Cells*. 2007;25(4):818-27.

[10] Planat-Benard V, Menard C, Andre M, et al. Spontaneous cardiomyocyte differentiation from adipose tissue stroma cells. *Circ. Res.* 2004;94(2):223-9.

[11] Lee JH, Kemp DM. Human adipose-derived stem cells display myogenic potential and perturbed function in hypoxic conditions. *Biochem. Biophys. Res. Commun.* 2006;341(3):882-8.

[12] Zuk PA, Zhu M, Mizuno H, et al. Multilineage cells from human adipose tissue: implications for cell-based therapies. *Tissue Eng.* 2001;7(2):211-28.

[13] Rodriguez AM, Pisani D, Dechesne CA, et al. Transplantation of a multipotent cell population from human adipose tissue induces dystrophin expression in the immunocompetent mdx mouse. *J. Exp. Med.* 2005;201(9):1397-405.

[14] Guilak F, Lott KE, Awad HA, et al. Clonal analysis of the differentiation potential of human adipose-derived adult stem cells. *J. Cell Physiol.* 2006;206(1):229-37.

[15] Zaragosi LE, Ailhaud G, Dani C. Autocrine fibroblast growth factor 2 signaling is critical for self-renewal of human multipotent adipose-derived stem cells. *Stem Cells.* 2006;24(11):2412-9.

[16] Bacou F, el Andalousi RB, Daussin PA, et al. Transplantation of adipose tissue-derived stromal cells increases mass and functional capacity of damaged skeletal muscle. *Cell Transplant.* 2004;13(2):103-11.

[17] Elabd C, Chiellini C, Massoudi A, et al. Human adipose tissue-derived multipotent stem cells differentiate in vitro and in vivo into osteocyte-like cells. *Biochem. Biophys. Res. Commun.* 2007;361(2):342-8.

[18] Planat-Benard V, Silvestre JS, Cousin B, et al. Plasticity of human adipose lineage cells toward endothelial cells: physiological and therapeutic perspectives. *Circulation.* 2004;109(5):656-63.

[19] Puissant B, Barreau C, Bourin P, et al. Immunomodulatory effect of human adipose tissue-derived adult stem cells: comparison with bone marrow mesenchymal stem cells. *Br. J. Haematol.* 2005;129(1):118-29.

[20] Di Nicola M, Carlo-Stella C, Magni M, et al. Human bone marrow stromal cells suppress T-lymphocyte proliferation induced by cellular or nonspecific mitogenic stimuli. *Blood.* 2002;99(10):3838-43.

[21] Gerdoni E, Gallo B, Casazza S, et al. Mesenchymal stem cells effectively modulate pathogenic immune response in experimental autoimmune encephalomyelitis. *Ann. Neurol.* 2007;61(3):219-27.

[22] Djouad F, Plence P, Bony C, et al. Immunosuppressive effect of mesenchymal stem cells favors tumor growth in allogeneic animals. *Blood.* 2003;102(10):3837-44.

[23] Karnoub AE, Dash AB, Vo AP, et al. Mesenchymal stem cells within tumour stroma promote breast cancer metastasis. *Nature.* 2007;449(7162):557-63.

[24] Miura M, Miura Y, Padilla-Nash HM, et al. Accumulated chromosomal instability in murine bone marrow mesenchymal stem cells leads to malignant transformation. *Stem Cells.* 2006;24(4):1095-103.

[25] Mariani O, Brennetot C, Coindre JM, et al. JUN oncogene amplification and overexpression block adipocytic differentiation in highly aggressive sarcomas. *Cancer Cell.* 2007;11(4):361-74.

[26] Delattre O, Zucman J, Plougastel B, et al. Gene fusion with an ETS DNA-binding domain caused by chromosome translocation in human tumours. *Nature.* 1992;359(6391):162-5.

[27] Tirode F, Laud-Duval K, Prieur A, Delorme B, Charbord P, Delattre O. Mesenchymal stem cell features of Ewing tumors. *Cancer Cell.* 2007;11(5):421-9.

[28] Sell S. Stem cell origin of cancer and differentiation therapy. *Crit. Rev. Oncol. Hematol.* 2004;51(1):1-28.

[29] Reya T, Morrison SJ, Clarke MF, Weissman IL. Stem cells, cancer, and cancer stem cells. *Nature.* 2001;414(6859):105-11.
[30] Vogelstein B, Kinzler KW. Cancer genes and the pathways they control. *Nat. Med.* 2004;10(8):789-99.
[31] Lobo NA, Shimono Y, Qian D, Clarke MF. The Biology of Cancer Stem Cells. *Annu. Rev. Cell Dev. Biol.* 2007.
[32] Hamburger AW, Salmon SE. Primary bioassay of human tumor stem cells. *Science.* 1977;197(4302):461-3.
[33] Bruce WR, Van Der Gaag H. A Quantitative Assay for the Number of Murine Lymphoma Cells Capable of Proliferation in Vivo. *Nature.* 1963;199:79-80.
[34] Bonnet D, Dick JE. Human acute myeloid leukemia is organized as a hierarchy that originates from a primitive hematopoietic cell. *Nat. Med.* 1997;3(7):730-7.
[35] Al-Hajj M, Wicha MS, Benito-Hernandez A, Morrison SJ, Clarke MF. Prospective identification of tumorigenic breast cancer cells. *Proc. Natl. Acad. Sci. USA.* 2003;100(7):3983-8.
[36] Jin L, Hope KJ, Zhai Q, Smadja-Joffe F, Dick JE. Targeting of CD44 eradicates human acute myeloid leukemic stem cells. *Nat. Med.* 2006;12(10):1167-74.
[37] Dalerba P, Dylla SJ, Park IK, et al. Phenotypic characterization of human colorectal cancer stem cells. *Proc. Natl. Acad. Sci. USA.* 2007;104(24):10158-63.
[38] Collins AT, Berry PA, Hyde C, Stower MJ, Maitland NJ. Prospective identification of tumorigenic prostate cancer stem cells. *Cancer Res.* 2005;65(23):10946-51.
[39] Prince ME, Sivanandan R, Kaczorowski A, et al. Identification of a subpopulation of cells with cancer stem cell properties in head and neck squamous cell carcinoma. *Proc. Natl. Acad. Sci. USA.* 2007;104(3):973-8.
[40] Li C, Heidt DG, Dalerba P, et al. Identification of pancreatic cancer stem cells. *Cancer Res.* 2007;67(3):1030-7.
[41] Goodison S, Urquidi V, Tarin D. CD44 cell adhesion molecules. *Mol. Pathol.* 1999;52(4):189-96.
[42] Shipitsin M, Campbell LL, Argani P, et al. Molecular definition of breast tumor heterogeneity. *Cancer Cell.* 2007;11(3):259-73.
[43] Singh SK, Hawkins C, Clarke ID, et al. Identification of human brain tumour initiating cells. *Nature.* 2004;432(7015):396-401.
[44] Lee JT, Herlyn M. Old disease, new culprit: Tumor stem cells in cancer. *J. Cell Physiol.* 2007;213(3):603-9.
[45] Uchida N, Buck DW, He D, et al. Direct isolation of human central nervous system stem cells. *Proc. Natl. Acad. Sci. USA.* 2000;97(26):14720-5.
[46] O'Brien CA, Pollett A, Gallinger S, Dick JE. A human colon cancer cell capable of initiating tumour growth in immunodeficient mice. *Nature.* 2007;445(7123):106-10.
[47] Peichev M, Naiyer AJ, Pereira D, et al. Expression of VEGFR-2 and AC133 by circulating human CD34(+) cells identifies a population of functional endothelial precursors. *Blood.* 2000;95(3):952-8.
[48] Yin S, Li J, Hu C, et al. CD133 positive hepatocellular carcinoma cells possess high capacity for tumorigenicity. *Int .J. Cancer.* 2007;120(7):1444-50.

[49] Hermann PC, Huber SL, Herrler T, et al. Distinct Populations of Cancer Stem Cells Determine Tumor Growth and Metastatic Activity in Human Pancreatic. *Cell Stem cell.* 2007;1(3):313-23.

[50] Kondo T, Setoguchi T, Taga T. Persistence of a small subpopulation of cancer stem-like cells in the C6 glioma cell line. *Proc. Natl. Acad. Sci. USA.* 2004;101(3):781-6.

[51] Hirschmann-Jax C, Foster AE, Wulf GG, et al. A distinct "side population" of cells with high drug efflux capacity in human tumor cells. *Proc. Natl. Acad. Sci. USA.* 2004;101(39):14228-33.

[52] Hess DA, Wirthlin L, Craft TP, et al. Selection based on CD133 and high aldehyde dehydrogenase activity isolates long-term reconstituting human hematopoietic stem cells. *Blood.* 2006;107(5):2162-9.

[53] Seigel GM, Campbell LM, Narayan M, Gonzales-Fernandez F. Cancer stem cell characteristics in retinoblastoma. *Molecular. Vision.* 2005;11:729-37.

[54] Dreesen O, Brivanlou AH. Signaling pathways in cancer and embryonic stem cells. *Stem Cell Rev.* 2007;3(1):7-17.

[55] Ruiz i Altaba A, Mas C, Stecca B. The Gli code: an information nexus regulating cell fate, stemness and cancer. *Trends Cell Biol.* 2007;17(9):438-47.

[56] Korkaya H, Wicha MS. Selective targeting of cancer stem cells: a new concept in cancer therapeutics. *BioDrugs.* 2007;21(5):299-310.

[57] James C, Ugo V, Le Couedic JP, et al. A unique clonal JAK2 mutation leading to constitutive signalling causes polycythaemia vera. *Nature.* 2005;434(7037):1144-8.

[58] Staerk J, Kallin A, Demoulin JB, Vainchenker W, Constantinescu SN. JAK1 and Tyk2 activation by the homologous polycythemia vera JAK2 V617F mutation: cross-talk with IGF1 receptor. *J. Biol. Chem.* 2005;280(51):41893-9.

[59] Bumm TG, Elsea C, Corbin AS, et al. Characterization of murine JAK2V617F-positive myeloproliferative disease. *Cancer Res.* 2006;66(23):11156-65.

[60] Vogelstein B, Lane D, Levine AJ. Surfing the p53 network. *Nature.* 2000;408(6810):307-10.

[61] Meletis K, Wirta V, Hede SM, Nister M, Lundeberg J, Frisen J. p53 suppresses the self-renewal of adult neural stem cells. *Development.* 2006;133(2):363-9.

[62] Dumble M, Moore L, Chambers SM, et al. The impact of altered p53 dosage on hematopoietic stem cell dynamics during aging. *Blood.* 2007;109(4):1736-42.

[63] van de Wetering M, Sancho E, Verweij C, et al. The beta-catenin/TCF-4 complex imposes a crypt progenitor phenotype on colorectal cancer cells. *Cell.* 2002;111(2):241-50.

[64] Katoh M. Comparative integromics on non-canonical WNT or planar cell polarity signaling molecules: transcriptional mechanism of PTK7 in colorectal cancer and that of SEMA6A in undifferentiated ES cells. *Int. J. Mol. Med.* 2007;20(3):405-9.

[65] Wielenga VJ, Smits R, Korinek V, et al. Expression of CD44 in Apc and Tcf mutant mice implies regulation by the WNT pathway. *Am. J. Pathol.* 1999;154(2):515-23.

[66] Kim BM, Mao J, Taketo MM, Shivdasani RA. Phases of canonical Wnt signaling during the development of mouse intestinal epithelium. *Gastroenterology.* 2007;133(2):529-38.

[67] Ricci-Vitiani L, Lombardi DG, Pilozzi E, et al. Identification and expansion of human colon-cancer-initiating cells. *Nature*. 2007;445(7123):111-5.

[68] Kinzler KW, Bigner SH, Bigner DD, et al. Identification of an amplified, highly expressed gene in a human glioma. *Science*. 1987;236(4797):70-3.

[69] Bale AE, Yu KP. The hedgehog pathway and basal cell carcinomas. *Hum. Mol. Genet.* 2001;10(7):757-62.

[70] Clement V, Sanchez P, de Tribolet N, Radovanovic I, Ruiz i Altaba A. HEDGEHOG-GLI1 signaling regulates human glioma growth, cancer stem cell self-renewal, and tumorigenicity. *Curr. Biol.* 2007;17(2):165-72.

[71] Chambers I, Smith A. Self-renewal of teratocarcinoma and embryonic stem cells. *Oncogene*. 2004;23(43):7150-60.

[72] Nichols J, Zevnik B, Anastassiadis K, et al. Formation of pluripotent stem cells in the mammalian embryo depends on the POU transcription factor Oct4. *Cell*. 1998;95(3):379-91.

[73] Hochedlinger K, Yamada Y, Beard C, Jaenisch R. Ectopic expression of Oct-4 blocks progenitor-cell differentiation and causes dysplasia in epithelial tissues. *Cell*. 2005;121(3):465-77.

[74] Ezashi T, Das P, Roberts RM. Low O2 tensions and the prevention of differentiation of hES cells. *Proc. Natl. Acad. Sci. USA*. 2005;102(13):4783-8.

[75] Sell S. Cancer and stem cell signaling: a guide to preventive and therapeutic strategies for cancer stem cells. *Stem Cell Rev*. 2007;3(1):1-6.

[76] Ventura A, Kirsch DG, McLaughlin ME, et al. Restoration of p53 function leads to tumour regression in vivo. *Nature*. 2007;445(7128):661-5.

[77] Xue W, Zender L, Miething C, et al. Senescence and tumour clearance is triggered by p53 restoration in murine liver carcinomas. *Nature*. 2007;445(7128):656-60.

[78] Bar EE, Chaudhry A, Lin A, et al. Cyclopamine-mediated hedgehog pathway inhibition depletes stem-like cancer cells in glioblastoma. *Stem Cells*. 2007;25(10):2524-33.